W9-CNE-548

For Reference

Not to be taken from this room

SALEM HEALTH
MAGILL'S
MEDICAL
GUIDE

SALEM HEALTH

MAGILL'S MEDICAL GUIDE

Sixth Edition

Volume II

Childhood infectious diseases — Flat feet

Medical Editors

Brandon P. Brown, M.D.
Indiana University School of Medicine

H. Bradford Hawley, M.D.
Wright State University

Margaret Trexler Hessen, M.D.
Drexel University College of Medicine

Clair Kaplan, A.P.R.N./M.S.N.
Yale University School of Nursing

Paul Moglia, Ph.D.
South Nassau Communities Hospital

Judy Mouchawar, M.D., M.S.P.H.
University of Colorado Health Sciences Center

Nancy A. Piotrowski, Ph.D.
Capella University and
University of California, Berkeley

Claire L. Standen, Ph.D.
University of Massachusetts Medical School

SALEM PRESS
Pasadena, California   Hackensack, New Jersey

Editor in Chief: Dawn P. Dawson
Editorial Director: Christina J. Moose
Project Editor: Tracy Irons-Georges
Copy Editors: Desiree Dreeuws, Connie Pollock
Editorial Assistant: Brett S. Weisberg

Photo Editor: Cynthia Breslin Beres
Production Editor: Andrea E. Miller
Acquisitions Editor: Mark Rehn
Page Design and Layout: James Hutson
Additional Layout: William Zimmerman

Illustrations: Hans & Cassidy, Inc., Westerville, Ohio

Magill's Medical Guide: Health and Illness, 1995
Supplement, 1996
Magill's Medical Guide, revised edition, 1998
Second revised edition, 2002
Third revised edition, 2005
Fourth revised edition, 2008
Sixth edition, 2011

∞ The paper used in these volumes conforms to the American National Standard for Permanence of Paper for Printed Library Materials, Z39.48-1992 (R1997).

Note to Readers

The material presented in *Magill's Medical Guide* is intended for broad informational and educational purposes. Readers who suspect that they suffer from any of the physical or psychological disorders, diseases, or conditions described in this set should contact a physician without delay; this work should not be used as a substitute for professional medical diagnosis or treatment. This set is not to be considered definitive on the covered topics, and readers should remember that the field of health care is characterized by a diversity of medical opinions and constant expansion in knowledge and understanding.

Library of Congress Cataloging-in-Publication Data

Magill's medical guide / Brandon P. Brown ... [et al.]. — 6th ed.
    p. cm. — (Salem health)
    Includes bibliographical references and index.
    ISBN 978-1-58765-677-4 (set : alk. paper) — ISBN 978-1-58765-679-8 (v. 2 : alk. paper) —
1. Medicine—Encyclopedias. I. Brown, Brandon P. II. Title: Medical guide.
    RC41.M34 2011
    610.3—dc22
                                                                                    2010031862

First Printing

Contents

COMPLETE LIST OF CONTENTS

VOLUME 1

VOLUME 2

VOLUME 3

VOLUME 4

VOLUME 5

VOLUME 6

SALEM HEALTH

MAGILL'S
MEDICAL
GUIDE

Childhood infectious diseases
Disease/disorder

Anatomy or system affected: Gastrointestinal system, immune system, lungs, muscles, musculoskeletal system, nose, respiratory system

Specialties and related fields: Bacteriology, epidemiology, family medicine, immunology, internal medicine, pediatrics, public health, virology

Definition: A group of diseases including diphtheria, tetanus, measles, polio, rubella (German measles), mumps, varicella (chickenpox), hepatitis, and pertussis (whooping cough).

Key terms:

anorexia: diminished appetite or aversion to food

conjunctivitis: inflammation of the conjunctiva, which lines the back of the eyelid, extends into the space between the lid and the globe of the eye, and goes over the globe to the transparent tissue covering the pupil

erythematous: related to or marked by reddening

malaise: a general feeling of discomfort, of being "out of sorts"

nuchal rigidity: stiffening of the back of the neck

oophoritis: inflammation of the ovary

orchitis: inflammation of the testis

photophobia: dread or avoidance of light

prodrome: a forewarning symptom of a disease

rhinitis: inflammation of the nasal mucous membrane

salivary glands: the glands that produce saliva

Causes and Symptoms

Acute communicable diseases occur primarily in childhood because most adults have become immune to such diseases, either by having acquired them as children or by having been inoculated against them. For example, prior to the use of vaccine for measles—a highly contagious disease found in most of the world—the peak incidence of the disease was in five- to ten-year-olds. Most adults were immune. Before a vaccine was developed and used against measles, epidemics occurred at two- to four-year intervals in large cities. Today, most cases are found in nonimmunized preschool children or in teenagers or young adults who have received only one dose of the vaccine.

A person infected with red measles (also known as rubeola) becomes contagious about ten days after exposure to the disease virus, at which time the prodromal stage begins. Typically, the infected person experiences three days of slight to moderate fever, a runny nose, increasing cough, and conjunctivitis. During the prodromal stage, Koplik's spots appear inside the cheeks opposite the lower molars. These lesions—grayish white dots about the size of sand particles with a slightly reddish halo surrounding them that are occasionally hemorrhagic—are important in the diagnosis of measles.

After the prodrome, a rash appears, usually accompanied by an abrupt increase in temperature (sometimes as high as 104 or 105 degrees Fahrenheit). It begins in the form of small, faintly red spots and progresses to large, dusky red confluent areas, often slightly hemorrhagic. The rash frequently begins behind the ears but spreads rapidly over the entire face, neck, upper arms, and upper part of the chest within the first twenty-four hours. During the next twenty-four hours, it spreads over the back, abdomen, entire arms, and thighs. When it finally reaches the feet after the second or third day of the rash, it is already fading from the face. At this point, the fever is usually disappearing as well.

The chief complications of measles are middle-ear infections, pneumonia, and encephalitis (a severe infection of the brain). There is no correlation between the severity of the case of measles and the development of encephalitis, but the incidence of the infection of the brain runs to only one or two per every thousand cases. Measles can also exacerbate tuberculosis.

The incubation period for rubella (German measles) lasts between fourteen and twenty-one days, and the disease occurs primarily in children between the ages of two and ten. Like the initial rash of measles, the initial rash of rubella usually starts behind the ears, but children with rubella normally have no symptoms save for the rash and a low-grade fever for one day. Adolescents may have a three-day prodromal period of malaise, runny nose, and mild conjunctivitis; adolescent girls may have arthritis in several joints that lasts for weeks. The red spots begin behind the ears and then spread to the face, neck, trunk, and extremities. This rash may coalesce and last up to five days. Temperature may be normal or slightly elevated. Complications from rubella are relatively uncommon, but if pregnant women are not immune to the disease and are exposed to the rubella virus during early pregnancy, severe congenital anomalies may result. Because similar symptoms and rashes develop in many viral diseases, rubella is difficult to diagnose clinically. Except in known epidemics, laboratory confirmation is often necessary.

The patient with mumps is likely to have fever, malaise, headache, and anorexia—all usually mild—but "neck swelling," a painful enlargement of the parotid gland near the ear, is the sign that often brings the child to a doctor. Maximum swelling peaks after one to three days and begins in one or both parotid glands, but it may involve other salivary glands. The swelling pushes the earlobe upward and outward and obscures the angle of the mandible. Drinking sour liquids such as lemon juice may increase the pain. The opening of the duct inside the cheek from the affected parotid gland may appear red and swollen.

The painful swelling usually dissipates by seven days. Abdominal pain may be caused by pancreatitis, a common complication but one that is usually mild. The most feared complication, sterility, is not as common as most believe. Orchitis rarely occurs in prepubertal boys and occurs in only 20 to 30 percent of older males. In 35 percent of patients with orchitis, both testes are involved, and a similar percentage of affected testes will atrophy. Surprisingly, impairment of fertility in males is only about 13 percent; absolute infertility is rare. Ovary involvement in women, with pelvic pain and tenderness, occurs in only about 7 percent of postpubertal women and with no evidence of impaired fertility. Mumps during early pregnancy may cause miscarriage, but this is a rare complication for females who have been immunized.

Hemophilus influenzae type B is the most common cause of serious bacterial infection in the young child. It is the leading cause of bacterial meningitis in children between the ages of one month and four years, and it is the cause of many other serious, life-threatening bacterial infections in the young child. Bacterial meningitis, especially from *Hemophilus influenzae* and pneumococcus, is the major cause of acquired hearing impairment in childhood.

Poliomyelitis (polio), an acute viral infection, has a wide range of manifestations. The minor illness pattern accounts for 80 to 90 percent of clinical infections in children. Symptoms, usually mild in this form, include slight fever, malaise, headache, sore throat, and vomiting but do not involve the central nervous system. Major illness occurs primarily in older children and adults. It may begin with fever, severe headache, stiff neck and back, deep muscle pain, and abnormal sensations, such as of burning, prickling, tickling, or tingling. These symptoms of aseptic meningitis may go no further or may progress to the loss of tendon reflexes and asymmetric weakness or paralysis of muscle groups. Fewer than 25 percent of paralytic polio patients suffer permanent disability. Most return in muscle function occurs

within six months, but improvement may continue for two years. Twenty-five percent of paralytic patients have mild residual symptoms, and 50 percent recover completely. A long-term study of adults who suffered the disease has documented slowly progressive muscle weakness, especially in patients who experienced severe disabilities initially.

Tetanus is a bacterial disease which, once established in a wound of a patient without significant immunity, will build a substance that acts at the neuromuscular junction, the spinal cord, and the brain. Clinically, the patient experiences "lockjaw," a tetanic spasm causing the spine and extremities to bend with convexity forward; spasms of the facial muscles cause the famous "sardonic smile." Minimal stimulation of any muscle group may cause painful spasms.

Diphtheria is another bacterial disease that produces a virulent substance, but this one attacks heart muscle and nervous tissue. There is a severe mucopurulent discharge from the nose and an exudative pharyngitis (a sore throat accompanied by phlegm) with the formation of a pseudomembrane. Swelling just below the back of the throat may lead to stridor (noisy, high-pitched breathing) and to the dark bluish or purplish coloration of the skin and mucous membranes because of decreased oxygenation of the blood. The result may be heart failure and damaged nerves; respiratory insufficiency may be caused by diaphragmatic paralysis.

Clinically, pertussis (whooping cough) can be divided into three stages, each lasting about two weeks. Initial symptoms resembling the common cold are followed by the characteristic paroxysmal cough and then convalescence. In the middle stage, multiple, rapid coughs, which may last more than a minute, will be followed by a sudden inspiration of air and a characteristic "whoop." In the final stage, vomiting commonly follows coughing attacks. Almost any stimulus precipitates an attack. Seizures may occur as a result of hypoxia (inadequate oxygen supply) or brain damage. Pneumonia can develop, and even death may occur when the illness is severe.

Varicella (chickenpox) produces a generalized itchy, blisterlike rash with low-grade fever and few other symptoms. Minor complications, such as ear infections, occasionally occur, as does pneumonia, but serious complications such as infection in the brain are rare. It is a very inconvenient disease, however, requiring the infected person to be quarantined for about nine days or until the skin lesions have dried up completely. Varicella, a herpes family virus, may lie dormant in nerve linings for years and suddenly emerge in the linear-grouped skin lesions identified as herpes zoster. These painful skin lesions follow the distribution of the affected nerve. Herpes zoster is commonly known as shingles.

Hepatitis type B is much more common in adults than in children, except in certain immigrant populations in which hepatitis B viral infections are endemic. High carrier rates appear in certain Asian and Pacific Islander groups and among some Inuits in Alaska, in whom perinatal transmission is the most common means of perpetuating the disease. Having this disease in childhood can cause problems later in life. An estimated five thousand deaths in the United States per year from cirrhosis or liver cancer occur as a result of hepatitis B. Carrier rates of between 5 and 10 percent result from disease acquired after the age of five, but between 80 and 90 percent will be carriers if they are infected at birth. The serious problems of hepatitis B occur most often in chronic carriers. For example, approximately, 15 to 40 percent of carriers will ultimately develop liver cancer. The virus is fifty to one hundred times more infectious than human immunodeficiency virus (HIV), the virus that causes acquired immunodeficiency syndrome (AIDS). Health care workers are at high risk of contracting hepatitis B, but virtually everyone is at risk for contracting this disease because it is so contagious.

Hepatitis type A is a virus that causes jaundice, fatigue, abdominal pain, nausea, diarrhea, and fever. Approximately 15 percent of those who have the disease will have relapsing symptoms for six to nine months. Hepatitis A is usually spread through fecal contamination, and during epidemic years over 35,000 cases are diagnosed in the United States.

TREATMENT AND THERAPY

The Centers for Disease Control and Prevention (CDC) and the U.S. Department of Health and Human Services recommend immunizing all infants soon after birth and again at age one to two months, with a final dose after the age of twenty-four weeks. The Committee on Infectious Diseases of the American Academy of Pediatrics recommends extending hepatitis B immunization to all adolescents, if possible. Based on field trials, the hepatitis B vaccine appears to be between 80 and 90 percent effective. The plasma-derived vaccine is protective against chronic hepatitis B infection for at least nine years. Newer, yeast-derived vaccines appear to be safe for administration to all, including pregnant

women and infants: Both the vaccine and a placebo evoke the same incidence of adverse reactions. These yeast-derived vaccines will be monitored to see if a booster dose is needed.

The incidence of infection with hepatitis B increases rapidly in adolescence, but teenagers are less likely to comply with immunization than are infants. Asking adolescents to participate in a three-dose immunization program over a six-month period is likely to result in high dropout rates. Therefore, the American Academy of Pediatrics has recommended combining vaccination at birth with vaccination of teenagers. Two states, Alaska and Hawaii, have implemented universal immunization of infants with hepatitis B vaccine, and so have twenty nations. Thirty-four states require vaccination for students before entry to middle school. Hepatitis A vaccine is recommended by the CDC for all children between twelve and twenty-three months of age. Two doses of the vaccine should be given, at least six months apart.

Primary vaccination with DTaP (diphtheria, tetanus, and acellular pertussis) vaccine is recommended at two months, four months, and six months of age, followed by boosters at fifteen to eighteen months and upon entry into school (at four to six years of age).

Once a child reaches fifteen months of age, only one dose of the *Hemophilus influenzae* type B vaccine is necessary, but vaccination should begin at two months of age. Three vaccines are licensed for use in infants. Depending upon which vaccine is used, shots are given at ages two, four, and six months, with a booster between twelve and fifteen months. These vaccines are safe and at least 90 percent effective in preventing serious illness, such as sepsis and meningitis, from influenza B.

At two and four months of age, infants should receive an inactivated poliovirus vaccination, with boosters between six and eighteen months and upon entry into school (four to six years of age).

MMR (measles, mumps, rubella) vaccination should take place at twelve and fifteen months and at four to six years of age. If the infant lives in a high-risk area, the first dose should occur at twelve months of age. While women who are pregnant or plan to become pregnant in the next three months should not receive MMR vaccination, children may receive the vaccine even if the mother is pregnant, since the viruses are not shed by immunized individuals.

Children who have not received the second dose should be vaccinated at eleven to twelve years. In the

1990's, researchers announced that they had developed a vaccine to prevent chickenpox. Preliminary trials show the vaccine to be safe and effective even in immunocompromised patients. Varicella vaccine should be given at or after twelve months of age to those children who have not had chickenpox.

Influenza vaccine, containing two strains of type A and one strain of type B, is now recommended to be administered to all children to prevent infection with seasonal influenza viruses. Annual vaccination is necessary as influenza viruses continually mutate, resulting in new strains not present in previous vaccines. Sometimes, special strains of influenza, such as H1N1 (swine) influenza, may necessitate adding a separate influenza vaccine. Vaccination is particularly important for children with chronic heart and lung disease, diabetes, HIV, sickle cell disease, and other chronic conditions that place them at greater risk for severe influenza.

Pneumococcal vaccine is now routinely given to children aged two to twenty-three months and to certain children aged twenty-four to fifty-nine months who are at risk of overwhelming pneumococcal infections. For example, children without spleens and children with sickle cell disease should be considered for vaccination against pneumococcal disease.

Meningococcal vaccine, which protects against bacteremia and meningitis caused by some strains of meningococci, should be given to children with certain immune deficiency states, including the absence of a functioning spleen. The vaccine may also be given if there is an outbreak of meningococcal disease caused by a strain included in the vaccine, or if the child is traveling to a part of the world where the disease is common.

Some parents refuse to have their children vaccinated against pertussis because of concerns about the vaccine's safety. Media focus on the safety of pertussis vaccines, as well as lawsuits, has frightened many physicians as well, the result being that they may be overly cautious in interpreting vaccine contraindications. Yet primary care physicians have also been sued for failing to give timely immunizations, which may result in complications from preventable disease. The Tennessee Medicaid Pertussis Vaccine Data should reassure them of the vaccine's safety. Other pertussis vaccine safety information is also available, including reports from the American Academy of Pediatrics Task Force on Pertussis and Pertussis Immunization. Some parents have feared that there is a link between vaccinations and neurological disorders such as autism, but studies have found no connection.

The means exist to prevent many serious illnesses from infectious diseases in childhood, but both parents and health care professionals must make the effort to vaccinate all children at the appropriate times in their lives.

PERSPECTIVE AND PROSPECTS

Some vaccines are more protective than others; effectiveness may hinge on a number of factors. In 1989, for example, 40 percent of people who developed measles had been vaccinated correctly under the old guidelines of one dose. Recommendations were therefore revised to include a booster dose. In the case of the hepatitis B vaccine, initial recommendations for administration of the vaccine established no injection site (only intramuscular), but studies revealed that there were fewer vaccine failures in recipients who were vaccinated in the deltoid region of the arm as opposed to the buttocks. The recommendation for injection site was therefore revised.

In the United States, vaccine coverage increased by the late 1990's after having been woefully inadequate during the 1980's: One state's department of health, in a 1987 study, discovered that only 64 percent of children who were two years old were adequately vaccinated with DTaP, oral polio, and MMR vaccines. However, by 2000, rates were closer to 80 percent. Undoubtedly, multiple and interacting factors have inhibited full vaccine coverage for all American children, including physicians' attitudes and practice behaviors. For parents, the cost of vaccination, lack of health insurance, and other barriers to health care frustrate their efforts to get their children immunized. Some parents, for ideological or other reasons, may even be disinterested in or opposed to vaccination. In today's highly mobile society, however, all persons should keep a standard personal immunization record to facilitate immunization coverage.

—*Wayne R. McKinny, M.D.;*
updated by Lenela Glass-Godwin, M.W.S.

See also Bacterial infections; Bacteriology; Bronchiolitis; Chickenpox; Common cold; Epidemics and pandemics; Epidemiology; Epiglottitis; Family medicine; Fifth disease; Giardiasis; Hand-foot-and-mouth disease; Hemolytic uremic syndrome; Hepatitis; Herpes; H1N1 influenza; Immunization and vaccination; Impetigo; Infection; Influenza; Kawasaki disease; Measles; Microbiology; Mononucleosis; Mumps; Noroviruses; Parasitic diseases; Pediatrics; Pinworms; Poliomyelitis; Rabies; Rheumatic fever; Roseola; Rotavirus; Roundworms; Rubella; Scarlet fever; Smallpox; Strep throat; Tapeworms; Tetanus; Tonsillitis; Tuberculosis; Viral infections; Whooping cough; Worms.

FOR FURTHER INFORMATION:

Beers, Mark H., et al., eds. *The Merck Manual of Diagnosis and Therapy.* 18th ed. Whitehouse Station, N.J.: Merck Research Laboratories, 2006. Published since 1899, this classic work is well indexed and easy to use. Discussions of the various infectious diseases of childhood are usually brief but thorough.

Behrman, Richard E., Robert M. Kliegman, and Hal B. Jenson, eds. *Nelson Textbook of Pediatrics.* 18th ed. Philadelphia: Saunders/Elsevier, 2007. This standard pediatrics textbook contains complete discussions of all common (and uncommon) causes of infectious disease in children. Many chapters are well written and easily understood by the nonspecialist.

Biddle, Wayne. *A Field Guide to Germs.* 2d ed. New York: Anchor Books, 2002. This comprehensive book is easily accessible to the nonspecialist and includes a discussion of nearly every virus, bacterium, and fungus known to cause human and nonhuman animal disease. The history of the microbe and the treatment of diseases are included.

Kimball, Chad T. *Childhood Diseases and Disorders Sourcebook: Basic Consumer Health Information About Medical Problems Often Encountered in Preadolescent Children.* Detroit, Mich.: Omnigraphics, 2003. Offers basic facts about common illnesses, serious diseases, and chronic conditions in children. Discusses frequently used diagnostic tests, surgeries, and medications. Also examines long-term care for seriously ill children.

Kumar, Vinay, Abul K. Abbas, and Nelson Fausto, eds. *Robbins and Cotran Pathologic Basis of Disease.* 8th ed. Philadelphia: Saunders/Elsevier, 2010. An excellent textbook that combines the clinical and the pathological beautifully.

Woolf, Alan D., et al., eds. *The Children's Hospital Guide to Your Child's Health and Development.* Cambridge, Mass.: Perseus, 2002. An authoritative and comprehensive guide to children's health, providing a guide to every common illness or condition that affects children and a carefully designed emergency section.

CHIROPRACTIC
SPECIALTY

ANATOMY OR SYSTEM AFFECTED: Back, bones, hips, musculoskeletal system, nervous system, spine

SPECIALTIES AND RELATED FIELDS: Neurology, orthopedics, preventive medicine

DEFINITION: The art and science of adjusting the spine and other bony articulations of the body to restore and maintain normal structure and function in the nervous system.

KEY TERMS:

adjustment: a thrust delivered into the spine or its articulations with the purpose of reestablishing normal joint and nerve function

nerve interference/pressure: chiropractic term that refers to a disturbance of normal nerve impulse transmission, usually via compression, stretch, or chronic irritation

neuromusculoskeletal: pertaining to the interrelationship between the nerves, muscles, and skeletal aspects of the body

palpation: the act of feeling with the hand; the application of the fingers with light pressure to the surface of the body for the purpose of determining the consistence of the parts beneath for physical diagnosis

subluxation: an incomplete or partial dislocation of a joint, which creates abnormal neurological and physiological symptoms in neuromusculoskeletal structures and/or other body systems via interference with nerve impulse transmission

SCIENCE AND PROFESSION

In the United States, chiropractic has the third largest patient base in the health care system, after medicine and dentistry. Licensed in every state, chiropractors are acknowledged as physicians along with medical doctors and osteopathic doctors, dentists, podiatrists, optometrists, and psychologists. Patients can consult with chiropractic physicians without referral. The scope of chiropractic practice varies from state to state, and reference must be made to specific state laws for exact information. The major premise of this field states that vertebrae of the spine can, and frequently do, become misaligned, causing interference in normal conduction of nerve impulses from the brain to the organs and tissues of the body. Although most spinal misalignments are corrected naturally through normal body movement, some become fixated. As a result, normal nerve transmission is impaired for long periods, and health suffers.

What distinguishes doctors of chiropractic from other health care professionals is that they work primarily to identify, analyze, and adjust the vertebrae and pelvis back to their correct positions. Treatment is directed at restoring and maintaining normal structure and mechanical function of the spine to reduce irritation of the spinal cord and spinal nerves. These irritations lead to pain and distress of the muscles and joints of the body. Less acknowledged and still in want of corroborating research is the relationship between the subluxation, the neuromusculoskeletal system, and internal organ dysfunction. Contrary to popular belief, the scope of chiropractic is recognized for its ability to promote the total health and integration of the body from the inside out. In addition to spinal adjusting, chiropractors encourage those whom they treat to take personal responsibility for their lives by teaching ways to preserve health rather than wait until symptoms of disease appear.

Doctors of chiropractic may examine, diagnose, analyze, and use X rays for diagnostic purposes according to generally recognized procedures taught in accredited chiropractic colleges. Clinical practice generally encompasses consultation and taking a history of the patient; physical, neurological, orthopedic, and chiropractic examinations; X-ray analysis of the spine and articulating structures; the administration of adjustments; physiotherapy; nutritional support; and the use of orthopedic supports. In most states, chiropractic practice does not include the prescription or administration of medicine or drugs, performance of surgery, practice of obstetrics, administration of radiation therapy, treatment of infectious or sexually transmitted diseases, performance of internal exams, reduction of fractures, or administration of anesthetics. Historically, chiropractic physicians practice either solo or in a group setting with other chiropractors and do not have hospital privileges. This is changing as some chiropractic physicians are entering into group practice settings with other health care specialists and gaining admittance to hospitals in a limited capacity.

Chiropractic history dates back to 1895 when D. D. Palmer experimented with a spinal adjustment on Harvey Lillard. Lillard, a janitor, had experienced a "popping sensation" in his upper spine caused by heavy lifting and subsequently had a loss of hearing. After treatment, Lillard's hearing improved and Palmer formulated early chiropractic scientific premise and philosophy: that illness is essentially functional in nature and becomes organic only as an end process. His

son, B. J. Palmer, is credited with refining and promoting the work of his father. Chiropractic can lay claim to a colorful and compelling history after its first century. From its humble beginnings, it has survived as a viable alternative health care system in America and has emerged as the second largest health care entity in the industry. The early educational program organized by D. D. Palmer was admittedly crude, abbreviated, and inadequate. As the profession grew and matured, however, so did the educational standards, to the current level, which is beyond reproach.

Chiropractic colleges are sanctioned as degree-granting institutions by the same regional accrediting agencies that regulate all other colleges and universities. Chiropractic colleges are accredited by the Council on Chiropractic Education, which is in turn approved by the United States Office of Education. Programs of study in chiropractic colleges parallel those in medical colleges except that chiropractic theory and practice replace surgery and medical theory. The medical curriculum is designed to prepare the medical student to diagnose and combat systemic diseases, with great emphasis on the use of drugs and surgery. The chiropractic curriculum, on the other hand, is designed to prepare the chiropractic student to evaluate and manage conservatively conditions from a holistic point of view, in which the various factors that affect a person's health are taken into consideration, including diet, nutritional supplementation, exercise, stress, and lifestyle.

Chiropractors have a full medical curriculum enabling them to make diagnoses. The education of a chiropractor begins with two years of preprofessional college study, with concentration in the human sciences. Although this prerequisite of two years is all that is required, the majority of students entering chiropractic college possess at least a bachelor's degree. The student then begins the doctor of chiropractic (D.C.) course of study at an accredited chiropractic college. The D.C. program is composed of four academic years of study most often divided into semesters or trimesters. The initial phase of study is much like any curriculum in the medical, dental, or veterinary schools, consisting of courses in the basic sciences: organic chemistry, biochemistry, anatomy of the musculoskeletal system (including limbs, trunk, and head), anatomy of the internal structures of the body (including all the organs, blood vessels, and internal systems), neuroanatomy (the anatomy of the brain, spinal cord, and entire nervous system), physiology (the study of how these systems function), neurophysiology, pathology (the study of disease), bacteriology, histology (the microscopic study of body tissues), and microbiology. The remainder of the courses are concentrated on the clinical sciences: X-ray physics, positioning, and interpretation; laboratory diagnosis (blood and urine studies); physical examination and diagnosis; neurology; orthopedics; cardiology; obstetrics and gynecology; pediatrics; geriatrics; dermatology; gastrointestinal and genitourinary systems; physical therapy nutrition; and chiropractic adjustment techniques.

During the later part of the student chiropractor's matriculation, he or she will see patients in a college-affiliated clinic as an "extern," which prepares the future doctor for patient care and management. In addition to the basic chiropractic curriculum, there are residencies available in both radiology and orthopedics. A chiropractic graduate may apply to study an additional three years in order to become either a chiropractic radiologist or a chiropractic orthopedist. The training received in these programs is highly specialized, and both of these chiropractic specialists are the equal of their medical counterparts in terms of diagnostic abilities. In addition, comprehensive 360-hour programs of study in orthopedics, neurology, radiology, and sports medicine exist; doctors completing such programs are eligible to sit for an examination to be awarded Diplomate status by chiropractic boards in the corresponding specialties. Postgraduate education for the practicing chiropractor includes seminars and workshops in soft tissue injuries, disk syndromes, low back pain, and other common and difficult conditions. Interdisciplinary seminars and conferences in nutrition, fitness, biochemical imbalances, and numerous other areas of common interest allow physicians from every discipline the opportunity to exchange views and perspectives.

The licensing procedure for the graduate chiropractic doctor varies from state to state. During the formal educational process, chiropractic students are exposed to thorough written examinations in all basic science and clinical subjects, which are administered by the National Board of Chiropractic Examiners. Successful completion of these written tests is a prerequisite to licensure in many states. Otherwise, completion of a written and practical examination administered by the respective state board is required, and in some states completion of the National Board Examinations and a state-administered written board are both required. The majority of states require doctors to attend certified ed-ucational seminars for continued licensure. The chiropractic profession is generally organized on a state basis through professional state associations and on a national basis through national organizations.

DIAGNOSTIC AND TREATMENT TECHNIQUES

To understand fully how chiropractic health care works, it is necessary to understand the spine and the role that it plays in overall body function. The nervous system—consisting of the brain, cranial nerves (nerves that originate in the head), the spinal cord, and thirty-one pairs of spinal nerves that branch out much as the limbs of a tree do—generates and regulates all activities in the body. While no one knows exactly how the nervous system functions, it is known that signals, or impulses, travel along the nerve fibers conveying information between the brain and the rest of the body. Since every tissue and organ of the body is connected to and controlled by nerves from the spinal cord and brain, removal of nerve interference can bring dramatic results. Interference with the transmission of these impulses results in alteration of normal body function. The cranium (skull) and spinal column, composed of twenty-four bones called vertebrae, house the brain and spinal cord. In addition to protecting the spinal cord, the spine is the core of the skeletal framework that supports upright posture, provides for organ and muscle attachment, and allows for the dynamics of human movement. Given this monumental job, the spine and its connecting framework are subject to much activity and abuse.

For the mechanics of body motion to occur properly, there must be full, free, and harmonious movement in every one of the spinal joints. The working unit of the spine is referred to as the motor unit. The motor unit is composed of two vertebrae joined by cartilage cushions called disks and four posterior joints called facet joints, two located to attach the superior vertebra and two to attach the inferior vertebra. The disks separate the vertebrae while allowing flexibility and shock absorption for the spine. They also maintain openings between the vertebrae that are necessary for the passage of the spinal nerves. The facet joints provide additional movement and are limited in their range of motion by ligaments. Restriction in any of them can be compensated for only by the other joints and adjoining structures (such as ribs, muscles, or tendons), thus producing strain in the compensating structures.

It is at the location of the facet joints of the spine where subluxation occurs—an alteration of the align-

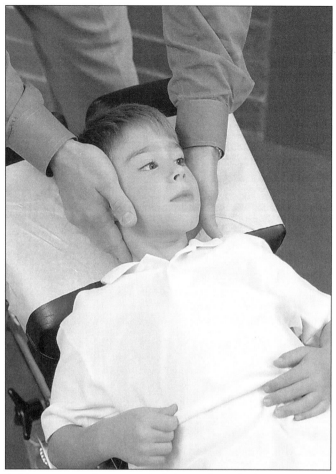

A chiropractor performs a manipulation on the neck of a young patient. (PhotoDisc)

instrument with the objective of mobilizing a fixated joint. It is a gentle but dynamic thrust applied to a specific joint in a way that generates joint movement in a specific direction. Basically, it is a way to "coax" a restricted joint into moving. Applied repeatedly over a period of time, spinal adjustments are capable of restoring mobility to even the most chronic spinal subluxations. Deep-rooted subluxations that have existed for several years typically require months of care. Fixations of lesser duration and severity respond in less time, often the mildest in one treatment. The procedure works because the restoration of the proper mechanics of spinal motion via the spinal adjustment improves joint function, corrects specific joint problems, and helps prevent injury through increased spinal strength brought about by spinal joints that function properly.

Chiropractic health care can be useful for the detection and correction of existing health problems and/or for preventive purposes. In lieu of concentrating on bacterial or viral infections or treating the end-symptoms of disease processes, chiropractors look for the reason that a patient's symptom developed, including such contributing factors as environmental conditions, lifestyle, systemic stress, and malfunction. For example, instead of giving medication to stop the pain of headache, the chiropractor analyzes possible irritating factors, including subluxation, that may be causing the headache and addresses that factor first. Thus, in many cases, the prescription of medication can be avoided.

PERSPECTIVE AND PROSPECTS

Chiropractic originated in the second half of the nineteenth century during a time when many theories of healing were being promulgated. Chiropractic and osteopathy shared their early beginnings amid the emergence of several alternatives to the regular school of healing (medicine), including the Thomsonian system (the use of botanicals), the Hygienic movement (the use of fresh fruits and vegetables, fresh air, exercise, and better food preparation), and homeopathy. Daniel David Palmer, born in 1845 in Canada, was involved in making and losing several small mercantile fortunes when he made his way to Iowa in 1886 to become a magnetic healer. Over the next decade, he would attract

ment and proper movement of the spinal joint resulting in irritation of the exiting spinal nerve via compression, stretch, or chronic (constant) irritation—and leads to alteration of normal body functions. Subluxations can result from various factors, including trauma, toxic irritation, muscular imbalance caused by disuse and/or repetitive tasks, ligamental weakening, organic dysfunction, and stress. The altered nerve impulse transmission, left uncorrected, results in accumulative dysfunction in the tissue cells of the body.

Spinal biomechanics, the basis of the chiropractor's evaluation, refers to the manner in which the spine works in movement. Restoration of spinal motion is the primary treatment on which chiropractors depend to alleviate patients' symptoms. The single most distinguishing element of chiropractic procedures is the spinal adjustment. This chiropractic adjustment is a technique of physically moving the spine by hand or by

patients from throughout the Midwest until one day in September, 1895, a janitor named Harvey Lillard came into his office, received an "adjustment," and regained his lost hearing. Soon afterward, the term "chiropractic" (Greek meaning "done by hand") was coined by Samuel Weed, a Palmer patient. D. D. Palmer began giving instruction at Dr. Palmer's School and Cure, later becoming Palmer Institute and Chiropractic Infirmary and finally Palmer Chiropractic College.

Brian Inglis, a distinguished British historian, commentator, and author of the two-volume work *The History of Medicine* (1965), has declared: "The rise of chiropractic . . . has been one of the most remarkable social phenomena in American history . . . yet it has gone virtually unexplored." In spite of its humble origins and formulative years, chiropractic has had a decided impact on the evolution of health care attitudes in the United States and to some degree in other parts of the Western world. For more than three-quarters of a century, it fought for its very survival, overcoming a strong medical lobby in 1977 when the American Medical Association (AMA) reversed its long-standing policy against professional interrelationships between medical doctors and chiropractors. In March, 1977, the AMA's Judicial Council announced:

A physician may refer a patient for diagnostic or therapeutic services to another physician, a limited practitioner, or any other provider of health care services permitted by law to furnish such services, whenever he believes that this may benefit the patient. As in the case of referrals to physician-specialists, referrals to limited practitioners should be based on their individual competence and ability to perform the services needed by the patient.

Despite the AMA's policy change toward chiropractic, however, complete acceptance by the medical profession has not occurred. This reluctance has not been attributable solely to the attitudes of the medical profession. Rather, it is the result of a combination of the continued opposition of the medical profession and the resistance of chiropractors to subordinate themselves to medical prescription, as with physical therapists who practice under medical supervision. Chiropractors have been independent practitioners for too long, functioning at a high level in the diagnosis and treatment of illness, for them to be willing to regress in status.

It is likely that the chiropractic profession will continue on its present course of becoming a health profession with parallels to medicine. Emphasizing the uniqueness of chiropractic treatment and the contrasting philosophical approaches of health maintenance and therapy, chiropractic has not only survived but also flourished. Whether used as a preventive means to ensure good health or as a way to help the body cure itself of disease, chiropractic has sometimes succeeded where other health care measures have failed.

—*Cindy Nesci, D.C.*

See also Alternative medicine; Anxiety; Bone disorders; Bones and the skeleton; Massage; Muscle sprains, spasms, and disorders; Muscles; Pain; Pain management; Physical rehabilitation; Spinal cord disorders; Spine, vertebrae, and disks; Stress; Stress reduction.

FOR FURTHER INFORMATION:
Bergmann, Thomas F., and David H. Peterson. *Chiropractic Technique: Principles and Procedures*. 3d ed. St. Louis, Mo.: Mosby/Elsevier, 2010. Traces the historical and scientific roots of chiropractic care and gives hands-on guidance to techniques.
Coulter, Ian Douglass. *Chiropractic: A Philosophy for Alternative Health Care*. Boston: Butterworth-Heinemann, 1999. Explores how chiropractic differs from orthodox medicine in its approach to health care and patient problems.
Haldeman, Scott, ed. *Principles and Practice of Chiropractic*. 3d ed. New York: McGraw-Hill, 2005. A collection of articles by leading authorities in the fields of history, sociology, neurophysiology, spinal biomechanics, and clinical chiropractic. Written with the purpose of presenting an accurate overview of the latest developments in the field.
Lenarz, Michael, and Victoria St. George. *The Chiropractic Way*. New York: Bantam, 2003. Explores the healing qualities of a rapidly growing alternative health field. Basic principles of spinal health, chiropractic techniques, and complementary diet, exercise, and stress-relief programs are covered.
Tousley, Dirk, and David M. Lees. *The Chiropractic Handbook for Patients*. 3d ed. Independence, Mo.: White Dove, 1985. This popular work on chiropractic is written with the general reader in mind. Contains information that will help patients understand their treatment.

CHLAMYDIA

DISEASE/DISORDER

ANATOMY OR SYSTEM AFFECTED: Eyes, genitals, lungs, lymphatic system, reproductive system, urinary system

SPECIALTIES AND RELATED FIELDS: Gynecology, microbiology

DEFINITION: The most common sexually transmitted bacterial disease in the United States, which primarily infects the reproductive tract and is caused by the bacterium *Chlamydia trachomatis*.

KEY TERMS:

contact tracing: also known as partner referral; a process that consists of identifying sexual partners of infected patients, informing the partners of their exposure to disease, and offering resources for counseling and treatment

screening procedures: tests that are carried out in populations which are usually asymptomatic and at high risk for a disease in order to identify those in need of treatment

sexually transmitted disease: an infection caused by organisms transferred through sexual contact (genital-genital, orogenital, or anogenital); transmission of infection occurs through exposure to lesions or secretions which contain the organisms

CAUSES AND SYMPTOMS

Chlamydia is the most common sexually transmitted bacterial disease in the United States, with a prevalence of about 10 percent in sexually active men and women. Chlamydia is caused by a bacterium, *Chlamydia trachomatis*, that infects cells on mucosal surfaces, such as the genital tract, urinary tract, anorectal tract, eyes, and throat. These infections cause inflammation of the cervix, urethra, prostate, or epididymis. In women, symptoms may include urinary discomfort, lower abdominal pain, and abnormal vaginal discharge. Women are commonly asymptomatic in early stages of the disease. In men, symptoms may involve urinary discomfort and unusual discharge from the urethra. Men may be asymptomatic in early stages of the disease.

Most cases of chlamydia are asymptomatic, and many patients are diagnosed based on screening procedures. Nevertheless, asymptomatic patients are able to infect others and can suffer serious consequences of chlamydia infection, such as pelvic inflammatory disease (PID) and infertility. PID occurs when chlamydia infection ascends the female reproductive tract to involve the uterus, Fallopian tubes, and pelvic cavity.

This infection of the upper reproductive tract can lead to scarring of these organs and puts the patient at increased risk of infertility and ectopic pregnancy.

In rare cases, chlamydia can travel to regional lymph nodes and cause abscesses, a condition termed lymphogranuloma venereum. This condition is commonly accompanied by systemic symptoms such as fever, chills, and muscle and joint aches.

An infant may contract chlamydia as it passes through the birth canal of an infected mother. The disease can lead to eye infection that results in visual impairment and blindness, as well as infection of the respiratory tract.

TREATMENT AND THERAPY

A patient receives antibiotic therapy if laboratory tests indicate infection with *C. trachomatis*. Uncomplicated chlamydia infection can be treated effectively with antibiotics such as doxycycline, azithromycin, erythromycin, or ofloxacin. A patient with risk factors for sexually transmitted diseases (STDs) or symptoms of the disease is treated presumptively with antibiotic therapy, even before the results of laboratory tests for chlamydia return.

Because chlamydia is associated with other STDs, such as gonorrhea, human immunodeficiency virus (HIV), syphilis, and hepatitis B and C, the patient should be advised to undergo testing for these diseases as well. Up to 50 percent of patients with gonorrhea also have chlamydia, so an antibiotic against chlamydia is given along with an antibiotic for gonorrhea, unless laboratory tests have declared the patient free of chlamydia. If chlamydia and gonorrhea are treated

---

INFORMATION ON CHLAMYDIA

CAUSES: Bacterial infection of mucosa (genital tract, urinary tract, anorectal tract, eyes, throat) through sexual transmission or childbirth

SYMPTOMS: Often none, but may include urinary discomfort, lower abdominal pain, abnormal discharge from vagina or urethra, complications such as pelvic inflammatory disease (PID) and infertility; in infants, eye infection, visual impairment, blindness, respiratory tract infection

DURATION: Chronic until treated

TREATMENTS: Antibiotics (doxycycline, azithromycin, erythromycin, ofloxacin)

early, complications such as PID or infertility can be avoided.

In addition to antibiotics, a key component of chlamydia treatment involves counseling in the prevention of STDs. To minimize future exposure to chlamydia and other STDs, patients are encouraged to use barrier methods such as condoms during intercourse and to avoid high-risk sexual behaviors.

Another key component to the treatment of chlamydia and other STDs is contact tracing, which occurs once the infection is confirmed with laboratory testing. With the cooperation of the patient, all sexual partners of the patient are notified regarding their exposure to disease. Partners are encouraged to seek medical attention, even if they have no symptoms themselves, in order to prevent reinfection of the patient during subsequent sexual encounters or further spread of the disease to other sexual partners.

In the United States, erythromycin eyedrops are given prophylactically to all newborns to prevent eye infections with chlamydia that could lead to visual impairment.

PERSPECTIVE AND PROSPECTS

Diseases caused by *C. trachomatis* have been described as early as ancient Egyptian times. It was not until 1907, however, that the bacterium was actually identified, and there was some controversy about whether it was a true bacterium because it requires host cells to live (obligate intracellular parasite). The organism favors cells that are more available on the cervix of young (versus older) women, which is partly why rates of chlamydia are so much higher in the young. In the 1960's, a clinically useful diagnostic test was developed that allowed screening of a large number of specimens within a few days. The development of a relatively easy test for chlamydia enabled clinicians to screen a large number of asymptomatic but at-risk patients (such as those under age twenty-five or those with multiple sexual partners).

A promising area of research is the search for a vaccine to *C. trachomatis*. This research focuses on identifying antigens on the bacterium that are important for its function, such as proteins responsible for bacterial attachment to or uptake into cells. The premise is to use these proteins to generate an immune response in patients so that when patients are exposed to chlamydia, their immune systems are prepared to respond against it.

—*Clair Kaplan, A.P.R.N./M.S.N.;*
additional material by Anne Lynn S. Chang, M.D.

See also Acquired immunodeficiency syndrome (AIDS); Antibiotics; Bacterial infections; Blindness; Conjunctivitis; Epidemiology; Genital disorders, female; Genital disorders, male; Gonorrhea; Gynecology; Hepatitis; Herpes; Human immunodeficiency virus (HIV); Infertility, female; Men's health; Pelvic inflammatory disease (PID); Reproductive system; Screening; Sexually transmitted diseases (STDs); Syphilis; Trachoma; Women's health.

FOR FURTHER INFORMATION:

Centers for Disease Control. "1998 Guidelines for the Treatment of Sexually Transmitted Diseases." *Morbidity and Mortality Weekly Report* 47, no. RR-1 (January, 1997): 1-115.

Holmes, King K., et al., eds. *Sexually Transmitted Diseases*. 4th ed. New York: McGraw-Hill Medical, 2008.

Kasper, Dennis L., et al., eds. *Harrison's Principles of Internal Medicine*. 16th ed. New York: McGraw-Hill, 2005.

Ryan, Kenneth J., and C. George Ray, eds. *Sherris Medical Microbiology: An Introduction to Infectious Diseases*. 4th ed. New York: McGraw-Hill, 2004.

CHOKING
DISEASE/DISORDER

ANATOMY OR SYSTEM AFFECTED: Chest, lungs, neck, respiratory system, throat

SPECIALTIES AND RELATED FIELDS: Emergency medicine

DEFINITION: A condition in which the breathing passage (windpipe) is obstructed.

CAUSES AND SYMPTOMS

A person who is choking may cough, turn red in the face, clutch his or her throat, or any combination of the above. If the choking person is coughing, it is probably best to do nothing; the coughing should naturally clear the airway. The true choking emergency occurs when a bit of food or other foreign object completely obstructs the breathing passage. In this case, there is little or no coughing—the person cannot make much sound. This silent choking calls for immediate action.

TREATMENT AND THERAPY

An individual witnessing a choking emergency should first call for emergency help and then perform the Heimlich maneuver. The choking person should never

INFORMATION ON CHOKING

CAUSES: Blockage of airway, injury
SYMPTOMS: Coughing, red face, grabbing at throat
DURATION: Acute
TREATMENTS: Heimlich maneuver, emergency care

be slapped on the back. The Heimlich maneuver is best performed while the choking victim is standing or seated. If possible, the person performing the Heimlich maneuver should ask the victim to nod if he or she wishes the Heimlich maneuver to be performed. If the airway is totally blocked, the victim will not be able to speak and may even be unconscious.

The individual performing the Heimlich maneuver positions himself or herself behind the choking victim and places his or her arms around the victim's waist. Making a fist with one hand and grasping that fist with the other hand, the rescuer positions the thumb side of the fist toward the stomach of the victim—just above the navel and below the ribs. The person performing the maneuver pulls his or her fist upward into the abdomen of the victim with several quick thrusts. This action should expel the foreign object from the victim's throat, and he or she should begin coughing or return to normal breathing.

The Heimlich maneuver is not effective in dislodging fish bones and certain other obstructions. If the airway is still blocked after several Heimlich thrusts, a finger sweep should be tried to remove the obstruction. First the mouth of the victim must be opened: The chin is grasped, and the mouth is pulled open with one hand. With the index finger of the other hand, the rescuer sweeps through the victim's throat, pulling out any foreign material. One sweep should be made from left to right, and a second sweep from right to left. The Heimlich maneuver may then be repeated if necessary.

—*Steven A. Schonefeld, Ph.D.*

See also Asphyxiation; Coughing; Cyanosis; First aid; Heimlich maneuver; Hyperventilation; Respiration; Resuscitation; Unconsciousness.

FOR FURTHER INFORMATION:
American College of Emergency Physicians. *Pocket First Aid*. New York: DK, 2003. An excellent reference guide illustrated with photographs and written in a clear, step-by-step format. Covers many first aid methods, from resuscitation of conscious and unconscious choking victims to how to deal with bleeding, shock, spinal injuries, poisoning, seizures, and fractures.

Castleman, Michael. "Life Saving Moves from EMS Experts." *Family Circle* 107, no. 4 (March 15, 1994): 37. Offers tips for the care of nine medical emergencies, including choking, bleeding, and shock. First aid help should be given with care, because certain injuries can be made worse with improper treatment.

Stern, Loraine. "Mom, I Can't Breathe!" *Woman's Day* 57, no. 6 (March 15, 1994): 18. Describes the various ailments that can cause breathing problems in children. The signs that could signal serious illness include inability to swallow, difficulty speaking or finishing a sentence, and breathing difficulties that rapidly become more severe.

CHOLECYSTECTOMY
PROCEDURE
ANATOMY OR SYSTEM AFFECTED: Abdomen, gallbladder, gastrointestinal system
SPECIALTIES AND RELATED FIELDS: General surgery
DEFINITION: The surgical removal of a diseased gallbladder.

INDICATIONS AND PROCEDURES
Cholecystectomy is indicated when the patient exhibits nausea, vomiting, and abdominal pain and examination reveals gallstones. Gallstones, which consist mostly of crystallized cholesterol and bile, form in the gallbladder and may lodge in the bile duct. The stones can be dissolved with medication or broken up with ultrasound and passed from the body. They can (and often do) form again, however, with renewed symptoms. Removal of the gallbladder is the method of choice to prevent the recurrence of symptoms. Surgery is performed under general anesthesia.

In open surgery, the abdomen is cleaned and a 7.5- to 15-centimeter (3- to 6-inch) incision made with a scalpel through the skin and abdominal tissues. The gallbladder is isolated from the liver. A duct and artery are tied off with surgical staples or sutures, and they are cut in order to free the gallbladder. The organ is removed, and the tissues are closed with sutures or staples.

In laparoscopic surgery, the surface is cleaned and the surgeon makes four small holes. A 1.3-centimeter (0.5-inch) cut is made at or near the navel and another just below the breastbone, as well as two small punctures to the right of the incisions. The laparoscope, with

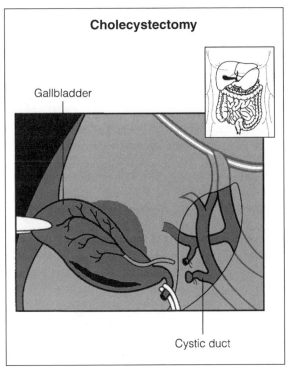

Cholecystectomy

Gallbladder

Cystic duct

The removal of the gallbladder may be indicated with severe infection of the organs or with repeated attacks of biliary colic caused by the presence of gallstones; the inset shows the location of the gallbladder.

a video camera and light, is inserted into the navel incision. Long, thin dissecting instruments are passed through the three punctures, and the gallbladder is cut free as in open surgery. The organ is removed through the navel incision, which is then closed with sutures or staples. The punctures are closed with small adhesive bandages.

USES AND COMPLICATIONS

Open surgery for cholecystectomy requires a hospital stay of five to eight days and a recovery time of four to six weeks. Complications occur in 1.0 to 9.4 percent of the surgeries and range from postoperative bleeding and diarrhea to intestinal obstruction. Rare but major complications include severing the common bile duct that connects the liver and small intestine, or puncturing a major blood vessel. Overall, the mortality rate is low: 0.2 to 0.6 percent.

Laparoscopic surgery may require an overnight stay and a recovery period of five to seven days. The complication rate is lower than the rate in open surgery, but this may be a reflection of the fact that sicker patients with more complex diseases and, therefore, greater risk

factors are generally referred for open surgery; not all patients are good candidates for the limited approach afforded by laparoscopy.

—*Albert C. Jensen, M.S.*

See also Cholecystitis; Gallbladder; Gallbladder cancer; Gallbladder diseases; Gastroenterology; Gastrointestinal system; Laparoscopy; Stone removal; Stones.

FOR FURTHER INFORMATION:

Chellappa, M. *Laparoscopic Cholecystectomy.* Teaneck, N.J.: World Scientific, 1994.

Dunn, David C., and Christopher J. E. Watson. *Laparoscopic Cholecystectomy: Problems and Solutions.* Cambridge, Mass.: Blackwell Science, 1992.

Parker, James N., and Philip M. Parker, eds. *The Official Patient's Sourcebook on Gallstones.* San Diego, Calif.: Icon Health, 2002.

Porter, Robert S., et al., eds. *The Merck Manual Home Health Handbook.* Whitehouse Station, N.J.: Merck Research Laboratories, 2009.

CHOLECYSTITIS

DISEASE/DISORDER

ANATOMY OR SYSTEM AFFECTED: Abdomen, gallbladder, gastrointestinal system, liver, pancreas

SPECIALTIES AND RELATED FIELDS: Emergency medicine, family medicine, gastroenterology, internal medicine, pathology

DEFINITION: An inflammation of the gallbladder.

CAUSES AND SYMPTOMS

There are basically two types of cholecystitis, calculous and acalculous, both of which could present as acute or chronic inflammation of the gallbladder. The calculous type is seen in 90 percent of cases and is caused by an obstruction of the neck of the gallbladder

---

INFORMATION ON CHOLECYSTITIS

CAUSES: Usually obstruction of gallbladder by gallstones; sometimes sepsis, severe trauma, severe burns

SYMPTOMS: Severe, progressive upper-right abdominal pain, with nausea, vomiting, fever, sometimes jaundice

DURATION: Often chronic, with acute episodes lasting one to three days

TREATMENTS: None (spontaneous resolution), sometimes gallbladder removal

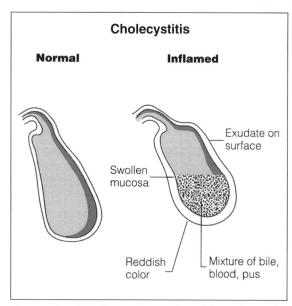

Cholecystitis

Normal   **Inflamed**

Exudate on surface

Swollen mucosa

Reddish color

Mixture of bile, blood, pus

A normal gallbladder and one inflamed by cholecystitis.

by gallstones, which are usually composed of cholesterol. The cholesterol stones may block the gallbladder neck and cause an acute attack of cholecystitis, or they may act as chemical irritants and result in chronic inflammation. About 10 percent of cases of cholecystitis are not the result of gallstones and are hence called acalculous. A variety of factors may precipitate an acute attack, such as sepsis, severe trauma, severe burns, and even the postpartum state. Approximately 75 percent of patients with acute cholecystitis are female.

Acute cholecystitis may first come to a medical attention in the emergency room, with the patient complaining of severe progressive right upper quadrant pain (biliary colic), which may be associated with nausea, vomiting, and fever and could radiate to the back. Jaundice (yellowish skin) may or may not be present, depending on the degree of obstruction of the gallbladder neck. The attack usually follows a large fatty meal and can last one to three days. Chronic cholecystitis is usually more insidious in onset and may be relatively asymptomatic; it also may be associated with a vague sensation of indigestion, which eventually progresses to mild, right-upper abdominal distress or long-standing pain.

Diagnosis is usually made with an ultrasound of the abdomen that demonstrates calcified gallstones. Obstruction of the gallbladder neck cannot be visualized, however, and thus requires another imaging test called a hepatobiliary iminodiacetic acid (HIDA) scan. An elevated white blood cell count is also seen in most cases.

TREATMENT AND THERAPY

Most acute attacks of cholecystitis may resolve spontaneously, but they should always be considered for surgery, as removal of the gallbladder (cholecystectomy) is the only definitive therapy for the disease. The gallbladder is usually removed using laparoscopic surgery, wherein small incisions are made in the abdomen through which surgical instruments and a fiber-optic camera are passed. In some cases, particularly if the gallbladder is highly inflamed, an open procedure is necessary. In acute attacks, it may also be necessary to maintain adequate nutrition and fluid replacement. A low-fat diet is usually recommended for these patients.

In those patients who decide against surgery, there is a risk of recurrent infections, pain, and even perforation of the gallbladder; the perforation of the gallbladder has a 25 percent mortality rate.

—*Rashmi Ramasubbaiah, M.D.,*
and Venkat Raghavan Tirumala, M.D., M.H.A.
See also Cholecystectomy; Gallbladder; Gallbladder diseases; Gastroenterology; Internal medicine; Stone removal; Stones.

FOR FURTHER INFORMATION:

American Medical Association. *American Medical Association Family Medical Guide.* 4th rev. ed. Hoboken, N.J.: John Wiley & Sons, 2004.

Frazier, Margeret Schell, and Jeanette Wist Drzymkowski. *Essentials of Human Diseases and Conditions.* 4th ed. St. Louis, Mo.: Saunders/Elsevier, 2009.

Kasper, Dennis L., et al., eds. *Harrison's Principles of Internal Medicine.* 16th ed. New York: McGraw-Hill, 2005.

Porter, Robert S., et al., eds. *The Merck Manual Home Health Handbook.* Whitehouse Station, N.J.: Merck Research Laboratories, 2009.

Rakel, Robert E., ed. *Textbook of Family Practice.* 6th ed. Philadelphia: W. B. Saunders, 2002.

CHOLERA

DISEASE/DISORDER

ANATOMY OR SYSTEM AFFECTED: Circulatory system, gastrointestinal system, intestines, kidneys

SPECIALTIES AND RELATED FIELDS: Environmental health, epidemiology, gastroenterology, internal medicine, microbiology, public health

DEFINITION: An acute bacterial disease transmitted by polluted water and contaminated food.

INFORMATION ON CHOLERA

CAUSES: Bacterial infection via contaminated food or water

SYMPTOMS: Diarrhea, vomiting

DURATION: Several days

TREATMENTS: Fluid and electrolyte replacement, antibiotics

CAUSES AND SYMPTOMS

The comma-shaped bacterium *Vibrio cholerae* causes the life-threatening disease cholera. The organism is spread when people ingest water or raw food contaminated with fecal matter. Studies have shown that the bacterium can live in both oceanic salt water and freshwater. In the ocean, it adheres to a type of zooplankton called copepods, which are eaten by certain types of shellfish. Therefore, people who consume shellfish grown in contaminated water can ingest the cholera organism. Also, people eating crops fertilized with human feces can ingest the organism.

Cholera affects particularly underdeveloped nations with poor sewage disposal and sanitation practices. It is endemic in Africa, Southeast Asia, the Indian subcontinent, and Central and South America. Even in developed nations, however, cholera may emerge after major disasters, such as hurricanes and earthquakes. Fewer than 250 cases were reported in the United States from 1996 to 2006, primarily around the Gulf Coast. Most of those cases were caused by the ingestion of contaminated raw shellfish.

After a person ingests contaminated food or water, between twenty-four and seventy-two hours elapse before the symptoms of cholera develop. Normally, between ten million to a billion *V. cholerae* bacteria must be present to cause infection, due to the large number that die in stomach acid. If an individual has taken antacids to neutralize stomach acid, however, then only about one thousand organisms are necessary to cause infection. Fewer organisms are also required if they enter the body via food, because the food protects some of the bacteria from the stomach acid.

The organisms that survive travel to the small intestine, attach to the epithelial cells there, and produce a toxin that causes a tremendous loss of water and electrolytes though extreme diarrhea and sometimes vomiting. Patients can lose more than twenty quarts of fluid per day. The extremely dilute feces are primarily a whitish liquid containing flecks of solid mucous mate-

rial resembling rice grains, and hence are commonly called rice-water stools. The tremendous loss of fluids and electrolytes can lead to hypotension (low blood pressure), an increase in both pulse and respiratory rates, cardiac arrhythmia, kidney failure, and the appearance of sunken eyes and cheeks. Shock, resulting from changes in blood acidity and extremely low blood volume, can lead to death within a few hours, especially in children.

Some strains of *V. cholerae* may produce almost no symptoms or only mild diarrhea in some individuals, but the majority of infected people experience very severe disease. Left untreated, approximately 60 percent of patients die; however, immediate rehydration therapy normally saves all but about 1 percent of patients. Nonfatal cases spontaneously resolve themselves after a few days, since both the organisms and the toxin that they produce are ejected from the patient's body in the diarrhea.

TREATMENT AND THERAPY

The best method for controlling cholera is prevention. Societies with adequate sanitation and sewage treatment are normally protected, except for contaminated seafood. Underdeveloped nations should be encouraged to improve their sanitation and sewage treatment practices and to cease using human feces as crop fertilizer. Also, especially in infected areas, raw foods and unpurified water should be avoided.

Although different vaccines have been developed, the immunity that they produce appears to be short-lived and not effective against all strains. Prophylactic antibiotic treatment for travelers entering affected areas has not been shown to be effective. Given the large number of bacteria needed for the disease to occur, however, proper hygienic practices alone should provide sufficient protection.

Treatment for cholera patients is primarily supportive, with rehydration and restoration of the electrolyte balance being paramount. Secondary treatment with antibiotics may reduce the presence of organisms and their production of toxin, thus ameliorating the symptoms. Because of the high volume of watery diarrhea, the antibiotic tends to be released from the body very rapidly. Doxycycline is usually the preferred drug, but trimethoprim-sulfamethoxazole or tetracycline have also been used. Unfortunately, certain strains of *V. cholerae* have been discovered to be resistant to the latter two antibiotics. Using antibiotics to more effectively eliminate the organism may be important, since it has been estimated that up to 20 percent of patients continue to carry *V. cholerae* asymptomatically for a time after recovery from the disease.

PERSPECTIVE AND PROSPECTS

Historically, cholera has been a very important epidemic pathogen credited with causing seven different pandemics. These pandemics have affected various areas, including Asia, the Middle East, and Africa. Between 1832 and 1836, two pandemics (the second and fourth) affected the North American continent, resulting in 200,000 American deaths. While studying and trying to limit the effects of the 1854 cholera epidemic in London, physician John Snow founded the science of epidemiology and introduced techniques that are still in use today. The seventh pandemic occurred in 1961, starting in Indonesia and spreading to South Asia, the Middle East, and portions of both Europe and Africa.

In 1991, Peru suddenly reported new cases after being free of cholera for more than a century. Contaminated bilge water discharged from a freighter into the Peru harbor has been hypothesized as being responsible for the disease's reappearance. The water supply in the capital city of Lima was not chlorinated, and the organism rapidly multiplied and infected the inhabitants. In two years, more than 700,000 cases and 6,323 deaths were recorded in South and Central America, and spread of this cholera strain continues today.

The 1961 pandemic strain has caused over five million cases of cholera and more than 250,000 deaths. In 1992, a genetic variant of this strain appeared in Bangladesh, causing an epidemic. This cholera strain spread to neighboring countries but has yet to initiate an eighth pandemic.

—*Steven A. Kuhl, Ph.D.*

See also Bacterial infections; Bacteriology; Diarrhea and dysentery; Environmental health; Epidemics and pandemics.

FOR FURTHER INFORMATION:

Ezzell, Carol. "It Came from the Deep." *Scientific American* 280 (June, 1999): 22-24.

Pennisi, Elizabeth. "Infectious Disease: Cholera Strengthened by Trip Through Gut." *Science* 296 (June, 2002): 1783-1784.

Reidl, Joachim, et al. *"Vibrio cholerae* and Cholera: Out of the Water and into the Host." *FEMS Microbiological Reviews* 26 (June, 2002): 125-139.

Wachsmuth, Kaye, et al. *"Vibrio cholerae" and Cholera: Molecular to Global Perspectives.* Washington, D.C.: American Society for Microbiology, 1994.

Zimmer, Carl. "Infectious Diseases: Taming Pathogens—An Elegant Idea, but Does It Work?" *Science* 300 (May, 2003): 1362-1364.

CHOLESTEROL

BIOLOGY

ANATOMY OR SYSTEM AFFECTED: Blood vessels, cells, circulatory system, gastrointestinal system

SPECIALTIES AND RELATED FIELDS: Biochemistry, cytology, family medicine, internal medicine, nutrition, preventive medicine, vascular medicine

DEFINITION: A lipid substance that is a structural component of cell membranes and that makes up the surface of lipoproteins.

KEY TERMS:

cholesterol: a lipid substance that is a component of cell membranes and the surface of circulating lipoproteins

cholesteryl ester: cholesterol linked to a fatty acid; it is stored in lipid droplets in the cytoplasm of cells and circulates in the core of lipoproteins

lipids: substances that are poorly soluble in water; in animal tissues, the principal lipids are triglycerides (fat), phospholipids, cholesterol, and cholesteryl esters

lipoproteins: lipid aggregates that transport fat and cholesteryl esters in the circulation; associated apolipoproteins determine how rapidly they are taken up by the liver or other tissues

sterols: a class of chemically related lipids; cholesterol is the principal sterol in vertebrates, but in plants its functions are served by related substances

STRUCTURE AND FUNCTIONS

Living cells are bounded by a cell membrane composed of a double layer of phospholipid, associated with and traversed by proteins that have catalytic, transportation, and signaling functions. Variable amounts of sterol are interspersed among the molecules of phospholipid in each membrane layer. Sterols are essential components in the membranes of fungal, plant, and animal cells (but not in bacteria). In vertebrates, the predominant sterol is cholesterol. There is little or no cholesterol in plant cell membranes; its place is taken by chemically related substances, chiefly sitosterol. This fact is of nutritional significance; only animal products add cholesterol to the diet.

In mammals, cholesterol is the precursor of steroid hormones, which are essential for mineral balance, adjustment of the body to stress, and normal reproductive function. It is also the precursor of bile acids, which are required for the absorption of dietary lipids. Bile acids play a role in cholesterol balance, since their formation and secretion by the liver, along with some free cholesterol, is the only significant pathway for removal of cholesterol from the body.

Cholesterol itself is required for normal functioning of the mammalian cell membrane. Cholesterol alters the membrane's fluidity—the ease with which proteins embedded in the membrane can move about and interact with one another—and also affects the activity of enzymes and transport proteins embedded in the membrane. Cultured cells that are prevented from making their own cholesterol will not grow unless it is provided in the medium.

Free cholesterol is confined to cellular membranes. Cholesterol content is highest (about one molecule of cholesterol for every one or two molecules of phospholipid) in the outer cell membrane that forms the boundary between a cell and its environment. It is much lower in intracellular membranes. Although cholesterol synthesis is completed within the endoplasmic reticulum, the ratio of cholesterol to phospholipid in this membrane is less than one to twenty. In a typical cell, it is estimated that between 80 and 90 percent of the total free cholesterol is located in the outer cell membrane.

Cholesterol in excess of normal proportions is coupled (esterified) to long-chain fatty acids. The resulting cholesteryl ester accumulates, along with triglyceride, in lipid droplets in the cytoplasm. The activity of the enzyme catalyzing this esterification is increased when cholesterol is imported into the cell in excess of its needs. The ability to esterify and sequester cholesterol defends the cell against excessive membrane concentration of the free sterol.

Free cholesterol and cholesteryl ester are carried in plasma in lipoproteins. Lipoproteins are aggregates of several thousand molecules of lipid and one or more molecules of specific proteins (apolipoproteins). Each lipoprotein particle consists of a core of triglyceride and cholesteryl ester surrounded by a single layer of phospholipid and free cholesterol. The apolipoproteins are embedded in the surface of the particle. Lipoproteins differ in size and relative lipid composition. In humans, about two-thirds of circulating cholesterol is contained in low-density lipoprotein (LDL), a core of cholesteryl ester with a single molecule of apolipoprotein B on the surface. LDL transports cholesterol from the liver to peripheral tissues. Most of the remaining circulating cholesterol is carried in high-density lipoprotein (HDL), which transports cholesterol from peripheral tissues back to the liver for disposal. Under normal conditions, LDL is the principal source of exogenous cholesterol available to a cell.

Uptake of LDL is mediated by a specific protein on the cell's surface, the LDL receptor, which is concentrated in pockets in the cell membrane termed coated pits. LDL receptors bind apolipoprotein B and particles such as LDL that contain this protein. Coated pits continually pinch off to form sealed vesicles (endosomes) inside the cell. At the same time, new coated pits form on the cell surface. When a coated pit pinches off, it carries with it LDL receptors and associated LDL. The fluid within the endosome is acidified, which causes LDL to dissociate from its receptor and float free. The LDL is transferred to lysosomes, where cholesteryl ester is cleaved to liberate cholesterol; along with the free cholesterol that formed part of the LDL surface, this liberated cholesterol is now available for use within the cell. The LDL receptor is returned to the cell surface, where it can again become associated with a coated pit and participate in a new round of LDL uptake.

The rate at which LDL is removed from the circulation depends on the concentration of LDL receptors in cells of the liver and other tissues. (Although there are other mechanisms for removing LDL, these are less efficient than uptake via the LDL receptor.) This process is subject to feedback regulation. When a cell contains an adequate supply of cholesterol, the synthesis of new LDL receptors is inhibited. This inhibition occurs at the transcriptional level: The rate at which the gene for the LDL receptor is copied into messenger ribonucleic acid (mRNA) is reduced. With less mRNA for this protein reaching the cytoplasm, the rate at which new copies of the protein are made also falls. Following normal turnover of existing receptors, the concentration of LDL receptors at the cell surface declines and the uptake of cholesterol is accordingly reduced.

The gene for the LDL receptor contains short stretches of deoxyribonucleic acid (DNA), termed sterol response elements (SREs), that make transcription sensitive to cholesterol-induced "down-regulation." These can be spliced out and inserted into another gene that codes for a bacterial protein. The foreign gene can be inserted into a mammalian cell, which will then begin to produce the corresponding protein. If the foreign gene does not contain an SRE, the rate of synthesis of the coded protein is unaffected by the cholesterol content of the recipient cell. When an SRE has been inserted into the gene in an appropriate location, however, excess cholesterol down-regulates transcription of the foreign gene just as it does that for the LDL receptor.

The signal that causes down-regulation of the cholesterol receptor has not been clearly identified. It is possible that an internal "regulatory" pool of cholesterol—such as the cholesterol content of certain internal membranes or the concentration of individual cholesterol molecules bound to some cytoplasmic protein carrier—is responsible. Some evidence, however, points to oxysterol analogues of cholesterol, rather than to cholesterol itself, as mediators of down-regulation. These analogues arise as minor metabolites of cholesterol and as intermediates and by-products of cholesterol synthesis. They are much more potent than cholesterol itself in inhibiting the synthesis of LDL receptors. A cytoplasmic oxysterol-binding protein has been identified whose affinity for different oxysterols parallels their relative potency in down-regulating the transcription of LDL receptor genes.

Mammalian cells also have the capacity to synthesize their own cholesterol. The enzymes catalyzing the successive reactions along this pathway are located in the cytoplasm and in the membranes of the endoplasmic reticulum. The starting material from which cholesterol is made is acetic acid in the form of acetyl coenzyme A (acetyl CoA). This material is generated in mitochondria as an intermediate in the oxidation of glucose and of fatty acids. To be utilized for synthesis of cholesterol, it must first be transported from the mitochondria to the cytoplasm; a specific shuttle exists for this purpose. The synthesis of fatty acids from acetyl CoA also takes place in the cytoplasm, and more of the translocated precursor is used for this purpose than to make cholesterol.

An early step on the pathway to cholesterol is the reduction of hydroxymethylglutaryl coenzyme A (HMG CoA) to mevalonic acid, catalyzed by HMG CoA reductase. The enzymatic capacity to catalyze this reaction is substantially lower than that for other steps on the pathway, so that the overall rate of cholesterol synthesis is largely determined by the activity of this enzyme. Both amount and activity are regulated to match the rates of cholesterol synthesis to the needs of the cell. When the cell has adequate supplies of cholesterol, HMG CoA reductase activity is low and, simultaneously, uptake via the LDL receptor is reduced. Conversely, when more cholesterol is needed, HMG CoA reductase activity and overall cholesterol synthesis are increased, as are expression of the LDL receptor and the uptake of cholesterol.

HMG CoA reductase activity is regulated at several points, including transcription of the gene, efficiency with which its mRNA is translated into protein, turnover of the enzyme protein, and inactivation by chemical modification. Regulation of the transcription of the HMG CoA reductase gene and regulation of the LDL receptor gene appear to have the same fundamental mechanism. The gene for HMG CoA reductase contains an SRE similar in sequence to those in the gene for the LDL receptor. Oxysterols that repress transcription of the LDL receptor exert the same effect on transcription of the gene for HMG CoA reductase, and with the same relative potency. Mutant cells that have lost the capacity to respond to oxysterols by repressing the synthesis of LDL receptors also fail to respond by repressing the synthesis of HMG CoA reductase.

Excess cholesterol also increases the rate at which HMG CoA reductase is broken down. This might be a response to changes in cholesterol concentration in the internal membranes in which HMG CoA reductase is embedded. When the gene for HMG CoA reductase is altered to remove the sequences that anchor it to the membrane and the altered gene is inserted into a recipient cell, the mutant protein is located unattached in the cytoplasm. In contrast to the native enzyme, the rate of turnover of the altered gene product is not affected by the cholesterol content of the recipient cell.

Phosphorylation (attachment of a phosphate to specific amino acid residues) of HMG CoA reductase is a third mechanism by which the synthesis of cholesterol is altered. This is best documented in the liver (which is also the principal site within the body for the synthesis of cholesterol). Liver cells contain an enzyme that phosphorylates and inactivates HMG CoA reductase; the same enzyme also phosphorylates and inactivates the enzyme catalyzing the rate-determining step in the synthesis of fatty acids, acetyl CoA carboxylase. The phosphorylation of both enzymes is promoted, and the synthesis of fatty acids and cholesterol is correspondingly inhibited, under fasting conditions. In the fed state, the reverse is true. These changes appear to be a response to circulating levels of the hormone insulin.

Most of the mevalonic acid that is produced by HMG CoA reductase activity is converted to cholesterol. Since its formation is the rate-determining step on the pathway, the addition of mevalonic acid itself to the cell results in much higher rates of cholesterol synthesis than can be achieved with acetyl CoA as starting material. Moreover, the synthesis of cholesterol from mevalonic acid is not controlled by feedback inhibition. Under these circumstances, expression of HMG CoA reductase and expression of the LDL receptor are maximally repressed.

Mevalonic acid is also the precursor of other substances needed by the cell. These include dolichol (a coenzyme needed for the addition of carbohydrate residues to proteins), ubiquinone (a participant in electron transport reactions in mitochondria), and isoprenyl side chains that are attached to specific proteins. Although their synthesis consumes only a minor portion of the mevalonic acid produced by HMG CoA reductase, these substances are essential to normal cell function. When HMG CoA reductase is inhibited by lovastatin, a drug that competes with the substrate HMG CoA for binding to the enzyme, cell growth is inhibited even when supplies of cholesterol in the medium are adequate. Resumption of cell growth requires the addition of small amounts of mevalonic acid as well as cholesterol. Mutant cell lines have been obtained that, even without lovastatin, are unable to grow unless mevalonic acid is present. The requirements of these cells can be met with a large amount of mevalonic acid in the medium or with a small amount of mevalonic acid plus a large amount of cholesterol.

The multiple roles of mevalonic acid are also reflected in the way that HMG CoA reductase activity is regulated. Although transcription of the HMG CoA reductase gene is reduced when cholesterol levels in the cell are high, some transcription continues to allow enough mevalonic acid to be produced to meet other needs of the cell. Adding small amounts of mevalonic acid further decreases the synthesis of HMG CoA reductase by decreasing the rate at which its mRNA is translated into protein. In contrast, expression of the LDL receptor is not under dual regulation; maximal suppression can be obtained with cholesterol alone.

DISORDERS AND DISEASES

Excessive levels of LDL cholesterol are associated with an increased risk of coronary heart disease and stroke. Efforts to reduce LDL cholesterol through changes in diet or through drugs take advantage of what is known about cholesterol balance in individual cells and in the body as a whole. The latter is determined by three factors: the dietary intake of cholesterol, the rate of cholesterol synthesis within the body (principally by the liver), and the rate of cholesterol disposal (also principally by the liver, through secretion of free sterol into the bile and by the conversion of cholesterol to bile acids). Accordingly, levels of LDL cholesterol can be diminished by limiting the intake and synthesis of new cholesterol, reducing cholesterol secretion by the liver (in the form of an LDL precursor particle), promoting LDL uptake by the liver (mediated by the LDL receptor), and increasing the formation and secretion of bile acids and free cholesterol.

The body can meet its need for cholesterol through synthesis; there is no dietary requirement. Cholesterol deficiency does not arise in humans even on a purely vegetarian (cholesterol-free) diet. The average Western diet, rich in meat and dairy products, contains between 250 and 500 milligrams of cholesterol per day. Small amounts of cholesterol in the diet are fairly well absorbed, but efficiency declines with larger quantities; on average, about half of the cholesterol consumed per day is assimilated. Absorption of cholesterol and other lipids in the small intestine requires the presence of bile acids. These mix with cholesterol and partially degraded dietary triglyceride to form small droplets that facilitate the absorption of lipids by the cells lining the small intestine. In the process, most of the bile acid (as well as cholesterol secreted in the bile) is reabsorbed and returned to the liver. The absorbed cholesterol is esterified and secreted into the lymph, along with triglyceride, in the core of chylomicrons. These large lipoproteins are reduced in size by removal of triglyceride in capillary beds, and the remnants, containing all the original cholesteryl ester, are taken up by the liver. Thus, the cholesterol absorbed in the intestine passes initially to the liver.

The liver is the most important site for cholesterol synthesis within the body. As explained above, hepatic synthesis of cholesterol is under feedback control. HMG CoA reductase activity and cholesterol synthesis are suppressed when large amounts of dietary cholesterol reach the liver and are augmented when the diet is cholesterol-free. Drugs such as lovastatin that inhibit

IN THE NEWS: CHOLESTEROL-LOWERING DRUGS

Since high cholesterol level contributes to major health problems including hypertension, heart disease, and stroke, it is essential that cholesterol levels be kept in check. While lifestyle changes including diet and exercise may help to lower cholesterol, most individuals with elevated cholesterol levels are placed on medication. These cholesterol-lowering medications fall into several different categories. Patients may be placed on one drug or on a combination of drugs. The major categories of cholesterol-lowering drugs are statins, selective cholesterol absorption inhibitors, bile acid sequestrants (resins), fibric acid derivatives (or fibrates), and nicotinic acid (niacin). The most commonly used of these medications are statins. These drugs work in the liver to inhibit the production of HMG CoA reductase, which controls the production of cholesterol. Statins have been found to decrease cholesterol levels between 20 and 60 percent by slowing the production of cholesterol, while increasing the ability of the liver to remove low-density lipoproteins (LDL) from the blood, and increasing high-density lipoproteins (HDL). This class of drugs includes Lipitor (atorvastatin), Crestor (rosuvastatin), Zocor (simvastatin), and Pravachol (pravastatin). Statins are contraindicated in people who are preganant or nursing, have liver damage, or have high alcohol intakes. A second category of cholesterol-lowering drugs are selective cholesterol absorption inhibitors. Drugs in this category interfere with the absorption of cholesterol in the intestines, allowing the body to eliminate more cholesterol, especially LDLs. Zetia (ezetimibe) is the most commonly used drug in this class. Resins also work in the intestines, although in a different manner. Resins bind to bile, so that it is eliminated and cannot be used in digestion, causing more bile to be produced. Cholesterol is used by the liver to produce bile, leaving less cholesterol in the bloodstream. Drugs in this category include Questran (cholestyramine) and WelChol (colesevelam Hcl). Fibrates are used to lower triglycerides, rather than LDLs, and may be used in combination with the statins. This category of drugs includes Lopid (gemffibrozil) and Tricor (fenofibrate). The final category of drug used to lower cholesterol is niacin, a nutritional supplement that is available over the counter and in prescription form. It acts in the liver to decrease cholesterol production. In prescription form, niacin can lower both LDL and triglycerides. Thus, physicians can use any of these medications, individually or in combination, to lower their patients' cholesterol.

—*Robin Kamienny Montvilo, R.N., Ph.D.*

the circulation. VLDL is secreted primarily to transport triglyceride to other tissues for use as a metabolic fuel or for storage. After serving this function, most of the VLDL remnants return to the liver. Those that escape hepatic reabsorption are transformed in the circulation into LDL. LDL is also taken up by the liver (and elsewhere), but at a much slower rate than VLDL remnant particles, so that this lipoprotein accumulates in the circulation. It is deposition of LDL in the lining of blood vessels that initiates the formation of atherosclerotic plaques—the beginning of atherosclerotic disease. Since cholesterol is required for the secretion of VLDL, HMG CoA reductase inhibitors that cause a partial depletion of cholesterol in liver cells reduce the rate at which it enters the bloodstream. By the same means, they also increase expression of LDL receptors in liver cells, which results in a more rapid removal of LDL from the circulation. Both mechanisms reduce circulating levels of LDL cholesterol.

Cholesterol in the liver may also be converted to bile acids and secreted in the bile. Although most of the secreted bile acid comes back to the liver, some escapes reabsorption in the small intestine. The bile acid that is lost must be replaced by the metabolization of more cholesterol. Bile acid sequestrants such as cholestyramine are also used to reduce circulating cholesterol. They act by forming complexes with bile acids in the small intestine and interfere with their reabsorption. A larger fraction of the secreted bile acid is thus lost by excretion, and the rate of conversion of cholesterol to bile acid in the liver is correspondingly increased.

HMG CoA reductase are useful in reducing cholesterol levels in the circulation, since they limit the ability of the liver to respond by making more cholesterol when the dietary intake is reduced.

Cholesterol within the liver may be incorporated into very low-density lipoprotein (VLDL) and secreted into

The liver secretes a large amount of free cholesterol into the bile. Most of this biliary cholesterol is reabsorbed and returned to the liver. Since bile acids are required for the intestinal uptake of cholesterol, a second beneficial action of bile acid sequestrants is to increase the fraction of biliary cholesterol that escapes reabsorption and is excreted. The combination of bile acid sequestrant and HMG CoA reductase inhibitor is especially effective in lowering blood levels of LDL cholesterol by limiting the uptake of cholesterol from the diet, limiting the synthesis of cholesterol in the liver, increasing the clearance of cholesterol from the blood by the liver, and increasing the conversion of hepatic cholesterol to bile acids.

Other drugs used to reduce circulating LDL cholesterol levels include nicotinic acid, fibiric acid derivatives, and probucol. Nicotinic acid (niacin) is also a vitamin, but the amounts required to affect plasma cholesterol levels are far in excess of the daily requirement for this compound as an essential nutrient. At these pharmacologic doses, side effects such as itching, facial flushing, and gastric distress are common. Nicotinic acid decreases the formation of VLDL triglyceride in the liver and therefore reduces the formation of LDL; it also promotes the uptake of LDL through LDL receptors and increases the concentration of HDL cholesterol (cholesterol being returned to the liver for disposal). The underlying mechanisms for these actions have not been determined. Fibric acid derivatives, such as gemfibrazole, also reduce VLDL secretion and promote LDL uptake by the liver; again the mechanism of drug action is uncertain. Probucol acts primarily to prevent chemical modification of LDL in the circulation that makes it more likely to be deposited in the walls of blood vessels.

Although high circulating levels of LDL cholesterol call for drug intervention, the risk of atherosclerotic disease can be reduced in most adults by attention to the dietary factors that affect cholesterol balance. Dietary studies have had a controversial history because of frequently contradictory findings. A few principles are, however, well supported by the data. First, eliminating cholesterol from the diet, with no other intervention, produces a significant drop in the levels of cholesterol in circulating LDL. Second, intake of calories beyond actual energy needs raises serum cholesterol. Excess fuel is stored as triglycerides, which to a large extent are formed in the liver and exported in VLDL. Since VLDL contains cholesterol, and since it is the precursor of LDL, high rates of triglyceride formation in the liver promote the accumulation of cholesterol in plasma LDL—which is especially likely to occur if the calories are ingested in the form of triglyceride. Not

only does this increase the requirement for the liver to secrete VLDL, but the fatty acids derived from triglyceride also stimulate cholesterol synthesis. Third, saturated fatty acids have the strongest tendency to elevate plasma cholesterol levels. This is the case even when these fatty acids are consumed as vegetable oils (such as palm oil and coconut oil) unaccompanied by cholesterol. The basis for this effect is not well understood but appears to result from decreased expression of LDL receptors in the liver. The American Heart Association recommends that not more than 200 milligrams per day of cholesterol be consumed in a diet which is matched to caloric need and in which not more than 30 percent of calories are consumed as fat (and not more than 10 percent as saturated fat).

PERSPECTIVE AND PROSPECTS

The average adult body contains about 150 grams of cholesterol. Less than 5 percent of this cholesterol is in circulating lipoproteins or trapped in atherosclerotic lesions. The remainder performs essential functions as a structural component of membranes and as the precursor of other vital substances. Although researchers have learned much about the subcellular distribution, the pathway for biosynthesis, and the mechanisms for transport of cholesterol, important questions remain. It is not known how cholesterol is transported within the cell or what determines its relative distribution among different cellular membranes. It is not known what signals suppress the synthesis of HMG CoA reductase and LDL receptors or how the message is transmitted to the nucleus to diminish transcription of these genes. Some product of mevalonic acid metabolism other than cholesterol also regulates the expression of HMG CoA reductase, but this factor has not yet been identified. It is not known why cholesterol is an absolute requirement for functioning of mammalian cell membranes. It is not known what determines the fraction of dietary cholesterol that is absorbed across the intestinal lining. Finally, there is much to learn about factors that regulate the secretion and reuptake of lipoproteins by the liver and that control the return to the liver of cholesterol in HDL.

These questions are of practical as well as academic interest. Coronary heart disease and other complications of atherosclerosis are the leading causes of death in the United States. Controlling and reversing this process is a serious medical challenge. While other factors such as hypertension, smoking, and diabetes mellitus contribute to the risk of atherosclerosis, reducing the level of cholesterol that circulates as a component of LDL and increasing the level transported in HDL have been shown to provide significant protection. Knowledge of how cholesterol is normally produced and assimilated has contributed to the design of drugs that reduce circulating levels by interfering with the absorption and synthesis of cholesterol and promoting its metabolism and excretion. This field of investigation continues to be a major concern of both basic and pharmaceutical scientists.

—Lauren M. Cagen, Ph.D.

See also Arteriosclerosis; Blood and blood disorders; Blood testing; Cells; Digestion; Food biochemistry; Heart disease; Hypercholesterolemia; Hyperlipidemia; Metabolism; Nutrition; Plaque, arterial; Preventive medicine; Strokes.

FOR FURTHER INFORMATION:

Dietschy, John M. "Physiology in Medicine: LDL Cholesterol—Its Regulation and Manipulation." *Hospital Practice* 25 (June 15, 1990): 67-78. An excellent nontechnical introduction to the subject of cholesterol balance and its regulation, by a major contributor to the field. The article discusses the effect of diet and of drug interventions.

Freeman, Mason W., with Christine Junge. *The Harvard Medical School Guide to Lowering Your Cholesterol.* New York: McGraw-Hill, 2005. Written for general readers, this book explains, among other topics, the differences between "good" and "bad" cholesterol, discusses cholesterol levels and managing those levels for prime health, and examines the use of cholesterol-lowering prescription drugs.

Grundy, Scott M. *Cholesterol and Atherosclerosis.* Philadelphia: J. P. Lippincott, 1990. The author provides a general overview of cholesterol balance, elevated plasma cholesterol, and its management by diet and drugs. Although intended for physicians, the book is written in a simple and direct style and is profusely illustrated.

Hirsch, Anita. *Good Cholesterol, Bad Cholesterol: An Indispensable Guide to the Facts About Cholesterol.* New York: Avalon, 2002. An easy-to-browse format that provides medical facts about cholesterol, lifestyle guidance to managing cholesterol levels, and recipes for low-cholesterol meals.

Leaf, David A. *Cholesterol Treatment: A Guide to Lipid Disorder Management.* 4th ed. Durant, Okla.: EMIS, 2000. The primary purpose of this book is to provide in a convenient reference much of the information that the practicing physician and supportive health care clinicians need to manage patients with lipid disorders.

McGowan, Mary P., and Jo McGowan Chopra. *Fifty Ways to Lower Cholesterol.* New York: McGraw-Hill, 2002. Advocates a multifaceted approach to lowering cholesterol levels, including diet, weight management, exercise, and medical intervention.

Nesto, N. W., and Lisa Christenson. *Cholesterol-Lowering Drugs: Everything You and Your Family Need to Know.* New York: William Morrow, 2000. Includes profiles of commonly used cholesterol-lowering prescription drugs and a discussion of side effects, interactions, and warnings. Includes special information for women, children, and seniors. Addresses the causes and dangers of high cholesterol; the effects of diet, exercise, and smoking; and age, gender, and genetic factors.

CHORIONIC VILLUS SAMPLING
PROCEDURE

ANATOMY OR SYSTEM AFFECTED: Reproductive system, uterus

SPECIALTIES AND RELATED FIELDS: Embryology, genetics, obstetrics, perinatology

DEFINITION: The collection of a small sample of chorionic villi tissue from the fingerlike projections of the placenta at the point of attachment to the uterine wall. These cells are examined for genetic and chromosomal abnormalities by means of karyotyping.

INDICATIONS AND PROCEDURES

Chorionic villus sampling can be performed between the tenth and twelfth weeks of pregnancy to detect genetic and chromosomal abnormalities. The procedure is recommended when there is increased risk of genetic disorders in the fetus such as Down syndrome, sickle cell disease, and muscular dystrophy.

Chorionic villus sampling involves collecting a small sample of the chorionic villi, the fingerlike projections on the developing placenta, which delivers food and oxygen to the fetus. A sample of chorionic villi can be obtained either by inserting a needle through the abdomen or by entering the cervix with a small flexible catheter through the vagina. The choice of approach depends on the position of the placenta. Ultrasound is used to locate the fetus and the placenta and its villi.

A 10- to 25-milligram sample is collected using a syringe, which is then purified and sometimes cultured. Since the chorionic villi originate from the same cell as the fetus, they normally have the same genetics. Results are available within days.

USES AND COMPLICATIONS

Along with exposing genetic and chromosomal disorders, chorionic villus sampling can be used to determine the sex of the embryo but should never be used for this purpose alone because of the risks involved. Testing can be done early in the pregnancy. Therefore, if the woman should choose to terminate her pregnancy, an easier first-trimester abortion can be performed. If the results from the test are favorable, the parents have an early peace of mind.

Possible complications from chorionic villus sampling include vaginal bleeding and cramping. More serious risks involve spontaneous abortion and even possible fetal injury. The rate of miscarriage is about 1 percent higher with chorionic villus sampling than with amniocentesis, performed after sixteen weeks and yielding the same information.

Some studies suggest that chorionic villus sampling itself may cause some birth defects; others do not. Also, the procedure can be inaccurate. Abnormalities may occur in some placental cells but not in the fetus. This might lead to aborting a healthy fetus. With the guidance of a physician, the risks and benefits should be compared with other available procedures.

—*Paul R. Boehlke, Ph.D., and Pavel Svilenov; updated by Robin Kamienny Montvilo, R.N., Ph.D.*

See also Abortion; Amniocentesis; Birth defects; Down syndrome; Embryology; Fetal surgery; Genetic counseling; Genetic diseases; Karyotyping; Miscarriage; Muscular dystrophy; Obstetrics; Perinatology; Pregnancy and gestation; Reproductive system; Sickle cell disease; Ultrasonography; Women's health.

FOR FURTHER INFORMATION:

Caughey, Aaron B., Linda M. Hopkins, and Mary E. Norton. "Chorionic Villus Sampling Compared with Amniocentesis and the Difference in the Rate of Pregnancy Loss." *Obstetrics and Gynecology* 108, no. 3 (September, 2006): 612-616.

Ettorre, Elizabeth, ed. *Before Birth: Understanding Prenatal Screening.* Brookfield, Vt.: Ashgate, 2001.

Filkins, Karen, and Joseph F. Russo, eds. *Human Prenatal Diagnosis.* 2d rev. ed. New York: Marcel Dekker, 1990.

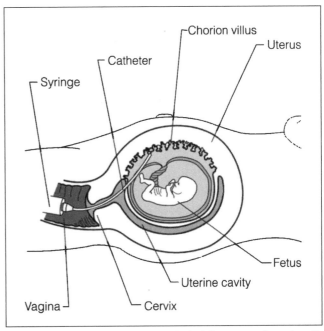

Chorionic villus sampling is one method of obtaining embryonic cells from a pregnant woman; examination of these cells helps physicians determine fetal irregularities or defects, which allows time to assess the problem and make recommendations for treatment.

Harper, Peter S. *Practical Genetic Counselling.* 6th ed. New York: Oxford University Press, 2004.

Lichtman, Ronnie, Lynn Louise Simpson, and Allan Rosenfield. *Dr. Guttmacher's Pregnancy, Birth, and Family Planning.* Rev. ed. New York: New American Library, 2003.

Moore, Keith L., and T. V. N. Persaud. *The Developing Human.* 8th ed. Philadelphia: Saunders/Elsevier, 2008.

Pierce, Benjamin A. *The Family Genetic Sourcebook.* New York: John Wiley & Sons, 1990.

CHROMOSOMAL ABNORMALITIES. *See* **BIRTH DEFECTS; GENETIC DISEASES.**

CHRONIC FATIGUE SYNDROME

DISEASE/DISORDER

ALSO KNOWN AS: Chronic fatigue and immune dysfunction syndrome

ANATOMY OR SYSTEM AFFECTED: Immune system, muscles, musculoskeletal system, psychic-emotional system

SPECIALTIES AND RELATED FIELDS: Family medicine, hematology, immunology, internal medicine, psychiatry

DEFINITION: Chronic fatigue syndrome is a multifaceted disease state characterized by debilitating fatigue.

KEY TERMS:

adenopathy: the enlargement of any gland (often the lymph gland)

cell-mediated immune response: an immune response that involves cells rather than antibodies, particularly T lymphocytes rather than B lymphocytes

cytokines: proteins secreted by immune cells which contribute to immune responses and inflammation

fibromyalgia: a condition of generalized chronic pain that shares many symptoms with chronic fatigue syndrome

infectious mononucleosis: acute self-limiting infection of lymphocytes by the Epstein-Barr virus

interleukin-2: a protein messenger that regulates T cell activity and differentiation during the immune response

lymphocytes: agranular leukocytes that differentiate into B lymphocytes and T lymphocytes and play a fundamental role in the immune response

polymerase chain reaction: a laboratory method used to increase the amount of DNA found in small quantities

suppressor T cell: a type of T lymphocyte that is believed to modulate the immune response

---

INFORMATION ON CHRONIC FATIGUE SYNDROME

CAUSES: Unknown; possibly microbial agents, stress, lifestyle factors, genetic makeup, immunological factors

SYMPTOMS: Debilitating fatigue, low-grade fever, sore throat, headache, muscle pain, painful lymph nodes, disturbed sleep patterns

DURATION: Chronic

TREATMENTS: None; alleviation of symptoms

CAUSES AND SYMPTOMS

Chronic fatigue syndrome is a heterogenous disease state that has been difficult to define, diagnose, and treat because of poorly understood cause-and-effect relationships. The disease can be best described in terms of long-lasting and debilitating fatigue, the etiology of which has been linked to such external factors as microbial agents, stress, and lifestyle as well as such internal factors as genetic makeup and the body's immune response. The fact that it is a physical disease with psychological components has also caused confusion in the medical community.

Among the many names that have been used for the disease, two that demonstrate the many factors that contribute to chronic fatigue syndrome are chronic Epstein-Barr virus syndrome and chronic fatigue immune dysfunction syndrome. Because of the marked immunological aspects of the disease and the fact that different viruses have been found in patients with chronic fatigue, the disease is referred to as chronic fatigue immune dysfunction syndrome by many involved in the study. The Centers for Disease Control and Prevention (CDC) continues to refer to it as chronic fatigue syndrome (CFS).

Although the disease is not specific by race, gender, or age group, there is demographic evidence that young white females make up two-thirds of the known cases. It is estimated by the CDC that between 1 and 10 of every 10,000 people in the United States have CFS. The disease has also been identified in Europe and Australia.

CFS can manifest itself in acute and chronic phases, although some patients do not remember an acute phase presentation. Acute phase symptoms are general and flulike, with a low-grade fever, sore throat, headache, muscle pain, painful lymph nodes, and overall fatigue. Unlike with a bout of influenza, the symptoms do not subside with time, instead intensifying into a chronic phase. The fatigue can become disabling, with severe muscle and joint pain, swollen and painful lymph nodes, and the inability to develop proper sleep patterns. The similarity of CFS to fibromyalgia, diffuse muscular pain throughout the body, has resulted in cross diagnosis by many physicians of the two syndromes. Some researchers blame psychological and emotional stress, with a viral infection having triggered the initial acute phase. Although the psychological description does not fit all cases, problems of concentration, attention, and depression have been implicated to the point that researchers recognize both psychological and physical components. The working definition from both a research and a clinical perspective requires that the fatigue cause at least 50 percent incapacitation and last at least six months. The ineffectiveness of treatment, compounded by the inability to provide a concrete diagnosis, further complicates the psychological aspects of the disease for the patient.

Although the environment provides an array of agents that could trigger the physical condition of CFS, the hypothesis for a viral cause is supported by the flulike symptoms, occasional clustering of cases, and presence of antiviral antibodies in the patient's serum. The involvement of the Epstein-Barr virus in some forms of CFS seems likely because of its role as the etiological agent of mononucleosis and Burkitt's lymphoma, which are similar diseases. In both of these diseases, the Epstein-Barr virus has a unique and harmful effect on the immune system because it directly invades B lymphocytes, the antibody-producing cells of the body, using them to grow new virus particles while disrupting the proper functioning of the immune system. Like CFS, mononucleosis is characterized by flulike symptoms and fatigue, but the disease is self-limiting and the patient eventually recovers.

Despite this seeming difference in outcome, the Epstein-Barr virus can cause a chronic condition. The viruses that infect humans can become dormant within the cells that they infect. The nucleic acid of a virus can become incorporated into the deoxyribonucleic acid (DNA) of its host cell, and the body no longer shows physical signs of its presence. A virus can become active at times of physical or emotional stress and can once again trigger the physical symptoms of disease. For example, herpes simplex virus 1 remains dormant in its host cell but periodically, in response to environmental factors, causes a cold sore lesion.

Immunological dysfunction has been observed in CFS patients because they demonstrate increased allergic sensitivity to skin tests when compared to individuals without CFS. Cells and cellular chemicals directly involved with protective immunity and the regulation of the immune response have been found in these patients in abnormal concentrations. For example, they have abnormal numbers of the natural killer cells and suppressor T cells that are essential to cell-mediated immunity. A variety of cytokines, such as gamma interferon, and various interleukins which regulate the activities of the cells in the cell-mediated and humoral immune responses are seen in abnormal concentrations in some CFS patients. Some of these cytokines are already known to mediate the immune response to viral infections. Infectious agents such as bacteria, viruses, yeast, intracellular parasites, and even cancer cells are eliminated from the body when humoral and cell-mediated immune systems are operating properly. The presence of abnormally high concentrations of these cytokines may contribute to inflammatory processes sometimes found in patients with CFS. When the immune system is not working properly, however, not

only is the body more susceptible to a variety of infectious agents but the immune system can begin to damage or destroy normal tissues as well. Such disease states are referred to as autoimmune diseases. Inflammation and allergic reactions are other examples of uncontrolled immune responses.

The psychological and emotional aspects of CFS are also in question. Some studies indicate that the brain is physically affected by inflammation and hormonal changes. Other studies demonstrate that some of the known viral infective agents can have neurological effects. Psychiatric studies give ample evidence that depression, memory loss, and concentration are significant problems for some CFS patients. The extent to which stress is a factor in the disease is unknown.

TREATMENT AND THERAPY

Defining and treating chronic fatigue syndrome has been difficult because it manifests itself as a systemic disease with confusing cause-and-effect relationships involving external factors such as infectious viruses, internal factors such as the immune response, and a psychological component that is difficult to assess in the light of the biological changes occurring in the body. The symptoms, provided by patient histories, physical examinations, and laboratory findings, involve neuromuscular, psychoneurological, and immunological changes that vary between patients. The variety of factors to consider has caused difficulty in establishing diagnostic criteria for primary care in a clinical setting or further definition of the disease and treatments in a research setting.

In 1988, the CDC established diagnostic criteria that are divided into two major criteria, eleven minor symptom criteria, and three minor physical criteria. The first major criterion defines chronic fatigue as lasting at least six months and causing debilitation to 50 percent of the patient's normal activity. The second major criterion requires that all other disease conditions that could fit the patient history, physical examination, and appropriate laboratory tests be ruled out. The categories of disease that might be similar to CFS are cancers, chronic degenerative disease, autoimmune disorders, microbial and parasitic disease, and chronic psychiatric disease. Combinations of some minor criteria that would fit a general flulike condition must be demonstrated.

In 1993, a meeting at the CDC attempted to evaluate what had been learned over the previous five-year period and to make recommendations regarding a case definition. It was suggested that the case definition format involve inclusion and exclusion criteria that would increase the number and range of cases being studied because of the heterogeneous nature of the disease. The cases should also be subcategorized to provide a homogeneity that would allow for subgroup identification and comparison. The inclusion evidence should be simple, with a descriptive interpretation of the fatigue being essential and having objective criteria to define a 50 percent reduction of physical activity. Symptoms that are specific to unexplained fatigue should be used, while the physical exam information should not be included. It was also suggested that exclusion of any cases should involve an in-depth history (both medical and psychiatric), a physical examination, and standardized testing that would involve medical, laboratory, and psychiatric information.

Because it appears that CFS overlaps with many other medical and psychiatric conditions that can be identified and treated, there is debate as to how to interpret CFS as it relates to patient care and research. Some believe that an in-depth history is fundamental to the understanding of CFS and that CFS could be the final pathway that occurs from a variety of biological and psychosocial insults to the body.

The minor criteria used to define CFS involve both symptom and physical criteria that have not been proved adequate to validate or define the condition. In fact, the conflicting data have only served to emphasize further the clinical heterogeneity of the disease and suggest a heterogeneity of cause. Suggestions have been made to drop the concept of minor criteria, use symptoms that are specific for the unexplained fatigue, and drop all physical examination criteria. The argument for eliminating physical criteria is that more specific criteria exist for a case definition. Because physical symptoms are inconsistent or periodic, it is believed that a documented patient history would provide more case-specific information.

Although symptom criteria have widespread support in the case definition of CFS, symptoms with the greatest sensitivity and specificity are also being debated. Night sweats, cough, gastrointestinal problems, and new and worsening allergies are not presently considered and are believed by some to be more specific than fever or chills and sore throat. Others have proposed that symptoms should be reduced to chills and fever, sore throat, neck or axilla adenopathy, and sudden onset of a main symptom complex. The most prevalent symptoms are believed to be muscle weakness and pain, problems in concentration, and sleep disturbance.

The importance of the psychiatric component in CFS continues to be a problem in case definition. Some believe that the neurological component is a major criterion in case definition and that behavior symptoms, including stress and psychiatric illness, must be emphasized in clinical diagnosis as well as in therapy. It has been recommended that objective neuropsychological testing be used to determine cognitive dysfunction and depression. There is agreement that CFS patients have impaired concentration and attention, but forgetfulness and memory problems are questioned. There is also evidence that the duration and severity of myalgia are closely associated with psychological distress and that psychotherapy improves physical symptoms. Finally, it has been argued that the psychiatric component of the case definition is essential because there is evidence that the disease directly affects the brain and that CFS can cause both isolation and limitation of the patient's normal lifestyle.

Whatever the case definition, the second major criterion will be expressed in some form. Proper patient care necessitates extensive evaluation in order to identify the biological or psychological reasons for the problem. Proper CFS patient care demands the elimination of other serious disease possibilities that may appear superficially similar. Primary care physicians may find it difficult to make a diagnosis without a team of specialists in the areas of hematology, immunology, and psychiatry. Numerous laboratory tests must be made available. Although there are no specific recommended tests, those that must be performed should be tailored to specific patients and used by the team of specialists for their care.

The possibility of infectious disease, either as part of CFS (as in the case of certain viral agents) or as an autonomous infection having no relation to CFS, requires a variety of antibody tests to detect such viruses as Epstein-Barr or HIV. Skin tests such as the purified protein derivative (PPD) test for tuberculosis are used. Polymerase chain reaction and tissue culture for cytopathic effects have been developed to detect certain retroviruses for ultimate use in diagnosis at the clinical level.

The immune system is so intimately interactive with the entire body that most disease conditions are affected by or affect its function. The measure of its components provides a clue to the identity of the disease that is operating because they indicate whether normal protection activity or immune dysfunction (or a combination) is occurring in the patient.

The components of the immune system can be measured in numerous ways, from methodologies used in standard clinical laboratory procedures to research protocols used to study immune function and disease treatment. Tests are available that can measure total antibody concentration and the various subgroups IgG, IgM, IgA, IgE, and IgD; cytokines such as interleukin-2 and gamma interferon; cellular components such as T cells and their subtypes (such as suppressor T cells and natural killer cells); and B cells.

Autoimmune diseases and allergies are immune dysfunction diseases in their own right. Because there is an immune dysfunction component to CFS, tests for these conditions are important considerations. An antinuclear antibody (ANA) test determines the presence of antibodies that attack the tissues of the patient, as in systemic lupus erythematosus. The type and extent of allergic reactions can be measured using the radioimmunosorbent (RIST) tests for total IgE concentration and radioallergosorbent (RAST) tests for IgE concentration for particular antigens.

Systemic disease states, including CFS, often involve generalized inflammation that is considered part of the body's protective response. While inflammation is important to the elimination of various infective agents, it is also involved in neurological and muscle tissue damage. C-reactive protein (CRP) and the erythrocyte sedimentation rate (ESR) tests measure the intensity of the inflammatory response. A variety of other tests provide information that indicates the extent of muscle, liver, thyroid, and other vital organ damage.

Although a diagnosis can be made for CFS, there is no standard treatment. Clinical treatment essentially takes the form of alleviating the symptoms. Antidepressants such as doxepin (Sinequan) are useful in the treatment of depression and are also used to control muscle pain, lethargy, and sleeping problems. Nonsteroidal anti-inflammatory drugs (NSAIDs) provide relief for headache and muscle pain. Two drugs that have demonstrated antiviral activities are acyclovir and ampligen; ampligen can also modulate the immune response.

An example of research to develop therapies that might alleviate other symptoms of CFS involves the treatment of a number of patients with dialyzable leukocyte extract and psychologic treatment in the form of cognitive-behavioral therapy. The patients' cell-mediated immune response after therapy was evaluated by peripheral blood T cell subset analysis and delayed hypersensitivity skin testing. Psychologic analysis was performed using numerous cognitive tests. Both therapies proved to be inconclusive.

Because of the systemic nature of the disease, including its psychoneurological component, consideration must be given to holistic medical treatment. Any treatment protocol must be able to address the interactive factors of CFS that are still being defined in terms of cause and effect. Some researchers believe that therapeutic treatment should comprise diet, exercise, vitamins, and homeopathic medicine. They further believe that psychoemotional treatment should allow patients to be responsible for their own recovery and help them to develop a personal lifestyle that provides general good health.

PERSPECTIVE AND PROSPECTS

The vague, often "flulike" symptoms used to define chronic fatigue syndrome have historically been associated with numerous infectious agents, such as *Brucella* (brucellosis), *Coxsiella*, Epstein-Barr virus infections (infectious mononucleosis), and other chronic viral diseases. In most cases, a specific etiological agent was discovered. Association with a specific agent allowed for treatment in many cases, or at the least a means to define the illness.

Since being linked with the Epstein-Barr virus, CFS has been the subject of many studies that support its definition as a heterogenous illness, including a category of postinfective fatigue syndromes that follow viral infections. The case definition provided by the CDC in 1988 has allowed the disease to be diagnosed and treated at the clinical level and to be identified and compared at the research level. The disease state has proven to be elusive, however, and the case definition too complex and open to interpretation. It is believed that the refinement of the case definition proposed by the CDC in 1993 will promote greater understanding of the problem at both clinical and research levels, particularly because more objective criteria to validate and define CFS have not emerged.

As indicated by its very definition, CFS has presented the health care system with a challenge whereby the primary care physician receives information provided by a team of specialists. Continued technological advances and research into both the immune system and the nature of viral infection will provide new insights into more traditional treatment protocols, including the role played by immune responses to the triggering agent. The neuropsychological components of the disease, as well as evidence demonstrating intimate ties between these components and the immune system, require a personal, active approach by the patient to achieving a healthy state. CFS provides a challenge to the patient to adapt to a personal lifestyle that will create a healthy mind and body.

CFS must also be considered in terms of the society in which it is manifest as a serious and genuine illness. Medical treatment and diagnostic testing can be costly as well as useless, particularly as the health care community continues to refine its understanding of the condition. Patients must remain vigilant regarding phony or trendy treatments that have no correlation to acceptable research findings; such treatments not only can be expensive but also could lead to deteriorating health. Furthermore, the definition and diagnosis of CFS have legal ramifications that have an impact on insurance and other forms of medical care compensation.

—*Patrick J. DeLuca, Ph.D.;*
updated by Richard Adler, Ph.D.

See also Autoimmune disorders; Epstein-Barr virus; Fatigue; Fibromyalgia; Immune system; Immunology; Mononucleosis; Multiple chemical sensitivity syndrome; Stress.

FOR FURTHER INFORMATION:

Afari, Niloofar, and Dedra Buchwald. "Chronic Fatigue Syndrome: A Review." *American Journal of Psychiatry* 160 (February, 2003): 221-236. Summary of the current state of knowledge addressing possible causes and treatment of CFS. The authors acknowledge that diagnosis is based upon symptoms rather than any specific pathology.

Berne, Katrina. *Chronic Fatigue Syndrome, Fibromyalgia, and Other Invisible Illnesses: The Comprehensive Guide.* 3d ed. Alameda, Calif.: Hunter House, 2002. Explores the interactions among the brain, emotions, and the immune system and reviews the current state of research.

Bested, Alison, and Alan Logan. *Chronic Fatigue Syndrome and Fibromyalgia.* Nashville: Cumberland House, 2006. Review of possible causes and treatments for chronic pain and fatigue. Addressed primarily to laypersons.

Centers for Disease Control and Prevention. Chronic Fatigue Syndrome. http://www.cdc.gov/cfs. This site provides evidence-based information concerning chronic fatigue syndrome, its manifestations, and treatment. Sections for patients and caregivers as well as health care professionals.

CFIDS Association of America. http://www.cfids.org.
A group dedicated to conquering chronic fatigue and immune dysfunction syndrome (CFIDS). Focuses on increasing the pace of CFIDS research, achieving public policy victories for people with CFIDS, and directing mainstream attention to the disease.

Englebienne, Patrick, and Kenny DeMeirleir, eds. *Chronic Fatigue Syndrome: A Biological Approach.* Boca Raton, Fla.: CRC Press, 2002. Reviews research advances in understanding the disease from the perspective of various fields of the biomedical sciences, such as protein biochemistry, virology, and pharmacology.

Friedberg, Fred. *Fibromyalgia and Chronic Fatigue Syndrome: Seven Proven Steps to Less Pain and More Energy.* Oakland, Calif.: New Harbinger, 2006. A layperson's directive on living with the clinical features of the illness as well as behaviors that might reduce any symptoms.

Patarca-Montero, Roberto. *Chronic Fatigue Syndrome and the Body's Immune Defense System.* New York: Haworth Medical Press, 2002. Patarca-Montero, a leading immunologist, examines the connections between the disease and immunology; reviews how therapeutic tools such as herbal medicine, vaccines, and cell therapy are being used in CFS research; and discusses the connection between CFS and fibromyalgia, Gulf War syndrome, sick building syndrome, and multiple chemical sensitivity.

Sticherling, Michael, and Enno Christophers, eds. *Treatment of Autoimmune Disorders.* New York: Springer, 2003. Explores the basic mechanisms of autoimmune disorders; neurological, gastrointestinal, ophthalmological, and skin diseases; and current and future therapeutic options.

CHRONIC OBSTRUCTIVE PULMONARY DISEASE (COPD)

DISEASE/DISORDER

ANATOMY OR SYSTEM AFFECTED: Lungs, respiratory system

SPECIALTIES AND RELATED FIELDS: Geriatrics and gerontology, public health, pulmonary medicine

DEFINITION: A progressive, irreversible disease of the lungs that causes expiratory airflow obstruction. The most common form of COPD is a combination of chronic bronchitis and emphysema.

KEY TERMS:

alpha 1 antitrypsin: a protein that protects the lungs

alveoli: air sacs in the lungs that exchange oxygen and carbon dioxide *barrel chest:* a rounded chest in which the anterior and posterior diameter is increased

bronchial tubes: branches in the airways in the lungs that allow for the exchange of oxygen and carbon dioxide

chronic bronchitis: a condition involving the inflammation and eventual scarring of the lining of the bronchial tubes and the production of excess mucus in the lungs

emphysema: airway disease involving permanent distension of distal airspaces and damage to alveolar walls of the lungs

exacerbation: worsening or intensifying

expiratory phase: exhalation, or breathing out

hypoxic: having low oxygen levels

pursed lip breathing: slow expirations from the abdomen against pursed lips

tachypnea: rapid breathing greater than twenty breaths per minute

---

> ### INFORMATION ON CHRONIC OBSTRUCTIVE PULMONARY DISEASE (COPD)
>
> **CAUSES:** Unknown; risk factors include smoking, air pollution, textile manufacturing, childhood respiratory infections
>
> **SYMPTOMS:** Chronic cough, shortness of breath, wheezing, limited physical activity
>
> **DURATION:** Chronic and progressive
>
> **TREATMENTS:** None; alleviation of symptoms (bronchodilators, antibiotics, steroids, oxygen therapy, vaccination against pneumonia and influenza, smoking cessation, pulmonary rehabilitation)

CAUSES AND SYMPTOMS

Patients suffering from chronic obstructive pulmonary disease (COPD), a combination of chronic bronchitis and emphysema, have a chronic cough and shortness of breath that progressively limits their tolerance for physical activity. A physical examination may appear normal in the early stages of COPD, but as the disease progresses, tachypnea and wheezing occur. Over time, the occasional cough becomes more frequent and greater effort is exerted to breathe. In later stages of COPD, the heart may be affected because the lungs can no longer supply an adequate amount of oxygen to the body. Other signs of COPD are a barrel chest, pursed lip breathing, and a prolonged expiratory phase of respirations. Coughing produces phlegm that becomes increasingly difficult to expel as it thickens. Persons with advanced COPD cannot lie flat to sleep and eventually may sit in an semiupright position in order to breathe.

The major risk factor for COPD is smoking. Other risk factors are air pollution (including exposure to mining), manufacturing (such as steel and cement), a history of childhood respiratory infections, and low socioeconomic status. In chronic bronchitis, the lining of the bronchial tubes become irritated, inflamed, and filled with mucus that blocks the airways, making it difficult to breathe. In emphysema, the alveoli become irritated, stiffen, and cannot transfer oxygen and carbon dioxide in the blood. Thus far, a deficiency of the enzyme alpha 1 antitrypsin is the only identified genetic cause of COPD.

COPD is an insidious disease that presents few symptoms until it is well developed in the lungs. It is usually not identified until the patient is fifty to sixty years old, although COPD caused by a deficiency of alpha 1 antitrypsin may be identified by thirty to forty years of age.

Confirmation of the diagnosis of COPD is made by pulmonary function tests (PFTs). PFTs are helpful in diagnosing COPD in its early stages and may be helpful in convincing patients to stop smoking, if necessary, so as to slow the progression of COPD. Spirometry measures the amount of air exhaled in one second, or forced expiratory volume (FEV1). The total amount of air exhaled, or forced vital capacity (FVC), is compared to the FEV1 to determine the extent of airway obstruction. A peak flow meter can show the severity of breathing impairment; after a deep breath, the patient blows into the instrument as forcefully and for as long as possible. Arterial blood gas tests measure the level of oxygen and carbon dioxide in the blood. Serum alpha-1-antitrypsin levels are measured by blood samples. Finally, chest X rays, pulmonary ventilation-perfusion scans, and chest magnetic resonance imaging (MRI) scans may all help to identify the degree of lung damage caused by COPD.

TREATMENT AND THERAPY

Since no cure exists for COPD, treatment focuses on decreasing symptoms and reducing complications. Bronchodilator medications, antibiotics, steroids, oxygen, and vaccination against pneumonia and influenza are used to treat or prevent symptoms, slow the progression of the disease, and manage any complications.

Smoking cessation is vitally important for slowing the progress of COPD. Nicotine replacement therapy, antidepressant therapy, and counseling are some of the methods used to assist in smoking cessation.

Patients with COPD who are hypoxic require long-term oxygen therapy to improve their functional status and rate of survival. The purpose of oxygen therapy is to maintain adequate oxygen levels to prevent respiratory difficulties.

Pulmonary rehabilitation can help reduce hospitalizations and improve the quality of life for those with COPD, improving their overall functional status. Pulmonary rehabilitation includes therapies to enhance breathing, physical training to improve muscle strength and stamina, and the pacing of activities to avoid overexertion. Pursed lip breathing helps to relieve abnormal breathing (dyspnea) and to slow respirations.

Lung transplantation and lung reduction surgery may be options for people who suffer from severe emphysema. Lung reduction surgery, which is still in the experimental stages, is the partial removal of the most damaged areas of the lungs in order to allow for better lung expansion of the normal areas of the lung. Gene therapy and alpha-1-antitrypsin replacement therapy are presently under evaluation as treatments for alpha-1-antitrypsin deficiency, but the long-term effects of these treatments are unknown.

PERSPECTIVE AND PROSPECTS

COPD costs in the United States exceed $32 billion annually. Between 80 and 90 percent of all cases are caused by smoking. COPD is the fourth leading cause of death in the United States. The incidence of this disease is increasing every year. Those with COPD are prone to recurrent respiratory infections, and their quality of life gradually declines as the disease worsens. Smoking cessation is the single most important prevention method.

—*Sharon W. Stark, R.N., A.P.R.N., D.N.Sc.*

See also Asbestos exposure; Aspergillosis; Bronchi; Bronchitis; Chest; Cyanosis; Emphysema; Environmental diseases; Environmental health; Geriatrics and gerontology; Influenza; Lungs; Nicotine; Occupational health; Oxygen therapy; Pneumonia; Pulmonary diseases; Pulmonary medicine; Respiration; Smoking; Wheezing.

FOR FURTHER INFORMATION:

American Lung Association. http://www.lungusa.org/lung-disease/copd. The American Lung Association site provides information on COPD and other lung diseases. Site sections include "COPD Management Tools," "Living with COPD," and "Connect with Others."

Barnett, Margaret. *Chronic Obstructive Pulmonary Disease in Primary Care*. New York: Wiley, 2006. Provides health professionals with practical advice and coping strategies for patients living with COPD.

Calverley, Peter M. A., et al., eds. *Chronic Obstructive Pulmonary Disease*. 2d ed. London: Hodder Arnold, 2003. Discusses the improvements in patient care and the development of new treatment methods.

Haas, François, and Sheila Sperber Haas. *The Chronic Bronchitis and Emphysema Handbook*. Rev. ed. New York: John Wiley & Sons, 2000. Provides an overview of the respiratory system; COPD symptoms and progression; smoking cessation; oxygen, drug, and alternative therapies; and surgical interventions for treating COPD.

Jenkins, Mark. *Chronic Obstructive Pulmonary Disease: Practical, Medical, and Spiritual Guidelines for Daily Living with Emphysema, Chronic Bronchitis, and Combination Diagnosis*. Center City, Minn.: Hazelden Information Education, 1999. Provides management techniques and references to resources for maintaining optimal physical and mental health during the course of COPD.

Parker, James N., and Philip M. Parker, eds. *The 2002 Official Patient's Sourcebook on Chronic Obstructive Pulmonary Disease*. San Diego, Calif.: Icon Health, 2002. Provides information for investigating a variety of topics related to COPD from multiple perspectives.

CHRONIC WASTING DISEASE (CWD)

DISEASE/DISORDER

ANATOMY OR SYSTEM AFFECTED: Brain, nervous system

SPECIALTIES AND RELATED FIELDS: Neurology

DEFINITION: A neurological disease of deer and elk caused by an infectious protein particle called a prion.

CAUSES AND SYMPTOMS

Chronic wasting disease (CWD) is an invariably fatal neurological disease that affects deer, elk, and moose in North America. The disease was first described in the late 1960's in captive animals in Colorado. As of 2006, CWD-infected animals—from either wild or captive populations—had been found in Colorado, Illinois, Kansas, Montana, Nebraska, New Mexico, New York, Oklahoma, South Dakota, Utah, West Virginia, Wisconsin, and Wyoming in the United States and in the provinces of Alberta and Saskatchewan in Canada. In the late stages of the disease, infected animals show progressive weight loss, listlessness, increased salivation and urination, increased water consumption, depression, and death.

The brains of dead animals show characteristic vacuoles, or holes, that give the brain the appearance of a sponge. This pathology is characteristic of all the transmissible spongiform encephalopathies (TSEs), including bovine spongiform encephalopathy (BSE) of cows (so-called mad cow disease), scrapie of sheep, and Creutzfeldt-Jakob disease (CJD) of humans. Although CWD is similar to these other diseases, it is not identical to them. These diseases appear to be caused by the misfolding of a small protein (prion) normally located in the membranes of neurons and other cells. The normal function of this protein is unknown, but when misfolded, it accumulates in the brain, resulting in the death of neurons. The misfolded, pathogenic prion appears to be able to direct the misfolding of any normal prion present in a cell, thus replicating its aberrant structure.

Prion diseases can be either inherited or transmitted. Humans can inherit CJD or contract it from contaminated blood or brain tissue. Evidence suggests that variant CJD in humans can result from consuming beef contaminated with the BSE prion. There is concern about whether the CWD prion in deer and elk can also "jump" the species barrier to humans in a manner similar to that of BSE. Recent research using monkeys suggests that there is a species barrier to humans, making it unlikely that CWD will be transmitted to humans despite contact with contaminated blood or tissues.

CWD is believed to be transmitted from animal to animal through contact with body fluids or feces. Research published in 2006 indicated that the disease is most easily transmitted via saliva and blood, although other modes of transmission have not been ruled out. Two recent studies found no strong clinical or epidemiological evidence that the disease can be transmitted to humans via the consumption of contaminated meat. Laboratory studies indicate that such transmission is possible, however. Because of the long incubation period for the disease, however, it is difficult to prove or disprove transmission from deer, elk, or moose to humans.

PERSPECTIVE AND PROSPECTS

Many states where CWD is prevalent have banned the baiting of deer and are thinning the deer population. Deer and elk in crowded populations, particularly captive herds, appear to be more susceptible to CWD.

Research efforts are focused on developing a sensitive field diagnostic test. Definitive diagnosis is made by autopsy, but tests based on tonsil biopsy and antibodies to detect prions in body fluids are also being developed. Transgenic mouse models of each of the known TSEs are also being created in order to learn more about transmission and pathology.

—Michele Arduengo, Ph.D.;
updated by David M. Lawrence

See also Brain; Brain disorders; Creutzfeldt-Jakob disease (CJD); Food poisoning; Nervous system; Neurology; Prion diseases.

FOR FURTHER INFORMATION:

Brown, David R., ed. *Neurodegeneration and Prion Disease.* New York: Springer, 2005.

Harris, David A., ed. *Prions: Molecular and Cellular Biology.* Portland, Oreg.: Horizon Scientific Press, 1999.

Prusiner, Stanley B., ed. *Prion Biology and Diseases.* 2d ed. Cold Spring Harbor, N.Y.: Cold Spring Harbor Laboratory Press, 2004.

Race, Brent, et al. "Susceptibilities of Nonhuman Primates to Chronic Wasting Disease." *Emerging Infectious Diseases* 15, no. 9 (2009): 1366-1376.

U.S. Geological Survey. "Chronic Wasting Disease." http://www.nwhc.usgs.gov/disease_information/chronic_wasting_disease.

CHRONOBIOLOGY

SPECIALTY

ANATOMY OR SYSTEM AFFECTED: All

SPECIALTIES AND RELATED FIELDS: Alternative medicine, endocrinology, neurology, preventive medicine

DEFINITION: The study of the biological cycles in the functioning of organisms; in humans, knowledge of such cycles as circadian rhythms may aid in the diagnosis and treatment of diseases.

KEY TERMS:

circadian rhythm: a cyclical variation in a biological process or behavior that has a duration of slightly greater than twenty-four hours

jet lag: the malaise, headache, fatigue, gastrointestinal disorders, and other symptoms that may result from traveling across several time zones within a few hours

melatonin: a hormone produced by the pineal gland within the epithalamus of the forebrain; it is usually released into the blood during the night phase of the light-dark cycle

period: the length of one complete cycle of a rhythm; ultradian rhythms are about twenty-four hours (twenty to twenty-eight hours), and infradian rhythms are longer than twenty-eight hours

seasonal affective disorder (SAD): a manic depression which undergoes a seasonal fluctuation as a result of various factors, both unknown and known

suprachiasmatic nuclei (SCN): two clusters of nerve cell bodies located in the hypothalamus of the forebrain; these structures display circadian rhythms and seem to be the source of rhythmicity for many of the body's other cycles

SCIENCE AND PROFESSION

Chronobiology refers to the study of various cycles or rhythms that are fundamental to living organisms, including human beings. Many of the early observations were made on plants and nonhuman animals, but the basic concepts also apply to human biology and medicine. In the twentieth century, early findings about cyclical changes in symptoms, body weight, pulse rate, and body temperature were substantiated and broadly expanded to include numerous aspects of human biology and medicine. Well-informed physicians now expect rhythms in their patients' behavior, physiology, and response to therapy. The extensive research on biological rhythms in diverse organisms makes up the specialized field called chronobiology. The presence of circadian, menstrual, weekly, seasonal, and other rhythms in humans necessitates a consideration of these cycles in any comprehensive approach to medical practice.

Despite their importance, the exact nature of these rhythms has not been resolved. Living organisms behave as though they have internal oscillators or biological clocks that time their activities. Some research provides evidence that many of the body's cells each have such internal timers. Until the exact causes for the various biological rhythms have been identified, there will be some limitations to the benefits derived from knowledge of their characteristics. An unsettled dispute concerns whether the actual timing information for circadian and other rhythms comes from within the organism (endogenous) or from the environment (exogenous). It is expected that travel to space beyond the moon may ultimately answer this question. Astronauts may have sufficient internal timing information to survive, or it may be necessary to create a rhythmic environment of change in light-dark cycles and perhaps magnetic field variations to provide vital timing information. In the meantime, there is much that is known in chronobiology.

In mammals, an important circadian timing mechanism resides in a cluster of cells called the suprachiasmatic nuclei, or SCN, which are located in the hypothalamus of the forebrain. From studies on laboratory mammals, it has been learned that removal of the SCN abolishes many of the body's circadian rhythms. In humans, chance tumors in this area are often found to disrupt the circadian rhythms of the patient. In laboratory mammals, it has been shown that there is a separate pathway from the eyes to the SCN that allows information about changes in the light-dark schedule to reach this part of the brain. Therefore, there is intense interest in learning more about the SCN and how they regulate circadian rhythms.

Additionally, the pineal gland, a small gland attached to the epithalamus of the forebrain, receives information from the SCN about the light-dark schedule. A hormone produced by the pineal gland called melatonin is released into the bloodstream at night and suppressed during daylight. Melatonin plays a significant role in the timing of body rhythms and sleep cycles. When melatonin levels rise, the brain interprets this as bedtime, a factor that has led to its increasing use as a treatment for jet lag.

The general physiology of the other tissues of the body is organized according to rhythmic processes.

The exact question of whether such rhythms are dependent on the SCN is still a point of controversy. Nevertheless, the greater application of chronobiology to medicine does not have to await the solution of such theoretical questions. Even now, a wide variety of examples can be cited of the utility of chronobiologic principles in medicine.

DIAGNOSTIC AND TREATMENT TECHNIQUES

Four medical applications of chronobiology will be discussed. One area from psychiatry is the treatment of seasonal affective disorder. Three from other areas of medicine are the chronobiological treatment of asthma, cancer, and jet lag.

Seasonal affective disorder, or SAD, is characterized by depression beginning each year as daylight shortens and fully remitting when days start to lengthen, sometimes switching to mania. The condition is related to where people live and the corresponding hours of sunlight; the condition remits in a few days when sufferers travel to sunnier climes and worsens as they travel to areas where the days are shorter. As many as one in four persons in the northern latitudes may suffer from SAD, and female sufferers outnumber male ones. Although the disorder has been recognized only recently, for years writers and poets have noted seasonal depression in themselves and others.

Some patients take a mid-winter vacation to a sunny climate to alleviate the condition. For those who cannot travel, the use of artificial lights has been introduced. Glow lights are placed in the homes of SAD patients and used early in the morning as well as after sunset to lengthen daylight hours. Morning lights appear to bring particularly prompt relief. Relapses have been reported when light is withdrawn. Research is currently under way to determine when during the day light is most effective, how much light is needed, and the mechanisms by which light works to fight SAD.

Some details are emerging about this process. The human forebrain contains a small organ about the size of a pea that produces the hormone melatonin according to a circadian schedule. Melatonin is usually released into the bloodstream during the night. The use of bright light therapy seems to inhibit the release of melatonin and thereby to cause other changes in the brain chemistry. In some mammals, this mechanism may be important in regulating their seasonal behavior. In humans, the situation is more complex, and an adequate theory for the neurochemical basis of SAD and other mental disorders has yet to be advanced.

Asthma sufferers have long known that their symptoms worsen at night. This increase in coughing, wheezing, and breathlessness at night has been identified only recently with circadian rhythms rather than environmental factors. At first, some researchers thought that asthma was worse at night because the patients were lying down. It has been shown, however, that the symptoms show their circadian periodicity whether the person is lying down or not. The normal nightly decrease in airway passage diameter in the lungs of normal persons is exaggerated in the asthmatic. The most dangerous hours for the asthmatic are the very early morning hours, a time when there are more deaths among asthmatics. Interestingly, asthmatics who become adapted to a nighttime work schedule shift their most severe asthma symptoms to the daytime sleep period.

Experts in the field such as Michael H. Smolensky of the University of Texas contend that much more research needs to be done on the role of circadian rhythms in asthma and its treatment. For example, adrenocortical hormones, which are powerful anti-inflammatory agents, have been used successfully to treat asthmatics. It was discovered that the time of day when the hormones were given was of great importance. If the hormones are given in the evening, the patient's own adrenal gland is inhibited. Therefore, the best time to give such hormones is in the early morning, near the time when they are normally released in the body.

Theophylline is a drug that has been very successful in ameliorating the symptoms of asthmatics. It has been found that certain types of sustained-release theophylline are effective in reducing the early morning symptoms if the drug is taken the night before. In the study of asthma, the benefit of considering chronobiology has become obvious, and any new products to treat asthma need to be evaluated chronobiologically before they are made available to the general public.

Cancer diagnosis and treatment are aspects of medicine that are receiving increased consideration by chronobiologists. The normal growth of tissues occurs by cell division, or mitosis, a rhythmic process that is normally precisely regulated. Cancer is essentially unregulated mitosis, resulting in the growth of a tumor that is no longer subject to the control mechanisms of the body. Yet even this breakdown in regulation has its seasons. In human males, some types of testicular cancer are more often diagnosed in the winter, and in females some types of cervical cancer have a peak occurrence in the summer.

The treatment of cancer involves the use of surgery, radiation, or chemotherapy in an attempt to remove or kill the cancerous cells without substantial damage to the normal tissues. Early studies in animal models demonstrated that there are often specific times of the day that these types of cancer treatment can be most effective. In a few cases, the tumor may have a rhythm of mitosis that is no longer synchronized to the rhythm of the surrounding tissue. In these cases, it may be possible to administer drugs or radiation that inhibits mitosis according to a schedule that will affect the cancer cells but will not harm the host tissue. More often, there will be a mixed effect of the timed treatment, so that some suppression of mitosis occurs along with some side effects.

The application of chronobiology to the treatment of breast cancer has raised hopes that there can be a marked improvement for survival rates of women who undergo breast surgery. William J. M. Hrushesky of Albany Medical College found that women who had breast surgery near the time of menses had a more than fourfold higher risk of recurrence and death than those patients who had surgery near the middle of the menstrual cycle. These findings are under review, and the final conclusions await the evaluation of more cases. It has also been observed that the diagnosis of breast cancer in the United States has a two-peaked seasonal rhythm in the spring and the fall. There is also evidence that the body temperature of the breast in normal women has a circadian rhythm along with perhaps an additional seven-day periodicity, whereas breasts with tumors have abnormal temperature rhythms of about twenty hours. This information may help in the early diagnosis of breast cancer if suitable automatic monitoring devices are used to measure breast temperature.

Jet lag may appear to be more of an inconvenience than a serious medical problem until one considers the disastrous consequences of a plane crash caused by pilot error or a poorly made decision by a diplomat in an international crisis. Wiley Post and Harold Gatty, on their 1931 plane trip around the world, were the first persons to suffer from this disorder. Essentially, the body is subjected to a shift in the day-night schedule, with sleep and meal times shifted earlier or later depending on the number of time zones crossed and the direction of the flight. The symptoms are general malaise, headaches, fatigue, disruptions of the sleep-wake cycle, and gastrointestinal disorders. There are individual differences in the time required to overcome jet lag. In general, younger and healthier people are better able to cope with such change.

A shift of six hours, such as a flight between New York and Paris, requires a substantial reorganization of one's circadian rhythms. It can take from two days to two weeks to resynchronize. Adaptation is slowest when one stays indoors and continues on a "home-time" schedule. Eastward flights are less easily tolerated than westward flights; the delays in resynchronization can take almost twice as long. The reason for the difference is that when one flies east, the sun comes up earlier relative to "home time." It is easier for most people to "advance" than to shift "backward"—that is, to go from day to night than to go backward from night to day. For this reason, it is suggested that travelers fly early in the day when flying east and later in the day when flying west.

Unfortunately, little consideration has been given to chronobiology in scheduling work time and time off. Pilots, diplomats, businesspersons, and other time zone travelers often perform poorly when their body rhythms are disturbed by jet lag. Similarly, people who must change their work shift every few weeks often find their performance level dropping. The rate at which work shifts should be rotated forward to increase worker effectiveness is now coming under considerable study.

It should be realized that the living body has myriad hormones, enzymes, and other important constituents that have rhythms of several different periods. Maintaining the correct time relationship between the rhythms can be critical for normal health. In the diagnosis of disease, chronobiology has to be taken into account. Erhard Haus of the St. Paul-Ramsey Medical Center has spent many years detailing the circadian and other rhythms that must be considered. What is normal for the morning hours may be pathological for the evening hours. These rhythmic values are yet to be determined for many important diagnostic measurements.

In 2005, a research study by the Feinberg School of Medicine and Northwestern University confirmed previous findings that school start times for adolescents are too early. In adolescents, melatonin, the hormone that helps induce sleep, increases later in the evening, causing melatonin levels to stay at high levels until approximately 8:00 A.M. There is no known way to change melatonin levels; for example, going to bed earlier does not cause melatonin to decrease earlier. The researchers encouraged parents and school districts to start later, as research consistently shows that adolescents have their poorest academic performance in the morning and have consistently better cognitive functioning later in the day. The researchers noted that school start times are easily modified. Many previous studies have shown the same effect, and some school districts have instituted later start times, with many schools reporting improved cognitive functioning and mood among students.

PERSPECTIVE AND PROSPECTS

One of the earliest written observations of a biological cycle was by Androsthenes, a soldier marching with Alexander the Great in the fourth century B.C.E., who recorded that the tamarind tree opens its leaves during the day and closes them at night. In experiments on similar leaf movements in other plants, the astronomer Jean Jacques d'Ortous de Mairan in 1729 found that plants held in the dark continued to open and close their leaves on a roughly twenty-four-hour schedule. Thus, circadian rhythms were shown not to be simple responses to the rising and setting of the sun but rather internal oscillations.

Early observers more interested in humans also identified rhythms. In the fifth century B.C.E., Hippocrates reported that his patients had twenty-four-hour fluctuations as well as longer-term rhythms in their symptoms. Herophilus of Alexandria in the third century B.C.E. observed a daily change in the human pulse rate. The Italian scientist Sanctorius in 1711 made repeated measurements of his own body weight and the turbidity of his urine, both of which he found to vary during the month. Later, he went to the extreme measure of constructing a giant scale and living on its huge pan so that a frequent record could be made of his changing weight. The French scientists Armand Seguin and Antoine-Laurent Lavoisier in 1790 did research that revealed circadian rhythms in the body weight of men. These researchers suggested that men who did not show such circadian rhythms in body weight should be suspected of being ill. The British scientist John Davy in 1845 reported that he had found both circadian and seasonal rhythms in his own body temperature.

The historical citations of persons taking an interest in chronobiology in past centuries were of only passing concern and did not, in most cases, help to establish this field. Chronobiology as a discipline has received attention from the medical community only since about the 1970's, and many of its contributions to improving health are yet to be realized. The foremost student of chronobiology as applied to medicine has been Franz Halberg of the University of Minnesota. He has repeatedly called the attention of the medical community to the importance of biological rhythms in maintaining health and in the diagnosis and treatment of disease. Halberg has promoted the use of "autorhythmometry," or the self-measurement of one's physiological variables to monitor one's changing health. It has been shown that this method can be used effectively even by groups of schoolchildren.

The phase or the timing of the peaks and troughs of circadian rhythms is germane in both diagnosis and treatment. The advent of portable automatic recording devices that store physiological data on computer chips is opening up a means of documenting a patient's circadian rhythms around the clock for weeks at a time. Eventually, when patients visit physicians there will then be a complete record of body temperature, blood pressure, and other physiological variables. This database will provide a much better basis for decisions than the limited data normally taken during infrequent medical visits.

The diagnosis of diabetes mellitus has been shown to depend to an extent on the time of day that the various tests, such as the glucose tolerance test, are administered. Some diabetics are "matinal" diabetics and do not have trouble regulating their blood glucose levels until the afternoon. These persons need to have glucose tolerance tests administered in the afternoon in order to reveal their diabetes. Many additional examples of the importance of chronobiology in diagnosis and treatment exist. As more physicians and health professionals become familiar with the concepts and application of chronobiology, the effectiveness of health care will be enhanced.

—John T. Burns, Ph.D.; Miriam Ehrenberg, Ph.D.;
updated by LeAnna DeAngelo, Ph.D.

See also Asthma; Cancer; Chemotherapy; Depression; Hormones; Light therapy; Melatonin; Metabolism; Physiology; Psychiatry; Seasonal affective disorder (SAD); Sleep disorders; Stress; Stress reduction.

FOR FURTHER INFORMATION:

Coleman, Richard M. *Wide Awake at 3:00 A.M.: By Choice or by Chance?* New York: W. H. Freeman, 1990. A popular presentation of the essentials of human chronobiology. Coleman is a former director of the Stanford University Sleep Disorders Clinic, and his coverage of this subspecialty is noteworthy. Shift work and jet lag are also discussed.

Columbus, Frank, ed. *Frontiers in Chronobiology Re-

search. New York: Nova Science, 2006. Covers topics from cell biology, developmental biology, ecology, endocrinology, genetics, molecular biology, neurobiology, and pharmacology. Focuses on circadian, tidal, seasonal, and annual rhythms.

Dunlap, Jay, Jennifer Loros, and Patricia Decourse, eds. *Chronobiology: Biological Timekeeping*. Sunderland, Mass.: Sinauer, 2003. Provides a general introduction. Compares the anatomy, physiology, genetics, and molecular biology of organisms with circadian clocks.

Endres, Klaus-Peter, and Wolfgang Schad. *Moon Rhythms in Nature: How Lunar Cycles Affect Living Organisms*. Translated by Christian von Arnim. Edinburgh, Scotland: Floris Books, 2002. A nonscientific introduction to the lunar influences on Earth's biosphere.

Palmer, John D. *The Living Clock: The Orchestrator of Biological Rhythms*. New York: Oxford University Press, 2002. An engaging exploration of a range of mammalian behavior affected by internal biological clocks.

Rosenthal, Norman E. *Winter Blues: Everything You Need to Know to Beat Seasonal Affective Disorder*. New York: Guilford Press, 2006. Written at the popular level, this book gives the layperson an overview of the symptoms and treatment of seasonal affective disorder.

Sehgal, Amita. *Molecular Biology of Circadian Rhythms*. Hoboken, N.J.: Wiley-Liss, 2004. Reviews research advances in understanding biological rhythms and discusses the linkages to the understanding of cell and body biochemistry, health, and aging, and the molecular control of behavior.

Waterhouse, J. M., et al. *Keeping in Time with Your Body Clock*. New York: Oxford University Press, 2003. Explains how the body clock works, how it can malfunction, and ways to optimize health and well-being.

CHYME

BIOLOGY

ALSO KNOWN AS: Chymus

ANATOMY OR SYSTEM AFFECTED: Gallbladder, gastrointestinal system, intestines, liver, pancreas, stomach

SPECIALTIES AND RELATED FIELDS: Gastroenterology, internal medicine

DEFINITION: The slurry-like mixture of food and digestive juices produced in the digestive tract.

STRUCTURE AND FUNCTIONS

Chewing and swallowing produces a bolus of food that descends through the esophagus into the stomach. There, the stomach walls secrete hydrochloric acid while waves of muscular contraction called peristalsis mix the stomach contents. The gastric juices break the bolus into small food particles, producing a thick fluid called chyme. Peristalsis causes the chyme to collect in the antrum, the lowest section of the stomach. The pyloric sphincter passes small portions of chyme into the duodenum at regular intervals.

Chyme is highly acidic because of the stomach acid. To protect the membrane lining the duodenum, the pancreas releases bicarbonate to neutralize the acid. In the duodenum, digestion continues. Bile produced in the liver is added to the chyme to emulsify fats into small globules. The pancreas contributes enzymes that break down fats, proteins, and carbohydrates so that nutrients, minerals, and salts can be absorbed through the membrane of the small intestine and into the bloodstream.

Over a period of three to five hours, peristalsis pushes the chyme through the small intestine and into the colon. There, bacteria convert some ingredients of the chyme into vitamin K and vitamin B, which the colon extracts along with excess water. Bacteria also produce various gases. These gases are mixed with the remaining waste matter, or feces.

DISORDERS AND DISEASES

Most disorders relating to chyme come from excessive food or water intake. When too much is eaten, the stomach distends and presses on the diaphragm. Peristalsis and the sheer bulk of the chyme can make breathing difficult and uncomfortable. When food contains a high proportion of fat, spices, or fibers and is eaten too quickly, the stomach can be overburdened. The churning of peristalsis may force some of the chyme back up the esophagus, causing a burning sensation there known as acid reflux or heartburn. This indigestion of the chyme, or dyspepsia, can make the stomach feel sour and achy and can lead to stomach ulcers. The stomach also may react to psychological stress by producing too much acid.

When the pancreas fails to produce enough bicarbonate to neutralize the acid in chyme after it enters the duodenum, the acid may burn through the mucosa in its wall and into tissue, producing a duodenal ulcer. Too much bile added to the chyme, if not reabsorbed in the distal small intestine, can lead to diarrhea, whereas too little bile can contribute to malabsorption of nutrients. Similarly, excessive water intake may leach sodium from the body or cause the intestine to process the chyme too quickly for all the nutrients to be removed from it.

—*Roger Smith, Ph.D.*

See also Acid-base chemistry; Acid reflux disease; Bile; Diarrhea and dysentery; Digestion; Enzymes; Food biochemistry; Gastroenterology; Gastroenterology, pediatric; Gastrointestinal disorders; Gastrointestinal system; Heartburn; Indigestion; Intestines; Malabsorption; Metabolism; Nutrition; Peristalsis; Ulcers; Vitamins and minerals.

FOR FURTHER INFORMATION:

Corcoran, Mary K., and Jef Czekaj. *The Quest to Digest.* Watertown, Mass.: Charlesbridge, 2006.

Parker, Steve. *The Human Body Book.* New York: DK Adult, 2001.

Seymour, Simon. *Guts: Our Digestive System.* New York: HarperCollins, 2005.

CIRCULATION

BIOLOGY

ANATOMY OR SYSTEM AFFECTED: Blood, blood vessels, circulatory system, liver

SPECIALTIES AND RELATED FIELDS: Cardiology, hematology, vascular medicine

DEFINITION: The flow of blood throughout the body; the circulatory system consists of the heart, lungs, arteries, and veins.

KEY TERMS:

aneurysm: a localized enlargement of a vessel, usually an artery

atherosclerosis: accumulation of plaque within the arteries

calcification: the deposit of lime salts in organic tissue, leading to calcium in the arterial wall

capillaries: hairlike vessels that connect the ends of the smallest arteries to the beginnings of the smallest veins

claudication: muscle cramps that occur when arterial blood flow does not meet the muscles' demand for oxygen

diastole: the period of relaxation in the cardiac cycle

hypertension: a blood pressure higher than what is considered to be normal

lumen: the space within an artery, vein, or other tube

stenosis: the constriction or narrowing of a passage

systole: the period of contraction in the cardiac cycle

thrombus: a blood clot that, commonly, obstructs a vein but may also occur in an artery or the heart

vasoconstriction: a decrease in the diameter of a blood vessel

vasodilation: an increase in the diameter of a blood vessel

STRUCTURE AND FUNCTIONS

The cardiovascular system is made up of the heart, arteries, veins, and lungs. The heart serves as a pump to deliver blood to the arteries for distribution throughout the body. The veins bring the blood back to the heart, and the lungs oxygenate the blood before returning it to the arterial system.

Contraction of the heart muscle forces blood out of the heart. This period of contraction is known as systole. The heart muscle relaxes after each contraction, which allows blood flow into the heart. This period of relaxation is known as diastole. A typical blood pressure taken at the upper arm provides a pressure reading during two phases of the cardiac cycle. The first number is known as the systolic pressure and represents the pressure of the heart during peak contraction. The second number is known as the diastolic pressure and represents the pressure while the heart is at rest. A typical pressure reading for a young adult would be 120/80. When blood pressure is abnormally elevated, it is commonly referred to as high blood pressure, or hypertension.

The heart is separated into two halves by a wall of muscle known as the septum. The two halves are known as the left and right heart. The left side of the heart is responsible for high-pressure arterial distribution and is larger and stronger than the right side. The right side of the heart is responsible for accepting low-pressure venous return and redirecting it to the lungs.

Because of these pressure differences from one side of the heart to the other, the vessel wall constructions of the arteries and the veins differ. Strong construction of the arterial wall allows tolerance of significant pressure elevations from the left heart. The arterial wall is made up of three major tissue layers, known as tunics. Secondary layers of tissue that provide strength and elasticity to the artery are known as elastic and connective tissues. As with the artery, the wall of the vein is made up of three distinct tissue layers. Compared to that of an artery, the wall of a vein is thinner and less elastic, which allows the wall to be easily compressed by surrounding muscle during contraction.

While the heart is at rest, between contractions, newly oxygenated arterial blood passes from the lungs and enters the left heart. Each time the heart contracts, blood is forced from the left heart into a major artery known as the aorta. From the aorta, blood is distributed throughout the body. Once depleted of nutrients and oxygen, arterial blood passes through an extensive array of minute vessels known as capillaries. A significant pressure drop occurs as blood is dispersed throughout the immense network of capillaries. The capillaries empty into the venous system, which carries the blood back to the heart.

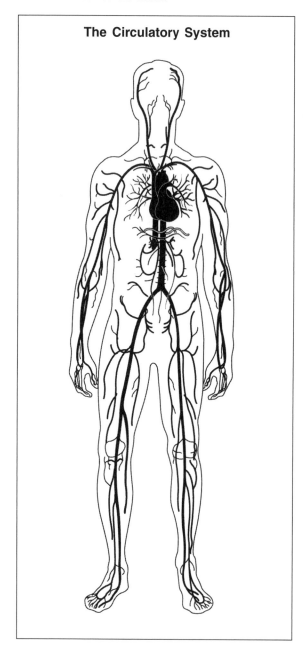

The Circulatory System

The primary responsibility of the venous system is to return deoxygenated blood to the lungs and heart. Much more energy is required from the body to move venous flow compared to arterial flow. Unlike the artery, the vein does not depend on the heart or gravity for energy to move blood. The venous system has a unique means of blood transportation known as the "venous pump," which moves blood toward the heart.

The components making up the venous pump include muscle contraction against the venous wall, intra-abdominal pressure changes, and one-way venous valves. Compression against the walls of a vein induces movement of blood. Muscle contraction against a vein wall occurs throughout the body during periods of activity. Activity includes every movement, from breathing to running. Variations in respiration cause fluctuations in the pressure within the abdomen, which produces a siphonlike effect on the veins, pulling venous blood upward. Valves are located within the veins of the extremities and pelvis. A venous valve has two leaflets, which protrude inward from opposite sides of the vein wall and meet one another in the center. Valves are necessary to prevent blood from flowing backward, away from the heart.

The venous system is divided into two groups known as the deep and superficial veins. The deep veins are located parallel to the arteries, while the superficial veins are located just beneath the skin surface and are often visible through the skin.

DISORDERS AND DISEASES

Numerous variables may affect the flow of blood. The autonomic nervous system is connected to muscle within the wall of the artery by way of neurological pathways known as sympathetic branches. Various drugs and/or conditions can trigger responses in the sympathetic branches and produce constriction of the smooth muscle in the arterial wall (vasoconstriction) or relaxation of the arterial wall (vasodilation). Alcohol consumption and a hot bath are examples of conditions that produce vasodilation. Exposure to cold and cigarette smoking are examples of conditions that produce vasoconstriction. Various drugs used in the medical environment are capable of producing similar effects. The diameter of the lumen of an artery influences the pressure and the flow of blood through it.

Another condition that alters the arterial diameter is atherosclerosis, a disease primarily of the large arteries, which allows the formation of fat (lipid) deposits to build on the inner layer of the artery. Lipid deposits are more commonly known as atherosclerotic plaque. Plaque accumulation reduces the diameter of the arterial lumen, causing various degrees of flow restriction. Plaque is similar to rust accumulation within a pipe which restricts the flow of water. A restriction of flow is referred to as a stenosis. The majority of stenotic lesions occur at the places where arteries divide into branches, also known as bifurcations. In advanced stages of plaque development, plaque may become calcified. Calcified plaque is hard and may become irregular, ulcerate, or hemorrhage, providing an environment for new clot formation and/or release of small pieces of plaque debris downstream.

An arterial wall may become very hard and rigid, a condition commonly known as hardening of the arteries. Hardened arteries may eventually become twisted, kinked, or dilated as a result of the hardening process of the arterial wall. A hardened artery which has become dilated is known as an aneurysm.

Normal arterial flow is undisturbed. When blood cells travel freely, they move together at a similar speed with very little variance. This is known as laminar flow. Nonlaminar (turbulent) flow is seen when irregular plaque or kinks in the arterial wall disrupt the smooth flow of cells. Plaque with an irregular surface may produce mild turbulence, while a narrow stenosis produces significant turbulence immediately downstream from the stenosis.

Many moderate or severe stenoses can be heard with the use of a standard stethoscope over the vessel of interest. A high-pitched sound can be heard consequent to the increased velocity of the blood cells moving through a narrow space. (A similar effect is produced when a standard garden hose is kinked to create a spray and a hissing sound is heard.) Medically, this sound is often referred to as a bruit. *Bruit* (pronounced "broo-ee") is a French word meaning noise.

Patients with significant lower extremity arterial disease will consistently experience calf pain and occasionally experience thigh discomfort with exercise. The discomfort is relieved when the patient stands still for a few moments. This is known as vascular claudication and occurs from a pressure drop as a consequence of a severely stenotic (reduced in diameter by greater than 75 percent) or occluded artery. If the muscle cannot get enough oxygen as a result of reduced blood flow, it will cramp, forcing the patient to stop and rest until blood supply has caught up to muscle demand. Alternate pathways around an obstruction prevent pain at

rest, when muscle demand is low. Alternate pathways are also referred to as collateral pathways. Small, otherwise insignificant branches from a main artery become important vessels when the body uses them as collateral pathways around an obstruction. Time and exercise help to collateralize arterial branches into larger, more prominent arterial pathways. If collateral pathways do not provide enough flow to prevent the patient from experiencing painful muscle cramps while performing a daily exercise routine or to heal a wound on the foot, it may be necessary to perform either a surgical bypass around the obstruction or another interventional procedure such as angioplasty, atherectomy, or laser surgery.

Claudication may also occur in the heart. The main coronary arteries lie on the surface of the heart and distribute blood to the heart muscle. Patients suffering from coronary artery disease (CAD) may experience tightness, heaviness, or pain in the chest subsequent to flow restriction to the heart muscle as a result of atherosclerotic plaque within the coronary arteries. These symptoms are known as angina pectoris, or simply angina, usually occurring with exercise and relieved by rest. Intensity of the symptoms is relative to the extent of disease. A myocardial infarction (heart attack) is the result of a coronary artery occlusion.

Unlike the arteries, the venous system is not affected by atherosclerosis. The primary diseases of the veins include blood clot formation and varicose veins. A varicose vein is an enlarged and meandering vein with poorly functioning valves. A varicosity typically involves the veins near the skin surface, the superficial veins, and is often visualized as an irregular and/or raised segment through the skin surface. Varicosities are most common in the lower legs.

Valve leaflets are common sites for development of a thrombus. Thrombosis is the formation of a clot within a vein, which occurs when blood flow is delayed or obstructed for many hours. Several conditions that may induce venous clotting include prolonged bed rest (postoperative patients), prolonged sitting (long airplane or automobile rides), and use of oral contraceptives. Cancer patients are at high risk of clot formation secondary to a metabolic disorder which affects the natural blood-thinning process.

Because numerous tributaries are connected to the superficial system, it is easy for the body to compensate for a clot in this system by rerouting blood through other branches. The deep venous system, however, has fewer branches, which promotes the progression of a thrombus toward the heart. A thrombus in the deep venous system is more serious because the risk of pulmonary emboli, commonly known as blood clots in the lungs, is much higher than superficial vein thrombosis. The further a thrombus propagates, the higher the risk to the patient.

Lower extremity venous return must take an alternate route via the superficial venous system when the deep system is obstructed by a thrombus. This is known as compensatory flow around an obstruction.

PERSPECTIVE AND PROSPECTS

Historically, the vasculature of the human body was evaluated by placing one's fingers on the skin, palpating for the presence or absence of a pulse, and making note of the patient's symptoms. Prior to the 1960's, treatment of the circulatory system was very limited or nonexistent, resulting in a high death rate and large numbers of amputations, strokes, and heart attacks. The development of arteriography (the angiogram), a procedure in which dye is injected into the vessels while X rays are obtained, revealed more about the vasculature and the nature of disease involving it. In conjunction with arteriography came corrective bypass surgery.

This period of development was followed by vast improvements in diagnostics, treatment, and knowledge of preventive maintenance. Today, synthetic bypass grafts are commonplace and are used to reroute flow around an obstruction. In many cases, procedures such as atherectomy and angioplasty, in which plaque or a thrombus is removed through a catheter inserted into the vessel, are often performed as outpatient procedures.

Diagnostic imaging of the cardiovascular system and the study of hemodynamics with the use of ultrasound have been useful for patient screening, the monitoring of disease progression, and the postoperative evaluation of surgical/interventional procedures. Ultrasound is a particularly valuable diagnostic tool because, compared to X rays or arteriography, it is less expensive; it is also quick, painless, and noninvasive (no radiation, needle, or dye is required).

In addition to technological advances, new medications have been made available to reduce the risk of graft rejection, hypertension, and clotting, and to lower blood cholesterol. Preventive measures, however, constitute the most effective approach to good health. Much new information has been made available to improve the knowledge of the general public regarding diet, exercise, and the avoidance of unhealthy habits as the way to create and maintain a healthier cardiovascular system.

—Bonnie L. Wolff

See also Aneurysmectomy; Aneurysms; Angina; Angiography; Angioplasty; Arteriosclerosis; Biofeedback; Bleeding; Blood and blood disorders; Blood testing; Blood vessels; Bypass surgery; Cardiopulmonary resuscitation (CPR); Catheterization; Chest; Cholesterol; Claudication; Coronary artery bypass graft; Cyanosis; Diabetes mellitus; Dialysis; Disseminated intravascular coagulation (DIC); Echocardiography; Edema; Embolism; Endarterectomy; Exercise physiology; Heart; Heart disease; Heat exhaustion and heatstroke; Hematology; Hematology, pediatric; Hemorrhoid banding and removal; Hemorrhoids; Hormones; Hypercholesterolemia; Hypertension; Ischemia; Kidneys; Lymphatic system; Phlebitis; Phlebotomy; Preeclampsia and eclampsia; Pulmonary hypertension; Shock; Shunts; Stents; Strokes; Systems and organs; Thrombolytic therapy and TPA; Thrombosis and thrombus; Transfusion; Transient ischemic attacks (TIAs); Varicose vein removal; Varicose veins; Vascular medicine; Vascular system; Vasculitis; Venous insufficiency.

FOR FURTHER INFORMATION:

Bick, Roger L., ed. *Disorders of Thrombosis and Hemostasis: Clinical and Laboratory Practice.* 3d ed. Philadelphia: Lippincott Williams & Wilkins, 2002. An excellent introduction to the diagnosis and management of clotting and bleeding disorders.

Guyton, Arthur C., and John E. Hall. *Human Physiology and Mechanisms of Disease.* 6th ed. Philadelphia: W. B. Saunders, 1997. A well-written text for medical students interested in learning the physiological effects of disease. Parts 3 and 4 pertain to the heart and circulation.

Marieb, Elaine N., and Katja Hoehn. *Human Anatomy and Physiology.* 9th ed. San Francisco: Pearson/Benjamin Cummings, 2010. Nonscientists at the advanced high school level or above will be able to understand this fine textbook. It includes a complete glossary, index, pronunciation guide, and other helpful features.

Saltin, Bengt, et al., eds. *Exercise and Circulation in Health and Disease.* Champaign, Ill.: Human Kinetics, 2000. This book is a compilation of integrated topics in cardiovascular regulatory physiology from more than forty authors.

Strandness, D. Eugene, Jr. *Duplex Scanning in Vascular Disorders*. 4th ed. London: Lippincott Williams & Wilkins, 2009. This book is written for medical vascular specialists and is somewhat technical in nature; however, it is well written. The beginning of each chapter defines the importance of that particular subject and the clinical presentation, treatment, and typical course of the vascular disease involved.

CIRCUMCISION, FEMALE, AND GENITAL MUTILATION
PROCEDURE

ANATOMY OR SYSTEM AFFECTED: Genitals, reproductive system

SPECIALTIES AND RELATED FIELDS: General surgery, gynecology, plastic surgery, psychiatry

DEFINITION: The partial or complete surgical removal of the clitoris, labia minora, or labia majora (or all) for cultural reasons. Often performed without anesthesia or sterilized instruments, and often performed on young females without assent or understanding.

KEY TERMS:

clitoridectomy: the removal of the entire clitoris, the prepuce, and adjacent labia

deinfibulation: an anterior episiotomy

episiotomy: the incision of the labia

infibulation: a clitoridectomy followed by the sewing up of the vulva

pharaonic circumcision: another term for infibulation

prepuce: the covering of the clitoris

sunna circumcision: the removal of the tip of the clitoris and/or the prepuce

INDICATIONS AND PROCEDURES

The various forms of female circumcision and female genital mutilation, although not universal to all cultures, have been practiced in numerous societies of the world for nearly two thousand years. Recorded evidence cites that female circumcision predates the advent of both Christianity and Islam and that early Christians, Muslims, and the Jewish group Falashas practiced circumcision on young girls. Historically, during the nineteenth century and until the 1940's, clitoridectomies were performed in Europe and America as a procedure to "cure" female masturbation, nervousness, and other specific types of perceived psychological dysfunction.

The 1989-1990 Demographic Health Survey of Circumcision stated that circumcision is still performed annually on an estimated 80 to 114 million women; 85 percent of these procedures involve clitoridectomy, while approximately 15 percent involve infibulation. Infibulation, or pharaonic circumcision, is the removal of the clitoris, the labia minora, and much of the labia majora; on occasion, the remaining sides of the vulva are stitched together to close up the vagina, except for a small opening maintained for the passage of blood and urine.

Certain contemporary cultures of Africa, the Middle East, and parts of Yemen, India, and Malaysia continue these practices. Contemporary Middle Eastern countries practicing female circumcision and genital mutilation are Jordan, Iraq, Yemen, Syria, and southern Algeria. In Africa, it is practiced in the majority of the countries, including Egypt, Ivory Coast, Kenya, Mali, Mozambique, Sudan, and Upper Volta. It has been estimated that 99 percent of northern Sudanese women aged fifteen to forty-nine are circumcised. In and around Alexandria, Egypt, 99 percent of rural and lower-income urban women are circumcised.

Cross-culturally, there are essentially four types of female genital circumcision and female genital mutilation. Circumcision, or sunna circumcision, is removal of the prepuce or hood of the clitoris, with the body of the clitoris remaining intact. Sunna means "tradition" in Arabic. Excision circumcision, or clitoridectomy, is the removal of the entire clitoris (both prepuce and glans) and all or part of the adjacent labia majora and the labia minora. Intermediate circumcision is the removal of the clitoris, all or part of the labia minora, and sometimes part of the labia majora.

All types of female genital mutilation frequently may create severe, long-term effects, such as pelvic infections that usually lead to infertility, chronic recurrent urinary tract infections, painful intercourse, obstetrical complications, and in some cases, surgically induced scars that can cause tearing of the tissue and even hemorrhaging during childbirth. In fact, it is not unusual for women who have been infibulated to require surgical enlargement of the vagina on their wedding night or when delivering children. Unfortunately, babies born to infibulated women may frequently suffer brain damage because of oxygen deprivation (hypoxia) caused by a prolonged and obstructed delivery. Babies may die during the painful birthing process because of a damaged birth canal. Other physical and psychological difficulties for the circumcised woman may be sexual dysfunction, delayed menarche, and genital malformation.

From a cultural perspective, there are numerous reasons or justifications given for these procedures. They are often described as rites of passage and proof of adulthood, and it is often argued that the procedures raise a woman's status in her community, because of both the added purity that circumcision brings and the bravery that initiates are called upon to demonstrate. The procedure also is believed to confer maturity and inculcate positive character traits, such as the ability to endure pain and to be submissive. In some cultures, the circumcision ritual is considered to be positive because the girl is the center of attention. She receives presents and moral instruction from her elders, creating a bond between the generations, as all women in the society must undergo the procedure; they thus share an important experience.

Furthermore, it is thought that a girl who has been circumcised will not be troubled by lustful thoughts or sensations or by physical temptations such as masturbation. Therefore, there is less risk of premarital relationships that can end in the stigma and social difficulties of illegitimate birth. The bond between husband and wife may be closer because one or both of them will never have had sex with anyone else. The relationship may be motivated by love rather than lust because there will be no physical drive for the wife, only an emotional one. There is little incentive for extramarital sex for the wife; hence, the marriage may be more secure. Children may be better cared for because the husband can be more confident that he is their father. Generally, a girl who is not circumcised is considered unclean by local villagers and therefore unmarriageable. In some societies, a girl who is not circumcised is believed to be dangerous, even deadly, if her clitoris touches a man's penis.

All of these arguments for female genital mutilation and female circumcision must be weighed against the pain and terror, the lack of consent, and the subjugation of girls and women that is inherent in the practice. The practice must also be weighed against the medical risks.

Female genital circumcision and female genital mutilation surgeries are invariably conducted in unsanitary conditions in which a midwife or close female relative uses unsterile sharp instruments, such as pieces of glass, razor blades, kitchen knives, or scissors. The induction of tetanus, septicemia, hemorrhaging, and even shock are not uncommon. Human immunodeficiency virus (HIV) can be transmitted. No anesthesia is used. These procedures usually are experienced by the girl at approximately three years of age, although the actual age depends upon the customs of the particular society or village. To minimize the risk of the transmission of viruses, countries such as Egypt have made it illegal for female genital mutilation to be practiced by anyone other than trained doctors and nurses in hospitals.

TREATMENT AND THERAPY

There is no information regarding the surgical restoration of severed or damaged genitals. Because of severe cultural sanctions by the participating groups, which continue to hold tenaciously to such practices, female genital circumcision is seldom discussed with outsiders. Those who follow these customs do not report their occurrence. Consequently, there are few data concerning the frequency of female genital circumcision and female genital mutilation within the United States, despite the knowledge that some immigrant groups from Africa, the Middle East, and Asia continue to practice these surgeries. Health care workers estimate that, within the United States, approximately ten thousand girls undergo these surgical procedures each year. Usually, the procedure is conducted in the home. Those who can pay physicians to perform the surgery may do so; in these cases, local anesthesia is used and the risk of infection is less.

PERSPECTIVE AND PROSPECTS

Because of the high number of female genital mutilations and the deaths that this procedure has caused, it is now prohibited in some communities in the United States, Great Britain, France, Sweden, and Switzerland, and in some countries of Africa, such as Egypt, Kenya, and Senegal. The National Organization of Circumcision Information Resource Centers (NOCIRC) is opposed to the procedures, as well as to male circumcision. The United Nations Children's Fund (UNICEF) and the World Health Organization (WHO) consider female genital mutilation to be a violation of human rights and recommend its eradication. In the United States, former representative Patricia Schroeder had introduced a bill that would outlaw female genital mutilation. The bill, called the Federal Prohibition of Female Genital Mutilation Act of 1995, was passed in 1996. The Canadian Criminal Code was enacted to protect children who are ordinarily residents in Canada from being removed from the country and subjected to female genital mutilation.

Both female genital circumcision and female genital mutilation perpetuate customs that seek to control female bodies and sexuality. It is hoped that with increasing legislation and attitude changes regarding bioethical issues, fewer girls and young women will undergo these mutilating surgical procedures. One problem in this campaign is the conflict between cultural self-determination and basic human rights. Feminists, physicians, and ethicists must work respectfully with, and not independently of, local resources for cultural self-examination and change.

—*John Alan Ross, Ph.D.*

See also Bleeding; Childbirth; Childbirth complications; Circumcision, male; Episiotomy; Ethics; Genital disorders, female; Gynecology; Infertility, female; Menstruation; Psychiatry; Reproductive system; Septicemia; Sexual dysfunction; Sexuality; Stillbirth; Women's health.

FOR FURTHER INFORMATION:

Benedek, Wolfgang, et al., eds. *The Human Rights of Women: International Instruments and African Experiences*. London: Zed, 2002. Examines a range of issues as they affect women around the globe. Female genital mutilation is discussed specifically.

"Female Genital and Sexual Mutilation." *WIN News* 26, no. 2 (Spring, 2000): 51-59. A look at the problem of female genital and sexual mutilation around the world. More than 149 million girls have been mutilated in Africa alone.

Female Genital Cutting Education and Networking Project. http://www.fgmnetwork.org. A Web-based clearinghouse for research and other information on female genital mutilation. Has a worldwide focus.

Galanti, Geri-Ann. *Caring for Patients from Different Cultures*. 4th ed. Philadelphia: University of Pennsylvania Press, 2008. The stated goal of this book is "to help the reader achieve cultural competence." Addresses the cultural misunderstandings and conflicts that arise between medical and health care professionals and their patients, which often lead to inferior care. Some discussion of female genital mutilation, including resources.

Gruenbaum, Ellen. *The Female Circumcision Controversy: An Anthropological Perspective*. Philadelphia: University of Pennsylvania Press, 2001. Argues that Western outrage over female circumcision often fails to appreciate the diversity of cultural contexts, the complex meanings, and the conflicting responses to change among citizens of developing nations, thus resulting in a strong backlash against Western intervention.

James, Stanlie M., and Claire C. Robertson, eds. *Genital Cutting and Transnational Sisterhood: Disputing U.S. Polemics*. Urbana: University of Illinois Press, 2002. In five essays, authors use a historical approach, feminist perspectives, and cultural relativism to argue that Western outrage over female circumcision is arrogant and ethnocentric.

Larsen, Ulla, and Sharon Yan. "Does Female Circumcision Affect Infertility and Fertility? A Study of the Central African Republic, Cote d'Ivoire, and Tanzania." *Demography* 37, no. 3 (August, 2000): 313-321. In Cote d'Ivoire and Tanzania, circumcised women had lower childlessness, lower infertility by age, and higher total fertility rates than women who were not circumcised; the reverse pattern prevailed in the Central African Republic.

Walker, Alice, and Pratibha Parmar. *Warrior Marks: Female Genital Mutilation and the Sexual Blinding of Women*. New York: Harcourt Brace, 1993. Describes Walker's journey around the world to interview a group of women trying to eliminate the traditional practice of female circumcision, a practice forced on women by the men of diverse societies, in a study that includes a new introduction offering an update on the issue.

Williams, Deanna Perez, William Acosta, and Herbert A. McPherson, Jr. "Female Genital Mutilation in the United States: Implications for Women's Health." *American Journal of Health Studies* 15, no. 1 (1999): 47-52. Female genital mutilation has become a public health concern in the United States because of an influx of immigrants from countries that practice it. The Centers for Disease Control estimates that 168,000 females in the United States are at risk for this procedure.

CIRCUMCISION, MALE
PROCEDURE

ANATOMY OR SYSTEM AFFECTED: Genitals, reproductive system

SPECIALTIES AND RELATED FIELDS: General surgery, pediatrics, urology

DEFINITION: The removal of the foreskin (prepuce) covering the head of the penis.

KEY TERMS:

chordee: the downward curvature of the penis, most apparent on erection, caused by the shortness of the skin on the downward side of the penile shaft

glans or *glans penis:* the head of the penis

necrosis: the death of one or more cells or a portion of a tissue or organ resulting from irreversible damage

phimosis: the narrowing of the opening of the skin covering the head of the penis sufficient to prevent retraction of the skin back over the glans

sepsis: an infection in the circulating blood

smegma: a pasty accumulation of shed skin cells and secretions of the sweat glands which collects in the moist areas of the foreskin-covered base of the glans

urinary tract infections: infections of the bladder, the kidneys, the urethra (which connects the bladder to the opening at the end of the penis), and the ureters (which connect the bladder to the kidneys); infection may be limited to one area of these organs or spread throughout the urinary tract

INDICATIONS AND PROCEDURES

Routine circumcision of the newborn male—in which the foreskin of the penis is stretched, clamped, and cut—is becoming an increasingly controversial procedure. Famed pediatrician Benjamin Spock once contended that circumcision is a good idea, especially if most of the boys in the neighborhood are circumcised; then a boy feels "regular." Yet, many wonder if that is justification for circumcision. Allowing routine circumcision of newborns as a religious and cultural rite still leaves the debate over medical necessity. The United States is the only country in the world that circumcises a majority of newborn males without a religious reason. In fact, circumcision has been termed a "cultural surgery."

True medical indications for the surgery are seldom present at birth. Such conditions as infections of the head and/or shaft of the penis may be indications for circumcision; an inability to retract the foreskin in the newborn (phimosis) is not an indication. Some argue that circumcision should be delayed until the foreskin has become retractable, making an imprecise surgical procedure presumably less traumatic. In 96 percent of infant boys, however, the foreskin is not fully retractable; it is normally so tight and adherent that it cannot be pulled back and the penis cleaned. By age three, that percentage decreases to 10 percent.

There are other definite contraindications to newborn circumcision. Circumcising infants with abnormalities of the penal head or shaft makes treatment more difficult because the foreskin may later be needed for use in reconstruction. Prematurity, instability, or a bleeding problem also preclude early circumcision. The foreskin is a natural protective membrane, representing 50 to 80 percent of the skin system of the penis, having 240 feet of nerve fibers, more than 1,000 nerve endings, and 3 feet of veins, arteries, and capillaries. It keeps the sensitive head protected, facilitating intercourse, and prevents the surface of the glans from thickening and becoming desensitized. Also, within the inner surface of the foreskin are a series of tiny ridged bands that contribute significantly to stimulating the glans.

The two most persistent arguments for the operation, however, are the risks of infection and cancer in the uncircumcised. Without circumcision, smegma accumulates beneath the base of the covered head of the penis. This cheeselike material of dead skin cells and secretions of the sweat glands is thought to be a cause of cancer of the penis and prostate gland in uncircumcised men and cancer of the cervix in their female partners. Doctors who argue against circumcision, however, say that the presence of smegma in the uncircumcised is simply a sign of poor hygiene and that poor sexual hygiene, inadequate hygienic facilities, and sexually transmitted diseases cause an increased incidence of cancer in ethnic groups or populations that do not practice circumcision. Doctors who argue against circumcision also point out that complete circumcision is found as often in male partners of women without cancer of the cervix as in male partners of women who have cervical cancer. In Sweden, moreover—where newborn circumcision is not routinely practiced but where good hygiene is practiced—the rates of these cancers are essentially the same as those found in Israel, where ritualistic circumcision is practiced.

The increased incidence of urinary tract infections and sexually transmitted diseases (STDs) in uncircumcised males sufficiently argues for circumcision, say its proponents. They warn that the intact foreskin invites bacterial colonization, which leads to urethral infection ascending to the bladder that ultimately may spread upward to the kidneys and sometimes cause permanent kidney damage. On the other hand, no proof exists that uncircumcised male infants who sustain urinary tract infections will have future urologic problems. Furthermore, the operation is not a simple procedure and is not without peril. Penile amputation, life-threatening infections, and even death have been well documented.

Slightly increased rates of infection with sexually transmitted diseases in the uncircumcised argue the case for some proponents, but it is acquired immunodeficiency syndrome (AIDS) that they most fear. In Africa, where circumcision is seldom practiced, the acquisition of AIDS by heterosexual men from infected women during vaginal intercourse is the most common mode of transmission.

Proponents say that infection with human immunodeficiency virus (HIV), the virus that leads to AIDS, depends on a break or an abrasion of the skin to gain entry. The intact foreskin provides a site for transfer of infected cervical secretions. In Africa, doctors at the University of Nairobi noted a relationship of HIV infection to genital ulcers and lack of circumcision. Uncircumcised men had a history of genital ulcers more often than did the circumcised, and they were more often HIV-positive. They were also more frequently HIV-positive even if they did not have a history of genital ulcer disease.

Every evaluation of circumcision, pro or con, should reflect the confounding genetic and environmental variables, as well as the actual increased risks and benefits. All the pros and cons should be explained to parents before informed consent is obtained.

USES AND COMPLICATIONS

In 1989, the American Academy of Pediatrics' Task Force on Circumcision concluded that "newborn circumcision has potential medical benefits and advantages as well as disadvantages and risks. When circumcision is being considered, the benefits and risks should be explained to the parents and informed consent obtained." This neutral statement does not lessen the anxiety of parents who are trying to weigh the pros and cons of routine newborn circumcision, but examination of the evidence does allow parents to weigh the individual benefits and risks and see if the scale tips in either direction.

Worldwide studies of predominantly uncircumcised populations have shown a higher incidence of urinary tract infection in boys during the first few months of life, which is the reverse of what is found in older infants and children, where girls predominate. In 1986, Brooke Army Medical Center in Fort Sam Houston, Texas, took a closer look. The doctors found the incidence of urinary tract infection in circumcised infant males to be 0.11 percent but 1.12 percent in the uncircumcised. Even without proof that the uncircumcised male infants who get urinary tract infections will have future urologic problems, the proponents for the surgical procedure claim about a 1 percent advantage.

The evidence for an increase in sexually transmitted diseases (such as genital herpes, gonorrhea, and syphilis) among the uncircumcised is conflicting. Furthermore, apparent correlations between circumcision status

and these diseases do not reflect confounding genetic and environmental variables. It is also difficult to factor in the risk from HIV infections. The studies from Africa do not look at any variables in the transmission of HIV except circumcision status and previous history of genital ulcers. The nutritional and economic status of the men was not examined, even though it is known that malnourishment suppresses the immune systems. Moreover, if everyone practiced safer sex, the argument for circumcision would be moot.

Almost all the surgical complications of circumcision can be avoided if doctors performing the procedure adhere to strict asepsis, are properly trained and experienced in the procedure, remove the appropriate and correct amount of tissue, and provide adequate hemostasis. The variety of circumstances, populations, and physicians affects the incidence of complications. In the larger, teaching hospitals, often the newest physicians with the least experience or supervision perform the operation. As a result, complications may arise. Excessive bleeding is the most frequent complication. The incidence of bleeding after circumcision ranges from 0.1 percent to as high as 35 percent in some reports. Most of the episodes are minor and can be controlled by simple measures, such as compression and suturing, but some of these efforts can lead to diminished blood supply to the head and shaft of the penis with necrosis of the affected part. Chordee can result if improper technique or bad luck intervenes, and such penile deformity begets the risk of emotional distress. The urethral opening on the end of the penis can become infected or ulcerated when the glans is no longer protected by foreskin; such infection rarely occurs in the uncircumcised. Finally, any surgical procedure runs the risk of infection. These localized infections rarely spread to the blood, but death from sepsis and its sequelae has been documented.

Overall, the surgical complication rate after circumcision runs around 0.19 percent, which could be lowered with strict protocols, meticulous technique, strict asepsis, and well-trained, experienced physicians. Strict protocols, it is hoped, would ensure that absolute contraindications to the procedure—such as anomalies of the penis, prematurity, instability, or a bleeding disorder—were honored.

Another human factor must be considered. Many insurance companies do not provide payment for newborn care, since it is considered preventive medicine. In 1997, a physician's fee for performing a circumcision ranged to approximately $400, with a nationwide average of $137. Interestingly, a growing number of circumcised men are undergoing expensive foreskin restoration procedures.

In part because of an additional cost that arises with anesthesia, the vast majority of infant circumcisions are performed without pain control. The surgery is painful, yet some physicians claim that the minute that the operation ends, the circumcised baby no longer cries and frequently falls asleep. Continuing pain, therefore, is probably not present.

Another perspective to examine is the experience of adult males, who are circumcised by their own choice. Many complain of at least a week's discomfort after the operation. The most compelling argument against adult circumcision, however, comes from their answer to "Would you do it again?" In one study of several hundred men who were circumcised as adults, they were asked five years later if they would do it again. All said no.

PERSPECTIVE AND PROSPECTS

Routine newborn circumcision originated in the United States in the 1860's, ostensibly as prophylaxis against disease. Some medical historians, however, believe that nonreligious circumcision was a deliberate surgical procedure to desensitize and debilitate the penis to prevent masturbation. During this era, and for nearly one hundred years afterward, most American physicians viewed masturbation as an inevitable cause of blindness, weak character, insanity, nervousness, tuberculosis, sexually transmitted disease, and even death. One physician maintained that a painful circumcision would have a salutary effect upon the newborn's mind, so that pain would be associated with masturbation. As late as 1928, the *American Medical Journal* published an editorial that justified male circumcision as an effective means of preventing the dire effects of masturbation. During World Wars I and II, soldiers were forcibly circumcised under threat of court martial, being told that the surgery was for reasons of hygiene and the prevention of epilepsy and other diseases.

Eventually, a general change in attitude occurred, notably in Great Britain and New Zealand, which virtually have abandoned routine circumcision. Rates of circumcision have also fallen dramatically in Canada, Australia, and even the United States. As recently as the mid-1970's, approximately 90 percent of U.S. male babies were circumcised. Not until 1971 did the American Academy of Pediatrics determine that circumci-

sion is not medically valid. By 2001, the incidence of newborn circumcision had declined to 55 percent.

In 1971, the American Academy of Pediatrics' Committee on the Fetus and Newborn issued an advisory that said, "There are no valid medical indications for routine circumcision in the neonatal period." In 1978, when the American College of Obstetricians and Gynecologists affirmed this statement, the circumcision rate had already declined to an estimated 70 percent of newborn males, compared to previous rates of between 80 and 90 percent.

Undoubtedly, the future will bring improved surgical techniques. More emphasis will be placed on avoiding surgical complications by more rigid monitoring of the operation and who performs the procedure. It is unlikely that circumcision will disappear completely.

Organizations such as Doctors Opposing Circumcision and the National Organization to Halt the Abuse and Routine Mutilation of Males, however, are actively proposing an end to routine neonatal circumcision. Some nursing groups and concerned mothers have formed local groups to oppose circumcision in male neonates. They argue that subjecting a baby to this procedure may impair mother-infant bonding. Another question posed by some physicians and parents is the ethics involved in the unnecessary removal of a functioning body organ, particularly without the patient's consent. Others claim that the baby's rights are being violated, noting that it is the child who must live with the outcome of the decision to perform a circumcision. As a result of these efforts, the rates of circumcision will probably continue to fall.

—Wayne R. McKinny, M.D.;
updated by John Alan Ross, Ph.D.

See also Circumcision, female, and genital mutilation; Ethics; Genital disorders, male; Men's health; Neonatology; Pediatrics; Reproductive system; Urology, pediatric.

FOR FURTHER INFORMATION:

Apuzzio, Joseph J., Anthony M. Vintzileos, and Leslie Iffy, eds. *Operative Obstetrics*. 3d ed. New York: Taylor & Francis, 2006. Examines obstetric surgical procedures, including the methods used in circumcision.

Behrman, Richard E., Robert M. Kliegman, and Hal B. Jenson, eds. *Nelson Textbook of Pediatrics*. 18th ed. Philadelphia: Saunders/Elsevier, 2007. This standard pediatric textbook briefly covers the medical risks and benefits of routine newborn circumcision fairly and without bias or excessive medical jargon. Draws no conclusions.

Bigelow, Jim. *The Joy of Uncircumcising! Exploring Circumcision—History, Myths, Psychology, Restoration, Sexual Pleasure, and Human Rights*. Rev. ed. Aptos, Calif.: Hourglass, 1998. This book provides an alternative view of this controversial procedure.

Gollaher, David L. *Circumcision: A History of the World's Most Controversial Surgery*. New York: Basic Books, 2000. Gollaher sets out to make "the strange familiar," but also "the familiar strange," in this book about the persistent practice of circumcision, which has been found in a variety of different cultures around the world.

King, Lowell R., ed. *Urologic Surgery in Neonates and Young Infants*. Philadelphia: W. B. Saunders, 1998. J. W. Duckett's contribution, "The Neonatal Circumcision Debate," is an excellent review of the controversies surrounding this operation. Although written for doctors, it is appropriate for laypersons as well.

Snyder, Howard M. "To Circumcise or Not." *Hospital Practice* 26 (January 15, 1991): 201-207. This widely available medical journal article examines in detail the medical evidence for and against circumcision. With a minimum of medical jargon, the author also states his own personal bias against the routine use of the procedure.

CIRRHOSIS

DISEASE/DISORDER

ANATOMY OR SYSTEM AFFECTED: Liver

SPECIALTIES AND RELATED FIELDS: Family medicine, internal medicine, psychology

DEFINITION: The formation of scar tissue in the liver, which interferes with its normal function.

CAUSES AND SYMPTOMS

The liver is a large, spongy organ that lies in the upper-right abdomen. Regarded as primarily part of the digestive system because it manufactures bile, the liver has many other functions, including the synthesis of blood-clotting factors and the detoxification of such harmful substances as alcohol.

Cirrhosis describes the fibrous scar tissue (or nodules) that replaces the normally soft liver after repeated long-term injury by toxins such as alcohol or viruses. The liver may form small nodules (micronodular cirrhosis), large nodules (macronodular cirrhosis), or a combination of the two types (mixed nodular cirrho-

sis). Cirrhosis is a frequent cause of death among middle-aged men, and increasingly among women. While alcoholism is the most common cause, chronic hepatitis and other rarer diseases can also produce the irreversible liver damage that characterizes cirrhosis.

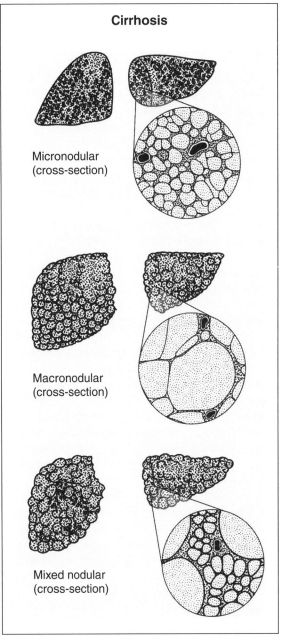

Cirrhosis

Micronodular (cross-section)

Macronodular (cross-section)

Mixed nodular (cross-section)

Cirrhosis appears in three forms, detectable under the microscope, each depending primarily on the cause of the liver damage. All are characterized by the replacement of normally soft, spongy tissue with hard, fibrous scarring. Alcohol-related cirrhosis usually produces the micronodular form.

INFORMATION ON CIRRHOSIS

CAUSES: Buildup of scar tissue in liver from toxins (alcohol, viruses)
SYMPTOMS: May include jaundice, fatigue, weakness, appetite loss, easy bruising
DURATION: Chronic
TREATMENTS: None

The resulting organ is shrunken and hard, unable to perform its varied duties. Because of its altered structure, the cirrhotic liver causes serious problems for surrounding organs, as blood flow becomes difficult. The barrier to normal circulation leads to two serious complications: portal hypertension (the buildup of pressure in the internal veins) and ascites (fluid leakage from blood vessels into the abdominal cavity).

TREATMENT AND THERAPY
Diagnosis is usually made from a history of alcoholism. A physical examination may reveal jaundice; a large nodular liver or a small shrunken one, depending upon the stage; or a fluid-filled abdomen (ascites). Laboratory studies may show elevated liver enzymes released from damaged cells and low levels of products that the liver normally produces (protein, clotting factors). A definitive diagnosis can be made only by biopsy, although radiographic methods such as computed tomography (CT) scanning and magnetic resonance imaging (MRI) can be quite conclusive.

The mortality rate is very high, as the damage is irreversible. Deaths from internal vein rupture and hemorrhage (the results of portal hypertension) and from kidney failure are most common. Repeated hospitalizations attempt to control the variety of complications that arise with agents that stop bleeding, bypass tubes that relieve pressure, the removal of the ascitic fluid, and nutritional support for malnutrition. Eventually, kidney failure ensues or one of these control measures fails, and death rapidly follows. Liver transplantation is considered in some cases. Cases of mild cirrhosis, where sufficient normal tissue remains, have a clearly better course.

—*Connie Rizzo, M.D., Ph.D.*

See also Alcoholism; Endoscopic retrograde cholangiopancreatography (ERCP); Hepatitis; Jaundice; Liver; Liver cancer; Liver disorders; Liver transplantation; Nonalcoholic steatohepatitis (NASH).

FOR FURTHER INFORMATION:
Fishman, Mark, et al. *Medicine.* 5th ed. Philadelphia: Lippincott Williams & Wilkins, 2004. A standard reference source that focuses on internal medicine. Includes bibliographical references and an index.
Goldman, Lee, and Dennis Ausiello, eds. *Cecil Textbook of Medicine.* 23d ed. Philadelphia: Saunders/Elsevier, 2007. This is a standard textbook of medicine. Although it is somewhat difficult, it is complete, beginning with normal conditions and progressing through disease process, diagnosis, and treatment.
Parker, James N., and Philip M. Parker, eds. *The Official Patient's Sourcebook on Primary Biliary Cirrhosis.* San Diego, Calif.: Icon Health, 2002.
_____. *The 2002 Official Patient's Sourcebook on Cirrhosis of the Liver.* San Diego, Calif.: Icon Health, 2002. Provides comprehensive information drawn from public, academic, government, and peer-reviewed research.
Zelman, Mark, et al. *Human Diseases: A Systemic Approach.* 7th ed. Upper Saddle River, N.J.: Pearson, 2010. This well-written and interesting book uses a case-oriented approach to explore the essential concepts of physiology and health.

CLAUDICATION
DISEASE/DISORDER
ANATOMY OR SYSTEM AFFECTED: Blood vessels, circulatory system, legs
SPECIALTIES AND RELATED FIELDS: Vascular medicine
DEFINITION: Pain in the calf or thigh muscle brought on by walking and relieved by rest.

CAUSES AND SYMPTOMS
Claudication is pain that develops in the calf or thigh muscle during walking. The pain increases if the patient continues walking and is relieved within a few minutes after walking is terminated. The medical term for this condition is intermittent claudication. The pain is caused by a narrowing in the arteries that supply the leg with blood. This narrowing is commonly caused by atherosclerosis, in which fatty material builds up on the inside wall of the artery. At first, as the fatty material accumulates in the artery, it creates no symptoms. Only after more than 50 percent of the artery is narrowed do symptoms occur. The first symptom is mild cramping or heaviness that develops during a long walk. Over time, the narrowing increases and the dis-

---

INFORMATION ON CLAUDICATION

CAUSES: Narrowing in leg arteries from atherosclerosis; risk factors include smoking, high blood pressure, heart disease, high cholesterol, advanced age

SYMPTOMS: Mild cramping or heaviness during long walks, progressing to leg pain at rest and sometimes amputation

DURATION: Chronic, progressive without treatment

TREATMENTS: Smoking cessation, lowering of cholesterol levels, program of long-distance walking, medications (pentoxifylline, cilostazol), surgery (angioplasty, bypass surgery, stents)

---

tance that the individual is able to walk decreases. If not treated, the narrowing of the artery may increase further and the pain will be present all the time, signaling a more serious condition called rest pain that may lead to limb loss.

Factors that may lead to this condition include smoking, high blood pressure, heart disease, high cholesterol, and advanced age. Elderly people are more likely to develop intermittent claudication, but younger individuals with multiple risk factors for vascular disease may develop this problem at any age. Sometimes a thrombus may obstruct an artery, causing claudication symptoms to occur suddenly instead of slowly as with atherosclerosis.

The diagnosis of claudication is fairly simple. Clinically, true intermittent claudication can be differentiated from a similar but unrelated condition by noting if the symptoms happen every time that the patient walks a similar distance. True claudication will develop every time, while pain from other conditions will occur at some times but not others.

To be more precise in diagnosing this condition, a Doppler study can be performed on an outpatient basis in a hospital or a doctor's office. The examination, called an ankle-brachial index (ABI), is simple and painless. Blood pressures are taken at the ankles and in the arms before and after exercise. If the pressure at the ankles drops with exercise and goes back to normal a few minutes later, then the diagnosis of intermittent claudication can be made. Ultrasound imaging or angiogram studies may be done to identify the exact location of the narrowing.

TREATMENT AND THERAPY
Treatment depends on the severity of the symptoms. Stopping smoking, lowering cholesterol levels, and beginning a program of long-distance walking may provide enough relief to allow some patients to return to near-normal routines. Medications such as pentoxifylline (Trental or Pentoxil) or cilostazol (Pletal) may provide limited relief from symptoms. More severe cases may require angioplasty, surgery to bypass the narrowed artery, or stenting of the diseased artery.

PERSPECTIVE AND PROSPECTS
Claudication has become more common in the United States as the population ages and sedentary lifestyles become more popular. Although some treatments are effective, it is a difficult problem to manage. Education programs are available to help those at risk for this condition make necessary lifestyle changes that may lessen their chances of developing this ailment. Those changes may include getting plenty of exercise (brisk walking being the best), not smoking, lowering cholesterol, and keeping diabetes under control.

—*Steven R. Talbot, R.V.T.*

See also Arteriosclerosis; Bypass surgery; Cholesterol; Circulation; Exercise physiology; Hypercholesterolemia; Lower extremities; Pain management; Plaque, arterial; Stents; Thrombosis and thrombus; Vascular medicine; Vascular system; Vasculitis.

FOR FURTHER INFORMATION:
Hershey, Falls B., Robert W. Barnes, and David S. Sumner, eds. *Noninvasive Diagnosis of Vascular Disease*. Pasadena, Calif.: Appleton Davies, 1984.
Rutherford, Robert B., ed. *Vascular Surgery*. 6th ed. Philadelphia: Saunders/Elsevier, 2005.
Zwiebel, William J., and John S. Pellerito, eds. *Introduction to Vascular Ultrasonography*. 5th ed. Philadelphia: Saunders/Elsevier, 2005.

CLEFT LIP AND PALATE
DISEASE/DISORDER

ANATOMY OR SYSTEM AFFECTED: Bones, musculoskeletal system

SPECIALTIES AND RELATED FIELDS: Neonatology, otorhinolaryngology, pediatrics, plastic surgery, speech pathology

DEFINITION: A fissure in the midline of the palate, resulting from the failure of the two sides to fuse during embryonic development; in some cases, the fissure may extend through both hard and soft palates into the nasal cavities.

Key terms:

alveolus: the bony ridge where teeth grow

ectrodactyly: a congenital anomaly characterized by the absence of part or all of one or more of the fingers or toes

hard palate: the bony portion of the roof of the mouth, contiguous with the soft palate

Logan's bow: a metal bar placed, for protection and tension removal, on the early postoperative cleft lip

obturator: a sheet of plastic shaped like a flattened dome which fits into the cleft and closes it well enough to permit nursing

soft palate: a structure of mucous membrane, muscle fibers, and mucous glands suspended from the posterior border of the hard palate

syndactyly: a congenital anomaly characterized by the fusion of the fingers or toes

uvula: the small, cone-shaped projection of tissue suspended in the mouth from the posterior of the soft palate

Causes and Symptoms

Cleft palate is a congenital defect characterized by a fissure along the midline of the palate. It occurs when the two sides fail to fuse during embryonic development. The gap may be complete, extending through the hard and soft palates into the nasal cavities, or may be partial or incomplete. It is often associated with cleft lip or "harelip." About one child in eight hundred live births is affected with some degree of clefting, and clefting is the most common of the craniofacial abnormalities.

Cleft palate is not generally a genetic disorder; rather, it is a result of defective cell migration. Embryonically, in the first month, the mouth and nose form one cavity destined to be separated by the hard and soft palates. In addition, there is no upper lip. Most of the upper jaw is lacking; only the part near the ears is present. In the next weeks, the upper lip and jaw are formed from structures growing in from the sides, fusing at the midline with a third portion growing downward from the nasal region. The palates develop in much the same way. The fusion of all these structures begins with the lip and moves posteriorly toward, then includes, the soft palate. The two cavities are separated by the palates by the end of the third month of gestation.

If, as embryonic development occurs, the cells that should grow together to form the lips and palate fail to move in the correct direction, the job is left unfinished.

Information on Cleft Lip and Palate

Causes: Congenital defect

Symptoms: Craniofacial abnormalities, greater susceptibility to colds, poor muscle reactivity, dental problems

Duration: Correctable, usually between seven and twelve months of age

Treatments: Surgery

Clefting of the palate generally occurs between the thirty-fifth and thirty-seventh days of gestation. Fortunately, it is an isolated defect not usually associated with other disabilities or with mental retardation.

If the interference in normal growth and fusion begins early and lasts throughout the fusion period, the cleft that results will affect one or both sides of the top lip and may continue back through the upper jaw, the upper gum ridge, and both palates. If the disturbance lasts only part of the time that development is occurring, only the lip may be cleft, and the palate may be unaffected. If the problem begins a little into the fusion process, the lip is normally formed, but the palate is cleft. The cleft may divide only the soft palate or both the soft and the hard palate. Even the uvula may be affected; it can be split, unusually short, or even absent.

About 80 percent of cases of cleft lip are unilateral; of these, 70 percent occur on the left side. Of cleft palate cases, 25 percent are bilateral. The mildest manifestations of congenital cleft are mild scarring and/or notching of the upper lip. Beyond this, clefting is described by degrees. The first degree is incomplete, which is a small cleft in the uvula. The second degree is also incomplete, through the soft palate and into the hard palate. Another type of "second-degree incomplete" is a horseshoe type, in which there is a bilateral cleft proceeding almost to the front. Third-degree bilateral is a cleft through both palates but bilaterally through the gums; it results in a separate area of the alveolus where the teeth will erupt, and the teeth will show up in a very small segment. When the teeth appear, they may not be normally aligned. In addition to the lip, gum, and palate deviations, abnormalities of the nose may also occur.

Cleft palate may be inherited, probably as a result of the interaction of several genes. In addition, the effects of some environmental factors that affect embryonic development may be linked to this condition. They might include mechanical disturbances such as an enlarged tongue, which prevents the fusion of the palate and lip. Other disturbances may be caused by toxins introduced by the mother (drugs such as cortisone or alcohol) and defective blood. Other associated factors include deficiencies of vitamins or minerals in the mother's diet, radiation from X rays, and infectious diseases such as German measles. No definite cause has been identified, nor does it appear that one cause alone can be implicated. It is likely that there is an interplay between mutant genes, chromosomal abnormalities, and environmental factors.

There are at least 150 syndromes involving oral and facial clefts. Four examples of cleft syndromes that illustrate these syndromes are EEC (ectrodactyly, ectodermal dysplasia, cleft lip/palate), popliteal pterygium syndrome, van der Woude's syndrome, and trisomy 13 syndrome. EEC and trisomy 13 both result in mental retardation as well as oral clefts, plus numerous other disabilities more serious than clefting. Popliteal pterygium has as its most common feature skin webbing (pterygium), along with clefts and skeletal abnormalities. Van der Woude's syndrome usually shows syndactyly as well as clefting and lower-lip pitting.

Problems begin at birth for the infant born with a cleft palate. The most immediate problem is feeding the baby. If the cleft is small and the lip unaffected, nursing may proceed fairly easily. If the cleft is too large, however, the baby cannot build up enough suc-

tion to nurse efficiently. To remedy this, the hole in the nipple of the bottle can be enlarged, or a plastic obturator can be fitted to the bottle.

Babies with cleft palate apparently are more susceptible to colds than other children. Since there is an open connection between the nose and mouth, an infection that starts in either location will easily and quickly spread to the other. Frequently, the infection will spread to the middle ear via the Eustachian tube. One end of a muscle is affixed to the Eustachian tube opening, and the other end is attached to the middle of the roof of the mouth (palate). Normal contraction opens the tube so that air can travel through the tube and equalize air pressure on both sides of the eardrum. As long as the eardrum has flexibility of movement, the basics for good hearing are in place. Children with cleft palates, however, do not have good muscle reactions; therefore, air cannot travel through the tube. If the tube remains closed after swallowing, the air that is trapped is absorbed into the middle-ear tissue, resulting in a vacuum. This pulls the eardrum inward and decreases its flexibility, and hearing loss ensues. The cavity of the middle ear then fills with fluid, which often breeds bacteria, causing infection. The infection may or may not be painful; if there is no pain, the infection may go unnoticed and untreated. The accumulated fluid can cause erosion of the tiny bones, which would decrease sound transmission to the auditory nerve. This conductive hearing loss is permanent. Persistent and prolonged

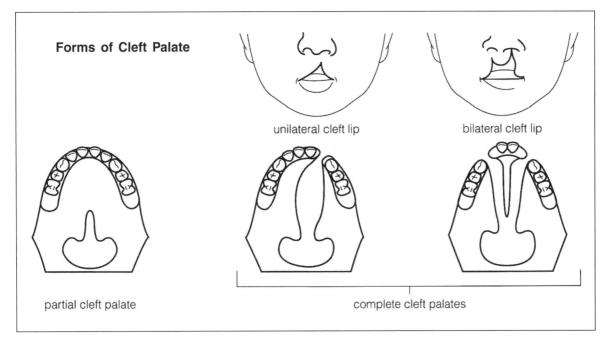

Forms of Cleft Palate

unilateral cleft lip

bilateral cleft lip

partial cleft palate

complete cleft palates

fluid buildup can also cause accumulation of dead matter, forming a tumorlike growth called a cholesteatoma.

Other problems associated with cleft palate are those related to dentition. In some children there may be extra teeth, while in others the cleft may prevent the formation of tooth buds so that teeth are missing. Teeth that are present may be malformed; those malformations include injury during development, fusion of teeth to form one large tooth, teeth lacking enamel, and teeth that have too little calcium in the enamel. If later in development and growth the teeth are misaligned, orthodontia may be undertaken. Another possible problem met by patients with a cleft palate is maxillary (upper jaw) arch collapse; this condition is also remedied with orthodontic treatment.

TREATMENT AND THERAPY

One of the first questions a parent of a child with a cleft palate will pose regards surgical repair. The purpose of surgically closing the cleft is not simply to close the hole—although that goal is important. The major purpose is to achieve a functional palate. Whether this can be accomplished depends on the size and shape of the cleft, the thickness of the available tissue, and other factors.

Cleft lip surgery is performed when the healthy baby weighs at least seven pounds; it is done under a general anesthetic. If the cleft is unilateral, one operation can accomplish the closure, but a bilateral cleft lip is often repaired in two steps at least a month apart. When the lip is repaired, normal lip pressure is restored, which may help in closing the cleft in the gum ridge. It may also reduce the gap in the hard palate, if one is present. Successive operations may be suggested when, even years after surgery, scars develop on the lip.

Surgery to close clefts of the hard and soft palate is typically done when the baby is at least nine months of age, unless there is a medical reason not to do so. Different surgeons prefer different times for this surgery. The surgeon attempts to accomplish three goals in the repair procedure. The surgeon will first try to ensure that the palate is long enough so that function and movement will result (this is essential for proper speech patterns). Second, the musculature around the Eustachian tube should work properly in order to cut down the incidence of ear infections. Finally, the surgery should promote the development of the facial bones and, as much as possible, normal teeth. This goal aids in eating and appearance. All of this may be accomplished in one operation, if the cleft is not too se-

vere. For a cleft that requires more procedures, the surgeries are usually spaced at least six months apart so that complete healing can occur. This schedule decreases the potential for severe scarring.

At one time, it was thought that if surgery were performed before the child began talking, speech problems would be avoided. In reality, not only did the surgery not remedy that problem, but the early closure often resulted in a narrowing of the upper jaw and interference with facial growth as well. Thus, the trend to put off the surgery until the child was four or five years of age developed; by this age, more than 80 percent of the lateral growth of the upper jaw has occurred. Most surgeons can perform the corrective surgery when the child is between one and two years of age without affecting facial growth.

Successful repair greatly improves speech and appearance, and the physiology of the oral and nasal cavities is also improved. Additional surgery may be necessary to improve appearance, breathing, and the function of the palate. Sometimes the palate may partially reopen, and surgery is needed to reclose it.

When the baby leaves the operating room, there are stitches in the repaired area. Sometimes a special device called a Logan's bow is taped to the baby's cheeks; this device not only protects the stitches but also relieves some of the tension on them. In addition, the baby's arms may be restrained in order to keep the baby's hands away from the affected area. (The child is fitted for elbow restraints before surgery; the elbows are encased in tubes that prevent them from bending.) A parent of a child that has just undergone cleft palate repair should not panic at the sight of bleeding from the mouth. To curb it, gauze may be packed into the repaired area and remain about five days after surgery. As mucus and other body fluids accumulate in the area, they may be suctioned out.

During the initial recovery, the child is kept in a moist, oxygen-rich environment (an oxygen tent) until respiration is normal. The patient will be observed for signs of airway obstruction or excessive bleeding. Feeding is done by syringe, eyedropper, or special nipples. Clear liquids and juices only are allowed. The child sits in a high chair to drink, when possible. After feeding, the mouth should be rinsed well with water to help keep the stitches clean and uncrusted. Peroxide mixed with the water may help, as well as ointment. Intake and output of fluids are measured. Hospitalization may last for about a week, or however long is dictated by speed of healing. At the end of this week, stitches are removed and the suture line covered and protected by a strip of paper tape.

An alternative to surgery is the use of an artificial palate known as an obturator. It is specially constructed by a dentist to fit into the child's mouth. The appliance, or prosthesis, is carefully constructed to fit precisely and snugly, but it must be easily removable. There must be enough space at the back so the child can breathe through the nose. While speaking, the muscles move back over this opening so that speech is relatively unaffected.

Speech problems are the most likely residual problems in the cleft palate patient. The speech of the untreated, and sometimes the treated, cleft palate patient is very nasal. If the soft palate is too short, the closure of the palate may leave a space between the nose and the throat, allowing air to escape through the nose. There is little penetrating quality to the patient's voice, and it does not carry well. Some cleft palate speakers are difficult to understand because there are several faults in articulation. Certainly not all cleft lip or palate patients, however, will develop communication problems; modern surgical procedures help ensure that most children will develop acceptable speech and language without necessitating the help of a speech therapist.

Genetic counseling may help answer some of the family's questions about why the cleft palate occurred, whether it will happen with future children, and whether there is any way to prevent it. There are no universal answers to these questions. The answers depend on the degree and type of cleft, the sex of the child, the presence of other problems, the family history, and the history of the pregnancy. Genetic counseling obtained at a hospital or medical clinic can determine whether the condition was heritable or a chance error and can establish the risk level for future pregnancies.

PERSPECTIVE AND PROSPECTS

Oral clefts, as well as other facial clefts, have been a part of historical records for thousands of years. Perhaps the earliest recorded incidence is a Neolithic shrine with a two-headed figurine dated about 6500 B.C.E. The origination and causative agent of such clefts remain mysterious today.

Expectant parents are rarely alerted prior to birth that their child will be born with a cleft, so it is usually in the hospital, just after birth, that parents first learn of the birth defect. Even if it is suspected that a woman is at risk for producing a child with a cleft palate, there is no way to determine if the defect is indeed present, as neither amniocentesis nor chromosomal analysis reveals the condition. When the baby is delivered, the presence of the cleft can evoke a feeling of crisis in the delivery room. Shocklike reactions may be caused by the unexpectedness of the event or can occur because the doctors and medical personnel in the room have had little exposure to the defect. The parents may feel personal failure.

The problems accompanying clefting may alter family morale and climate, increasing the complexity of the problem. A team of specialists usually works together to help the patient and the family cope with these problems. This team may include a pediatrician, a speech pathologist, a plastic surgeon, an orthodontist, a psychiatrist, a social worker, an otologist, an audiologist, and perhaps others.

The cooperating team should monitor these situations: feeding problems, family and friends' reactions to the baby's appearance, how parents encourage the child to talk or how they respond to poor speech, and whether the parents are realistic about the long-term outcome for their child. The grief, guilt, and shock that the parents often feel can be positively altered by how the professional team tackles the problem and by communication with the parents. Usually the team does not begin functioning in the baby's life until he or she is about a month old. Some parents have confronted their feelings, while others are still struggling with the negative feeling that the birth brought to bear. Therefore, the first visit that the parents have with the team is important, because it establishes the foundation of a support system which should last for years.

If the cleft were only a structural defect, the solution would simply be to close the hole. Yet, problems concerning feeding and health, facial appearance, communication, speech, dental functioning, and hearing loss, as well as the potential for psychosocial difficulties, may necessitate additional surgical, orthodontic, speech, and otolaryngological interventions. In other words, after the closure has been made, attention is focused on aesthetic, functional, and other structural deficits.

—Iona C. Baldridge

See also Birth defects; Cleft lip and palate repair; DiGeorge syndrome; Oral and maxillofacial surgery; Speech disorders.

FOR FURTHER INFORMATION:

Berkowitz, Samuel, ed. *Cleft Lip and Palate: Diagnosis and Management.* 2d ed. New York: Springer, 2006. A review of treatment approaches. Offers facial and palatal growth studies.

Cleft Palate Foundation. http://www.cleftline.org. Web site is divided into two sections, one for patients and families and one for professionals. The group offers publications, Cleftline (a toll-free phone number for information and support), and annual research grants.

Clifford, Edward. *The Cleft Palate Experience*. Springfield, Ill.: Charles C Thomas, 1987. This author writes from the perspective of a cleft palate team participant and incorporates the value of the team in his chapters. Much space is given to the child's development of a positive self-image and the parents' role, from birth, in forming this image.

Gruman-Trinker, Carrie T. *Your Cleft-Affected Child: The Complete Book of Information, Resources, and Hope*. Alameda, Calif.: Hunter House, 2001. An excellent guide to cleft disorders, including topics such as surgical procedures, financial assistance, emotional impact, and forming support groups.

Lorente, Christine, et al. "Tobacco and Alcohol Use During Pregnancy and Risk of Oral Clefts." *American Journal of Public Health* 90, no. 3 (March, 2000): 415-419. This study examines the relationship between maternal tobacco and alcohol consumption during the first trimester of pregnancy and oral clefts. Multivariate analyses showed an increased risk of cleft lip with or without cleft palate associated with smoking and an increased risk of cleft palate associated with alcohol consumption.

Stengelhofen, Jackie, ed. *Cleft Palate*. New York: Churchill Livingstone, 1988. Explores the various communication problems met by those with a cleft palate. An appeal to the entire team of professionals treating the patient and their partnership with parents. Case histories are discussed.

Wyszynski, Diego F., ed. *Cleft Lip and Palate: From Origin to Treatment*. New York: Oxford University Press, 2002. An excellent reference covering all aspects of cleft lip and palate formation, etiology, treatment, and prevention.

Cleft lip and palate repair

Procedure

Anatomy or system affected: Bones, gums, mouth, musculoskeletal system, skin

Specialties and related fields: General surgery, neonatology, otorhinolaryngology, pediatrics, plastic surgery

Definition: The surgical closure of cleft lip and cleft palate, deformities of the mouth that are often described as either the failure of tissue migration to allow fusion or the failure of tissue ingrowth (filling in).

Indications and Procedures

Cleft lip is more common in males than in females. Additionally, males tend to have more severe cleft deformities than females. Cleft lip repair is classically performed according to the rule of tens: The infant should be ten weeks old, weigh at least ten pounds, and have a white blood cell count under ten thousand (no infections) and a hemoglobin count of ten grams (not anemic). Today, many surgeons prefer to perform repairs earlier in healthy, full-term newborns ranging in age from one day to fourteen days. Cleft lip repairs typically involve making flaps around the lip area and

The Repair of Cleft Lip

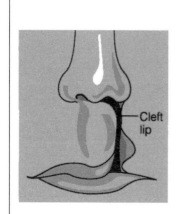
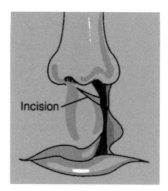
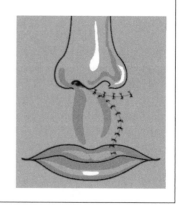

A cleft lip, a congenital deformity in which the tissues between the lip and nostril have failed to fuse, can be corrected surgically through realignment and suturing.

merging the gaping sides. The muscular layer around the mouth must be sealed into a functional unit, as must the skin.

Cleft palate is more prevalent in females than males by a 2:1 ratio. A cleft palate may involve only the soft palate, or it may involve both the hard and the soft palates. Suckling can be a greater challenge with a cleft palate than with cleft lip. Moreover, middle-ear disease and infections are a greater problem for an infant with a cleft palate, because the reflux of fluids or solids into the nasal or middle-ear regions can occur. Surgical closure of a cleft palate usually is performed on infants between nine months and one year of age; delays can permanently retard speech and phonation development, while premature closure can stunt facial bone growth and contribute to dentition problems. Typically, if both the hard and the soft palates are open, they will be surgically closed at the same time. Closure of the soft palate occurs in a three-layer manner, while closure of the hard palate is done in a two-layer approach.

Cleft lip coupled with cleft palate is more common in males and tends to be left-sided more often than right-sided. Combined cleft lip and palate repair follows the same plans as described above, but there is greater concern about the well-being of an infant with the combined deformity.

—*Mary C. Fields, M.D.*

See also Birth defects; Bones and the skeleton; Cleft lip and palate; Oral and maxillofacial surgery; Pediatrics; Plastic surgery; Surgery, pediatric.

FOR FURTHER INFORMATION:

Berkowitz, Samuel, ed. *Cleft Lip and Palate: Diagnosis and Management.* 2d ed. New York: Springer, 2006.

Clifford, Edward. *The Cleft Palate Experience.* Springfield, Ill.: Charles C Thomas, 1987.

Dronamraju, Krishna R. *Cleft Lip and Palate.* Springfield, Ill.: Charles C Thomas, 1986.

Gruman-Trinker, Carrie T. *Your Cleft-Affected Child: The Complete Book of Information, Resources, and Hope.* Alameda, Calif.: Hunter House, 2001.

Watson, A. C. H. *Management of Cleft Lip and Palate.* Philadelphia: Whurr, 2001.

Wynn, Sidney K., and Alfred L. Miller. *A Practical Guide to Cleft Lip and Palate Birth Defects.* Springfield, Ill.: Charles C Thomas, 1984.

Wyszynski, Diego F. *Cleft Lip and Palate: From Origin to Treatment.* New York: Oxford University Press, 2002.

CLINICAL TRIALS

PROCEDURE

ANATOMY OR SYSTEM AFFECTED: All

SPECIALTIES AND RELATED FIELDS: All

DEFINITION: Research studies that test new drugs or treatments on human subjects to determine whether and at what dosage they are safe, effective, and better than similar products already in use.

KEY TERMS:

blinded or *single-blind:* a study in which the patients are not told whether they are in an experimental or control group

control group: a group of patients receiving either a standard treatment or a placebo, allowing comparison with the experimental treatment

double-blind: referring to a study in which neither the patients nor the research staff knows which patients are receiving which treatment

informed consent: consent for treatment by a patient who has been educated fully about the purpose, benefits, and risks of a clinical trial

Institutional Review Board (IRB): a committee that oversees informed consent, reviews the progress of clinical trials, and safeguards participants' rights

placebo: an inactive substance resembling the experimental drug that might be given to a control group, especially when no standard treatment exists

protocol: a lengthy, technical document outlining the rules for inclusion in, scientific rationale of, and procedures for a clinical trial

randomization: assigning, by chance, patients with similar characteristics to either the experimental or the control group in a clinical trial

INDICATIONS AND PROCEDURES

Clinical trials offer the most reliable process for bringing new drugs and medical treatments into public use. The process has features that can protect human participants, avoid biases, ensure that patient improvements are due to the experimental treatment and not to other factors, and allow accurate comparison of the experimental treatment with others on the market. Clinical trials are usually initiated and managed by academic institutions (often with grant funding), pharmaceutical companies, or government research agencies, such as the National Cancer Institute.

In 1998, it was estimated that the cost of developing a new drug was, on average, $500 million, and the process could take twelve to fifteen years—from discovery and laboratory testing, through clinical trials, to Food and Drug Administration (FDA) approval, and finally getting the drug to market. By the late 1990's, a new drug might go through sixty-eight clinical trials. The average number of patients enrolled in a trial was 3,800.

Clinical trials fit into one of four types. Phase I trials, which usually involve only twenty to one hundred seriously ill patients, try to determine how to administer a new drug, the maximally tolerated dose (MTD), how the human body processes the drug, and any significant side effects. Phase II trials, which are usually randomized, treat up to several hundred patients who all have measurable rates of disease. These trials study the effectiveness of the drug. Phase III trials, which are usually randomized and blinded and which treat hundreds or thousands of patients, have more relaxed criteria for inclusion and are usually multicenter (held simultaneously at more than one site). These trials try to determine whether the new drug is better than current, standard ones. Phase IV trials, conducted once a drug is on the market, are often informal. Pharmaceutical companies may simply ask physicians to submit reports on how their patients are responding to the drug.

USES AND COMPLICATIONS

The 1979 Belmont Report detailed three ethical principles to guide clinical trials. They include respect for persons (abiding by their opinions and choices as autonomous agents), beneficence (doing no harm and maximizing the possible benefits while minimizing possible harm), and justice (distributing the benefits and burdens of research fairly).

Two standard features of clinical trials help ensure that ethical principles are being followed. First, all clinical trials in the United States must be approved and monitored by an Institutional Review Board (IRB), which includes both scientists and laypersons. Multicenter trials must also have a data safety and monitoring board composed of independent experts. This group monitors data from the trial regarding the treatment's effectiveness and any adverse reactions. Second, the detailed informed consent document that patients must carefully consider and sign gives a number of categories of information. Most important, anticipated physical risks and discomforts are explained, as are financial risks.

PERSPECTIVE AND PROSPECTS

In October, 1948, *The British Medical Journal* published an article reporting on what was probably the first study using all the methodological features of the randomized clinical trial. Since then, the randomized clinical trial has come to be regarded as perhaps the most important medical achievement of the twentieth century. It transformed biomedical research and allowed physicians to make treatment choices based on scientific evidence rather than personal opinion and experience.

The National Cancer Institute (NCI) and other sources reported a small participation rate in clinical trials—ranging in the late 1990's from 3 to 20 percent of patients. One of many causes was that insurance companies and managed care providers frequently refused payment for experimental treatments. Their concerns were that they might be liable for adverse reactions or additional care after the trial ends and that clinical trials are more costly than conventional treatments. Because so many insurers would not cover the costs of clinical trials, researchers had trouble finding patients willing to participate, thus slowing the development of more effective drugs and treatments. Insurers gradually realized that more widespread coverage of the costs of trials might speed the development of better drugs, which could ultimately save them money. In 1998, states began to pass laws requiring insurers to cover the routine medical costs (such as tests and office visits) of treatment in clinical trials of drugs for life-threatening diseases.

Criticism has been leveled at clinical trials for insufficient inclusion of women, children, people of color, and the aged. When these groups are underrepresented, there is no certainty that a drug will be effective or without side effects for them.

In June, 2000, the FDA added a regulation that would place a clinical hold on a phase I trial of a drug or treatment for a life-threatening disease affecting both women and men if either gender was excluded because of risk to their reproductive potential. That same month, President Bill Clinton signed an executive memorandum directing Medicare to reimburse senior citizens for routine medical costs incurred in clinical trials. A major impetus for this change came from reports that only 33 percent of cancer clinical trial participants were over sixty-five, while 63 percent of all cancer patients are over sixty-five.

—*Glenn Ellen Starr Stilling, M.A., M.L.S.*

See also Animal rights vs. research; Cancer; Clinics; Death and dying; Disease; Ethics; Food and Drug Administration (FDA); Iatrogenic disorders; Invasive tests; National Cancer Institute (NCI); Noninvasive tests; Over-the-counter medications; Pharmacology; Pharmacy; Screening; Terminally ill: Extended care.

For Further Information:

CenterWatch Clinical Trials Listing Service. http://www.centerwatch.com.

ClinicalTrials.gov. http://www.clinicaltrials.gov.

Finn, Robert. *Cancer Clinical Trials: Experimental Treatments and How They Can Help You.* Sebastopol, Calif.: O'Reilly, 1999.

Green, Stephanie, Jacqueline Benedetti, and John Crowley. *Clinical Trials in Oncology.* 2d ed. Boca Raton, Fla.: Chapman & Hall, 2003.

Harrington, David P. "The Randomized Clinical Trial." *Journal of the American Statistical Association* 95, no. 449 (March, 2000): 312-315.

Malay, Marilyn. *Making the Decision: A Cancer Patient's Guide to Clinical Trials.* Sudbury, Mass.: Jones and Bartlett, 2002.

Quinn, Susan. *Human Trials: Scientists, Investors, and Patients in the Quest for a Cure.* Cambridge, Mass.: Perseus, 2002.

Clinics

Health care system

Definition: Organizations that provide outpatient care to specific types of patients; they can be in-hospital or out of hospital, usually consist of a physical space with reception and examination rooms, and are staffed by doctors, nurses, and other health care professionals.

Key terms:

ambulatory surgery center: a facility providing day surgery outside a hospital setting

clinic: a site for outpatient care

hospital: an inpatient care facility that provides overnight care and in many cases intensive care, emergency care, and surgical services

inpatient care: overnight patient treatment at a hospital

outpatient care: patient treatment not requiring an overnight stay at a hospital

provider: the medical practitioner within a clinic or hospital; providers may be physicians, nurses, dentists, or other licensed health care professionals

Organization and Functions

There are three main types of patient care facilities in North America: hospitals, ambulatory surgery centers, and clinics. Hospitals care for patients who require overnight care, emergency care, or intensive care treatment. Hospital emergency rooms are not usually considered a clinic due to the highly specialized equipment needed and the fact that many patients who are treated in the emergency room are then admitted for overnight stay at a hospital. Ambulatory surgery centers provide outpatient surgery. Clinics provide outpatient nonsurgical care. In some cases, minor procedures are performed in clinics; however, a clinic does not provide outpatient surgery.

A clinic will usually consist of at least a waiting room and patient exam rooms. The number of examination rooms and size of the clinic will depend on the number of providers and the clinic type. Clinics can range in size from a solo practice with a very small office to very large multispecialty outpatient clinics such as the Mayo Clinic or Cleveland Clinic. Specialized equipment may be part of a clinic, such as in a dental clinic. Clinics may be located within a hospital, in a private building, or in a public building. Clinics can be owned and operated by a single practitioner, a group of practitioners, a private group, a public or nonprofit group, a hospital, or a government agency.

Clinics will most often have regular business hours and are not usually open overnight. Some urgent care walk-in clinics may have extended hours. Most clinics will be closed on major holidays. Some smaller solo practitioner clinics may close for one or more weeks per year when the provider is on vacation. Some clinics will have an answering service or after-hours coverage for emergency calls.

Clinic administration will depend on the ownership of the clinic. A solo private practitioner may do administration as well as provision of care. Hospital-based clinics will generally have a clinic manager who works within the administrative system of the hospital. Some clinics may be part of a publicly held company and will have an office manager who reports to a board. Most clinics will have a clinic manager and a medical director. Larger clinics will have more administrative staff, including human resource staff and marketing staff.

Each clinic serves a specific patient population that will be determined by the primary provider or providers within the clinic. For example, a solo family practice physician will serve children and adults for treatment of common illnesses and conditions. In contrast, a pediatric clinic will see only children, and some public health clinics may provide only immunization services. There are as many clinics as there are health care specialties. Some providers will work in groups, such as a multidiscipline group that may contain internal medicine, pediatrics, and dermatology.

Clinics may accept direct fee-for-service payment, insurance, or government funding such as Medicare, Veterans Administration, or Indian Health Service. In Canada, most clinics will accept fee-for-service payment, provincial health insurance payment, or both.

A large number of combinations are possible in terms of specific services offered, number of providers, payment types accepted, clinic size, and clinic location. No matter what the combination of these features, all clinics have in common the provision of nonsurgical outpatient health care services.

STAFF AND SERVICES

A health care clinic will generally be staffed by a primary provider and support staff. The primary provider will often be a medical doctor but can be another type of provider such as physical therapist, chiropractor, optometrist, dentist, or naturopath. Support staff will include nurses, physician assistants, technicians, office staff, and, in some cases, specialized paraprofessionals. Providers and other specialized staff who provide direct patient care will have licensing requirements that are specific to the state or province and that will vary depending on the field. For example, physicians and dentists will have different licensing requirements.

Depending on the clinic, patients may require referral from a physician. Other clinics such as urgent care clinics will accept walk-ins without referral. Walk-in clinics may refer patients to family practice clinics or other clinics for ongoing care of chronic disease.

Services will depend on the clinic providers. For example, a family practice clinic will provide physical examination, diagnosis, and treatment recommendations for people of all ages for general nonsurgical outpatient medical care. Diagnosis might include giving a patient requisitions to have laboratory or radiology (X-ray) or other specialized tests done at a laboratory or radiology facility. Some family practice clinics may have the capacity to do some simple laboratory tests such as a dip urinalysis or electrocardiography (ECG or EKG). Treatment may include advice, prescription for medications, or treatment of minor injuries.

Another example of a clinic would be a physical therapy clinic. This type of clinic would have one or more physical therapists as providers. These providers would provide limited physical examination, usually of the musculoskeletal system. Diagnosis would be based on the physical examination. Physical therapists would not usually order specialized testing such as X rays or magnetic resonance imaging (MRI) but might comanage a patient with a physician provider if these additional diagnostic tests were needed. Treatment within a physical therapy clinic will usually consist of specialized exercises, massage therapy, heat or cold treatment, specialized physical therapy maneuvers, and, in some cases, acupuncture.

Specialized clinics will treat only specific groups of patients. For example, an obstetrics clinic will provide care only to pregnant women. Pediatrics clinics will treat only children. Ophthalmology clinics will treat both children and adults but will care only for vision and other eye-related problems. Similarly, an orthopedic clinic will be focused on musculoskeletal disorders, and sports medicine clinics will treat sports-related injuries.

Urgent care clinics are designed to treat minor illnesses and minor injuries. More significant illness or injury would be treated in a hospital emergency room. Most urgent care clinics will operate on a walk-in basis due to the nature of the clinic focus. Some hospitals have both an urgent care clinic and an emergency room to keep the emergency room available for the more seriously ill or injured.

The Mayo Clinic and the Cleveland Clinic are examples of clinics that have grown to become very large multidisciplinary clinics that provide outpatient care. These large clinics are affiliated with hospitals that provide inpatient and surgical care.

Some clinics receive public funding to serve low-income populations. This type of clinic may operate on a sliding scale for fee payment. Often this type of clinic will be located in an urban area and may serve homeless populations as well. These clinics are sometimes staffed by volunteers, including volunteer providers.

Regardless of the clinic type, the usual practice is to have the patient check in at a desk in the reception area. Patients may have to wait in the reception area until the appropriate staff is ready and until an exam or treatment room is available. Each patient will have a paper or computerized chart that will record the examinations, diagnosis, and treatment recommendations. The patient will then be taken to the exam room, where a nurse or other specialized staff will often do some preliminary testing such as blood pressure and a preliminary history to determine what services are needed. If the chart is a paper chart, then it will be taken along with the patient to the exam room. The provider will often go from one exam room to the next to examine and treat patients. The support staff will clean each exam room as it is vacated and then room the next patient. This system allows for more efficiency for the provider. Once the provider is done with examination, diagnosis, and treatment, the patient is directed back to the reception area to book additional appointments or testing, if necessary, and is then dismissed from the clinic.

A patient who comes to a clinic with a life-threatening condition or serious injury will be directed to the nearest emergency room. In some cases, an ambulance will be called to transport a patient who is in need of inpatient care, emergency treatment, or immediate surgery.

PERSPECTIVE AND PROSPECTS

The word "clinic" is derived from the Greek word for bed, *kline*. Evidence exists for the use of herbs and other natural substances for the treatment of medical conditions even in prehistoric times. The provision of health care has been historically linked with religious and spiritual beliefs. In some cases, religious leaders such as shamans or monks were the providers of health care, and illness was attributed to demons or witchcraft.

Ancient Egypt has been credited with having organized houses of medicine, and Herophilos (335-280 B.C.E.) is considered the founder of the medical school in Alexandria, Egypt. The knowledge of human anatomy was very limited, there was no understanding of sterile technique, no understanding of germ theory, and few treatment options were available; however, these early institutions served to further medical knowledge. In the Middle Ages, medical care was provided in monasteries, which in some cases had hospitals attached.

Licensing standards vary across the world, and in some places the provision of health care is still largely unregulated. There are some areas in which the only clinics in existence are provided by volunteer organizations, and in some areas these clinics are in the form of mobile trailers.

The Mayo Clinic is one of the best known multidisciplinary clinics. It was established in the aftermath of a destructive tornado in Rochester, Minnesota, in 1883. William Mayo and his sons Charles and William joined the Sisters of St. Francis to establish a hospital and clinic to care for tornado victims. It grew to be the first and largest nonprofit multispecialty clinic serving more than one-half million patients annually at its three locations.

—*E. E. Anderson Penno, M.D., M.S., FRCSC*

See also Emergency care; Emergency rooms; Hospitals; Nursing; Physician assistants.

FOR FURTHER INFORMATION:

Fauci, Anthony, et al. *Harrison's Principles of Internal Medicine*. 17th ed. New York: McGraw-Hill, 2008. Chapter 1, "The Practice of Medicine," outlines the standards for providing health care in the United States and discusses inpatient care, outpatient care, and different levels of care within hospitals.

Gonzalez-Crussi, F. *A Short History of Medicine*. New York: Modern Library, 2007. A compendium of medical care from ancient times to the early twenty-first century.

Kennedy, Michael. *A Brief History of Disease, Science, and Medicine from the Ice Age to the Genome Project*. Mission Viejo, Calif.: Asklepiad Press, 2004. History of medicine and disease.

CLONING

PROCEDURE

ALSO KNOWN AS: Nuclear transplantation
ANATOMY OR SYSTEM AFFECTED: Cells
SPECIALTIES AND RELATED FIELDS: Biotechnology, embryology, ethics, genetics
DEFINITION: From a scientific perspective, the term "clone" signifies an exact genetic copy of a segment of deoxyribonucleic acid (DNA), cell, or organism. Cloning is a procedure conducted by teams of molecular biologists, geneticists, and embryologists to introduce the genetic information from one cell into another for the purpose of producing a clone.

KEY TERMS:

blastocyst: the stage during early embryonic development, just prior to implantation in the uterus, in which the cells form a large hollow ball; at this point, the cells are undifferentiated

complementary DNA (cDNA): DNA that is made from messenger ribonucleic acid (mRNA) and thus represents the genes actively being expressed in a cell at a given time

eukaryotic: referring to a type of cell that contains a nucleus and membrane-bound organelles; all animal cells are eukaryotic, as are those of plants and fungi

parthenogenesis: the development of an adult from an unfertilized egg

pluripotent: a description for stem cells that have begun differentiation and are capable of forming limited cell types

totipotent: an undifferentiated cell that still retains the ability to form any other cell type of the adult organism; cells of this type are commonly referred to as stem cells

transduction: the incorporation of a piece of DNA into the genome of a bacterium using a virus as a vector

transformation: the incorporation into a cell of cell-free DNA from the environment

transgenic: referring to an organism that contains genetic material from two or more species

vector: a system that is used to carry a fragment of DNA for molecular cloning

Uses and Complications

Scientists use the word "cloning" to indicate an experimental process by which an exact genetic duplicate is made of a molecule, cell, or organism. It is frequently divided into two general categories. Molecular cloning involves copying genes, short segments of DNA, or cells (sometimes also called cellular cloning) for the purpose of producing multiple copies of a molecule or cell for further scientific study. The cloning of DNA is commonly called recombinant DNA technology or genetic engineering. Cloning at the organismal level, also called nuclear transplantation, has been used to create genetically identical organisms and has the potential to produce genetically identical tissues and organs from a donor.

The procedure for molecular cloning involves choosing a vector for the study of the target DNA. The choice of the vector depends on the size of the genetic information being studied and whether it is genomic DNA or complementary DNA (cDNA). Common vectors include plasmids (small circular pieces of bacterial DNA), viruses, and artificial chromosomes. For example, if the length of the DNA being studied is small, then the researcher may choose to insert it into a plasmid. By the process of transformation, the selected plasmid is moved into the bacteria (usually *E. coli*), and as the bacteria divide, cells are produced that are clones for the DNA in the plasmid vector. If the researcher is unsure what area contains the gene to be cloned, then the genome is first fragmented and individual fragments are placed into viruses, or bacteriophages. This creates a library of genetic information. Each bacteriophage vector then infects a bacterium by a process called transduction. The infected bacterium is allowed to divide, producing a colony of bacteria that are clones for the information contained within the bacteriophage vector. These colonies may then be screened using molecular techniques to isolate a colony that contains the desired section of DNA.

If the DNA fragment is larger, as is frequently the case with studies of genomic DNA, then the researcher

may decide to create an artificial chromosome. The purpose is to create a small pseudo-chromosome that is replicated by the host cell prior to cell division. Bacterial artificial chromosomes (BACs) and yeast artificial chromosomes (YACs) are commonly used, but the formation of human artificial chromosomes (HACs) has recently been announced. In all cases, the purpose is to create cells that are genetically identical, or cloned, for a specific stretch of DNA. While this is a useful technique, molecular cloning is not able to produce an entire organism that is genetically identical to the original.

In eukaryotic organisms, the result of sexual reproduction is to produce offspring that contain new combinations of the parents' genomes. While this provides variability to the species, it complicates medical research since it effectively shuffles the genome every generation. Identical, or monozygotic, twins are the closest thing to clones in humans, but between even their cells small genetic differences exist. For scientific studies of development and cell biology, large numbers of cloned cells are needed.

The process of nuclear transplantation, or cloning as it is commonly called, has the ability to create large numbers of genetically identical cells. In theory, cloning is not a difficult process: Simply remove the DNA from the host cell, replace it with the DNA from the donor cell, and encourage the new cell to divide. Procedures such as this have been performed on amphibians since the 1950's, but nuclear transplantation in mammals is slightly more complicated. For example, mammalian egg cells, called oocytes, are vastly smaller than those of amphibians.

Technological advances in microscopy and embryology helped to remedy this problem. In mammalian nuclear transplantation, a researcher, frequently an embryologist, uses a microscope equipped with a micropipette. The micropipette is effectively a microscopic needle that is controlled remotely by the researcher. During the procedure, the egg is held in place by a second pipette to allow for greater control. The researcher then inserts the needle from the first pipette into the oocyte through the zona pellucida (outer covering of the oocyte) and gently removes the genetic material from the cell. At this stage, the oocyte contains only the zona pellucida, cytoplasm, and the internal organelles of the cell, such as the mitochondria. The researcher then inserts a donor cell, complete with DNA, into the area between the oocyte and the zona pellucida. At this point, there are effectively two cells alongside each other—one containing nothing but cytoplasm, the other containing the donor DNA. To form a single cell, the plasma membranes of the two cells must be fused. This is done using a process called electrofusion, in which a small current is applied to the cells, temporarily disrupting the membranes and allowing the cytoplasm of the two cells (and the donor DNA) to mix. The end result is an egg cell than contains the DNA of a second cell.

However, this is not yet technically a clone. To produce a group of cells that are identical to the original donor cell, the oocyte must be persuaded to divide. In some systems, the first cell divisions occur naturally in response to electrofusion, but this is not always the case. Frequently, growth factors or other chemical signals need to be applied to make the cell divide. As the cells divide, they form a blastocyst, in which all cells are clones of one another and the DNA in the original donor cell.

The development of improved technologies in nuclear transplantation has enabled scientists to create organisms that are genetically the same. In the media, the use of the term "clone" usually signifies an organism produced by this procedure. To create a cloned organism, the researcher must insert the blastocyst into the uterus of a surrogate mother, who will carry the organism to term. To do this, scientists have adapted the techniques of in vitro fertilization. During in vitro fertilization, eggs are fertilized by sperm cells in the laboratory and then transferred into the uterus of the female. Cloning does not require the fertilization step, since the blastocyst contains the ball of cloned cells. Theoretically, once implanted, the cloned blastocyst should develop in the same manner as an embryo from a natural fertilization event.

An additional form of cloning is gathering significant attention from the scientific community: therapeutic cloning. The purpose of therapeutic cloning is to generate a large number of stem cells that have been cloned from a donor's DNA for the purpose of treating a disease. The idea is that since embryonic stem cells are totipotent, or have the ability to produce all cell types, then if they are reintroduced into the donor the stem cell theoretically has the ability to take the place of damaged or diseased cells. Only embryonic stem cells are totipotent, however, so the key is to introduce a donor's DNA into an oocyte by nuclear transplantation, allowing it to divide and form a blastocyst. Within the blastocyst forms a group of cells called the inner cell mass (ICM) that contains totipotent stem cells. These cells can then be harvested and grown under laboratory conditions that persuade the cells to develop into new tissues, such as nerves or skin cells.

Recently, researchers have proposed a new technique to generate these stem cells involving parthenogenesis, or the development of an unfertilized egg. Parthenogenesis is common in amphibians and insects, but it does not occur naturally in humans. If a female egg cell could be chemically persuaded to form blastocysts without having to go through the process of nuclear transplantation, then the resulting stem cells could be used to generate new organs or tissues for the female. The process could not be done the same way in males, since sperm cells lack the cytoplasmic components found in egg cells.

INDICATIONS AND PROCEDURES

By definition, the purpose of cloning is to produce genetically identical cells or individuals for scientific studies. Yet even identical, or monozygotic, twins, whose cells are derived from the same fertilized egg, are not truly identical. For example, monozygotic twins do not have the same fingerprint pattern, even though they possess the same genes for ridges on the fingers. The reason for this difference is environmental. For twins, the genes establish a general pattern, but it is the touch of the fingers on the inner wall of the uterus that establishes the final pattern of fingerprints. Environment plays a significant role in the development of the embryo, and this fact has presented a challenge for scientists who wish to produce identical genetic clones.

Dolly, a cloned ewe, was not an exact copy of her donor, even though she possessed the same genetic information as the donor ewe. The reason is that Dolly was raised in the uterus of a surrogate mother and thus was exposed to the minor, but important, environmental variations specific to the surrogate mother. It is known that, by a process called genomic imprinting, the mother can override certain traits in the embryo and impose her own traits, regardless of the genes present in the embryo. The mother also provides all the nutrients needed for the developing embryo, and thus any metabolic problems with the surrogate mother may inhibit proper development in the cloned embryo.

Another problem with nuclear transplantation is that not all the DNA in the cell is located within the nucleus. Mitochondria, the energy factories of a cell, contain small circular pieces of DNA. The genes on this DNA are inherited along with the mother's cytoplasm, so that individuals receive all mitochondrial DNA from the maternal line. During nuclear transplantation, mitochondria are not removed from the host cell, so once transplantation is complete the new cell contains donor DNA but both host cell and donor cell mitochondria. Because mitochondrial genetic disorders exist, it is known that the genes in the mitochondria contribute to the characteristics of the organism.

Cells age and have a finite life span. This appears to be at least partially controlled by the length of the chromosome, specifically the ends of the chromosome called the telomeres. After each cell division, the telomeres shorten like a genetic fuse, until the cell is no longer able to divide. A prime concern among those involved with cloning is whether the cloned cells inherit the telomere length (and thus age) of the donor cell or whether the telomere length is reset in the blastocyst. Claims have been made that support both ideas, and research is ongoing in this area. What is important, however, is the fact that the cloned cell, although totipotent, may not be perfect and may bring with it the genetic flaws of the donor cell.

One of the greatest challenges facing the process of cloning is ethical, which involves the opinion of the general public regarding the cloning of mammals and, potentially, humans. Some consider the cloning of organisms to be an unnatural event, while others question the source of embryonic stem cells. The greatest concern among the general public is the debate on the cloning of humans and the moral right of people to create life by artificial processes. Many of these same debates occurred when in vitro fertilization was introduced. The arguments both for and against human cloning appear to be endless and will continue into the foreseeable future. What should be noted is that the majority of scientists involved in cloning research are interested in either the therapeutic benefits of cell cloning or the study of embryonic development and cell differentiation, not the creation of a cloned human.

Perspective and Prospects

While for many people the history of cloning may appear to have begun in 1996, when Ian Wilmut of the Roslin Institute in Scotland introduced the world to Dolly the cloned ewe, the reality is that the cloning of organisms had been going on for some time. The making of cloned plants had been occurring for decades and now represents a common occurrence in agriculture. If one restricts the discussion to animals, then Dolly does not really even represent the first cloned mammal, but rather the first adult animal cloned from the cells of another adult animal.

The cloning of animals by nuclear transplantation has its roots in the late nineteenth century, when early embryologists were studying cell division in the eggs of invertebrate animals. The first experiments that transferred a nucleus from one cell to another in a vertebrate animal were conducted in the early 1950's by Robert Briggs and Thomas King. Briggs and King worked with nuclear transplantation in amphibians. These researchers were not interested in the creation of a cloned frog but rather the question of nuclear programming, or whether the cells isolated from the blastocyst had the genetic ability to form a new adult frog. These experiments examined the use of embryonic cells to produce a functionally adult organism.

In later experiments, researchers, including Briggs and King, set out to determine at what age of embryonic development cells differentiate to the point where they cannot be used to produce a functioning adult. In essence, they were studying the potency of the cells and beginning to distinguish between totipotent cells and pluripotent cells. For the next several decades, scientists perfected methods of nuclear transplantation in a variety of organisms, including mammals such as mice and rabbits.

In 1996, the researchers at the Roslin Institute used tissue from the mammary gland of an adult ewe in a nuclear transplantation experiment. The result was Dolly, the first mammal to be cloned from an adult cell. Although this experiment was widely reported as producing the first cloned mammal, its real importance was the demonstration that the genes of an adult cell could be expressed in an embryo to produce a living organism. For decades, scientists had debated whether adult cells were capable of being used in cloning. Adult cells are highly specialized, and many of their developmental genes are inactivated. The experiments with Dolly demonstrated that, under the right conditions, the environment within the blastocyst allows DNA from adult cells to be used. In other words, the DNA from differentiated tissue can be used to create undifferentiated stem cells. This remains a major advance in the understanding of cellular processes.

The question may then be asked as to why scientists pursue experiments involving the cloning of organisms. Since public opinion is against the cloning of humans and no immediate need exists to clone an individual, then research in this area would appear to be at an impasse. The reality, however, is that the process of nuclear transplantation and organism cloning gives scientists the ability to answer some important questions about cellular differentiation, especially during embryonic development, and the patterns of expression of genes within cells during development.

Furthermore, while the cloning of humans may not be morally acceptable, cloning can serve society in many other ways, such as in studies using transgenic organisms and in tissue and organ transplantation. Scientific research frequently involves the use of transgenic organisms for study. In the study of human genetics and biochemistry, mice are frequently used as a model system. The ability to study the effects of a particular gene in a transgenic organism is dependent on that organism being genetically pure (homozygous) for that trait. In animals, it can take up to fifteen generations of inbreeding to develop a pure line. For organisms with long gestation periods or a small number of offspring per generation, this becomes both cost- and time-prohibitive. The cloning of new organisms, which are at least genetically the same as the donor, can facilitate research with transgenics.

Organ transplantation in humans is a difficult process. Recipients of organ transplants must be carefully matched with donors for a variety of biochemical factors to ensure that the new organ is not rejected by the recipient's immune system. Even when a match is close, the use of immunosuppressant drugs increases the chances of infection in the recipient. The process of nuclear transplantation may alleviate some of these problems. Rather than being matched with a donor, a patient would contribute genetic material for nuclear transplantation. Stem cells could then be harvested and chemically induced to form the required tissue, or someday even the entire organ. Experiments are currently under way to manufacture skin for burn victims using this type of procedure. The applications of nuclear transplantation are almost endless, and developments in this area of research have the potential to influence directly the lives of the majority of people alive today.

—Michael Windelspecht, Ph.D.;
updated by Jeffrey A. Knight, Ph.D.

See also Assisted reproductive technologies; Cells; Conception; Embryology; Ethics; Fetal tissue transplantation; Gene therapy; Genetic diseases; Genetic engineering; Genetics and inheritance; Genomics; In vitro fertilization; Law and medicine; Multiple births; Pregnancy and gestation; Transplantation.

FOR FURTHER INFORMATION:

Cibelli, Jose, Robert Lanza, Michael West, and Carol Ezzell. "The First Human Cloned Embryo." *Scientific American* 286 (January, 2002): 44-51. Discusses the process by which clones are generated for therapeutic purposes, as well as a new strategy for producing cloned cells using only unfertilized eggs. Illustrations of cloning procedures are included.

McKinnell, Robert, and Marie Di Berardino. "The Biology of Cloning: History and Rationale." *Bioscience* 49 (November, 1999): 875-885. Reviews the history of cloning from the nineteenth century onward, including the scientific experiments that led to the cloning of amphibians and the advances in mammalian cloning.

National Institutes of Health. Department of Health and Human Services. *Regenerative Medicine 2006.* Bethesda, Md.: NIH Press, 2006. A collection of articles describing advances in stem cell and cloning technologies since this resource was first published in 2001.

Nussbaum, Martha, and Cass Sunstein, eds. *Clones and Clones: Facts and Fantasies About Human Cloning.* New York: W. W. Norton, 1999. A series of contributed essays on all aspects of human cloning, including science, ethics, and legal issues.

Pasternak, Jack J. *An Introduction to Human Molecular Genetics.* 2d ed. Hoboken, N.J.: Wiley-Liss, 2005. An excellent primer on many technologies as applied to humans, including genetic engineering, stem cell research, cloning, and gene therapy.

Wilmut, Ian, Keith Campbell, and Colin Tudge. *The Second Creation: Dolly and the Age of Biological Control.* New York: Farrar, Straus and Giroux, 2000. Coauthored by one of the creators of Dolly, this book examines the process of cloning and the steps that led to the cloning of the first mammal. It also provides insight into the reason that Dolly was cloned.

CLOSTRIDIUM DIFFICILE INFECTION
DISEASE/DISORDER

ALSO KNOWN AS: *C. difficile* disease, *C. difficile*-associated infection, *C. diff.*

ANATOMY OR SYSTEM AFFECTED: Gastrointestinal system

SPECIALTIES AND RELATED FIELDS: Family medicine, gastroenterology, infectious diseases

DEFINITION: An acute, contagious gastrointestinal infection caused by the anaerobic, gram-positive, spore-forming bacillus, *Clostridium difficile.*

CAUSES AND SYMPTOMS

The bacteria *Clostridium difficile* that cause *C. difficile* infection are transmitted through the fecal-oral route. These bacteria are shed from feces of a colonized or infected person. When shed, they form spores as a protective mechanism when they enter the environment. They are able to survive in this form for many months on environmental surfaces. *C. difficile* infection is spread through contact with an infected or colonized patient, the environment, or the contaminated hands of a health care worker. The incubation period of *C. difficile* is unknown; however, one study suggests that it might be less than seven days.

The major risk factors for *C. difficile* infection include advanced age, hospitalization, and antibiotic use. Nearly every antibiotic has been implicated in *C. difficile* infection but clindamycin, cephalosporins, and floroquinolones are associated with a higher risk. When a patient receiving antibiotics ingests *C. difficile* spores, they germinate in the small intestine, where the normal flora has been altered. The spores multiply, flourish, and produce toxins. The toxins, toxin A and B, cause inflammation and mucosal damage leading to colitis. In severe infection, *C. difficile* can cause toxic megacolon, septic shock, and death.

When a patient becomes infected with *C. difficile*, fever, abdominal pain or tenderness, anorexia, nausea, and watery diarrhea commonly occur. In severe infection, the patient may develop pseudomembranous colitis, which may progress to toxic megacolon, a toxic dilation of the colon. If the patient develops toxic megacolon, then sepsis and death may quickly follow.

TREATMENT AND THERAPY

Some cases may resolve in two to three days after discontinuing current antibiotic use. However in most cases a ten-day course of metronidazole or vancomycin orally is effective. Surgical intervention may be necessary in severe *C. difficile* infection if pseudomembranous colitis or perforation develop.

PERSPECTIVE AND PROSPECTS

Before the mid 1970's, pseudomembranous colitis, an inflammatory process in the colon caused by bacterial toxins, was associated with the use of certain antibiotics; mainly lincomycin and clindamycin. It was not until 1978 that *C. difficile* was identified as the causative agent of antibiotic-associated pseudomembranous colitis. Since that time, *C. difficile* has become the leading cause of antibiotic-associated diarrhea. The incidence

---

> ## INFORMATION ON *CLOSTRIDIUM DIFFICILE* INFECTIONS
>
> **CAUSES:** Bacterial infection
> **SYMPTOMS:** Fever, abdominal pain or tenderness, anorexia, nausea, watery diarrhea
> **DURATION:** Acute
> **TREATMENTS:** Antibiotics, sometimes IV fluids to prevent dehydration

---

of *C. difficile* infection in discharged patients has doubled over the last several years. Moreover, a hyper-virulent strain called BI/NAP1/027 has emerged. This strain produces a type of toxin not previously seen in other strains; it is also highly resistant to the fluoroquinolone antibiotics.

—*Collette Bishop Hendler, R.N., M.S., C.I.C.*

See also Antibiotics; Bacterial infections; Bacteriology; Drug resistance; Emerging infectious diseases; Hospitals.

FOR FURTHER INFORMATION:

Carrico, Ruth, et al. *Guide to the Elimination of "Clostridium difficile" in Healthcare Settings*. Washington, D.C.: APIC, 2008.

"*Clostridium difficile:* Information for Healthcare Providers." http://www.cdc.gov/ncidod/dhqp/id_Cdiff FAQ_HCP.html.

Professional Guide to Diseases. 9th ed. Ambler, Pa.: Lippincott Williams & Wilkins, 2008.

CLUB DRUGS

DISEASE/DISORDER

ALSO KNOWN AS: Designer drugs, psychedelics

ANATOMY OR SYSTEM AFFECTED: All

SPECIALTIES AND RELATED FIELDS: Alternative medicine, critical care, emergency medicine, pharmacology, preventive medicine, psychiatry, psychology, public health, toxicology

DEFINITION: A slang term for a variety of substances of abuse that generally are used in social situations, have hallucinogenic properties, and may either excite or sedate the user.

KEY TERMS:

amnesia: a diverse condition where there is complete or partial loss of memory for specific periods of time, for specific types of information, or both

blackout: memory loss, usually as a result of taking substances known to disrupt memory, in which the affected person may function as if aware of what is happening, despite having no memory of activities

psychedelic drugs: substances that cause alterations in perception and thinking, such as changes in awareness or sense of self and hallucinations

raves: social gatherings that are distinguished by long periods of music, dancing, and often a percentage of individuals using psychedelic drugs and other substances of abuse

synergistic effects: the combined effects of drugs interacting with one another, such that the effects of the drugs together have a compounded effect, greater than that of any one alone

CAUSES AND SYMPTOMS

Less expensive, easily accessible, intoxicating drugs can often be attractive to persons wanting a momentary high or psychedelic experience, when they are at a rave, dance party, or bar with friends. This desire, combined with a belief that club drugs seem safe, leads people to trying club drugs and sometimes using them regularly. Club drugs are often first used in dance clubs or with friends. The belief that such drugs are natural forms of prescription drugs or are not necessarily always illegal fuels a misconception of their safety. Because these drugs are psychedelic, the reactions that individual users have can vary quite significantly depending on the user's emotional state, concurrent use of other substances, underlying psychiatric conditions, personality, and past experience with the drug. Additionally, as they are street drugs, usually subject to some variability in their contents (such as being mixed with less expensive drugs), their quality may vary substantially. Finally, the individual situations where the substances are used can pose a variety of dangers of varying levels.

Club drugs go by many different names. They include substances such as gamma-hydroxybutyrate (GHB, Georgia Home Boy, Liquid X), ketamine hydrochloride (ketamine, special K), lysergic acid diethylamid (LSD, acid, blotter), methylenedioxymethamphetamine (MDMA, Adam, ecstasy, X), and rohypnol (roofies, roach, roche). They also include herbal ecstasy (herbal X, cloud nine, herbal bliss), which is a drug made from ephedrine or pseudoephedrine and caffeine. These substances vary in their effects but as a group cause a variety of positive reactions, including euphoria, feelings of well-being, emotional clarity, a decreased sense of personal boundaries, and feelings of empathy and closeness to others. They also can cause, however, significant negative reactions, including panic,

impaired judgment, amnesia, impaired motor control, insomnia, paranoia, irrational behavior, flashbacks, hallucinations, rapid heartbeat, high blood pressure, chills, sweating, tremors, respiratory distress, convulsions, and violence. It is not uncommon for individuals to mix these drugs with alcohol, prescription drugs, and illegal drugs. Taken in combination, these substances can make these very dangerous reactions even worse.

TREATMENT AND THERAPY

The effects of club drugs vary somewhat by substance; as such, treatment also varies by substance. In general, though, club drugs may tend to be seen more in emergency care settings than in primary health care settings. This is due to the fact that some of the problems that they cause, as a group, are often of an emergency nature. For instance, overdose, strokes, allergic shock reactions, blackouts, loss of consciousness, and accidents related to these conditions may require emergency care. Similarly, dehydration and heat exhaustion can result from prolonged periods of dancing or other physical exertion, as can occur in rave situations, and result in a need for emergency care. Finally, because date rapes have been known to occur with these drugs, particularly rohypnol, injuries due to sexual assault also may need attention.

Certainly the long-term impact of problems like those described above may require some type of psychotherapy. In addition, problems related to the abuse of or dependence upon club drugs would be addressed in much the same manner as for other substances of abuse. General addiction treatment would be advised. A special area of treatment may also include exploration of what it is like to deal with blackouts, amnesia, and flashbacks, as these are features that are commonly reported with psychedelic drugs.

PERSPECTIVE AND PROSPECTS

Club drugs emphasize that there is a continuing need for the social awareness of the dangers of substances that may otherwise seem harmless. Just because a substance is not listed as an illegal drug does not mean that it cannot be dangerous. Any drug, whether sold over the counter, by prescription, or any other place, can be misused and can be dangerous. Where drugs are used, how much is used, with whom they are used, and with what they are used can all make a difference.

Club drugs are also a reminder that in efforts to find ways of joining with each other, finding community, and discovering themselves and their relationships, people will sometimes resort to experimenting with substances. While the experimental use of psychedelic substances for psychotherapeutic work continues and may prove beneficial to certain groups of patients, such work is balanced by investigations into neurology, physiology, psychopharmacology, and psychology to ensure that the benefits do not outweigh the risks. Continued exploration of the neuronal, developmental, social, and other health effects of using club drugs is likely, as they pose a significant danger to public health, particularly that of younger populations.

—*Nancy A. Piotrowski, Ph.D.*

See also Addiction; Amnesia; Emergency medicine; Hallucinations; Herbal medicine; Intoxication; Marijuana; Panic attacks; Paranoia; Pharmacology; Seizures; Substance abuse; Tremors.

FOR FURTHER INFORMATION:

Holland, Julie, comp. *Ecstasy: The Complete Guide—A Comprehensive Look at the Risks and Benefits of MDMA.* Rochester, Vt.: Inner Traditions International, 2001.

Jansen, Karl. *Ketamine: Dreams and Realities.* Ben Lomond, Calif.: Multidisciplinary Association for Psychedelic Studies, 2004.

Kuhn, Cynthia, et al. *Buzzed: The Straight Facts About the Most Used and Abused Drugs from Alcohol to Ecstasy.* 3d ed. New York: W. W. Norton, 2008.

O'Neill, John, and Pat O'Neill. *Concerned Intervention: When Your Loved One Won't Quit Alcohol or Drugs.* Oakland, Calif.: New Harbinger, 2003.

Stafford, Peter. *Psychedelics.* Berkeley, Calif.: Ronin, 2003.

CLUSTER HEADACHES

DISEASE/DISORDER

ANATOMY OR SYSTEM AFFECTED: Blood vessels, brain, head, nerves, nervous system

SPECIALTIES AND RELATED FIELDS: Neurology

DEFINITION: The most severe headache syndrome, characterized by paroxysmal onset of one side of the head, short duration, and episodic occurrence. Cluster headaches are often confused with migraine headaches, which are a similar syndrome but with different causes, patterns, and treatments.

KEY TERMS:

alarm clock headaches: an earlier term for cluster headaches, emphasizing the characteristic awakening of sufferers during the night

circadian rhythm: the biological clockwise regularity associated with many body processes; most suffer-

ers of cluster headaches have attacks at the same time of day during the same season of the year

cluster period: a time period, from two weeks to four months, during which cluster headaches occur; they usually disappear, or "enter remission," after the cluster period ends

paroxysmal: having a sudden, spasmlike, and painful onset

trigeminal-autonomic reflex pathway: the nerve pathway at the base of the brain activated during cluster attacks; the trigeminal nerve, the most important facial nerve for sensations such as temperature and pain, causes the "hot-poker-in-the-eye" pain typical of cluster headaches

unilateral: occurring only on one side (for example, on one side of the head or behind one eye)

CAUSES AND SYMPTOMS

Cluster headache is a well-defined, rare, but often misdiagnosed syndrome characterized by excruciatingly severe unilateral headaches that last from a half hour to three hours, with an average duration of forty-five minutes. Its features include paroxysmal onset of one side of the head, a short duration, and episodic occurrence. The pain often wakes sufferers one to two hours after they fall asleep. "Cluster" refers to the original perception that the headaches emerged in groups over a period of time (called the cluster period) lasting weeks to months, followed by periods that are free of pain and attacks (called remission or interim periods). The International Headache Society divides cluster headaches into episodic cluster and chronic cluster, with chronic further subclassified into primary and secondary variants. Chronic cluster headaches do not have a cessation, or interim, period but recur for years.

The precise cause of cluster headaches is unknown, although the season of the year is the most common trigger. Because they usually begin with spring or autumn, cluster headaches are often misattributed to seasonal allergies (such as hay fever) or seasonal-related stress (such as the beginning of school, final examinations, or the height of business cycles).

Positron emission tomography (PET) scanning has revealed that in cluster headaches the hypothalamus activates the trigeminal nerve, which is responsible for most of the severe pain. Located deep in the brain, the hypothalamus is also responsible for the internal biological clock that regulates the approximately twenty-four-hour sleep-wake cycle. The production and activity of the neurotransmitter serotonin, which is important in

INFORMATION ON CLUSTER HEADACHES

CAUSES: Unknown; may be seasonal

SYMPTOMS: Sudden headache on one side of head, with intense pain behind one eye often spreading to teeth, jaw, neck, or temple; occasionally preceded by visual aura

DURATION: Recurrent, with acute episodes occurring one to six times a day and lasting a half hour to three hours each during cluster periods

TREATMENTS: For symptom alleviation, oxygen therapy, injections of sumatriptan or dihydroergotamine, zolmitriptan tablets, intranasal lidocane, ergotamine; for prevention, verapamil, ergotamine, lithium, methysergide, prednisone, valproic acid, divalproex

the self-regulation of these circadian rhythms, is also altered during attacks. Cluster headache is not related to the development of tumors or lesions.

Cluster headaches are rare. No more than .03 percent of the population ever experiences them. Men suffer them more than women do, although with improvements in epidemiological techniques the known ratio has been changed from 7:1 to 2:1. The age of onset is usually in the late twenties. As with migraine headaches, cluster headaches tend to run in families, with a fourteenfold increase in the chances of having them if a first-degree relative (mother, father, son, daughter, brother, or sister) suffers from the syndrome. In addition, a statistically significant incidence of migraine headaches exists in families with a cluster headache sufferer.

Cluster headache attacks, which are excruciatingly severe, debilitating, and dramatic, are almost always unilateral and occur from one to six times a day. They are most intense in, around, or behind one eye. Because the pain, commonly described as "boring" or "stabbing," often spreads into the upper teeth, jaw, neck, or temple, the headaches can be misdiagnosed as coming from dental or sinus problems. The attacks are rapid, peaking in five to ten minutes, and are occasionally, but not frequently, preceded by a visual aura. Attacks are much more likely to occur if tobacco and/or alcohol have been recently used, and they even more frequently will awaken sufferers during their first hour of napping or sleeping.

While migraine headache sufferers seek quiet, darkened places and try to remain still, cluster headache suf-ferers feel more pain if they try to lie down or recline in a chair. Typically, cluster headache sufferers are restless, pacing back and forth, or want to sit upright, holding their heads with their hands. A sufferer may even bang his or her head against a wall to obtain relief.

TREATMENT AND THERAPY

Treatments are oriented either toward abortive therapies or prophylactic therapies. Abortive approaches attempt to shorten the duration and/or intensity of an individual attack. Prophylactic approaches attempt to shorten or prevent the cluster periods themselves. While a fortunate characteristic of the attacks is their brevity, this feature also limits the range of abortive measures that can be undertaken; by the time that some agents are metabolized, the attack is over.

Although not always practical, a successful and safe abortive treatment is simply breathing 100 percent oxygen for ten to twenty minutes through a nonrebreathing mask. Also not always practical but effective are subcutaneous injections of sumatriptan (Imitrex) or intravenous, intramuscular, or subcutaneous injections of dihydroergotamine (Migranal). Other effective first-line therapies for acute intervention include zolmitriptan (Zomig) tablets, intranasal lidocane, or ergotamine (Cafergot).

Prophylactic, or preventive, treatments prevent attacks or at least lessen their intensity. All cluster headache sufferers should be on a prophylactic regimen (unless their cluster periods are less than two weeks, which is rarely the case). Verapamil (marketed as Calan, Covera, Isoptin, Tarka, and Verelan) is the most commonly prescribed medication because its mechanism as a calcium-channel blocker is well understood and it is usually effective. Occasionally, higher-than-typical doses must be employed. For those who do not respond well or receive sufficient relief on verapamil alone, a second medication such as ergotamine, lithium, methysergide (Sansert), or prednisone is often added. Sometimes, these second medications are effectively used alone, as are valproic acid and divalproex (Depakote).

In the event that pharmacology proves ineffective, several surgical or radiation techniques can block the trigeminal-autonomic reflex pathway. The benefits of these, or any, invasive treatments must be weighed against potential harm. For example, corneal anesthesia, needed to carry out these procedures, can put the eye at risk.

PERSPECTIVE AND PROSPECTS

People have suffered from cluster headaches as long as people have suffered from headaches, although the rarity, seasonal occurrence, and symptoms of cluster headaches have made their recognition as a distinct syndrome difficult. Through PET scanning, neurovascular research has identified three areas of the brain particularly affected by cluster headaches. Because two of these areas are affected every time any sort of pain is felt, research is being concentrated on the third area, hypothalamic gray matter. Researchers expect that probes here will resolve their biggest debate: Is the vasodilation associated with cluster headache the primary problem or the result of activation of the trigeminal vascular system? Researchers do agree that cluster headaches, while distinct, belong to a family of related conditions, the cranial neuralgias.

—*Paul Moglia, Ph.D.*

See also Brain; Brain disorders; Head and neck disorders; Headaches; Migraine headaches; Pain; Pain management; Stress.

FOR FURTHER INFORMATION:

Dalessio, Donald J. "Relief of Cluster Headache and Cranial Neuralgias." *Postgraduate Medicine* 109, no. 1 (January, 2001): 69-78.

Kudrow, L. "Cluster Headache: Diagnosis and Management." *Headache* 19 (1979): 141-148.

Newman, Lawrence C., Peter Goadsby, and Richard B. Lipton. "Cluster and Related Headaches." In *Headache*, edited by Ninan T. Mathew. Philadelphia: W. B. Saunders, 2001.

COCCIDIOIDOMYCOSIS

DISEASE/DISORDER

ALSO KNOWN AS: San Joaquin Valley fever, valley fever

ANATOMY OR SYSTEM AFFECTED: All

SPECIALTIES AND RELATED FIELDS: Dermatology, family medicine, general surgery, internal medicine, microbiology, pulmonary medicine

DEFINITION: A fungal infection acquired by inhaling the spores of particular soil-based fungi. It initially attacks the lungs and often resolves without causing symptoms, but it can cause pneumonia and disseminate throughout the body.

KEY TERMS:

arthroconidia: asexual fungal spores that are made by the segmentation of preexisting fungal hyphae

endospores: tiny, round cells produced by spherules as

they divide into smaller and smaller cells that are released upon rupture

erythema nodosum: inflammation of the fatty layer of the skin that results in red, painful bumps, usually located on the front of the legs

hyphae: the long, filamentous, often branching cells of many fungi

mycelium: a body of the fungal organism that consists of a collection of hyphae

mycetoma: a progressive and chronic fungal or bacterial infection that causes overgrowth of the infected tissue and the formation of sinuses filled with the infecting organism

pulmonary nodules: small, round growths on the lung that contain either trapped microorganisms or cancer cells

spherules: a thick-walled, spherical structure that is the tissue-specific form of *Coccidioides* species

CAUSES AND SYMPTOMS

Coccidioidomycosis is an infection caused by the soil-based fungi *Coccidioides immitis* (*C. immitis*) and *Coccidioides posadasii* (*C. posadasii*). These fungi are found only in the Western hemisphere, and they prefer dry, alkaline soils. *C. immitis* and *C. posadasii* are endemic to the Southwestern United States (south-central California, Nevada, Arizona, New Mexico, and western Texas), those regions of Mexico that border the western United States, parts of Central America (Guatemala, Honduras, and Nicaragua), and the desert regions of South America (Argentina, Paraguay, and Venezuela).

While in the soil, *Coccidioides*, like most fungi, grows as thin, branching filaments called hyphae. A collection of hyphae is called a mycelium. When it rains, the mycelium grows quite rapidly, but once the soil dries out, it forms resting cells called arthrospores. If disturbed by wind, earthquakes, or soil excavation, these arthrospores become airborne and, if inhaled, can cause coccidioidomycosis.

Once inhaled, the arthrospore transforms into a thick-walled, spherical structure called a spherule that divides itself into hundreds of small endospores. When the spherule ruptures, it releases the endospores, which grow into spherules that form more endospores.

About 60 percent of patients show no symptoms, and the disease resolves spontaneously. Those patients who show symptoms suffer from fever, sore throat, headache, cough, fatigue, painful bumps on the skin (erythema nodosum), and chest pain approximately one to three weeks after inhaling arthrospores. About 95 percent of symptomatic patients recover without further problems after several weeks. If symptoms persist beyond three months, however, then the patient has chronic progressive coccidioidal pneumonia. Between 5 and 7 percent of those patients with coccidioidal pneumonia form pulmonary nodules, which are areas of the lung where the immune system has walled-off the organism from the rest of the lung. On an X ray, these nodules can look exactly like cancerous masses in the lung. A biopsy is often necessary to distinguish between lung cancer and coccidioidal pulmonary nodules. In 5 percent of patients with coccidioidal pulmonary nodules, the nodules enlarge to form pulmonary cavities that can become infected, rupture, and bleed, causing the release of pus between the lungs and the ribs (empyema). Small cavities (less than 2.5 centimeters) can heal after one to two years, but larger cavities can persist and cause the patient to spit up blood (hemoptysis) and allow the growth of fungi throughout the cavity (mycetoma).

A minority of patients develop disseminated coccidioidomycosis, in which the organism penetrates blood vessels, invades the bloodstream, and infects any organ in the body. Disseminated coccidioidomycosis occurs weeks or months after the primary pneumonia and can even develop in cases where there is no previous evidence of respiratory disease. Particular ethnic groups such as Filipinos and African Americans show increased risk of developing disseminated disease, as do pregnant women in the third trimester of their pregnancy, infants younger than one year old, diabetics, patients with acquired immunodeficiency syndrome (AIDS), or those taking drugs or suffering from diseases that suppress the immune system.

TREATMENT AND THERAPY
Asymptomatic or symptomatic infections are usually self-limited and require little more than supportive care. Patients with coccidioidal pneumonia require fluconazole or itraconazole treatment for at least twelve months and intravenous amphotericin B for stubborn cases. Pulmonary nodules are typically not treated, but they may require surgery. Pulmonary cavities are only treated with antifungal drugs if the patient shows symptoms. Surgical removal might also be warranted if the infection resists treatment. Disseminated coccidioidomycosis requires higher doses of fluconazole, and very sick patients may require amphotericin B or a combination of fluconazole and amphotericin B.

INFORMATION OF COCCIDIOIDOMYCOSIS

CAUSES: Fungal infection
SYMPTOMS: Chest pains, chills, cough, fever, headache, spitting up blood, loss of appetite, muscle aches and stiffness, night sweats, rash, light sensitivity, excessive sweating, weight loss, wheezing
DURATION: Up to three months or more
TREATMENTS: Antifungal drugs

Amphotericin B is preferred for pregnant women, since other drugs harm the developing fetus.

PERSPECTIVE AND PROSPECTS
Coccidioidomycosis was first described in 1892 by Roberto Johann Wernicke and Alejandro Posadas in South America. The first case in the United States was reported in California in 1894. Two years later, Emmet Rixford and Thomas Caspar Gilchrist reported several clinical infections that were caused by an organism that, they thought, resembled the protozoan *Coccidia*. Therefore they named it *Coccidioides*, which means "*Coccidia*-like." In 1905, William Ophüls described the fungal life cycle and pathology of *C. immitis*. Charles E. Smith studied the epidemiology of coccidioidomycosis in the San Joaquin Valley of California and went on to develop the coccidioidin skin test and serological testing for the disease.

New treatments under investigation for coccidioidomycosis include posaconazole, voriconazole, caspofungin, and a new lipid-dispersal formulation of amphotericin B that reduces its kidney toxicity. Nikkomycin A is another experimental agent that is very active against *Coccidioides* in culture and infected animals.
—*Michael A. Buratovich, Ph.D.*

See also Acquired immunodeficiency syndrome (AIDS); Aspergillosis; Candidiasis; Environmental diseases; Environmental health; Fungal infections; Immune system; Immunodeficiency disorders; Immunology; Immunopathology; Lungs; Microbiology; Mold and mildew; Pneumonia; Pulmonary diseases; Pulmonary medicine; Respiration.

FOR FURTHER INFORMATION:
Anstead, Gregory M., and John R. Graybill. "Coccidioidomycosis." *Infectious Disease Clinics of North America* 20, no. 3 (September, 2006): 621-643.

Galgiani, John N. "Changing Perceptions and Creating Opportunities for Its Control." *Annals of the New York Academy of Sciences* 1111 (September, 2007): 1-18.

Kwon-Chung, K. J., and John E. Bennett. *Medical Mycology.* Philadelphia: Lea and Febiger, 1992.

Parish, James, M., and James E. Blair. "Coccidioidomycosis." *Mayo Clinic Proceedings* 83, no. 3 (March, 2008): 343-348.

COGNITIVE DEVELOPMENT

DEVELOPMENT

ANATOMY OR SYSTEM AFFECTED: Brain, nervous system, psychic-emotional system

SPECIALTIES AND RELATED FIELDS: Environmental health, genetics, pediatrics, psychology

DEFINITION: The growth and age-related changes that occur over time in children's mental processes and in activities related to the faculties of attending, learning, perceiving, problem solving, thinking, and remembering.

KEY TERMS:

adaptation: change or adjustment made to create a balance between existing thought structures and the environment

assimilation: the process of attempting to explain a new experience in terms of existing schemes

cognition: the activity of knowing and the processes through which knowledge is acquired and used

cognitive equilibrium: a term used by psychologist Jean Piaget to describe the balanced relationship between an individual's mental processes and the environment

conservation: understanding that an object's properties remain unchanged when its appearance is altered

egocentrism: seeing the world only from one's own point of view; being unable to acknowledge or recognize different perspectives

equilibration: the process of adapting or adjusting one's existing knowledge or mental structures to the new situation, thus constructing more complex and sophisticated structures

miseducation: the tendency to hurry and pressure children to perform activities and tasks for which they are not cognitively or physically ready

reflexive: referring to an automatic response to external stimuli

reversibility: the ability to negate an action by mentally reversing it or imagining its opposite

scheme: a pattern of thought constructed by the child to organize experience in a meaningful way

PHYSICAL AND PSYCHOLOGICAL FACTORS

The mental capabilities and skills of humans develop gradually over a period of time during childhood and adolescence. The quality of the processes by which an individual responds to and adapts thinking to particular situations and evaluates, plans, and solves problems also changes over time.

In childhood, the brain develops very rapidly. At birth, the human brain already weighs about 25 percent of its adult weight. By six months of age, this figure is 50 percent. By the age of five, the child's brain has achieved 90 percent of its eventual weight. While the basic structure of the brain is genetically and biologically determined, environment and experience play a significant role in the growth of cognition. Children's biological constitutions may affect the way in which they interact with and respond to their environment.

According to the Swiss psychologist Jean Piaget, the cognitive growth of all children follows a universal or holistic pattern of development through infancy, childhood, and adolescence. The thought processes of young children are less mature and complex than those of older children, and as children grow and experience life, their cognitive structures become more sophisticated, as well as qualitatively different from those of children in earlier or later stages of development. Cognitive structures, or "schemes" as Piaget called them, are thought patterns that children construct to explain, understand, or interpret their experiences. When children's schemes or thought processes are in harmony with their environment, they experience cognitive equilibrium. When children encounter new and puzzling events or objects, they are in a state of imbalance or disequilibrium and must achieve equilibrium via a process called equilibration. This process consists of adapting or adjusting one's existing knowledge or mental structures to the new situation, thus constructing more complex and sophisticated structures. Adaptation takes place through the processes of assimilation and accommodation.

Assimilation refers to the process of attempting to explain a new experience in terms of existing schemes. For example, a child who sees a pony for the first time may call it a "kitty" because a cat is the existing model of that child for four-legged animals. Noticing that there are differences between the scheme of a cat and the reality of the pony, however, the child soon attempts to modify existing mental structures to fit the new experience. This process of modification is accommodation. Through assimilation and accommodation, children organize their knowledge into schemes which better explain their world.

Piaget's theory of cognitive development, with its emphasis on continuous and active organization and adaptation involving assimilation and accommodation, implies that children actively construct their own knowledge. This construction is based on the child's current stage of cognitive development: Piaget proposed that all children in a specific, universal cognitive stage construct similar interpretations of similar experiences.

According to Piaget, cognitive development can be divided into four major stages. The order in which these stages occur is universal, and all individuals must experience each stage. No stage can be skipped, although the rates at which children go through a stage may vary. The basis for Piaget's insistence on the unvarying sequence of cognitive stages is a concept known as epigenesis, which he used to explain the gradual development of thinking processes. Each new structure or cognitive skill is based on and develops from an earlier one. Hence, each stage, and each structure within each stage, is necessary for the development of new, more advanced structures. Piaget called this feature of development "hierarchization."

The four stages of cognitive development identified by Piaget are the sensorimotor stage (up to age two), the preoperational stage (two to seven years of age), the concrete operations stage (seven to eleven years of age), and the formal operations stage (age eleven and up).

During the sensorimotor stage, children act upon their environment and acquire knowledge of it through their senses and motor activities. In the first two years, cognition progresses from reflexive actions, such as sucking and grasping, to primitive symbolic functions or representation, such as language use and symbolic play. The sensorimotor stage can be further divided into six substages. Substage 1 lasts from birth to one month and centers on exercising basic reflexes, including eye movements, sound orientation, and vocalization, and assimilating and accommodating objects into reflexive schemes. Substage 2, from one to four months, consists of simple repetitive actions, such as thumb sucking, which are discovered by chance and acquired through repeated trials. Piaget called these actions primary circular reactions. Substage 3 appears between four and eight months of age. Piaget named this period secondary circular reactions. Infants notice stimulating events in the environment beyond their bodies—such as a noise made by squeezing a toy or a movement caused by touching an object—and attempt to re-create the events.

Between eight and twelve months of age, infants experience substage 4, or the coordination of secondary schemes. This means that infants can use two already acquired schemes to reach a simple goal. For example, they are able to remove an object to grasp a hidden toy. These early coordinations reflect intentional behavior and simple problem solving. Tertiary circular reactions are characteristic of substage 5, appearing between the ages of twelve and eighteen months. Infants display curiosity, experiment actively, and find new ways of solving problems. Their behaviors are goal-directed but are carried out through trial and error. Substage 6, from eighteen to twenty-four months, reflects inner experimentation or new mental combinations. The infant now displays symbolic functioning through language, imagery, and symbolic play. Children also begin to acquire a sense of cause and effect.

During the sensorimotor stage, children develop the ability to imitate. Piaget believed that novel actions could be imitated by infants around eight to twelve months of age and needed much practice. The ability to imitate absent models, called deferred imitation, appears between twelve and twenty-four months of age.

Another important milestone of the sensorimotor stage is the development of a sense of object permanence. Before the age of four months, objects are of interest to infants only if they can be experienced by the senses. They lose interest in objects that are hidden; such objects no longer exist for them. Between four and eight months of age, they may retain interest in partially hidden objects, and by twelve to eighteen months of age, the concept of objects is stronger. The idea that objects have permanence even when not seen appears around the age of eighteen months, when children can represent objects mentally.

The preoperational stage, the second of Piaget's stages of cognitive development, occurs between the ages of two and seven. During this stage, children increase their use of words and images to represent objects and experiences. Piaget called this stage "preoperational" because he believed that children had not yet achieved "operations," or cognitive schemes to think logically. The preoperational stage can further be divided into a preconceptual period (two to four years of age) and an intuitive period (four to seven years of age).

Characteristics of the preconceptual period include growth of symbolic representation, expressed through developing language and pretend play. Children in this stage demonstrate animism; that is, they attribute life to nonliving things. They are egocentric, seeing the world as revolving around themselves and having difficulty in seeing other points of view.

Although still egocentric during the intuitive period, children are less so than before. Piaget argued that they also display centered thinking, or the capacity to classify objects according to one feature or attribute even though several may be evident. Children in this stage find it hard to conserve, or understand that a substance or object's properties can remain unaltered even when its appearance changes. They cannot reverse actions mentally, such as realizing that water poured from a tall glass into a flat dish is the same amount of water and would look as high as before if poured back into the glass.

In the concrete operations stage, between the ages of seven and eleven, children's cognitive structures develop to include operations that help them think more competently and logically about objects and events experienced. Children are less egocentric; are able to classify, sequence, and quantify more efficiently; and display skills of conservation and reversibility. Piaget believed, however, that children are still unable to hypothesize or think about abstract concepts during this stage.

From eleven years onward, children enter the formal operations stage. They can hypothesize and reason inductively about abstract concepts such as religion, goodness, or beauty. According to Piaget, this transition from concrete to formal operations is very gradual. He also suggested that many adults reason at the formal operations level only if a problem is important or interesting to them.

Another approach to cognitive development compares individuals as information-processing systems to computers. The hardware in this system consists of physical components such as the brain, the sensory receptors, and the nervous system. The software consists of the mental processes and strategies used to store, interpret, access, and analyze information. The information-processing mechanisms of young children are elementary and immature. As children grow, as their nervous systems and brains develop, their information-processing strategies improve and become more sophisticated, like modern computers.

Humor and the appreciation of humor have also been associated with an individual's level of cognitive development. A child whose mental structures and language acquisition have developed enough to enable the child to notice incongruities or deviations from the usual and expected can perceive humor in incongruous situations. To a two-year-old, calling a bird a cat may seem hilarious or making barking sounds and pretending to be a dog may provoke much laughter. A picture of a fish in a tree will amuse a three-year-old. Seven-year-olds who can understand the double meanings inherent in language will laugh at puns and "knock-knock" jokes and can create riddles. As children's understanding of language ambiguities matures and becomes more sophisticated, they are able to appreciate more complex humor.

SOCIOCULTURAL FACTORS

The Russian psychologist Lev Vygotsky believed that cognition is sociocultural, that it is influenced by values and beliefs of cultures as well as by the specific tools that each culture uses for adaptation and problem solving. Children are born with simple mental processes like attention, memory, perception, and sensation. These processes develop into what Vygotsky called higher mental functions, or more competent ways of using intellectual capabilities. The strategies and tools for thinking are taught to children by their culture and develop as young children interact and collaborate with capable adults or peers, who guide and model problem-solving techniques that encourage cognitive development. Vygotsky called the difference between children's level of achievement when working independently and their potential development when guided by a competent adult the zone of proximal development.

For Vygotsky, language plays an important role in cognitive growth. Adults use language to transmit the culture's ways of thinking to the child. The child uses language to plan and regulate activities and behavior and to solve problems. Language helps children organize thought and reach objectives. Younger children verbalize phrases and words aloud during this process, but older children and adults internalize speech that, although no longer uttered aloud, still organizes and guides thinking and action.

DISORDERS AND EFFECTS

The importance of experience on the cognitive development of children implies that when children live in intellectually impoverished environments, their cognitive development may be stunted or fail to reach its potential. Studies show the children whose parents play and interact in a variety of ways with them and provide stimulating materials to engage their interest and attention do better in school than children who lack this cognitive stimulation. Verbal interactions between parents and children, collaborative activities with competent peers, and guided activities with adults have been found to help children improve their thinking and planning abilities. Mary Ainsworth's research on mother-infant attachment showed that mothers who interacted with their infants had securely attached children who, in turn, felt confident enough to explore their environment more independently than less securely attached infants. In this way, cognitive growth was affected by social functioning. Some longitudinal studies have found that securely attached children demonstrated more cognitive competence through childhood and adolescence than children who did not have secure attachments. Parental support and responsiveness encouraged cognitive growth over time.

The effects of the curriculum within programs and schools for children can maximize or discourage cognitive development. The Cognitively Oriented Curriculum, developed at the High/Scope Institute by David Weikart and his associates, focused on active learning. It was based on Piagetian principles and involved children in planning and other cognitively oriented activities. The games that children play can also affect their thinking and can be utilized in the curriculum. Research by Constance Kamii and Rheta DeVries has shown how the use of games and play-oriented activities can help children develop numerical thinking, language competency, and other cognitive abilities, while promoting autonomy or the ability to think independently and enhancing cooperative and social skills.

As an understanding of the negative effects of poverty and lack of enriching experiences increased during the 1950's and 1960's, initiatives such as Head Start and various other compensatory early childhood programs were established in the United States to reverse the effects of early cognitive deprivation. Initial studies on the effects of such programs were extremely encouraging, and gains in intelligence quotient (IQ) scores and cognitive performance were found to be significant. It was later discovered, however, that such gains could be lost if intellectual stimulation was not maintained. The need to continue to provide stimulating educational experiences was recognized. It was found that positive attitudes toward schooling and a sense of self-esteem also occur when compensatory education and enrichment programs are provided.

The increasing evidence of brain research concerning the importance to the developmental process of stimulating experiences during the first few years of life, as well as knowledge about the growth and weight of the brain in infancy, suggests the need to provide such experiences from a very early age. Prenatal experiences and their impact on cognitive and other areas of development are also being studied.

The concept of cognitive development as a highly active process that occurs in a series of stages has certain implications for the education and well-being of children. One implication is that children in a particular stage of development should not be hurried but should be allowed to develop and mature at their own pace. Hurrying children beyond their developmental capacity can cause mental and emotional damage. David Elkind uses the term "miseducation" to refer to the tendency to hurry and pressure children to perform activities and tasks for which they are not cognitively or physically ready. He believes that miseducation is an increasingly common problem in the United States.

Another implication of the active nature of cognitive development is that children should be given numerous opportunities to explore materials and the environment, and thus acquire knowledge for themselves. Materials, equipment, and knowledge to be discovered should be appropriate to the stage of the child and should be based on the child's existing structures and schemes.

Perspective and Prospects

The cognitive and intellectual development of children was not studied seriously or scientifically until the late nineteenth century in Europe and America. G. Stanley Hall was the first person to develop an instrument—the questionnaire—to study the minds of children. The twentieth century saw the emergence of developmental theories such as the psychoanalytic theory of Sigmund Freud and the psychosocial theory of Erik Erikson. Behaviorism, which viewed children's learning and development as passive and therefore controllable, dominated much of the earlier part of the century. John Watson proposed that children were like blank tablets on which anything could be written. In other words, children's development was shaped by their environment and by the people around them. This view had been held in the seventeenth century by the philosopher John Locke. Watson's theory was extended by B. F. Skinner, who evolved a learning theory based on the use of reinforcement and external stimuli to influence and control behavior. Albert Bandura's theory of social cognition departed from the earlier passive learning theories of Watson and Skinner. He believed that individuals actively process information. Bandura also emphasized the role of observational learning, or learning by observing others and thinking about outcomes, in the process of children's development.

During the 1950's, a cognitive revolution occurred as the theory and research of Jean Piaget became known. Piaget was interested in how children think, in their "wrong" answers as indicators of their stage of cognitive development, and in their active construction of knowledge. He observed his own children's early interactions and explorations. He also utilized the clinical method, in which he interviewed children of different ages to understand the nature of their hypotheses and problem-solving strategies. The questions in this method were flexible and depended on the responses given by the child.

Piaget's theories were later criticized and were seen to underestimate children's abilities. His assumption of the heterogeneity or universality of cognitive stages was also questioned. Critics charged that Piaget did not give enough credit to the role of cultural and social factors in cognitive development. The impact of culture and social interaction on the child's thinking and use of strategies as culturally transmitted tools of thought was studied by Lev Vygotsky. In the last decades of the twentieth century, Vygotsky's ideas aroused much interest. The difference in learning styles was also studied, and it was recognized that learning styles vary across cultures as well as from individual to individual.

Many neo-Piagetian theories attempted to integrate some Piagetian assumptions with information-processing approaches. These approaches examined cognitive processes such as memory and attention and demonstrated their influence on children's cognitive development.

The influence of the environment and various activities cannot be overemphasized in its importance to cognitive development. As technologies continue to develop for use by children, ranging from toys to educational tools, it will be crucial to consider all aspects of development carefully. One example is recent research evaluating the impact on brain development of frequent video game and computer use by children. The research suggested that activities which encourage vision and movement skills, to the exclusion of other skills important to development, may be problematic. The concern is that some capacities may become overused, while others may not receive enough stimulation to encourage adequate development. More research is certainly needed to examine the potential impact of new technologies and exposure to diverse stimuli. Important lessons can be learned from history in an effort to guard against anything that impoverishes a child's learning environment.

—Nillofur Zobairi, Ph.D.;
updated by Nancy A. Piotrowski, Ph.D.

See also Bonding; Developmental disorders; Developmental stages; Learning disabilities; Mental retardation; Motor skill development; Psychiatric disorders; Psychiatry, child and adolescent; Reflexes, primitive.

For Further Information:

Berk, Laura E. *Child Development*. 8th ed. Boston: Pearson/Allyn & Bacon, 2009. A text that reviews theory and research in child development, cognitive and language development, personality and social development, and the foundations and contexts of development.

Berk, Laura E., and Adam Winsler. *Scaffolding Children's Learning: Vvgotsky and Early Childhood Education*. Washington, D.C.: National Association for the Education of Young Children, 1995. The authors examine Lev Vygotsky's life and the key concepts of his developmental approach, which stresses the strong links between a child's social, cognitive, and psychological existence, in a clear and understandable way. Implications for early childhood education are discussed.

Bjorklund, David F. *Children's Thinking: Developmental Function and Individual Differences*. 4th ed. Belmont, Calif.: Thomson/Wadsworth, 2005. The book provides a detailed description of theory and research in the field of cognitive development. It includes discussions on the biological foundations of cognition, individual differences, and the impact of culture and schooling.

Elkind, David. *Miseducation: Preschoolers at Risk.* New York: Alfred A. Knopf, 1987. The author discusses the many pressures on modern children, explaining how their physical and emotional health may be at risk when schools and parents attempt to "miseducate" them before they are developmentally ready. Elkind's examples can be appreciated by both professionals and laypeople.

Nathanson, Laura Walther. *The Portable Pediatrician: A Practicing Pediatrician's Guide to Your Child's*

Growth, Development, Health, and Behavior from Birth to Age Five. 2d ed. New York: HarperCollins, 2002. An engaging, easy-to-read guide for parents to assess their child's development, medical symptoms, and behavioral problems.

Shore, Rima. *Rethinking the Brain: New Insights into Early Development.* Rev. ed. New York: Families and Work Institute, 2003. The author summarizes research on the brain and discusses implications for development, especially in the first three years of life. The material is presented in a readable and understandable style.

COLD SORES

DISEASE/DISORDER

ALSO KNOWN AS: Fever blisters

ANATOMY OR SYSTEM AFFECTED: Mouth, skin

SPECIALTIES AND RELATED FIELDS: Family medicine

DEFINITION: An infectious disease characterized by thin-walled vesicles around the mouth.

CAUSES AND SYMPTOMS

Cold sores are an infectious disease caused by the herpes simplex virus. Cold sores and fever blisters are two terms used for sores that develop around the mouth. They are among the most common disorders around the mouth area, causing pain and annoyance to millions of Americans. An estimated 45 to 80 percent of adults and children in the United States have had at least one cold sore. There are two types of herpes simplex. Type 1 usually causes oral herpes, or fever blisters, while type 2 usually causes genital herpes. About 95 percent of the fever blisters located on the mouth are caused by herpes simplex type 1.

Fever blisters are highly contagious, more so in the first day or two of an eruption. Once the blister has formed a dry scab, transmission is low and the herpes simplex virus usually cannot be recovered from the site. The virus can spread to others through touch; frequently, infection spreads through kissing. The chance of infection is higher if the body's defenses are weakened by stress, illness, or injury.

Once a person is infected with oral herpes, the virus remains in the nerve located near the fever blister. It may stay dormant at this site for years. People who have had fever blisters in the past can sometimes predict when an outbreak is going to occur. The appearance of cold sores may be preceded by a few hours of a tingling, burning, or itching sensation, a phenomenon

> ## INFORMATION ON COLD SORES
>
> **CAUSES:** Infection by herpes simplex virus
>
> **SYMPTOMS:** Sores around mouth that dry to form scabs; preceded by tingling, burning, or itching sensation
>
> **DURATION:** Chronic, with acute outbreaks lasting from three to ten days
>
> **TREATMENTS:** Keeping area clean and dry, avoidance of sore irritation or stress; prevention through antiviral compounds (acyclovir, valacyclovir, foscarnet)

called a prodrome. Typically, the sores erupt in a small cluster, with each blister about the size of a large pimple. The blisters quickly dry to form a scab. Generally, no scarring or loss in sensation occurs. Outbreaks usually last from three to ten days.

TREATMENT AND THERAPY

Treatment includes keeping the area clean and dry to prevent bacterial infection. The patient should avoid irritating the sores, as touching them may spread the virus. For example, if a person rubs the sore and then rubs an eyelid, a new sore may appear on the eyelid in a few days. When the fever blister is contagious, kissing should be avoided. People whose cold sores appear in response to stress should try to avoid stressful situations. Some investigators have suggested that adding L-lysine to the diet or eliminating certain foods (such as nuts, chocolate, and seeds) may help, although no research studies have validated these suggestions. Even sunlight has been linked as a trigger for fever blisters. The National Institute of Dental and Craniofacial Research recommends the use of sunscreen on the lips to prevent sun-induced recurrences of herpes.

Antiviral therapy of mucocutaneous herpes simplex virus infection is rarely curative, but is given for treatment of severe cases and to prevent or ameliorate recurrences. Treatment can also decrease viral shedding, making transmission to other people less likely. Available antiviral compounds include nucleoside analogues, which selectively interfere with viral deoxyribonucleic acid (DNA) replication. Oral acyclovir (Avirax or Zovirax) and valacyclovir (Valtrex), antiviral drugs that keep the virus from multiplying, can be taken to prevent recurrence. Acyclovir applied locally has also been found effective, and foscarnet (Foscavir) is useful in treating acyclovir-resistant infections. Two topical preparations, Zovirax and penciclovir (Vectavir), have been shown to influence the eruption and duration of cold sores when applied during the prodromal stage. Antibiotics may be used in treating secondary infections. An ophthalmologist should treat any eye lesions.

Some cold sore treatments that have been successful in selected people are solvents such as ether, alcohol, povidone iodine, and antiseptic mouthwash. Other patients have applied ice or toothpaste to the sores. While none of these treatments has scientific backing, eating an ice pop or applying an ice cube to the blister may relieve the discomfort.

Perspective and Prospects

Future research is aimed at determining the precise form and location of the inactive herpesvirus in nerve cells. This information might allow scientists to design antiviral drugs that can attack the virus while it lies dormant in nerves. Researchers are also trying to learn more about how sunlight, injury, and stress act as triggers so that the cycle of recurrences can be stopped. An experimental new herpes treatment derived from an herb known as *Prunella vulgaris* may one day help prevent and treat both types of herpes.

—*Janet Mahoney, R.N., Ph.D., A.P.R.N.*

See also Blisters; Canker sores; Herpes; Lesions; Skin; Skin disorders; Stress; Stress reduction; Ulcers; Viral infections.

For Further Information:

Ignatavicius, Donna D., and M. Linda Workman, eds. *Medical-Surgical Nursing: Critical Thinking for Collaborative Care*. 5th ed. Philadelphia: Saunders/Elsevier, 2006.

Lewis, Sharon Mantik, et al., eds. *Medical-Surgical Nursing: Assessment and Management of Clinical Problems*. 7th ed. 2 vols. St. Louis, Mo.: Mosby/Elsevier, 2007.

National Institutes of Health. National Institute of Dental Research. *Fever Blisters and Canker Sores*. Rev. ed. Bethesda, Md.: Author, 1992.

Smeltzer, Suzanne C., and Brenda G. Bare, eds. *Brunner and Suddarth's Textbook of Medical-Surgical Nursing*. 12th ed. Philadelphia: Wolters Kluwer/Lippincott Williams & Wilkins, 2010.

Colic

Disease/disorder

Anatomy or system affected: Gastrointestinal system, intestines, psychic-emotional system

Specialties and related fields: Gastroenterology, pediatrics

Definition: As a general term, a paroxysm of acute abdominal pain caused by spasm, obstruction, or twisting of a hollow abdominal organ. As a specific entity, infantile colic is a group of behaviors displayed by young infants including crying, facial grimacing, drawing-up of the legs over the abdomen, and clenching of the fists.

Key terms:

flatulence: the presence of excessive gas in the stomach and intestines, which is expelled from the body

irritability: a state of general overreaction to external stimuli

spasm: an involuntary muscle contraction; a painful spasm is called a cramp

Causes and Symptoms

As a general term, colic can arise from any site in the abdomen. For example, cramplike pain caused by a stone obstructing the bile ducts or a stone obstructing the urinary tract are known as biliary colic or renal colic, respectively. More specifically, the term "colic," when unmodified, generally refers to infantile colic.

The crying of colicky infants tends to be more prominent in the evening, although they cry more than other infants at other times of day. The "rule of threes" of infantile colic holds that infants with colic cry for more than three hours per day for more than three days per week for more than three weeks. The associated gestures suggest to some that the infant is experiencing abdominal pain and is responsible for the use of the term "colic" to describe the condition.

Several causes of infantile colic have been postulated, but conclusive evidence is lacking for any of them. This combination of behaviors has been interpreted as abdominal pain, leading to the idea that cramping somewhere in the intestine is the cause. Neurobehavioral explanations have been offered. The most common is that colic represents a state of agitation that may not require a noxious stimulus for agitation and crying to continue. Rarely is colic the result of organic disease, and the prevailing opinion is that it is a variant of normal infant behavior. It appears to be unrelated to caregiving style or intensity. Other proposed mechanisms include difficult temperament, sleep disturbance, diarrhea, child abuse, and irritable bowel syndrome (IBS). Some theories ascribe colic to hypersensitivity to dietary protein—usually proteins derived from cow's milk, which can be secreted in breast milk—thus explaining the occurrence of colic in breast-fed infants. Intestinal gas, either from air swallowed during feeding or from fermentation of incompletely absorbed carbohydrates in the colon, has also been implicated. Parents of colicky infants frequently describe flatulence as an associated symptom.

TREATMENT AND THERAPY

The medical treatment of the infant with colic begins with a thorough medical history and a careful physical examination. While the likelihood of finding a cause of the infant's symptoms are slight, the thoroughness of this approach provides an effective basis for reassurance and demonstrates that the parents' complaint is taken seriously.

Infantile colic virtually always resolves spontaneously, leaving the infant healthy and thriving. The essentials of therapy are demystification, reassurance, and support for the haggard and anxious parents. Demystification is the explanation of the source of the infant's distress, which alleviates the anxiety attendant on diagnostic hypotheses that occur to or are suggested to the parents. It is important for pediatricians to deal with the anxiety aroused by the infant's symptoms with reassurance, pointing out that the baby will be fine; the only risk of lasting damage is to the parents.

Quick, superficial attempts to solve the problem with formula changes or medications, particularly when not accompanied by patient demystification and reassurance, reinforce the parents' suspicion that there is something wrong with the child, ultimately increasing parental perception of the child's vulnerability. The results of studies in the medical literature investigating the usefulness of switching formulas and using agents such as simethicone to deal with intestinal gas are

---

INFORMATION ON COLIC

CAUSES: Unknown; abdominal pain suspected
SYMPTOMS: Crying for long periods of time, facial grimacing, drawing of legs over abdomen, clenching of fists
DURATION: Typically one to three months
TREATMENTS: Switching formulas, swaddling, mimicking of in utero motion, medications

---

mixed. Dicyclomine, an anticholinergic medication used in the past, should not be given to infants under six months of age because of the possibility that it will interfere with the baby's breathing.

More frequent, smaller feedings may help, as may increased carrying (called "walking the floor") and rocking. One theory holds that mimicking the environment in the womb is reassuring, which can be achieved through closeness to a warm person with a detectable heartbeat (sometimes called "kangaroo care"), swaddling (wrapping the baby in a blanket to restrict movement of the extremities), and rhythmic stimulation provided by background music and car or stroller rides. One commonly used method involves placing the baby in an infant seat on top of a running washer or dryer, thus exposing the infant to constant vibration. Care must be taken to stay with the baby or to secure the infant seat to prevent injury resulting from a fall off the appliance. Most colicky infants have excessive gas, and gas pains have long been suspected as being responsible for colic. Since virtually all the gas in the intestine is swallowed air, minimizing air swallowing and maximizing burping after feedings are important measures in reducing colic. The use of cereal to ease the infant's hunger and decrease the vigor with which he or she sucks on the nipple results in less air being swallowed. Unfortunately, many parents are advised to put cereal in a bottle; this increases the negative pressure required to suck the slurry of milk and cereal and increases the amount of air swallowed.

PERSPECTIVE AND PROSPECTS

One theory holds that infantile colic is related to a familial prevalence of irritable bowel syndrome, also called irritable colon or spastic colon. IBS is viewed in this context as a familial abnormality in the regulation of intestinal motility that produces different symptoms at different ages. According to this theory, if one is born into an "irritable colon" family, one proceeds through distinct, age-related symptom complexes, the first of which is infantile colic. Between six months and three years of age, irritable colon syndrome of infancy (also called chronic nonspecific diarrhea or toddler diarrhea) is prominent, manifesting as recurrent, watery diarrhea with no other symptoms and no repercussions on growth and development. Recurrent, periumbilical abdominal pain, frequently exacerbated by meals in schoolchildren between five and twelve years of age, is the third of these symptom complexes. It is followed by the development of similar symptoms in adulthood, usually accompanied by alternating diarrhea and constipation. In fact, infants with irritable bowel syndrome of infancy have a higher-than-normal incidence of having had prolonged or severe infantile colic, and several studies show that children with symptoms of irritable colon have a higher-than-normal prevalence of other family members with symptoms of irritable colon. It is useful to identify other members of the family with such symptoms to aid in demystifying the illness.

—*Wallace A. Gleason, Jr., M.D.*

See also Bonding; Colon; Diarrhea and dysentery; Gastroenterology, pediatric; Gastrointestinal system; Irritable bowel syndrome (IBS); Lactose intolerance; Neonatology; Pediatrics.

FOR FURTHER INFORMATION:

Barr, Ronald G. "Changing Our Understanding of Infant Colic." *Archives of Pediatrics and Adolescent Medicine* 156, no. 12 (December, 2002): 1172-1175. Argues that many of the symptoms of colic, including a pattern of repeated crying, are now understood to be behaviors likely universal to normal infant development.

Brazelton, T. Berry. *Calming Your Fussy Baby: The Brazelton Way.* Cambridge, Mass.: Perseus, 2002. Brazelton, a well-known pediatrician, offers advice for calming infants and covers colic and effective ways of addressing it.

Lampe, John B. "Infantile Colic: Follow-up at Four Years of Age." *Clinical Pediatrics* 29, no. 10 (October, 2000): 620. A now four-year-old group of formerly colicky infants and controls was reexamined with respect to possible persistent differences in behavior, temperament, eating and sleeping habits, psychosomatic complaints, growth, and family atmosphere.

McCormick, David P. "The Challenge of Colic." *Clinical Pediatrics* 39, no. 7 (July, 2000): 401-402. McCormick offers his reaction to a study on colic by Susan Levitzky, a pediatrician, and Robyn Cooper, a psychologist, published in the same issue.

Thompson, June. "Infantile Colic: What Is It and Are There Effective Treatments?" *Community Practitioner* 73, no. 9 (September, 2000): 767. Infantile colic, also called three month colic and evening colic, has been studied extensively, and many possible causes and factors have been suggested. Thompson reviews some of the research on the etiology and effectiveness of treatments for this phenomenon.

_____. "Low Birth Weight and Colic 'Linked.'" *Community Practitioner* 73, no. 8 (August, 2000): 727. It has been hypothesized that depletion of nutrition during critical stages of organ development influences organ function, and impaired fetal growth has been associated with a large number of diseases. This study aimed to describe how fetal growth and gestational age affect infantile colic while considering other potential risk factors.

Walling, Anne D. "Diagnosing Biliary Colic and Acute Cholecystitis." *American Family Physician* 62, no. 6 (September 15, 2000): 1386. Approximately 500,000 cholecystectomies are performed annually in the United States. Symptomatic gallstones are the most common indication for cholecystectomy.

Waltman, Alicia Brooks. "The Crying Game." *Parenting* 14, no. 3 (April, 2000): 128-132. Waltman offers information about the latest research on colic and the best ways to soothe a crying baby. For many babies, a surefire soother is a breast or a bottle.

White, Barbara Prudhomme, et al. "Behavioral and Physiological Responsivity, Sleep, and Patterns of Daily Cortisol Production in Infants with and Without Colic." *Child Development* 71, no. 4 (July/August, 2000): 862-877. To describe the behavioral and physiological responses associated with colic, the responses of twenty two-month-old infants with and twenty without colic were studied during a physical examination.

COLITIS

DISEASE/DISORDER

ANATOMY OR SYSTEM AFFECTED: Abdomen, gastrointestinal system, intestines, stomach

SPECIALTIES AND RELATED FIELDS: Gastroenterology, internal medicine

DEFINITION: A potentially fatal but manageable disease of the colon that inflames and ulcerates the bowel lining, occurring in both acute and chronic forms.

KEY TERMS:

diarrhea: persistent liquid or mushy, shapeless stool

dysentery: bloody diarrhea caused by infectious agents affecting the colon

ileum: the last section of the small bowel, which passes food wastes to the colon through the ileocecal valve

inflammation: swelling caused by the accumulation of fluids and chemical agents

mucosa: the membrane of cells that lines the bowel; admits fluids and nutrients but also serves as the first-line protection against infectious agents and other materials foreign to the body

procedure: any medical treatment that entails physical manipulation or invasion of the body

stoma: an opening, formed by surgery, from the bowel to the exterior surface of the body

stool: the food wastes mixed with fluid, bacteria, mucus, and dead cells that exit the body upon defecation

ulcer: an area of the mucosa that has been abraded or dissolved by infection or chemicals, creating an open sore

CAUSES AND SYMPTOMS

The colon is the section of the lower bowel, or intestines, extending from the ileocecal valve to the rectum. It is wider in diameter than the small bowel, although shorter in length at about one meter. From behind the pelvis, the colon rises along the right side of the body (ascending colon), turns left to cross the upper abdominal cavity (transverse colon), and then turns down along the left side of the body (descending colon) until it joins the sigmoid (S-shaped) colon. The sigmoid colon empties into the rectum, a pouch that stores the waste products of digestion that are excreted through the anus. The colon absorbs most of the fluid passed to it from the small bowel, so that wastes solidify; meanwhile, bacteria in the colon break down undigested proteins and carbohydrates, creating hydrogen, carbon dioxide, and methane gases in the process.

A key structure in colonic activity is its mucosa. This thin sheet of cells lining the bowel wall permits passage of fluids and certain nutrients into the bloodstream but resists bacteria and toxins (poisonous chemical compounds). When the mucosa is torn or worn away, bacteria and toxins enter, infecting the bowel wall. The body responds to infection by rushing fluids and powerful chemicals to the endangered area to confine and kill the infecting agents. In the process, the tissues of the bowel wall swell with the fluids; this is known as inflammation. The medical suffix denoting this response is *itis*; when it occurs in the colon, physicians call it colitis.

A variety of agents can cause colitis, which is divided into two major types depending on the duration of the disease: acute colitis and chronic ulcerative colitis. Acute colitis is a relatively brief, single episode of inflammation. It is often caused by bacteria or parasites. For example, *Giardia lamblia*, a bacterium in many American streams, is a common infectious agent in colitis, and the amoebas in polluted water supplies are responsible for the type of colitis known as amebic

> ### INFORMATION ON COLITIS
>
> **CAUSES:** Unknown; possibly bacterial or viral infection, genetic factors, exposure to antibiotics, autoimmune reaction
>
> **SYMPTOMS:** Swelling of bowel lining, ulcers, bloody diarrhea, pain, fever, severe weight loss, anemia, lack of energy, dehydration, uncontrollable urge to defecate
>
> **DURATION:** Chronic, with acute episodes
>
> **TREATMENTS:** Medications (anti-inflammatory agents), surgery, dietary restrictions

dysentery. Some medicines, however, especially antibiotics, can also induce colitis. Acute colitis either disappears on its own or can be cured with drugs. Untreated, however, it may be fatal.

Chronic ulcerative colitis and Crohn's disease constitute a category of serious afflictions called inflammatory bowel disease (IBD) whose primary physical effects include swelling of the bowel lining, ulcers, and bloody diarrhea. Although some medical researchers think that these afflictions may be two aspects of the same disease, ulcerative colitis affects only the colon, whereas Crohn's disease can involve the small bowel as well as the colon. Moreover, colitis chiefly involves the colonic mucosa, but Crohn's disease delves into the full thickness of the bowel wall.

Chronic ulcerative colitis is a permanent disease that manifests itself either in recurring bouts of inflammation or in continuous inflammation that cannot be cleared up with drugs. It is commonly called ulcerative colitis because ulcers, open sores in the mucosa, spread throughout the colon and rectum, where the disease usually starts. Researchers have not yet discovered the causes of chronic ulcerative colitis, although there are many theories, of which three are prominent. The first is bacterial or viral infection, and many agents have been proposed as the culprit. Because such a multitude of organisms commonly reside in or pass through the colon, researchers have enormous difficulty separating out a specific kind in order to show that it is always present during colitis attacks. Second is autoimmune reaction. Research in other diseases has shown that sometimes the body's police system, enforced by white blood cells, mistakes native, healthy tissue for a foreign agent and attacks that tissue in an attempt to destroy it. Yet no testing in chronic ulcerative colitis has yet proven the theory. Third is a combination of foreign infection and autoimmune response; it is as if the immune system overreacts to an infectious agent and continues its attack even after the agent has been neutralized. Many researchers have suspected that the disease is inherited, because certain families have higher rates of the disease than others. This genetic theory is not universally accepted, however, because it is just as likely that family members share infection rather than having passed on a genetic predisposition for the disease. Other theories propose food allergies as the cause; even toothpaste has been considered.

Regardless of the cause, there is no doubt that colitis is a painful, disabling, bewildering disease. When the bowel inflames, the tissues heat up and fever results. Cramps are common, and sufferers feel an urgent, frequently uncontrollable urge to defecate. When they reach the toilet (if they do so in time), they have soft, loose stool or diarrhea, which can seem to explode from the anus. They may have as many as ten to twenty bowel movements a day. Because ulcers often erode blood vessels, blood can appear in the stool, as well as mucus and pus from the bowel wall. Severe weight loss, anemia, lack of energy, dehydration, and anorexia often develop as the colitis persists. The symptoms may clear up on their own only to recur months or years later; attacks may come with increasing frequency thereafter. The first attack, if it worsens rapidly, is fatal in about 5 to 10 percent of patients, although the death rate can rise to 25 percent among first-time sufferers who are more than sixty years old.

Complications from colitis can be life-threatening. These include perforation of the bowel wall, strictures, hemorrhaging, and toxic megacolon (hyperinflation of the colon, an emergency medical condition). Furthermore, studies show that patients who have had ulcerative colitis for more than ten years have about a 20 percent chance of developing cancer in the colon or rectum.

Because colitis is a relapsing, embarrassing disease, patients often suffer psychological turmoil. In *Colitis* (1992), Michael P. Kelly reports the results of his study of forty-five British colitis patients. According to Kelly, they typically denied that early symptoms were the signs of serious illness, passing them off as the result of overeating or influenza. The denial continued until the continual, desperate urge to defecate made them despair of controlling their bowels without help. Often, they suffered embarrassment because they had to flee family gatherings or work in order to find a toilet or because they passed stool inadvertently in public.

Many feared being beyond easy access to a toilet, shunned public places, and felt humiliated. Only then did some visit a physician, and even after chronic ulcerative colitis was diagnosed, a portion hoped they could still cope on their own. When they could not, they grew depressed, insomniac, angry at their fate, or antisocial. Even with treatment, the strain of enduring the disease can be debilitating.

TREATMENT AND THERAPY

Fortunately, medical science has several well-tested methods of controlling or curing colitis. In the case of acute colitis, patients usually resume normal bowel functions on their own and emerge as healthy as they were before the onset of symptoms. For chronic ulcerative colitis patients, however, the body is rarely the same again, and they must adjust to the effects of medication, surgery, or both—an adjustment that some authors claim is essentially a redefinition of the self.

After interviewing a patient and assessing the reported symptoms, the physician suspecting colitis orders a stool sample to check for blood, bacteria, parasites, and pus. If any of these are present, the physician directly examines the rectum and colon by inserting a fiberoptic endoscope into the rectum and up the colon. Early in the disease, the mucosa looks granular with scattered hemorrhages and tiny bleeding points. As the disease progresses, the mucosa turns spongy and has many ulcers that ooze blood and pus. An X ray often helps determine the extent of inflammation, and tissue samples taken by endoscopic biopsy can establish if it is ulcerative colitis or infection, and not Crohn's disease, that is present.

There is no easy treatment for chronic ulcerative colitis. Dietary restrictions—especially the elimination of fibrous foods such as raw fruits and vegetables or of milk products—may reduce the irritation to the inflamed colon, and symptoms then may improve if the disease is mild. Antidiarrheal drugs can firm the stool and reduce the patient's urgency to defecate, although such drugs must be used very cautiously to avoid dangerous dilation of the bowels.

Such nonspecific measures are seldom more than delaying tactics, and drugs are needed to counteract the colon's inflammation. Two types are most common. The first, sulfasalazine, is a sulfa drug developed in the 1940's. It is an anti-inflammatory agent that is most effective in mild to moderate ulcerative colitis and helps prevent recurrence of inflammation. Corticosteroids, the second type, behave like the hormones produced by the adrenal gland that suppress inflammation. The drug works well in relieving the symptoms of moderate to moderately severe attacks. Both types of drugs have serious side effects, so physicians must carefully tailor dosages for each patient and check repeatedly for reactions. In some patients, sulfasalazine induces nausea, vomiting, joint pain, headaches, rashes, dizziness, and hepatitis (liver inflammation). The effects of corticosteroids include sleeplessness, mood swings, acne, high blood pressure, diabetes, cataracts, thinning of the bones (especially the spine), and fluid retention and swelling of the face, hands, abdomen, and ankles. Women may grow facial hair, and adolescents may have delayed sexual maturation. In most cases, the side effects clear up when patients stop taking the drugs.

With medication, people who suffer mild or moderate chronic ulcerative colitis can control it for years, often for the rest of their lives. Severe colitis requires surgery, and sometimes patients with milder forms choose to have surgery rather than live with the disease's unpredictable recurrence or the ever-present side effects of drugs. In any case, surgery is the one known cure for chronic ulcerative colitis, although fewer than one-third of patients undergo surgical procedures. Several types of these surgeries have high success rates.

Because ulcerative colitis eventually spreads throughout the colon, complete removal of the large bowel and rectum is the surest way to eliminate the disease. This "total proctocolectomy" takes place in three steps. The surgeon first cuts through the wall of the abdomen, the incision extending from the mid-transverse colon to the rectum, and removes the colon. Next, the end of the ileum is pulled through a hole in the abdomen to form a stoma (a procedure called an ileostomy). Finally, the rectum is removed and the anus sutured shut. Thereafter the patient defecates through the stoma. Either of two arrangements prevents stool from simply spilling out unchecked. Most patients affix plastic bags around their stomas into which stool flows without their control; when full, the bag is either emptied and reattached or thrown away and replaced. To avoid external bags, some patients prefer a "continent ileostomy," so called because it allows them to control defecation. The surgeon constructs a pouch out of a portion of the ileum and attaches it right behind the stoma, a procedure called a Kock pouch after its inventor, Nils Kock of Sweden. When this pouch is full, the patient empties it with a catheter inserted through the stoma. Some patients can choose to have an ileoanal anastomosis. In this procedure, the surgeon forms the end of the ileum

into a pouch, which is attached to the anus and collects wastes in place of the rectum. The patient continues to defecate through the anus rather than through a stoma.

None of these surgical procedures is free of problems, and all require extensive recovery in the hospital and rehabilitation. Moreover, both infections and mechanical failures can occur. If healthy portions of the colon are left intact, they often flare with colitis later, and more operations become necessary. Patients with stomas are vulnerable to bacterial inflammation of the small intestine, resulting in diarrhea, vomiting, and dehydration. Stomas and pouches sometimes leak or close up, and even after successful operations patients lose some capacity to absorb zinc, bile salts, and vitamin B_{12}, although food supplements can make up for these deficiencies.

Any major surgery is an emotional trial. One that leaves a basic function of the body permanently altered, as with proctocolectomy or ileostomy, is difficult to accept afterward, even when the surgery was an emergency measure to save the patient's life. Patients must live with a bag of stool on their abdomen or a pouch that they must empty with a plastic straw—bags and pouches that sometimes leak stool or gas and that, even when functioning smoothly, are not pleasant to handle. They must pay close attention to body functions that they rarely had to think about before the ulcerative colitis began. The changes can severely depress patients, who then may need psychiatric help and antidepressant drugs to recover their spirits. Patients with anastomoses, who continue to defecate through their anus, also find their bowel functions changed, although not so severely. For example, it takes many months before normal stool forms, and diarrhea plagues these patients.

After their operations, patients have access to considerable help in addition to physicians and surgeons. Special nurses train patients to care for their stomas, check regularly for infection or malfunction, and generally ease them into their new lives. Formal support groups and informal networks are common, through which the afflicted can get information and reassurance. In the United States, the National Foundation for Ileitis and Colitis arranges many support groups, as well as sponsoring medical research and education programs.

PERSPECTIVE AND PROSPECTS

Acute forms of colitis, especially amebic dysentery, have long been recognized as among the endemic diseases of polluted water, and until the development of antibiotics, they regularly killed significant portions of local populations, especially the young and elderly. Chronic ulcerative colitis was first described in 1859, but no effective treatment for it existed until the 1940's. At that time, Nana Svartz of Sweden noticed that when rheumatoid arthritis patients were given sulfasalazine, the bowel condition of those who had colitis improved as well. J. Arnold Bargen, an American physician, confirmed Svartz's observation in a formal clinical trial, and sulfasalazine soon was mass-produced for distribution in the United States and later throughout the world. Since the 1940's, medications and surgical techniques for ulcerative colitis have proliferated, although none restores a patient's original state of health.

Because the agents causing ulcerative colitis are unknown, the historical and geographical origin of the disease likewise cannot be determined. Nevertheless, three somewhat odd social facets of the disease are recognized.

Evidence suggests that ulcerative colitis is a disease of urban industrial society. Along with Crohn's disease, colitis appears to be entrenched in Scandinavia, the United States, Western Europe, Israel, and England. It rarely occurs in rural Africa, Asia, or South America, despite the poor nutrition and sanitation in some of these areas. Yet the disease does not appear to vary solely by racial type or nationality, although Jewish people tend to fall ill with it more often than any other group. For example, African Americans, whether from families long-established in the United States or recently immigrated, show an incidence of colitis as high as residents of European descent.

Furthermore, ulcerative colitis strikes the young. It most often begins between the ages of fifteen and thirty; men and women are equally likely to come down with it. This fact, taken with the high rate of inflammatory bowel disease (IBD) sufferers who have family members also with the disease (20 to 25 percent), has led some researchers to believe that a genetic factor creates a susceptibility for IBD.

Finally, IBD patients bear some social stigma, or at least believe they do. Ulcerative colitis involves bowel incontinence and often ends with surgical replacement of the anus with a stoma; in such cases, bowel movements can dominate a patient's life and become obvious to family members, coworkers, and even strangers. Because the subject of stool is taboo to many and the odor offends most people, patients can feel severe embarrassment and come to see themselves as pariahs.

Even though the causes of ulcerative colitis remain obscure and the treatment is often distressing, modern medicine saves people who otherwise would die.

—Roger Smith, Ph.D.

See also Amebiasis; Colon; Colorectal cancer; Colorectal surgery; Crohn's disease; Diarrhea and dysentery; Diverticulosis and diverticulitis; Gastroenterology; Gastrointestinal disorders; Gastrointestinal system; Giardiasis; Intestinal disorders; Intestines; Irritable bowel syndrome (IBS); Rectum; Ulcers.

FOR FURTHER INFORMATION:

Beers, Mark H., et al., eds. *The Merck Manual of Diagnosis and Therapy.* 18th ed. Whitehouse Station, N.J.: Merck Research Laboratories, 2006. This is a reference work for physicians, and the nomenclature can be daunting. It is best consulted after more general introductory reading. The sections on colitis describe the physical symptoms, tests, and treatments systematically and thoroughly.

Brandt, Lawrence J., and Penny Steiner-Grossman, eds. *Treating IBD: A Patient's Guide to the Medical and Surgical Management of Inflammatory Bowel Disease.* Reprint. Philadelphia: Lippincott-Raven, 1996. One of the most thorough introductions to ulcerative colitis and Crohn's disease. Illustrations, tables, and very helpful glossaries accompany the text.

Crohn's and Colitis Foundation of America. http://www.ccfa.org. Provides support groups and a wide range of educational publications and programs on Crohn's and ulcerative colitis.

Kalibjian, Cliff. *Straight from the Gut: Living with Crohn's Disease and Ulcerative Colitis.* Cambridge, Mass.: O'Reilly, 2003. Shares numerous personal stories from those suffering from colitis and offers advice on all aspects of living with the disease.

Kelly, Michael P. *Colitis.* New York: Routledge, 1992. Kelly begins his book with a description of symptoms and treatments, but his is primarily a sociological study. Based on interviews with forty-five patients, the work discusses typical effects that the disease had on their lives and how they coped with the treatments, especially surgical procedures.

Parker, James N., and Philip M. Parker, eds. *The 2002 Official Patient's Sourcebook on Ulcerative Colitis.* San Diego, Calif.: Icon Health, 2002. Draws from public, academic, government, and peer-reviewed research to provide a wide-ranging reference about the causes, treatments, and risk factors of colitis.

Saibil, Fred. *Crohn's Disease and Ulcerative Colitis: Everything You Need to Know.* Rev. ed. Toronto, Ont.: Firefly Books, 2009. A leading expert on IBD, Saibil covers topics such as signs and symptoms, how the gastrointestinal system works normally and how IBD affects it, procedures and instruments used to diagnose IBD, effects of diet, children and IBD, and effects on sexual activity and child-bearing.

Sklar, Jill, Manual Sklar, and Annabel Cohen. *The First Year—Crohn's Disease and Ulcerative Colitis: An Essential Guide for the Newly Diagnosed.* 2d ed. New York: Marlowe, 2007. A unique guide for patients with specific gastrointestinal disorders, setting expectations and answering questions related to the first week of diagnosis, the first months, and the first year. Topics include treatment options, dietary choices, fertility issues, and holistic alternatives.

Steiner-Grossman, Penny, Peter A. Banks, and Daniel H. Present, eds. *The New People, Not Patients: A Source Book for Living with Inflammatory Bowel Disease.* Rev. ed. Dubuque, Iowa: Kendall/Hunt, 1997. Written to help IBD patients live with the disease, this book combines very practical information—about support groups and patients' rights, for example—with overviews of symptoms and treatments.

COLLAGEN

BIOLOGY

ANATOMY OR SYSTEM AFFECTED: All, especially joints, ligaments, musculoskeletal system, skin, tendons

SPECIALTIES AND RELATED FIELDS: Biochemistry, rheumatology

DEFINITION: A fibrous protein that is the main component of most connective tissues; the most common protein in animals.

STRUCTURE AND FUNCTIONS

Collagen is a complex protein made up of three separate polypeptide chains that form a triple helix. These polypeptides are unusual because every third amino acid is a glycine and because prolines make up an additional 17 percent of the chains. There are at least twenty-eight types of collagen made up of forty-three distinct polypeptide chains, each coded for by a different gene. For example, type I collagen, the most common type, has two chains classified as alpha-1 and alpha-2. These peptides are initially produced on the rough endoplasmic reticulum (ER) and then processed in the ER lumen, where sequences at the ends are removed and hydroxyl groups are added to many of the chains' prolines and lysines. The triple helix then formed is called procollagen. Further processing, including preparation for secretion, takes place in the Golgi bodies. Once secreted, more end sequences are cleaved off to form collagen (also called tropocollagen). In the extracellular region, collagen molecules associate into collagen fibrils and eventually collagen fibers.

Collagen is a flexible but not stretchable protein that is an important component of most connective tissues. It is the primary component of tendons and ligaments, giving them the requisite strength to connect muscles to bones and bones to other bones or organs. Cartilage found at joints and in many other structures is mostly collagen. The connective tissues found in the dermal layer of the skin, the capsules surrounding internal organs, and blood vessels are also primarily made of collagen. Bones are initially formed from collagen, which then serves as a matrix for calcium phosphate deposition. (Collagen fragments have even been extracted from fossilized dinosaur bones.) During healing, excess collagen production can lead to scar tissue formation. Collagen can be heat treated to produce gelatin or animal-based glues, and injected collagen is often used to plump lips and smooth out wrinkles.

DISORDERS AND DISEASES

Collagen is associated with many disorders. Osteogenesis imperfecta (brittle bone disease) is caused by mutations in the gene for the alpha-1 protein in type I collagen. An inherited form of osteoporosis is caused by a defect in the same gene. Ehlers-Danlos syndrome, which results in hyperextensible joints and fragile, stretchable skin, is caused by defects in types III and V collagen. An early-onset form of osteoarthritis is caused by a lack of functional type VI collagen, and in all forms of osteoarthritis cartilage is lost from the ends of bones at joints. In rheumatoid arthritis, modification of type II collagen forms new antigens that are attacked by the immune system. Vitamin C deficiency decreases activity of the enzymes that add hydroxyl groups to proline, thus leading to lowered amounts of functional type I collagen, which causes scurvy.

—*Richard W. Cheney, Jr., Ph.D.*

See also Arthritis; Cartilage; Connective tissue; Joints; Ligaments; Osteoarthritis; Osteogenesis imperfecta; Rheumatoid arthritis; Rheumatology; Scurvy; Tendon disorders; Tendon repair; Wrinkles.

FOR FURTHER INFORMATION:

Fratzl, Peter. *Collagen: Structure and Mechanics.* New York: Springer, 2008.

Myllyharju, Joahanna, and Kari Kivirkko. "Collagen and Collagen-Related Diseases." *Annals of Medicine* 33 (2001): 7-21.

Whitford, David. *Proteins: Structure and Function.* Hoboken, N.J.: John Wiley & Sons, 2005.

COLON

ANATOMY

ALSO KNOWN AS: Large intestine, large bowel, large gut

ANATOMY OR SYSTEM AFFECTED: Abdomen, gastrointestinal system, intestines, nervous system

SPECIALTIES AND RELATED FIELDS: Alternative medicine, biochemistry, gastroenterology, general surgery, histology, internal medicine, nutrition, oncology, osteopathic medicine, pathology, pediatrics, pharmacology

DEFINITION: The section of the gastrointestinal system where the absorption of water, sodium, and some vitamins occurs and where residual chyme is converted to semisolid feces before expulsion through the anal canal. It is connected to the small intestine through the ileo-cecal valve and is populated by commensal bacteria.

KEY TERMS:

chyme: food in a semifluid state that reaches the large intestine after digestion in the upper gastrointestinal tract

epithelium: tissue made up of tightly adherent cells, usually lining the surfaces of the body and organs

STRUCTURE AND FUNCTIONS

In the average adult man, the large intestine is about 1.5 to 1.8 meters long. It is divided into the cecum; the ascending, transverse, descending, and sigmoid colon; and the rectum, and it ends in the anus. Its wall contains both circular and longitudinal layers of smooth muscle and innervation that controls its motility. The longitudinal musculature runs along the outside of the colon in three separate bands, called teniae coli, which converge around the sigmoid colon and the rectum. The inner layer of the large intestine consists of mucosa with sparse or no villi but with numerous invaginations (glands); it is lined with simple columnar epithelium. The glands contain goblet cells, endocrine cells, and absorptive cells. There are no digestive enzymes linked to the inner surface of the colon.

The main function of the colon is to absorb water from the chyme, and to process it into feces for elimination. Most nutrients and about 90 percent of water are absorbed in the small intestine. When it reaches the large intestine, chyme still contains some electrolytes (sodium, magnesium, and chloride) and indigestible food components, such as fiber.

An abundant and varied bacterial population colonizes the human colon shortly after birth and resides in the large intestine for life. Bacteria digest fiber and produce short-chain fatty acids (acetate, propionate, and butyrate). Short-chain fatty acids promote the integrity of the colonic epithelial cells, prevent inflammation, and provide some protection against potential pathogens.

The large intestine absorbs some vitamins (mainly vitamin K) and electrolytes but mainly water—up to 5 liters of water per day. Water moves passively with sodium, which is mostly absorbed in the distal colon. Water absorption is in part regulated by aldosterone, a hormone that increases the absorption of sodium in response to volume depletion. Water absorption solidifies the chyme into stools.

The motility of the colon allows mixing the contents and retaining them for prolonged periods. Periodically, the colon is swept with propulsive contractions (peristalsis) that move its contents toward the rectum. The gastrocolic reflex causes mass peristalsis after a meal. The sigmoid colon and rectum serve as a reservoir and participate in defecation.

DISORDERS AND DISEASES

A number of disorders are associated with the colon. Appendicitis is the inflammation of the vermiform appendix. It requires surgery. Constipation is the failure to empty the bowels regularly and easily. It can be linked to diet, stress, and a variety of conditions and medications. It is treated with dietary fiber and laxatives. Diarrhea involves frequent loose or liquid bowel movements. It may have many different causes and is treated mainly with loperamide or bismuth salicilate.

Diverticulitis refers to the development of outpouchings in the colon. A low-fiber diet and age are risk factors. Symptoms are linked to inflammation (diverticulosis) and mostly treated with antibiotics. Complications may require surgical removal of the outpouchings. Hirschsprung's disease (congenital aganglionic megacolon) involves the complete absence of neuronal ganglion cells (which make the intestinal muscles contract, so the stool is pushed forward) from a segment of the intestine, usually the distal colon. It requires surgery.

Inflammatory bowel disease (IBD) is a general name for diseases that cause intestinal swelling. They include ulcerative colitis (inflammation and ulcers in the top layer of the lining of the large intestine) and Crohn's disease (all layers of the intestine may be involved; healthy bowel segments alternate with affected segments). Treatment varies widely, but the condition will recur. Irritable bowel syndrome (IBS) is a functional disorder of the colon of unknown cause. Its symptoms are abdominal pain, abnormal bowel habit, bloating, and either constipation, diarrhea, or both alternating. It is worsened by stress. IBS may be linked to hypersensitivity of intestinal muscles and nerves. Its treatment varies according to symptoms.

Colorectal polyps are growths on the lining of the colon or rectum. In time, they can develop into colorectal cancer. They are removed with endoscopic microsurgery. Colorectal cancer refers to cancerous growths in the colon, rectum and appendix, mostly thought to arise from adenomatous polyps in the colon. It requires surgery.

PERSPECTIVE AND PROSPECTS
The intuition that the colon is associated with waste accumulation and release dates to antiquity. Ancient Egyptian physicians also viewed "intestinal putrefaction" as the basic cause of disease, a concept later incorporated into the humoral doctrine of disease by ancient Greeks. This concept of autointoxication lasted throughout the centuries with few adaptations. In the nineteenth century, early studies showed the presence and activity of bacteria in the colon. It was then thought that colonic bacteria generate toxic amines that shorten life span. This theory was finally abandoned by the 1920's. Current research is about the molecular mechanisms of water and electrolyte movements and their regulation and about the pathways that modulate the secretory and absorptive functions of the colon. Recent developments in genetics and immunology have allowed a deeper understanding of inflammatory diseases of the colon. The advent of endoscopic techniques has vastly improved microsurgery and cancer prevention.

—*Donatella M. Casirola, Ph.D.*

See also Abdomen; Abdominal disorders; Anus; Appendicitis; Colitis; Colonoscopy and sigmoidoscopy; Colorectal cancer; Colorectal polyp removal; Colorectal surgery; Constipation; Crohn's disease; Diarrhea; Digestion; Diverticulitis and diverticulosis; Endoscopy; Enemas; Gastroenterology; Gastroenterology, pediatric; Gastrointestinal disorders; Gastrointestinal system; Hirschsprung's disease; Internal medicine; Intestinal disorders; Intestines; Irritable bowel syndrome (IBS); Laparoscopy; Nutrition; Obstruction; Peristalsis; Proctology; Rectum; Small intestine.

FOR FURTHER INFORMATION:
Bäckhed, Fredrik, et al. "Host-Bacterial Mutualism in the Human Intestine." *Science* 307 (March 25, 2005): 1915-1920. An article in a scientific magazine about commensal bacteria in the human colon, within a special section about the gut.
Barrett, Kim E. "Functional Anatomy of the GI Tract and Organs Draining into It." In *Gastrointestinal Physiology.* New York: McGraw-Hill, 2006. A chapter in a textbook for biomedical students that requires basic knowledge of gastrointestinal functions.
Sherwood, Lauralee. "The Digestive System." In *Human Physiology: From Cells to Systems.* 7th ed. Belmont, Calif.: Brooks/Cole/Cengage Learning, 2010. A chapter in a textbook for undergraduate students, easily accessible to the nonspecialist.

COLON THERAPY
TREATMENT
ALSO KNOWN AS: Colonic irrigation, colon hydrotherapy
ANATOMY OR SYSTEM AFFECTED: Abdomen, anus, gastrointestinal system, intestines
SPECIALTIES AND RELATED FIELDS: Alternative medicine
DEFINITION: Irrigation of the colon, or large intestine, with water in order to detoxify it.

INDICATIONS AND PROCEDURES
Colon therapy involves washing out the entire approximately 5-foot length of the colon with pure water in order to dislodge any impacted fecal material. Some practitioners believe that the colon may not function properly because of poor dietary habits, insufficient fluid intake, and physical or emotional stress or illness. Such malfunction can lead to a buildup of hardened, impacted fecal material, which may stagnate and decay in the colon. Bacterial decomposition of the material may create toxins that are absorbed into the bloodstream. This in turn could cause other body organs to overwork themselves as they attempt to detoxify the waste materials and could lead to a variety of illnesses, from colds to cardiovascular disease.

During this procedure, a flexible tube is inserted into

the rectum and water is slowly pumped into the intestine. The pressure is regulated in order to avoid injury. Alternation of warm and cool water leads to contraction and relaxation of the intestinal walls, which helps to remove impacted pieces of dry feces from the walls. Feces, gas, mucus, and bacteria exit through the same tube. A cleaner internal surface of the colon provides more surface area for the absorption of nutrients and water. Approximately 20 gallons of water are used in the procedure, which lasts about one hour.

USES AND COMPLICATIONS

Irrigation of the entire colon came into prominence during the late nineteenth century in Russia. In the United States, John Harvey Kellogg espoused colonic irrigation along with other health and fitness regimes at his sanatorium in Battle Creek, Michigan, in the early twentieth century. The procedure fell into obscurity during the late 1940's, when medical research indicated no benefit to the procedure. Renewed interest in colonics in the late twentieth century led to the establishment of the International Association for Colon Hydrotherapy, which provides training and certification for practitioners. While colon therapy regained enthusiastic followers, mainstream physicians point out that waste products in the colon cannot "toxify" the body. They also believe that colonics may interfere with the natural balance of helpful bacteria that keep the intestines functioning normally.

After a procedure, some patients report feeling energized and lighter, while others report nausea, headaches, or flulike symptoms. These symptoms generally subside within a few hours. Other side effects may include diarrhea and a loss of necessary intestinal bacteria.

—*Karen E. Kalumuck, Ph.D.;*
updated by LeAnna DeAngelo, Ph.D.

See also Alternative medicine; Colon; Gastrointestinal system; Hydrotherapy; Intestines; Preventive medicine.

FOR FURTHER INFORMATION:

Collings, Jillie. *Principles of Colonic Irrigation: The Only Introduction You'll Ever Need.* New York: Thorsons, 1996.

Goldberg, Burton, John Anderson, and Larry Trivieri, eds. *Alternative Medicine: The Definitive Guide.* 2d ed. Berkeley, Calif.: Celestial Arts, 2002.

Jonas, Wayne, ed. *Mosby's Dictionary of Complementary and Alternative Medicine.* St. Louis, Mo.: Mosby/Elsevier, 2005.

COLONOSCOPY AND SIGMOIDOSCOPY

PROCEDURES

ANATOMY OR SYSTEM AFFECTED: Gastrointestinal system, intestines

SPECIALTIES AND RELATED FIELDS: Gastroenterology, general surgery

DEFINITION: The insertion of a flexible tube into the rectum to look at the inside surface of the colon.

KEY TERMS:

biopsy: removal of a piece of tissue for examination under a microscope

colitis: inflammation of the inner surface of the colon

lumen: the space inside a tubelike structure such as the colon

mucosa: the layer of tissue that lines the inside of a tubelike structure such as the colon

polyp: a small piece of tissue that extends from the surface of the colon into the lumen

INDICATIONS AND PROCEDURES

Colonoscopy and sigmoidoscopy are common procedures to evaluate the lower part of the gastrointestinal tract. Colonoscopy refers to examination of the entire large bowel, whereas sigmoidoscopy examines only the part closest to the rectum (known as the sigmoid colon). The advantage of sigmoidoscopy is that it is less time-consuming and can be performed without sedation. Since sigmoidoscopy evaluates only part of the colon, however, full colonoscopy is often preferred. The most common reason for having a colonoscopy is to screen for colon cancer. If sigmoidoscopy is used for this purpose, it must be combined with a barium enema and an X ray to evaluate the upper part of the colon.

Prior to colonoscopy, the bowel must be cleaned of stool to enable the physician to see the underlying mucosa. Patients are often asked to go on a diet of clear liquids (such as chicken broth, gelatin, and juice) for one to three days prior to the procedure. The night before the procedure, patients ingest a purgative to clear out any residual stool. The two most common preparations are polyethylene glycol (GoLytely) and a sodium phosphate mix (Fleet Phospho-Soda). Following ingestion of these solutions, patients should have clear or very light-colored liquid bowel movements. Regular medications that may cause excessive bleeding from biopsy sites, such as aspirin, warfarin, and nonsteroidal anti-inflammatory drugs (NSAIDs), are often discontinued prior to the procedure. Patients should also discontinue iron supplements, since they may create a black coating

IN THE NEWS: RISKS OF FLAT LESIONS IN INTESTINAL LINING

Approximately 0.3 percent to 0.9 percent of patients develop colon cancer a few years after having a successful colonoscopy or sigmoidoscopy. Doctors, once puzzled by this response, now attribute at least some cancer occurrence to undetected or inadequately removed flat or depressed lesions in the intestinal lining. These lesions were previously thought to be harmless. However, a study published in March, 2008, in the *Journal of the American Medical Association* cautioned that flat or depressed growths are five times more likely to be cancerous than other more easily identified lesions such as polyps.

Flat or depressed lesions are often smaller than polyps and the same color as the colon. Consequently, they innocently blend right into the surrounding healthy colon tissue. These growths also occur infrequently, comprising only 15 percent of the total lesions detected in males. They occur even less often in the female population. The danger of flat or depressed lesions makes it even more imperative that patients follow the pretest cleansing routine carefully. Remaining waste, no matter how small, may cover and hide a serious growth.

To detect flat or depressed lesions, physicians must be trained to do the test slowly, carefully look for the growths, and inject a blue dye into the colon to define the lesion. Doctors must also learn new techniques to ensure that the growths are completely removed. Physicians are encouraged to track their own success rate in detecting these difficult lesions.

Increasingly popular virtual or relatively noninvasive colonoscopies use computed tomography (CT) to detect polyps that rise from the colon wall. However, CT is not sensitive enough to detect flat or depressed lesions. Promising new techniques to readily identify these growths include narrow-band imaging, a novel illumination technology, zoom magnification, and high-definition processor technology.

—*Renée Euchner, R.N.*

colonoscope also has channels to administer air or water, as well as a suction channel. Air is introduced to expand the walls of the colon, enabling better viewing. Water is used to remove residual stool that may obstruct the view of the colon. The colonoscope is advanced to the cecum (the first part of the large bowel) or even the terminal ileum (the last part of the small bowel). The instrument is then slowly withdrawn while any abnormalities in the mucosa are noted. Following the procedure, patients are often observed for a period of time to make sure that no complications occur. If sedative medications were used, patients should not drive or operate machinery for the rest of the day.

USES AND COMPLICATIONS

In addition to screening for colon cancer, colonoscopy and sigmoidoscopy can be used to evaluate blood in the stool, chronic diarrhea or other changes in bowel habits, and unexplained abdominal pain. Common findings include polyps, which may be biopsied. It is common practice to remove a polyp completely, in case it turns out to be the precancerous type (known as an adenomatous polyp). Other findings include diverticula, small outpouchings of the colon which have very thin walls and are prone to spontaneous bleeding. They may also become infected, resulting in a condition known as diverticulitis. Other findings during colonoscopy may be useful in establishing the presence of a particular disease. Yellowish pseudo-membranes line the gut in colitis associated with the bacterium *Clostridium difficile*. A dusky hue is often seen in cases of ischemic colitis caused by diminished blood supply to the colon. Characteristic findings are also seen in inflammatory bowel disease.

Colonoscopy is a very safe procedure. One common aftereffect is abdominal discomfort as a result of the air used to distend the colon. This condition usually re-

that makes it difficult for the physician to see the mucosa.

When patients enter the colonoscopy suite, they are given an intravenous (IV) catheter to administer fluids, as well as sedative and analgesic medications. Patients are asked not to eat or drink anything the day of the procedure. Sedative medications sometimes cause nausea, and any food that is present in the stomach may be vomited. Blood pressure, pulse, and oxygen saturation are monitored throughout the procedure. The patient is positioned on his or her left side, and a colonoscope is inserted through the rectum into the colon. The colonoscope is a long, flexible tube with a fiber-optic channel connected to a camera. The image of the inside of the colon is transmitted to a television screen. The

solves over a few hours as the air is passed. The most serious complications of colonoscopy are perforation and bleeding. Perforation refers to a hole in the colon. It is an extremely rare occurrence, but it can be deadly. Patients with perforations often have severe abdominal pain and a rigid abdomen. If it is large and results in free air in the abdomen, a perforation requires emergency surgery. Rarely, very small perforations can be treated with observation and antibiotics. Bleeding is a risk if a biopsy is taken during the procedure. Most of the time, the bleeding stops by itself, but in some cases repeat colonoscopy may be required to control the bleeding. Rarely, bleeding may occur a few hours to several days after colonoscopy, so patients should report these symptoms to their physician. Whenever sedation is used, there is a risk of too much being given, which can lead to respiratory or cardiac arrest. Other possible complications include pain and inflammation at the site of the catheter and allergic reactions to sedative or analgesic medications.

—*Ahmad Kamal, M.D.*

See also Colon; Colorectal cancer; Colorectal polyp removal; Colorectal surgery; Diverticulitis and diverticulosis; Endoscopy; Enemas; Gastroenterology; Gastrointestinal system; Intestines; Invasive tests; Oncology; Proctology; Screening; Tumor removal; Tumors.

FOR FURTHER INFORMATION:

Church, James M. *Endoscopy of the Colon, Rectum, and Anus.* New York: Igaku-Shoin, 1995.
Drossman, Douglas A., et al., eds. *Handbook of Gastroenterologic Procedures.* 4th ed. Philadelphia: Lippincott Williams & Wilkins, 2005.
Waye, Jerome D., Douglas K. Rex, and Christopher B. Williams, eds. *Colonoscopy: Principles and Practice.* 2d ed. Malden, Mass.: Blackwell, 2009.

COLOR BLINDNESS
DISEASE/DISORDER

ANATOMY OR SYSTEM AFFECTED: Eyes
SPECIALTIES AND RELATED FIELDS: Brain, optometry
DEFINITION: An inability to distinguish certain colors resulting from an inherited defect in the light receptor cells in the retina of the eye.

CAUSES AND SYMPTOMS

The retina of the eye is a thin, fragile membrane that contains millions of photoreceptor cells. They convert light energy into an electrical signal, which is transmitted to the brain via the optic nerve. On a microscopic

---

INFORMATION ON COLOR BLINDNESS

CAUSES: Genetic defect resulting in photoreceptor deficiency
SYMPTOMS: Inability to distinguish between certain colors (red, orange, yellow, green)
DURATION: Lifelong
TREATMENTS: None

---

scale, the structure of the retina is like a carpet with its many fibers sticking upward. There are two types of photoreceptor cells, called rods and cones because of their distinctive shapes. Only the cones are important for color vision. There are three varieties of cones with peak sensitivities for red, green, and blue, respectively. The shades and tints of all other colors are mixtures of these three.

Color blindness involves a deficiency in these photoreceptor cells. A deficiency of green photoreceptor cells is much more common than a deficiency of red photoreceptors. Some people are totally color-blind, which means that they are completely unable to distinguish among red, orange, yellow, and green. Color blindness is quite rare in females (less than 1 percent of the population) but is more prevalent in males (about 8 percent).

Diagnostic tests are available to determine the extent of color blindness. The Ishihara color test, named after a Japanese ophthalmologist, consists of a mosaic of colored dots containing a letter of the alphabet made up of dots of a different color—for example, yellow dots in a background of green ones. Color-blind individuals would be unable to distinguish the letter because yellow and green look the same to them.

A more precise diagnostic test makes use of the Nagel anomaloscope, which has two colored light sources whose brightness can be adjusted. The patient tries to match a given color by superimposing the two light beams while varying their intensities. For normal eyes, red and green lights of similar intensities can be superimposed to create yellow. However, a patient who requires a considerably larger green component to create yellow evidently has a deficiency of green photoreceptor cells.

TREATMENT AND THERAPY

Color blindness is a genetic defect from birth, not a disease. No procedure is known by which it can be corrected. Color-blind people must find ways to counter the effects of their condition. For example, they can obtain driver's licenses because they learn that stoplights are always red on top, yellow in the middle, and green on the bottom. Color-blind individuals may need help, however, with tasks such as clothing selection. Good color discrimination is required for some occupations, such as interior decorating, graphic design, advertising, or airplane piloting. Fortunately, color blindness is not a deterrent for most jobs.

—Hans G. Graetzer, Ph.D.

See also Eye infections and disorders; Eyes; Genetic diseases; Vision; Vision disorders.

FOR FURTHER INFORMATION:

Cameron, John R., James G. Skofronick, and Roderick M. Grant. *Medical Physics: Physics of the Body.* Madison, Wis.: Medical Physics, 1992.

Kasper, Dennis L., et al., eds. *Harrison's Principles of Internal Medicine.* 16th ed. New York: McGraw-Hill, 2005.

"Vision." In *Encyclopaedia Brittanica.* 15th ed. Chicago: Encyclopaedia Britannica, 2002.

COLORECTAL CANCER
DISEASE/DISORDER

ALSO KNOWN AS: Large bowel cancer

ANATOMY OR SYSTEM AFFECTED: Abdomen, anus, gastrointestinal system, intestines, lymphatic system

SPECIALTIES AND RELATED FIELDS: Gastroenterology, genetics, immunology, oncology, proctology

DEFINITION: Cancer occurring in the large intestine, which is the second deadliest type of this disease.

CAUSES AND SYMPTOMS

With an estimated sixty thousand deaths per year in the United States, cancer of the colon and rectum is the second most deadly cancer, ranking only behind lung cancer. About 90 percent of colorectal cancers arise from the glandular epithelium lining the inner surface of the large bowel and are termed adenocarcinomas. The cells of this layer are constantly being replaced by new cells. This fairly rapid cell division, along with the relatively hostile environment within the bowel, promotes internal cellular errors that lead to the formation of aberrant cells. These cells can become disordered and produce abnormal growths or tumors. Often, colorectal tumors protrude into the lumen (the spaces within the bowel), forming growths called polyps. Some polyps are be-

---

INFORMATION ON COLORECTAL CANCER

CAUSES: Hereditary and/or environmental factors, dietary habits, colon polyps, long-standing ulcerative colitis

SYMPTOMS: Fatigue, weakness, shortness of breath, change in bowel habits, narrow stools, diarrhea or constipation, red or dark blood in stool, weight loss, abdominal pain, cramps, bloating

DURATION: Chronic

TREATMENTS: Surgery, chemotherapy, radiation

---

nign and do not spread to other parts of the body, but they may still disturb normal bowel functions. Other polyps become malignant by forming more aggressive cell types, which allows them to grow larger and spread to other organs. The cancer can grow through the layers of the colon wall and extend into the body cavity and nearby organs such as the urinary bladder. Cancer cells can also break away from the main tumor and spread (metastasize) through the blood or lymphatic vessels to other organs, such as the lungs or liver. If not controlled, the spreading cancer eventually causes death by impairment of organ and system functions.

The tendency to develop colorectal polyps and cancer can be inherited; this genetic predisposition may be responsible for about 5 to 7 percent of all colorectal cancers. One example is an inherited disorder called familial adenomatous polyposis (FAP), in which multiple polyps develop in the colon; it often leads to colorectal cancer. Some of the defective genes that cause this and other types of colorectal cancers have been identified and are being studied to determine their role. The interplay between the various oncogenes (mutated cell division and growth genes) and tumor suppressor genes (cell division and growth inhibitor genes) has been determined. Whether inherited or caused by carcinogens, damage to these specific genetic regions disrupts the delicate balance that regulates orderly and perfectly timed cell reproduction and development, producing cancer cells. Irritable bowel syndrome (IBS) and exposure to certain occupational carcinogens are also known to increase the risk.

TREATMENT AND THERAPY

The chances for survival are greatly increased when colorectal cancer is detected and treated at an early stage. Early detection in the general population is possible with the use of a number of available medical tests: digital rectal examination, in which the physician checks the inner surface of the rectal wall with a gloved finger for abnormal growths; fecal occult blood test, in which a stool sample is tested for hidden blood that may have emanated from a cancerous growth; sigmoid-oscopy, in which the physician examines the rectal and lower-colon inner lining with a narrow tubular optical instrument inserted through the anus; colonoscopy, in which an optical instrument, inserted through the anus, assesses more of the colon and can remove tissue for pathological examination; virtual colonoscopy, which is a noninvasive test to assess the colon through use of X rays; and double contrast barium enema, in which X rays are taken after a liquid containing barium is put into the rectum. Newer screening tests, called fecal DNA testing, continue to be under study. These tests look for early genetic changes in the colon cells that are sloughed off into the stool.

Once cancer is suspected, further tests will be done to arrive at a diagnosis. These tests may include a computed tomography (CT) scan, double-contrast barium enema X-ray series, and colonoscopy. The CT scan and contrast X rays reveal abnormal growths, and colo-noscopy is similar to sigmoidoscopy but uses a longer, flexible tube in order to inspect the entire colon. During sigmoidoscopy and colonoscopy, the physician can re-move polyps and obtain tissue samples for biopsy. Mi-croscopic examination of the tissue samples by a pa-thologist can determine the stage or extent of growth of the cancer. This is important because it helps determine the type of treatment. In one type of staging, the follow-ing criteria are used: stage 0 (cancer confined to epithe-lium lining of the bowel), stage 1 (cancer confined to the bowel wall), stage 2 (cancer penetrating through all layers of the bowel wall and possibly invading adjacent tissues), stage 3 (cancer invading lymph nodes and/or adjacent tissues), and stage 4 (cancer spreading to dis-tant sites, forming metastases).

Surgery is the primary treatment for colorectal can-

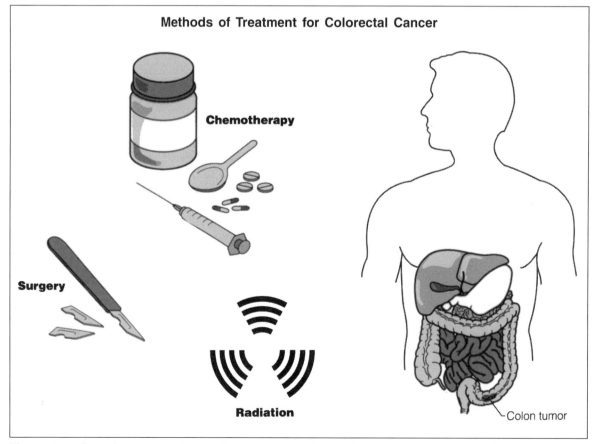

Methods of Treatment for Colorectal Cancer

Chemotherapy

Surgery

Radiation

Colon tumor

The presence of a malignant tumor in the colon requires some form of treatment or a combination of treatments, usually beginning with its surgical removal and followed by radiation therapy and/or chemotherapy (the use of anticancer drugs).

cer. Very small tumors in stage 0 can be removed surgically with the colonoscope. Tumors in more advanced stages require abdominal surgery in which the tumor is removed along with a portion of the bowel and possibly some lymph nodes. For cases in which the bowel cannot be reconnected, an opening is created through the abdominal wall (colostomy). This is usually a temporary procedure, and the hole will be closed when the bowel can be rejoined. Some advanced cancers cannot be cured by surgery alone. Adjuvant therapies—chemotherapy, radiation therapy, and biological therapy—may be used in combination with surgery. Chemotherapy drugs kill spreading cancer cells. The most common is 5-fluorouracil (5-FU), a chemical that interferes with the production of deoxyribonucleic acid (DNA) in dividing cells. 5-FU is more effective when given together with leucovorin (a compound similar to folic acid) and levamisole (an immune system stimulant).

In 2002, the Food and Drug Administration (FDA) approved the use of the Eloxatin injection in combination with 5-FU and leucovorin for the treatment of patients whose cancer has recurred or become worse following initial drug therapy. This approach was shown to shrink tumors in some patients and delay resumed tumor growth. Levamisole and other treatments that reinforce the immune system are forms of biological therapy. Radiation therapy, given either before or after surgery, is helpful in killing undetected cancer cells near the site of the tumor.

Perspective and Prospects

More than 150,000 new cases of colorectal cancer are diagnosed in the United States each year, or roughly 15 percent of all cancers. The incidence of colorectal cancer is lower among females than males and rises dramatically after the age of fifty. Colorectal cancer is more common in developed countries such as the United States and in densely populated, industrialized regions. American mortality rates from colorectal cancer are higher in the Northeast and north-central regions of the country than in the South and Southwest. Populations moving from low-risk parts of the world, such as Asia or Africa, to high-risk areas, such as the United States or Europe, take on the higher risk within a generation or two, and vice versa.

Research is ongoing in discerning the risk factors of and creating treatments for colorectal cancers. Recent epidemiological evidence has supported the use of nonsteroidal anti-inflammatory drugs (NSAIDs) as a means of reducing the risk of cancers of the colon and rectum, as well as the risk of intestinal cancers resulting from exposure to carcinogens. The studies focused only on the daily use of aspirin, but similar results have been reported following long-term use of sulindac and indomethacin. Sulindac has shown an ability to induce regression of colon polyps in patients with familial adenomatous polyposis. Researchers are still working on finding the right balance in dose and frequency since sulindac has potentially severe side effects and aspirin may induce bleeding if high doses are maintained on a daily basis.

—*Rodney C. Mowbray, Ph.D.;*
updated by Connie Rizzo, M.D., Ph.D.

See also Biopsy; Cancer; Chemotherapy; Colon; Colon therapy; Colonoscopy and sigmoidoscopy; Colorectal polyp removal; Colorectal surgery; Ileostomy and colostomy; Intestinal disorders; Intestines; Malignancy and metastasis; National Cancer Institute (NCI); Oncology; Radiation therapy; Rectum; Stomach, intestinal, and pancreatic cancers; Tumor removal; Tumors.

For Further Information:

Adrouny, Richard. *Understanding Colon Cancer.* Jackson: University Press of Mississippi, 2002. An excellent lay guide to the disease, offering information on topics such as diagnosis, prognosis, treatment, demographics, high-risk conditions, the sequence from bowel polyps to cancer, the warning signs, the stages of the disease, and theories of how colon cancer spreads.

American Cancer Society (ACS). http://www.cancer.org. Web site is divided into sections for patients, family, and friends; survivors; health information seekers; ACS supporters; and professionals. Information on all cancers is wide ranging.

Bub, David S., et al. *One Hundred Questions and Answers About Colorectal Cancer.* Sudbury, Mass.: Jones and Bartlett, 2003. Provides authoritative answers to questions about treatment options, posttreatment quality of life, and sources of support.

De Vita, Vincent T., Jr., Samuel Hellman, and Steven A. Rosenberg, eds. *Cancer: Principles and Practice of Oncology.* 8th ed. Philadelphia: Lippincott Williams & Wilkins, 2008. This thoroughly revised and updated classic reflects the latest breakthroughs in every aspect of oncology, from molecular biology, to multimodality treatment, to new data on cancer prevention by drugs and diet.

Dollinger, Malin, et al. *Everyone's Guide to Cancer Therapy.* 5th ed. Kansas City, Mo.: Andrews McMeel, 2008. An excellent source of medical information about cancer, written for the general public. Describes various cancer sites in the body. Includes a helpful glossary of medical terminology.

Eyre, Harmon J., Dianne Partie Lange, and Lois B. Morris. *Informed Decisions: The Complete Book of Cancer Diagnosis, Treatment, and Recovery.* 2d ed. Atlanta: American Cancer Society, 2002. The American Cancer Society endorses this excellent book, which provides a complete consumer reference for cancer diagnosis, treatment, and recovery. From assessing different therapy options and coping with stress and depression, this provides an excellent all-around survey of cancer's special decision-making requirements.

Goldman, Lee, and Dennis Ausiello, eds. *Cecil Textbook of Medicine.* 23d ed. Philadelphia: Saunders/Elsevier, 2007. This is a standard textbook of medicine. Although it is somewhat difficult, it is complete, beginning with normal conditions and progressing through disease process, diagnosis, and treatment.

Levin, Bernard, et al., eds. *American Cancer Society's Complete Guide to Colorectal Cancer.* Atlanta: American Cancer Society, 2006. An accessible guide with a foreword by journalist Katie Couric.

Miskovitz, Paul, and Marian Betancourt. *What to Do If You Get Colon Cancer: A Specialist Helps You Take Charge and Make Informed Choices.* New York: Wiley, 1997. Designed for patients and families of patients with colon cancer, this volume has three sections: discovery, treatment, and recovery. The appendixes are useful, containing information on financial aid and insurance considerations.

Parker, James N., and Philip M. Parker, eds. *The Official Patient's Sourcebook on Colon Cancer.* San Diego, Calif.: Icon Health, 2002. Draws from public, academic, government, and peer-reviewed research to provide a wide-ranging reference about the causes, treatments, and risk factors of colon cancer.

COLORECTAL POLYP REMOVAL

PROCEDURE

ANATOMY OR SYSTEM AFFECTED: Abdomen, anus, gastrointestinal system, intestines

SPECIALTIES AND RELATED FIELDS: Gastroenterology, general surgery, proctology

DEFINITION: The surgical removal of overgrowths of the tissue lining the rectum and colon.

INDICATIONS AND PROCEDURES

Rectal and colon polyps are growths of tissue that occur in the mucous membranes lining the colon and rectum. They are usually not malignant. Common types of colorectal polyps are juvenile polyps, Peutz-Jeghers polyps (hamartomas), hyperplasias, adenomas, and mixed hyperplastic-adenomatous polyps. Adenomas are both the most dangerous and the most common type of colon polyp.

Rectal or colon polyps are removed when they are found, even if they cause no symptoms, because identifying the kind of polyp helps doctors determine whether cancer is likely to develop. The type of polyp is determined in the laboratory after surgical removal, using microscopic techniques.

The presence of polyps does not mean that a patient has cancer, although larger polyps (greater than 1 centimeter) indicate a higher risk for cancer than do smaller ones. Certain types of polyps also are more likely than others to develop into cancer. Hyperplasias are polyps with no potential to develop into cancer. Juvenile polyps and Peutz-Jeghers polyps are associated with inherited disorders that indicate an increased risk for colon cancer, but they do not always develop into malignant tumors. Colorectal adenomas are particularly dangerous when they occur in conjunction with a genetic condition known as familial adenomatous polyposis (FAP). In patients with FAP, untreated colorectal adenomas develop into colon cancer virtually 100 percent of the time. Mixed hyperplastic-adenomatous polyps, although not as risky as pure adenomas, can develop into colon cancer, and patients with a diagnosis of this type of polyp should be closely monitored.

Colon polyps often cause no symptoms. They are usually detected by routine screening for colorectal cancers. The most common symptoms, when they occur, are bleeding from the anus (visible on underwear or toilet paper), constipation or diarrhea lasting more than a week, and blood in the stool, which can appear as red streaks or an overall darkening of fecal matter. The fecal occult blood test will detect blood that is not visible.

When polyps are suspected, the physician will perform a rectal examination or special tests such as barium enema X rays, flexible sigmoidoscopy, or colonoscopy. In a rectal examination, the doctor feels the rectal tissue with his fingers, looking for abnormalities. Barium makes healthy intestinal tissue look white on an X ray, and polyps appear dark against the white background. The sigmoidoscope is a flexible fiber-optic tube that can be inserted through the anus. The tube has a light and small video camera so that the doctor can visualize the lower third of the large intestine. Colonoscopy is similar to sigmoidoscopy, but the colonoscope allows the physician to visualize the entire intestine.

Removal is most commonly accomplished using colonoscopy to visualize the polyps and specialized forceps to detach and remove the growths. Snare forceps can be used to surround a polyp and cut it from the lining of the colon or rectum. Other methods of removal include a laser beam, burning, or ultrasound, depending on the size of the polyp. Bleeding during the procedure can be controlled with electrocautery forceps, which use heat to sever the polyp from the surrounding healthy tissue and seal off blood vessels, or by pressing epinephrine-soaked gauze against the removal site.

Special precautions must be taken during surgery to remove gas from the colon so that the combustion of hydrogen or methane gas does not occur. These gases are normally produced by bacteria that inhabit the colon.

A polyp in the lower portion of the colon may be removed using similar procedures during the sigmoidoscopy. In some cases, the patient may undergo surgery to remove the polyp through the abdomen.

USES AND COMPLICATIONS

Since colonoscopy is somewhat uncomfortable for the patient, sedatives are usually given, but general anesthesia is usually not necessary. Rectal and colon polyp removal is typically done as an outpatient procedure.

Because of the gas that enters the intestine during the procedure, patients may experience bloating, pressure, and intestinal cramps in the twenty-four hours following removal. This discomfort subsides as the gas passes out of the intestine.

Repeat colonoscopy should be performed so that recurrent polyps can be removed and examined for malignancy. Colorectal cancer is the second leading cause of cancer deaths in the United States, and the majority of these cancers arise from colorectal polyps.

—*Matthew Berria, Ph.D.,*
and Douglas Reinhart, M.D.;
updated by Caroline M. Small
See also Biopsy; Cancer; Colon; Colonoscopy and sigmoidoscopy; Colorectal cancer; Colorectal surgery; Electrocauterization; Endoscopy; Enemas; Gastroenterology; Gastrointestinal system; Hemorrhoid banding and removal; Hemorrhoids; Intestinal disorders; Intestines; Oncology; Polyps; Proctology; Rectum; Screening.

FOR FURTHER INFORMATION:

American Cancer Society. *American Cancer Society's Complete Guide to Colorectal Cancer.* New York: Author, 2005.
Burke, Carol, and James Church, eds. *Hereditary Colorectal Cancer Syndromes.* New York: Blackwell, 2007.
Corman, Marvin L. *Colon and Rectal Surgery.* 5th ed. Philadelphia: Lippincott Williams & Wilkins, 2005.
Longo, Walter E., and John M. A. Northover, eds. *Reoperative Colon and Rectal Surgery.* New York: Martin Dunitz, 2003.
National Institutes of Health. National Cancer Institute. *Cancer of the Colon and Rectum.* Rev. ed. Bethesda, Md.: Author, 1991.
_____. *What You Need to Know About Cancer of the Colon and Rectum.* Rev. ed. Bethesda, Md.: Author, 1999.
Zollinger, Robert M., Jr., and Robert M. Zollinger, Sr. *Zollinger's Atlas of Surgical Operations.* 8th ed. New York: McGraw-Hill, 2003.

COLORECTAL SURGERY
PROCEDURE

ANATOMY OR SYSTEM AFFECTED: Abdomen, anus, gastrointestinal system, intestines

SPECIALTIES AND RELATED FIELDS: Gastroenterology, general surgery, proctology

DEFINITION: Surgery that is required to correct pathologies of the colon, rectum, and anus.

KEY TERMS:
abscess: a pocket of infection or inflammation
acute: referring to a short, immediate disease state
chronic: referring to an enduring disease state
ulcer: a lesion that destroys tissue

INDICATIONS AND PROCEDURES

The large intestine, or colon, is shaped like an inverted *U.* It starts at the lower right side of the pelvis, where the small intestine empties into the cecum. The colon rises from the cecum to the center of the abdomen, crosses to the left, and descends to the S-shaped sigmoid colon, the rectum, and the anus. Common disorders of the colon, rectum, and anus that require surgery are hemorrhoids, Crohn's disease, ulcerative colitis, cancer, diverticulosis, and diverticulitis.

Hemorrhoids are swollen veins in the lower part of the rectum and the anus. They protrude as nodes or lumps that can cause severe pain, itching, and inflammation. Hemorrhoids can be tied off with tiny rubber bands. After a few days, they fall off painlessly. Medications can shrink internal hemorrhoids, or hemorrhoidal tissue can be removed by photocoagulation, a process that uses electromagnetic energy to eradicate affected tissues. Sometimes, a hemorrhoidectomy is required. This procedure involves the extensive excision of hemorrhoidal tissue and can be quite painful.

Crohn's disease and ulcerative colitis are chronic inflammatory bowel diseases (IBDs) that can affect the colon. Crohn's disease usually occurs in the small intestine, although it may be limited to the colon. When Crohn's disease is severe and restricted to the colon, the surgeon may perform a colectomy and ileostomy. This procedure involves removing the entire lower intestine, rectum, and anus. The anal opening is closed, and a new opening, or stoma, is made in the abdominal wall. The ileum, the lower end of the small intestine, is then attached to the opening. A removable pouch is sealed to the opening to collect fecal matter, which must be emptied manually.

Ulcerative colitis may exist with no symptoms other than an occasional flare-up, or it can be a chronic, serious, or life-threatening disease. It is characterized by a series of ulcers on the inner wall of the colon. Bloody diarrhea, abdominal pain, and painful bowel movements are symptoms. In severe cases, there is danger of perforation of the colon wall or of swelling (toxic megacolon), either of which can be life-threatening. Ulcerative colitis may also be a precursor of colon cancer. In severe cases of ulcerative colitis, surgery is required. Colectomy and ileostomy are the surgical procedures usually performed, but recently developed is a procedure called ileoanal anastomosis. As in ileostomy, the surgeon removes the entire colon and rectum but leaves the anal sphincter muscles. The ileum is then attached to the anus. This procedure allows the patient to have natural bowel movements and avoids the necessity of the ileostomy pouch.

Cancers of the colon or rectum, called colorectal cancers, are major causes of morbidity and mortality. The possibility of colon cancer is often signaled by the presence of polyps on the lower intestinal wall. Symptoms such as mucus or blood in the stool may alert the physician to look for polyps and determine whether they are likely to become cancerous. Benign polyps are usually removed surgically.

When polyps are likely to become cancerous, and in the presence of actual colorectal cancer, surgery is usually performed to remove diseased tissue. This often requires excising part or all of the colon. Sometimes a colectomy and colostomy are performed, an operation similar to an ileostomy. In this procedure, the diseased sections of the colon, the rectum, and the anus are removed. The anal opening is sealed, and the remaining colon is brought to an opening in the abdominal wall. This opening, or stoma, is fitted with a removable colostomy bag or pouch to collect fecal matter.

Diverticula are small, saclike pouches that develop in the colon wall, most often in the sigmoid colon. Their presence is known as diverticulosis. These sacs can collect stagnant fecal matter and become inflamed, resulting in diverticulitis. Abscesses and infection may develop. As inflammation progresses or recurs, the wall of the colon thickens, reducing the width of the passage and increasing the possibility of obstruction and distension of the colon. Perforations in the colon wall may develop and cause peritonitis (infection of the membrane that covers the abdomen).

In severe cases, it may be necessary to perform a temporary colostomy. The diseased section of colon is removed, and the rectum and anus are closed. A stoma is made in the abdominal wall and attached to the remaining colon and covered by a pouch to collect fecal matter. After the bowel has healed, the rectum and anus can be reopened and attached to the colon.

Uses and Complications

Patients with permanent ileostomies and colostomies have a hole in their abdomens that is often 5 or more centimeters (2 or more inches) in diameter. Patients are required to wear removable pouches sealed to their stomas to collect fecal matter so that it can be eliminated. The apparatus is cumbersome, and the entire process can be unpleasant enough to cause serious depression in the patient. Patients' spouses and other family members are often involved in changing and emptying the bags, particularly with older, infirm persons. Ileoanal anastomosis solves some of these problems because it allows natural bowel movements, but it is useful only in certain conditions.

Perspective and Prospects

Current surgical procedures are often effective in serious colorectal conditions. The success rate of these surgeries for the treatment of cancer is quite high if the cancer is caught before it spreads to other parts of the body. Nevertheless, patients may have to endure the inconvenience of ostomy bags and paraphernalia for the rest of their lives. Ostomy equipment has been improved: Better sealing adhesives are now in use so that the bags do not slip or leak as they once did. The configuration of belts, bags, and other appliances has been altered to make them more convenient and easier to live with. New surgical procedures that could maintain normal bowel function for more patients, however, would be a major advancement.

—*C. Richard Falcon*

See also Abdomen; Abdominal disorders; Biopsy; Cancer; Colitis; Colon; Colonoscopy and sigmoidoscopy; Colorectal cancer; Colorectal polyp removal; Crohn's disease; Diverticulitis and diverticulosis; Electrocauterization; Endoscopy; Enemas; Fistula repair; Gastroenterology; Gastrointestinal system; Hemorrhoid banding and removal; Hemorrhoids; Hernia repair; Hernias; Ileostomy and colostomy; Intestinal disorders; Intestines; Oncology; Proctology; Rectum; Tumor removal; Tumors.

FOR FURTHER INFORMATION:

Feldman, Mark, Lawrence S. Friedman, and Lawrence J. Brandt, eds. *Sleisenger and Fordtran's Gastrointestinal and Liver Disease: Pathophysiology, Diagnosis, Management.* New ed. 2 vols. Philadelphia: Saunders/Elsevier, 2010. A comprehensive textbook of gastrointestinal diseases and physiology. Contains excellent chapters on all disorders mentioned in the text, as well as some beautiful endoscopic photographs.

Kapadia, Cyrus R., James M. Crawford, and Caroline Taylor. *An Atlas of Gastroenterology: A Guide to Diagnosis and Differential Diagnosis.* Boca Raton, Fla.: Pantheon, 2003. Provides a fully illustrated, nonspecialist understanding of myriad gastrointestinal diseases, including heartburn, dyspepsia, diarrhea, irritable bowel syndrome, and pancreatitis. Includes bibliographic references and an index.

Litin, Scott C., ed. *Mayo Clinic Family Health Book.* 4th ed. New York: HarperResource, 2009. Perhaps the best general medical text for the layperson, this book covers the entire medical field. While the information is derived from a wide variety of highly technical sources, the articles are written to be easily understood by a general audience.

Phillips, Robert H. *Coping with an Ostomy: A Guide to Living with an Ostomy for You and Your Family.* Wayne, N.J.: Avery, 1986. Writing for soon-to-be ostomates, Phillips summarizes types of operations and their typical causes, then concentrates on the emotional and social aspects of living with a stoma.

Zollinger, Robert M., Jr., and Robert M. Zollinger, Sr. *Zollinger's Atlas of Surgical Operations.* 8th ed. New York: McGraw-Hill, 2003. A comprehensive examination of surgery. Covers basic surgical anatomy and vascular, gynecologic, gastrointestinal, and miscellaneous abdominal procedures.

COMA

DISEASE/DISORDER

ANATOMY OR SYSTEM AFFECTED: Brain, head, nervous system, psychic-emotional system

SPECIALTIES AND RELATED FIELDS: Critical care, emergency medicine

DEFINITION: A loss of consciousness from which a person cannot be aroused; a symptom signifying a variety of causes.

KEY TERMS:

alcoholic coma: coma accompanying severe alcohol intoxication

apoplectic coma: coma induced by cerebral, cerebellar, or brain-stem hemorrhage, as well as by embolism or cerebral thrombosis

brain death: irreversible brain damage so extensive that the organ enjoys no potential for recovery and can no longer maintain the body's internal functions

coma: a loss of consciousness from which the patient cannot be aroused

conscious: having an awareness of one's existence

hepatic coma: coma accompanying cerebral damage caused by the degeneration of liver cells (especially that associated with cirrhosis of the liver)

traumatic coma: coma following a head injury

CAUSES AND SYMPTOMS

Consciousness is defined by the normal wakeful state, with its self-aware cognition of past events and future anticipation. Disease or dysfunction that impairs this state usually causes readily identifiable conditions such as coma. The self-aware, cognitive aspects of consciousness depend largely on the interconnected neural networks of the cerebral hemispheres. Normal conscious behavior depends on the continuous, effective interaction of these systems. Loss of consciousness from medical causes can be brief (a matter of minutes to an hour or so) or it can be sustained for many hours, days, or sometimes even weeks. The longer the duration of the comatose state, the more likely it is to reflect

---

INFORMATION ON COMA

CAUSES: Head injury, disease, brain tumor, brain abscess, intracerebral hemorrhage, drug overdose, hypoxia, acute alcoholic intoxication

SYMPTOMS: No response to external stimulation (such as shouting or pinching)

DURATION: Ranges from minutes to several weeks or months

TREATMENTS: Maintenance of oxygenation and circulation, intravenous administration of glucose or thiamine, control of generalized seizures, restoration of blood acid-base and osmolar balance

---

structural damage to the brain rather than a transient alteration in its function.

The word "coma" comes from the Greek *koma*, meaning to put to sleep or to fall asleep. This state of unarousable unresponsiveness results from disturbance or damage to areas of the brain involved in conscious activity or the maintenance of consciousness—particularly parts of the cerebrum (the main mass of the brain), upper parts of the brain stem, and central regions of the brain, especially the limbic system. A wide spectrum of specific conditions can injure the brain and cause coma. The damage to the brain may be the result of a head injury or of an abnormality such as a brain tumor, brain abscess, or intracerebral hemorrhage. Often there has been a buildup of poisonous substances that intoxicates brain tissues. This buildup can occur because of a drug overdose, advanced kidney or liver disease, or acute alcoholic intoxication. Encephalitis (inflammation of the brain) and meningitis (inflammation of the brain coverings) can also cause coma, as can cerebral hypoxia (lack of oxygen in the brain, possibly attributable to the impairment of the blood flow to some areas). Whatever the underlying mechanism, coma indicates brain failure, and the high degree or organization of cerebral biochemical systems has been disrupted. Coma is easily distinguishable from sleep in that the person does not respond to external stimulation (such as shouting or pinching) or to the needs of his or her body (such as a full bladder).

Comas are classified according to the event or condition that caused the comatose state. Some of the most frequently encountered types of comas are traumatic coma, alcoholic coma, apoplectic coma, deanimate coma, diabetic coma, hepatic coma, metabolic coma, vigil coma, pseudo coma, and irreversible coma. Traumatic coma follows a head injury. It enjoys a somewhat more favorable outcome than that of comas associated with medical illness. About 50 percent of patients in a coma from head injuries survive, and the recovery is closely linked to age: The younger the patient, the greater the chance for recovery. Alcoholic coma refers to the coma accompanying severe alcohol intoxication, usually more than 400 milligrams of alcohol per 100 milliliters of blood. This coma is marked by rapid, light respiration, usually with tachycardia and hypotension. Apoplectic coma is induced by cerebral, cerebellar, or brain-stem hemorrhage, as well as by embolism or cerebral thrombosis. The term "deanimate coma" refers to a deep coma with loss of all somatic and autonomic reflex activity. The maintenance of life depends wholly upon such supportive measures as assisted respiration, and cardiac arrest will quickly follow if the respirator is stopped; this may be a transient or irreversible state. Diabetic coma is the coma of severe diabetic acidosis. Hepatic coma is the coma accompanying cerebral damage resulting from degeneration of liver cells, especially that associated with cirrhosis of the liver. "Metabolic coma" is the term applied to the coma occurring in any metabolic disorder in the absence of a demonstrable macroscopic physical abnormality of the brain. Vigil coma is defined as a state of stupor in which the patient is mute and shows no verbal or motor responses to stimuli although the eyes are open and give a false impression of alertness. Pseudo coma refers to states resembling acute unconsciousness but with self-awareness preserved. Irreversible coma, or brain death, occurs when irreversible brain damage is so extensive that the organ enjoys no potential for recovery and can no longer maintain the body's internal functions.

TREATMENT AND THERAPY

Of the acute problems in clinical medicine, none is more difficult than the prompt diagnosis and effective management of the comatose patient. The difficulty exists partly because the causes of coma are so many and partly because the physician possesses only a limited time in which to make the appropriate diagnostic and therapeutic judgment.

Measurements of variations in the depth of coma are important in its assessment and treatment. Varying depths of coma are recognized. In less severe forms, the person may respond to stimulation by, for example, moving an arm. In severe cases, the person fails to respond to repeated vigorous stimuli. Yet even deeply comatose patients may show some automatic responses, as they may continue to breathe unaided or may cough, yawn, blink, or show roving eye movement. These actions indicate that the lower brain stem, which controls these responses, is still functioning.

Assessment of the patient in a coma includes an evaluation of all vital signs, the level of consciousness, neuromuscular responses, and reaction of the pupils to light. In most hospitals, a printed form for neurologic assessment is used to measure and record the patient's responses to stimuli in objective terms. The Glasgow coma scale also provides a standardized tool that aids in assessing a comatose patient and eliminates the use of ambiguous and easily misinterpreted terms such as "unconscious" and "semicomatose." Additional assessment data should include evaluation of the gag and corneal reflexes. Abnormal rigidity and posturing in response to noxious stimuli indicate deep coma.

The definitive treatment of altered states of consciousness requires removing, correcting, or halting the specific process responsible for the state to whatever degree possible. Often, accurate diagnosis and specific therapy require time, and the first priority is to protect the brain from permanent damage.

General treatment measures that apply to all patients include the following: assurance of an adequate airway passage and oxygenation; maintenance of proper circulation; intravenous administration of glucose or thiamine if the patient is undernourished; any measures necessary to stop generalized seizures; the restoration of the blood acid-base and osmolar balance; the treatment of any detected infection; the treatment and control of extreme body temperatures; the administration of specific antidotes for situations such as drug overdoses; control of agitation; and the protection of the corneas.

In the absence of the gag reflex, regurgitation and aspiration are potential problems. Tube feeding, if necessary, must be done slowly and with the head of the bed raised during the feeding and for about half an hour later. Absence of the corneal reflex can inhibit blinking and natural moistening of the eye. The cornea cannot be allowed to dry, since blindness can result; therefore, artificial tears are instilled in the eyes to keep them moist.

Once the cause leading to the comatose state has been determined, the appropriate steps should be taken to minimize or eliminate it whenever possible. For many causes of coma, rapid intervention and treatment can mean recuperation for the patient, such as in the cases of diabetes, removable hematomas, and drug overdose.

Comatose patients are predisposed to all the hazards of immobility, including impairment of skin integrity and the development of ulcers, contractures and joint disabilities, problems related to respiratory and circulatory status, and alterations in fluid and electrolyte balance. All these factors must be taken into consideration when dealing with the comatose patient.

The outcome from severe medical coma depends on its cause and, with the exception of depressant drug poisoning, on the initial severity and extent of neurologic damage. Depressant drug poisoning reflects a state of general anesthesia, and, barring severe complications, almost all patients who survive drug intoxication can recover physically unscathed.

The clinical tests most valuable for estimating the capacity for recovery after medical coma are identical to those used in making the initial diagnosis. Within a few hours or days after the onset of coma, many patients show neurologic signs that can differentiate, with a high probability, the future extremes of either no improvement or the capacity for good recovery. After a period of about six hours (except for patients on drugs), certain neurological findings begin to correlate with the potential for neurologic recovery and can predict the outcome of about one-third of patients who will do badly. By the end of the first day, tests can predict the two-thirds of the patients who will do well. With each successive day, the signs develop greater predictive power. Persistence of coma in an adult for more than four weeks is almost never associated with later complete recovery.

PERSPECTIVE AND PROSPECTS

Attempts to define "coma" must give at least brief consideration to the concepts of consciousness. Consciousness involves not only the reception of stimuli but also the emotional implications of such stimuli, as well as the construction of intricate mental images.

Since the days of the ancient Greeks, people have known that normal conscious behavior depends on intact brain function and that disorders of consciousness are a sign of cerebral insufficiency. The range of awake and intelligent behavior is so rich and variable, however, that clinical abnormalities are difficult to recognize unless there are substantial deviations from the norm. Impaired, reduced, or absent conscious behavior implies the presence of severe brain dysfunction and demands urgent attention if recovery is to be expected.

The brain can tolerate only a limited amount of physical or metabolic injury without suffering irreparable harm, and the longer the failure lasts, the narrower the margin between recovery and the development of permanent neurologic invalidism.

Since such researchers as Pierre Mollaret and Maurice Goulon first examined the question in 1959, many others have tried to establish criteria that would accurately and unequivocally determine that the brain is dead, or about to die no matter what therapeutic measures one undertakes. In 1968, the Harvard Medical School Ad Hoc Committee to Examine the Definition of Brain Death established criteria for determining irreversible coma, or brain death. These criteria are often used to complement the traditional criteria for determining death. All other existing guidelines, such as the Swedish, British, and United States Collaborative Study Criteria, include nearly identical clinical points but contain some differences as to the duration of observation necessary to establish the diagnosis as well as the emphasis to be placed on laboratory procedures in diagnosis.

Techniques such as computed tomography (CT) scanning and electroencephalography (EEG) have transformed the process of diagnosis in clinical neurology, with technology sometimes replacing clinical deduction. The art of diagnosis, however, is to comprehend the whole picture—where the lesion is, what it comprises, and above all, what it is doing to the patient.

Advances in resuscitative medicine have made obsolete the traditional clinical definition of death, that is, the cessation of heartbeat. Cardiac resuscitation can salvage patients after periods of asystole lasting up to several minutes. Cardiopulmonary bypass machines permit the patient's heartbeat to cease for several hours with full clinical recovery after resuscitation. While respiratory depression formerly meant death within minutes, modern mechanical ventilators can maintain pulmonary oxygen exchange indefinitely. Such advances have permitted many patients with formerly lethal cardiac, pulmonary, and neuromuscular disease to return to relatively full and useful lives. Abundant clinical evidence, however, demonstrates that severe damage to the brain can completely destroy the organ's vital functions and capacity to recover, even when the other parts of the body still live. The result has been to switch the emphasis in defining death to a cessation of brain function. Brain death occurs when brain damage is so extensive that the organ has no potential for recovery and cannot maintain the body's internal functions. Countries worldwide have adopted the principle that death occurs when either the brain or the heart irreversibly fails in its functions. In the United States, the time of brain death has been accepted as the time of the person's death in legal terms.

The determination of whether a comatose patient is brain-dead or can possibly recuperate is extremely important. Issues such as organ transplant programs that require donation of healthy organs and the economic and emotional expense involved in the treatment and care of a comatose patient make it critical to know when to fight for life and when to diagnose death.

In carrying out the many details of the physical care and assessment of the comatose patient, health care personnel must not lose sight of the fact that the patient is a fellow human being and a member of a family. One cannot always be sure exactly how much the patients are aware of what is being said or done as care is given. Whatever the level of awareness and response, comatose patients should be told what will be done to and for them, as they deserve the same respect afforded alert and aware patients.

—Maria Pacheco, Ph.D.

See also Brain damage; Concussion; Death and dying; Ethics; Euthanasia; Intensive care unit (ICU); Living will; Unconsciousness.

FOR FURTHER INFORMATION:

Bongard, Frederick, and Darryl Y. Sue, eds. *Current Critical Care Diagnosis and Treatment.* 3d ed. New York: McGraw-Hill Medical, 2008. A medical text that combines medical and surgical perspectives with diagnostic and treatment knowledge. Covers forty topics in critical care basics, medical critical care, and essentials of surgical intensive care and includes information on pregnancy, psychiatric disorders, imaging procedures, and transport, among other topics.

Goldman, Lee, and Dennis Ausiello, eds. *Cecil Textbook of Medicine.* 23d ed. Philadelphia: Saunders/Elsevier, 2007. Offers detailed coverage of numerous medical conditions and a comprehensive presentation of the comatose state. The discussion is technical, however, and requires a good science background.

Leikin, Jerrold B., and Martin S. Lipsky, eds. *American Medical Association Complete Medical Encyclopedia.* New York: Random House Reference, 2003. A concise presentation of numerous medical terms and illnesses. A very good general reference.

Miller, Benjamin F., Claire Brackman Keane, and Marie T. O'Toole. *Miller-Keane Encyclopedia and Dictionary of Medicine, Nursing, and Allied Health.* Rev. 7th ed. Philadelphia: Saunders/Elsevier, 2005. Contains a concise presentation of the topic of coma.

Plum, Fred, and J. B. Posner. *The Diagnosis of Stupor and Coma.* 3d ed. New York: Oxford University Press, 2000. An excellent book dealing in detail with the diagnosis, treatment, and management of the comatose patient. Well organized and easy to read, it also includes an excellent bibliography for individuals who are interested in more specific presentations of the topic.

Ropper, Alan H., et al. *Neurological and Neurosurgical Intensive Care.* 4th ed. Philadelphia: Lippincott Williams & Wilkins, 2004. Covers a range of topics related to neurologic injury, including comas, head injury, myasthenia, electrophysiologic monitoring, and metabolic derangements.

COMMON COLD
DISEASE/DISORDER

ANATOMY OR SYSTEM AFFECTED: Chest, lungs, nose, respiratory system

SPECIALTIES AND RELATED FIELDS: Family medicine, internal medicine, otorhinolarnygology, public health, virology

DEFINITION: A class of viral respiratory infections that form the world's most prevalent illnesses.

KEY TERMS:

acute: referring to a disease process of sudden onset and short duration

chronic: referring to a disease process of long duration and frequent recurrence

coronavirus: a microorganism causing respiratory illness; one of the most prevalent causes of the common cold

pathogen: any disease-causing microorganism

rhinovirus: a microorganism causing respiratory illness; one of the most prevalent causes of the common cold

virus: an extremely small pathogen that can replicate only within a living cell

CAUSES AND SYMPTOMS

One of the reasons that no cure has ever been found for the common cold is that it is caused by literally hundreds of different viruses. More than two hundred distinct strains from eight genera have been identified, and no doubt more will be discovered. Infection by one of

INFORMATION ON COMMON COLD

CAUSES: Viral infection
SYMPTOMS: Fatigue, runny or congested nose, muscle aches, sore throat, coughing, fever
DURATION: Typically several days
TREATMENTS: Bed rest, limiting physical stress, alleviation of symptoms via medications (antihistamines, decongestants, analgesics, cough medicines, etc.)

these viruses may confer immunity to it, but there will still be scores of others to which that individual is not immune. The common cold is usually restricted to the nose and surrounding areas—hence its medical name, rhinitis (*rhin* meaning "nose" and *itis* meaning "inflammation").

Children get the most colds, averaging six to eight per year until they are six years old. From that age, the number diminishes until, for adults, the rate is three to five colds per year. Colds and related respiratory diseases are the largest single cause of lost workdays and school days. Colds and related respiratory diseases are probably the world's most expensive illnesses. In the United States, about a million and a half person-years are lost from work each year; this figure accounts for one-half of all absences. Worldwide, the costs of lost workdays, medications, physician's visits, and the complications that may require extensive medical care are incalculable.

Among the virus types that cause the common cold are rhinovirus, coronavirus, influenza virus, parainfluenza virus, enterovirus, adenovirus, respiratory syncytial virus, and coxsackie virus. They are not all equally responsible for cold infections. Rhinoviruses and coronaviruses between them are thought to cause 25 to 60 percent of all colds. Rhinoviruses appear to be responsible for colds that occur in the peak cold seasons of late spring and early fall. Coronaviruses appear to be responsible for colds that occur when rhinovirus is less active, such as in the late fall, winter, and early spring. Enteroviruses are the most common cause of the "summer cold." During the summer months up to 20 percent of children may be shedding one of these viruses and thus are infective.

A respiratory syncytial virus can cause the common cold in adults; in children it causes much more severe diseases, including pneumonia and bronchiolitis (inflammation of the bronchioles, small air passages in the lungs). Similarly, influenza and parainfluenza viruses, adenoviruses, and enteroviruses can be responsible for rhinitis and sore throat, but they are also capable of causing more serious illnesses such as pneumonia and meningitis.

Viruses are the smallest of the invading microorganisms that cause disease, so small that they are not visible using ordinary microscopes. They can be seen, however, with an electron microscope, and their presence in the body can be detected through various laboratory tests.

Viruses vary enormously in their size and structure. Some consist of three or four proteins with a core of either deoxyribonucleic acid (DNA) or ribonucleic acid (RNA); some have more than fifty proteins and other substances. Viruses can replicate only within living cells. They invade the body and produce disease conditions in different ways. Some travel through the body to find their target host cells. A good example is the measles virus, which enters through the mucous membranes of the nose, throat, and mouth and then finds its way to target tissues throughout the body. Some, such as the viruses that cause the common cold, enter the body through the nasal passages and settle directly into nearby cells.

Rhinoviruses are members of the Picornaviridae family (*pico-* from "piccolo," meaning "very small"; *rna* from RNA, the genetic material that it contains; and

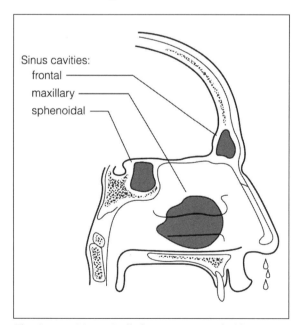

The sinus cavities typically become congested with mucus as the body fights the virus that has caused the cold.

Sinus cavities:
  frontal
  maxillary
  sphenoidal

viridae denoting a virus family). Coronaviruses are members of the Coronaviridae family, and they also contain RNA. Most viruses that are pathogenic to humans can thrive only at the temperature inside the human body, 37 degrees Celsius (98.6 degrees Fahrenheit). Rhinoviruses prefer the cooler temperatures found in the nasal passages, 33 to 34 degrees Celsius (91.4 to 93.2 degrees Fahrenheit). More than one hundred different rhinovirus types have been identified.

Exactly how a patient contracts a cold is better understood than it once was. Exposure to a cold environment—for example, getting a chill in winter weather—does not cause a cold unless the individual is exposed to the infecting virus at the same time. Fatigue or lack of sleep does not increase susceptibility to the cold virus, and even the direct exposure of nasal tissue to cold viruses does not guarantee infection.

A group in England, the Medical Research Council's Common Cold Unit, studied the disease from 1945 to 1990 and made many fundamental discoveries—even though the researchers never found a cure, or, for that matter, any effective methods to prevent the spread of the disease. As part of their research, they put drops containing cold virus into the noses of volunteers. Only about one-third of the subjects thus inoculated developed cold symptoms, showing that direct exposure to the infecting agent does not necessarily bring on a cold.

What appears to be essential in the spread of the disease is bodily contact, particularly handshaking or touching. The infected individual wipes his or her nose or coughs into his or her hand, getting nasal secretions on the fingers. These infected secretions are then transferred to the hand of another person who, if susceptible, can become infected by bringing the hand up to the mouth or nose. Sneezing and coughing also spread the disease. Many viral and bacterial diseases are transmissible through nasopharyngeal (nose and throat) secretions; these include measles, mumps, rubella, pneumonia, influenza, and any number of other infections.

One or more individuals in a group become infected and bring the disease to a central place, such as a classroom, office, military base, or day care center. In the case of the common cold, transferring infected particles by touch exposes another person to the infection. In other respiratory diseases, breathing, sneezing, or coughing virus-laden particles into the air will spread the disease. The infected individual then becomes the means by which the disease is brought into the home. By far, the largest number of colds are brought into the family by children who have contracted the infection in classrooms or day care centers.

The pathogenesis of the common cold—that is, what happens when an individual is exposed to the cold virus—is not fully understood. It is believed that the virus enters the nasal passages and attaches itself to receptors on a cell of the nasal mucous membrane and then invades the cell. Viruses traveling freely in the blood or lymphatic system are subject to attack by white blood cells called phagocytes in what is part of the body's nonspecific defense system against invading pathogens.

Once inside the host cell, the virus replicates itself by stealing elements of the protoplasm of the cell and using them to build new viruses under the direction of the RNA component. These new viruses are released by the host cell to infect other cells. This process can injure or kill the host cell, activating the body's specific immune response system and starting the chain of events that will destroy the invading virus and create immunity to further infection from it.

In response to cell death or injury, certain chemicals are released that induce inflammation in the nasal passages. Blood vessels in the nasal area enlarge, increasing blood flow to the tissues and causing swelling. The openings in capillary walls enlarge and deliver lymphocytes, white blood cells that produce antibodies to fight the virus, as well as other specialized white blood cells.

Nasal mucosa swell and secretions increase, a condition medically known as rhinorrhea (-rrhea meaning "flowing," denoting the runny nose of the common cold). During the first few days of infection, these secretions are thin and watery. As the disease progresses and white blood cells are drawn to the area, the secretions become thicker and more purulent, that is, filled with pus. A sore throat is common, as is laryngitis, or inflammation of the larynx or voice box. Fever is not a usual symptom of the common cold, but a cough will often develop as excess mucus or phlegm builds up in the lungs and windpipe.

As mucus accumulates and clogs nasal passages, the body attempts to expel it by sneezing. In this process, impulses from the nose travel to the brain's "sneeze reflex center," where sneezing is triggered to help clear nasal passages. Similarly, as phlegm accumulates in the windpipe and bronchial tree of the lungs, a message is sent to the "cough reflex center" of the brain, where coughing is initiated to expel the phlegm.

The common cold is self-limiting and usually resolves within five to ten days, but there can be complications in some cases. Patients who have asthma or chronic bronchitis frequently develop bronchoconstriction (narrowing of the air passages in the lungs) as a result of a common cold. If severe purulent tracheitis and bronchitis develop, there may be a concomitant bacterial infection. In some patients, the infection may spread to other organs, such as the ears, where an infection called otitis media can develop. Sinusitis, infection of the cavities in the bone of the skull surrounding the nose, is common. If the invading organism spreads to the lungs, bronchitis or pneumonia may develop.

Other possible complications of the common cold depend on the individual virus. Rhinoviruses, usually limited to colds, may infrequently cause pneumonia in children. Coronaviruses, also usually limited to colds, infrequently cause pneumonia and bronchiolitis. A respiratory syncytial virus causes pneumonia and bronchiolitis in children, the common cold in adults, and pneumonia in the elderly. Parainfluenza virus, which causes croup and other respiratory diseases in children, can cause sore throat and the common cold in adults and, rarely, may cause tracheobronchitis in these patients. Influenza B virus, an occasional cause of the common cold, also causes influenza and, infrequently, pneumonia.

Another condition that can closely resemble the common cold, but which is not caused by a virus, is allergic rhinitis. The major form of allergic rhinitis is hay fever. It has many of the same symptoms as the common cold: sneezing, runny nose, nasal congestion, and, sometimes, sore throat. In addition, the hay fever victim may suffer from itching in the eyes, nose, mouth, and throat. Hay fever is an allergic reaction to certain pollens. Because the pollens that cause hay fever are abundant at certain times of the year, it may be prevalent at the same times as some colds. Spring is a peak season for the common cold and also for hay fever, because of the many tree pollens that are carried in the air. In the fall, weed pollens, such as those of ragweed, affect hay fever sufferers during another peak period for colds. Colds occur less frequently in summer, but summer is another peak season for hay fever.

TREATMENT AND THERAPY

The nose is the first barrier of defense against the bacteria and viruses that cause upper respiratory infections. The nasal cavity is lined with a thin coating of mucus, a thick liquid that is constantly replenished by the mucous glands. Inner nasal surfaces are filled with tiny hairs, or cilia. Dust, bacteria, and other foreign matter are trapped by the mucus and moved by the cilia toward the nasopharynx to be expectorated or swallowed.

The blood vessels in the nasopharyngeal bed respond automatically to stimulation from the brain. Certain stimuli cause the vessels to constrict, widening air passages and at the same time reducing the flow of mucus. Other stimuli, such as those that are sent in response to a viral infection, allergen, or other irritant, cause blood vessels to dilate and increase the flow of mucus. Nasal passages become swollen, and airways are blocked.

The mucus-covered lining of the nasal passages contains various substances that help ward off infection and irritation by allergens. Lysozyme (lyso meaning "dissolution" and zyme from "enzyme," a catalyst that promotes an activity) attacks the cell walls of certain bacteria, killing them. It also attacks pollen granules. Mucus also contains glycoproteins that temporarily inhibit the activity of viruses. Mucus has small amounts of the antibodies immunoglobulin IgA and IgC that also may inhibit the activity of invading viruses.

Bed rest is usually the first element of treatment. Limiting physical stress may help keep the cold from worsening and may avoid secondary infections. The medications used to treat the common cold are directed at relieving individual symptoms: There is nothing available that will kill the viruses that cause it. Most cases of the common cold are treated at home with over-the-counter cold preparations. Children's colds and the complications that may arise from colds, such as bacterial and viral superinfection, may require the services of a physician.

Many medications for the common cold contain antihistamines. Histamine is a naturally occurring chemical in the body that is released in response to an allergen or an infection. It is a significant cause of the inflammation, swelling, and runny nose of hay fever. When these symptoms are seen with the common cold, however, they are probably caused by the body's inflammatory defense system rather than by histamine.

When antihistamines were first discovered, it was thought that they could inhibit the inflammatory defense against a cold. Patients were advised to take antihistamines at the first sign of a cold, in the hope of avoiding a full infection. Current thinking is that antihistamines have little value in the treatment of the common cold. They may have a minor effect on a runny nose, but there are better agents for this purpose. Antihistamines are usually highly sedative—most over-the-counter sleeping pills are antihistamines—so they may cause drowsiness. Patients taking many antihistamines are cautioned to avoid driving or operating machinery that could be dangerous.

The mainstays of therapy for the common cold are the decongestants that are applied topically (that is, directly to the mucous membranes in the nose) or taken orally. They are also called sympathomimetic agents because they mimic the effects of certain natural body chemicals that regulate many body processes. A group of these, called adrenergic stimulants, regulate vasoconstriction and vasodilation—in other words, they can narrow or widen blood vessels, respectively. Their vasoconstrictive capability is useful in managing the common cold, because it reduces the size of the blood vessels in the nose, reduces swelling and congestion, and inhibits excess secretion.

Topical decongestants are available as nasal sprays or drops. The sprays are squirted up into each nostril. The patient is usually advised to wait three to five minutes and then blow his or her nose to remove the mucus. If there is still congestion, the patient is advised to take another dose, allowing the medication to reach farther into the nasal cavity. Nose drops are taken by tilting the head back and squeezing the medication into the nostrils through the nose-dropper supplied with the medication. Clearance of nasal congestion is prompt, and the patient can breathe more easily. Nasal irritation is reduced, so there is less sneezing. Some nasal sprays and drops last longer than others, but none works around-the-clock, so applications must be repeated throughout the day.

Patients who use nasal sprays and drops are advised to follow the manufacturer's directions exactly. Applied too often or in too great a quantity, these preparations can cause unwanted problems, such as rhinitis medicamentosa, or nasal inflammation caused by a medication (also called rebound congestion). As the vasoconstrictive effect of the drugs wears down, the blood vessels dilate, the area becomes swollen, and secretions increase. This reaction may be attributable to the fact that the drug's vasoconstrictive effect has deprived the area of blood, and thus excited an increased inflammatory state, or it may simply be attributable to irritation by the drug. Use of sprays or drops should be limited to three or four days.

Oral decongestants are also effective in reducing swelling and relieving a runny nose, although they do not have as great a vasoconstrictive effect concentrated in the nasal area as sprays or drops. Because they circu-

such as monoamine oxidase inhibitors (MAOIs), guanethidine, bethanidine, or debrisoquin sulfate.

Three kinds of coughs may accompany colds: coughs that produce phlegm or mucus; hyperactive nagging coughs, which result from overstimulation of the cough reflex; and dry, unproductive coughs. If the phlegm or mucus collecting in the lungs is easily removed by occasional coughing, a soothing syrup, cough drop, or lozenge may be all that the patient requires. If the cough reflex center of the brain is overstimulated, there may be hyperactive or uncontrollable coughing and a cough suppressant, such as dextromethorphan, may be needed. Dextromethorphan works in the brain to raise the level of stimulus that is required to trigger the cough reflex. Some antihistamines, such as diphenhydramine hydrochloride, are effective cough suppressants. If coughing is unproductive—that is, if the mucus has thickened and dried and is not easily removed—an expectorant should be taken. Currently, the only expectorant used in over-the-counter drugs is guaifenesin. It helps soften and liquefy mucus deposits, so that coughs become productive. When the cough of a cold is serious enough for a physician to be consulted, prescription drugs may have to be used, such as codeine to stop hyperactive coughing and potassium iodide for unproductive coughs.

For allergic rhinitis or hay fever, avoidance of allergens is recommended but is not always possible. For hay fever outbreaks, antihistamines are the mainstays of therapy, with other agents added to relieve specific symptoms. For example, topical and oral decongestants may be required to relieve a runny nose.

late throughout the body, their vasoconstrictive effects may be seen in other vascular beds. There are many patients who are warned not to use oral decongestants unless they are under the care of a physician. These people include patients with high blood pressure, diabetics, heart patients, and patients taking certain drugs

Perspective and Prospects

Viruses are among the most intriguing and baffling challenges to medical science. Great progress has been made in preventing some virus diseases, such as by immunization against smallpox and hepatitis B. There has been only limited success, however, in finding agents to cure viral diseases, and so far nothing has been found to prevent or cure the common cold. Vaccines have been developed against certain rhinoviruses, and no doubt many more could be developed. Yet because the common cold is caused by so many different types of virus—more than two hundred—and vaccines against one virus are not necessarily effective against others, it is questionable whether such vaccines would ever be useful. A helpful vaccine would be one that could immunize against an entire family of viruses such as rhinoviruses or coronaviruses, the two leading causes of the common cold.

The search goes on for agents to cure the common cold. Substances, such as interferons, have been found that are effective against a wide range of viruses. One of the interferons was used by the British Medical Research Council's Common Cold Unit. Those researchers reported that interferon applied as an intranasal spray was highly effective in protecting subjects from cold infection. After some years, however, experimentation with interferon in the common cold was abandoned because the agent had significant side effects, nasal congestion among them.

The science of virology only began in the 1930's, so it is not surprising that viruses continue to hide their mysteries. Nevertheless, many fundamental discoveries have been made and one can predict increasing success. As scientists unravel the intricacies of viral infections, they find clues that help them devise ways of interfering with virus life processes. In some cases, effective drugs have been developed, such as the interferons, acyclovir for herpes simplex, and amantadine for the influenza virus. It is likely that the cure for the common cold will continue to be elusive, unless a broad-spectrum antiviral agent could be developed that works against multiple viral infections in the way that broad-spectrum antibiotics work against multiple bacterial infections.

—*C. Richard Falcon*

See also Allergies; Antihistamines; Bronchitis; Coughing; Decongestants; Fever; Influenza; Nasopharyngeal disorders; Nausea and vomiting; Noroviruses; Otorhinolarnygology; Pneumonia; Rhinitis; Rhinoviruses; Sinusitis; Sore throat; Viral infections.

For Further Information:

American Pharmaceutical Association. *Handbook of Nonprescription Drugs*. 15th ed. Washington, D.C.: Author, 2006. The section on drugs for colds, coughs, and allergies contains a thorough background discussion of these conditions. All major over-the-counter medications are listed.

Biddle, Wayne. *A Field Guide to Germs*. 2d ed. New York: Anchor Books, 2002. This comprehensive book is easily accessible to the nonspecialist and includes a discussion of nearly every virus, bacterium, and fungus known to cause human and nonhuman animal disease. The history of the microbe and the treatment of diseases are included.

Gallo, Robert. *Virus Hunting*. New York: Basic Books, 1991. Gallo gives a good general account of viruses—how they live and how modern medical science is trying to combat them.

Kimball, Chad T. *Colds, Flu, and Other Common Ailments Sourcebook*. Detroit, Mich.: Omnigraphics, 2001. A comprehensive guide for general readers covering treatment issues and controversies surrounding common ailments and injuries. Includes discussions on ailments of the nose, throat, lungs, ears, eyes, and head; common injuries; alternative therapies; choosing a doctor; and buying drugs and finding health information online.

Litin, Scott C., ed. *Mayo Clinic Family Health Book*. 4th ed. New York: HarperResource, 2009. One of the most thorough and accessible medical texts for the layperson.

Woolf, Alan D., et al., eds. *The Children's Hospital Guide to Your Child's Health and Development*. Cambridge, Mass.: Perseus, 2002. An authoritative and comprehensive guide to children's health, providing a guide to every common illness or condition that affects children and a carefully designed emergency section.

Young, Stuart H., Bruce Dobozin, and Margaret Miner. *Allergies*. Rev. ed. New York: Plume, 1999. A useful book that covers the treatment of allergic coldlike conditions, such as hay fever, and gives advice on how to manage them.

COMPUTED TOMOGRAPHY (CT) SCANNING
PROCEDURE

ALSO KNOWN AS: Computed axial tomography, CAT scan

ANATOMY OR SYSTEM AFFECTED: Circulatory system, endocrine system, gastrointestinal system, musculoskeletal system, nervous system, reproductive system, respiratory system

SPECIALTIES AND RELATED FIELDS: Biotechnology, cardiology, emergency medicine, endocrinology, gastroenterology, internal medicine, oncology, preventive medicine, psychiatry, radiology, vascular medicine

DEFINITION: The use of X rays and a computer to produce detailed cross-sectional images of most body regions to aid in diagnosis.

KEY TERMS:

cathode: an electrode that produces electrons

cathode-ray tube (CRT): a vacuum tube whose cathode emits electrons accelerated through a high voltage anode, focused on a fluorescent image screen

slice: a CT cross section of a body part

soft tissue: tissue other than bone

tomogram: the three-dimensional image of a CT slice

X ray: high-energy electromagnetic radiation

INDICATIONS AND PROCEDURES

Computed tomography (CT) scanning collects X-ray data and uses a computer to produce three-dimensional images, called tomograms, of body cross sections, or slices. The noninvasiveness of CT scanning yields easy and safe body part analysis based on varying tissue opacity to X rays. Bone absorbs X rays well and appears white. Air absorbs them poorly, so the lungs are dark. Fat, blood, and muscle absorb X rays to varying extents, yielding different shades of gray. Tumors and blood clots, for example, appear as areas of abnormal shades in normal tissue.

CT scanning is used to analyze disorders of the brain (brain CT) and most body parts (body CT), yielding tomograms that are hundreds of times more definitive than conventional X rays. For example, conventional abdominal X rays show bones and faintly outline the liver, kidneys, and stomach. Tomograms clearly depict all abdominal organs and large blood vessels.

Physicians call CT scanning the most valuable diagnostic method because, without it, the symptoms that patients describe may not be identified clearly as minor, serious, or life-threatening. For example, a subjective description of repeated headache does not reveal whether the cause is tension, stroke, or brain cancer. Before CT scanning, an accurate diagnosis often required complex or dangerous identification methods.

A CT patient changes into a hospital gown, removes any metal possessions, and lays on a table that can be raised, lowered, or tilted. During a scan, the patient enters a doughnut-shaped scanner that holds an X-ray source, detectors, and computer hookups. In brain CT, the patient's head is in the scanner. Some CT patients have experienced claustrophobia, which can be prevented with faster scanner speeds and less-enclosed scanners. A patient who must stay still for an extended time may be given a sedative. If small anomalies are foreseen, then contrast materials are given before or during the procedure. These materials include barium salts and iodine, X-ray blockers that allow better visualization of specific tissues. Subjects may take the materials orally, by enema, or intravenously.

The CT scanner generates a continuous, narrow X-ray beam while moving in a circle around the patient's head or body. The beam is monitored by X-ray detectors sited around the aperture through which the patient passes. Slices are produced as the scanner circles the head or body. Between slices, the table moves through the scanner. Slices become tomograms seen on a cathode-ray tube (CRT) and are stored in a computer. The procedure used to take twenty to forty minutes in a standard scanner. However, in the newer spiral CT, which is now standard in most hospitals, a patient is

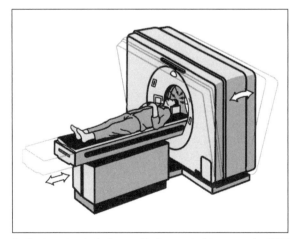

In the imaging technique called computed tomography (CT) scanning (formerly known as a CAT scan), multiple X-ray pictures are taken as the scanner tilts and rotates around the patient. These images are then assembled by a computer to create a three-dimensional view of a body part, such as the head.

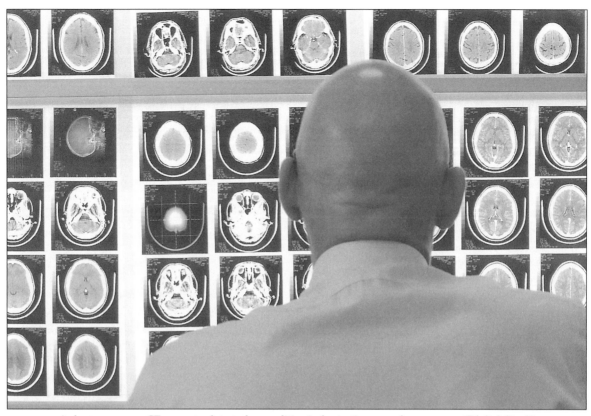

A doctor can use CT scans to detect abnormalities in brain tissue, such as tumors. (Digital Stock)

scanned rapidly as the x-ray tube rotates in a spiral. There are no gaps, as with slices, and tissue-volume tomograms are produced. A simple spiral scan is completed while the patient holds his or her breath, aiding the detection of small lesions and decreasing scan artifacts. Spiral CT, twenty times faster than standard CT, is useful in all patients, from restless children to the critically ill.

USES AND COMPLICATIONS

CT scanning detects organ abnormalities, and a major use is in diagnosing and treating brain disease. Even the earliest scanners could distinguish tumors from clots, aiding in the diagnosis of cancer, stroke, and certain birth defects. Furthermore, brain CT saves lives as physicians avoid risky methods requiring opening of the brain for pretreatment diagnosis. In addition, post-surgical scans can find recurrences or metastases.

Body CT allows for better damage appraisal of broken bones than does conventional X-ray analysis. Another use of body spiral CT is in the diagnosis of pulmonary embolism; it is safer than using pulmonary angiography, which maneuvers a catheter from the heart to the pulmonary artery. CT scans can also guide surgery, biopsy, and abscess drainage and can help fine-tune radiation therapy. Speed and excellent soft tissue elucidation make CT scanning invaluable for trauma detection in emergency rooms.

There are few side effects to CT scanning. Preparation for a scan may be mildly uncomfortable, but it is rarely dangerous. Before body CT, subjects often fast, take enemas to clear the bowels, and receive contrast materials through enemas or IVs. If contrast materials are used, then physicians must be told of allergies, especially to iodine. Contrast materials—enhancers of specific tissue CT—may cause hot flashes. Barium enemas for lower gastrointestinal tract scans cause full feelings and urges to defecate.

PERSPECTIVE AND PROSPECTS

British engineer Godfrey Hounsfield and American physicist Alan Cormack won the 1979 Nobel Prize in Physiology or Medicine for the theory and development of computed tomography. CT scanning was first used in 1972, after Hounsfield made a brain scanner holding an X-ray generator, a scanner rotated around a circular chamber, a computer, and a CRT. The patient laid on a gurney, head in the scanner, and emitter detectors rotated 1 degree at a time for 180 degrees. At each position, 160 readings entered the computer, so 28,800 readings were processed.

CT scanning is essential to radiology, which began in 1885 after Wilhelm Conrad Röntgen discovered X rays. The rays soon became medical aids, and for years broad X-ray beams were sent through body parts to exit onto film, yielding conventional X-ray images. Bones absorb X rays well, appearing white, and conventional images can show bone fractures and give some soft tissue data. However, soft tissue evaluation is poor, the tissues superimpose, and estimating their condition is difficult. CT scans allow convenient, noninvasive analysis.

CT scans and stereotaxic neurosurgery, later joined, have improved diagnosis and treatment. For example, the implantation of electrodes in a brain can be monitored using CT, enhancing accuracy. Similar techniques are used in breast biopsy. Current progress in CT scans includes thinner slices, spiral scans, and fast-operating standard scanners. Because complex scans expose patients to more radiation than do conventional X rays, fast scans are preferred to minimize patient risk.

—*Sanford S. Singer, Ph.D.*

See also Brain; Brain disorders; Headaches; Imaging and radiology; Magnetic resonance imaging (MRI); Neuroimaging; Noninvasive tests; Nuclear medicine; Positron emission tomography (PET) scanning; Single photon emission computed tomography (SPECT); Strokes; Tumors; Ultrasonography.

FOR FURTHER INFORMATION:

Durham, Deborah L. *Rad Tech's Guide to CT: Imaging Procedures, Patient Care, and Safety.* Malden, Mass.: Blackwell Scientific, 2002. Contains useful information for CT technicians and general readers.

Hsieh, Jiang. *Computed Tomography: Principles, Design, Artifacts, and Recent Advances.* 2d ed. Bellingham, Wash.: SPIE Press, 2009. Illustrated. Covers the title issues and provides an index and a bibliography.

Kalender, Willi A. *Computed Tomography: Fundamentals, System Technology, Image Quality, Applications.* 3d ed. Weinheim, Germany: Wiley VCH, 2009. Covers history and principles, spiral CT, applications, and future prospects. Illustrated and indexed, with a bibliography.

Slone, Richard M., et al., eds. *Body CT: A Practical Approach.* New York: McGraw-Hill, 2000. Covers CT techniques and protocols for many tissues. Illustrated. Contains a bibliography and an index.

CONCEPTION

BIOLOGY

ANATOMY OR SYSTEM AFFECTED: Cells, reproductive system, uterus

SPECIALTIES AND RELATED FIELDS: Embryology, gynecology, obstetrics

DEFINITION: The process of creating new life, encompassing all the events from deposition of sperm into the female to the first cell divisions of the fertilized ovum.

KEY TERMS:

cervix: the lowest part of the uterus in contact with the vagina; contains an opening filled with mucus through which sperm can pass

ejaculation: the reflex activated by sexual stimulation that results in sperm mixed with fluid being expelled from the male's body

fertilization: the union of the sperm and the ovum, which usually occurs in the female's oviduct

menstruation: the process of shedding the lining of the uterus that occurs about once a month

oviduct: the thin tube that leads from near the ovary to the upper part of the uterus; also called the Fallopian tube

ovulation: the process by which the mature ovum is expelled from the ovary

ovum: the round cell produced by the female that carries her genetic material; also called the egg

sperm: the motile cells produced within the male that carry his genetic material

uterus: the organ above the vagina through which the sperm must pass on their way to the ovum; also called the womb

vagina: the stretchy, tube-shaped structure into which the male's penis is inserted during intercourse; the site of sperm deposition

PROCESS AND EFFECTS

The process of conception begins with the act of intercourse. When the male's penis is inserted into the female's vagina, the stimulation of the penis by movement within the vagina triggers a reflex resulting in the ejaculation of sperm. During ejaculation, involuntary muscles in many of the male reproductive organs contract, causing semen, a mixture of sperm and fluid, to

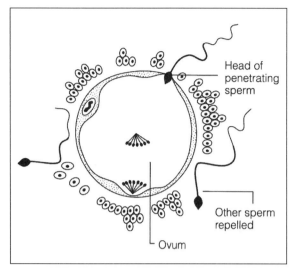

Male sperm cells propel themselves toward the ovum (female egg) by the swimming movements of their tails; fertilization occurs when a sperm cell penetrates the layers surrounding the ovum and fuses its membrane with the membrane of the ovum.

move from its sites of storage out through the urethra within the penis.

The average volume of semen in a typical human ejaculation is only 3.5 milliliters, but this small volume normally contains two hundred million to four hundred million sperm. Other constituents of semen include prostaglandins, which cause contractions of involuntary muscles in both the male and the female; the sugar fructose, which provides energy to the sperm; chemicals that adjust the activity of the semen; and a number of enzymes and other chemicals.

In a typical act of intercourse, the semen is deposited high up in the woman's vagina. Within a minute after ejaculation, the semen begins to coagulate, or form a clot, because of the activation of chemicals within the semen. Sperm are not able to leave the vagina until the semen becomes liquid again, which occurs spontaneously fifteen to twenty minutes after ejaculation.

Once the semen liquefies, sperm begin moving through the female system. The path to the ovum (if one is present) lies through the cervix, then through the hollow cavity of the uterus, and up through the oviduct, where fertilization normally occurs. The sperm are propelled through the fluid within these organs by the swimming movements of their tails called flagella, as well as by female organ contractions that are stimulated by the act of intercourse and by prostaglandins contained in the semen. It is not necessary for the woman to

experience orgasm, a pleasurable climax, for these contractions to occur. The contractions allow sperm to reach the oviduct within five minutes after leaving the vagina, a rate of movement that far exceeds their own swimming abilities.

Although some sperm can reach the oviduct quite rapidly, others never enter the oviduct at all. Of the two hundred million to four hundred million sperm deposited in the vagina, it is estimated that only one hundred to one thousand enter the oviducts. Some of the other millions of sperm may be defective, lacking the proper swimming ability. Other apparently normal sperm may become lost within the female's organs, possibly trapped in clefts between cells in the organ linings. The damaged and lost sperm will eventually be destroyed by white blood cells produced by the female.

Sperm movement through the female system is enhanced around the time of ovulation. For example, at the time of ovulation, the hormones associated with ovulation cause changes in the cervical mucus that aid sperm transport. The mucus at that time is extremely liquid and contains fibers that align themselves into channels, which are thought to be used by the sperm to ease their passage through the cervix. The hormones present at the time of ovulation also increase the contractions produced by the uterus and oviduct, and thus sperm transport through the structures is enhanced as well.

During transport through the female, sperm undergo a number of important chemical changes, collectively called capacitation, that enable them to fertilize the ovum successfully. Freshly ejaculated sperm are not capable of penetrating the layers surrounding the ovum, a fact that was uncovered when scientists first began to experiment with in vitro fertilization (the joining of sperm and ovum outside the body). Capacitation apparently occurs during transport of the sperm through the uterus and possibly the oviduct, and it is presumably triggered by some secretion of the female. With in vitro fertilization, capacitation is achieved by adding female blood serum to the dish that contains the sperm and ovum. Capacitation is not instantaneous; it has been estimated that this process requires an hour or more in humans. Even though the first sperm may arrive in the vicinity of the ovum within twenty minutes after ejaculation, fertilization cannot take place until capacitation is completed. In 2003, scientists discovered that sperm has a type of chemical sensor that causes the sperm to swim vigorously toward concentrations of a chemical attractant. While researchers long have known that chemical signals are an important component of conception, the 2003 findings were the first to demonstrate that sperm will respond in a predictable and controllable way, a fact promising for future contraception and infertility research.

The site where ovum and sperm typically come together is within the oviduct. At the time of ovulation, an ovum is released from the surface of the ovary and drawn into the upper end of the oviduct. Once within the oviduct, the ovum is propelled by contractions of the oviduct and possibly by wavelike motions of cilia, hairlike projections that line the inner surface of the oviduct. It takes about three days for the ovum to travel the entire length of the oviduct to the uterus, and since the ovum only remains fertilizable for twelve to twenty-four hours, successful fertilization must occur in the oviduct.

Upon reaching the ovum, the sperm must first penetrate two layers surrounding it. The outermost layer, called the corona radiata, consists of cells that break away from the ovary with the ovum during ovulation; the innermost layer, the zona pellucida, is a clear, jellylike substance that lies just outside the ovum cell membrane. Penetration of these two layers is accomplished by the release of enzymes carried by the sperm. Once through the zona pellucida, the sperm are ready to fertilize the ovum.

Fertilization occurs when a sperm fuses its membrane with the membrane of the ovum. This act triggers a protective change in the zona pellucida that prevents any additional sperm from reaching the ovum and providing it with extra chromosomes. Following fusion of the fertilizing sperm and ovum, the chromosomes of each become mingled and pair up; the resulting one-celled zygote contains a complete set of chromosomes, half contributed by the mother and half by the father.

It is at the moment of fertilization that the sex of the new child is decided. Genetic sex is determined by a pair of chromosomes denoted X and Y. Female body cells contain two X's, and each ovum produced contains only one X. Male body cells contain an X and a Y chromosome, but each sperm contains either an X or a Y chromosome. Men usually produce equal numbers of X- and Y-type sperm. The sex of the new individual is determined by which type of sperm fertilizes the ovum: If it is a Y-bearing sperm, the new individual will be male, and if it is an X-bearing sperm, the new individual will be female. Since entry of more than one sperm is prohibited, the first sperm to reach the ovum is the one that will fertilize it.

Following fertilization, the zygote or early embryo begins a series of cell divisions while it travels down the oviduct. When it arrives at the uterus about three days after ovulation, the zygote will be in the form of a hollow ball of cells called a blastocyte. Initially, this ball of cells floats in the fluid-filled cavity of the uterus, but two or three days after its arrival in the uterus (five to six days after ovulation), it will attach to the uterine lining. Researchers in 2003 made an exciting discovery when they identified how embryos stop and burrow into the lining of a woman's uterus. A protein, called L-selectin, on the surface of the embryo acts like a puzzle piece when it touches and quickly locks to carbohydrate molecules found on the uterine surface. This implantation process must occur in exact synchrony during a very short time in a woman's cycle. (If it occurs outside the uterus, usually in one of the Fallopian tubes, then the result is an ectopic pregnancy, which is often a medical emergency.) Over the next nine months, the body of the embryo will take on a human form and develop the ability to live independently outside the uterus.

COMPLICATIONS AND DISORDERS

Three factors limit the time frame in which conception is possible: the fertilizable lifetime of the ovulated ovum, estimated to be between twelve and twenty-four hours; the fertilizable lifetime of ejaculated sperm in the female tract, usually assumed to be about forty-eight hours; and the time required for sperm capacitation, which is one hour or more. The combination of these factors determines the length of the fertile period, the time during which intercourse must occur if conception is to be achieved. Taking the three factors into account, the fertile period is said to extend from forty-eight hours prior to ovulation until perhaps twenty-four hours after ovulation. For example, if intercourse occurs forty-eight hours before ovulation, the sperm will be capacitated in the first few hours and will still be within their fertilizable lifetime when ovulation occurs. On the other hand, if intercourse occurs twenty-four hours after ovulation, the sperm will still require time for capacitation, but the ovum will be near the end of its viable period. Thus the later limit of the fertile period is equal to the fertilizable lifetime of the ovum, minus the time required for capacitation.

Obviously, a critical factor in conception is the timing of ovulation. In a typical twenty-eight-day menstrual cycle, ovulation occurs about halfway through the cycle, or fourteen days after the first day of menstrual bleeding. In actuality, cycle length varies widely from month to month. It appears that generally the first half of the cycle is more variable in length, with the second half more stable. Thus, no matter how long the entire menstrual cycle is, ovulation usually occurs fourteen days prior to the first day of the next episode of menstrual bleeding. Therefore, it is relatively easy to determine when ovulation occurred by counting backward, but difficult to predict the time of ovulation in advance.

Assessment of ovulation time in women is notoriously difficult. There is no easily observable outward sign of ovulation. Some women do detect slight abdominal pain about the time of ovulation; this is referred to as *Mittelschmerz*, which means, literally, pain in the middle of the cycle. This slight pain may be localized on either side of the abdomen and is thought to be caused by irritation of the abdominal organs by fluid released from the ovary during ovulation. Other signs of ovulation are an increased volume of the cervical mucus and flexibility of the cervix and a characteristic fernlike pattern of the mucus when it is dried on a glass slide. There is also a slight rise in body temperature after ovulation, which again makes it easier to determine the time of ovulation after the fact rather than in advance. It is also possible to measure the amount of luteinizing hormone (LH) in urine or blood; this hormone shows a marked increase about sixteen hours prior to ovulation. Home test kits to detect LH levels are available for urine samples. There are additional signs of the time of ovulation, such as a slight opening of the cervix and a change in the cells lining the vagina, that can be used by physicians to determine the timing and occurrence of ovulation.

Since ovulation time is so difficult to detect in most women on an ongoing basis, most physicians would counsel that, to achieve a pregnancy, couples should plan on having intercourse every two days. This frequency will ensure that sperm capable of fertilization are always present, so that the exact time of ovulation becomes unimportant. A greater frequency of intercourse is not advised, since sperm numbers are reduced when ejaculation occurs often. Approximately 85 to 90 percent of couples will achieve pregnancy within a year when intercourse occurs about three times a week.

Couples often wonder if it is possible to predetermine the sex of their child by some action taken in conjunction with intercourse. Scientists have found no consistent effect of diet, position assumed during intercourse, timing of intercourse within the menstrual cycle, or liquids that are introduced into the vagina to kill one type of sperm selectively. In the laboratory, it is possible to achieve partial separation of sperm in a semen sample by subjecting the semen to an electric current or other procedure due to the physical difference of X- and Y-containing sperm. The separated sperm can then be used for artificial insemination (the introduction of semen through a tube into the uterus). This method is not 100 percent successful in producing offspring of the desired sex and so is available only on an experimental basis.

Some couples have difficulty in conceiving a child, in a few cases as a result of some problem associated with intercourse. For example, the male may have difficulty in achieving erection or ejaculation. The vast majority of these cases are caused by psychological factors such as stress and tension rather than any biological problem. Fortunately, therapists can teach couples how to overcome these psychological problems.

About 15 percent of couples in the United States suffer from some type of biological infertility—that is, infertility that persists when intercourse occurs successfully. In 10 percent of the cases of infertility, doctors are unable to establish a cause. In another 20 percent of couples, both partners are infertile. In the remaining 70 percent of cases, about half the problems are in the male and half in the female.

In men, the most commonly diagnosed cause of infertility is low sperm count. Sometimes low sperm count is caused by a treatable imbalance of hormones. If not treatable, this problem can sometimes be circumvented by the use of pooled semen samples in artificial insemination or through in vitro fertilization. In vitro fertilization may also be a solution for men who produce normal numbers of sperm but whose sperm lack swimming ability. Another cause of male infertility is blockage of the tubes that carry the semen from the body, which may be caused by a previous infection. Surgery is sometimes successful in removing such a blockage.

In women, a common cause of infertility is a hormonal problem that interferes with ovulation. Treatment with one of a number of so-called fertility drugs may be successful in promoting ovulation. Fertility drugs, however, have some disadvantages: They have a tendency to cause ovulation of more than one ovum, thus raising the possibility of multiple pregnancy, which is considered risky; and they may alter the environment of the uterus, making implantation of a resulting embryo less likely.

Another common cause of female infertility is blockage of the oviducts resulting from scar tissue formation in the aftermath of some type of infection. Because surgery is not always successful in opening the oviducts, this condition may require the use of in vitro fertilization or the new technique of surgically introducing ova and sperm directly into the oviduct at a point below the blockage.

Finally, some cases of infertility result from biological incompatibility between the man and the woman. It may be that the sperm are unable to penetrate the cervical mucus, or perhaps that the woman's body treats the sperm cells as foreign, destroying them before they can reach the ovum. Techniques such as artificial insemination and in vitro fertilization offer hope for couples experiencing these problems.

PERSPECTIVE AND PROSPECTS

For most of history, the events surrounding conception were poorly understood. For example, microscopic identification of sperm did not occur until 1677, and the ovum was not identified until 1827 (although the follicle in which the ovum develops was recognized in the seventeenth century). Prior to these discoveries, people held the belief espoused by early writers such as Aristotle and Galen that conception resulted from the mixing of male and female fluids during intercourse.

There was also confusion about the timing of the fertile period. Some early doctors thought that menstrual blood was involved in conception and therefore believed that the fertile period coincided with menstruation. Others recognized that menstrual bleeding was a sign that pregnancy had not occurred; they assumed that the most likely time for conception to result was immediately after the menstrual flow ceased. It was not until the 1930's that the first scientific studies on the timing of ovulation were completed.

Since there was little scientific understanding of the processes involved in conception, medical practice for most of human history was little different from magic, revolving around the use of rituals and herbal treatments to aid or prevent conception. Gradually, people rejected these practices, often because of religious teachings. By the twentieth century, conception had been established as an area of intense privacy, thought by physicians and the general public to be unsuitable for medical intervention.

In the early part of the twentieth century, the role of physicians in aiding conception was mostly limited to educating and advising couples finding difficulty in conceiving. There were few techniques, other than arti-

ficial insemination and fertility drug treatment, available to assist in conception at that time.

The situation changed with the first successful in vitro fertilization in 1978. This event ushered in an era of intense medical and public interest in assisting conception. Other methods to aid conception were soon introduced, including embryo transfer, frozen storage of embryos, and surgical placement of ova and sperm directly into the oviduct.

Paralleling the development of these techniques has been demand on the part of society for medicine to apply them. Infertility rates in the United States have been gradually increasing. One reason for increased infertility has been the increasing age at which couples decide to start a family, since the fertility of women appears to undergo a decline past the age of thirty. Another factor affecting fertility rates of both men and women has been an increased incidence of various sexually transmitted diseases, which can result in chronic inflammation of the reproductive organs and infertility caused by scar tissue formation.

People's attitudes toward medical intervention in conception have also changed. The earlier religious taboos against interference in conception have been somewhat relaxed, although some churches still do not approve of certain methods of fertility management. Although there remain ethical issues to be resolved, the general public seems to have accepted the idea that medicine should provide assistance to those who wish to, but cannot, conceive children.

—*Marcia Watson-Whitmyre, Ph.D.;*
updated by Alexander Sandra, M.D.

See also Assisted reproductive technologies; Childbirth; Cloning; Contraception; Gamete intrafallopian transfer (GIFT); Gynecology; In vitro fertilization; Infertility, female; Infertility, male; Menstruation; Multiple births; Obstetrics; Pregnancy and gestation; Reproductive system; Sperm banks; Uterus.

FOR FURTHER INFORMATION:

Doherty, C. Maud, and Melanie M. Clark. *Fertility Handbook: A Guide to Getting Pregnant.* Omaha, Nebr.: Addicus Books, 2002. The authors, a reproductive endocrinologist and a former infertility patient, combine their experiences to explore infertility options and treatments. Addresses the causes, getting diagnoses, choosing a fertility specialist, and utilizing new assisted reproductive technology.

Harkness, Carla. *The Infertility Book: A Comprehensive Medical and Emotional Guide.* Rev 2d ed.

Berkeley, Calif.: Celestial Arts, 1992. A comprehensive guide to problems of infertility that combines medical and emotional perspectives. Contains anecdotal accounts in the patients' own words.

Jones, Richard E., and Kristin H. Lopez. *Human Reproductive Biology.* 3d ed. Burlington, Mass.: Academic Press/Elsevier, 2006. This college-level textbook provides comprehensive coverage of all biological aspects of human reproduction. There is a separate chapter on fertilization; information on the timing of ovulation, contraception, and infertility treatment is also presented.

Kearney, Brian. *High-Tech Conception: A Comprehensive Handbook for Consumers.* New York: Bantam Books, 1998. An increasing number of specialists are responding to the predicament of childless couples by offering procedures requiring the removal of eggs from the ovaries. Kearney's handbook provides potential high-tech customers with information for critically assessing the potentials and risks of the various techniques.

Weschler, Toni. *Taking Charge of Your Fertility.* Rev. ed. New York: Collins, 2006. An excellent book that encourages women to become responsible for their own reproductive health. Includes discussions of infertility, natural birth control, and achieving pregnancy.

Wisot, Arthur L., and David R. Meldrum. *Conceptions and Misconceptions: The Informed Consumer's Guide Through the Maze of In Vitro Fertilization and Other Assisted Reproduction Techniques.* 2d ed. Point Roberts, Wash.: Hartley & Marks, 2004. Written by two leading fertility experts, this book is an excellent guide. Includes a thorough discussion of the basic physiology of conception and reproduction.

CONCUSSION

DISEASE/DISORDER

ANATOMY OR SYSTEM AFFECTED: Brain, head, nerves, nervous system

SPECIALTIES AND RELATED FIELDS: Critical care, emergency medicine, neurology, sports medicine

DEFINITION: Mild brain injury that briefly impairs neurological functions.

KEY TERMS:

amnesia: memory loss

disorientation: lack of comprehension of reality

unconsciousness: lack of awareness of one's surroundings

CAUSES AND SYMPTOMS

Annually in the United States, 1.4 million people suffer concussions, with 75 percent of those conditions being considered mild in nature. Concussions can be caused by a variety of traumatic events: motor vehicle accidents, penetrating injuries, sports injuries, and falls. Recent studies indicate that the number of concussions from motor vehicle accidents and falls have decreased, while penetrating injuries (gunshot wounds) and sports-related injuries are on the increase. Concussion is a common athletic injury experienced by approximately 300,000 youths each year. Recent information suggests that children heal more slowly than adults following head trauma. Although concussions are the mildest traumatic brain injuries, they can result in irreversible damage or death if a person suffers another head trauma prior to recovering fully from the initial injury.

People experiencing head trauma that disrupts brain activity and sometimes causes brief unconsciousness, ranging from several seconds to minutes immediately after an impact, are considered to have sustained a concussion. Direct, sudden, powerful blows to the head or an impact to the body that jars the head causes the brain to bounce inside the skull and suffer tissue bruising. Nerve fibers tear, and chemical reactions are altered.

Concussions are described as mild, moderate, or severe, though there is a lack of standardized definitions for each type of concussion. A mild concussion may or may not involve a brief period of unconsciousness; the brain generally recovers quickly and without long-term damage. However, approximately 15 percent of those injured will continue to experience symptoms one year after the initial injury. These symptoms may range from headaches to emotional or behavioral problems. The Centers for Disease Control and Prevention (CDC) and the National Center for Injury Prevention and Control have developed recommendations for standardized terminology, treatment, and prevention of mild traumatic brain injuries. A severe concussion is considered an emergency and requires an extended time for recovery.

Headache, dizziness, nausea, and disorientation immediately following the injury are considered risk factors for long-term complications from the head injury. Each person's brain and injury are unique. Therefore, a wide variety of symptoms may occur. Patients may experience double vision and suffer hearing problems. People with concussions also report becoming uncoordinated and sensitive to light and noises, and they may

INFORMATION ON CONCUSSION

CAUSES: Brain trauma from car accidents, falls, sports injuries, etc.

SYMPTOMS: Unconsciousness, memory loss, headache, dizziness, nausea, disorientation, double vision, hearing problems, lack of coordination, sensitivity to light and noises, sensory changes in smell and taste

DURATION: Ranges from several seconds to minutes immediately after impact

TREATMENTS: Dependent on severity; none (mild), rest and alleviation of symptoms (moderate), neck immobilization and hospitalization (severe)

experience sensory changes in smell and taste. Patients may become moody, cognitively impaired, unable to concentrate, and fatigued.

Researchers have determined that the major neuropsychological complications of concussion may occur in the brain's memory, learning, and planning functions. Some concussion patients taking tests, such as the Wechsler Abbreviated Scale of Intelligence, have revealed decreased concentration, reaction, and processing skills in performing intellectual tasks. Their strategies to solve problems are impaired when compared to people who have not suffered concussions.

Medical professionals assess patients with a head injury by physical examination, radiological tests, and a standardized scale that measures level of consciousness called the Glasgow Coma Scale. Computed tomography (CT) and magnetic resonance imaging (MRI) scans may be used. The American Academy of Neurology emphasizes the duration of loss of consciousness to determine the degree of concussions. Evaluations also consider orientation and posttraumatic amnesia. Medical professionals assess patients' responses to stimuli and memory of incidents before their injury, defining the concussion according to the level of confusion, amnesia, and duration of loss of consciousness. Physicians ask patients questions about who and where they are and about the time and date. The duration of amnesia after the brain trauma helps medical professionals determine the extent of the injury and treatments that would be most effective to heal the brain. The Colorado Medical Society developed a popular system, assigning Grades 1 (mild), 2 (moderate), and 3 (severe) to concussions, to guide athletic

personnel in examining players who suffer concussions during games and deciding how long they must refrain from participation in order to prevent additional damage.

Brain damage and death can result from serial concussions. Postconcussion complications may include second impact syndrome: If a patient suffers another concussion before healing is complete following the first injury, then the second concussion can be the catalyst for rapid cerebral swelling that causes increased pressure within the rigid structure of the brain. This pressure can cause the brain to press on the brain stem and result in respiratory failure and death. This condition is usually fatal.

More common is postconcussive syndrome (PCS), which consists of such cognitive and physical symptoms as headache, anxiety, vertigo, nausea, and hallucinations. An estimated 30 percent of professional football players suffer from PCS. Researchers have determined that people who experience several concussions, such as athletes and soldiers, are more vulnerable to becoming clinically depressed.

TREATMENT AND THERAPY

Research has found that patients who rest for one week following a concussion, with a slow return to previous activities to allow the brain to heal, have fewer long-term complications than do those patients who resume activities more quickly. Specific medications and therapies might be prescribed to alleviate symptoms and assist patients in resuming normal behaviors. Although most patients recover, some experience long-term concussion-related conditions, such as memory loss and neurological impairment.

Severe concussions with increased brain pressure require hospitalization, often in a neurological intensive care unit. The patient's head is maintained in a neutral position. The patient is at risk for stopped breathing due to increased brain pressure. This risk is decreased by placing the patient on a mechanical ventilator. The patient may have suffered internal bleeding in the brain because of the injury, and blood clots can form there. Surgery may be required to remove these clots. Patients with preexisting conditions such as epilepsy and diabetes may develop complications related to those diseases and require longer recovery times.

Physicians recommend wearing helmets to absorb shocks sustained during athletic activities involving the risk of head injury in order to prevent or minimize concussions. The American Academy of Neurology has demanded a ban on boxing because the sport involves knocking out opponents by inflicting concussions. Boxers often suffer permanent brain damage and are at a heightened risk for neurological diseases.

PERSPECTIVE AND PROSPECTS

Muslim physician Rhazes (850-923) was the first person known to describe concussion. He differentiated between a head injury that caused neurological symptoms from those injuries that resulted in lesions and structural damage. In the nineteenth century, medical researchers developed hypotheses, often controversial, regarding the physical and emotional influences of concussion symptoms. Since then, investigators have studied the impact of concussions on neuropsychological functioning and have addressed cognitive impairment and potential and the duration of recovery. Second impact syndrome was first defined in 1984.

The development of sports medicine increased the interest in studying concussions. The understanding of the internal brain damage involved in concussions did not significantly advance, however, until imaging technologies such as CT scanning and magnetic resonance imaging (MRI) were developed in the late twentieth century. In the twenty-first century, medical professionals utilize those techniques to view brain tissues and to observe the physiological reactions to concussion-causing trauma. Positive emission tomography (PET) has been developed to measure chemical changes in the brain. In the case of concussion, the PET scan can be used to evaluate changes that signal areas of injury in the brain.

—*Elizabeth D. Schafer, Ph.D.;*
updated by Amy Webb Bull, D.S.N., A.P.N.

See also Amnesia; Bleeding; Brain; Brain damage; Brain disorders; Coma; Dizziness and fainting; First aid; Head and neck disorders; Nausea and vomiting; Nervous system; Neuroimaging; Neurology; Sports medicine; Subdural hematomas; Unconsciousness.

FOR FURTHER INFORMATION:

Evans, Randolph W., ed. *Neurology and Trauma.* 2d ed. New York: Oxford University Press, 2006.

Kennedy, Jan, Robin Lumpkin, and Joyce Grissom. "A Survey of Mild Traumatic Brain Injury Treatment in the Emergency Room and Primary Care Medical Clinics." *Military Medicine* 171, no. 6 (June, 2006): 516-521.

Kerr, Mary, and Elizabeth Crago. "Acute Intracranial Problems." In *Medical-Surgical Nursing,* edited by Sharon Lewis, Margaret Heitkemper, and Shannon Dirksen. 6th ed. St. Louis, Mo.: Mosby, 2004.

Metzl, Jordan. "Concussion in the Young Athlete." *Pediatrics* 117, no. 5. (May, 2006): 1813.

National Center for Injury Prevention and Control. *Report to Congress on Mild Traumatic Brain Injury in the United States: Steps to Prevent a Serious Public Health Problem.* Atlanta: Centers for Disease Control and Prevention, 2003. Also available at http://www.cdc.gov/ncipc/tbi/mtbi/report.htm.

Shannon, Joyce Brennfleck, ed. *Sports Injuries Sourcebook.* 2d ed. Detroit, Mich.: Omnigraphics, 2002.

Wrightson, Philip, and Dorothy Gronwall. *Mild Head Injury: A Guide to Management.* New York: Oxford University Press, 1999.

CONGENITAL ADRENAL HYPERPLASIA
DISEASE/DISORDER

ALSO KNOWN AS: Adrenogenital syndrome, 21-hydroxylase deficiency

ANATOMY OR SYSTEM AFFECTED: Endocrine system, genitals, reproductive system

SPECIALTIES AND RELATED FIELDS: Endocrinology, genetics, urology

DEFINITION: A family of genetic conditions that affect hormone production by the adrenal glands.

KEY TERMS:

adrenal glands: endocrine glands located above the kidneys that produce glucocorticoid, mineralocorticoid, and androgenic hormones

aldosterone: a mineralocorticoid that controls sodium retention

androgens: hormones that regulate sexual differentiation, development, and maintenance of male sex characteristics

cortisol: a glucocorticoid that raises blood sugar levels; elevated in response to physical or psychological stress

glucocorticoids: drugs or hormones that regulate carbohydrate metabolism

hydrocortisone: a pharmaceutical term for cortisol

mineralocorticoids: hormones that regulate the balance of water and electrolytes

salt-wasting: a condition in which there is an inappropriately large excretion of salt; symptoms include poor feeding, weight loss, vomiting, dehydration, and hypotension and can progress to adrenal crisis and death

virilization: the development of masculine sex characteristics in a female

CAUSES AND SYMPTOMS

Congenital adrenal hyperplasia (CAH) is a family of autosomal recessive conditions that affect the production of hormones by the adrenal glands. It is caused by an inherited deficiency in one of the enzymes that is necessary to convert cholesterol to cortisol. About 95 percent of cases of CAH are caused by a deficiency in the enzyme 21-hydroxylase, but deficiencies in 3-beta hydroxysteroid dehydrogenase, 11-beta-hydroxylase, 17-alpha-hydroxylase, or cholesterol desmolase can also cause the condition.

If an individual has a mutation in one copy of the gene that codes for one of these enzymes, then he or she will not have any clinical symptoms but is considered a carrier of CAH. If both parents are carriers, then there is a 25 percent chance that their child will inherit both of these mutations. Individuals with two mutated copies of a gene will have a deficiency of the corresponding enzyme and will be clinically affected with CAH.

Individuals with CAH have reduced levels of cortisol production. They may also have decreased aldosterone production and increased production of androgens, such as testosterone.

Girls who are born with classic CAH often have virilized or ambiguous external genitalia, while boys may have enlarged penises. Affected infants may also experience weight loss, dehydration, vomiting, and salt-wasting crises. If left untreated, affected individuals may experience very early puberty, irregular menstrual cycles, infertility, and short stature in adulthood. There is also a nonclassic form of CAH that is less severe and develops in late childhood or early adulthood.

A diagnosis of CAH is usually made based on biochemical testing. Affected individuals typically have decreased serum levels of cortisol, aldosterone, sodium, chloride, and total carbon dioxide. They also have elevated levels of the steroid hormone 17-hydroxyprogesterone (17-OHP) and serum DHEA sulfate (an androgen). Genetic testing for CAH is also available. Newborn screening for CAH is routine and is done by measuring the concentration of 17-OHP on a filter paper blood spot sample.

TREATMENT AND THERAPY

The principal treatment for CAH is lifelong hormone replacement therapy. The aim of this therapy is to replace deficient glucocorticoid, reduce the production of androgens, prevent the development of secondary male sex characteristics in females, optimize growth, and promote fertility.

INFORMATION ON CONGENITAL ADRENAL HYPERPLASIA

CAUSES: Genetic defect in hormone production
SYMPTOMS: Ambiguous genitalia in girls, enlarged penis, salt-wasting, very early puberty, irregular menstrual cycles, infertility
DURATION: Lifelong; can be fatal during infancy if untreated
TREATMENTS: Hormone therapy, genital reconstructive surgery

In children, oral hydrocortisone is usually given in two to three daily doses. Individuals with the salt-wasting form of CAH may also need supplemental sodium chloride and mineralocorticoids. Serum concentrations of 17-OHP and other hormones must be checked regularly to assess hormonal control. Overtreatment with glucocorticosteroids can result in elevated cortisol levels and can lead to Cushing's syndrome. Signs of Cushing's syndrome include an accumulation of fat between the shoulders; a full, rounded face; muscle weakness; stretch marks on the skin of the abdomen, thighs, and breasts; high blood pressure; and bone loss.

Girls with virilization or genital ambiguity may need corrective surgery to ensure proper urinary, sexual, and reproductive functioning. Males are at risk for testicular adrenal rest tumors and require periodic imaging of the testes with ultrasound or magnetic resonance imaging (MRI).

If a couple is known to be at risk for having a pregnancy affected with CAH, then oral dexamethasone can be given to the mother during pregnancy to prevent virilization of a female fetus. To be effective, however, treatment must be started early in the pregnancy, before testing can be done to determine the sex of the fetus or if the fetus is affected with CAH. This often results in unnecessary treatment of a male or unaffected fetus.

PERSPECTIVE AND PROSPECTS

Luigi De Crecchio, an Italian anatomist, is credited with the earliest known description of a case of probable CAH. In 1865 he wrote an account of Joseph Marzo, a man who had passed away following an episode of vomiting and diarrhea. Although Marzo had a male appearance, he had ambiguous external genitalia and internal female reproductive organs.

J. Phillips helped to identify CAH as a genetic condition when he reported in 1887 the case of a family with four children who had been born hermaphrodites and passed away in early infancy with wasting disease. Then, in 1905, J. Fibiger noted that some infants with prolonged vomiting and dehydration had enlarged adrenal glands.

Lawson Wilkins, a researcher at Johns Hopkins Medical School, concluded that the impaired ability to produce cortisol led to adrenal hyperplasia and over-production of adrenal androgens in individuals with CAH. In 1950, he reported that adrenal cortical extracts could be used to treat children with CAH. By the late 1950's, hydrocortisone, fludrocortisone, and predni-sone were available and could be used for treatment. By 1990, many of the causative genes and enzymes had been identified.

Research continues on improving the hormone re-placement regimen for individuals with CAH. Excess adrenal androgen secretions need to be suppressed while still allowing for normal growth and develop-ment. There is also continuing research on the psycho-logical effects of CAH. The degree to which prenatal androgen exposure may affect psychosexual develop-ment in females with CAH is an ongoing subject of re-search.

—*Laura Garasimowicz, M.S.*

See also Corticosteroids; Cushing's syndrome; Endocrine disorders; Endocrinology; Endocrinology, pediatric; Genetic diseases; Hormones; Hyperplasia.

For Further Information:

Hsu, C. Y., and Scott A. Rivkees. *Congenital Adrenal Hyperplasia: A Parents' Guide.* Bloomington, Ind.: AuthorHouse, 2005.

Kliegman R. M., et al. "Congenital Adrenal Hyper-plasia and Related Disorders." In *Nelson Textbook of Pediatrics.* 18th ed. Philadelphia: Saunders/El-sevier, 2007.

Parker, Philip M. *Congenital Adrenal Hyperplasia: A Medical Dictionary, Bibliography, and Annotated Research Guide to Internet References.* San Diego, Calif.: ICON Group, 2004.

Congenital disorders

Disease/disorder

Anatomy or system affected: All

Specialties and related fields: Genetic coun-seling, genetics, neonatology, obstetrics, pediatrics

Definition: An abnormality present at birth, which may be due to a genetic defect, exposure to a toxic or infectious agent in utero, or a deficiency or lack of a substance necessary for fetal development.

Key terms:

amniocentesis: withdrawal of fluid from the amniotic sac for genetic analysis

aneuploidy: an abnormal number of chromosomes

chorionic villus sampling (CVS): removal of a small portion of chorionic villi (placental tissue) for ge-netic analysis

chromosomes: paired structures that contain genetic material (DNA)

Down syndrome: a highly studied genetic defect caused by an extra twenty-first chromosome

genetics: the study of the hereditary transmission of characteristics

triple test: a blood test that screens for genetic defects

trisomy: the presence of an extra chromosome; for ex-ample, Down syndrome is trisomy 21

Causes and Symptoms

Congenital disorders can be the result of genetic fac-tors, environmental exposure, infection during preg-nancy, or a deficiency or lack of a substance required for proper fetal development.

Genetic defects include defective genes, extra chro-mosomal material, and missing chromosomal material. Examples of defects from a single gene include Hun-tington's disease, cystic fibrosis, and Tay-Sachs dis-ease. Huntington's disease is caused by an autosomal dominant gene (inheritance of the disease from one parent will produce the disease). Cystic fibrosis and Tay-Sachs disease are autosomal recessives (inheri-tance of the gene from both parents is necessary for ex-pression of the disease). Huntington's disease is a pro-gressive and fatal deterioration of the central nervous system with an onset in middle age. Patients with cys-tic fibrosis produce excessive mucus in their lungs, pancreas, and other secretory organs. The secretions in the lungs clog respiratory passages, causing pulmonary damage, and subject the patient to life-threatening in-fection. Secretions in the pancreas prevent the flow of enzymes into the intestines and damage the pancreatic islet cells, resulting in diabetes. Tay-Sachs disease is a fatal disorder in which a fatty substance known as ganglioside G_{M2} builds up in tissues and nerve cells in the brain. Even with meticulous medical care, death usually occurs by age four.

In some types of defects due to recessive genes, the possession of one abnormal gene can be detrimental. One example is sickle cell disease and sickle cell trait,

Information on Congenital Disorders

Causes: Vary; genetic abnormality, exposure to toxic or infectious agent in utero, deficiency or lack of substance necessary for fetal development

Symptoms: Vary from mild to profound, can affect one or more organ systems

Duration: Often lifelong; some defects correctable through surgery or medication

Treatments: Vary by specific disorder

which is an abnormality of the red blood cells. Individuals with two defective genes are much more severely affected than those with one. Some defective genes reside on the sex chromosomes. Females have two X chromosomes, and males have one X and one Y chromosome. The Y chromosome is shorter than the X chromosome and has less genetic material. A defective gene on an X chromosome in the area with no corresponding material on the Y chromosome will always express itself; therefore, these diseases affect males much more frequently than females. An example of an X-linked disease is red-green color blindness, in which individuals cannot distinguish between red and green.

Ethnicity is a factor in the inheritance of a genetic disorder. For example, Tay-Sachs disease is most common among Eastern European Jews (Ashkenazi), sickle cell disease is most common among individuals of African descent, and thalassemia (a blood disease) is most common among people of Mediterranean descent.

A number of genetic defects are the result of aneuploidy, which is the presence of extra or missing chromosomes. The normal human complement is 22 pairs of autosomes and one pair of sex chromosomes (X and Y). A number of defects due to extra chromosomal material are trisomies. Two examples of trisomies are Down syndrome (trisomy 21) and Edwards syndrome (trisomy 18). Down syndrome is characterized by mental retardation and physical deformities (such as an enlarged tongue, poor muscle tone, and cardiac abnormalities). Trisomy 18 is characterized by profound physical deformities and mental retardation; about 95 percent of affected fetuses die in the uterus before birth, and those that live rarely survive beyond infancy. Turner syndrome is an example of aneuploidy due to a missing chromosome. Affected individuals have one

X chromosome and no Y chromosome. They are sterile and have short stature, a webbed neck, and other abnormalities.

Toxic substances ingested by the mother during pregnancy can affect the developing fetus, often to a much greater extent than the mother. Examples of toxin exposure include the fetal alcohol syndrome, cocaine abuse, and smoking. Fetal alcohol syndrome is characterized by mental retardation, low birth weight, and facial deformities. The syndrome has occurred in infants of mothers who reportedly consumed as little as two drinks per day (one drink equivalent is 1.25 ounces of 80 proof liquor, twelve ounces of beer, or six ounces of wine). Infants born of mothers who use cocaine may have low birth weight and disproportionately small heads. They may have learning difficulties; some research suggests that a variety of birth defects are prevalent in these children. Mothers who smoke during pregnancy are more likely to deliver a low birth weight infant and/or one with respiratory problems. Although most congenital disorders due to toxic effects are related to maternal exposure, paternal exposure is a factor in some cases. For example, cocaine use by the father at the time of conception has been reported to affect the fetus. This is thought to be the result of the lodging of the cocaine molecule on the spermatozoa head; these molecules are passed to the ovum during fertilization. In general, use of a toxic substance increases the risk of fetal loss and premature birth.

Infectious agents that cause congenital defects include rubella, HIV/AIDS, and syphilis. A pregnant woman who becomes infected with the rubella virus, particularly during the first trimester (three months), may give birth to an infant with the rubella syndrome. The syndrome is characterized by auditory, cerebral, cardiac, and ophthalmic defects. Symptoms range from mild to severe. Without treatment during pregnancy, the transmission of human immunodeficiency virus (HIV) to the fetus is likely. Infants born with congenital syphilis may appear normal at birth; however, they can subsequently develop central nervous system, bone, teeth, and eye disorders.

Poor nutrition in pregnancy can result in a congenital disorder. Folic acid deficiency has been implicated in the development of neural tube defects such as spina bifida, anencephaly, and encephalocele. Spina bifida is caused by failure of the spinal column to close during fetal development. The severity of symptoms depends on the location and size of the defect. Affected infants may have varying degrees of paralysis of the lower extremities as well as problems with bowel and bladder control. Anencephaly is due to the lack of the formation of a cranium (skull cap); as a result, the brain does not form at all or in major part. This disorder is always fatal. An encephalocele is a skull defect that exposes a portion of the brain. This disorder may be fatal or result in varying degrees of mental disability.

TREATMENT AND THERAPY

As is the case with all disorders, prevention is preferable to treatment. Avoidance of harmful substances during pregnancy (mind-altering drugs, alcohol, and tobacco) is essential; adequate nutrition, including vitamin supplements, is extremely important. Exposure to infectious agents (rubella, HIV, syphilis) should be avoided. Certain medications can increase the risk of birth defects, such as isotretinoin (Accutane) and etretinate (Tegison) for the treatment of acne and phenytoin (Dilantin) and carbamezapine (Tegretol) for the treatment of epilepsy. Any woman who is pregnant or contemplating pregnancy should consult a health care professional in regard to any medication, prescription or nonprescription.

Screening tests such as the triple test are blood tests that can screen for genetic abnormalities. Chorionic villus sampling (CVS) and amniocentesis can definitively diagnose genetic abnormalities. These tests can diagnose disorders such as Down syndrome and trisomy 18. Single-gene defects can also be diagnosed with CVS or amniocentesis, particularly in cases where a family history of the defect is present. Prenatal diagnosis allows the parents the ability to choose whether to continue with the pregnancy. If they opt to continue with the pregnancy, it gives them time to seek counseling and join support groups to help them cope with caring for a child with a genetic abnormality.

Treatment for congenital disorders ranges from nonexistent to complete. For example, anencephaly has no known treatment. Phenylketonuria (PKU) is a metabolic defect that leads to mental retardation. It is caused by an inability to metabolize phenylalanine. A special low-phenylalanine diet can markedly reduce progression of the disease. Surgery can correct some congenital disorders such as cardiac defects related to Down syndrome and spinal defects associated with spina bifida.

Advances in medical science and supportive therapy have greatly improved the longevity of patients with genetic disorders. For example, a few decades ago, many children with cystic fibrosis died in childhood.

Currently, according to the Cystic Fibrosis Foundation, the average life expectancy is thirty-seven years.

PERSPECTIVE AND PROSPECTS

Genetic disorders have been recognized for centuries; however, the genetic basis was not understood until the latter half of the twentieth century. Down syndrome and cystic fibrosis are two typical examples. English physician John Down noted that Down syndrome was a specific type of mental disability with distinct physical features. For centuries, the foreheads of children with cystic fibrosis were licked; if a salty taste was noted, the child was deemed to be bewitched and expected to die soon. It was not until the 1990's that the mutated gene that caused the disease was identified.

In addition to Down syndrome and cystic fibrosis, rapid progress has been made in the past two decades in regard to genetic abnormalities. The locations of defective genes have been mapped, and alleles (different forms of a gene) have been identified. Research is ongoing for the treatment of genetic abnormalities. Currently, treatment is mainly limited to surgical correction of defects (correction of a cardiac abnormality in a child with Down syndrome), medical therapy (enzyme therapy for a child with cystic fibrosis), and supportive care (pulmonary therapy to loosen secretions in a child with cystic fibrosis). The most promising treatment for specific gene defects rests in the field of stem cell research. Single-gene defects may be curable via gene therapy in the near future. To date, most of the studies have been animal or in vitro (laboratory) studies.

The outlook is much poorer for defects such as trisomies, which involve a significant amount of extra chromosomal material. The outlook is extremely poor for severe defects such as trisomy 18 and virtually hopeless for abnormalities such as anencephaly. In these cases, the best option at present is early diagnosis via CVS or amniocentesis and pregnancy termination.

There now exists an increased public awareness of the impact of exposure to toxins and infections on pregnancy. This increased awareness has the potential to reduce these preventable disorders. It also can reduce the incidence of defects caused by a deficiency. For example, awareness of the benefits of folic acid can reduce the incidence of neural tube defects. Aggressive therapy for children with a disorder due to exposure of a toxin can sometimes reverse the damage. For example, speech therapy and other behavioral support can reverse central nervous disorders resulting from congenital cocaine exposure. The therapy must be initiated promptly when symptoms are recognized, while the developing brain is in its formative phase. Therapy is most effective before the age of five.

—*Robin L. Wulffson, M.D.*

See also Amniocentesis; Batten's disease; Birth defects; Breast cancer; Cardiology, pediatric; Cerebral palsy; Childbirth; Childbirth complications; Chorionic villus sampling; Cleft lip and palate; Cleft lip and palate repair; Colon cancer; Color blindness; Congenital heart disease; Congenital hypothyroidism; Cornelia de Lange syndrome; Cystic fibrosis; Diabetes mellitus; DiGeorge syndrome; DNA and RNA; Down syndrome; Dwarfism; Embryology; Endocrinology, pediatric; Environmental diseases; Enzymes; Fetal alcohol syndrome; Fetal surgery; Fragile X syndrome; Fructosemia; Gaucher's disease; Gene therapy; Genetic counseling; Genetic diseases; Genetic engineering; Genetics and inheritance; Genomics; Gigantism; Glycogen storage diseases; Hemochromatosis; Hemophilia; Huntington's disease; Hydrocephalus; Immunodeficiency disorders; Klinefelter syndrome; Klippel-Trenaunay syndrome; Laboratory tests; Leukodystrophy; Maple syrup urine disease (MSUD); Marfan syndrome; Mental retardation; Metabolic disorders; Mucopolysaccharidosis (MPS); Multiple sclerosis; Muscular dystrophy; Mutation; Neonatology; Neurofibromatosis; Niemann-Pick disease; Obstetrics; Oncology; Pediatrics; Phenylketonuria (PKU); Polycystic kidney disease; Porphyria; Prader-Willi syndrome; Pregnancy and gestation; Premature birth; Progeria; Proteomics; Rubinstein-Taybi syndrome; Screening; Severe combined immunodeficiency syndrome (SCID); Sickle cell disease; Spina bifida; Tay-Sachs disease; Teratogens; Thalassemia; Thalidomide; Thrombocytopenia; Turner syndrome; Von Willebrand's disease; Wilson's disease; Wiskott-Aldrich syndrome.

For Further Information:

American Pregnancy Association. http://www.american pregnancy.org.

Amniocentesis Report. http://www.amniocentesis.org.

Cummings, Michael. *Human Heredity: Principles and Issues*. 8th ed. Belmont, Calif.: Brooks/Cole, 2008. A comprehensive yet accessible introduction to all aspects of human genetics.

Cystic Fibrosis Foundation. http://www.cff.org.

Lewis, Ricki. *Human Genetics*. 8th ed. New York: McGraw-Hill, 2007. A basic human genetics reference text written by a practicing genetics counselor.

March of Dimes. http://www.marchofdimes.com.

Rapp, Rayna. *Testing Women, Testing the Fetus: The Social Impact of Amniocentesis in America*. New York: Routledge, 2000. Examines the social impact and cultural meaning of currently available prenatal tests.

Scriver, Charles. *The Metabolic and Molecular Bases of Inherited Disease*. 8th ed. 4 vols. New York: McGraw-Hill, 2007. A comprehensive reference indispensable to those in the field, as well as a much broader audience.

Congenital heart disease
Disease/disorder

Anatomy or system affected: Chest, circulatory system, heart

Specialties and related fields: Cardiology, neonatology, pediatrics, vascular medicine

Definition: Conditions resulting from malformations of the heart that occur during embryonic and fetal development, accounting for about 25 percent of all congenital defects.

Key terms:

atria: heart chambers that receive blood, the left from the lungs and the right from the body

great arteries and veins: large vessels channeling blood into and out of the heart, including the aorta (to the body), the pulmonary artery (to the lungs), the vena cava (from the body), and the pulmonary veins (from the lungs)

heart failure: the inability of the heart to pump adequate amounts of blood to maintain the organs and tissues of the body; often results in tissue fluid retention and congestion

murmur: a sound made by the heart other than the normal two-step beat; murmurs are caused by the turbulent movement of blood and may indicate a heart defect

septum: a membrane that serves as a wall of separation; in the heart, the interatrial septum divides the two atria and the interventricular septum divides the two ventricles

ventricles: heart chambers that pump blood out of the heart, the left to the body and the right to the lungs

Causes and Symptoms

Congenital heart disease collectively includes various structural and functional defects of the heart and blood vessels resulting from errors that occur during embryonic development. The defects may cause heart murmurs, high or low blood pressure, congestive heart failure, cyanosis (blue skin), abnormal heart rhythms and rates, and incidences of low oxygen (hypoxia). Congenital heart disease is detected in about 0.7 percent of live births and 2.7 percent of stillbirths. Some babies born with congenital heart disease have difficulty during the first few weeks of life. Some problems, however, are not easily detected at the time of birth and are discovered at various stages of life. Heart defects may be inherited from parents, induced by environmental agents such as drugs, or caused by an interaction of genetic and environmental factors. Defects are more common in children with genetic disorders such as Down syndrome. With intensive treatment, including surgery, many forms of congenital heart disease can be corrected, allowing those affected to lead normal lives.

Knowledge of normal heart development will help in understanding how congenital heart disease occurs and will provide a means for categorizing these defects. Near the end of the third week of embryonic development, the heart begins to form from two cords of tissue that hollow out and fuse to form a primitive heart tube. This tube undergoes some constrictions and dilations to form the early divisions of the heart, including a receiving chamber, the atrium, and a pumping chamber, the ventricle, which exits into a muscular tube called the truncus arteriosus. At about twenty-two days, the heart begins to contract and pump blood. A day later, it bends or loops upon itself to form an S shape, with the atrium on one side, the truncus arteriosus on the other side, and the ventricle in the middle. If it bends to the left instead of to the right, a rare heart defect called dextrocardia results. The heart will be displaced to the right side of the body and may have some accompanying abnormalities.

During the fourth and fifth week of development, the heart begins to divide into four chambers by first forming a septum (dividing membrane) in the canal between

---

INFORMATION ON CONGENITAL HEART DISEASE

CAUSES: Genetic and environmental factors
SYMPTOMS: Shortness of breath, fatigue, sweating while eating, inability to gain weight, lung congestion, altered blood pressure, hypoxia, congestive heart failure
DURATION: Ranges from short-term to lifelong
TREATMENTS: Surgery, medications, insertion of balloon catheter

---

the atrium and the ventricle. This septum is formed by heart tissue called the endocardial cushions. Failure of this septum to form properly causes atrioventricular canal defects. These are often associated with Down syndrome. During the fifth week of development, a spiral septum forms in the truncus arteriosus which divides it into two vessels: the pulmonary artery, which connects to the right ventricle, and the aorta, which connects to the left ventricle. The formation of this septum and the ventricular connections are subject to error and may result in a group of anomalies called conotruncal defects.

As these large arteries are forming, a shunt (bypass) develops between them called the ductus arteriosus. This short vessel allows the blood to be diverted away from the nonfunctional fetal lungs into the aorta and on to the placenta, where it will receive oxygen and nutrients. Persistence of this shunt after birth is responsible for a defect called patent ductus. A septum dividing the atrium into right and left halves also forms during the fourth and fifth weeks of development; however, blood is allowed to pass from the right atrium to the left atrium through a small hole in this septum called the foramen ovale. This hole normally closes after birth but is necessary during fetal life to shunt blood away from the fetal lungs and toward the placenta in a manner similar to that of the ductus arteriosus. At about the same time, a septum forms from the floor of the ventricle and divides it into right and left halves. Failure of the atrial and ventricular septa to form properly and to close at the time of birth results in septal defects.

After the appearance of the four chambers, two pairs of valves form in the heart to prevent the backflow of blood and to ensure greater efficiency in pumping. The semilunar valves (also called the pulmonary and aortic valves) form between the ventricles and their respective outlet arteries (pulmonary artery and aorta), and the atrioventricular valves (bicuspid or mitral on the left and tricuspid on the right) form between the atria and the ventricles. Improperly formed valves can lead to flow defects. During development, the heart also makes connections with veins returning from the general circulation and the lungs. Errors in these connections and other structural errors cause several other less common congenital heart defects.

The most common congenital heart defects are the septal defects and patent ductus, which together account for about 37 percent of all heart defects. After birth, because the pressure becomes higher in the left side of the heart, blood moves from left to right through the openings in the heart that come with such defects, causing too much to flow to the lungs and a mixing of systemic and pulmonary blood. The child's lungs will be congested, causing difficulty in breathing and eventually heart failure.

About 29 percent of congenital heart defects are categorized as right-heart and left-heart flow defects. These defects impede the flow of blood from either the right or the left side of the heart to its normal destination. Right-heart flow defects include bicuspid pulmonary valve (a valve with two cusps instead of three), pulmonary valve stenosis (a narrowing of the valve), dysplastic pulmonary valve (a malformed valve), peripheral pulmonary stenosis (a narrowing of the walls of the pulmonary artery), infundibular pulmonary stenosis (a narrowing below the valve), and hypoplastic right ventricle (incomplete formation of the valve). These defects impede blood flow to the lungs, which results in poor oxygenation of the blood (cyanosis). Left-heart flow defects include bicuspid aortic valve, aortic valve stenosis, coarctation of the aorta (narrowing), aortic atresia (a blocked aorta), and hypoplastic left ventricle. These defects impede blood flow to the body and often result in altered blood pressure, hypoxia of body tissues, and congestive heart failure.

The principal conotruncal defects, which account for about 17 percent of heart defects, are tetralogy of Fallot and transposition of the great arteries. Tetralogy of Fallot includes four defects that result in cyanosis: pulmonary stenosis, a ventricular septal defect, an overriding or displaced aorta, and hypertrophy or enlargement of the right ventricle. With transposition of the great arteries, the aorta connects to the right ventricle and the pulmonary artery to the left ventricle, the opposite of the normal formation. The blood is not properly oxygenated, and survival is not possible without medical intervention or a natural shunt such as patent ductus. Other rare conotruncal defects include double outlet right ventricle (the aorta and the pulmonary artery attached to right ventricle), truncus arteriosus (failure of the truncus to separate into the aorta and the pulmonary artery), and aortopulmonary window (an opening between the aorta and the pulmonary artery).

Defects resulting from improper fusion of the endocardial cushions and surrounding tissues cause atrioventricular defects, which affect about 9 percent of patients with congenital heart disease. Complete atrioventricular canal defect occurs in about 20 percent of Down syndrome cases, but it is rare outside this group. The defect produces a large open space in the

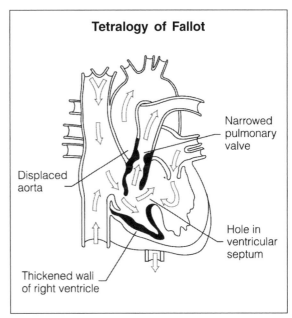

Tetralogy of Fallot

Narrowed pulmonary valve

Displaced aorta

Hole in ventricular septum

Thickened wall of right ventricle

A relatively common congenital heart defect, tetralogy of Fallot comprises four defects: an overriding or displaced aorta, pulmonary stenosis (a narrowed pulmonary valve), a ventricular septal defect (a hole in the ventricular septum), and a thickened, or enlarged, right ventricle. These together result in cyanosis: poor blood oxygenation.

center of the heart, allowing blood to intermix freely between the right and left sides of the heart. The defect is sometimes accompanied by hypoplastic ventricle. If the condition is not treated, the heart will fail. Patent foramen primum or ostium primum is a milder form of atrioventricular canal defect in which the atrial septum fails to fuse with the endocardial cushions, resulting in a problem similar to atrial septal defect. In addition, the mitral valve is usually deformed.

Other less common defects include looping defects such as dextrocardia, in which the apex of the heart points to the right instead of to the left. This change in symmetry normally does not affect heart function, but some looping defects are associated with other problems such as transposition of the great arteries. Another less common defect is anomalous venous return, in which the veins returning blood to the heart from the lungs attach to the right atrium or return to the right atrium by attaching to other large veins rather than to the left atrium. Errors in the coronary artery connections may also occur, causing poor circulation of blood to the heart muscles. Very rarely, the heart may protrude through the chest wall at birth, causing a difficult-to-treat problem called ectopia cordis.

Treatment and Therapy

Congenital heart disease can often be diagnosed shortly after birth, especially if the baby experiences certain symptoms such as cyanosis, shortness of breath, fatigue and sweating while eating, and inability to gain weight. A physical examination by a physician will include checking the heart and breathing rates for abnormalities and listening to the heart for possible murmurs. Heart murmurs are whooshing sounds caused by turbulent movement of blood that may indicate faulty valves, patent ductus, and other heart defects. A cardiologist will make the definitive diagnosis by administering such tests as the electrocardiogram, the Doppler-echocardiogram, and the cardiac catheterization. The electrocardiogram measures the rhythmic electrical signal that passes through the heart with each beat. An abnormal signal will often indicate problems with a particular region of the heart and is especially useful in identifying rhythm disorders. The echocardiogram produces visual images of the heart by sending out ultrasound waves that bounce off and return to a receiving device. Most structural heart defects can be detected with this technique, and many are discovered prenatally with routine fetal ultrasound monitoring. At the same time, a second receiving device (the Doppler) analyzes ultrasound signals from blood moving through the heart and is able to provide information about the speed and direction of blood flow within the heart. This helps detect abnormal functions such as reverse blood flow. The Doppler-echocardiogram has revolutionized congenital heart disease diagnosis and in most cases provides enough information to define the patient's problem accurately.

If the cardiologist believes it to be necessary, then further tests can be done. A chest X ray may be taken to determine if there is any lung involvement in the disorder. Cardiac catheterization can add information about the internal heart blood pressures and blood oxygen levels and can help visualize some defects better with the administration of contrast dyes in combination with X-ray analysis. Special monitors can be used to record the electrocardiogram for one or two days to check for intermittent rhythm irregularities, and older children can be monitored while exercising to see how the heart performs under stress. These and other tests allow physicians to assess the seriousness of the problem and to recommend timely and appropriate treatment.

Serious heart malformations need to be treated immediately upon diagnosis. Often these include defects that cause cyanosis, including transposition of the great arteries, left-heart flow defects such as coarctation of the aorta, and defects that cause heart failure, such as truncus arteriosus. Immediate emergency surgery may be needed to save the life of the newborn infant. Additional follow-up surgeries may also be required to correct the defect completely. For example, one way of correcting transposition of the great arteries is by performing an atrial switch operation in which systemic blood returning from the body is diverted to the left side of the heart (so it can be pumped to the lungs) and pulmonary blood from the lungs is diverted to the right side of the heart (so it can be pumped to the body). This is accomplished by first enlarging the foramen ovale with a balloon catheter, a procedure called Rashkind balloon atrial septostomy. A second operation several months later enlarges the opening between the two atria further and installs a flap to enhance the cross flow of blood. This is known as a Mustard or Senning atrial switch operation. A more recently developed procedure for correcting this defect requires only one operation. The misplaced aorta and pulmonary artery are both cut and then reattached to the correct heart chamber; this is called a Jatene arterial switch operation. At the same time, the coronary arteries are moved to the new aorta.

Some defects require no surgery but can be treated with drugs and other less traumatic procedures, such as the balloon catheter. Drugs are also used to help improve heart performance before and after surgery. When fluid accumulates in the lungs or other body tissues, the heart has problems pumping all the blood that returns to it because of the congestion. The overworked heart suffers under this stress, and thus the condition is called congestive heart failure. Diuretics such as Lasix (furosemide) improve the kidneys' ability to remove the excess fluid and relieve the congestion. Another drug, digitalis, can be helpful in treating congestive heart failure by slowing the heart rate and causing the heart to beat more forcefully. An open ductus is beneficial to children born with cyanotic heart defects because it allows a more even distribution of oxygenated blood. Treatment with prostaglandin E1 helps keep the ductus open until corrective surgery can be performed. Indomethacin has the opposite effect and is often used to promote closing of a patent ductus in premature babies. As in adults, drugs such as digitalis, beta-blockers, and calcium channel blockers can be used to treat abnormal heart rhythms (arrhythmia) in children with congenital heart disease. The balloon catheter is used in a nonsurgical technique to enlarge narrow vessels and passages and has been used successfully to treat pulmonary and aortic valve stenosis in a technique called balloon valvuloplasty.

Types of surgery done later in infancy or childhood include closed heart operations such as repair of a patent ductus and partial treatment of some types of cyanosis with a Blalock-Taussig shunt (connecting the subclavian artery to the pulmonary artery to bring more blood to the lungs). Open heart surgery is used to repair defects inside the heart such as septal defects. A heart-lung machine is used to bypass the heart and lungs while the operation is under way, and the body is cooled so that the brain and other tissues require less oxygen. Children with very serious heart defects such as hypoplastic right or left ventricles may require a series of corrective surgical operations, and for some the only hope is a heart transplant. For example, children with hypoplastic right ventricle are given a Blalock-Taussig shunt shortly after birth to improve blood flow to their lungs and then are later given the Fontan operation, which involves closing off the Blalock-Taussig shunt and connecting the pulmonary artery to the right atrium so that blood returning from the body will flow directly to the lungs, completely bypassing the defective right ventricle.

Some heart defects require no treatment. For example, most small septal defects close on their own during the first one or two years of life. Also, mild disorders such as benign valve defects usually require no treatment, and many children with heart murmurs have no detectable problems.

Perspective and Prospects

In the late nineteenth and early twentieth centuries, physicians were beginning to understand that certain congenital heart defects such as patent ductus could be diagnosed by listening to the heart. Treatment, however, was not possible at that time. The *Atlas of Congenital Cardiac Disease* was published in 1936 by Maude Abbot of McGill University. This work greatly assisted other physicians in recognizing and diagnosing congenital heart disease. In 1939, Robert Gross of Boston repaired a patent ductus, and in 1944, Alfred Blalock and Helen Taussig developed and performed their famous shunt operation in order to treat children with tetralogy of Fallot. Open heart surgery had to wait until the mid-1950's, when the heart-lung machine was perfected. Even then, open heart surgery could be performed only on older children. These operations were pioneered by Walton Lillehei of the University of Minnesota and John Kirlin of the Mayo Clinic. Open heart

surgery on newborn infants was developed in the 1970's by Brian Barratt-Boyes of New Zealand.

During the period while heart surgery was being developed, cardiac catheterization was also advancing. It was used primarily for diagnosis, but in 1966, William Rashkind of Philadelphia began to use the balloon catheter to enlarge openings in the atrial septum in order to treat transposition of the great arteries. Microsurgical catheters are currently being developed to repair patent ductus and other heart defects without the need for major surgery. The echocardiogram was pioneered by Inge Edler in the 1950's, and the Doppler-echocardiogram came into widespread use as a diagnostic tool in the 1980's. This instrument has greatly reduced the need for other diagnostic tests that were used in the past.

The modern strategy for treatment of congenital heart defects is to perform the corrective surgery as early in infancy as possible. This eliminates the need for numerous hospitalizations and diagnostic tests and reduces the need for extensive drug treatment. Children with multiple defects may still need more than one surgery. Modern treatment also emphasizes the roles of the child, the family, and health care personnel in fostering an understanding of the condition, treatment, and outcome. Even children who have been successfully treated will sometimes have physical limitations. These children need to be encouraged and supported by their families and allowed to pursue their goals to the fullest extent possible. Overcoming congenital heart disease is now possible for the vast majority of those who are afflicted.

—*Rodney C. Mowbray, Ph.D.*

See also Arrhythmias; Birth defects; Blue baby syndrome; Bypass surgery; Cardiology; Cardiology, pediatric; Congenital disorders; Cyanosis; DiGeorge syndrome; Echocardiography; Genetic diseases; Heart; Heart disease; Heart failure; Heart transplantation; Mitral valve prolapse; Neonatology; Shunts.

For Further Information:

American Heart Association. http://www.americanheart .org. A group dedicated to reducing disability and death from cardiovascular diseases and stroke. Offers thorough information on a wide range of cardiovascular diseases, referrals to emergency cardiovascular care classes, and research statistics and articles.

Beers, Mark H., et al., eds. *The Merck Manual of Diagnosis and Therapy.* 18th ed. Whitehouse Station, N.J.: Merck Research Laboratories, 2006. Contains complete medical descriptions of the common congenital heart defects and appropriate methods of diagnosis and treatment.

Gersh, Bernard J., ed. *The Mayo Clinic Heart Book*. 2d ed. New York: William Morrow, 2000. One of the most respected texts for laypeople on heart disease. Covers all aspects of anatomy, physiology, diagnosis, treatment, and prevention.

Koenig, Peter, Ziyad M. Hijazi, and Frank Zimmerman, eds. *Essential Pediatric Cardiology*. New York: McGraw-Hill, 2004. An excellent text for the nonspecialist that covers cardiac disorders in the neonate, child, and adolescent.

Kramer, Gerri Freid, and Shari Mauer. *Parent's Guide to Children's Congenital Heart Defects: What They Are, How to Treat Them, How to Cope with Them*. New York: Three Rivers Press, 2001. Experts in pediatric cardiology provide easy-to-understand answers to help parents coping with a child's heart disease. Includes the latest information on diagnosis, treatment options, surgery, aftercare, and growing up with heart defects, as well as stories from parents who have lived through the ordeal.

Moore, Keith L., and T. V. N. Persaud. *The Developing Human*. 8th ed. Philadelphia: Saunders/Elsevier, 2008. An outstanding textbook on human embryonic development. Includes discussion of the development of the circulatory system. The diagrams and descriptions allow the reader to compare normal and abnormal development and to see exactly how errors in development result in congenital heart defects.

Neill, Catherine A., Edward B. Clark, and Carleen Clark. *The Heart of a Child: What Families Need to Know About Heart Disorders in Children*. 2d ed. Baltimore: Johns Hopkins University Press, 2001. A comprehensive work on heart disease affecting children, written for the layperson by medical professionals. The authors give a thorough description of all congenital heart defects and explain their developmental basis.

Park, Myung K. *The Pediatric Cardiology Handbook*. 4th ed. St. Louis, Mo.: Mosby/Elsevier, 2010. A text for the medical specialist with discussion of all congenital heart defects, including atrial septal defects, ventricular septal defects, cushion defects, coarctation, and interrupted aortic arch.

Sherwood, Lauralee. *Human Physiology: From Cells to Systems*. 7th ed. Pacific Grove, Calif.: Brooks/Cole/Cengage Learning, 2010. This college textbook contains useful biological information about embryonic development and genetic defects.

Congenital hypothyroidism
Disease/disorder

Also known as: Infantile hypothyroidism, cretinism

Anatomy or system affected: Endocrine system, musculoskeletal system, neck, nervous system

Specialties and related fields: Endocrinology, internal medicine, perinatology, preventive medicine

Definition: Retardation of mental and physical growth arising from prenatal or neonatal hypothyroidism.

Key terms:

goiter: the sometimes gross enlargement of the thyroid gland in an effort to produce hormones when insufficient iodine is available

L-thyroxine (T4): a less potent thyroid hormone than the T_3 form that can be converted in the cells to T_3

L-triiodothyronine (T3): the most potent of the thyroid hormones

thyroid gland: the endocrine gland in humans that produces the hormones that control metabolism

Causes and Symptoms

In humans, the thyroid gland consists of two connected lobes in the front of the neck, on either side of the thyroid cartilage or Adam's apple. It produces the thyroid hormones, the most important of which are L-triiodothyronine (T_3) and L-tetraiodothyroxine or L-thyroxine (T_4). These compounds circulate in the blood serum to the body's cells and regulate virtually all metabolism: the production and consumption of proteins, carbohydrates, fats, and vitamins and the generation of energy that makes body heat. In these activities, the T_3 molecule (which can be derived in the cells from T_4) has two to four times the effectiveness of T_4. Because of the high iodine content of both T_3 and T_4, sufficient dietary iodine must be supplied to maintain normal thyroid function.

Abnormal levels of T_3 and T_4 have a profound effect on all bodily functions. In adults, the low production of T_3 and T_4, or hypothyroidism, leads to reduced mental and physical activity, weight gain, general weakness, and other symptoms. Elevated thyroid activity, or hyperthyroidism, produces restlessness and irritability, weight loss, and symptoms generally the opposite of those seen with hypothyroidism. When either of these conditions develops in adults, surgery or drug regimens, or both, are available to control them and to produce normal metabolism in the patient. When these conditions occur in utero, however, there is almost no way to counteract their effects.

A child born with congenital hypothyroidism (CH) is mentally retarded with little or no chance of improvement and, unless immediately treated with thyroid hormones, also physically disabled or dwarfed, with the bone ends not growing or maturing normally. The typical infant with CH can show a variety of symptoms: low body temperature, poor appetite, decreased activity, flabbiness, low pulse rate, delayed union of bones of the skull, feeding difficulties even to the point of choking and cyanosis (turning blue from lack of oxygen), and thickened, off-color skin.

TREATMENT AND THERAPY

For the child born with CH, no treatment is available for the mental damage that has taken place. Thyroid replacement therapy from birth, using either natural or synthetic hormones, will avert most physical effects, but the mental retardation is irreversible.

The most effective way to avoid this problem is to ensure that a pregnant woman consumes enough iodine to be made into the T_3 and T_4 molecules by her fetus. The thyroid hormones do not transfer readily from the placental blood supply to that of the fetus, but the iodide ion does. This alone is enough, when made available before the end of the second trimester of pregnancy, to allow the fetal thyroid gland to develop normally and the unborn fetus to have proper neurological and musculoskeletal function. Iodide ions are most easily supplied in iodized salt, but they can also be given as an injection of iodized oil or by the oral administration of a number of iodine-containing medicines, such as Lugol's iodine solution.

When hypothyroidism develops in the older child or adolescent—often appearing as a goiter, in addition to the other symptoms described above—iodine therapy is sometimes sufficient to return thyroid function to normal levels. Oddly, such therapy can also be counterproductive. The complex mechanisms that maintain proper hormone levels in blood serum can be misled by artificially high iodine concentrations and may close down hormone production because it appears high. For this condition, only thyroid hormone administration is effective.

PERSPECTIVE AND PROSPECTS

Hypothyroidism, goiter, and CH are worldwide health problems because of the body's dependence on dietary

---

INFORMATION ON CONGENITAL HYPOTHYROIDISM

CAUSES: Thyroid disorder
SYMPTOMS: Mental retardation, low body temperature, poor appetite, decreased activity, flabbiness, low pulse rate, delayed union of skull bones, feeding difficulties, off-color skin
DURATION: Lifelong
TREATMENTS: Thyroid replacement therapy from birth

---

iodine. Many places on Earth have low soil levels of iodine, leading to low iodine levels in crops and thus inadequate iodine intake from food. Such areas include high mountain country, such as the Himalayas, where glacial meltwater leaches iodine from the soil with no replacement from higher geologic formations; and the Ganges River basin, where the sheer volume of water removes iodine from crop lands. Some mountainous areas of the United States—such as the hill country of West Virginia, Kentucky, and Tennessee—have been, historically, centers of endemic goiter formation. Supplying iodine to inhabitants of these areas is a medical necessity but, like so many such problems, is complicated by logistic and political considerations.

—*Robert M. Hawthorne, Jr., Ph.D.*

See also Birth defects; Congenital disorders; Dwarfism; Endocrine system; Endocrinology, pediatric; Growth; Hashimoto's thyroiditis; Malnutrition; Mental retardation; Nutrition; Thyroid disorders; Thyroid gland; Vitamins and minerals.

FOR FURTHER INFORMATION:

"Another Reason for Iodine Prophylaxis." *The Lancet* 335, no. 8703 (June 16, 1990): 1433-1434. Despite iodine supplementation programs, severe iodine deficiency persists in several parts of Europe and the developing countries. The failure of iodine supplementation programs is discussed in an editorial.

Cao, Xue-Yi, et al. "Timing of Vulnerability of the Brain to Iodine Deficiency in Endemic Cretinism." *New England Journal of Medicine* 331, no. 26 (December 29, 1994). Iodine was administered to children from birth to three years of age and women at each trimester of pregnancy in an iodine-deficient area of the Xinjiang region of China. According to the results, iodine treatment protects the fetal brain from the effects of iodine deficiency.

Gomez, Joan. *Thyroid Problems in Women and Children*. Alameda, Calif.: Hunter House, 2003. Discusses current research, incorporates case studies, and includes special chapters for pregnant women and about babies and children with the disease.

Hetzel, Basil S. "Iodine and Neuropsychological Development." *Journal of Nutrition* 130, no. 2S (1999): 493S-495S. The establishment of the essential link among iodine deficiency, thyroid function, and brain development has emerged from a fascinating combination of clinical, epidemiologic, and experimental studies.

Kronenberg, Henry M., et al., eds. *Williams Textbook of Endocrinology*. 11th ed. Philadelphia: Saunders/Elsevier, 2008. Text that covers the spectrum of information related to the endocrine system, including thyroid disorders, diabetes, endocrinology and aging, female reproduction and fertility control, sexual function and dysfunction, kidney stones, and endocrine hypertension.

Maberly, Glen F. "Iodine Deficiency Disorders: Contemporary Scientific Issues." *Journal of Nutrition* 124, no. 8 (August, 1994): 1473-1478S. Iodine deficiency is the leading cause of preventable intellectual impairment and is associated with a spectrum of neurologic pathology. Although some 1 billion people are at risk, developing fetuses and infants are most susceptible to the intellectual impairment caused by iodine deficiency.

March of Dimes. http://www.marchofdimes.org. Web site offers a range of excellent fact sheets on myriad birth defects, information about prenatal testing, and special sections for pregnant women and for researchers and professionals.

Rosenthal, M. Sara. *The Thyroid Sourcebook*. 5th ed. New York: McGraw-Hill, 2009. A wide-ranging examination of thyroid disorders from hyperthyroidism to cancer.

Woeber, K. A. "Iodine and Thyroid Disease." *Medical Clinics of North America: Thyroid Diseases* 75, no. 1 (January, 1991): 169-178. Environmental iodine deficiency continues to be a significant public health problem worldwide, compounded in some regions by the presence of other goitrogens in some staple foods.

CONGESTIVE HEART FAILURE. *See* **HEART FAILURE.**

CONJUNCTIVITIS
DISEASE/DISORDER

ALSO KNOWN AS: Pinkeye

ANATOMY OR SYSTEM AFFECTED: Eyes, immune system

SPECIALTIES AND RELATED FIELDS: Bacteriology, family medicine, microbiology, ophthalmology, optometry, virology

DEFINITION: An acute inflammatory disease of the eye caused by infection or irritation.

CAUSES AND SYMPTOMS

Conjunctivitis, or pinkeye, is one of the most common eye disorders. The conjunctiva is a thin translucent membrane that overlies the white part of the eye and the inner surface of the eyelids. It protects the eye from foreign objects and infection.

The conjunctiva may become inflamed through infection with a virus or bacterium, allergic reactions, and exposure to certain chemicals. Inflammation of the conjunctiva brings increased blood flow to the eye, producing a red, or bloodshot, appearance. Conjunctivitis causes a feeling of irritation, burning, or mild pain. A discharge often occurs, which may form a crust on the eyelids when it dries. Conjunctivitis does not cause visual loss, fever, or severe pain. It is typically mild and short-lived, lasting from a few days to a few weeks.

Most conjunctivitis is caused by infection and is highly contagious, spreading quickly from one eye to the other and from person to person by touch. Viral conjunctivitis will resolve without treatment, although symptoms may persist as long as a few weeks. Upper-respiratory symptoms often occur simultaneously, since similar viruses cause the common cold. These viruses may live on surfaces for several hours and can be transmitted in poorly chlorinated swimming pools. Bacterial conjunctivitis causes a thicker discharge and more severe crusting. It is caused by various bacteria, and all respond well to topical antibiotics.

Allergic conjunctivitis may be stimulated by a reac-

INFORMATION ON CONJUNCTIVITIS

CAUSES: Viral or bacterial infection, allergic reactions, exposure to chemicals or irritants

SYMPTOMS: Red or bloodshot eye, burning sensation, mild pain, discharge forming crust on eyelids

DURATION: Ranges from a few days to a few weeks

TREATMENTS: None or topical antibiotics

tion to dust, mold, animal dander, or pollen. It causes burning or itching in both eyes and occurs in a seasonal pattern. Chemicals, wind, dust, smoke, and chronic dry eyes can also cause direct irritation of the conjunctiva.

TREATMENT AND THERAPY

For viral conjunctivitis, no therapy is required, but the patient may be contagious for as long as two weeks. Common bacterial conjunctivitis resolves quickly with antibiotic eyedrops or ointment. A person remains contagious with bacterial conjunctivitis until after twenty-four hours of antibiotic treatment. The spread of infection can be prevented by washing one's hands frequently, using separate towels, and isolating an infected child from interaction with other children for the first twenty-four hours of treatment. For allergic conjunctivitis, avoiding the offending allergen and using topical antihistamines or artificial tears are effective treatments.

PERSPECTIVE AND PROSPECTS

Conjunctivitis in the United States is generally benign and rarely causes permanent injury. Elsewhere in the world, however, conjunctivitis is a leading cause of blindness. In areas of extreme poverty, repeated infections with trachoma, a bacterial infection spread by flies, lead to permanent scarring of the eyes. Newborns may also contract severe bacterial conjunctivitis from the mother's cervix during birth. For this reason, most developed nations require that all newborns receive antibiotic eyedrops at birth.

—Christopher D. Sharp, M.D.

See also Allergies; Bacterial infections; Blindness; Childhood infectious diseases; Eye infections and disorders; Eyes; Keratitis; Trachoma; Viral infections; Vision; Vision disorders.

FOR FURTHER INFORMATION:

Johnson, Gordon J., et al., eds. *The Epidemiology of Eye Disease.* 2d ed. New York: Oxford University Press, 2003.

Kasper, Dennis L., et al., eds. *Harrison's Principles of Internal Medicine.* 16th ed. New York: McGraw-Hill, 2005.

Parker, James N., and Philip M. Parker, eds. *The Official Patient's Sourcebook on Conjunctivitis.* San Diego, Calif.: Icon Health, 2002.

Stoffman, Phyllis. *The Family Guide to Preventing and Treating One Hundred Infectious Illnesses.* New York: John Wiley & Sons, 1995.

Turkington, Carol, and Bonnie Lee Ashby. *The Encyclopedia of Infectious Diseases.* 2d ed. New York: Facts On File, 2003.

CONNECTIVE TISSUE
ANATOMY

ANATOMY OR SYSTEM AFFECTED: Blood, bones, ligaments, musculoskeletal system, tendons

SPECIALTIES AND RELATED FIELDS: Biochemistry, hematology, orthopedics, rheumatology

DEFINITION: A category of tissue composed of adipose (fat), blood, bone, cartilage, ligaments, and tendons; the function of connective tissue is to connect, support, bind, protect, and store materials.

STRUCTURE AND FUNCTION

Cells, the structural and functional units of life, are organized into tissue, a group of different types of cells and their nonliving intracellular matrix, or glue, that performs a specialized function. The four groups of tissues are epithelial (covering and lining tissue; also glands); connective (adipose, blood, bone, cartilage, ligament, and tendon); muscle (skeletal, cardiac, and smooth); and nervous (brain and spinal cord).

Connective tissue typically has cells widely scattered throughout a large amount of intraceliular matrix (that is, a substance in which the cells are embedded), unlike epithelial tissue that typically has cells arranged in an orderly manner and has a limited amount of intracellular matrix.

Connective tissues are categorized as loose (aerolar), dense, and specialized. Some connective tissues are difficult to classify, with the distinction between "loose" and "dense" not clearly defined. Also, dense connective tissue may be called fibrous connective tissue because of the large amount of collagen or elastin fibers contained.

Because a tissue is defined as a collection of different cells, several types of cells that may be found in various types of connective tissue: fibroblasts, which secrete collagen and other elements of the extracellular matrix, thereby creating and maintaining the matrix; adipocytes, which store excess caloric energy in the form of fat; and mast cells, macrophages, leukocytes, and plasma cells, which have immune functions and, therefore, an active role in inflammation. The components of the matrix are different in the different types of connective tissue and may include fibers, amorphous ground substances (glycoproteins, proteins, and proteoglycans), and tissue fluid. Each type of connective tissue has a characteristic pattern of cells and a distinctive amount and type of matrix. For example, bone matrix includes minerals, while blood has plasma for a matrix.

Loose connective tissue is the most common type of connective tissue; it holds organs in place and attaches epithelial tissue to underlying tissues. Loose connective tissue can be further categorized based on the type of fibers and how the fibers are arranged: collagenous fibers, which are composed of collagen and are arranged as coils; elastic fibers, which are composed of elastin and are able to stretch; and reticular fibers, which join connective tissue to other tissues. Loose connective tissue has a relatively large amount of cells, matrix, or both, and a relatively small amount of fibers. Loose connective tissue is found in the hypodermis and fascia (the connective tissue that loosely binds structures to one another).

Dense connective tissue is identified by the high density of fibers in the tissue and a low density of cells and matrix. The type of fiber that predominates determines the type of dense connective tissue. Dense collagenous connective tissue, for example, contains an abundance of collagen fibers and is found in structures where tensile strength is needed, such as the sclera (white) of the eye, tendons, and ligaments. Dense elastic connective tissue contains an abundance of elastin fibers and is found in structures where elasticity is needed (for example, the aorta).

Specialized connective tissues include adipose tissue, cartilage, bone, and blood. Adipose tissue is a form of loose connective tissue that stores fat. It is found in the fatty layer around the abdomen, in bone marrow, and around the kidneys. Cartilage is a form of fibrous connective tissue. It is composed of closely packed collagenous fibers embedded in a gelatinous intracellular matrix called chondrin. While the skeleton of human embryos are composed of cartilage, cartilage does not become bone but rather is replaced by bone. The replacement is not universal; cartilage provides flexible support for ears (external pinnae), nose, and trachea.

Blood too, is a type of specialized connective tissue. Blood may seem to be an unlikely connective tissue, but it fits the definition: different cells widely dispersed in intracellular matrix, working together to perform a specific function. Unlike other connective tissues, blood has no fibers. Blood does have several types of cells: red blood cells or erythrocytes, white blood cells or leukocytes (with subdivisions of monocytes, macrophages, eosinophils, lymphocytes, neutrophils, and basophils), and platelets or thrombocytes. The matrix is liquid and contains enzymes, hormones, proteins, carbohydrates, and fats.

DISORDERS AND DISEASES

Connective tissue, like any other tissue, is subject to disorders and diseases. Some disorders are inherited (passed from one generation to the next by means of DNA in chromosomes), while other disorders are related to the environment (such as a lack of specific nutrients).

Some inherited connective tissue disorders are Marfan syndrome and osteogenesis imperfecta. In Marfan syndrome, connective tissue grows outside the cell, having deleterious effects on the lungs, heart valves, aorta, eyes, central nervous system, and skeletal system. People with Marfan syndrome are often unusually tall with long, slender arms, legs, and fingers. In osteogenesis imperfecta, or brittle bone disease, the quantity and quality of collagen is insufficient to produce healthy bones. People with this disorder have multiple spontaneous bone breaks. Other connective tissue diseases are environmental, such as scurvy, which is caused by a lack of vitamin C required for the production and maintenance of collagen. Without sufficient vitamin C in the diet, and subsequent lack of collagen, the patient will develop spots on the skin, particularly the legs and thighs; will be tired and depressed; and may lose teeth. Osteoporosis has many factors, but lack of vitamin D and calcium in the diet will lead to a thinning of the bone, subjecting the patient to fractures, primarily of the hip, spine, and wrist.

Connective tissue diseases may also be classified as systemic autoimmune disease and may have both genetic and environmental causes. In these situations, the immune system is spontaneously overactivated and extra antibodies are produced. Examples of systemic autoimmune diseases include systemic lupus erythromatosus and rheumatoid arthritis. Systemic lupus erythromatosus can damage the heart, joints, skin, lungs, blood vessels, liver, kidneys, and nervous system. More woman than men are diagnosed with lupus, and more black women than other groups. Rheumatoid arthritis is caused when immune cells attack the membrane around joints and destroys the cartilage of the joint; it can also affect the heart and lungs and interfere with vision.

—M. A. Foote, Ph.D.

See also Blood and blood disorders; Bones and the skeleton; Cartilage; Ligaments; Tendon disorders.

FOR FURTHER INFORMATION:

Lundon, Katie. *Orthopedic Rehabilitation Science: Principles for Clinical Management of Nonmineralized Connective Tissue.* Boston: Butterworth-Heinemann, 2003.

Price, Sylvia Anderson, and Lorraine McCarty Wilson, eds. *Pathophysiology: Clinical Concepts of Disease Processes.* St. Louis: Mosby, 2003.

Royce, Peter M., and Beat Steinmann, eds. *Connective Tissue and Its Heritable Disorders: Molecular, Genetic, and Medical Aspects.* New York: Wiley-Liss, 2002.

CONSTIPATION

DISEASE/DISORDER

ANATOMY OR SYSTEM AFFECTED: Abdomen, gastrointestinal system, intestines

SPECIALTIES AND RELATED FIELDS: Family medicine, gastroenterology, internal medicine

DEFINITION: The slow passage of feces through the bowels or the presence of hard feces.

CAUSES AND SYMPTOMS

People of every age group, from infants to the elderly, can experience the unpleasant symptoms of constipation, which is characterized primarily by discomfort. Certain disease states such as diabetes mellitus, paralysis of the legs, colon cancer, and hypothyroidism predispose a person to constipation. Possible causes of constipation are medications, iron supplements, toilet training procedures, pregnancy, lack of adequate fluids, a low-fiber diet, and lack of physical activity.

TREATMENT AND THERAPY

Most cases of constipation can be treated by the patient at home. Drinking adequate fluids makes it easier for fecal material to pass through the large intestine. Without adequate hydration, a person may experience small, pelletlike stools. Eight to ten glasses of liquids per day are recommended, including water, milk, cocoa, fruit juice, herbal tea, and soup. Once adequate hydration is achieved, a high-fiber diet can gradually be started. Without enough fluids, a high-fiber diet can worsen the problems of constipation. A high-fiber diet adds bulk to the bowel movement (increasing stool volume, decreasing pressure within the colon, and decreasing the intestinal transit time of foods) and thus can lead to more regular bowel habits and partial relief of the symptoms. One can increase fiber in the diet by eating prunes, high-fiber breakfast cereals, beans or le-

---

INFORMATION ON CONSTIPATION

CAUSES: Lack of fiber or adequate fluids in diet, certain medications, iron supplements, pregnancy, lack of physical activity, aging

SYMPTOMS: Uncomfortable passage of stools, bloating, abdominal discomfort

DURATION: Ranges from short-term to chronic

TREATMENTS: Adequate hydration, high-fiber diet, exercise, laxatives

---

gumes, raw fruits and vegetables, and whole-grain breads. To minimize gastrointestinal discomforts such as increased flatulence (gas), it is recommended to increase one's fiber consumption gradually.

In addition to adequate liquids and a high-fiber diet, exercise is important in treating constipation. Any sort of physical activity, such as walking, running, tennis, or swimming, can help to stimulate the activity of the large intestine.

Laxatives and enemas should not be used until after a discussion with a physician. Mineral oil should also not be used because many essential fat-soluble vitamins (such as vitamins A, D, E, and K) may be excreted as well. Persistent constipation should be evaluated by a physician.

—*Martha M. Henze, M.S., R.D.*

See also Colon; Diarrhea and dysentery; Enemas; Fiber; Gastroenterology; Gastroenterology, pediatric; Gastrointestinal disorders; Gastrointestinal system; Hemorrhoid banding and removal; Hemorrhoids; Indigestion; Intestinal disorders; Intestines; Obstruction; Over-the-counter medications; Rectum.

FOR FURTHER INFORMATION:

Berkson, D. Lindsey. *Healthy Digestion the Natural Way.* New York: Wiley, 2000.

Capasso, Francesco. *Laxatives: A Practical Guide.* New York: Springer, 1997.

Gitnick, Gary, and Karen Cooksey. *Freedom from Digestive Distress.* New York: Crown, 2000.

Parker, James N., and Philip M. Parker, eds. *The Official Patient's Sourcebook on Constipation.* San Diego, Calif.: Icon Health, 2002.

Peikin, Steven R. *Gastrointestinal Health.* Rev. ed. New York: Quill, 2001.

Wexner, Steven D., and Graeme S. Duthie, eds. *Constipation: Etiology, Evaluation, and Management.* 2d ed. London: Springer, 2006.

Whorton, James C. *Inner Hygiene: Constipation and the Pursuit of Health in Modern Society.* New York: Oxford University Press, 2000.

CONTRACEPTION

PROCEDURE

ANATOMY OR SYSTEM AFFECTED: Genitals, reproductive system, uterus

SPECIALTIES AND RELATED FIELDS: Gynecology, obstetrics, urology

DEFINITION: The use of techniques to prevent pregnancy, which may interfere with ovulation, sperm transport, or implantation of an embryo.

KEY TERMS:

barrier method: a contraceptive that physically prevents sperm from meeting an egg

cervix: the entrance to the uterus from the vagina

ejaculation: the release of semen from the male's body during sexual activity

hormone: a chemical signal carried in the blood that allows distant body parts to coordinate their actions

implantation: the process in which the embryo attaches to the uterine lining

ovulation: the monthly release of a mature egg from the ovary

spermicide: a chemical that kills sperm after they are ejaculated

toxic shock syndrome: an infection normally caused by staphylococci that can develop rapidly into severe untreatable shock, which can be fatal

uterus: the organ that supports the embryo during its development

vagina: the tube-shaped cavity of the female into which the male's penis is inserted during intercourse

vas deferens: the tubes in the male reproductive system that carry sperm

METHODS AND EFFECTIVENESS

Contraception is defined as the avoidance of conception by either natural means (abstinence) or artificial means (physical barriers, chemicals, hormones). Pregnancy can be prevented by interfering with the process of conception at any number of sites in the male or female anatomy.

Barrier methods. A male condom, or prophylactic, is a thin sheath made to fit an erect penis. It can be made of latex (a type of rubber), polyurethane (a type of plastic), or natural products such as lamb's intestines. A condom prevents semen, which contains sperm, from entering a woman's vagina during intercourse. The latex or polyurethane condom is one of the few forms of contraception that can also protect against sexually transmitted diseases (STDs). Men who are not allergic to latex should use latex condoms, as they are the best at preventing pregnancy and STDs. Polyurethane condoms break more easily, and natural condoms are not as effective at preventing STDs.

Male condoms should be used any time a man has intercourse with his partner and desires to prevent STDs or pregnancy. If the condom does not have space at the end called a sperm repository, then 0.25 inches of the condom should be left at the tip of the penis to collect semen. To increase the protective birth control value, spermicidal foam or jelly can be used in addition to the condom. According to the American College of Obstetricians and Gynecologists, this combination is 99 percent effective. Vaseline or other types of petroleum jelly, lotion, or oils should not be used as a lubricant with condoms because they weaken the latex rubber. Non-oil-based lubricants or even water can be used with latex condoms. Condoms come in a variety of sizes and can be purchased over the counter at drugstores and pharmacies and in coin machines in many public restrooms. There is no age restriction on buying condoms.

The female condom is a lubricated, thin polyurethane or nitrile tube that has a flexible ring that facilitates insertion and an outside ring that helps keep the condom in place around the vulva. The closed end of the tube is inserted into the vagina, and the other end remains outside the vagina, slightly covering the labia and providing some enhanced protection against skin-borne infections. With proper use, the female condom is similar to the male condom in effectiveness, and it may be more accepted by male partners who do not wish to wear a condom. Female condoms, however, are more expensive and harder to find. Recent introduction of a new nitrile female condom, FC2, has lowered the price, and many public health and reproductive health advocates are working to make the method more accepted and widely available. Like the male condom, the female condom should be used only once per intercourse, and female and male condoms should not be used together.

A diaphragm is a dome-shaped rubber disk with a flexible rim, which covers the cervix so that sperm are unable to enter the uterus. A diaphragm, which must be prescribed and sized by a health care professional, is designed to be used with a spermicide that is applied inside the dome and around the rim. The diaphragm provides birth control protection up to six hours after insertion. A new application of spermicide should be inserted into the vagina with an applicator and with the diaphragm in place for repeated intercourse. To be effective, the diaphragm must remain in the vagina six hours after the last intercourse, but never longer than twenty-four hours because of the risk of toxic shock syndrome. The diaphragm is approximately 83 percent effective as a birth control method.

The cervical cap is a soft rubber or plastic cup with a round rim, which fits snugly over the cervix. As with a diaphragm, it must be fitted by a health care professional. The cervical cap should be used in combination with a spermicidal cream or jelly for optimal effectiveness. It can provide birth control protection for up to forty-eight hours. The cervical cap should be removed after forty-eight hours because of a low risk of toxic shock syndrome. It does not provide any protection against STDs.

Vaginal spermicides include creams, jellies, films, foams, suppositories, and tablets. They contain sperm-killing chemicals and act somewhat as a barrier to sperm entering the uterus. Spermicides used by themselves are up to 79 percent effective for birth control, but when used properly with condoms, they are up to 99 percent effective. They are available without a prescription. For spermicides to be effective, they should be inserted into the woman's vagina up to twenty minutes before intercourse and stay in the vagina at least eight hours. A new application of spermicide should be applied for repeated intercourse. Spermicides do not protect against STDs unless they are used in combination with condoms.

Hormonal methods. Oral contraceptives or birth control pills, often simply called "the pill," are the most popular form of reversible birth control in the United States. They contain synthetic hormones that interact with a woman's natural hormones to prevent pregnancy. There are two types of birth control pills, combination estrogen-progestin and progestin alone.

Combination birth control pills stop the ovaries from releasing eggs. Available only by prescription, combination pills come in packages of twenty-one or twenty-eight pills per month, although there are new pills designed for continuous or extended cycling that come in packages with more than a month's supply. There are twenty-one active pills in the twenty-one-day pack. The twenty-eight-day pack contains twenty-one active pills and seven placebo or sugar pills, with the exception of some newer formulations that extend the active

pill cycle to more than twenty-one pills, reducing the number of inactive or placebo pills. Menstruation occurs during the week with no pills or inactive pills, although extended or continuous cycling involves a longer or continuous regimen of active pills and delays menstruation until a pill-free interval.

Some other form of contraception should be used for the first month in addition to the birth control pill. By the second month, the pill should provide the needed birth control. Pills should be taken at the same time of the day each day. Oral contraceptives are 98 to 99 percent effective in providing birth control, but they provide no protection against STDs. Oral contraceptives can be taken safely by most women, but they are not recommended for women over thirty-five who smoke. A benefit of oral contraceptives is that they can make

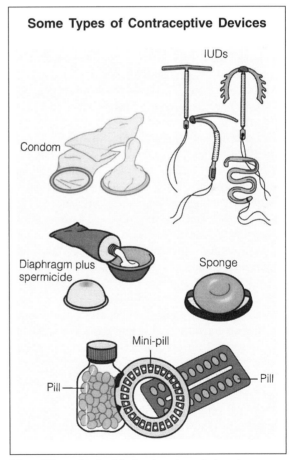

Some Types of Contraceptive Devices

Many different kinds of devices have been designed to prevent pregnancy, from barrier methods such as condoms and diaphragms to hormonal methods such as birth control pills. Each method has its own advantages, disadvantages, and failure rates.

a woman's menstrual cycle regular and lighter, and they are protective against pelvic inflammatory disease (PID), ovarian cancer, and endometrial cancer.

The second form of oral contraception is the mini-pill. It contains only one hormone, progestin, and works by thickening the cervical mucus so that sperm is unable to reach the egg. Progestin also changes the lining of the uterus so that implantation cannot occur. Mini-pills are 95 percent effective in preventing pregnancy, but their effectiveness diminishes if they are not taken on time. The pill taken more than two hours from the set time for a daily dose constitutes a missed pill and significantly raises the chance of unintended pregnancy.

Ortho Evra is a thin patch that releases a combination of estrogen and progestin. It is worn on the upper outer arm, upper torso (excluding the breast), buttocks, or abdomen. Once attached, it delivers hormones through the skin and into the bloodstream. The patch will remain in place during exercise or bathing and in humid conditions. It is worn for three weeks, then removed for one week before a new patch is worn. The patch offers approximately 99 percent birth control protection, but no protection from STDs. It has been found to be significantly less effective in women weighing more than 198 pounds.

NuvaRing is a transparent flexible ring that is inserted into the vagina, and normally stays around the cervix. The ring releases estrogen and progestin into the vagina to stop ovulation, to thicken cervical mucus, and to prevent implantation if fertilization occurs. The ring is worn for three weeks, followed by a week off, during which menstruation occurs. Vaginal rings must be replaced each month. If the ring slips out of the vagina, the patient can wash the ring with cold to luke-warm water (avoiding hot water) and reinsert it. The chance of pregnancy is increased if the ring is outside the vagina for more than three hours; if this occurs, the woman should use a backup method for another seven days to obtain maximum protection against pregnancy. Both NuvaRing and Ortho Evra share the same contraindications and benefits as combined oral contraceptives.

Depo-Provera (depo-medroxyprogesterone acetate, or DMPA) contains only the hormone progestin and is given by a health care provider as an injection every twelve weeks. DMPA comes in two formulations and can be given by intramuscular or subcutaneous injection. Patients need to be aware that irregular bleeding (which may include brownish spotting) and probable lack of normal menses is an expected side effect of DMPA, not a sign of a serious adverse affect. For some women who discontinue using DMPA, delayed fertility can last up to one year beyond the end of the injections. DMPA works in the same way as the mini-pill.

Those who use DMPA should be cautious, as both adolescents and adults have experienced a significant loss of bone density. This bone loss is thought to correct itself when the injections are discontinued, with the exception of women in perimenopause, who may not have enough time to reclaim bone mass before menopause. Furthermore, DMPA leads to weight gain in some women, through increased appetite. Women should be cautioned against overeating once beginning DMPA as their birth control method.

Emergency contraceptive pills can be used after a sexual assault, after intercourse without contraception, after finding that a condom broke during or after sex, or after the failure of some other method. Emergency contraception can be performed through a progestin-only formulation that involves taking two pills as soon as possible after unprotected sex, but within seventy-two hours (based on strong evidence, some clinical practices recommend emergency contraception as effective for up to five days after unprotected intercourse). A woman should have her menstrual cycle within ten to twenty-one days of taking emergency contraception pills, and thereafter her cycle should return to normal. These pills prevent conception, rather than causing a miscarriage, by thickening the cervical mucus, thus preventing sperm from fertilizing the egg. In 2003, a Food and Drug Administration (FDA) panel recommended that these morning-after pills, as they came to be known, be made available over the counter. They are now available over the counter to girls and women seventeen years of age and older. Girls under the age of seventeen need a prescription from a health care provider to obtain emergency contraception. Additional but less widely used methods of emergency contraception include the Yuzpe method, involving high doses of combined oral contraceptives, and insertion of an IUD following unprotected intercourse.

Intrauterine devices (IUDs). The IUD is a small device that is inserted into a woman's uterus by a health care provider in a simple office procedure. Two IUDs are currently available in the United States. Both are shaped like a capital *T*, and both have a silky or plastic thread that extends out into the cervix, allowing for easy removal. The ParaGard T 380A contains copper, but no hormones, and can be kept in the uterus for ten years. Mirena is an IUD that contains a progestin that

IN THE NEWS:
NEW CONTRACEPTION OPTION IMPLANON

Implanon, an etonogestrel-releasing implant effective for up to three years, was approved in July, 2006. Implanon has advantages over Norplant, a contraceptive implant no longer available in the United States. It requires implantation of one rod into the upper arm instead of Norplant's six, making insertion and removal easier. Additionally, blood levels appear to vary less with Implanon. Fertility is regained within a few days following removal. Implanon is highly associated with irregular bleeding. Other side effects are similar to those from oral contraceptives. Because the product is progestin-only, it may be appropriate for some women who cannot use estrogens. Trial data suggest that Implanon in combination with injectable testosterone may be effective as a male contraceptive. Further study is needed for this indication.

—*Karen M. Nagel, R.Ph., Ph.D.*

releases slowly throughout the time that the device is in place. It can be kept in the uterus for five years. While ParaGard may result in some increased bleeding, a woman will have regular menses. Mirena greatly decreases menstrual flow but can result in irregular spotting, especially in the first three months of insertion, and some women stop having menses altogether. An IUD is thought to prevent pregnancy because it is a foreign object whose presence causes the woman's uterus to function improperly. The IUD interferes with sperm reaching the egg and prevents the egg from implanting in the uterus. IUDs that contain copper are thought to work by releasing of copper ions into the uterus. The copper in the uterine cavity stops sperm from moving through the vagina and into the uterus. IUDs are 97 to 99 percent effective in preventing pregnancy but provide no protection from STDs.

Sterilization. Essure is a sterilization device shaped much like a spring. The device is threaded through a thin tube through the vagina and into the Fallopian tubes. Two Essure devices are inserted, one in each Fallopian tube. Once they are in place, a meshlike substance inside the devices irritates the Fallopian tubes, causing scarring of the Fallopian tubes over time. The scarring finally causes permanent closing of the tube. Since this process of blockage in the tubes takes time, women are advised to use another form of birth control for the first three months after the insertion of Essure. The device then provides more than 99 percent effectiveness as birth control. It provides no protection from STDs.

Female sterilization through tubal ligation is one of the most common forms of contraception in the United States. An estimated 700,000 women undergo tubal ligation each year. The procedure involves surgically sealing the Fallopian tubes in order to prevent eggs from being released into the uterus. This surgery also prevents a male's sperm from entering the Fallopian tube, where fertilization normally occurs. The procedure is performed in a hospital or an outpatient surgical clinic under general anesthesia. One or two small incisions are made in a woman's abdomen, and a laparoscope is inserted. Instruments are also inserted and used to burn or seal the passages into the Fallopian tubes. Patients are usually able to return home a few hours after surgery. This procedure is more than 99 percent effective as birth control but provides no protection from STDs.

Male sterilization through vasectomy can be performed in a doctor's office. Local anesthesia is applied and a small incision is made in the upper part of the scrotum. The vas deferens is cut and sealed. This simple operation prevents sperm from traveling out of the testes. There is also a nonsurgical technique in which the doctor locates the vas deferens and holds it in place with a small clamp. A tiny puncture is made in the skin, and the opening is stretched so that the vas deferens can be cut and tied. This procedure requires no stitches because the punctures heal quickly on their own. With either of these methods, a man is able to return home immediately after the procedure and usually needs only a day of rest before resuming his normal activities. It is recommended that another form of birth control be used during the first nine or ten ejaculations to ensure that the seminal fluid no longer contains sperm. This method is 99 to 100 percent effective in preventing pregnancy; however, it provides no protection against STDs.

PERSPECTIVE AND PROSPECTS
Even though highly effective contraceptive techniques are available both over the counter and through health care providers, almost 60 percent of pregnancies in the United States are not planned, and many are unwanted. The contraception and reproductive branch of the National Institute of Child Health and Human De-

velopment (NICHD), which has as one of its goals to prevent acquired immunodeficiency syndrome (AIDS) and other STDs, is looking into the development of new microcides with spermicidal activity that can provide birth control as well as simultaneous protection against major STDs. One of the top objectives is to link contraceptive technology to HIV-AIDS prevention.

—Clair Kaplan, A.P.R.N./M.S.N.;
additional material by Toby R. Stewart, Ph.D.

See also Abortion; Conception; Ethics; Gynecology; Hormones; Hysterectomy; Men's health; Menstruation; Over-the-counter medications; Pregnancy and gestation; Reproductive system; Semen; Sterilization; Tubal ligation; Uterus; Vasectomy; Women's health.

FOR FURTHER INFORMATION:

Connell, Elizabeth B. *The Contraception Sourcebook.* Chicago: Contemporary Books, 2002. Provides a history and explanation of contraception, from oral contraceptives to male contraception.

Global Campaign for Microbicides. http://www.global -campaign.org. An organization working to combine birth control with protection against STDs.

Keyzer, Amy Marcaccio. *Family Planning Sourcebook.* Detroit, Mich.: Omnigraphics, 2001. Contains excellent information on all types of contraception and family planning.

Porter, Robert S., et al., eds. *The Merck Manual Home Health Handbook.* Whitehouse Station, N.J.: Merck Research Laboratories, 2009. A comprehensive book of medical knowledge, including information on contraception.

Thornton, Yvonne S. *Woman to Woman: A Leading Gynecologist Tells You All You Need to Know About Your Body and Your Health.* New York: E. P. Dutton, 1998. Divided into six sections covering topics from female physiology to contraception.

CORNEAL TRANSPLANTATION

PROCEDURE

ANATOMY OR SYSTEM AFFECTED: Eyes

SPECIALTIES AND RELATED FIELDS: General surgery, ophthalmology

DEFINITION: A delicate surgical operation involving the removal and replacement of the cornea, the transparent outer covering of the eye.

KEY TERMS:

endothelium: the inner surface of the cornea, which is separated from the rest of the eye by an essential layer of transparent fluid

keratoplasty: surgery on the cornea

lamellar keratoplasty: the partial removal or transplantation of a portion of the cornea; usually possible in younger patients or those with less advanced disorders

penetrating keratoplasty: the surgical transplantation of the entire thickness of the cornea, which is made up of four distinct layers of tissue

trephine: a specialized surgical instrument that is used to cut a perfectly vertical incision to remove corneas from both the donor and the recipient

INDICATIONS AND PROCEDURES

The cornea, which has four distinct layers, is the transparent outer coating of the eye. It serves both to protect the eye and to provide the main refracting surface as light reaches the eye and is transmitted to the lens and retina. Its total thickness is approximately 0.52 millimeter. The layers of specialized tissue are the epithelium, the stroma, Descemet's membrane, and the endothelium, or inner surface of the cornea.

Several types of corneal disorders may lead to a decision to perform partial or total keratoplasty. Most of these fall under the general term "corneal dystrophy." The most common, or classical, cases of corneal dystrophy involve the deposit of abnormal material in the cornea, resulting in irritation and eventually damage. Frequently, such disorders stem from genetic factors, making it possible to diagnose the dystrophy during the patient's childhood and perform a lamellar keratoplasty. Other dystrophies include granular dystrophy and macular dystrophy. The former involves lesions in the center of the cornea, which may multiply and coalesce. At that stage, they may extend into the deeper layers of the stroma, the second layer of the cornea. Macular dystrophy actually begins in the stroma, causing all layers to become opaque.

Entirely different types of disorders that may call for corneal transplantation are interstitial keratitis (a type of inflammation) and trachoma. The latter condition can reach near epidemic levels in underdeveloped areas of the world, where low levels of hygiene allow the implantation and rapid multiplication of bacteria in the cornea. The effect is a breakdown of tissue accompanied by the discharge of mucus.

Whether the cornea has been affected by disease or injury, the goal of corneal transplantation is to eliminate any opacity that can hamper vision. The graft operation itself may be described in only a few stages, each marked by the need for a high degree of technical skill to increase the likelihood of success. First, the surgeon must calculate the exact size of the graft in question. This is done through the use of a special tool called a trephine, which will make the cuts to remove both the donor and the host eye corneas. Some trephines are equipped with transparent lenses to give the surgeon maximum levels of accuracy. When the two vital incisions are made, great care is taken to obtain a perfectly vertical cut.

Beginning with this initial stage, the surgeon may add a bubble of air through the incision to protect the endothelium and reduce the likelihood of an immune system reaction once the donor cornea has been transplanted. As the transfer occurs, another air bubble is introduced. After suturing, this bubble will be replaced by a balanced salt solution called acetylcholine.

This suturing, which must be very precise, almost always begins with four sutures at the cardinal points to ensure even tension. The last stage of the operation involves checking the wound for leakage of acetylcholine. This step is necessary not only to avoid infection but also to guard against rejection of the cornea by the host organ.

USES AND COMPLICATIONS

Significant differences in the healing process following corneal transplantation occur according to the method of suturing. A choice is made between a continuing or an interrupted series of sutures around the circumference of the cornea. Interrupted sutures may be preferred if there is a chance of uneven healing of the wound, something the physician may judge following examination of the degree of vascularization in particular corneal graft beds. In some cases, surgeons may opt for double suturing.

The chief complication that can follow corneal transplantation is rejection by the immune system. Surgeons try to obviate this risk by close study of the factors that can affect the receptivity of the eye to a new cornea. Earlier literature on corneal transplantation tended to assume that there was a lack of antigenicity—the production of disease-fighting antigens, or antibodies, as a defense system against viruses, bacteria, or foreign tissues—in the cornea. As ophthalmologists developed a fuller understanding of the immunological role of blood vessels and the lymphatic system, however, the need to give considerable attention to the degree of vascularization of the graft bed zone became more obvious. One method that surgeons can use to reduce antigen activity and enhance host acceptance is part of the

transplantation operation itself: constant maintenance of a liquid layer between the host tissue and the new cornea tissue being transplanted. In the late 1990's, researchers at the University of Texas Southwestern Medical Center at Dallas announced the creation of an oral vaccine that may prevent rejection. Processed corneal cells in liquid form fed to laboratory mice produced a marked reduction in rejection rates. Current studies focus on the success of the vaccine with humans.

Although the period for healing and suture removal varies from patient to patient, the surgeon looks for the normal development of a gray-tinged scar tissue in the incision area as a sign of success. Failure, if discovered in time, may lead to a second transplantation attempt.

PERSPECTIVE AND PROSPECTS

The first attempts to perform corneal transplantation— all unsuccessful—date from the nineteenth century. In the 1820's, German doctor F. Reisinger experimented with corneal grafts using rabbits and chickens. In the 1830's, Samuel Bigger of Ireland and R. S. Kissam of the United States tried to pioneer surgical grafts on humans, but both made the error of trying to replace human corneas with animal corneas. Success with living tissue (as opposed to the application of a glass product) finally came in 1905 when Moravian doctor Edward Zirm transplanted a child donor's cornea to the eye of a chemical burn victim. Zirm's success was based on cumulative medical knowledge of antiseptics, anesthesia, and technical aids such as the ophthalmoscope and the trephine. After a long period without major changes, in 1935 a Russian scientist named Filatov experimented with two innovations that were copied in other countries: the use of egg membrane to enhance a firm fix and the insertion of a delicate spatula between the cornea and lens to protect the intraocular tissues.

The greatest advances were made soon after antibiotics and steroids were introduced in the 1940's. By the 1950's, the use of extremely delicate surgical needles helped reduce postsurgical rejection rates. Major contributions to the development of delicate surgical instruments were made by the Spanish ophthalmologist Ramón Castroviejo, who performed many operations in the United States. By the 1980's, Castroviejo was urging others to follow the example of Townley Paton, who founded New York's first eye bank some two decades earlier.

By the turn of the twenty-first century, forty thousand people in the United States had received corneal transplants using cells taken from the eyes of donors who had died. However, many patients with severe corneal damage cannot be helped by conventional cornea transplants. Two research teams, one in Taiwan, at the University of Taoyuan, and one at the University of California at Davis School of Medicine, used stem cells to continually produce new corneal cells within the eye. In Taiwan, stem cells were placed on amniotic membrane, taken from placentas, to grow the tissue. In California, cells were first grown in laboratory dishes and then placed on the amniotic membrane to produce the tissue, which was transplanted to the damaged corneas. The use of this kind of tissue showed improved or restored vision for patients with corneal damage. While these procedures hold great potential for worldwide application, they have been called "investigational" and by no means eliminate the need for cornea donors.

The prospects for increasingly higher success rates in the field of corneal transplantation are linked to technical progress in donor organ conservation and the level of precision that can be achieved in carrying out transplantation operations.

—Byron D. Cannon, Ph.D.

See also Eye infections and disorders; Eye surgery; Eyes; Grafts and grafting; Keratitis; Ophthalmology; Trachoma; Transplantation; Vision; Vision disorders.

FOR FURTHER INFORMATION:

Brightbill, Frederick S., ed. *Corneal Surgery.* 3d ed. St. Louis, Mo.: Mosby, 1999. This rather technical text is divided into sections in which the authors discuss their specific areas of expertise.

Foster, C. Stephen, Dimitri T. Azar, and Claes H. Dohlman, eds. *Smolin and Thoft's The Cornea: Scientific Foundations and Clinical Practice.* 4th ed. Philadelphia: Lippincott Williams & Wilkins, 2005. This covers some cornea-related topics that either are absent from standard texts (for example, congenital anomalies) or reflect recent surgical advances (for example, corneal surgery to make refractive corrections to reduce or remove myopia).

Parker, James N., and Philip M. Parker, eds. *The Official Patient's Sourcebook on Corneal Transplant Surgery.* San Diego, Calif.: Icon Health, 2002. Draws from public, academic, government, and peer-reviewed research to provide a wide-ranging handbook for patients facing corneal transplant surgery.

Spaeth, George L., ed. *Ophthalmic Surgery: Principles and Practice.* 3d ed. Philadelphia: W. B. Saunders, 2003. The subsections of this text deal with all aspects of eye surgery, including corneal surgery and operations to correct glaucoma, cataracts, and retinal displacement.

Sutton, Amy L., ed. *Eye Care Sourcebook: Basic Consumer Health Information About Eye Care and Eye Disorders.* 3d ed. Detroit, Mich.: Omnigraphics, 2008. A complete guide to eye care that includes such topics as eye anatomy, preventive vision care, refractive disorders and eye diseases, surgical treatment, current research and clinical trials, and a list of organizations.

CORNELIA DE LANGE SYNDROME
DISEASE/DISORDER

ALSO KNOWN AS: Amsterdam dwarfism, Brachmann-de Lange syndrome

ANATOMY OR SYSTEM AFFECTED: Arms, brain, ears, eyes, feet, hair, hands, head, heart, immune system, legs, mouth, nose, teeth

SPECIALTIES AND RELATED FIELDS: Genetics, neurology, pediatrics, physical therapy

DEFINITION: A disorder with distinctive physical abnormalities and mental retardation usually apparent at birth.

CAUSES AND SYMPTOMS

Cornelia de Lange syndrome occurs at an estimated rate of 1 per 10,000 to 30,000 live births. Sometimes siblings have this syndrome, reinforcing the hypothesis that it is hereditary. Although the precise causation is unknown, researchers are investigating the possibility that a mutated gene on chromosome 3 is responsible.

The physical appearance of children with this syndrome is significantly altered. Patients are smaller in size and weight than average infants, and their growth and motor development are usually delayed. Upper limbs are often deformed, with missing tissues. Although legs attain average size and development appropriate to patients' age, sometimes toes are webbed. Hands tend to be tiny. Patients share similar facial characteristics. Heads are abnormally small with upturned nostrils and thin lips and eyebrows. Heavy body hair often grows.

Intellectual development is impeded, particularly affecting vocalization. Hearing and vision sometimes are affected. Patients often suffer heart abnormalities, cleft palate, reflux, and convulsions. They are vulnerable to infections because of impaired immune systems.

Prenatal ultrasounds can reveal if fetuses have physi-

INFORMATION ON CORNELIA DE LANGE SYNDROME

CAUSES: Unknown, possibly genetic
SYMPTOMS: Low size and weight, delayed growth and motor development, deformed upper limbs, webbed toes, small hands, small head, heavy body hair, heart abnormalities, cleft palate, reflux, convulsions, impaired immune system
DURATION: Lifelong
TREATMENTS: Incubation to monitor respiration and nutrition, antibiotics, surgical procedures for specific ailments, physical therapy, auditory devices, prosthetics

cal deficiencies that might be associated with Cornelia de Lange syndrome. Physicians identify the syndrome by observing characteristics evident in infants and toddlers. Genetic professionals confirm diagnoses, especially in patients whose symptoms are less obvious.

TREATMENT AND THERAPY

Many newborns with Cornelia de Lange syndrome require incubation to monitor respiration and nutrition. Antibiotics and other medications, as well as surgical procedures, are administered to treat specific ailments affecting these individuals. Physical therapy, auditory devices, and prosthetics can aid children. Some patients have shortened life spans and are unable to live autonomously. Heart conditions cause most of the deaths associated with this syndrome.

Although no known cure or prevention exists, medical awareness and treatment of this syndrome can extend the life span and enhance the quality of life for many patients. Some patients with milder conditions survive to average life expectancies. Adults with this syndrome attain a height from four to five feet and undergo puberty at normal ages. Various therapies can assist patients who exhibit aggressive and self-destructive behaviors and improve communication and social skills.

PERSPECTIVE AND PROSPECTS

In 1916, Winfried R. Brachmann became the first physician to document this syndrome's characteristics in an infant. Dutch pediatrician Cornelia C. de Lange clinically described two patients in 1933 and discussed her work at neurological conferences. By the early twenty-first century, researchers had established a Cornelia de Lange syndrome database to coordinate information. Geneticists, particularly Ian Krantz and his colleagues, conducted molecular investigations to determine the genetic causation of this syndrome. A mutation in a gene known as NIPBL is now known to be one cause of this relatively rare disorder. This gene provides direction for the making of a protein, delangin, which is very important in developmental regulation of a number of body parts in the fetus. In the United States, the Cornelia de Lange Syndrome-USA Foundation provides support for affected families.

—Elizabeth D. Schafer, Ph.D.;
updated by Lenela Glass-Godwin, M.W.S.
See also Birth defects; Congenital disorders; Dwarfism; Genetic diseases; Genetics and inheritance; Mental retardation.

FOR FURTHER INFORMATION:

Benson, M. "Cornelia de Lange Syndrome: A Case Study." *Neonatal Network* 21, no. 3 (April, 2002): 7-13.

Berg, J. M., et al. *The De Lange Syndrome*. New York: Pergamon Press, 1970.

Cornelia de Lange Syndrome-USA Foundation. http://www.cdlsusa.org.

Gardner, R. J. M. "Another Explanation for Familial Cornelia de Lange Syndrome." *American Journal of Medical Genetics* 118A, no. 2 (April 15, 2003): 198.

Gilbert, Patricia. *Dictionary of Syndromes and Inherited Disorders*. 3d ed. Chicago: Fitzroy Dearborn, 2000.

CORNS AND CALLUSES

DISEASE/DISORDER
ANATOMY OR SYSTEM AFFECTED: Feet, hands, skin
SPECIALTIES AND RELATED FIELDS: Dermatology, podiatry
DEFINITION: Areas of thickened skin that form as a result of constant pressure or friction over a bony prominence.

CAUSES AND SYMPTOMS

Both corns (clavi) and calluses (tylomas or tyloses) occur when chronic pressure or friction causes hypertrophy of the dermal skin layer and a proliferation of keratin as a protective response. Both corns and calluses usually occur on the feet. Corns develop from pressure on normally thin skin. Calluses develop over areas where the skin is normally thicker. They commonly de-

INFORMATION ON CORNS AND CALLUSES

CAUSES: Constant pressure or friction over bony prominence, often from improperly fitting shoes
SYMPTOMS: Pain, inflammation, rough skin
DURATION: Typically short-term, occasionally chronic
TREATMENTS: Better-fitting footwear, over-the-counter medications, occasionally surgery

velop on the plantar (sole) surface of the foot and on the palmar (palm) surface of the hand. Corns are frequently painful, whereas calluses usually are not painful. Corns are small, flat, or slightly elevated lesions with a smooth, hard surface. Calluses cover a larger area than corns and are less well demarcated.

There are two classifications of corns: hard and soft. Hard corns have a conical structure composed of keratin, with the point of the cone directed inward, causing pain when pressed into the soft, underlying tissue. Hard corns have a circumscribed border that demarcates the lesions from the surrounding soft tissue. Hard corns usually develop on the top or sides of the toes, where shoes press on the interphalangeal joints of the toes, or the plantar surface of the foot, where pressure is exerted against bony prominences.

Soft corns develop in areas where a bony prominence causes constant pressure against soft tissue, resulting in a blanched thickening of the skin. Because soft corns commonly develop on interdigital surfaces, such as between the fourth and fifth toe, they are characteristically moist and macerated and can become inflamed.

Calluses develop as a protection against continual pressure. They do not have the central core of keratin and as a result are not sensitive to pressure. Normal skin markings are present over callused areas. Calluses usually develop on weight-bearing areas of the foot under the metatarsal heads and the heel. Calluses on the palm are frequently the result of manual occupations.

TREATMENT AND THERAPY

Treatment of corns and calluses depends on symptoms. Since corns and calluses are caused by chronic pressure, preventive measures include removing the source of friction or pressure. Well-fitting shoes that do not crowd the toes relieve pressure on interdigital areas.

Soft, sufficiently wide or open-toed shoes are good choices. Soft insoles and properly fitting stockings also reduce pressure. Wrapping lamb's wool or other padding over pressure points can increase air circulation and reduce pressure and discomfort. Corns and calluses can be treated with over-the-counter keratolytic agents. Salicylic acid plasters are used to soften the tissue, which can then be removed with a pumice stone. When corns, or occasionally calluses, become inflamed or painful, they can be removed by paring or trimming. This should be done by a health care provider, especially in patients with compromised circulation to the feet. In rare circumstances, surgery may be required if a corn or callus becomes infected or if the chronic pressure on particular areas is caused by a structural abnormality of the foot, such as a hammertoe.

—*Roberta Tierney, M.S.N., J.D., A.P.N.*

See also Bedsores; Bunions; Dermatology; Feet; Foot disorders; Hammertoe correction; Hammertoes; Hypertrophy; Podiatry; Skin; Skin disorders.

FOR FURTHER INFORMATION:

Copeland, Glenn, and Stan Solomon. *The Foot Doctor: Lifetime Relief for Your Aching Feet.* Rev. ed. Toronto, Ont.: Macmillan Canada, 1996.

Lippert, Frederick G., and Sigvard T. Hansen. *Foot and Ankle Disorders: Tricks of the Trade.* New York: Thieme, 2003.

Lorimer, Donald L., et al., eds. *Neale's Disorders of the Foot.* 7th ed. New York: Churchill Livingstone/ Elsevier, 2006.

Mackie, Rona M. *Clinical Dermatology.* 5th ed. New York: Oxford University Press, 2003.

CORONARY ARTERY BYPASS GRAFT

PROCEDURE

ANATOMY OR SYSTEM AFFECTED: Circulatory system, heart

SPECIALTIES AND RELATED FIELDS: Cardiac surgery, cardiology

DEFINITION: A surgical procedure in which a healthy blood vessel is taken from another part of the body and grafted into a segment of a coronary artery in order to bypass a blockage.

KEY TERMS:

angina: pain in the chest caused by insufficient blood flow to the heart muscle

angioplasty: surgical procedure to reduce blockages in a coronary artery that uses a catheter

atherosclerosis: a process in which plaque builds up on the walls of blood vessels

catheter: a flexible tube inserted into a small opening or incision in the body

heart-lung bypass machine: equipment that pumps and oxygenates the blood during heart surgery

ischemia: insufficient blood flow to a part of the body

plaque: fat deposits on the blood vessel walls

saphenous vein: a vein from the upper leg often used to bypass a blocked coronary artery

INDICATIONS AND PROCEDURES

Atherosclerosis is a disease in which fat deposits called plaque accumulate on the walls of arteries and restrict blood flow. Although plaque can form in any arteries in the body, the effect is most noticeable in the coronary arteries, which supply blood to the heart muscle. Since the heart must pump continuously, it needs a steady supply of oxygenated blood. When the plaque in a coronary artery gets too thick, an area of the heart muscle will not receive enough blood, resulting in a condition called ischemia. The result is often chest pain called angina. Patients with angina are high risk for having a heart attack.

To alleviate angina and restore sufficient blood flow to the heart muscle, coronary artery bypass graft surgery may be performed. The patient is given general anesthesia for the procedure. The breastbone or sternum is sawed in two, and the chest is opened to expose the heart. At the same time, an assistant removes a healthy vein from an arm or leg. Most commonly, the saphenous vein from the upper leg is used. The heart is stopped and the patient is put on a heart-lung bypass machine that pumps the blood during the surgery. While the heart is stopped, the surgeon cuts the coronary artery above the blockage, and the healthy vessel which was removed from another part of the body is attached. Then the coronary artery is cut below the blockage and the other end of the healthy vessel is attached. This procedure effectively reroutes the blood flow through the grafted vessel and around the blockage, thereby giving it the name bypass graft. Because the normal blood flow is restored, the angina is alleviated and the risk of heart attack is decreased. Another approach is to use the internal mammary artery, which is already attached to the aorta, for a blood source. Only one incision below the blockage needs to be made to establish good blood flow. After the bypass is completed, the heart is restarted and the machine is removed. The sternum is wired together and the incision is sutured.

USES AND COMPLICATIONS

Coronary artery bypass surgery is used to restore sufficient blood flow through a coronary artery that is narrowed or blocked with plaque. In patients with coronary artery disease it is common to have more than one artery narrowed or blocked. In this case, multiple bypasses may be completed in one surgery. Double, triple, and quadruple bypass surgeries are common. In these cases, the grafting procedure is repeated as many times as necessary to bypass all narrowed or blocked arteries.

One major problem for postoperative cardiac patients who have had bypass surgery is the threat of additional blockages developing. Sometimes patients need to have additional bypass surgeries several years later to bypass new blockages that have developed. Therefore, after surgery most patients will be referred to a cardiac rehabilitation program, or cardiac rehab. In cardiac rehab, patients learn to exercise safely, eat right, and manage stress better. By making lifestyle changes patients can delay or prevent the development of additional plaque obstructions.

PERSPECTIVE AND PROSPECTS

Bypass graft surgery is one way to restore blood flow through a blocked coronary artery. It has been widely used since the 1970's and has been safe and effective. However, it is a major surgical procedure that causes great discomfort to the patient. With advances in technology that are less invasive, such as cardiac catheters, other options are now available.

A procedure that competes with coronary artery bypass surgery is angioplasty. Instead of a major incision through the chest, angioplasty uses a catheter inserted through a small incision in an arm or the groin. The catheter is run through the blood vessels and into the heart. When the catheter reaches the narrowed area, the surgeon inflates a small balloon that compresses the plaque against the wall of the artery. Like bypass surgery, this procedure also improves blood flow to the heart muscle. Unfortunately, not all patients are good candidates for angioplasty and the more invasive bypass surgery must be used. As technology continues to improve, however, more patients will be able to have angioplasty.

—Bradley R. A. Wilson, Ph.D.

See also Angina; Angioplasty; Arteriosclerosis; Bypass surgery; Cardiac surgery; Cardiology; Cardiology, pediatric; Circulation; Heart; Heart disease; Heart valve replacement; Vascular medicine; Vascular system.

FOR FURTHER INFORMATION:

Chizner, Michael A. *Clinical Cardiology Made Ridiculously Simple.* Miami: MedMaster, 2008.

Rippe, James M. *Heart Disease for Dummies.* Hoboken, N.J.: Wiley, 2004.

Sheridan, Brett C., et al. *So You're Having Heart Bypass Surgery.* Hoboken, N.J.: John Wiley & Sons, 2003.

CORONAVIRUSES

DISEASE/DISORDER

ANATOMY OR SYSTEM AFFECTED: Immune system, lungs, lymphatic system, respiratory system

SPECIALTIES AND RELATED FIELDS: Environmental health, epidemiology, immunology, public health, pulmonary medicine, virology

DEFINITION: Viruses frequently infecting the upper respiratory system and capable of producing either the common cold or severe acute respiratory syndrome (SARS).

KEY TERMS:

common cold: an acute respiratory tract infection including stuffy or running nose, sore throat, sneezing, fever, wheezing, and nasal pressure headache

epidemiology: the study of epidemic disease; that which determines the onset, distribution, and course of disease within populations

rhinoviruses: spherical, non-enveloped, positive single-strand RNA viruses with a diameter of about thirty nanometers and the most common viral agent infecting humans; infection results in upper respiratory distress

severe acute respiratory syndrome (SARS): a deadly, novel coronavirus disease originating in China in 2002 that became a global epidemic in 2003

virion: a single virus particle

CAUSES AND SYMPTOMS

Coronaviruses are spherical, enveloped virion particles sixty to two hundred nanometers in diameter with twenty-nanometer-long surface projections looking like ball-topped points of a crown. Coronaviruses are positive-strand ribonucleic acid (RNA) viruses with nonsegmented genomes containing roughly thirty thousand nucleotides. Coronaviruses are widespread in the environment and exist in a large range of hosts including humans, dogs, cats, mice, cattle, swine, turkeys, and chickens, and may also be present in rats and rabbits.

The dominant mode of coronavirus transmission is uncertain, usually contact with infected carrier animals who act as vectors for the virus without becoming ill themselves or contact with surfaces or body fluids contaminated with the virus. Depending on environmental conditions, the virus can survive minutes to hours on exposed surfaces or within discharged fluids.

In humans, two to ten days after exposure, symptoms appear, including fever with high temperature, headache, nasal discharge, cough and sore throat, general lethargy, diarrhea, and breathing difficulties; in severe cases collapsed lungs, massively reduced white blood cell count, depleted platelet reserves, blood cells leaking into glands and major organs, and dead tissue in glands and major organs. In animals, symptoms of coronavirus infection include stresses to digestive, respiratory, reproductive, renal, and central nervous systems.

TREATMENT AND THERAPY

It is not possible to distinguish coronavirus infections from rhinovirus infections based on symptoms alone. Diagnosis of a coronavirus infection requires laboratory tests including organ or cell cultures, electron microscopy, immunofluorescence, nucleic acid hybridization, reverse transcription-polymerase chain reaction, and serology, the most effective method being an enzyme-linked immunoassay. Though there is presently no direct line of evidence linking back to respiratory infection, coronaviruses are tenuously implicated in a number of nonrespiratory diseases including highly infectious mononucleosis, pancreatitis, thyroiditis, nephropathy, pericarditis, and multiple sclerosis.

Besides the common cold, the most notable coronavirus infection is associated with highly contagious severe acute respiratory syndrome (SARS), which pro-

---

INFORMATION ON CORONAVIRUSES

CAUSES: Usually contact with infected carrier animals or with surfaces or body fluids

SYMPTOMS: High fever, headache, nasal discharge, cough, sore throat, general lethargy, diarrhea, breathing difficulties; in severe cases, collapsed lungs, massively reduced white blood cell count, depleted platelet reserves, blood cells leaking into glands and major organs, dead tissue in glands and major organs

DURATION: Two to eighteen days

TREATMENTS: Fever-reducing drugs, extra oxygen, ventilator support (if needed), some antiviral drugs

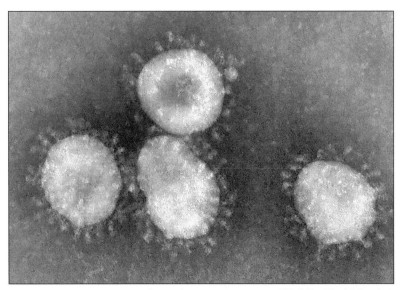

Coronavirus virions seen with an electron microscope. (CDC/Dr. Fred Murphy)

duces an atypical pneumonia and a resulting high death rate.

Coronaviruses have an incubation period of two days to two weeks. There are two to eighteen days of active infection, and reinfections are common.

Treatment consists of fever-reducing drugs, extra oxygen, ventilator support if needed, and some antiviral drugs.

PERSPECTIVE AND PROSPECTS

Human coronaviruses were first identified in 1965, and continuing epidemiological research suggests coronaviruses are prime agents of respiratory illness in humans, though the viruses can also infect nerve cells and immune system cells as well. Coronaviruses are second only to rhinoviruses as causes of upper respiratory illnesses collectively known as the common cold: coronaviruses are likely responsible for 30 percent of such infections. Most people have endured at least one bout of coronavirus infection before reaching adulthood. Coronaviruses may also result in severe secondary infections to the lower respiratory system if the patient has an existing health condition such as asthma.

The first identified case of SARS can be traced back to November 16, 2002, in Foshan, China. The patient was diagnosed with pneumonia and sent home to recover. Soon a large number of people in the area became ill with the same symptoms of respiratory distress. Chinese authorities took no action to contain the disease. By February, 2003, the disease had spread to Hong Kong, and guests at the Metropole Hotel began to fall ill. Many international guests of the hotel, showing no symptoms, boarded planes and traveled home only to become symptomatic after arriving at their destinations. As more and more people in Hong Kong, and then in distant locations, became severely ill, an intense effort was mounted to find the cause: a coronavirus.

The coronavirus responsible for SARS was traced back to specific locations in China where wild mammals were being sold in meat markets as exotic food. While the carrier animals were immune to the virus, a mutation in the virus's genes allowed it to infect humans and then spread from person to person. The global spread of SARS was precipitated by air travel from China, initiating outbreaks in a number of countries in a matter of days. Once the source of the outbreak was identified and scientists discovered the infection was caused by a coronavirus, efforts to stop the spread of SARS were initiated worldwide. The World Health Organization (WHO) and the U.S. Centers for Disease Control and Prevention issued global alerts. Airports and rail stations in many countries set up infrared scanners to detect travelers with fevers and quarantine them until they were screened for the virus. In some cities with identified cases of SARS, entire blocks, districts, and buildings were quarantined: sporting events, school attendance, international conferences, and religious services were canceled. Within four months of its outbreak, SARS had spread to twenty-four nations on four continents.

Eventually, the SARS epidemic was suppressed by breaking the chain of human transmission with quarantines. Globally, diagnosed SARS cases reached 8,098 with 774 deaths. There is no effective treatment for SARS beyond supporting the patient toward recovery. In May, 2005, WHO declared SARS eradicated. SARS and smallpox are the only two diseases to be listed as eradicated.

—*Randall L. Milstein, Ph.D.*

See also Common cold; Environmental diseases; Environmental health; Epidemiology; Microbiology; Pneumonia; Pulmonary diseases; Pulmonary medicine; Severe acute respiratory syndrome (SARS); Viral infections; Zoonoses.

For Further Information:

Kleinman, A., and J. Watson, eds. *SARS in China: Prelude to Pandemic?* Stanford, Calif.: Stanford University Press, 2006.

Peiris, M., et al., eds. *Severe Acute Respiratory Syndrome.* Malden, Mass.: Blackwell, 2005.

Schmidt, A., M. H. Wolff, and O. Weber, eds. *Coronaviruses with Special Emphasis on First Insights Concerning SARS.* Boston: Birkhäuser, 2005.

Siddell, Stuart G., ed. *The Coronaviridae.* New York: Plenum Press, 1995.

Corticosteroids

Biology

Also known as: Glucocorticoids, mineralocorticoids

Anatomy or system affected: Endocrine system, immune system

Specialties and related fields: Biochemistry, endocrinology, family medicine, immunology

Definition: Steroid hormones such as cortisol and aldosterone synthesized and secreted by the adrenal cortex, or their synthetic equivalents.

Key terms:

Addison's disease: a disease characterized by hypoadrenalism caused by cortisol deficiency

cortisol: a steroid hormone of the adrenal cortex that has many physiological actions

Cushing's syndrome: a disease characterized by hyperadrenalism caused by an excess secretion or exogenous administration of cortisol

glucocorticoid: a steroid hormone such as cortisol from the adrenal cortex that has many physiological actions, including the regulation of glucose metabolism

mineralocorticoid: a steroid hormone from the adrenal cortex that regulates salt and water balance

Structure and Functions

Corticosteroids are steroid hormones produced by the cortex of the adrenal glands. They have several physiological actions, including regulation of glucose, lipid and protein metabolism, regulation of inflammation and the immune response, maintenance of homeostasis during stress, and control of water and electrolyte balance and blood pressure.

Corticosteroids that have their primary effects on glucose metabolism are glucocorticoids, whereas those that have the control of electrolyte and water balance as their main functions are mineralocorticoids. Cortisol is the primary glucocorticoid, although significant amounts of corticosterone and cortisone are secreted. Aldosterone is the primary mineralocorticoid.

Glucocorticoids promote an increase in blood glucose by stimulating the synthesis of glucose (gluconeogenesis). They also stimulate the catabolism of lipids and proteins. Thus, glucocorticoids increase blood glucose and are antagonistic to insulin.

The synthesis of corticosteroids is controlled by adrenocorticotropic hormone (ACTH) produced by the pituitary gland. Corticotropin-releasing hormone (CRH) produced by the hypothalamus controls the secretion of ACTH. A feedback loop exists so that when cortisol levels are high, the release of CRH and ACTH is inhibited, and when cortisol levels are low, CRH and ACTH are released.

Aldosterone is primarily responsible for the control of salt and water balance by promoting the excretion of potassium and the retention of sodium and water. Through its effect on salt and water balance, aldosterone can increase blood pressure. Plasma levels of aldosterone are controlled by a variety of mechanisms, including plasma volume and potassium ion concentration.

Disorders and Diseases

Addison's disease results from adrenal insufficiency (hypocortisolism). Although most cases are caused by a disorder of the adrenal glands (primary adrenal insufficiency), some cases are caused by a disorder of the pituitary gland (secondary adrenal insufficiency). An autoimmune disorder that destroys the adrenal cortex is the major cause of primary adrenal insufficiency. Secondary adrenal insufficiency is usually caused by a lack of ACTH. Pituitary tumors, surgical removal of the pituitary, and loss of blood flow to the pituitary are the major causes of secondary adrenal insufficiency. Major symptoms of adrenal insufficiency include loss of appetite, weight loss, fatigue, muscle weakness, and hypotension. Addison's disease can be diagnosed by administering ACTH and monitoring the adrenal gland's response by measuring serum and urine cortisol levels. Adrenal insufficiency is treated by oral administration of hydrocortisone, a synthetic form of cortisol. If aldosterone is also deficient, then fludrocortisone is administered.

Adrenal insufficiency is often caused by a mutation in one of the enzymes synthesizing cortisol. These cases are referred to as congenital adrenal hyperplasia (CAH). Since serum cortisol is low or absent, the pituitary gland stimulates the adrenal gland to produce more cortisol. The precursor steroids and their metabolic products that accumulate can cause varying degrees of virilization of female fetuses and infants. Replacement therapy is the treatment of choice. Surgery to reconstruct the genital organs may be necessary in severe cases.

Hypercortisolism can lead to Cushing's syndrome. Major symptoms include obesity, osteoporosis, fatigue, hypertension, hyperglycemia, and amenorrhea (absence of menstruation). Cushing's syndrome may be caused by prolonged use of glucocorticoids or by an overproduction of glucocorticoids by the adrenal glands. The major causes of an overproduction of glucocorticoids are pituitary and adrenal tumors. Diagnosis of Cushing's syndrome is most commonly made by determining the amount of cortisol in the urine. Cushing's syndrome can be treated by reducing administered glucocorticoids or by treatment of the tumor causing the disease through surgical removal, radiation, and/or chemotherapy.

Hypoaldosteronism is a condition in which the adrenal cortex does not produce an adequate amount of aldosterone, which results in an inability to control and regulate blood volume and blood pressure. Blood pressure can fall to dangerously low levels.

Synthetic corticosteroids such as prednisone, prednisolone, methylprednisolone, hydrocortisone, and dexamethasone have an immunosuppressive effect and are used to treat a variety of chronic autoimmune and inflammatory diseases. They can reduce the pain, swelling, itching, inflammation, and redness associated with arthritis, bursitis, asthma, dermatitis, eczema and psoriasis, lupus erythematosus, Crohn's disease, and various ear, eye, and skin infections and allergic reactions.

Prolonged use of corticosteroids can lead to medically induced Cushing's syndrome, suppression of the immune system, hypertension, hypokalemia (low serum potassium), and hypernatremia (high serum sodium).

PERSPECTIVE AND PROSPECTS

In 1855, Thomas Addison became the first physician to describe the clinical symptoms of adrenal insufficiency. In the early 1930's, Frank Hartman, Wilbur Swingle, and Joseph Pfiffner were the first to prepare active adrenal extracts capable of treating the symptoms of adrenal insufficiency. By the mid-1930's, Pfiffner, Edward Calvin Kendall, Oskar Wintersteiner, and Tadeus Reichstein had isolated and crystallized

some of the adrenal hormones. In 1944, Lewis Sarett became the first to synthesize cortisone. In the late 1940's, Philip Showalter Hench discovered that the administration of cortisone could alleviate the symptoms of arthritis.

In recent years, it has been shown that corticosteroids express their effect by modulating the expression of a variety of genes involved in many physiological functions, including metabolism and the immune or inflammatory response.

—*Charles L. Vigue, Ph.D.*

See also Addison's disease; Adrenal glands; Adrenalectomy; Cushing's syndrome; Endocrine disorders; Endocrine glands; Endocrinology; Endocrinology, pediatric; Glands; Hormones; Kidneys; Osteonecrosis; Steroids.

FOR FURTHER INFORMATION:
Griffin, James E., and Sergio R. Ojeda, eds. *Textbook of Endocrine Physiology.* 5th ed. New York: Oxford University Press, 2004. An examination of endocrine physiology with several chapters devoted to adrenal physiology and disorders. Each chapter is by a different expert in the field.
Lüdecke, Dieter K., George P. Chrousos, and George Tolis, eds. *ACTH, Cushing's Syndrome, and Other Hypercortisolemic States.* New York: Raven Press, 1990. The proceedings of a 1989 conference. Several contributors are specialists in adrenal disorders.
Vaughan, Darracott E., and Robert M. Carey. *Adrenal Disorders.* New York: Thieme Medical, 1989. Specifically addresses the various disorders of the adrenal gland. Several specialists have contributed chapters.
Vinson, Gavin P., Barbara Whitehouse, and Joy Hinson. *The Adrenal Cortex.* Englewood Cliffs, N.J.: Prentice Hall, 1992. Addresses the adrenal cortex and its associated disorders.

COSMETIC SURGERY. *See* PLASTIC SURGERY.

COUGHING
DISEASE/DISORDER
ANATOMY OR SYSTEM AFFECTED: Chest, immune system, lungs, respiratory system
SPECIALTIES AND RELATED FIELDS: Family medicine, internal medicine, pulmonary medicine
DEFINITION: A physiological act in which air is forcibly expelled from the lungs.

CAUSES AND SYMPTOMS

The energy that is consumed during the breathing process is used to stretch the chest cavity and allow air to flow into the lungs. This amounts to about 1 percent of the basic energy requirements of the body but increases considerably during periods of exercise or respiratory system illness.

When the respiratory tract is invaded by irritants (such as smoke, perfume, and pollen) or there is an excessive accumulation of secretions, coughing takes place. It arises via a reflex mechanism that starts with the stimulation of the nerves that supply the larynx, trachea (windpipe), and bronchial tubes. The pressure within the chest cavity is increased by the action of chest muscles and the diaphragm. The glottis, the opening of the windpipe at the back of the mouth, remains closed in order to allow the pressure to rise. Within a few seconds, the glottis opens again and a rapid, noisy release of air is allowed through the bronchial tubes and the windpipe. Any invading foreign substance is expelled through the mouth.

TREATMENT AND THERAPY

Coughing is an important symptom of diseases that affect any part of the respiratory system, such as the nasal cavities, the pharynx (throat), the larynx, the trachea, the bronchi, and lung tissue. Sputum formation during coughing is an important evidence of a disease, such as bronchitis. In this case, the lining of the bronchi enlarges dramatically and sputum production may increase to 60 milliliters per day. An irritative cough without sputum may be due to the extension of the disease to the bronchial tube and eventually to nearby organs. The use of antibiotics and anti-inflammatory agents to reduce the discomfort is part of the standard treatment.

The presence of blood in the sputum (called hemoptysis) is important and should alert patients or their caregivers to call a doctor. This symptom often arises from an existing infection, inflammation, or tumor. It is also a sign of tuberculosis. In this case, extensive and reliable tests will identify the real cause of the bleeding.

Polluted air increases the possibility of chronic bronchitis. Common air pollutants include vehicle exhaust, chemical fumes, smoke, smog, molds, and pollen. They are all responsible for a decrease in arterial oxygen and an increase in carbon dioxide tension in the lungs. The use of air-conditioning, air filters, and inhalers and an increased-oxygen environment can provide relief for people with respiratory problems.

—*Soraya Ghayourmanesh, Ph.D.*

INFORMATION ON COUGHING

CAUSES: Various diseases, allergens, lung infection, environmental factors
SYMPTOMS: Breathlessness, chest and lung pain
DURATION: Ranges from short-term to chronic
TREATMENTS: Antibiotics, anti-inflammatory drugs

See also Allergies; Asbestos exposure; Aspergillosis; Avian influenza; Bronchi; Bronchitis; Choking; Common cold; Croup; Cystic fibrosis; Diphtheria; Immune system; Influenza; Laryngitis; Lung cancer; Lungs; Otorhinolaryngology; Over-the-counter medications; Pneumonia; Pulmonary diseases; Pulmonary medicine; Pulmonary medicine, pediatric; Respiration; Sore throat; Tuberculosis; Wheezing; Whooping cough.

FOR FURTHER INFORMATION:

Adelman, Daniel C., et al., eds. *Manual of Allergy and Immunology.* 4th ed. Philadelphia: Lippincott Williams & Wilkins, 2002.

Braga, Pier Carlo, and Luigi Allegra, eds. *Cough.* New York: Raven Press, 1989.

Chung, Kian Fan, John G. Widdicombe, and Homer A. Boushey, eds. *Cough: Causes, Mechanisms, and Therapy.* Malden, Mass.: Blackwell, 2008.

Glenn, Jim. *Colds and Coughs.* Springhouse, Pa.: Springhouse, 1986.

Kimball, Chad T. *Colds, Flu, and Other Common Ailments Sourcebook.* Detroit, Mich.: Omnigraphics, 2001.

Korpás, Juraj, and Z. Tomori. *Cough and Other Respiratory Reflexes.* New York: S. Karger, 1979.

Woolf, Alan D., et al., eds. *The Children's Hospital Guide to Your Child's Health and Development.* Cambridge, Mass.: Perseus, 2002.

CRANIOSYNOSTOSIS

DISEASE/DISORDER

ANATOMY OR SYSTEM AFFECTED: Bones, head
SPECIALTIES AND RELATED FIELDS: Orthopedics, plastic surgery
DEFINITION: The premature closing of the open areas between the bones in an infant's skull.

CAUSES AND SYMPTOMS

Craniosynostosis is an important craniofacial abnormality that occurs in a variety of forms. The skull of a newborn infant contains several open areas between the bones that make up the skull. These areas, called fontanelles, allow the skull to expand as the child's brain grows. Craniosynostosis is the premature closure of one or more of these open areas, resulting in the abnormal shaping of the head and face. Craniosynostosis may occur alone or in association with other defects.

INFORMATION ON CRANIOSYNOSTOSIS

CAUSES: Birth defect
SYMPTOMS: Abnormal head and face shape
DURATION: Typically correctable, with side effects of surgery lasting several months
TREATMENTS: Fronto-orbital advancement

TREATMENT AND THERAPY

During the 1960's the French surgeon Paul Tessier developed improved techniques for treating craniosynostosis. Treatment of craniosynostosis is often done with a surgical procedure known as fronto-orbital advancement. This technique involves cutting the skull in such a way that the frontal bone (the portion of the skull behind the forehead) and the supraorbital rim (the portion of the skull above and to the sides of the eyes) can be moved forward. These portions of the skull are then attached to the rest of the skull in their new positions with surgical wire. For some types of craniosynostosis, it may also be necessary to cut the frontal bone and the supraorbital rim down the middle to allow them to be reshaped. Fronto-orbital advancement usually takes place after the patient is three months old.

Correction of craniosynostosis is a complicated procedure, requiring the patient to be monitored in a special hospital bed for at least four or five days after surgery. After the plastic surgery, the patient will experience severe swelling of the eyelids and scalp. Most patients will be unable to open their eyes until several days after surgery, and the swelling may not completely disappear for a few months. Care must be taken to keep the incision clean.

—*Rose Secrest*

See also Birth defects; Bone disorders; Bones and the skeleton; Growth; Surgery, pediatric.

FOR FURTHER INFORMATION:

Cohen, M. Michael, Jr., and Ruth E. MacLean, eds. *Craniosynostosis: Diagnosis, Evaluation, and Management.* 2d ed. New York: Oxford University Press, 2000.

Galli, Guido, ed. *Craniosynostosis.* Boca Raton, Fla.: CRC Press, 1984.

Hayward, Richard, et al., eds. *The Clinical Management of Craniosynostosis.* New York: Cambridge University Press, 2004.

McCarthy, Joseph G., ed. *Distraction of the Craniofacial Skeleton.* New York: Springer, 1999.

Moore, Keith L., and T. V. N. Persaud. *The Developing Human.* 8th ed. Philadelphia: Saunders/Elsevier, 2008.

Sadler, T. W. *Langman's Medical Embryology.* 11th ed. Philadelphia: Lippincott Williams & Wilkins, 2009.

Turvey, Timothy A., Raymond J. Fonseca, and Katherine W. Vig, eds. *Facial Clefts and Craniosynostosis: Principles and Management.* Philadelphia: W. B. Saunders, 1996.

CRANIOTOMY

PROCEDURE

ANATOMY OR SYSTEM AFFECTED: Brain, head
SPECIALTIES AND RELATED FIELDS: Critical care, neurology
DEFINITION: A means of exposing or gaining access to the brain and cranial nerves so that intracranial disease can be treated surgically.

INDICATIONS AND PROCEDURES

Problems requiring craniotomy include tumors, abscesses, hematomas, and vascular lesions. The cranium may also be opened to excise an area of cortex or to disrupt various nerves and fiber tracts for the relief of pain, seizures, tremors, or spasms that do not respond to pharmacologic therapy. Skull fractures and other traumatic head wounds may be repaired by opening the cranium. Bony defects, dural tearing, bleeding, and removal of penetrating objects are also treated with this procedure. In case of a neoplasm (tumor), the goal of surgery is to remove the pathology completely while preserving the normal neural and vascular structures.

In craniotomy, the skin is cut to the skull bone. Small bleeding arteries are sealed with electric current, and the skin is pulled back. Three burr holes are drilled into the skull, and a fine-wire Gigli's saw is used to connect the holes. The skull piece is hinged open, and the dura mater, a tough membrane covering the brain, is dissected away. After the required procedure on the brain is completed, the dura mater is stitched together, the bone flap is replaced and secured with soft wire, and the scalp incision is closed.

An intracranial operation can be considered a planned head injury, and the complications are similar. Postoperatively, the degree of impairment depends on the extent of damage to neural tissue caused both by the neurological disorder and by surgical manipulation. Damage may be transient or permanent.

USES AND COMPLICATIONS

With craniotomy, complications include cerebral edema (swelling), which is a normal reaction to the manipulation and retraction of brain tissue. Periorbital edema and ecchymosis (bleeding under the skin) usually follow frontal and temporal surgery. Focal motor deficits result from cerebral edema and are transitory. Permanent focal motor deficits may occur and are a direct and predictable consequence of the surgical procedure or the result of a complication such as stroke. Hematomas are the most devastating and dreaded complication. The clots may be extradural, intradural, or both and usually are caused by a single bleeding vessel rather than a generalized bleed.

Pain and discomfort are expected following cranial surgery, with headache being most common. Pain control may be accomplished with mild analgesics. Fever may occur following operations in the region of the upper brain stem and hypothalamus, and it requires vigorous treatment. Infection may occur, with the risk being greater following open head trauma and if a cerebrospinal fluid leak is present. Postoperative seizure risk is related to the underlying pathological condition and the degree of damage caused by surgery. Diabetes insipidus and the syndrome of inappropriate antidiuretic hormone (SIADH) secretion are also possible complications of craniotomy. These endocrine disorders may be transient or permanent. If unchecked, either may be life-threatening because of the severity of the fluid and electrolyte imbalance precipitated.

A cerebrospinal fluid leak may occur immediately following surgery but usually appears later in the postoperative course. Fluid seeps from the wound edges. Discharge from the nose (rhinorrhea) or ears (otorrhea) of cerebrospinal fluid is frequent with basal skull fractures, but these conditions may also occur following surgery in the frontal sinus or mastoid cavity. Anosmia (loss of sense of smell) frequently occurs following head injury or frontal craniotomy. Visual loss may be caused by damage to the optic nerve, resulting in blindness and lack of response to direct light. Hydrocephalus may develop as a result of postoperative adhesions secondary to blood sealing the subarachnoid space. Postoperative meningitis, abscess formation, and osteomyelitis of the bone flap occur as complications of a break in sterility or the introduction of organisms as a result of a contaminated open wound.

—*Jane C. Norman, Ph.D., R.N., C.N.E.*

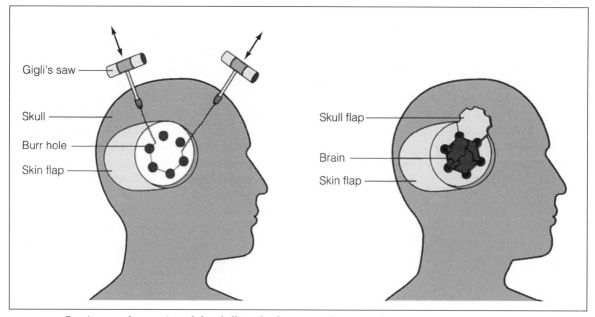

Craniotomy, the opening of the skull, is the first step taken to perform neurosurgery on the brain.

See also Bones and the skeleton; Brain; Brain disorders; Hydrocephalus; Neuroimaging; Neurology; Neurology, pediatric; Neurosurgery.

FOR FURTHER INFORMATION:

Aminoff, Michael J., David A. Greenberg, and Roger P. Simon. *Clinical Neurology.* 7th ed. New York: McGraw-Hill Medical, 2009.

Bakay, Louis. *An Early History of Craniotomy: From Antiquity to the Napoleonic Era.* Springfield, Ill.: Charles C Thomas, 1985.

Rowland, Lewis P., ed. *Merritt's Textbook of Neurology.* 12th ed. Philadelphia: Lippincott Williams & Wilkins, 2010.

Samuels, Martin A., ed. *Manual of Neurologic Therapeutics.* 7th ed. New York: Lippincott Williams & Wilkins, 2004.

CRETINISM. *See* CONGENITAL HYPOTHYROIDISM.

CREUTZFELDT-JAKOB DISEASE (CJD)
DISEASE/DISORDER

ANATOMY OR SYSTEM AFFECTED: Brain, nervous system

SPECIALTIES AND RELATED FIELDS: Environmental health, epidemiology, microbiology, neurology, public health, virology

DEFINITION: Creutzfeldt-Jakob disease (CJD) is a human central nervous system disorder that is characterized by distinctive lesions in the brain, progressive dementia, lack of coordination, and eventual death. Although uncommon, it is the most prevalent of the human spongiform encephalopathies, inherited or transmissible illnesses of uncertain etiology associated with proteinaceous molecules called prions. Mad cow disease is a spongiform encephalopathy that affects cattle but may be transmissible to humans, leading to a new variant of CJD. It is important to note, however, that the new form variant of CJD is different from classic CJD.

KEY TERMS:

dementia: an organic mental disorder characterized by personality disintegration, confusion, disorientation, stupor, deterioration of intellectual function, and impairment of memory and judgment

encephalopathy: any abnormality in the structure or function of the brain

knockout mouse: a mouse in which a specific gene has been inactivated or "knocked out"

myoclonus: involuntary twitching or spasm of muscle
spongiform: shaped like or resembling a sponge

CAUSES AND SYMPTOMS

Spongiform encephalopathies are inherited or transmissible neurological diseases that are associated with abnormalities in proteinaceous molecules called prions, which can aggregate, leading to spongelike lesions in the brain and causing disruptions in brain function. Prions are found in all species from yeast to humans, but their normal role is not known. Their evolutionary persistence in so many species implies an important purpose, although knockout mice lacking prions do not appear to be deleteriously affected.

Inherited spongiform encephalopathies are primarily attributed to mutations in the prion gene, producing abnormal prions that adopt an unusual conformation and clump together over time to cause the brain pathology and neurological symptoms characteristic of this type of disease. The diseases can be transmitted to a susceptible animal by inserting a fragment or extract from diseased tissue into the brain or blood or, much less efficiently, by oral ingestion. The infectious agent seems to be the abnormal prion itself, which apparently recruits normal prions in the brain to adopt the abnormal conformation, leading to their aggregation and the disruption of brain function. This is an unorthodox etiology, in that the infectious agent appears to be devoid of nucleic acid (RNA or DNA); its mode of action is not fully understood, nor is this etiology universally accepted.

Creutzfeldt-Jakob disease (CJD), known since the 1920's, is the major spongiform encephalopathy in humans, although it occurs in only one per million persons worldwide. It has different forms, namely sporadic, inherited, infectious, and, recently, new variant.

The sporadic form has no known basis, accounts for 85 percent of the cases, and usually affects individuals aged fifty-five to seventy years of age. The pathologic findings are limited to the central nervous system, although the transmissible agent can be detected in many organs. Researchers noted in 2002 that psychiatric and neurological symptoms are often present within four months of the disease's onset. Common symptoms include withdrawal, anxiety, irritability, insomnia, and a loss of interest. Within a few weeks or months, a relentlessly progressive dementia becomes evident, and myoclonus is often present at some point. Deterioration is usually rapid, with 90 percent of victims dying within one year. CJD patients do not have fevers, and their

> ## INFORMATION ON CREUTZFELDT-JAKOB DISEASE (CJD)
>
> **CAUSES:** Prion disease; can be acquired through ingestion of infected cow tissue
> **SYMPTOMS:** Dementia, lack of coordination, personality change
> **DURATION:** Weeks to months; death typically occurs within one year
> **TREATMENTS:** None

blood and cerebrospinal fluid are normal.

The inherited or familial form has been noted in some one hundred extended families, accounting for 15 percent of the cases of CJD. At least seven different point mutations and one insertion mutation in the prion gene have been identified. Some prion mutations result in slightly different symptoms and are classified as different diseases. Other mutations may lead to the sporadic, infectious, or new variant forms.

The infectious form is rare and generally has been associated with medical procedures, such as organ transplants, inadvertent infection from contaminated surgical instruments, or treatment with products derived from human brains. Because the infectious agent is highly resistant to denaturation, thorough decontamination of surgical instruments has proven essential in minimizing transmission. A number of cases occurred in individuals receiving growth hormone extracts derived from human pituitary glands, a practice discontinued in the United States in 1985. The infectious form also appears to be the basis for kuru, a disease previously endemic among the Fore people of the eastern highlands of Papua New Guinea. Typically, it was characterized by cerebellar dysfunction, dementia, and progression to death within two years. Evidence indicates that the kuru agent was transmitted through the ritual handling and consumption of affected tissues, especially brains, from deceased relatives. With discontinuation of these cultural practices, kuru has virtually disappeared.

A new variant CJD (nvCJD) was first reported in Britain in 1996. It differed from sporadic CJD in affecting younger persons (aged sixteen to thirty-nine) and in its behavioral symptoms, pathology, and longer course. This variant followed the British epidemic of bovine spongiform encephalopathy (BSE), known as mad cow disease. Contaminated beef consumption was suspected as the source of nvCJD, which has subsequently been shown to have a molecular signature similar, if not identical, to that for BSE. Furthermore, nvCJD has been observed only in countries with BSE.

BSE first appeared in Britain in 1986 and has subsequently been diagnosed in nine other European countries. It occurs in adult cattle between two and eight years of age and is fatal. In the course of the disease, the animals lose coordination and show extreme sensitivity to sound, light, and touch. While it may be transmitted from mother to calf, the major cause of the BSE epidemic in Britain is attributed to feed containing contaminated ruminant-derived protein. Following a ban on incorporating such protein into cattle feed, the incidence has decreased. Since the beginning of the epidemic, a total of 200,000 cattle have been diagnosed with the disease; fewer than 1,000 new cases are currently reported per year. In the United States, a surveillance program is in effect, importation of beef from affected countries is prohibited, and incorporating ruminant-derived protein into cattle feed has been banned. Nevertheless, an infected cow was discovered in 2003 on a farm in Washington State. It had been imported from Canada.

When the British BSE outbreak occurred, concern arose for its human health implications, despite the fact that scrapie, the comparable condition in sheep, was long known not to be a risk to human consumers. A surveillance unit was established in 1990, and ten cases of the new variant form of CJD were reported in 1996. In 2000, twenty-eight cases were recorded in Britain. The numbers began to slow soon afterward, but fears of another epidemic remained.

TREATMENT AND THERAPY

Research on experimental animals has been crucial to understanding the unusual etiology of these diseases. Brain tissue from patients dying of kuru was inoculated into the brains of chimpanzees that, after a prolonged incubation period, developed a similar disease. CJD, BSE, and scrapie have been similarly transmitted to a wide variety of laboratory animals. Mouse models have been particularly useful. Knockout mice lacking their normal prion gene are not susceptible to transmissible disease, indicating the importance of endogenous brain prions in the etiology. Transgenic mice, whose own prions have been replaced with those from other species or with specific mutations, exhibit different susceptibilities to various infectious particles.

Because none of the spongiform encephalopathies stimulates a specific immune response, diagnosis of these diseases in living persons or animals is difficult. Postmortem identification of brain lesions is necessary to verify the diagnosis. The use of antibodies to prions is permitting rapid confirmation of the diagnosis from specimens obtained by brain biopsy or postmortem examination. As of 2010, no effective treatment was available for these diseases, which are uniformly fatal. Although these diseases can be transmitted to health care workers and others having contact with CJD patients, the risk is no higher than for the general population. Isolation of patients is not suggested, but reasonable care should be exercised. No organs, tissues, or tissue products from these patients or others with an ill-defined neurologic disease should be used for transplantation, replacement therapy, or pharmaceutical manufacturing.

PERSPECTIVE AND PROSPECTS

Clinically, Creutzfeldt-Jakob disease can be mistaken for other disorders that cause dementia in the elderly, especially Alzheimer's disease. CJD, however, usually has a shorter clinical course and includes myoclonus. While nvCJD has a longer clinical course, it generally affects younger persons.

Continued monitoring of CJD and especially nvCJD in Britain is warranted. In addition, surveillance of the food supply in the United States and other countries should persist to prevent meat from BSE cattle from reaching consumers. Above all, further research into the etiology of these pathologies is needed. Research into prion biology and disease epidemiology, including studies of nvCJD clusters, must be pursued until the progression of these diseases is fully understood. Early detection and effective treatment await this understanding.

—James L. Robinson, Ph.D.

See also Brain; Brain disorders; Dementias; Food poisoning; Prion diseases; Viral infections; Zoonoses.

FOR FURTHER INFORMATION:

Balter, Michael. "Tracking the Human Fallout from Mad Cow Disease." *Science* 289 (September, 2000): 1452-1453. This news report presents the history, status, and future prospects of nvCJD, the new variant of Creutzfeldt-Jacob disease that is associated with consumption of cattle affected by mad cow disease.

Bloom, Floyd E., M. Flint Beal, and David J. Kupfer, eds. *The Dana Guide to Brain Health.* New York: Dana Press, 2006. An easy-to-understand health guide to the brain from neuroscience, neurology, and psychiatry perspectives. More than seventy psychiatric and neurological disorders, their diagnoses, and their treatments are covered.

Dana.org. http://www.dana.org. A nonprofit organization of neuroscientists, which was formed to provide information about the personal and public benefits of brain research. The Web site is research oriented and gives excellent information and links on current brain studies, new diagnosis and treatment technology, and brain-related news stories.

Marieb, Elaine N., and Katja Hoehn. *Human Anatomy and Physiology.* 9th ed. San Francisco: Pearson/ Benjamin Cummings, 2010. Several chapters explore the fundamentals of the nervous system and nervous tissue, the central nervous system, and neural integration. Well illustrated and includes many applications in the fields of physical education and medical science.

Nolte, John. *Human Brain: An Introduction to Its Functional Anatomy.* 6th ed. Philadelphia: Mosby/ Elsevier, 2009. Text covering major concepts and structure-function relationships in the human neurological system.

Prusiner, Stanley B. "The Prion Diseases." *Scientific American* 272, no. 1 (January, 1995): 48-57. The author explains the history and basis for the prion theory, which he developed and for which he was awarded a Nobel Prize in 1997.

_____, ed. *Prion Biology and Diseases.* 2d ed. Cold Spring Harbor, N.Y.: Cold Spring Harbor Laboratory Press, 2004. The originator of the prion theory edited this book, which presents the latest scientific information about prions and the diseases with which they are associated.

Schwartz, Maxime. *How the Cows Turned Mad.* Translated by Edward Schneider. Berkeley: University of California Press, 2003. Traces the history of mad cow disease and related infectious brain diseases of livestock and people, and outlines advances in understanding the disease.

Spencer, Charlotte A. *Mad Cows and Cannibals: A Guide to the Transmissible Spongiform Encephalopathies.* Upper Saddle River, N.J.: Prentice Hall, 2004. Explores the biology of and issues surrounding mad cow disease and related conditions, including discussions of ritualistic cannibalism in New Guinea and modern agricultural feeding practices that triggered the mad cow disease epidemic in Great Britain.

Transmissible Spongiform Encephalopathies in the United States. Ames, Iowa: Council for Agricultural Science and Technology, 2000. This report of a scientific task force organized to evaluate mad cow disease and related disorders provides a factual, balanced, and succinct summary of these conditions.

CRITICAL CARE
SPECIALTY
ANATOMY OR SYSTEM AFFECTED: All

SPECIALTIES AND RELATED FIELDS: Anesthesiology, cardiology, emergency medicine, gastroenterology, geriatrics and gerontology, neurology, nursing, obstetrics, pharmacology, pulmonary medicine, radiology, sports medicine, toxicology

DEFINITION: The care of patients who are experiencing severe health crises—short-lived or prolonged, accidental or anticipated—that require continuous monitoring.

KEY TERMS:

asphyxia: an impaired exchange of oxygen and carbon dioxide in the lungs; if prolonged, this condition leads to death

aspirate: to suck fluid or a foreign body into an airway of the lungs, which frequently leads to aspiration pneumonia

debridement: the excision of bruised, injured, or otherwise devitalized tissue from a wound site

electrocardiogram (EKG or ECG): a graphic record of the electrical activity of the heart, obtained with an electrocardiograph and displayed on a computer screen or paper strip

emphysema: an increase in the size of air spaces at the terminal ends of bronchioles in the lungs; this damage reduces the ability of the lungs to exchange oxygen and carbon dioxide

esophagus: the portion of the digestive system connecting the mouth and stomach; it is muscular, propelling food during the act of swallowing

hypothermia: a subnormal body temperature; clinically, it is a sustained cooling of the body to lower-than-normal temperatures

resuscitation: the restoration to life after apparent death; the methods used to restore normal organ functioning, primarily referring to the heart

sternum: the breastbone; found in the midline of the chest cavity and lying over the heart

trauma: an injury caused by rough contact with a physical object; it can be accidental or induced

SCIENCE AND PROFESSION

Critical care is the branch of medicine that provides immediate services, usually on an emergency basis. It also encompasses some forms of ongoing care provided in a hospital setting for patients who are so sick that they are medically unstable and must be monitored constantly. Such patients are at an ongoing high risk for disastrous complications.

Critical care personnel must be specially trained, and standards for training and evaluation in this field have been prepared for physicians, nurses, and other hospital personnel. Ninety percent of hospitals in the United States with fewer than two hundred beds have a single critical care unit, usually called an intensive care unit (ICU). Only 9 percent of these hospitals have a second intensive care facility, typically dedicated solely to the care of heart attack victims. In total, 7 to 8 percent of all hospital beds in the United States are used for intensive care. Because ICU facilities are at a premium and are expensive to operate, patients are transferred to a regular hospital bed as quickly as possible, given their specific medical condition. Of the physicians who are certified in critical care, most are anesthesiologists, followed by internists. A shortage of trained critical care physicians has existed in the United States for many years.

Critical care facilities are available in several varieties, providing specialized care to particular patients. The most common type of ICU is for individuals who require care for medical crises. These patients frequently have a short-term condition or disease that can be treated successfully. Others are admitted to a medical ICU for multiple organ system failure. These people are often very sick with conditions that overwhelm even the best available care and equipment. Heart attack victims are often admitted to a coronary ICU, which has specialized equipment for support and resuscitation if needed. Once medically stable, coronary ICU patients are transferred to a regular hospital bed.

Larger hospitals may have an ICU for surgical patients. Typically, these individuals are admitted to the surgical ICU from the operating room after a procedure. In the ICU, they are stabilized while the effects of anesthesia wear off. They, too, are transferred to a normal hospital room as soon as is medically safe. Neonatal ICUs exist in some larger hospitals to provide care for premature and very sick infants. Such infants may stay in neonatal ICUs for extended periods of time (weeks to months) depending on their specific condition. There may also be a pediatric ICU specially designed for very sick children.

DIAGNOSTIC AND TREATMENT TECHNIQUES

Critical care is synonymous with immediate care: Swift action is required on an emergency basis to sustain or save a life. The most immediate of critical care needs are to establish and maintain a patent airway for ventilation and to maintain sufficient cardiac functioning to provide minimal perfusion or blood supply to critical organs of the body.

Resuscitation is the support of life by external means when the body is unable to maintain itself. Basic life support is for emergency situations and consists of delivering oxygen to the lungs, maintaining an airway, inflating the lungs if necessary, and assisting with circulation. These methods are collectively known as cardiopulmonary resuscitation (CPR). Oxygen can be transferred from one mouth to another by forceful breathing or by the means of pumps and pure oxygen from a container. The airway is commonly maintained by positioning the head and neck so as to extend the chin and open the trachea. It is also possible to make an incision in the trachea, insert a tube, and provide oxygen through the tube. The lungs may be inflated by using the force of exhaled air from one person breathing into another's mouth or by utilizing a machine that inflates the lungs to a precise level and delivers oxygen in accurate, predetermined amounts. When a victim's heart is not working, the circulation of blood is provided by external compression of the chest. This action squeezes the heart between the sternum and the spine, forcing blood into the circulatory system.

Advanced life support includes attempts to restart a nonfunctioning heart. This goal is commonly accomplished by electrical means (defibrillation). The heart is given a brief shock that is sufficient to start it beating on its own. Drugs can also be used to restore spontaneous circulation in cardiac arrest. Epinephrine (adrenaline) is the most commonly used drug, although sodium bicarbonate is used for some conditions. A heart can be restarted by manual com-pression. This technique requires direct access to the heart and is limited to situations in which the heart stops beating during a surgical procedure involving the thorax, when the heart is directly accessible.

Prolonged life support is administered after the heart has been restarted and is concerned chiefly with the brain and other organs such as the kidneys that are sensitive to oxygen levels in the blood. Drugs and mechanical ventilation are used to supply oxygen to the lungs. Prolonged life support uses sophisticated technology to deliver oxygenated blood to the organs continuously. The body can be maintained in this manner for long periods of time. Once begun, prolonged life support is continued until the patient regains consciousness or until brain death has been certified by a physician. A patient's state of underlying disease may be determined to be so severe that continuing prolonged life support becomes senseless. The factors entering into a decision to terminate life support are complex and involve a patient's family, the physician, and other professionals.

Individuals who are critically ill must be closely

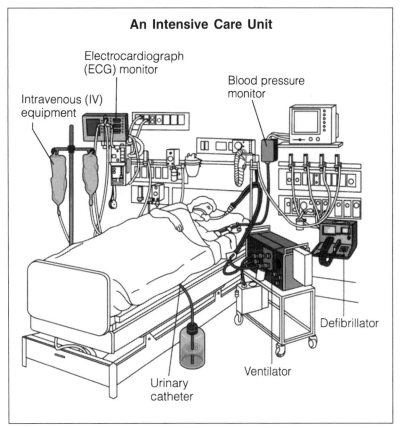

An Intensive Care Unit

Electrocardiograph (ECG) monitor

Blood pressure monitor

Intravenous (IV) equipment

Defibrillator

Ventilator

Urinary catheter

Critical care involves the constant monitoring of patients with life-threatening conditions. This care is usually provided in an intensive care unit (ICU).

monitored. Many of the advancements in the care of these patients have been attributable to improvements in monitoring. While physiologic measurements cannot replace the clinical impressions of trained professionals, monitoring data often provide objective information that reinforces clinical opinions. More people die from the failure of vital organs than from the direct effects of injury or disease. The most commonly monitored events are vital signs: heart rate, blood pressure, breathing rate, and temperature. These are frequently augmented by electrocardiograms (ECGs or EKGs). Other, more sophisticated electronic methods are available for individuals in intensive care units.

Vital signs are still frequently assessed manually, although machinery is available to accomplish the task. Modern intensive care units are able to store large amounts of data that can be analyzed by computer programs. Data can be transmitted to distant consoles, thus enabling a small number of individuals to monitor several patients simultaneously. Monitoring data can also be displayed on computer screens, allowing more rapid evaluation. Automatic alarms can be used to indicate when bodily functions fall outside predetermined parameters, thus rapidly alerting staff to critical or emergency situations.

Breathing—or, more correctly, ventilation—can be monitored extensively. The volume of inspired air can be adjusted to accommodate different conditions. The amount of oxygen can be changed to compensate for emphysema or other loss of oxygen exchange capacity. The rate of breathing can also be regulated to work in concert with the heart in order to provide maximum benefit to the patient. The effectiveness of pulmonary monitoring is itself monitored by measuring the amount of oxygen in arterial blood. This, too, can be accomplished automatically, with adjustments made by instruments.

Common situations that require critical care are choking, drowning, poisoning, physical trauma, psychological trauma, and environmental disasters.

Choking. Difficulty in either breathing or swallowing is termed choking. The source of the obstruction may be either internal or external. Internal obstructions can result from a foreign body becoming stuck in the mouth (pharynx), throat (esophagus or trachea), or lungs (bronchi). The blockage may be partial or total. A foreign body that is caught in the esophagus will create difficulty in swallowing; one that is caught in the trachea will obstruct breathing. Any foreign body may become lodged and create a blockage. Objects that com-

monly cause obstructions include teeth (both natural and false), food (especially meat and bones from fish), and liquids such as water and blood.

Obstructions can occur externally. Examples of external causes of choking include compression of the larynx or trachea as a result of blunt trauma (a physical blow or other injury sustained in an accident), a penetrating projectile such as a bullet or stick, and toys or small items of food that are swallowed accidentally. Foods such as nuts or candy are frequently aspirated as the result of trying to catch one in the mouth after tossing it in the air. An object that becomes stuck in the lungs frequently does not cause an acute shortage of breath, but this situation can lead to aspiration pneumonia, which is extremely difficult to treat.

The symptoms of choking are well known: gagging, coughing, and difficulty in breathing. Pain may or may not be present. Frequently, there is a short episode of difficulty in breathing followed by a period when no symptoms are experienced. The foreign body may be moved aside or pushed deeper into the body by the victim's initial frantic movements. A foreign body lodged in the esophagus will not interfere with breathing but may cause food or liquids to spill into the trachea and become aspirated; as with an object in the lungs, this usually leads to pneumonia or other serious respiratory conditions.

Drowning. Drowning is defined as the outcome (usually death) of unanticipated immersion into a liquid (usually water). Consciousness is an important determinant of how an individual reacts to immersion in water. A person who is conscious will attempt to escape from the fluid environment, which involves attempts to regain orientation and not to aspirate additional liquids. An unconscious person has none of these defenses and usually dies when the lungs fill rapidly with water. Normal persons can hold their breath for thirty seconds or more. Frequently, this is sufficient time for a victim to escape from immersion in a fluid environment. When a victim exhales just prior to entering water, this time period is not available; indeed, panic frequently develops, and the victim aspirates water.

Most but not all victims of drowning die from aspirating water. Approximately 10 percent of drowning victims die from asphyxia while underwater, possibly because they hold their breath or because the larynx goes into spasms. The brain of the average person can survive without oxygen for about four minutes. After that time, irreversible damage starts to occur; death follows in a matter of minutes. After four minutes, survival is possible but unlikely to be without the permanent impairment of mental functions.

The physical condition of the victim exerts a profound influence on the outcome of a drowning situation. Physically fit persons have a far greater chance of escaping from a drowning environment. Individuals who are in poor condition, who are very weak, or who have handicaps must overcome these conditions when attempting to escape from a drowning situation; frequently, they are unable to remove themselves and die in the process.

Another physical condition such as exhaustion or a heart attack may also be present. An exhausted person is weak and may not have the physical strength or endurance to escape. A person who experiences a heart attack at the moment of immersion is at a severe disadvantage. If the heart is unable to deliver blood and nutrients to muscles, even a physically fit person is weakened and may be less likely to escape a drowning situation.

The temperature of the water is critical. Immersing the face in cold water (below 20 degrees Celsius or 56 degrees Fahrenheit) initiates a reflex that slows the person's heart rate and shunts blood to the heart and brain, thus delaying irreversible cerebral damage. Immersion in water even colder leads to hypothermia (subnormal body temperature). In the short term, hypothermia reduces the body's consumption of oxygen and allows submersion in water for slightly longer periods of time. There have been reports of survival after immersion of ten minutes in warm water and forty minutes in extremely cold water. Age is also a factor: Younger persons are more likely to tolerate such conditions than older persons.

Poisoning. Whether intentional or accidental, poisoning demands immediate medical care. Intoxication can also initiate a crisis that requires critical care. Alcohol is the most common intoxicant, but a wide range of other substances are accidentally ingested. Accidental poisoning is the most common cause of death in young children. When an individual is poisoned, the toxic substance must be removed from the body. This removal may be accomplished in a variety of ways and is usually done in a hospital. Supportive care may be needed during the period of acute crisis. The brain, liver, and kidneys are usually at great risk during a toxic crisis; steps must be taken to protect these organs.

Physical trauma. In the United States, more than 1.5 million persons are hospitalized each year as a result of trauma; some 100,000 of these patients die. Trauma is the leading cause of death in persons under the age of forty and, overall, is the third most common cause of death. Approximately three million people have died as a result of motor vehicle accidents alone in the United States; the first such death occurred in 1899. Trauma is commonly characterized as either blunt or penetrating.

Blunt trauma occurs when an external force is applied to tissue, causing compression or crushing injuries as well as fractures. This force can be applied directly from being hit with an object or indirectly through the forces generated by sudden deceleration. In the latter event, relatively mobile organs or structures continue moving until stopped by adjacent, relatively fixed organs or structures. Any of these injuries can result in extensive internal bleeding. Damage may also cause fluids to be lost from tissues and lead to shock, circulatory collapse, and ultimately death.

The most frequent sources for penetrating wounds are knives and firearms. A knife blade produces a smaller wound; fewer organs are likely to be involved, and adjacent structures are less likely to sustain damage. In contrast, gunshot wounds are more likely to involve multiple tissues and to damage adjacent structures. More energy is released by a bullet than by a knife. This energy is sufficient to fracture a bone and usually leads to a greater amount of tissue damage.

The wound must be repaired, typically through surgical exploration and suturing. Extensively damaged tissue is removed in a process called debridement. Any visible sources of secondary contamination must also be removed. With both knife and firearm wounds often comes contamination by dirt, clothing, and other debris; this contamination presents a serious threat of infection to the victim and is also a problem for critical care workers. The wound is then covered appropriately, and the victim is given antibiotics to counteract bacteria that may have been introduced with the primary injury.

Psychological trauma. Critical care is often required in situations that lead to psychological stress. Individuals taking drug overdoses require critical supportive care until the drug has been metabolized by or removed from the body. Respiratory support is needed when the drug depresses the portion of the brain that controls breathing. Some drugs cause extreme agitation, which must be controlled by sedation.

Severe trauma to a loved one can initiate a psychological crisis. Psychological support must be provided to the victim; frequently, this is done in a hospital setting. An entire family may require critical care support for brief periods of time in the aftermath of a catastrophe. Severe trauma, disease, or the death of a child may require support by outsiders. Most hospitals have professionals who are trained to provide such support. In addition, people with psychiatric problems sometimes fail to take the medications that control mental illness. Critical care support in a hospital is often needed until these people are restabilized on their medications.

Environmental disasters. The need for psychological support, as well as urgent medical care, is magnified with natural or environmental disasters such as earthquakes, hurricanes, floods, or tornadoes. Environmental disasters seriously disrupt lives and normal services; they arise with little or no warning. The key to providing critical care in a disaster situation is adequate prior planning.

Responses to disasters occur at three levels: institutional (hospital), local (police, fire, and rescue), and regional (county and state). The plan must be simple and evolve from normal operations; individuals respond best when they are asked to perform tasks with which they are familiar and for which they are trained. The response must integrate all existing sources of emergency medical and supportive services. Those who assume responsibilities for overall management must be well trained and able to adapt to different conditions that may be encountered. Because no two disasters are ever alike, such flexibility is essential. Summaries of individual duties and responsibilities should be available for all involved individuals. Finally, the disaster plan should be practiced and rehearsed using specific scenarios. Experience is the single best method to ensure competency when a disaster strikes.

Environmental disasters such as earthquakes, hurricanes, floods, or tornadoes cause loss of life and extensive loss of property. Essential services such as water, gas, electricity, and telephone communication are often lost. Victims must be provided food, shelter, and medical care on an immediate basis. Critical care is usually required at the time of the disaster, and the need for support may continue long after the immediate effects of the disaster have been resolved.

PERSPECTIVE AND PROSPECTS

One of the most important issues with regard to critical care is sometimes controversial: when to discontinue life support. Life-support equipment is usually withdrawn as soon as patients are able to function independent of the machinery. These patients continue to recover, are discharged from the hospital, and complete their recovery at home. For some, however, the outcome is not as positive. Machines may be used to assist breathing. For a patient who does not improve, or who deteriorates, there comes a point in time when a decision to stop life support must be made. This is not an easy decision, nor should it be made by a single individual.

The patient's own wishes must be paramount. These wishes, however, must have been clearly communicated while the individual was in good health and had unimpaired thought processes. A patient's family is entitled to provide input in the decision to terminate care, but others are also entitled to provide input: the patient's physician, representatives of the hospital or institution, a representative of the patient's religious faith, and the state.

Medical science has developed criteria for death. The application of these criteria, however, is not uniform. The final decision to terminate life support is frequently a consensus of all the parties mentioned above. When there is a dispute, the courts are often asked to intervene. Extensive disagreements exist concerning the ethics of terminating critical care. It is beyond the scope of this discussion to provide definitive guidelines. This logical extension of critical care may not have a uniform resolution; the values and beliefs of each individual determine the outcome of each situation.

—*L. Fleming Fallon, Jr., M.D., Ph.D., M.P.H.*

See also Accidents; Aging: Extended care; Choking; Coma; Critical care, pediatric; Death and dying; Disease; Drowning; Electrocardiography (ECG or EKG); Electroencephalography (EEG); Emergency medicine; Ethics; Euthanasia; Hospice; Hospitals; Hyperbaric oxygen therapy; Intensive care unit (ICU); Living will; Nursing; Palliative medicine; Paramedics; Poisoning; Psychiatric disorders; Respiration; Resuscitation; Surgery, general; Terminally ill: Extended care; Tracheostomy; Unconsciousness; Wounds.

FOR FURTHER INFORMATION:

Bongard, Frederick, and Darryl Y. Sue, eds. *Current Critical Care Diagnosis and Treatment.* 3d ed. New York: McGraw-Hill Medical, 2008. A medical text that combines medical and surgical perspectives with diagnostic and treatment knowledge. Covers forty topics in critical care basics, medical critical care, and essentials of surgical intensive care and includes information on pregnancy, psychiatric disorders, imaging procedures, and transport, among other topics.

Fink, Mitchell P., et al. *Textbook of Critical Care.* 5th

ed. Philadelphia: Saunders/Elsevier, 2005. This medical text, written by experts in the field, represents the views of the Society of Critical Care Medicine. The general reader will find it interesting but may elect to skip some sections containing highly technical details.

Hogan, David E., and Jonathan L. Burstein. *Disaster Medicine*. 2d ed. Philadelphia: Lippincott Williams & Wilkins, 2007. Examines a wide range of relevant topics including natural, industrial, transportation, and conflict-related disasters; and infectious diseases, winter storms, fires and mass burn care, intentional chemical disasters, and mass shootings.

Markovchick, Vincent J., and Peter T. Pons. *Emergency Medicine Secrets*. 4th ed. Philadelphia: Mosby/Elsevier, 2006. A clinical reference book that covers decision making in emergency medicine, hematology and oncology, metabolism and endocrinology, infectious disease, environmental emergencies, neonatal and childhood disorders, toxicologic emergencies, and behavioral emergencies, among many other topics.

Safar, Peter, and Nicholas G. Bircher. *Cardiopulmonary Cerebral Resuscitation: Basic and Advanced Cardiac and Trauma Life Support—An Introduction to Resuscitation Medicine*. 3d ed. Philadelphia: W. B. Saunders, 1988. A text that completely describes the process of cardiopulmonary resuscitation (CPR). The general reader can learn much from it but is cautioned to take a training course taught by the Red Cross or American Heart Association before attempting to use CPR.

CRITICAL CARE, PEDIATRIC
SPECIALTY

ANATOMY OR SYSTEM AFFECTED: All

SPECIALTIES AND RELATED FIELDS: Anesthesiology, cardiology, emergency medicine, gastroenterology, neonatology, neurology, nursing, pediatrics, pharmacology, pulmonary medicine, radiology, toxicology

DEFINITION: The hospital care of seriously ill or injured infants and children.

KEY TERMS:

computed tomography (CT) scanning: a radiographic technique using computer-enhanced X-ray images to show the anatomy of cross sections of the body

magnetic resonance imaging (MRI): a technique using strong electromagnets to show the anatomy of cross sections of the body in great detail

SCIENCE AND PROFESSION

When a serious illness or injury occurs to children, they cannot simply be treated as small adults. The serious illnesses from which they suffer are different from those of adults. Children's bodies respond differently to illness and injuries and require different types of resuscitative fluids and medications. The critical care pediatrician is specially trained to provide this special care.

A critical care pediatrician has undergone, in addition to four years of medical school, three years of pediatric residency and three years of fellowship training in the care of critically ill or injured children. Critical care pediatricians usually practice in large referral hospitals or children's hospitals.

The care of a seriously ill or injured child requires many skills, including the resuscitation and stabilization of the patient's condition, consultation with other specialists, and the establishment and execution of a plan of action. The plan is often complicated, especially if more than one organ system is involved. The critical care pediatrician coordinates the work of the patient's health team.

Resuscitation usually begins in the emergency room and is directed by the emergency room physician. The critical care pediatrician may take over care in the emergency room or when the patient is moved from there or from the operating room to the intensive care unit (ICU).

On the patient's arrival at the hospital, the team first ensures that the patient is able to breathe adequately, and, if not, begins to ventilate the patient's lungs. The patient's cardiac output is quickly evaluated, and chest compression is begun if it is inadequate. The degree of shock is evaluated next and is treated with intravenous fluid. As this resuscitation is being carried out, the critical care pediatrician obtains a history of the illness or injury and conducts a thorough examination of the patient. Based on this information, the physician orders appropriate laboratory and radiographic tests and calls on other specialists, as needed, for help and advice.

Once the patient arrives in the ICU, the critical care pediatrician must continue to treat the initial problem as well as any complications and difficulties added by surgery or other therapies. The physician must be able to relate these problems to his or her knowledge of anatomy and physiology. A quick and accurate assessment of a large number of factors is required, as is the ability to gain an overview of all the conditions faced in the care of the patient.

The critical care pediatrician's day is largely spent in

a hospital emergency room and its intensive care areas. This type of specialist does not usually practice in a clinic except for occasional follow-up examinations of patients who have been discharged from the hospital.

DIAGNOSTIC AND TREATMENT TECHNIQUES
The critical care pediatrician utilizes a wide variety of diagnostic techniques. Complete blood counts, blood chemistry tests, and cultures of blood, urine, and cerebrospinal fluid are initially helpful, especially in looking for bacterial infections. These tests must be performed periodically to assess the patient's progress. Depending on the patient's problem, more specific tests may be necessary. Imaging studies, such as X rays, ultrasonography, and computed tomography (CT) or magnetic resonance imaging (MRI) scans, are often critical to this evaluation.

Besides closely monitoring the patient's condition, the critical care pediatrician must be able to perform a number of procedures. One is the management of ventilators, machines that can breathe for a child who is too ill or injured to breathe adequately on his or her own. The critical care physician is also expert at inserting a number of intravascular devices, such as central intravenous catheters, for intravenous (IV) fluids and for monitoring the function of the heart, and intra-arterial catheters, for monitoring blood pressure and conducting blood gas tests, which are used to evaluate the function of the lungs.

A complicated form of cardiopulmonary support for some critically ill children is called extracorporeal membrane oxygenation (ECMO). It is the circulation of the child's blood through an artificial lung machine using large intravenous tubes, generally inserted in the neck. This machine adds oxygen to and removes carbon dioxide from the child's circulation. ECMO requires a team of highly trained technicians. Its use is overseen by the critical care pediatrician when the patient is older than a newborn. ECMO is available only in the largest referral hospitals.

The care of critically ill children requires much emotional maturity on the part of the physician. The child's family is frightened and anxious, and the child is under great emotional stress. The team of caregivers feels the stress of working with these children as well. The critical care pediatrician must be able to provide empathetic support to all people involved in the health crisis. Despite its share of tragedies, critical care pediatrics is a richly rewarding field. The outcome for critically ill children is better than that for equally ill adults.

PERSPECTIVE AND PROSPECTS
While there have always been pediatricians with an interest in critical pediatric care, fellowships in the specialty were first developed in the last quarter of the twentieth century. Critical care was recognized as a subspecialty of pediatrics in 1987. By 1994, there were only sixty-five pediatricians who had been accepted as fellows of the American College of Critical Care Medicine. By then, there was a rapidly increasing demand for these specialists, with four to six positions being advertised for pediatric critical care doctors for every one adult position.

—*Thomas C. Jefferson, M.D.*

See also Accidents; Choking; Coma; Critical care; Death and dying; Disease; Drowning; Electrocardiography (ECG or EKG); Electroencephalography (EEG); Emergency medicine; Ethics; Euthanasia; Hospitals; Intensive care unit (ICU); Nursing; Paramedics; Pediatrics; Poisoning; Psychiatric disorders; Respiration; Resuscitation; Surgery, pediatric; Terminally ill: Extended care; Tracheostomy; Unconsciousness; Wounds.

FOR FURTHER INFORMATION:
Behrman, Richard E., Robert M. Kliegman, and Hal B. Jenson, eds. *Nelson Textbook of Pediatrics.* 18th ed. Philadelphia: Saunders/Elsevier, 2007. Text covering all medical and surgical disorders in children with authoritative information on genetics, endocrinology, aetiology, epidemiology, pathology, pathophysiology, clinical manifestations, diagnosis, prevention, treatment, and prognosis.

Fuhrman, Bradley P., and Jerry J. Zimmerman, eds. *Pediatric Critical Care.* 3d ed. Philadelphia: Mosby/Elsevier, 2006. A manual of pediatric intensive and emergency care. Includes bibliographical references and an index.

Merenstein, Gerald B., and Sandra L. Gardner, eds. *Merenstein and Gardner's Handbook of Neonatal Intensive Care.* 7th ed. Maryland Heights, Mo.: Mosby/Elsevier, 2011. A text covering clinical issues such as nutritional and metabolic support and diseases of the neonate.

Todres, I. David, and John H. Fugate, eds. *Critical Care of Infants and Children.* Boston: Little, Brown, 1996. Written from the necessarily pragmatic point of view of the busy clinician, this invaluable volume is filled with practical information without digressions into obscure basic science. A comprehensive section of procedures opens the book, with systems forming its basic organization.

CROHN'S DISEASE

DISEASE/DISORDER

ALSO KNOWN AS: Regional enteritis

ANATOMY OR SYSTEM AFFECTED: Gastrointestinal system, intestines

SPECIALTIES AND RELATED FIELDS: Gastroenterology, immunology, nutrition, pediatrics

DEFINITION: A chronic disease process in which the bowel becomes inflamed, leading to scarring and narrowing of the intestines.

KEY TERMS:

abscess: a localized collection of pus (dead cells and a mixture of live and dead bacteria)

antigen: a foreign substance in the body causing an immunological response that produces antibodies

fissure: a break in the surface tissue of the anal canal or the wall of the gastrointestinal tract

fistula: an abnormal connection between two hollow structures or between a hollow structure and the skin surface

CAUSES AND SYMPTOMS

Crohn's disease is a chronic disease of the digestive system. It is one of two diseases labeled as inflammatory bowel disease (IBD); the other is ulcerative colitis. With both diseases, patients suffer from diarrhea, abdominal pain, bleeding from the rectum, and fever. The cell lining of the bowel (usually the small intestine) becomes inflamed, leading to erosion of tissues and bleeding.

Crohn's disease may affect areas of the gastrointestinal system from the mouth to the exit of the body, the anus. The inflammatory process may spread to include the joints, skin, eyes, mouth, and sometimes liver. In children, IBD involves a substantial risk of slow or interrupted growth.

The most common early sign is abdominal pain, often felt over the navel or on the right side. Diarrhea and subsequent weight loss often follow. Other early signs of Crohn's disease include sores in the anal area (skin tabs), hemorrhoids, fissures (cracks), fistulas (abnormal openings from the intestines to the skin surface or other organs), abscesses (uncommon in children), and nausea and vomiting, especially in young children. Children as young as ten may develop this disease; however, in the majority of cases the onset is between the ages of sixteen and twenty-five. Some sources report that Crohn's disease is slightly more common in females. The incidence is greater in persons of Jewish ethnic origin.

Diagnosis often is made after a series of abdominal X rays, an upper gastrointestinal series, or a colonoscopy (visual inspection of the intestines with a camera). The gastrointestinal (GI) tract is best pictured as a continuous tube that begins at the mouth and ends at the anus. The mucosal layer of intestine that absorbs nutrients contains immune cells that act as defenders of the body (antibodies). Sometimes, this mucosal layer breaks down, and harmful bacteria enter the deep layers of the intestine. The resulting inflammatory process can entail swelling (edema), increased blood flow, and ulcerations (disruptions in the intestinal lining). In Crohn's disease, these ulcerations involve the full thickness of the intestinal lining.

When the inflamed intestine heals, it may become scarred around the areas previously inflamed. This may lead to a narrowing of the bowel, or stricture, which can lead to partial or total blockage of the intestinal flow (bowel obstruction).

TREATMENT AND THERAPY

Crohn's disease is a baffling, unpredictable disease for which a truly successful treatment has not been found. Some of the medications used in treatment are corticosteroids, such as prednisone and adrenocorticotropic hormone (ACTH), and sulfasalazine-type drugs, such as Azulfidine. Both have limited benefits and some side effects. Prednisone-type drugs reduce tissue inflammation and thereby relieve symptoms such as diarrhea, rectal bleeding, abdominal pain, and fever. They may cause side effects including rounding of the face, increased facial hair, fluid retention, bone loss (osteoporosis), high blood pressure, and high blood sugar levels. These drugs also may cause mood swings. They are prescribed conservatively by most doctors. Sulfasalazine contains two active ingredients, a sulfa preparation (sulfapyridine) and an aspirin-like drug (5-aminosalicylic acid, or 5-ASA), which are bonded together. The 5-ASA

INFORMATION ON CROHN'S DISEASE

CAUSES: Infection

SYMPTOMS: Diarrhea, abdominal pain, rectal bleeding, fever, weight loss, anal sores, hemorrhoids, fissures, fistulas, abscesses, nausea, vomiting

DURATION: Chronic

TREATMENTS: Medications for symptom alleviation

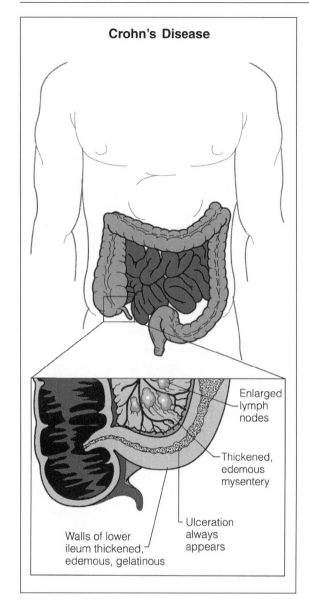

Crohn's Disease

Enlarged lymph nodes

Thickened, edemous mysentery

Ulceration always appears

Walls of lower ileum thickened, edemous, gelatinous

Crohn's disease can cause inflammation and ulceration within any region of the digestive tract, but most often in the ileum.

medication is thought to act on the surface of the lining of the intestine, suppressing tissue inflammation.

The drug 6-mercaptopurine, or 6-MP, is an immunosuppressive, a substance that alters the body's normal immune response to a disease or antigen. Immunosuppressive drugs have been used to treat autoimmune diseases, conditions in which the body literally attacks itself, among them Crohn's disease. It is believed that these drugs can stop the mechanism that causes the body to attack itself.

Drugs can offer relief of symptoms, but no drug has yet been found to alter the long-term progression or natural course of Crohn's disease. Surgical removal of the diseased intestine is usually reserved for cases in which medical treatment has failed. The recurrence rates of Crohn's disease following surgery are high.

PERSPECTIVE AND PROSPECTS

Unlike ulcerative colitis, which affects only the inner lining of the intestines, Crohn's disease affects the full thickness of the bowel wall. Both types of IBD occur in predominantly Western or developed countries, especially Scandinavia, England, Western Europe, Israel, and the United States. In recent years, IBD has been reported in Japan. IBD is seen rarely in Africa, most of Asia, and parts of South America. IBD seems to cluster in families, suggesting a genetic factor. Up to 20 percent of people with IBD have one or more blood relatives with the disease.

American gastroenterologist Burrill B. Crohn first identified Crohn's disease in 1932. The prognosis for sufferers was poor, and their quality of life was limited. Surgical removal of the diseased colon or small colon was the only treatment. Prednisone was the first of the above-mentioned medications to be used to treat Crohn's disease. Investigation into the causes and treatment of IBD continues in many areas, including genetic studies. Current research offers reason for optimism that the causes of IBD will be found and that a cure will follow.

—Lisa Levin Sobczak, R.N.C.

See also Colitis; Colon; Diarrhea and dysentery; Gastroenterology; Gastroenterology, pediatric; Gastrointestinal system; Immune system; Intestinal disorders; Intestines; Irritable bowel syndrome (IBS); Nausea and vomiting.

FOR FURTHER INFORMATION:

Brandt, Lawrence J., and Penny Steiner-Grossman, eds. *Treating IBD: A Patient's Guide to the Medical and Surgical Management of Inflammatory Bowel Disease.* Reprint. Philadelphia: Lippincott-Raven, 1996. One of the most thorough introductions to ulcerative colitis and Crohn's disease. Writing for patients, the authors, who are all medical experts, present technical information and guidelines on symptoms, drugs, surgical procedures, nutritional management, psychotherapy, and counseling.

Crohn's and Colitis Foundation of America. http://www.ccfa.org. Provides support groups and a wide range of educational publications and programs on Crohn's and ulcerative colitis.

Kalibjian, Cliff. *Straight from the Gut: Living with Crohn's Disease and Ulcerative Colitis*. Cambridge, Mass.: O'Reilly, 2003. Shares numerous personal stories from those suffering from colitis and offers advice on all aspects of living with the disease.

Murray, Michael T. *Stomach Ailments and Digestive Disturbances: How You Can Benefit from Diet, Vitamins, Minerals, Herbs, Exercise, and Other Natural Methods*. Rocklin, Calif.: Prima, 1997. Chronic stomach ailments affect many Americans, and the number can only increase as the population ages. Murray counters that trend with practical information and sensible advice for getting well and staying well naturally.

Saibil, Fred. *Crohn's Disease and Ulcerative Colitis: Everything You Need to Know*. Rev. ed. Toronto, Ont.: Firefly Books, 2009. A leading expert on IBD, Saibil covers topics such as signs and symptoms, how the gastrointestinal system works normally and how IBD affects it, procedures and instruments used to diagnose IBD, effects of diet, children and IBD, and effects on sexual activity and childbearing.

Sklar, Jill, Manuel Sklar, and Annabel Cohen. *The First Year—Crohn's Disease and Ulcerative Colitis: An Essential Guide for the Newly Diagnosed*. 2d ed. New York: Marlowe, 2007. A unique guide for patients with specific gastrointestinal disorders, setting expectations and answering questions related to the first week of diagnosis, the first months, and the first year. Topics include treatment options, dietary choices, fertility issues, and holistic alternatives.

Steiner-Grossman, Penny, Peter A. Banks, and Daniel H. Present, eds. *The New People, Not Patients: A Source Book for Living with Inflammatory Bowel Disease*. Rev. ed. Dubuque, Iowa: Kendall/Hunt, 1997. Written to help IBD patients live with the disease, this book combines very practical information—about support groups and patients' rights, for example—with overviews of symptoms and treatments. Its main strength, however, lies in case histories of patients from different walks of life.

Zonderman, Jon, and Ronald S. Vender. *Understanding Crohn Disease and Ulcerative Colitis*. Jackson: University Press of Mississippi, 2000. Crohn's patient Zonderman and Vender, his gastroenterologist, base their presentation of the medical and psychological aspects of two inflammatory bowel diseases on solid medical evidence. They deal with related medical conditions and how Crohn's disease and ulcerative colitis can affect persons of different ages differently.

CROSSED EYES. *See* STRABISMUS.

CROUP
DISEASE/DISORDER

ALSO KNOWN AS: Viral croup, spasmodic croup, laryngotracheobronchitis

ANATOMY OR SYSTEM AFFECTED: Lungs, respiratory system, throat

SPECIALTIES AND RELATED FIELDS: Emergency medicine, otorhinolaryngology, pediatrics, preventive medicine, virology

DEFINITION: An inflammation of the larynx, throat, and upper bronchial tubes causing hoarseness, cough, and difficult breathing.

KEY TERMS:

cortisone: a steroid hormone used to reduce inflammation

epiglottis: a small piece of cartilage that covers the entry to the windpipe during swallowing

epiglottitis: a serious condition caused by a bacterial infection sometimes confused with croup

larynx: the voice box

stridor: the characteristic noisy, labored breathing present with croup

trachea: the windpipe

CAUSES AND SYMPTOMS

Croup is an inflammation of the larynx, trachea, and upper bronchial tubes of the lungs affecting children between the ages of six months and generally no more than five years. Two-year-olds seem to be the most commonly affected. The inflammation of the trachea causes a narrowing of the child's already small airways, making breathing difficult. Technically, croup is a syndrome, or collection of symptoms associated with several different kinds of infections. These symptoms include hoarseness, a distinctive cough most often described as "barky" and noisy, and labored breathing known as stridor.

Croup occurs in three different forms. The first, viral croup, usually begins with a cold and is most commonly caused by parainfluenza viruses. Indeed, studies indicate that the parainfluenza viruses are responsible for about 70 to 75 percent of croup cases. Viral croup is often accompanied by a low-grade fever. A second type of croup is called spasmodic croup. This condition

INFORMATION ON CROUP

CAUSES: Viral or bacterial infection, allergens, change in environment (seasonal change)
SYMPTOMS: Hoarseness, "barking" cough, difficulty breathing
DURATION: Acute
TREATMENTS: Medications (cortisone, antibiotics), humidifier; if severe, emergency care and oxygen tent

tends to occur with changes of the weather and/or seasons, and the child does not usually run a fever. Allergies are often thought to be responsible for this kind of croup. A third, but rare, form is a bacterial infection caused by mycoplasma. This form can be very serious and is often identified by the extreme difficulty that the child experiences with breathing.

Studies indicate that attacks of croup most commonly occur in October through March and generally strike at night. In general, boys are somewhat more likely to be affected by croup than are girls.

A serious, but rare, condition known as epiglottitis can sometimes be mistaken for croup. In this condition, the epiglottis, the flap that covers the windpipe during swallowing, becomes inflamed and swollen, potentially cutting off the child's air supply. The symptoms of epiglottitis are similar to those of croup, but the child's difficulty in breathing is much more severe, and the child will often run a high fever, drool, and be unable to make voiced sounds. Epiglottitis develops quickly; a child's life can be in jeopardy in only a few hours. Consequently, this condition must be treated as an emergency, requiring hospital care.

TREATMENT AND THERAPY

A number of treatments are generally used to bring relief to the child suffering from viral or spasmodic croup. The use of a cool mist humidifier can ward off an attack in the child who exhibits a tendency toward developing croup. A mild attack can also be alleviated through use of the humidifier. If the attack of croup is well under way or if it is severe, however, a cool mist humidifier may not be adequate. Many doctors recommend that after an attack of croup, a cool mist humidifier should be run in the child's room for the next three or four evenings. Another commonly used treatment is to take the child, properly dressed, outside at night. Usually the cold, damp air will soothe the child's inflamed airways.

Still another technique reported to relieve the symptoms of croup is to fill the bathroom with steam by running a hot shower. Setting the child in the steam-filled room for fifteen to twenty minutes often eases the child's breathing. The most successful use of this treatment requires that the child be held, not placed on the floor, because steam rises.

Neither cough syrups nor antibiotics are appropriate treatments for croup. Cough syrups prevent the expulsion of phlegm, while antibiotics have no effect on viral infections. Croup caused by mycoplasma, however, is treated with an antibiotic, generally erythromycin.

Pediatricians recommend that the child's doctor be called in the event of a croup attack. Serious attacks are generally treated in a hospital emergency room. There, the child may be given cortisone by injection or by mouth. In addition, hospitals can administer breathing treatments.

Bacterial croup is also treated at a hospital with antibiotics and an oxygen tent as needed. Indeed, immediate emergency room treatment is called for if there is a whistling sound in the breathing that seems to grow louder, if the child does not have enough breath to speak, or if the child is struggling to breathe.

PERSPECTIVE AND PROSPECTS

Accounts of croup can be found in medical literature dating back to the eighteenth century. Membranous croup, also known as diphtheria, was a great killer of children and adults alike in the past. Immunization made this kind of croup extremely rare, however, by the mid-twentieth century.

During the last quarter of the twentieth century, doctors continued to research the uses of corticosteroids in the treatment of croup, as well as the most effective way to deliver the drugs.

—*Diane Andrews Henningfeld, Ph.D.*

See also Bacterial infections; Bronchi; Bronchitis; Childhood infectious diseases; Coughing; Diphtheria; Epiglottitis; Laryngitis; Lungs; Respiration; Sore throat; Trachea; Viral infections; Wheezing.

FOR FURTHER INFORMATION:

American Medical Association. *American Medical Association Family Medical Guide.* 4th rev. ed. Hoboken, N.J.: John Wiley & Sons, 2004. An excellent reference for the beginner. The scientific accuracy of the text is not compromised by its accessibility.

Nathanson, Laura Walter. "Coping with Croup." *Par-*

ents 70, no. 9 (September, 1995): 29-31. Offers practical advice for treating the scary-sounding cough known as croup. Although home remedies can help alleviate croup, special medications allow a child to breathe easier and recover faster.

Niederman, Michael S., George A. Sarosi, and Jeffrey Glassroth. *Respiratory Infections.* 2d ed. Philadelphia: Lippincott Williams & Wilkins, 2001. Text that covers a range of respiratory problems, including croup.

Shelov, Steven P., et al. *Caring for Your Baby and Young Child: Birth to Age Five.* 5th ed. New York: Bantam Books, 2009. Offers a comprehensive discussion of illnesses that commonly affect young children.

Spock, Benjamin, and Robert Needlman. *Dr. Spock's Baby and Child Care.* 8th ed. New York: Pocket Books, 2004. For more than a half century, this book has been a virtual bible for parents seeking trustworthy information on child care. Informative, easy to use, and responsive to the changes in society, this revised and updated edition makes a classic work more essential than ever.

West, John B. *Pulmonary Pathophysiology: The Essentials.* 7th ed. Philadelphia: Wolters Kluwer/ Lippincott Williams & Wilkins, 2008. Examines lungs afflicted with obstructive, restrictive, vascular, and environmental diseases.

Woolf, Alan D., et al., eds. *The Children's Hospital Guide to Your Child's Health and Development.* Cambridge, Mass.: Perseus, 2002. An authoritative and comprehensive guide to children's health, providing a guide to every common illness or condition that affects children and a carefully designed emergency section.

CROWNS AND BRIDGES
TREATMENT

ALSO KNOWN AS: Restorative dentistry, indirect restorations

ANATOMY OR SYSTEM AFFECTED: Mouth, teeth

SPECIALTIES AND RELATED FIELDS: Dentistry

DEFINITION: Structures that restore the function of the mouth after teeth have been broken or lost. A crown covers and protects a single tooth, while a bridge is a false tooth suspended between two crowns to replace a missing tooth.

KEY TERMS:

abutment: a tooth protected by a crown that serves to anchor one end of a bridge

indirect restoration: a restoration that is fabricated outside the mouth, such as a crown or bridge

restoration: an item or material that is used to restore the structure and function of a compromised tooth

root canal: treatment in which the nerve and pulp of a damaged or infected tooth are removed

INDICATIONS AND PROCEDURES

A crown may be needed to protect a tooth from cracking or breaking, especially one that already has a large filling. It may also be used to cover a tooth that has already broken, become infected, and required endodontic treatment (commonly called a root canal). A crown provides a whole new chewing surface, so it must be able to withstand tremendous jaw pressure. Crowns are indirect restorations that may be made of porcelain, which is tooth-colored, or metal (preferably gold), or a combination of the two. In this combination, the porcelain is fused to gold, palladium, or platinum. In all-metal crowns, gold is preferable because it can be cast accurately for a tight fit and it will not corrode.

The first step in the preparation of a crown is to modify the tooth to receive a crown. Then an impression of the tooth is made and from this, a mold is made in which to cast the crown. Once produced, the crown is polished and contoured to approximate a natural tooth. Any porcelain is colored and glazed to match the shade of the patient's natural teeth. Once the crown is finished, the dentist adjusts its fit in the patient's mouth and cements the crown in place. This process is usually accomplished in two visits; the patient is given a temporary crown, usually acrylic, to wear while the permanent one is being made.

A bridge is indicated when one or several teeth in a row are missing and there are stable teeth on either side of the gap to serve as abutments. It is important to fill the gap to maintain optimal function for chewing and speaking by preventing the remaining teeth from shifting and losing their proper alignment.

Models of the patient's mouth are made that indicate the shapes and positions of the abutting teeth that will receive crowns to support the bridge and the gap to be filled by the artificial tooth or teeth. The components of the bridge may be made of metal or porcelain or a combination of the two. The dentist will indicate to the bridge fabricator what shade from a standard color system to make the porcelain to best match the patient's natural teeth. Once the bridge is made, the dentist adjusts the fit in the patient's mouth and cements the bridge in place. The entire process may require several visits; the patient is given a temporary acrylic bridge to protect the area while the permanent one is being made.

USES AND COMPLICATIONS

Because the preparation of crowns and bridges involves drilling on teeth, the dentist provides local anesthetic to numb the area. This numbness may last a while, and the patient must be careful not to bite the lips or tongue.

While the permanent restoration is being fabricated, the patient wears a temporary piece that is held in place with a light adhesive so it may be easily removed later. However, it may become dislodged before the next dental appointment. It is important that the temporary crown or bridge is replaced as soon as possible to keep the prepared teeth protected and stable. Should their shape or position change, the finished restoration would no longer fit properly.

Fabricating and fitting indirect restorations requires skill and patience. Any excess space inadvertently left between the tooth and the crown or bridge increases the risk of decay or infection because food may become trapped. This is especially problematic for teeth that have not had root canal treatment because a painful abscess may form under the crown. Excess space in bridgework creates the possibility of teeth shifting, which the bridge was originally designed to avoid.

When the crown or bridge is delivered, it might feel high and contact the teeth on the opposite jaw sooner than expected. The dentist will make adjustments at the time of delivery, but a return visit may be necessary if further discomfort is felt.

The teeth involved may be somewhat sensitive to cold following delivery of the restoration. This sensitivity may last for weeks, but it typically resolves on its own.

PERSPECTIVE AND PROSPECTS

Indirect restorations were initially unattractive but functional metal structures. Later, fabrication with porcelain allowed for a less obvious appearance. Advances in materials science have led to the development of stronger, more fracture-resistant ceramics. These contribute to longer lasting, more aesthetically pleasing restorations.

Technology is partnering with dentistry to generate computer-aided design and computer-aided manufacturing (CAD/CAM) for use in crown and bridge fabrication. Dentists and dental lab technicians are using CAD/CAM technology to increase the precision of individual restorations by capturing each tooth's exact size, shape, and position. Digital impressions are more comfortable for the patient and less technique-dependent than customary alginate impressions. The resulting three-dimensional image appears on a computer screen, and the dentist can electronically draw the restoration design on the image instead of sculpting wax on a stone model. The details can then be transmitted digitally without distortion to the dental lab technician, who uses a CAD/CAM machine to mill a ceramic material into a detailed replica of the drawing. By looking at the same electronic image before manufacturing, the dentist and the dental lab technician can clearly communicate their needs and expectations for an accurate preparation that will result in a quality custom restoration.

—*Bethany Thivierge, M.P.H., E.L.S.*

See also Aging; Bone disorders; Cavities; Dental diseases; Dentistry; Dentures; Teeth.

FOR FURTHER INFORMATION:

Christensen, Gordon J. "Salvaging Crowns and Fixed Prostheses: When and How to Do It." *Journal of the American Dental Association* 139 (December, 2008): 1679-1682.

Jacobsen, Peter. *Restorative Dentistry: An Integrated Approach.* Malden, Mass.: Blackwell, 2008.

Walmsley, A. Damien, et al. *Restorative Dentistry.* 2d ed. New York: Churchill Livingstone/Elsevier, 2007.

CRYOSURGERY

PROCEDURE

ALSO KNOWN AS: Cryotherapy

ANATOMY OR SYSTEM AFFECTED: All

SPECIALTIES AND RELATED FIELDS: Dermatology, family medicine, general surgery, gynecology, neurology, oncology, otorhinolaryngology, plastic surgery, urology

DEFINITION: The destruction of undesired or abnormal body tissues by exposure to extreme cold.

KEY TERMS:

cryogenic agent: a substance (such as liquid nitrogen) that produces low temperatures

cryoprobe: a liquid nitrogen-cooled, probelike tool used in cryosurgery

lesion: abnormal or diseased tissue

INDICATIONS AND PROCEDURES

Cryosurgery, the therapeutic use of extreme cold, is used to remove minor skin lesions such as freckles and

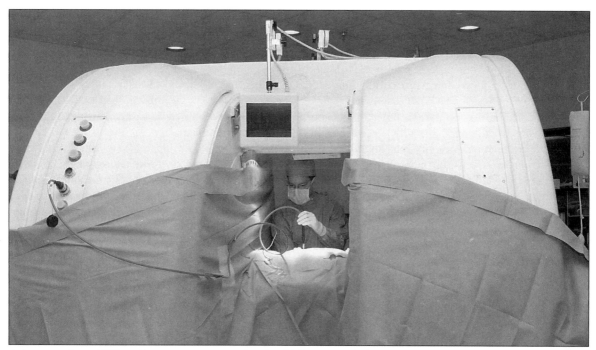

A doctor performs MRI renal cryosurgery, a procedure in which a surgical tube with a freezing tip at the end is used to destroy cancerous kidney tumors while the patient is monitored with MRI. (AP/Wide World Photos)

warts as well as cancers of the skin and other tissues. Skin heals well after cold injury, and skin pathologies were among the first lesions treated cryosurgically. Although cryosurgery is not the first treatment choice for all skin problems, it is a popular one because of the availability of liquid nitrogen, the main cryogenic agent. In addition, cryosurgery is inexpensive, compared to other procedures, and can be performed without surgical facilities. For example, family physicians and dermatologists use it to treat minor skin lesions at their offices.

Cryosurgery kills tissue via extracellular and intracellular ice. When cells freeze, extracellular ice squeezes them together and changes their extracellular/intracellular volumes. Thawing causes similar, opposite changes that break cell membranes. The rapid temperature drops used in cryosurgery produce intracellular ice, another major source of cell destruction. The result is altered solute concentrations in tissue fluid, electrolyte loss from cells, disrupted membranes, and protein inactivation and transmigration. Reversed temperature gradients cause more destruction during thawing.

Cryosurgery results in tissue hyperemia, discoloration, and ice buildup. On thawing, edema (swelling) develops, yielding necrosis (cell death) in four days. Dead tissue sloughs off in three more days. Within a month, it is replaced by granulation tissue, which yields normal tissue.

Cryosurgery uses between one and five freeze-thaw cycles (FTCs). The freeze speed is 300 degrees Celsius per minute with a drop from 37 degrees Celsius to −196 degrees Celsius followed by crash (about ten-second), short (one-minute), medium (about three-minute), or long (ten-minute) thaws, depending on the type of lesion treated.

For external tissue treatment, liquid nitrogen (at −196 degrees Celsius) may be applied by swab or in a spray. More often, liquid nitrogen-cooled cryoprobes are pressed on lesions. Cryoprobes are cylindrical, with flat contact surfaces. The duration of cryoprobe use depends on the lesion size and type. For example, genital warts of the cervix are treated by quick freeze, a several-minute thaw, and refreezing.

Treating cancer is more complex. In treating internal cancer, liquid nitrogen is circulated through a cryoprobe touching the lesion. Its position and cell freezing are monitored by ultrasound, which also minimizes the destruction of healthy tissue and identifies the extent of cancer death. The size of the cryoprobe depends on the size of the lesion. If a lesion is not destroyed entirely, then the number of FTCs and the treatment time can be lengthened at follow-up visits.

USES AND COMPLICATIONS

The complexity of cryosurgery varies. Cervical warts require one FTC and a cryoprobe, without any anesthetic. Because of the possibility of postoperative fainting, patients are observed for twenty minutes and should arrange for a ride home. Mild abdominal cramps or vaginal discharge may occur. The surgeon should be contacted about prolonged bleeding, infection, or cramps lasting more than twenty-four hours.

Most skin cancers, most often basal and squamous cell carcinomas, can be treated cryosurgically. Often, three or four FTCs are used. Ear, eyelid, and nose cartilage sites are good targets because scarring and necrosis of surrounding tissue are rare. Superficial basal cell carcinoma exhibits a near 100 percent cure rate, as do nose and ear lesions, because these cancers rarely enter cartilage. Squamous cell carcinoma often does, however, and is harder to treat without creating scars. Cryosurgery is the treatment of choice for facial Bowen's squamous cell carcinoma, with a cure rate near 100 percent, and for cancers of the cervix or penis; removing these cancers does not leave scars. Treating lesions on the eyelids, however, may cause them to swell shut.

Cryosurgery can also be used for localized prostate cancer. Warm saline is passed through a urethral catheter to prevent freezing. Cryoprobe placement is achieved through incisions between the anus and scrotum, guided by ultrasound. As with conventional surgery, anesthesia is needed for pain. The appearance of prostate tissue changes during cryosurgery, and damage to healthy tissue can be minimized through the observation of ultrasound images. The prostate gland swells postoperatively, and a catheter in the bladder is used to prevent urination stoppage. This complication and bruises from probe insertion sites can result in hospital stays. However, cryosurgery causes less bleeding, shorter hospitalization and recovery periods, and less pain than does surgical removal of the prostate. Assurance of complete cancer destruction requires follow-up with radiation or chemotherapy.

Cryosurgery is also used to treat liver, pancreas, and breast cancers, and the applicability of cryosurgery to bone, brain, and spinal cancers is under study. In these cases, cryosurgery is part of a mixed treatment, including conventional surgery and radiation or chemotherapy. Initial reports are encouraging, but the long-term effectiveness here is unknown. When standard treatments fail or are unusable in primary or secondary liver cancer, cryosurgery may be used alone. If the surgical removal of cancer from other internal organs is impossible, then cryosurgery may be used to increase symptom-free survival time.

With all cryosurgeries, the discoloration of treated areas and minor scarring may occur. The skin can lose pigment, sweat glands, and hair follicles. Therefore, cryosurgery is less desirable for dark skin and is not suggested for lesions at sites where alopecia (hair loss) would be a problem.

PERSPECTIVE AND PROSPECTS

The first use of cryosurgery was in the early twentieth century through liquid air freezing for skin cancer treatment and cosmetic surgery. In the mid-1950's, improved cryotools began the expansion of cryosurgery to its modern state. This progress was enhanced by the availability of liquid nitrogen, which enabled clinicians to work at temperatures of −196 degrees Celsius.

Cryosurgery is a standard method used in cosmetic surgery and the treatment of skin cancers and is accepted for use with other cancers, including prostate, liver, pancreatic, uterine, lung, and brain cancers. Cryosurgery is employed alone and with other treatments (such as traditional surgery), or when other methods fail. After cryosurgery, many patients regain a high quality of life and are pain-free. Moreover, they are often outpatients, spend little time in surgery, have short hospitalizations, and recuperate rapidly. Scarring is minimal, and cure rates are high.

Cryosurgery has side effects, though they are less severe than those of traditional surgery. In treatment of the liver, cryosurgery may damage bile ducts or blood vessels, causing hemorrhage or infection. In the treatment of prostate cancer, it may cause incontinence and impotence. The main disadvantage, unclear long-term value in internal cancer surgery, is sure to be addressed.

—*Sanford S. Singer, Ph.D.*

See also Cancer; Cervical procedures; Dermatology; Electrocauterization; Lesions; Melanoma; Moles; Prostate cancer; Skin; Skin cancer; Skin disorders; Skin lesion removal; Tumor removal; Tumors; Warts.

FOR FURTHER INFORMATION:

Dehn, Richard W., and David P. Asprey, eds. *Clinical Procedures for Physician Assistants*. Philadelphia: W. B. Saunders, 2002. The chapter on cryosurgery provides useful information for patients and general readers.

Jackson, Arthur, Graham Colver, and Rodney Dawber. *Cutaneous Cryosurgery: Principles and Clinical Practice*. 3d ed. New York: Taylor & Francis, 2006.

An illustrated handbook that provides the information needed for running a cryosurgery clinic.

Korpan, Nikolai N., ed. *Basics of Cryosurgery.* New York: Springer, 2001. Discusses cryosurgery from cosmetic work to major surgery. Indexed, with references and illustrations.

Lask, Gary P., and Ronald L. Moy, eds. *Principles and Techniques of Cutaneous Surgery.* New York: McGraw-Hill, 1996. A classic text with a chapter on cryosurgery.

CT SCANNING. *See* COMPUTED TOMOGRAPHY (CT) SCANNING.

CULDOCENTESIS

PROCEDURE

ANATOMY OR SYSTEM AFFECTED: Abdomen, reproductive system

SPECIALTIES AND RELATED FIELDS: General surgery, gynecology

DEFINITION: A diagnostic procedure in which fluid in the cul-de-sac of Douglas, the space behind the uterus and in front of the rectum, is removed using a needle inserted through the vagina.

INDICATIONS AND PROCEDURES

Culdocentesis is indicated in cases where a woman is suspected of having fluid in the abdomen or pelvis with an unclear cause. The patient may have an acutely painful and tender abdomen. Culdocentesis can identify the presence of fluid in the pelvis as well as distinguish whether the fluid is the result of active bleeding, infection, a perforated organ, or other causes.

For culdocentesis, the patient lies on her back with her legs in stirrups, as for a pelvic examination. A speculum is inserted into the vagina to visualize the cervix, and the cervix is gently lifted with a grasping instrument. A long, thin needle is inserted through the vagina, behind the cervix, and into the cul-de-sac of Douglas. Any fluid in this cul-de-sac is aspirated, and analysis of the fluid is subsequently performed.

USES AND COMPLICATIONS

Culdocentesis is not common, as noninvasive imaging modalities such as pelvic ultrasound with vaginal transducer have replaced this procedure to evaluate fluid collections in the abdomen and pelvis. Nevertheless, culdocentesis can yield useful information regarding the nature of abdominal or pelvic fluid, and hence it can assist in diagnosis and treatment decisions. For in-

stance, nonclotted bloody fluid can be consistent with active bleeding, such as from a ruptured ectopic pregnancy or hemorrhagic ovarian cyst. Either of these conditions may require immediate surgery to stop the bleeding. The fluid aspirated from the cul-de-sac may be bile or bowel contents, indicating perforation of the gastrointestinal tract and possible need for urgent surgery. Infected fluid suggests pelvic inflammatory disease (PID) or abscess, for which surgery may not be the first line of treatment. Nonbloody, noninfected fluid may be caused by the rupture of a benign ovarian cyst, which would not require intervention.

Complications associated with culdocentesis are very rare. They include perforation of internal organs, such as the bowel or uterus, with the needle. In almost all cases, no serious aftereffects occur from these perforations, as the needle used is thin, but there are case reports of bleeding from organ perforations that require surgical intervention. Other examples of risks involved with culdocentesis are infection and bleeding from the puncture site.

—*Anne Lynn S. Chang, M.D.*

See also Abdomen; Abscess drainage; Abscesses; Cyst removal; Cysts; Ectopic pregnancy; Gynecology; Invasive tests; Pelvic inflammatory disease (PID); Rectum; Reproductive system; Uterus; Women's health.

FOR FURTHER INFORMATION:

Doherty, Gerard M., and Lawrence W. Way, eds. *Current Surgical Diagnosis and Treatment.* 12th ed. New York: Lange Medical Books/McGraw-Hill, 2006.

Rock, John A., and Howard W. Jones III, eds. *Te Linde's Operative Gynecology.* 10th ed. Philadelphia: Wolters Kluwer/Lippincott Williams & Wilkins, 2008.

Stenchever, Morton A., et al. *Comprehensive Gynecology.* 5th ed. St. Louis, Mo.: Mosby/Elsevier, 2007.

CUSHING'S SYNDROME

DISEASE/DISORDER

ANATOMY OR SYSTEM AFFECTED: Abdomen, back, blood, bones, endocrine system, glands, hair, muscles, skin

SPECIALTIES AND RELATED FIELDS: Endocrinology, family medicine, immunology, internal medicine, nutrition, radiology, urology

DEFINITION: A hormonal disorder caused primarily by chronic exposure of body tissues to excessive levels of cortisol.

INFORMATION ON CUSHING'S SYNDROME

CAUSES: Chronic exposure of body tissues to excess cortisol from overproduction by adrenal glands (tumor) or steroid use

SYMPTOMS: Rounded face, fat trunk with thin arms and legs, fat pads over neck and shoulders, purple stretch marks, easy bruising, muscle weakness, poor wound healing, fractures, high blood pressure, diabetes mellitus, emotional instability

DURATION: Chronic until treated

TREATMENTS: Restoration of hormonal balance, surgical removal of tumor, discontinuance of steroid use

CAUSES AND SYMPTOMS

Cushing's syndrome is a group of abnormalities that result from either excessive levels of hormones produced by the outer layer of the adrenal glands or from the taking of steroid hormones. The primary source of the disorder is the hormone cortisol. This condition is typically triggered by an excess production of adrenocorticotropic hormone (ACTH) from the pituitary gland. ACTH in turn stimulates the adrenal glands to produce hormones, particularly cortisol. Excessive production of ACTH may result from a pituitary gland tumor or a tumor associated with other organs or as a side effect from taking steroid hormones used to treat asthma, rheumatoid arthritis, and other serious diseases. Adrenal gland tumors also produce excess amounts of cortisol. Though extremely rare, an inherited tendency to develop endocrine gland tumors is another cause of Cushing's syndrome.

Since the hormones produced by the adrenal glands regulate processes throughout the body, excess production can cause widespread disorders. Some of the more common symptoms of Cushing's syndrome are a rounded face, a fat trunk with thin arms and legs, fat pads over the neck and shoulders, purple stretch marks on the skin, easy bruising, muscle weakness, poor wound healing, fractures in weakened bones, high blood pressure, diabetes mellitus, emotional instability, and severe fatigue. Men can experience diminished desire for sex, while women have increased hairiness, acne, and decreased or absent menstrual periods. Children are usually obese, and their growth rate is slow.

TREATMENT AND THERAPY

Cushing's syndrome is treated by restoring the hormonal balance within the body, which may take several months. If Cushing's syndrome is left untreated, it can lead to death. The disease is diagnosed through blood and urine tests to determine excess amounts of cortisol. Pituitary tumors and tumors at other locations in the body that have been diagnosed as producing ACTH are surgically removed, when possible, or are treated with radiation or chemotherapy. Cortisol replacement therapy is provided after surgery until cortisol production resumes. Lifelong cortisol replacement therapy may be necessary. If steroids are not being used to control a life-threatening illness, however, then they should be discontinued.

Adrenal and pituitary tumors are always surgically removed. The remaining adrenal gland, which has usually diminished in size as a result of inactivity, will return to its normal size and function. As it is doing so,

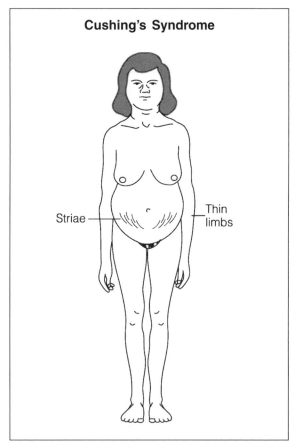

Cushing's Syndrome

Striae

Thin limbs

An adrenal disorder, Cushing's syndrome causes symptomatic fatty deposits, striae, and thin limbs and may be associated with a variety of mild to serious conditions.

steroid hormones are administered to supply the needed cortisol and then tapered off over time. Some tumors may recur after surgical excision.

PERSPECTIVE AND PROSPECTS

The first diagnosis of Cushing's syndrome was made by Harvey Cushing in 1912. In 1932, he linked the disease to an abnormality in the pituitary gland that stimulated an overproduction of cortisol from the adrenal glands. Pituitary tumors cause approximately 70 percent of the disease. Cushing's syndrome is more frequent in women than in men, with most cases occurring between the ages of twenty-five and forty-five. The disease can be very serious, possibly even fatal, unless diagnosed and treated early.

—*Alvin K. Benson, Ph.D.; updated by Sharon W. Stark, R.N., A.P.R.N., D.N.Sc.*

See also Addison's disease; Adrenal glands; Corticosteroids; Endocrine disorders; Endocrine glands; Endocrinology; Endocrinology, pediatric; Hormones; Tumors.

FOR FURTHER INFORMATION:

Endocrine and Metabolic Diseases Information Service. National Institute of Diabetes and Digestive and Kidney Diseases (NIDDK). National Institutes of Health. *Cushing's Syndrome.* http://endocrine .niddk.nih.gov/pubs/cushings/cushings.htm. A comprehensive overview of Cushing's syndrome and its diagnosis and treatment.

Fox, Stuart Ira. *Human Physiology.* 11th ed. Boston: McGraw-Hill, 2010. A college-level human physiology textbook that is well written and richly illustrated.

Kronenberg, Henry M., et al., eds. *Williams Textbook of Endocrinology.* 11th ed. Philadelphia: Saunders/ Elsevier, 2008. Comprehensive information regarding endocrine diseases, pathophysiology, diagnoses, treatment, and prognoses.

MedlinePlus. *Cushing's Syndrome.* Edited by Nikheel S. Kolatkar. http://www.nlm.nih.gov/medlineplus/ ency/article/000410.htm. General information regarding Cushing's syndrome, diagnosis, treatment, complications, expectations, and prevention.

CYANOSIS

DISEASE/DISORDER

ANATOMY OR SYSTEM AFFECTED: Blood, skin

SPECIALTIES AND RELATED FIELDS: Hematology, internal medicine, pulmonary medicine, toxicology

DEFINITION: Dark blue discoloration of the skin and nail beds resulting from decreases in the oxygenation of hemoglobin in the red blood cells in the arteries.

KEY TERMS:

arterial blood: blood from an artery receiving blood from the left ventricle; usually bright red

hemoglobin: the protein in red cells that combines reversibly with oxygen to form oxyhemoglobin; also referred to as reduced hemoglobin or deoxyhemoglobin

hemoglobin saturation: the portion of total hemoglobin that is combined with oxygen, usually expressed as a percentage

methemoglobin: oxidized hemoglobin, which is present normally as up to 1 percent of total hemoglobin; it does not combine reversibly rapidly with oxygen and cannot serve in oxygen transport

oxyhemoglobin: a reversibly oxygenated form of hemoglobin

sulfhemoglobin: the reaction product of hemoglobin with certain toxic agents (oxidants)

venous blood: blood from a vein conducting blood to the right ventricle, before passage through the lungs

CAUSES AND SYMPTOMS

Cyanosis, a dark blue discoloration of the skin and nail beds, is a sign of a disorder, not a disease in itself, and it may have several causes. It is also not a symptom sensed by a patient but a physical finding. To appear, cyanosis requires a concentration in arterial blood of 4 to 5 grams per deciliter of reduced hemoglobin. Anemic patients may not show cyanosis even though their hemoglobin saturations are low. Its presence indicates one or more of the following: inadequate oxygenation of arterial blood (a decrease of oxygen saturation to 85 percent or less), the presence of a normal constituent (methemoglobin) in increased concentration, or the presence of an abnormal constituent (sulfhemoglobin).

Inadequate oxygenation of normally circulating blood. The obstruction of large airways (the tracheobronchial system) can occur from external compression or the aspiration of solid or semisolid materials (foodstuffs, particularly ground meat). Laryngospasm may be a factor. The aspiration of aqueous fluids, as

INFORMATION ON CYANOSIS

CAUSES: Inadequate oxygenation of hemoglobin in arterial blood from various injuries, illnesses, and disorders
SYMPTOMS: Dark blue discoloration of skin and nails
DURATION: Chronic until treated
TREATMENTS: Oxygen administration, treatment of underlying disorder

in drowning in freshwater, can fill the alveoli and decrease or prevent the contact of inspired air with the blood in the pulmonary capillaries. Freshwater can pass rapidly into the blood and eventually free the alveoli for gas exchanges. Drowning in seawater is usually accompanied by marked laryngospasm. If the hypertonic seawater reaches the alveoli, then water will cross from the blood into the alveoli and produce even more fluid and froth in the lungs (pulmonary edema).

The inhalation of certain toxic agents, available industrially or used in warfare, can damage the alveoli and the pulmonary capillaries and produce pulmonary edema. Typical agents are chlorine and phosgene. Smoke inhalation is another possible cause of lung damage. Pulmonary edema from cardiac failure can occur as a result of increased pressure in the alveolar capillaries. Respiratory distress syndrome, or noncardiogenic pulmonary edema, occurs probably as the end result of a variety of initiators (shock, sepsis) culminating in the production of damaging free radicals.

Pharmacologically active agents such as heroin and morphine injected intravenously, as by drug abusers, can produce fulminating pulmonary edema extremely rapidly, possibly as the result of alpha-adrenergic discharge. Substances such as ethchorvynol (Placidyl) can also produce this condition if injected intravenously, although they may be innocuous if taken orally.

Pulmonary infections such as pneumococcal pneumonia can cause edema through the perfusion of alveoli which are filled with fluid, that is, nonventilated. This condition is essentially venous admixture, and it can occur when three or more lobes of the lungs are involved. Chronic obstructive pulmonary disease (COPD) can produce cyanosis because of destruction of lung tissue (emphysema) and because of obstruction to air movement. Oxygenation is incomplete, and cyanosis is a common feature of advanced disease.

Low oxygen concentration in ambient atmosphere occurs with ascent to high altitudes. In certain caves, oxygen may be displaced by carbon dioxide. Incorrect gas mixtures may be administered to patients under anesthesia or on artificial respiration. The oxygen of the ambient atmosphere may be decreased in closed environments such as submarines. Polycythemia (increased numbers of red blood cells per unit volume of blood) may occur as a result of chronic exposure to high altitudes or as a spontaneous problem (polycythemia vera). The oxygen content of the blood may be normal or high, but the unoxygenated portion may be increased so that a ruddy cyanosis may be present.

Admixture of venous and arterial blood flows. Patent ductus arteriosus is a heart defect that produces blue baby syndrome. It offers a classic example of the direct entry of venous blood into the arterial system, as the lungs are partially bypassed. Other cardiopulmonary abnormalities, such as right-to-left shunts, can also produce cyanosis.

Localized circulatory problems. Frostbite and Raynaud's phenomenon are examples of localized occurrence of cyanosis. In these conditions, vascular changes limit blood flow, leading to congestion and unsaturation.

Increased concentrations of methemoglobin or sulfhemoglobin. Naturally occurring methemoglobin is present at about the 1 percent level in blood. From 0.5 to 3 percent of the total hemoglobin is oxidized each day and returned to deoxyhemoglobin through enzymatic reductase activity. In congenital forms of methemoglobinemia, cyanosis appears when the concentration of methemoglobin approaches 10 percent of the total (about 1.4 grams per deciliter).

Acquired increased concentration can be caused by a variety of agents (such as sodium perchlorate, Paraquat, nitroglycerine, and inhaled butyl and isobutyl nitrites) by oxidizing hemoglobin to methemoglobin through the formation of free radicals. Nitrates, absorbed by mouth, are transformed into nitrites in the gut and also produce methemoglobin. Sulfhemoglobin can also be formed and produces cyanosis at concentrations of 0.5 gram per deciliter.

TREATMENT AND THERAPY
Treatment is directed not to the cyanosis itself but to the underlying problem. Oxygen administration is crucial in many but not all cases.

For airway obstruction, the Heimlich maneuver may be lifesaving, as may an emergency tracheostomy. Drowning requires artificial respiration, positioning of the body so that drainage of fluid from the lungs is facilitated, and administration of oxygen, if available. Full cardiopulmonary resuscitation (CPR) may be indicated. Pulmonary edema from cardiac failure or respiratory distress syndrome calls into use a variety of approaches, but oxygen is almost always provided. Artificial respiration and oxygen are usually required in heroin, morphine, and ethchlorvynol pulmonary edema. COPD and emphysema are chronic, progressive disorders in which oxygen, bronchodilators, antibiotics, steroids, and surgical interventions (lung volume reduction) may be used. In methemoglobinemia, the congenital forms may not require any treatment. If the cyanosis is the result of exposure to nitrites and other potential oxidants, then methylene blue is usually effective.

PERSPECTIVE AND PROSPECTS

Cyanosis has been recognized for centuries as a sign or indicator of an underlying problem. The focus of investigations has been on identifying these problems. The properties of the hemoglobins have been investigated by physiologists and hematologists, leading to an understanding of their structures and functions. Surgical correction of the vascular abnormalities of so-called blue babies by Alfred Blalock and Helen Taussig led to the opening of the field of cardiovascular surgery. Molecular biology has provided knowledge of the enzymatic and genetic factors involved in the development of methemoglobinemia.

—*Francis P. Chinard, M.D.*

See also Accidents; Altitude sickness; Asphyxiation; Blood and blood disorders; Blue baby syndrome; Cardiac surgery; Cardiology; Cardiology, pediatric; Choking; Chronic obstructive pulmonary disease (COPD); Circulation; Congenital heart disease; Edema; Emphysema; Frostbite; Heart; Heart failure; Heimlich maneuver; Hyperbaric oxygen therapy; Lungs; Poisoning; Pneumonia; Pulmonary diseases; Pulmonary medicine; Pulmonary medicine, pediatric; Respiration; Respiratory distress syndrome; Toxicology; Vascular system.

FOR FURTHER INFORMATION:

Dickerson, Richard E., and Irving Geis. *Hemoglobin: Structure, Function, Evolution, and Pathology.* Menlo Park, Calif.: Benjamin/Cummings, 1983.

Icon Health. *Cyanosis: A Medical Dictionary, Bibliography, and Annotated Research Guide to Internet References.* San Diego, Calif.: Author, 2004.

Nagel, Ronald L., ed. *Hemoglobin Disorders: Molecular Methods and Protocols.* Totowa, N.J.: Humana Press, 2003.

Weibel, Ewald R. *The Pathway for Oxygen: Structure and Function in the Mammalian Respiratory System.* Cambridge, Mass.: Harvard University Press, 1984.

CYST REMOVAL
PROCEDURE

ANATOMY OR SYSTEM AFFECTED: Breasts, genitals, glands, joints, reproductive system, skin

SPECIALTIES AND RELATED FIELDS: Dermatology, general surgery, gynecology, plastic surgery

DEFINITION: A surgical procedure to remove a fluid-filled nodule, performed in a physician's office or a hospital depending on the type and location of the cyst.

KEY TERMS:

aspirate: to remove a substance using suction; a cyst can be aspirated using a needle and syringe to withdraw its contents

cyst: a sac containing a fluid or semifluid substance

incision: a cut made with a scalpel during a surgical procedure

laparoscope: a small surgical tube which can be inserted through a small incision into the abdominal cavity to view and perform surgery on abdominal organs

INDICATIONS AND PROCEDURES

Many types of cysts can develop in the body. The vast majority of them are noncancerous, although in rare cases small areas of cancerous tissue may be found within a cyst. The indications and procedures for removing cysts depend on the type of cyst, its location, and whether it is causing symptoms. Examples of common types of cysts are Baker's, Bartholin's, ovarian, sebaceous, thyroglossal, and breast cysts.

Baker's cysts are small lumps that form behind the knee. Fluid-filled sacs found around joints, known as bursas, normally protect the moving joint from causing damage to overlying skin, tendons, and muscles. When the bursas behind the knee accumulate excess fluid, they can expand and form a Baker's cyst. This fluid accumulation often occurs if the knee is arthritic. Physicians usually apply pressure bandages to reduce the bursal swelling. If this does not work, then the cyst must be excised surgically.

Bartholin's gland cysts are formed when the Bartholin's glands found in the female genital area (specifically the vulva) become occluded and swollen with fluid. Infections can occur in the ducts of these glands, causing pain and scarring. Bartholin's cysts are treated with conservative measures such as warm water soaks, antibiotics, and placement of a Word's catheter, which continuously drains the cyst. If these methods fail, then the cyst may be incised in the operating room and then marsupialized, a procedure which sutures the inner cyst wall to the vulvar skin and keeps the cyst open and draining.

Ovarian cysts do not usually need to be removed, and many of them are physiologic and come and go with the menstrual cycle. When an ovarian cyst becomes large (greater than 6 centimeters in diameter), it may cause the ovary to twist, a condition called ovarian torsion. A twisted ovary is at risk for necrosis, since its blood supply is cut off. In this case, the ovarian cyst would need to be removed. Other reasons for removing an ovarian cyst include a cyst that is persistent and growing with time and a cyst with characteristics upon ultrasound examination that suggest malignancy.

If an ovarian cyst is thought to be noncancerous, then it can usually be removed through the abdomen using a laparoscope. The laparoscope enables visualization of the cyst, while manipulation of the ovary and cyst is accomplished through incisions and tools placed on the sides of the abdomen. The cyst is usually shelled out from the remainder of the ovary using blunt dissection, and the remaining ovary is inspected for areas of bleeding, which may be cauterized. Many patients do not need to be hospitalized if the surgery is straightforward. If there is a concern about cancer within an ovarian cyst, then an open abdominal surgery is indicated. In this case, the abdomen is opened surgically and the cyst is removed, along with any other abnormal-appearing tissue surrounding the cyst.

A sebaceous cyst may develop when a duct from a sebaceous gland in the skin becomes blocked and the oily fluid is unable to escape. These glands, which are associated with hair follicles, secrete sebum to lubricate the hair and skin. If the sebaceous cyst is very large or infected with bacteria, then surgical removal is usually indicated. This operation can be done in a physician's office under local anesthesia. A small incision is made in the skin, and the entire cyst is removed or drained. The complete wall of the cyst is removed in order to prevent recurrence. A few sutures are usually placed to close the wound.

Thyroglossal cysts usually arise because of a con-

genital defect in which the duct that connects the base of the tongue to the thyroid gland fails to disappear. If a cyst develops in this area, a noticeable swelling will occur above the thyroid cartilage (Adam's apple). This cyst nearly always becomes infected and thus should be removed surgically. This procedure involves an incision just above the thyroid cartilage and gland. The surgeon then separates surrounding tissue up to the base of the tongue to gain access to the cyst. The cyst can then be removed and the skin sutured.

Breast cysts are common and can come and go with the menstrual cycle. They are usually detected as a breast lump on physical examination. If they are persistent, then they can be visualized on ultrasound (or mammogram) to confirm that they are fluid-filled (rather than solid, which could be indicative of cancer). Breast cysts can be drained using a needle and the fluid sent for pathological analysis. If the fluid is benign, then no further procedures are indicated.

Uses and Complications

The uses of cyst removal in general are to relieve pain and discomfort, minimize the chance of infection, and preserve the normal anatomy and function of surrounding organs. In addition, the cyst can be sent for pathological analysis after it is removed, in order to determine if any portions suggest cancer.

Complications common to all cyst removal procedures include bleeding at the site where the cyst has been removed, damage to organ structures surrounding the cyst during the excision process, and risk of infection from the excision procedure itself, as foreign instruments are introduced into the field. Another complication is that the cysts may recur, necessitating further intervention. In addition, each type of cyst removal has its own specific risks. For instance, thyroglossal cyst removal surgery may inadvertently remove thyroid tissue, which can lead to thyroid hormone deficiency and the need for thyroid medication for replacement.

—Matthew Berria, Ph.D.,
and Douglas Reinhart, M.D.;
updated by Anne Lynn S. Chang, M.D.

See also Abscess drainage; Abscesses; Biopsy; Breast biopsy; Breast disorders; Breasts, female; Colorectal polyp removal; Colorectal surgery; Cysts; Dermatology; Fibrocystic breast condition; Ganglion removal; Genital disorders, female; Glands; Gynecology; Hydroceles; Laparoscopy; Myomectomy; Nasal polyp removal; Ovarian cysts; Ovaries; Polyps; Reproductive system; Skin; Skin disorders; Skin lesion removal.

For Further Information:

Doherty, Gerard M., and Lawrence W. Way, eds. *Current Surgical Diagnosis and Treatment.* 12th ed. New York: Lange Medical Books/McGraw-Hill, 2006.

Icon Health. *Ovarian Cysts: A Medical Dictionary, Bibliography, and Annotated Research Guide to Internet References.* San Diego, Calif.: Author, 2004.

Kasper, Dennis L., et al., eds. *Harrison's Principles of Internal Medicine.* 16th ed. New York: McGraw-Hill, 2005.

Tierney, Lawrence M., Stephen J. McPhee, and Maxine A. Papadakis, eds. *Current Medical Diagnosis and Treatment 2007.* New York: McGraw-Hill Medical, 2006.

Cystic fibrosis

Disease/disorder

Anatomy or system affected: Chest, lungs, respiratory system, most bodily systems

Specialties and related fields: Genetics, neonatology, pediatrics, pulmonary medicine

Definition: A disease that affects the exocrine glands and, secondarily, most physical systems, resulting in death usually between the ages of sixteen and thirty.

Key terms:

chloride transport: the movement of one of the ions found in ordinary salt across a membrane from the inside of a cell to the outside; this transport is common in human cells and is critical for many important metabolic functions

cystic fibrosis transmembrane-conductance regulator (CFTR): the protein product of the cystic fibrosis gene and a chloride transport channel

meconium ileus: the puttylike plug found in the intestines of some cystic fibrosis babies when they are born

mutation: an alteration in the deoxyribonucleic acid (DNA) sequence of a gene, which usually leads to the production of a nonfunctional enzyme or protein and thus a lack of a normal metabolic function

recessive genetic disease: a disease caused by mutated genes that must be inherited from both parents for that individual to show its symptoms

secretory epithelium: tissues or groups of cells that have the ability to move substances, such as chloride ions, from the inside of cells to a duct or tube

Causes and Symptoms

Genetic diseases are inherited, rather than caused by any specific injury or infectious agent. Thus, unlike many other types of diseases, genetic diseases range throughout a person's lifetime and often begin to exert their debilitating effects prior to birth. Since in many cases the primary defect or underlying cause of the disease is unknown, treatment is difficult or impossible and is usually restricted to treating the symptoms of the disease. Genetic diseases include sickle cell disease; thalassemia; Tay-Sachs disease; some forms of muscular dystrophy, diabetes, and hemophilia; and cystic fibrosis.

In each disease, a specific normal function is missing because of a defect in the individual's genes. Genes are sequences of deoxyribonucleic acid (DNA) contained on the chromosomes of an individual that are passed to the next generation via ova and sperm. Usually, the primary defect in a genetic disease is the inability to produce a normal enzyme, the class of proteins used to speed up, or catalyze, the chemical reactions that are necessary for cells to function. A defective gene, also called a mutation, may not allow the production of a necessary enzyme; therefore, some element of metabolism is missing from an individual with such a mutation. This lack of function leads to the symptoms associated with a genetic disease, such as the lack of insulin production in juvenile diabetes or the inability of the blood to clot in hemophilia. In the 1940's and 1950's, when the understanding of basic cellular metabolism made clear the relationship between genes, enzymes, mutant genes, and lack of enzyme function, the modern definition of genetic disease came into routine medical use.

Cystic fibrosis, one such genetic disease, has several major effects on an individual. These effects begin before birth, extend into early childhood, and become progressively more serious as the affected individual ages. The primary diagnosis for the disease is a very simple test that looks for excessive saltiness in perspiration. Although the higher-than-normal level of salt in the perspiration is, of itself, not life-threatening, the associated symptoms are. Because these other symptoms may vary from one individual to the next, the perspiration test is a very useful early diagnostic tool.

Major symptoms of cystic fibrosis include the blockage of several important internal ducts. This blockage occurs because the cystic fibrosis mutation has a critical effect on the ability of certain internal tissues called secretory epithelia to transport normal amounts of salt and water across their surfaces. These epithelia are often found in the ducts that contribute to the digestive and reproductive systems.

The blockage of ducts resulting from the production and export of overly viscous secretions reduces the delivery of digestive enzymes from the pancreas to the intestine; thus, proteins in the intestine are only partly digested. Fat-emulsifying compounds, called bile salts, are often blocked as well on their route from the pancreas to the intestine, so the digestion of fats is often incomplete. These two conditions often occur prior to birth. Approximately 10 percent of newborns with cystic fibrosis have a puttylike plug of undigested material in their intestines called the meconium ileus. This plug prevents the normal movement of foods through the digestive system and can be very serious.

Because of their overall inefficiency of digestion, young children with cystic fibrosis can seem to be eating quite normally yet remain severely undernourished. They often produce bulky, foul-smelling stools as a result of the high proportion of undigested material. This symptom serves as an indicator of the progress of the disease, as such digestive problems often increase as the affected child ages.

As individuals with cystic fibrosis grow older, their respiratory problems increase because of the secretion of a thick mucus on the inner lining of the lungs. This viscous material traps white blood cells that release their contents when they rupture, which makes the mucus all the more thick and viscous. The affected individuals constantly cough in an attempt to remove this material. Of greater importance is that the mucus forms an ideal breeding ground for many types of pathogenic bacteria, and the affected individual suffers from continual respiratory infections. Male patients are almost always infertile as a result of the blockage of the ducts of the reproductive system, while female fertility is sometimes reduced as well.

Traditional treatments for cystic fibrosis have improved an individual's chance of survival and have dramatically affected the quality of life. In the 1950's, a child afflicted with cystic fibrosis usually lived only a year or two. Thus, cystic fibrosis was originally described as a children's disease and was intensively studied only by pediatricians. Today, aggressive medical intervention has changed survival rates dramatically. Affected individuals are treated by a package of therapies designed to alleviate the most severe symptoms of the disease, and taken together, they had extended the median age of survival of cystic fibrosis patients to thirty-two years by 1999. In fact, since this figure contains many individuals who were born before many of the effective treatments were developed and so did not benefit from them throughout their entire lifetimes, the true average life expectancy may be as high as forty years.

The available treatments, however, do not constitute a cure for the disease. The major roadblock to developing a cure was that the primary genetic defect remained

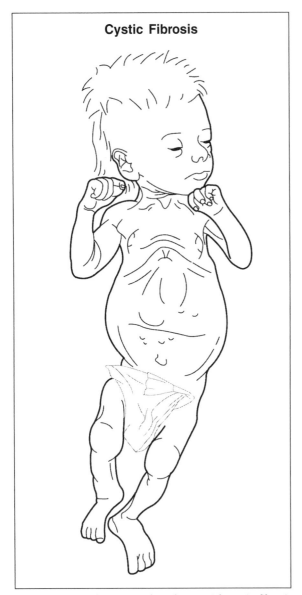

Cystic Fibrosis

Approximately 10 percent of newborns with cystic fibrosis have a puttylike plug of undigested material in their intestines called the meconium ileus, which results in emaciation with a distended abdomen.

INFORMATION ON CYSTIC FIBROSIS

CAUSES: Genetic defect
SYMPTOMS: Severe malnutrition, production of bulky stools, chronic respiratory infections, constant coughing, compromised fertility
DURATION: Chronic and progressive
TREATMENTS: Alleviation of symptoms with dietary supplements, balanced diet, backslapping to break up mucus, antibiotics

unknown. All that was clear until the mid-1980's was that many of the secretory epithelia had a salt and water transport problem. By the late 1980's, the defect was further restricted to a problem in the transport of chloride ions, one of the two constituents of ordinary salt and a critical chemical in many important cellular processes. Because individuals who had severe forms of cystic fibrosis could still live, however, this function was deemed important but not absolutely essential for survival. Furthermore, only certain tissues and organs in the body seemed to show abnormal functions in a cystic fibrosis patient, while other organs—the heart, brain, and nerves—seemed to function normally. Thus, the defect was not uniform.

The pattern of inheritance of cystic fibrosis was relatively easy to determine. The disease acts as a recessive trait. Humans, like most animals, have two copies of each gene: one that is inherited on a chromosome from the egg, and the other on a similar chromosome from the sperm. There is a gene in all humans that controls some normal cellular function related to the transport of chloride from the inside of a cell to the outside. If this function is missing or impaired, the individual shows the symptoms of cystic fibrosis.

A recessive trait is one that must be inherited from both the mother and the father in order to take effect. Inheriting only a single copy of the mutation from one parent does not have a deleterious effect on an individual, who would not demonstrate any of the disease symptoms. Such a person, however, is a carrier of the disease and can still pass that mutation on to his or her own children. Thus, genetic diseases caused by recessive mutations, such as cystic fibrosis, can remain hidden in a family for many generations. When two carriers of the disease procreate, their children at risk. The rules of genetics, as first described by Gregor Mendel in the nineteenth century, predict that in such a union, approximately one in four children will have cystic fi-

brosis. Another one-fourth will be normal, and the remaining half will be carriers of the disease like their parents. Because the production of eggs and sperm involves a random shuffling of genes and chromosomes, however, the occurrence of normal individuals, carriers, and affected individuals cannot be predicted; only average probabilities can be discussed.

TREATMENT AND THERAPY

The treatment of cystic fibrosis typically focuses on preventing or delaying lung damage and optimizing growth and nutrition. Traditional treatments usually include dietary supplements which contain the digestive enzymes and bile salts that cannot pass through the blocked ducts; this is a daily requirement. Individuals with cystic fibrosis are also placed on special balanced diets to ensure proper nutrition despite their difficulties in digesting fats and proteins. One characteristic of cystic fibrosis treatment is the long daily ritual of backslapping, which is designed to help break up the thick mucus in the lungs. Aggressive antibiotic therapy can keep infections of the lungs from forming or spreading. In the 1990's, an additional therapy was begun using a special enzyme which when inhaled can break down DNA in the lung mucus. Many white blood cells rupture while trapped in the thick mucus lining of the lungs, and the release of their DNA adds to the high viscosity of the mucus. Genetically engineered deoxyribonuclease (DNase), an enzyme produced from bacteria, has been found to be helpful in degrading this extra DNA, thus making it easier to break up and cough out the mucus found in the lungs of affected patients.

Another treatment approach for cystic fibrosis focused on determining the nature of the primary genetic defect. The ultimate goal was to determine which of the thousands of human genes was the one that, when defective, led to cystic fibrosis. Once accomplished, the next step would be to determine the normal function of this gene so that therapies designed to replace this function could be developed.

The classic approach to studying any genetic phenomenon involves mapping the gene. First, it must be determined which of a human's twenty-three chromosomes contains the DNA that makes up the gene. By studying the inheritance of the disease, along with other human traits, the gene was located on chromosome number 7. To localize the gene more precisely, however, modern molecular techniques had to be applied. Success came when two independent groups announced that they had identified the location of the gene in 1989. The groups were led by Lap-Chee Tsui of the Hospital for Sick Children in Toronto, Canada, and Francis Collins of the University of Michigan in Ann Arbor. The groups not only located the exact chromosomal location of the gene but also purified the gene from the vast amount of DNA in a human cell so that it could be studied in isolation. Then the structure of the normal form of the gene was compared to the DNA structure found in individuals with the disease.

DNA from more than thirty thousand individuals with cystic fibrosis was analyzed, and to the surprise of most, more than 230 differences between these defective cystic fibrosis genes and normal genes were found. Although about 70 percent of the affected individuals did have a single type of DNA difference or mutation, the other 30 percent had a tremendous variety of differences. Thus, unlike sickle cell disease, which seems to be attributable to the same defect in every affected individual, cystic fibrosis is a widely varying group of differences, which accounts for the range in severity of its symptoms. More important, this enormous diversity of defects makes developing a single, simple DNA-based screening procedure difficult. The only thing that all these individuals had in common was that, in each case, the same gene and gene product were affected.

Tsui's and Collins's groups, as well as several others, tried to determine the normal function of the protein that was coded by the cystic fibrosis gene. This protein was called cystic fibrosis transmembrane-conductance regulator (CFTR) because it was soon shown to create a channel or passage by which cells move chloride ions across their membranes. In an individual afflicted with cystic fibrosis, this channel does not work properly; both the salt and the water balance of the affected cell, and ultimately of the whole tissue, is disturbed. The thick mucus buildup in the lungs is a direct consequence of this disturbance, as is the higher-than-normal salt concentration in the patient's perspiration.

Remarkably, CFTR is an enormous protein that is embedded in the membrane of cells found in the lungs, pancreas, and reproductive tracts. CFTR contains 1,480 amino acids linked end to end. The CFTR found in 70 percent of individuals with cystic fibrosis contains the same amino acids as normal genes, with one exception: The 508th amino acid found in a normal individual is missing. Thus, the extensive debilitating symptoms of this disease result from the mere omission of one amino acid from a long chain containing 1,479 identical ones. The other mutations affect different parts of this protein and, in all cases, reduce the ability of the CFTR protein to carry out its normal function.

In the cases of several other genetic diseases, screening programs have been developed to help patients make informed choices about having children. For Tay-Sachs disease, a fatal neurological disease found in 1 in 3,600 Ashkenazi Jews, a screening program coupled with a strong educational program combined to reduce the incidence of the disease from approximately 100 births a year in the 1970's to an average of 13 by the early 1980's. Similar screening programs have been developed for a rare genetic disease called phenylketonuria (PKU). A screening program for cystic fibrosis, however, would be much more difficult for several reasons.

First, the population at risk for cystic fibrosis is much larger; hence, the costs and scope of the program would be enormous. Second, since there are many different mutations that can affect the gene responsible for causing cystic fibrosis, it may not be easy to develop a simple test which could detect this enormous variation accurately without missing affected individuals or falsely concluding that some normal individuals are affected. Finally, the symptoms shown by individuals affected with cystic fibrosis range from quite severe to nearly normal, thus making it even more difficult to provide definitive genetic counseling. For such counseling to be truly effective, large numbers of individuals from groups known to be at risk for the disease would have to undergo screening and counseling. Furthermore, a prenatal diagnostic test would need to be available to allow couples at risk to ascertain with some degree of certainty whether any particular child is going to be born with the disease. Developing these tests and coupling them with widely available, low-cost counseling remain major challenges to the medical community.

Therapies for cystic fibrosis, like those of any genetic disease, once consisted solely of ways to treat the symptoms. Since every cell in the affected individual lacked a particular metabolic function as a result of the disease, there was no easy way to replace these functions. For cystic fibrosis, this problem was exacerbated by the lack of understanding of the primary defect. The work of Tsui's and Collins's teams allowed a more direct assault on the actual defect. Gene therapy involves either replacing a defective gene with a normal one in affected cells, or adding an additional copy or copies of the normal gene to affected cells, in an attempt to restore the same functional enzymes and thus reestablish a normal metabolic process. In the case of cystic fibrosis, animal studies have shown that it is possible to produce normal lung function when either genes or genetically engineered viruses containing normal genes are sprayed into the lungs of affected animals. Yet since there is no similar direct route for getting engineered viruses or purified genes to the pancreas or reproductive system, because of their location deep within the body, other procedures will need to be developed. In the case of the lung cells, only those cells that actually receive the purified gene change, becoming normal. Since the cells lining the lung are continuously being replenished, lung gene therapy would need to be an ongoing process.

PERSPECTIVE AND PROSPECTS

Patients with the symptoms of cystic fibrosis were first described in medical records dating back to the eighteenth century. The disease was initially called mucoviscidosis and later cystic fibrosis of the pancreas. It was not clear that these symptoms were related to a single specific disease, however, until the work of Dorothy Anderson of Columbia University in the late 1930's. Anderson studied a large number of cases of persons who died with similar lung and pancreas problems. She noticed that siblings were sometimes affected and thus suspected that the disease had a genetic cause. Anderson was responsible for naming the disease on the basis of the fibrous cysts on the pancreas that she often saw in autopsies performed on affected individuals.

In the United States, cystic fibrosis is the most prevalent lethal genetic disease among Caucasians. Estimates vary, but most are in the range of 1 affected child in every 2,000 births. In the early 1990's, there were approximately 25,000 affected Americans and more than 50,000 affected people worldwide. The incidence of cystic fibrosis among Asian American and African American populations is considerably lower, ranging from 1 in 17,000 births for African Americans and less than 1 in 80,000 births for certain Asian American groups. What is particularly striking about this disease is that approximately 1 in 25 Caucasians is a carrier. Such individuals do not show disease symptoms but can have affected children if they procreate with another carrier.

Since this rate is so high, a premium has been placed on the development of inexpensive and accurate diagnostic procedures, which along with good genetic counseling could greatly reduce the incidence of cystic fibrosis in the population. Yet, since carriers are perfectly normal and often do not realize that they are in-

deed carrying the gene, conventional genetic counseling cannot easily reduce the incidence of the mutation in human populations at risk. Only the widespread use of a DNA-based diagnostic procedure could serve to identify the large population of carriers, but even then, since three-fourths of the children of a marriage between two carriers would be normal, counseling would be fraught with severe ethical problems. Why such a deleterious gene remains in such high frequencies in the population remains a mystery.

—*Joseph G. Pelliccia, Ph.D.*

See also Birth defects; Congenital disorders; Coughing; Genetic counseling; Genetic diseases; Lungs; Respiration; Wheezing.

FOR FURTHER INFORMATION:

Cystic Fibrosis Foundation (CFF). http://www.cff.org. Web site gives comprehensive information about the disease, locations of local CFF chapters and care centers, research and clinical trials, and living with the disease.

Harris, Ann, and Anne H. Thompson. *Cystic Fibrosis: The Facts.* 4th ed. New York: Oxford University Press, 2008. An excellent overview of the disease, its symptoms, and its treatment in a readable text.

Kepron, Wayne. *Cystic Fibrosis: Everything You Need to Know.* Buffalo, N.Y.: Firefly Books, 2004. A comprehensive guide that draws on current research to discuss symptoms, diagnosis, complications arising from the disease, treatments (including lung transplants), and the transition to adulthood.

Orenstein, David. *Cystic Fibrosis: A Guide for Patient and Family.* 3d ed. Philadelphia: Lippincott Williams & Wilkins, 2004. An accessible guide that examines a host of issues surrounding the disease including day-to-day concerns, physiological effects, and long-term issues.

Parker, James N., and Philip M. Parker, eds. *The Official Patient's Sourcebook on Cystic Fibrosis.* Rev. ed. San Diego, Calif.: Icon Health, 2002. Draws from public, academic, government, and peer-reviewed research to provide a wide-ranging reference about the causes, treatments, and risk factors of cystic fibrosis.

Pierce, Benjamin A. *The Family Genetic Sourcebook.* New York: John Wiley & Sons, 1990. Contains good background reading on genetics and genetic diseases. Cystic fibrosis is not the main focus of the text, but it is discussed.

Tsui, Lap-Chee. "Cystic Fibrosis, Molecular Genetics." In *The Encyclopedia of Human Biology*, edited by Renato Dulbecco. 2d ed. Vol. 2. New York: Academic Press, 1997. The pursuit of the cystic fibrosis gene is documented, along with some discussion of the function of the CFTR. Readable by someone with a strong high school science background.

U.S. Congress. Office of Technology Assessment. *Cystic Fibrosis and DNA Tests: Implications of Carrier Screening*. Washington, D.C.: Government Printing Office, 1992. An excellent overview of the scientific, ethical, social, economic, and political issues involved with screening for cystic fibrosis or for any genetic disease.

_____. *Genetic Counseling and Cystic Fibrosis Carrier Screening: Results of a Survey-Background Paper*. Washington, D.C.: Government Printing Office, 1992. This government survey looks at issues related to genetic screening for cystic fibrosis.

Yankaskas, James R., and Michael R. Knowles, eds. *Cystic Fibrosis in Adults*. Philadelphia: Lippincott-Raven, 1999. This volume covers the veritable explosion of information about cystic fibrosis in the late twentieth century, ranging from the discovery and characterization of the cystic-fibrosis transmembrane regulator (CFTR) gene and protein, to new therapeutic approaches such as anti-inflammatory, mucolytic, and inhaled antibiotic therapies.

CYSTITIS

DISEASE/DISORDER

ANATOMY OR SYSTEM AFFECTED: Bladder, urinary system

SPECIALTIES AND RELATED FIELDS: Bacteriology, gynecology, urology

DEFINITION: An inflammation of the bladder, primarily caused by bacteria and resulting in pain, a sense of urgency to urinate, and sometimes hematuria (blood in the urine).

KEY TERMS:

cytoscopy: a minor operation performed so that the urologist can examine the bladder

dysuria: painful urination, usually as a result of infection or an obstruction; the patient complains of a burning sensation when voiding

Escherichia coli: bacteria found in the intestines that may cause disease elsewhere

hematuria: the abnormal presence of blood in the urine

perineum: the short bridge of flesh between the anus and vagina in women and the anus and base of the penis in men

ureters: the two tubes that carry urine from the kidneys to the bladder

urethra: the tube carrying urine from the bladder to outside the body

CAUSES AND SYMPTOMS

The term "cystitis" is a combination of two Greek words: *kistis*, meaning hollow pouch, sac, or bladder, and *itis*, meaning inflammation. Cystitis is often used generically to refer to any nonspecific inflammation of the lower urinary tract. Specifically, however, it should be used to refer to inflammation and infection of the bladder. Three true symptoms denote cystitis: dysuria, frequent urination, and hematuria. In a given year, about two million people are afflicted with cystitis; most of them are women. Fifteen percent of those affected will be struck again.

The symptoms of cystitis may appear abruptly and, often, painfully. One of the trademark symptoms signaling an onset is dysuria (burning or stinging during urination). It may precede or coincide with an overwhelming urge to urinate, and very frequently, although the amount passed may be extremely small. In addition, some sufferers may experience nocturia (sleep disturbance because of a need to urinate). In many cases there may be pus in the urine. Origination of hematuria (blood in the urine), which often occurs with cystitis, may be within the bladder wall, in the urethra, or even in the upper urinary tract. These painful symptoms should be enough to spur one to seek medical attention; if left untreated, the bacteria may progress up the ureters to the kidneys, where a much more serious infection, pyelonephritis, may develop. Pyelonephritis can cause scarring of the kidney tissue and even life-threatening kidney failure. Usually kidney infections are accompanied by chills, high fever, nausea and/or vomiting, and back pain that may radiate downward.

Acute cystitis can be divided into two groups. One is when infection occurs with irregularity and with no recent history of antibiotic treatments. This type is commonly caused by the bacteria *Escherichia coli*. Types of bacteria other than *E. coli* that can cause cystitis are *Proteus, Klebsiella, Pseudomonas, Streptococcus, Enterobacter*, and, rarely, *Staphylococcus*. The second group of sufferers have undergone antibiotic treatment; those bacteria not affected by the antibiotics can cause infection. Most urinary tract infections are precipitated by the patient's own rectal flora. Once bacteria enter the bladder, whether they will cause infection depends on how many bacteria invade the bladder, how well

INFORMATION ON CYSTITIS

CAUSES: Bacterial infection
SYMPTOMS: Pain and burning upon urination, sense of urgency to urinate, sometimes blood in urine
DURATION: Acute
TREATMENTS: Antibiotics

the bacteria can adhere to the bladder wall, and how strongly the bladder can defend itself. The bladder's inherent defense system is the most important of the factors.

One of the natural defense mechanisms employed by the bladder is the flushing provided by regular urination at frequent intervals. If fluid intake is sufficient—most urologists consider this amount to be eight 8-ounce glasses daily—there will be regular and efficient emptying of the bladder, which can wash away the bacteria that have entered. This large volume of fluid also helps dilute the urine, thereby decreasing bacterial concentration. Another defense mechanism is the low pH of the bladder, which also helps control bacterial multiplication. It may be, too, that the bladder lining employs some means to repel bacteria and to inhibit their adherence to the wall. Others theorize that genetic, hormonal, and immune factors may help determine the defensive capability of the bladder.

Many women experience their first episode of cystitis as they become sexually active. So-called honeymoon cystitis, that related to sexual activity, comes about because intercourse may massage bacteria into the bladder, as can repeated thrusts of the penis, penetration of the vagina by fingers or other objects, or manual stimulation of the clitoris. Bacteria are boosted into and forced upward through the urethra. Also, a change in position—from back to front but not from front to back—may precede an attack of cystitis. When intercourse from the rear occurs, the penis may be contaminated with bacteria from the anal region, which then are transferred to the urethra. From the urethra, it is a short trip to the bladder for the bacteria. Unless they are voided upon conclusion of intercourse, they may multiply, causing inflammation and infection. Sex late in the day may be particularly hazardous if the perineal area has not been thoroughly cleansed after a bowel movement. Bathing after intercourse is too late to prevent the *E. coli* from being pushed into the urethral opening. Some instances of cystitis may be reduced if there is ad-

equate vaginal lubrication prior to intercourse and vaginal sprays and douches are avoided.

Women who use a diaphragm as birth control are more than twice as likely to develop urinary tract infections than other sexually active women. The reason for this increased likelihood may be linked to the more alkaline vaginal environment in diaphragm users, or perhaps to the spring in the rim of the diaphragm that exerts pressure on the tissue around the urethra. Urine flow may be restricted, and the stagnant urine is a good harbor for bacterial growth.

When urine remains in the bladder for an extended period of time, its stagnation may allow for the rapid growth of bacteria, thereby leading to cystitis. Besides the use of a diaphragm, urine flow may be restricted by an enlarged prostate or pregnancy. Diabetes mellitus may also lead to cystitis, as the body's resistance to infection is lowered. Infrequent voiding for whatever reason is associated with a greater likelihood of cystitis.

Less frequently, cases have been linked to vaginitis as a result of *Monilia* or *Trichomonas*. Yeasts such as these change the pH of the vaginal fluid, which will allow and even encourage bacterial growth in the perineal region. Sometimes, it is an endless cycle: A patient takes antibiotics for cystitis, which kills her protective bacteria and allows the overgrowth of yeasts. The yeasts cause vaginitis, which may promote another case of cystitis, and the cycle continues. In fact, recurrent cystitis may be a result of an inappropriate course of antibiotic treatment; the antibiotic is not specific to the bacteria. More rarely, recurrent cases may be a result of constant seeding by the kidneys or a bowel fistula. The most common cause of recurrent cystitis, however, is new organisms from the rectal area that invade the perineal area. This new pool may be inadvertently changed by antibiotic treatment.

A less common but often more severe kind of cystitis is interstitial cystitis, an inflammation of the bladder caused by nonbacterial causes, such as an autoimmune or allergic response. With this type of cystitis, there may be inflammation and/or ulceration of the bladder, which may result in scarring. These problems usually cause frequent and painful urination and possible hematuria. What separates interstitial cystitis from acute cystitis is that it primarily strikes women in their early to mid-forties and that, while urine output is normal, soon after urination, the urge to void again is overwhelming. Delaying urination may cause a pink tinge to appear in the urine. This minimal bleeding is most often a result of an overly small bladder being stretched so that minute tears in the bladder wall bleed into the urine. This form is often hard to diagnose, as the symptoms may be mild or severe and may appear and disappear or be constant.

TREATMENT AND THERAPY

Medical students are typically underprepared to deal with the numerous cases of cystitis. The student is told to test urine for the presence of bacteria, prescribe a ten-day course of antibiotics, sometimes take a kidney X ray and/or perform a cytoscopy, and then perhaps prescribe more antibiotics. If the patient continues to complain, perhaps a painful dilation of the urethra or cauterizing (burning away) of the inflamed skin is performed. None of these procedures guarantees a cure.

Diagnosis of cystitis should be relatively easy; however, in a number of cases it is misdiagnosed because the doctor has failed to identify the type of bacteria, the patient's history of past cases, and possible links between cystitis and life factors (sexual activity, contraceptive method, and diet, for example). A more appropriate antibiotic given at this point might lower the risks of frequent recurrences. Diagnosis of urinary tract infection takes into account the medical history, a physical examination of the patient, and performance of special tests. The history begins with the immediate complaints of the patient and is completed with a look back at the same type of infections that the patient has

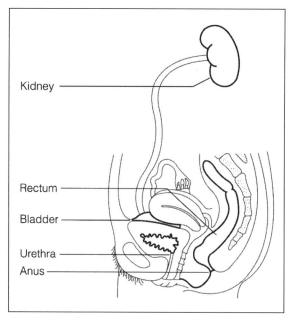

Cystitis, an inflammation of the bladder, may progress to the kidneys if left untreated.

had from childhood to the present. The physician should conduct urinalysis but be cognizant that, if the urine is not examined at the right time, the bacteria may not have survived and thus a false-negative reading may occur.

One special test, a cytoscopy, is used to diagnose some of the special characteristics of cystitis. These include redness of the bladder cells, enlarged capillaries with numerous small hemorrhages, and in cases of severe cystitis, swelling of bladder tissues. Swelling may be so pronounced that it partially blocks the urethral opening, making incomplete emptying of the bladder likely to occur. Pus pockets may be visible.

In a woman who first experiences cystitis when she becomes sexually active, the doctor usually instructs the patient to be alert to several details. She should wash or shower before intercourse and be warned that contraceptive method and position during intercourse may increase her chances of becoming infected. To decrease the chance of introducing the contamination of bowel flora to the urethra, wiping after urination and defecation from front to back is advised.

Children are not immune to attacks of cystitis; in fact, education at an early age may aid children in lowering their chances of developing cystitis. Some of the following may be culprits in causing cystitis and maintaining a hospitable environment for bacteria to grow: soap or detergent that is too strong, too much fruit juice, overuse of creams and ointments, any noncotton underwear, shampoo in the bath water, bubble bath, chlorine from swimming pools, and too little fluid intake. Once children reach the teenage years, many of the above remain causes. Added to them are failure to change underwear daily, irregular periods, use of tampons, and the use of toiletries and deodorants. Careful monitoring of these conditions can greatly reduce the risk of recurrent infections.

The symptoms of cystitis are often urgent and painful enough to alert a sufferer to visit a physician as quickly as possible. Such a visit not only makes the patient feel better but also decreases the chances that the bacteria will travel toward and even into the kidney, causing pyelonephritis. Antibiotic therapy is the typical mode of treating acute or bacterial cystitis. The antibiotics chosen should reach a high concentration in the urine, should not cause the proliferation of drug-resistant bacteria, and should not kill helpful bacteria. Some antibiotics used to treat first-time sufferers of cystitis with a high success rate (80 to 100 percent) are TMP-SMX, sulfisoxazole, amoxycillin, and ampicillin. Typically, a three-day course of therapy not only will see the patient through the few days of symptoms but also will not change bowel flora significantly. When *E. coli* cause acute cystitis, there is a greater than 80 percent chance that one dose of an antibiotic such as penicillin will effectively end the bout, and again, the bowel flora will not be upset. Such antibiotics, when chosen carefully by the physician to match the bacteria, are useful in treating cystitis because they act very quickly to kill the bacteria. Sometimes, enough bacteria can be killed in one hour that the symptoms begin to abate immediately.

Yet antibiotics are not without their drawbacks: They may cause nausea, loss of appetite, dizziness, diarrhea, and fatigue and may increase the likelihood of yeast infections. The most common problem is the one posed by antibiotics that destroy all bacteria of the body. When the body's normal bacteria are gone, yeasts may proliferate in the body's warm, moist places. In one of the areas, the vagina, vaginitis causes a discharge which can seep into the urethra. The symptoms of cystitis may begin all over again.

For those suffering from recurrent cystitis, the treatment usually is a seven- to ten-day course of antibiotic treatment that will clear the urine of pus, indicating that the condition should be cured. If another bout recurs fairly soon, it is probably an indication that treatment was ended too quickly, as the infective bacteria were still present. To ensure that treatment has been effective, the urine must be checked and declared sterile.

Because cystitis is so common, and because many are frustrated by the inadequacies of treatment, self-treatment has become very popular. Self-treatment does not cure the infection but certainly makes the patient more comfortable while the doctor cultures a urine specimen, determines the type of bacteria causing the infection, and prescribes the appropriate antibiotic. Monitoring the first signs that a cystitis attack is imminent can save a victim from days of intense pain.

Those advocating home treatment do not all agree, however, on the means and methods that reduce suffering. All agree that once those first sensations are felt, the sufferer should start to drink water or water-based liquids; there is some disagreement on whether this intake should include fruit juice, especially cranberry juice. Some believe that the high acidic content of the juice may act to kill some of the bacteria, while others believe that the acid will only decrease the pH of the urine, causing more intense burnings as the acidic urine passes through the inflamed urethra. Through an in-

creased fluid intake, more copious amounts of urine are produced. The excess urine acts to leach the bacteria from the bladder and, by diluting the urine, decreases its normal acidity. More dilute urine will relieve much of the burning discomfort during voiding. If a small amount of sodium bicarbonate is added to the water, it will aid in alkalinizing the urine. The best self-treatment is to drink one cup of water every twenty minutes for three hours; after this period, the amount can be decreased. A teaspoonful of bicarbonate every hour for three or four hours is safe (unless the person suffers from blood pressure problems or a heart condition). Additionally, the patient may wish to take a painkiller, such as acetaminophen. If lifestyle permits, resting will enhance the cure, especially if a heating pad is used to soothe the back or stomach. After the frequent visits to the toilet, cleaning the perineal area carefully can reduce continued contamination.

Diagnosis of interstitial cystitis can be made only using a cytoscope. Since the cause is not bacterial, antibiotics are not effective in treating this type of cystitis. To enhance the healing process of an inflamed or ulcerated bladder as a result of interstitial cystitis, the bladder may be distended and the ulcers cauterized; both procedures are done under anesthesia. Corticosteroids may be prescribed to help control the inflammation.

PERSPECTIVE AND PROSPECTS

Writings throughout history indicate that people have always suffered from bladder problems, including cystitis, although the prevalence probably was not as high. The first urologists likely were the Hindus of the Vedic era, about 1500 B.C.E. They were considered experts in removing bladder stones and relieving obstructions of the urinary tract.

The recorded incidence of cystitis was possibly lower because the topic would have been taboo; women in particular would not have mentioned the problem. Couples of generations past would not have participated in intercourse as frequently; both sexes wore so many clothes and had so many children underfoot or servants around that daytime sexual activity would have been rare. Without contraception, intercourse was often for procreation; once there were several children, the couple might choose to inhabit separate bedrooms. Life spans were clearly shorter; women frequently died in childbirth. Thus, the primary causes of cystitis were not common until the twentieth century.

Those forebears did not have antibiotics, but apparently those who suffered from cystitis recovered. The treatment they did use, though, has some merit. They drank copious amounts of herb teas—chamomile, mint, and parsley. They probably added some belladonna for pain relief. All this fluid would have served to help quench the "fire." It would also have had the benefit of helping flush the bacteria from the bladder.

Infection in males is far less frequent than in females; in fact, cystitis occurs ten times more often in females than in males, and it affects about 30 percent of women at some time in their lives. Unfortunately, most urologists are better-versed in male problems. Female specialists, gynecologists, treat the reproductive system but may not have studied female urinary dysfunction. If a male suffers from urinary dysfunction, he should seek the services of a urologist. A woman who has interstitial cystitis should also see a urologist, specifically one who knows about this form of cystitis. If a female is experiencing recurrent cystitis, she is probably already seeing a gynecologist or an internist; however, if she is not getting relief, she should avail herself of a urologist, especially one specializing in female urology, if possible.

A strong social stigma is associated with bladder dysfunction, which may create an obstacle when treatment is necessary. From the time of infancy, some children are taught that anything to do with bladder or bowel function is shameful or dirty. Therefore, when dysfunction occurs, self-esteem may be decreased. As a result, the sufferer may fail to ask for help. Such a reaction must be overcome if there is to be significant progress in treating and conquering cystitis.

—*Iona C. Baldridge*

See also Antibiotics; Bacterial infections; Hematuria; Kidneys; Urethritis; Urinalysis; Urinary disorders; Urinary system; Urology; Urology, pediatric; Women's health.

FOR FURTHER INFORMATION:

Chalker, Rebecca, and Kristene E. Whitmore. *Overcoming Bladder Disorders.* New York: HarperCollins, 1990. This book was written to inform the general public about bladder disorders. It is meant to aid in diagnosis and in the selection of the right physician. Diagrams and a glossary help make this work easy to read.

Cohen, Barbara J. *Memmler's The Human Body in Health and Disease.* 11th ed. Philadelphia: Wolters Kluwer Health/Lippincott Williams & Wilkins, 2009. This textbook offers a clear presentation of how human systems maintain homeostasis through their interactions. Integral to the discussion of each system is a detailed list of the conditions that produce disease.

Gillespie, Larrian, with Sandra Blakeslee. *You Don't Have to Live with Cystitis.* Rev. ed. New York: Quill, 2002. A popular work on cystitis and women's health.

Parker, James N., and Philip M. Parker, eds. *The Official Patient's Sourcebook on Urinary Tract Infection.* San Diego, Calif.: Icon Health, 2002. Draws from public, academic, government, and peer-reviewed research to provide a wide-ranging handbook for patients with recurring urinary tract infections.

Schrier, Robert W., ed. *Diseases of the Kidney and Urinary Tract.* 8th ed. Philadelphia: Wolters Kluwer Health/Lippincott Williams & Wilkins, 2007. Covers the full range of the biochemical, structural, and functional correlations in the kidney, as well as hereditary diseases, urological diseases and neoplasms of the genitourinary tract, acute renal failure, nutrition, and drugs, among many additional topics.

CYSTOSCOPY

PROCEDURE

ANATOMY OR SYSTEM AFFECTED: Bladder, reproductive system, urinary system

SPECIALTIES AND RELATED FIELDS: Gynecology, oncology, urology

DEFINITION: An endoscopic procedure that utilizes a water or carbon dioxide distension system to visualize the urethra and bladder.

INDICATIONS AND PROCEDURES

Cystoscopy is indicated in patients for whom visual inspection of the urethra, bladder mucosa, and ureteral orifices is likely to yield a diagnosis. This includes patients who have hematuria (blood in the urine), incontinence, and irritative bladder symptoms for whom all obvious causes have been ruled out. In addition, patients who have undergone difficult abdominal or pelvic surgery may receive cystoscopy to verify that the bladder and the ureters, the tubes that carry urine from the kidneys to the bladder, are intact.

Cystoscopy is performed with the patient in a supine position with legs in stirrups. The cystoscope consists of a small metal tube, through which distension medium is passed. The light source, which enables visualization, also passes through this tube. The cystoscope can be attached to a video screen, or the clinician can visualize the urethral and bladder mucosas directly through the cystoscope. The cystoscope may be angled at 0 degrees, 30 degrees, or 70 degrees to facilitate visualization of different parts of the bladder. The procedure involves passing the cystoscope into the urethra and then the bladder under direct visualization. Cystoscopy is performed in a systematic fashion to ensure complete coverage of the urethral and bladder mucosas. Abnormal areas can be biopsied. The ureteral orifices can be visualized using the cystoscope, and the presence of urine flow from the orifices confirms patency (lack of obstruction) of the ureters.

Uses and Complications

Cystoscopy can be used to diagnose a variety of benign and malignant conditions of the lower urinary tract. Among the benign conditions commonly found through cystoscopy are endometriosis of the bladder, interstitial cystitis, foreign bodies, and anatomic abnormalities such as fistulas (communicating tracts between the bladder and another organ such as the bowels) or diverticula (small outpouchings of the bladder or urethra). By filling the bladder with distension fluid during cystoscopy, it is also possible to perform limited bladder function tests. Malignant conditions that may be found on cystoscopy include bladder cancers and cancers of adjacent pelvic organs, such as the cervix, which may invade the bladder.

Cystoscopy is an extremely safe procedure. Theoretical risks include the possibility of bladder injury or perforation from the cystoscope.

—*Anne Lynn S. Chang, M.D.*

See also Bladder cancer; Bladder removal; Cervical, ovarian, and uterine cancers; Cystitis; Diverticulitis and diverticulosis; Endometriosis; Endoscopy; Fistula repair; Hematuria; Incontinence; Invasive tests; Urethritis; Urinalysis; Urinary disorders; Urinary system; Urology; Urology, pediatric.

For Further Information:

Doherty, Gerard M., and Lawrence W. Way, eds. *Current Surgical Diagnosis and Treatment.* 12th ed. New York: Lange Medical Books/McGraw-Hill, 2006.

Miller, Brigitte E. *An Atlas of Sigmoidoscopy and Cystoscopy.* Boca Raton, Fla.: Parthenon, 2002.

Rock, John A., and Howard W. Jones III, eds. *Te Linde's Operative Gynecology.* 10th ed. Philadelphia: Wolters Kluwer/Lippincott Williams & Wilkins, 2008.

Stenchever, Morton A., et al. *Comprehensive Gynecology.* 5th ed. St. Louis, Mo.: Mosby/Elsevier, 2007.

Cysts

Disease/disorder

Anatomy or system affected: All

Specialties and related fields: All

Definition: A walled-off sac that is not normally found in the tissue where it occurs. To be a true cyst, a lump must have a capsule around it. Cysts usually contain a liquid or semisolid core (center) and vary in size from microscopic to very large. They may occur in any tissue of the body in a person of any age.

Key terms:

asymptomatic: not causing any symptoms

benign: not malignant; noncancerous

capsule: the wall that encloses a cyst

computed tomography (CT) scan: a technique that generates detailed pictures from a series of X rays

genetic: inherited

magnetic resonance imaging (MRI): a radiologic technique that uses radio signals and magnets and a computer to produce highly detailed images of tissues

malignant: cancerous; able to spread into and destroy nearby tissues and to spread to distant areas

renal: pertaining to the kidney

sebaceous: pertaining to glands in the skin that secrete an oily substance called sebum

ultrasonography: the use of sound waves to create an image of the soft tissues of the body

Causes and Symptoms

Cysts can be caused by a many different processes, including infections, defects in the development of an embryo during pregnancy, various obstructions to the flow of body fluids, tumors, a number of different inflammatory conditions, and genetic diseases.

Cysts may have no symptoms at all, or they may be quite noticeable, depending on their size and location. For example, a person with a cyst in the skin or breast will most likely be able to feel the lump. On the other hand, a cyst on an internal organ may not produce any symptoms unless it becomes so large that it keeps the organ from functioning properly or presses on another organ. Many times, internal cysts are discovered by chance on an X ray, computed tomography (CT) scan, magnetic resonance imaging (MRI) scan, or ultrasound for an unrelated condition.

It is impossible to list all the different types of cysts that might form in the body, but they are usually benign. Only very rarely are cysts associated with cancer or with serious infection. Some of the common types of cysts include sebaceous cysts, which are found in the oil-secreting glands of the skin. They may become quite large and contain a foul-smelling, cheesy substance within the capsule. Breast cysts are filled with fluid and may enlarge and recede with the changing hormones of the menstrual cycle. Just before menses, breast cysts may be quite tender. Ganglion cysts occur over joints and on the tendons of the body. A chalazion, or cyst in the eyelid, is usually not painful but can be quite irritating.

Some cyst development is part of a particular disease or disorder. For example, cysts form on the ovaries in a disorder called polycystic ovary syndrome. There are also a number of different renal diseases that involve the development of cysts on the kidney.

TREATMENT AND THERAPY

The treatment for cysts depends on their size and location and whether they are causing symptoms. A small, asymptomatic cyst is often simply monitored.

When surgery is performed to remove a cyst, it is usually "shelled out" so that the entire capsule and its contents are removed. (If the capsule is left intact, then it might simply fill up again.) Depending on the location of the cyst, this may be performed in an office using local anesthesia or in the operating room of a hospital. When cancer is a possibility, the cell wall and any fluids are evaluated microscopically to determine whether any malignant cells are present.

Aspiration is another technique for treating cysts. A needle is inserted into the middle of the cyst, and any fluid is removed (aspirated) through the needle. If the cyst is deep within the body, then the aspiration may be guided by ultrasound or another radiologic technique. Aspiration may make the cyst disappear, or it may fill up again.

Some cysts are treated by incision and drainage. An opening is made in the cyst, and all the material in the core is removed. The cyst is then packed with gauze to ensure that the surgical incision does not close and allow the cyst to fill up again. The gauze is replaced periodically until healing takes place.

Ganglion cysts on tendons or joints may be successfully treated by injection with a steroid. If the cyst is part of another medical condition such as polycstic ovary syndrome, then any treatment is usually aimed at the medical condition rather than the cyst itself.

—*Rebecca Lovell Scott, Ph.D., PA-C*

See also Abscess removal; Abscesses; Acne; Bone disorders; Bones and the skeleton; Breast disorders; Breasts, female; Cyst removal; Fibrocystic breast condition; Ganglion removal; Hydroceles; Kidney disorders; Kidneys; Ovarian cysts; Ovaries; Plastic surgery; Reproductive system; Skin; Skin disorders; Tendon disorders.

FOR FURTHER INFORMATION:

American Medical Association. *American Medical Association Family Medical Guide.* 4th rev. ed. Hoboken, N.J.: John Wiley & Sons, 2004.

Komaroff, Anthony, ed. *Harvard Medical School Family Health Guide.* New York: Free Press, 2005.

Stoppard, Miriam. *Family Health Guide.* London: DK, 2006.

CYTOLOGY

SPECIALTY

ANATOMY OR SYSTEM AFFECTED: Cells, immune system

SPECIALTIES AND RELATED FIELDS: Bacteriology, hematology, histology, immunology, oncology, pathology, serology

DEFINITION: The study of the appearance of cells, usually with the aid of a microscope, to diagnose diseases.

KEY TERMS:

cell: a tiny baglike structure within which the basic functions of the body are carried out

chromosomes: rodlike cell parts made up of the genes that are the blueprints for every feature of the body; located in the nucleus of almost all cells

electron: a tiny particle with an electronic charge; a component of an atom

enzyme: a protein that is able to speed up a particular chemical reaction in the body

membranes: sheetlike structures that enclose each cell and separate the various organelles from one another *nucleus:* the "control center" of plant and animal cells; a large spherical mass occupying up to one-third of the volume of a typical cell

organelles: specialized parts of cells

pathologist: a physician who is specially trained to use cytology and related methods to diagnose disease

protein: an abundant kind of molecule found in cells; proteins have many functions, from acting as enzymes to forming mechanical structures such as tendons and hair

SCIENCE AND PROFESSION

Cytology is the study of the appearance of cells, the fundamental units that make up all living organisms. Cells are complex structures constructed from many different subcomponents that must work together in a precisely regulated fashion. Each cell must also cooperate with neighboring cells within the organism. A cell is like a complex automobile: Many separate components must be synchronized, and the cell (or car) must follow a strict order of function to coordinate successfully with its neighbors. Because illness results from the malfunction of cells, physicians must be able to measure key cell functions accurately. The normal and abnormal function of cells can be evaluated in many different ways; cytology is the study of cells using microscopes. A sophisticated collection of cytological techniques is available to pathologists; with these a precise diagnosis of cellular malfunction is possible.

All cells share several basic features. They are surrounded by a membrane, a flexible, sheetlike structure which encloses the fluid contents of the cell but allows required materials to move into the cell and waste products to move out of it. The complex salty fluid contained by the membrane is the cytoplasm; the other subcomponents of the cell, called organelles, are suspended in this substance. Each cell contains a set of genes, located on chromosomes, which function as blueprints for all other structures of the cell; the genes are inherited from one's parents. In plant and animal cells, the chromosomes are contained in a prominent organelle called the nucleus, which is surrounded by its own membrane inside the cell. Cells must also have a collection of enzymes used to convert food into energy to power the cell. In the cells of animals and plants, these enzymes are packaged into organelles called mitochondria. Membranes, the nucleus, and the mitochondria are the most prominent parts of a cell that are visible with a microscope, but cells also contain a variety of other specialized parts that are required for them to function properly. In addition, cells can also export (secrete) a variety of materials. For example, secreted materials make up bone, cartilage, tendons, mucus, sweat, and saliva.

Despite these basic features, the different types of cells have very distinct appearances. The cells of bacteria, plants, and animals are easily distinguishable from one another using a microscope. Bacterial cells are simplified, lacking organized nuclei and mitochondria. Different kinds of bacteria can be precisely distinguished; for example, strep throat is caused by spherical bacteria that form chains, like beads of a necklace. Some dangerous bacteria can be colored with dyes that do not stain harmless bacteria. Because so many human diseases are caused by bacteria, highly accurate procedures have been developed for their identification.

The adult human body is made up of several trillion individual cells. Although much larger than bacteria, all of these are far too small to be seen with the naked eye (typically about 20 microns in diameter). Each organ of the body—the brain, liver, kidney, skin, and so on—is made up of several kinds of cells, specialized for particular functions. They must cooperate closely: Mistakes in the activities of any of these many cells can cause disease. A pathologist is able to recognize small changes in the appearance of each of many different cell types.

A few of the characteristic cell types in the human body include nerve, muscle, secretory, and epithelial cells. Nerve cells are designed to pass information throughout the nervous system. The nerve cells function much like electrical wires, so they have slender wirelike extensions that can be several feet long. Defects in the wiring circuits, for example in patients with Alzheimer's disease, can be readily detected. Muscle cells are easily identified because they are elongated cylinders packed with special fibers that cause muscular contraction. Secretory cells produce and release such substances as digestive enzymes. Such cells are often filled with membrane-bound packets of their specialized product, ready to be released from the cell. The skin and the surfaces of various internal organs are encased in a cell type called epithelium. Epithelial cells are tilelike and are often fastened tightly to neighboring epithelial cells by special kinds of connectors. Numerous other specialized cell types are found in the body as well, but these four types represent the most common cell designs.

Cells are sophisticated and delicate structures that carry out specific functions efficiently. The structure and function of normal cells are stable and predictable. If significant numbers of cells are somehow damaged, disease is the result. Such defective cells change in their appearance in characteristic ways. Therefore, cytology is an important element in the diagnosis of many diseases and for monitoring the cellular response to therapy.

Many different types of stress can cause cell damage. One of the most common stresses is oxygen deprivation, known as hypoxia. Even a brief interruption of oxygen can cause irreversible damage to cells because it is needed for energy production. Since oxygen is transported in the blood, the most common cause of hypoxia is loss of blood supply, which can occur with blockage by blood clots or narrowed blood vessels and with several kinds of lung or heart problems. Carbon monoxide poisoning results from interference with the blood's ability to absorb and carry oxygen, while the poison cyanide interferes with a cell's ability to make use of oxygen.

Poisons such as cyanide can damage cells in many other ways, as can drugs. Prolonged use of barbiturates or alcohol can damage liver cells. These cells are also sensitive to common chemicals such as carbon tetrachloride, once used widely as a household cleaning agent. The liver is where foreign chemicals are changed to harmless forms, which explains why the liver cells are often damaged. Even useful chemicals, however, can cause harm to cells in some circumstances. Constant high levels of glucose, a sugar used by all cells, may overwork certain cells of the pancreas to the point where they become defective. Some foods (especially fats) and certain food additives, if they are eaten in excess, can interfere with how cells work.

Physical damage to cells—caused, for example, by blows to the body—can dislocate parts of cells, preventing their proper coordination. Extreme cold can interfere with the blood supply, causing hypoxia; extreme heat can cause cells to speed up their rate of metabolism, again exceeding the oxygen-carrying capacity of the circulatory system. The "bends," the affliction suffered by surfacing deep-sea divers, results from tiny bubbles of nitrogen that block capillaries. Various kinds of radiant energy, such as radioactivity or ultraviolet light, can damage specific chemicals of cells, causing them to malfunction. Electrical energy generates extreme local heat within the body, which can damage cells directly.

Many small living organisms can interfere with cellular function as well. Viruses are effective parasites of cells, using cells for their own survival. This relationship can result in cell death, as in poliomyelitis; in depressed cell function, as in viral hepatitis; or in abnormal cell growth, as in some cancers. Bacteria can also live as parasites, releasing toxins that interfere with cellular function in a variety of ways. Malaria is caused by a single-celled animal that damages blood cells, athlete's foot is caused by a fungus, and tiny worms called nematodes can invade cells and cause them to work improperly.

All cell types are not equally sensitive to damage by each agent. Liver cells are particularly sensitive to damage by toxic chemicals. Nerve and muscle cells are the first to be injured by hypoxia. Kidney cells are also easily damaged by loss of blood supply. Lung cells are affected by anything that is inhaled.

DIAGNOSTIC AND TREATMENT TECHNIQUES

Before cells can be successfully observed, they must be prepared through several steps. First, it is necessary to select a relatively small sample of a particular organ for closer scrutiny. Such a sample is called a biopsy when it is collected by a physician who wishes to test for a disease. The biopsy must then be preserved, or fixed, so that its parts will not deteriorate. Next, the specimen must be encased within a solid substance so that it can be handled without damage. Most often, the fixed specimen is soaked in melted paraffin, which then is allowed to solidify in a mold. For some kinds of microscopes, harder plastic materials are used. Next, the specimen must be thinly sliced so that the internal details can be seen. The delicate slices are mounted on a support, typically a thin glass slide for light microscopy. Finally, the parts of the cell must be colored, or stained. Without this coloring, the cell parts would be transparent and thus unobservable.

The basic tool of the cytologist is the light microscope. It can magnify up to about seven hundred times. Numerous sophisticated methods are used with light microscopy. Specific stains have been developed for distinguishing the different molecules that make up cells. For example, Alcian blue is a dye that stains a type of complex sugar that accumulates outside certain abnormal cells, making it easier to identify these cells. Also, specially prepared antibodies can recognize particular proteins within cells. Disease-causing proteins, including the proteins of dangerous viruses and bacteria, can be precisely identified in this way.

A major advance in cytology is the electron microscope. It forms images in essentially the same way as a light microscope does, but using electrons rather than visible light. Because of the properties of electrons, this type of microscope can magnify tens of thousands of times beyond life size. A wide range of new cell features has been revealed with the electron microscope. The details of how genes work, how materials enter and leave cells, how energy is produced, and how molecules are synthesized have been made clearer. The steps for preparing specimens for electron microscopy are delicate, time-consuming, and demanding. Furthermore, the electron microscope itself is complex and expensive. Considerable skill is required to use it effectively. For these reasons, electron microscopy is not commonly used for routine medical diagnoses.

Cell injury causes predictable changes in cells that can be interpreted by a pathologist to suggest the underlying cause of the damage and how best to treat it. Almost all forms of reversible injury cause changes in the size and shape of cells. Cellular swelling is an obvious symptom that almost always reflects a serious underlying problem. Such cells also have a characteristic cloudy appearance. Swelling and cloudiness indicate loss of energy reserves and abnormal uptake of water into the cell through improperly functioning cell-surface membranes. An indication of serious damage is the accumulation within the cell of vacuoles—small, fluid-filled sacs that have a characteristic clear appearance when viewed through a microscope. More severe

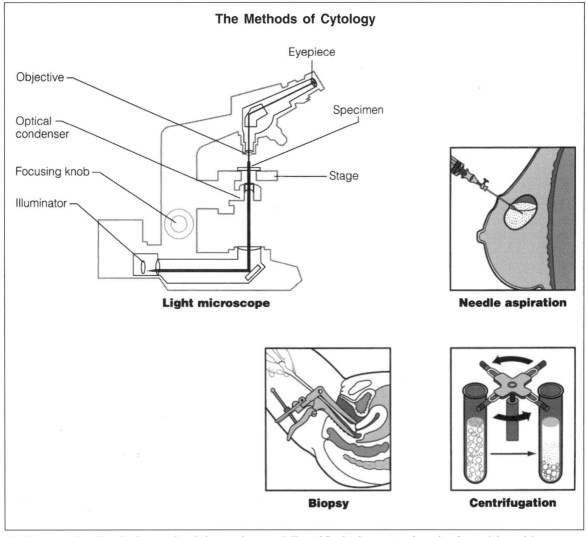

Cytologists study cells in both normal and abnormal states. Cells and fluid to be examined may be obtained through biopsy, separated by centrifugation, and studied under a light microscope.

injury can cause the formation of vacuoles that contain fat, giving the cells a foamy appearance. Such damage is most often seen in cells of the heart, kidneys, and lungs. These changes appear to reflect both membrane abnormalities and the defective metabolism of fats.

Cells that are damaged beyond the point of repair will die, a process called necrosis. The two key processes in necrosis are the breakdown and mopping up of cellular contents, and large changes in structure of cellular proteins in ways that can be identified using a microscope. The most conspicuous and reliable indicators of necrosis are changes in the appearance of the nucleus, which can shrink or even break into pieces and which eventually disappears completely. Ultimately, the entire cell disappears.

Cancer provides a good illustration of how cytology is employed in the diagnosis of a specific disease. A skilled cytologist can detect cells at an early stage of cancer development and, with accuracy, can gauge how dangerous a cancer cell is or is likely to become. Cancer is a disease of abnormal growth. Cancer cells may have few abnormal features other than their improper growth; tumors made up of such cells are generally not dangerous and so are labeled benign. Malignant tumor cells, on the other hand, are highly abnormal. They can damage and invade other parts of the body, making these cells much more dangerous.

The cells of benign tumors may have nearly the same appearance as the cells of the normal tissue from which they arose. Benign cancers of skin, bone, muscle, and nerve keep the obvious structures that allow these highly specialized cell types to carry out their normal functions. Ironically, however, continued normal function can itself become a problem, because there are too many cells producing specialized products. For example, tumors in tissues that produce hormones can result in massive excesses of such hormones, causing severe imbalances in the function of the body's organs. Malignant tumor cells, on the other hand, have lost some or all of the functional and cytological features of their parent normal cells. They have a simpler and more primitive appearance, termed anaplasia by pathologists. The degree of anaplasia is one of the most reliable hallmarks of how malignant a cell has become.

Almost any part of the cell can become anaplastic. A common change is in the chromosomes of a cancer cell. The number, size, and shape of chromosomes change, and detailed analysis of these changes is often important in diagnosis, as in leukemia. Many malignant tu-

mor cells secrete enzymes that attack surrounding connective tissue, changing its appearance in characteristic ways. Membrane systems of anaplastic cells are also abnormal, with serious consequences. The movement of materials in and out of cells becomes defective, and energy production mechanisms are upset, causing the characteristic changes in appearance described above. A general feature of tumors made up of anaplastic cells is the variability among individual cells. Some cells can appear virtually normal, while other tumor cells nearby can appear highly abnormal in several ways.

The cells of benign tumors remain where they arose. The cells of malignant tumors, however, have the ability to spread through the body (metastasize), penetrating and damaging other organs in the process. These abilities, to invade and metastasize, have serious effects on the rest of the body. Invading cells often can be identified easily with a microscope. Extensions of the tumor cells may reach into surrounding normal organ parts. Tumor cells can be observed penetrating into blood and lymph vessels and other body cavities, such as the abdominal cavity and air pockets in the lung. Small clusters of tumor cells can be found in blood and identified in distant organs. These cells can begin the process of invasion all over again, producing so-called secondary tumors in other organs. How malignant cancer cells can cause so much harm becomes clear.

PERSPECTIVE AND PROSPECTS

Of the diagnostic procedures that are available to physicians, cytologic techniques are among the most popular. Because the cells being examined are so tiny, the microscopes used must be able to magnify the cells enough to allow observation of their characteristics. Historically, the use of cytology in medical practice has closely paralleled the development of adequate microscopes and methods for preparing specimens.

Magnifying lenses by themselves lack the power required for observing cells. A microscope of adequate power must use several such lenses stacked together. The first crude microscopes with this design appeared late in the sixteenth century. During the next several hundred years, microscopes were mostly used to observe cells of plant material because the woody parts of plants can be thinly sliced and then observed directly, without the need for further preparation. The word "cell" was first employed by Robert Hooke (1635-1703) in a paper published in 1665. He observed small chambers in pieces of cork, which were where cells had been located in the living cork tree. These chambers reminded Hooke of monks' cells in a monastery, hence the name.

The great anatomist Marcello Malpighi (1628-1694) may have been the first to observe mammalian cells, within capillaries. The real giant of this era, however, was the Dutch microscopist Antoni van Leeuwenhoek (1632-1723), who greatly improved the quality of microscopes and then used them to observe single-celled animals, bacteria, sperm, and the nuclei within certain blood cells. Although most progress continued to be made with plants, numerous observations accumulated during the seventeenth and eighteenth centuries which suggested that animals are made up of tiny saclike units, and Hooke's word "cell" was applied to describe them. This concept was clearly stated in 1839 by Theodor Schwann (1810-1882); his idea that all animals are composed of cells and cellular products quickly gained acceptance. At this time, however, there was essentially no comprehension of how cells work. Without an understanding of normal cell function, cytology was still of little use in identifying and understanding disease.

During the late nineteenth and early twentieth centuries, the appearance of different cell types was carefully described. The main organelles of cells were identified, and such fundamental processes as cell division were observed and understood. At last it was possible to utilize cytology for medical purposes. The principles of medical cytology were established by the great pathologist Rudolf Virchow (1821-1902), who suggested for the first time that diseases originate from changes in specific cells of the body.

Rapid progress in cytology was made in the 1940's and 1950's, for two reasons. First, improved microscopes were developed, allowing greater accuracy in observing cell structure. The second reason—rapid progress in genetics and biochemistry—greatly increased the knowledge of how cells function and of the significance of specific changes in their appearance. Because cells are the basic units of life, scientists will continue to study them in detail, and the medical world will benefit directly from further, improved understanding in this field.

—*Howard L. Hosick, Ph.D.*

See also Bacterial infections; Bacteriology; Biopsy; Blood and blood disorders; Blood testing; Cancer; Cells; Cytopathology; Diagnosis; Gram staining; Hematology; Hematology, pediatric; Histology; Karyotyping; Laboratory tests; Malignancy and metastasis; Microbiology; Microscopy; Oncology; Pathology; Prognosis; Serology; Urinalysis; Viral infections.

FOR FURTHER INFORMATION:
Kumar, Vinay, et al., eds. *Robbins Basic Pathology.* 8th ed. Philadelphia: Saunders/Elsevier, 2007. Presents a reasonably concise overview of the entire field of pathology, but the emphasis is on cytology. The chapter on disease at the cellular level is excellent and readable. The authors are unusually adept at explaining the facts in a simple and interesting way.
Taylor, Ron. *Through the Microscope.* Vol. 22 in *The World of Science.* New York: Facts On File, 1986. A fine introduction to the wonders of microscopy, recommended for all readers. In a large format with more than one hundred beautiful photographs. The clear, simple, and brief text explains how microscopes work and what is being seen. The section "Microscopes, Health, and Disease" is particularly relevant, explaining cytological detective work.
Wolfe, Stephen L. *Cell Ultrastructure.* Belmont, Calif.: Wadsworth, 1985. This book presents electron microscope photographs of the important structures of viruses, bacteria, and plant and animal cells. Included for most structures are three-dimensional drawings that are particularly useful for visualizing how cells are put together.

CYTOMEGALOVIRUS (CMV)
DISEASE/DISORDER

ANATOMY OR SYSTEM AFFECTED: Blood, brain, cells, ears, eyes, gastrointestinal system, immune system, liver, lungs

SPECIALTIES AND RELATED FIELDS: Family medicine, gastroenterology, hematology, immunology, obstetrics, pediatrics, virology

DEFINITION: A viral disease normally producing mild symptoms in healthy individuals but severe infections in the immunocompromised. Congenital infection may lead to malformations or fetal death.

KEY TERMS:
hepatitis: inflammation of the liver; usually caused by viral infections, toxic substances, or immunological disturbances
hepatosplenomegaly: enlargement of the liver and spleen such that they may be felt below the rib margins
heterophil antibodies: antibodies that are detected using antigens other than the antigens that induced them
jaundice: yellow staining of the skin, eyes, and other tissues and excretions with excess bile pigments in the blood

latency: following an acute infection by a virus, a period of dormancy from which the virus may be reactivated during times of stress or immunocompromise

microcephaly: a congenital condition involving an abnormally small head associated with an incompletely developed brain

Causes and Symptoms

Cytomegalovirus (CMV) is a member of the herpesvirus group that includes such viruses as the Epstein-Barr virus, which causes infectious mononucleosis, and the varicella-zoster virus, which causes chickenpox. CMV is a ubiquitous virus that is transmitted in a number of different ways. A newly infected woman may transmit the virus across the placenta to her unborn child. Infection may also occur in the birth canal or via mother's milk. Young children commonly transmit CMV by means of saliva. Sexual transmission is common in adults. Blood transfusions and organ transplants may also transmit cytomegalovirus to recipients. More than 80 percent of adults worldwide have antibodies indicating exposure to cytomegalovirus.

Congenital cytomegaloviral infection is universally common and especially prevalent in developing nations. Approximately 1 percent of live births in the United States are infected. Most congenitally infected infants exhibit no symptoms. Normal development may follow, but some infants suffer problems such as deafness, visual impairment, and/or mental retardation. Approximately 10 to 20 percent exhibit clinically obvious evidence of cytomegalic inclusion disease: hepatosplenomegaly, jaundice, microcephaly, deafness, seizures, cerebral palsy, and blood disorders such as thrombocytopenia (a decrease in platelets) and hemolytic anemia (in which red blood cells are destroyed). Giant cells having nuclei containing large inclusions are found in affected organs. Cytomegalovirus is a leading cause of mental retardation and responsible for about 10 percent of cases of microcephaly.

In immunocompetent adults and older children, cytomegalovirus can cause heterophil-negative mononucleosis, an infectious mononucleosis in which no heterophil antibodies are formed. Such antibodies are found in infectious mononucleosis caused by the Epstein-Barr virus. Heterophil-negative mononucleosis is characterized by fever, hepatitis, lethargy, and abnormal lymphocytes in blood.

Severe systemic cytomegalovirus infections are frequently seen in the immunocompromised. Transplant patients are intentionally immunosuppressed to reduce the likelihood of graft rejection, making them vulnerable to infection by cytomegalovirus either by reactivation or by acquisition of the virus from the donor organ. Resulting systemic infections are manifested in diseases such as pneumonia, hepatitis, and retinitis. In addition to these CMV diseases, acquired immunodeficiency syndrome (AIDS) patients suffer from infections of the central nervous system and gastrointestinal tract. Their blood cells may also be affected, resulting in disorders such as thrombocytopenia. AIDS patients frequently have intestinal CMV infections leading to chronic diarrhea. Cytomegalovirus retinitis in AIDS patients is particularly serious and may lead to retinal detachment and blindness. This is the most common sight-damaging opportunistic eye infection found in AIDS patients.

Treatment and Therapy

Ganciclovir, valganciclovir, foscarnet, and cidofovir are all antiviral agents which have been found useful in treating CMV infections in immunocompromised patients. Toxic properties, however, can limit their long-term administration. Ganciclovir exhibits hematopoietic toxicity; that is, it has an adverse affect on blood cells that may result in neutropenia, a decrease in the number of neutrophils in the blood. Foscarnet has more side effects than ganciclovir. It is a nephrotoxic substance, which means that it may damage the kidneys and thus cannot be used in patients with renal failure.

Valganciclovir, the oral form of ganciclovir, has been used effectively to prevent CMV infection in transplant recipients. It is administered to CMV-seronegative transplant patients receiving an organ from a CMV-seropositive donor as well as in CMV-seropositive recipients who will be undergoing immunosuppression to prevent rejection of the transplanted

---

Information on Cytomegalovirus (CMV)

Causes: Viral infection spread during childbirth or through body fluid exchange

Symptoms: Deafness, visual impairment, mental retardation, jaundice, microcephaly, seizures, cerebral palsy, blood disorders, infectious mononucleosis

Duration: Varies

Treatments: Antiviral drugs (ganciclovir, foscarnet)

organ. Another material employed as a prophylaxis for bone marrow and renal transplant recipients is intravenous cytomegalovirus immune globulin.

Therapy for CMV retinitis involves intravenous treatment with either ganciclovir, foscarnet, or cidofovir plus oral probenecid or oral valganciclovir. Alternatively, an intraocular ganciclovir implant may be used along with one of the systemic treatments mentioned above. Therapy of retinitis as well as other types of CMV infection in AIDS patients should be accompanied by highly effective antiretroviral therapy (HAART) to treat the human immunodeficiency virus and improve the immune function in the the the patient. Successful HAART may allow the CMV antiviral therapy to be discontinued, but the patient must be carefully monitored for relapse of the CMV infection.

Retinal detachment is another complication arising from cytomegalovirus retinitis. It may occur even in those undergoing successful antiviral treatment. Surgical intervention is required to restore functional vision in these cases.

Perspective and Prospects

The term "cytomegalia" was first used in 1921 to describe the condition of an infant with intranuclear inclusions in the lungs, kidney, and liver. This condition in an adult was first attributed to a virus of the herpes group in 1925. Twenty-five cases of apparent cytomegalic inclusion disease had been described by 1932. Cytomegalovirus was pursued and isolated in the mid-1950's by Margaret Smith in St. Louis. Around the same time, independently and serendipitously, groups in Boston and in Bethesda, Maryland, also isolated the virus.

Development of new antiviral drugs and measures to reduce the immunocompromised state should continue to progress and improve the outcomes for patients infected with CMV.

—Nancy Handshaw Clark, Ph.D.;
updated by H. Bradford Hawley, M.D.
See also Acquired immunodeficiency syndrome (AIDS); Birth defects; Epstein-Barr virus; Eye surgery; Eyes; Hepatitis; Herpes; Immune system; Immunodeficiency disorders; Immunology; Mental retardation; Mononucleosis; Pregnancy and gestation; Stillbirth; Transplantation; Viral infections; Vision disorders.

For Further Information:

Bellenir, Karen, and Peter D. Dresser, eds. *Contagious and Noncontagious Infectious Diseases Sourcebook.* Detroit, Mich.: Omnigraphics, 1996. A handy reference source on infectious diseases. Includes bibliographical references and an index.

Roizman, Bernard, ed. *Infectious Diseases in an Age of Change: The Impact of Human Ecology and Behavior on Disease Transmission.* Washington, D.C.: National Academy Press, 1995. This book reports on major infectious diseases on the rise today, such as sexually transmitted diseases, Lyme disease, human cytomegalovirus, diarrheal diseases, dengue fever, hepatitis viruses, HIV, and malaria.

Roizman, Bernard, Richard J. Whitley, and Carlos Lopez, eds. *The Human Herpesviruses.* New York: Raven Press, 1993. A helpful text discussing all aspects of the herpesvirus and offering information on vaccination against the disease. Includes bibliographical references and an index.

Scheld, W. Michael, Richard J. Whitley, and Christina M. Marra, eds. *Infections of the Central Nervous System.* 3d ed. Philadelphia: Lippincott Williams & Wilkins, 2004. This comprehensive multiauthor book covers viral infections, with six separate chapters on one herpesvirus group: herpes simplex, varicella zoster, cytomegalovirus, Epstein-Barr virus, human herpesvirus 6, and B virus.

Wagner, Edward K., and Martinez J. Hewlett. *Basic Virology.* 3d ed. Malden, Mass.: Blackwell Science, 2008. A very readable undergraduate text covering issues of virology and viral disease, properties of viruses and virus-cell interaction, working with viruses, and replication patterns of specific viruses.

Cytopathology

Specialty

Anatomy or system affected: Cells, immune system

Specialties and related fields: Bacteriology, cytology, forensic pathology, hematology, histology, oncology, pathology, serology

Definition: The medical field that deals with changes in cell structure or physiology as a result of injuries, infectious agents, or toxic substances.

Science and Profession

The profession of cytopathology deals with the search for lesions or abnormalities within individual cells or groups of cells. Generally speaking, a pathologist is a physician trained in pathology, the study of the nature of diseases. Observations of tissue or cell lesions are utilized in the diagnosis of disease or other agents associated with damage to cells.

Cell damage may result from endogenous phenomena, including the aging process, or from exogenous agents such as biological organisms (viruses or bacteria), chemical agents (bacterial toxins or other poisons), and physical agents (heat, cold, or electricity). For example, particular biological agents produce recognizable lesions that may be useful in the diagnosis of disease, such as the crystalline structures characteristic of certain viral infections.

The type of necrosis, or cell death, encountered is useful in diagnosing the problem. For example, certain types of enzymatic dissolution of cells, which result in areas of liquefaction, are the result of bacterial infection. Gangrenous necrosis often follows the restriction of the blood supply, because of either infection or a blood clot.

Pathologic changes within the cell can also help pinpoint the time of death. Organelles degenerate at a rate dependent on their use of oxygen. For example, mitochondria, which utilize significant amounts of oxygen, are among the first organelles to degenerate.

DIAGNOSTIC AND TREATMENT TECHNIQUES

The diagnosis and treatment of cancer are prime examples of the use of cytopathology. The extent of pleomorphism in cell size and shape, irregularity of the nucleus, and presence (or absence) of organelles all provide the basis for the choice of treatment and help determine the ultimate prognosis. Specific organelles are stained with characteristic histochemicals, followed by microscopic observation. A preponderance of large, irregularly shaped cells provides for a poorer prognosis than if cells appear more normally differentiated. The nuclei in highly malignant tumors show a greater variation in size and chromatin pattern, as compared with those of cells from benign growths. Such differences lead directly to decisions on the choice of treatment: surgical removal, chemotherapy, or radiation.

—*Richard Adler, Ph.D.*

See also Bacteriology; Biopsy; Blood and blood disorders; Blood testing; Cancer; Cells; Cytology; Diagnosis; Gram staining; Hematology; Hematology, pediatric; Histology; Laboratory tests; Malignancy and metastasis; Microbiology; Microscopy; Oncology; Pathology; Prognosis; Serology; Toxicology; Tumors; Urinalysis.

FOR FURTHER INFORMATION:

Geisinger, Kim R., et al. *Modern Cytopathology.* Philadelphia: Churchill Livingstone/Elsevier, 2004.

Kumar, Vinay, et al., eds. *Robbins Basic Pathology.* 8th ed. Philadelphia: Saunders/Elsevier, 2007.

Lewin, Benjamin, et al., eds. *Cells.* Sudbury, Mass.: Jones and Bartlett, 2007.

Majno, Guido, and Isabelle Joris. *Cells, Tissues, and Disease: Principles of General Pathology.* 2d ed. New York: Oxford University Press, 2004.

Silverberg, Steven G., ed. *Silverberg's Principles and Practice of Surgical Pathology and Cytopathology.* 4th ed. New York: Churchill Livingstone/Elsevier, 2006.

DEAFNESS
DISEASE/DISORDER

ALSO KNOWN AS: Hearing loss, hearing impairment, presbycusis

ANATOMY OR SYSTEM AFFECTED: Ears, nervous system

SPECIALTIES AND RELATED FIELDS: Audiology, geriatrics and gerontology, speech pathology

DEFINITION: Deafness is either partial or complete loss of hearing. Hearing loss occurs most often in older adults, but people may be born deaf or become deaf at young ages.

KEY TERMS

acquired: not present at birth; developing after birth

auditory: pertaining to hearing

cerumen: earwax produced by specialized glands to protect and lubricate the ear canal

cochlea: the organ of hearing in the inner ear that takes the vibrations from the middle ear organs and converts them into nerve impulses for the brain to interpret

congenital: present at birth

eighth cranial nerve: also known as the auditory nerve or the vestibulocochlear nerve; the nerve running between the ear and the brain, involved with hearing and balance

genetic: inherited

ossicles: the chain of tiny bones in the middle ear which carry the vibrations of the tympanic membrane to the cochlea

ototoxic: toxic or harmful to the ears

tympanic membrane: also called the eardrum; a thin membrane that separates the external or outer ear from the middle ear

CAUSES AND SYMPTOMS

To understand deafness, it is first necessary to understand how sound is heard. The sound waves produced by any noise travel through the air and are funneled down the ear canal by the external ear, which is specially shaped for this function. The sound waves then cause the tympanic membrane to vibrate, which in turn causes the chain of tiny ossicles to vibrate. This mechanical energy of vibration is then transformed by the cochlea into nerve impulses which travel along the eighth cranial nerve to the spinal cord. These impulses are transmitted to the auditory cortex (center) of the brain, where they are interpreted. The ability to hear depends on all these elements working properly.

Deafness can occur when any particular part of this hearing pathway is not functioning as it should. If the ear canal is blocked with cerumen, a foreign body, fluid, or the products of infection or inflammation, then the sound waves are unable to travel to the eardrum. If the eardrum has ruptured or if it has become stiff (sclerosed), then it cannot vibrate. If the ossicles have been damaged in any way, then they cannot vibrate. If the middle ear is filled with fluid from inflammation or infection, then the eardrum and ossicles cannot work properly. If the cochlea, auditory nerve, or both have been damaged through trauma or use of an ototoxic drug or disease, then they cannot do their job of converting vibration into nerve impulses and transmitting them to the brain. If the auditory center of the brain is damaged, then it cannot interpret the nerve impulses correctly.

Hearing loss is classified by the cause: conductive, sensory, and neural. Conductive losses are those that affect the conduction of sound waves; they involve problems with the external ear, ear canal, tympanic membrane, and ossicles. The sensory and neural causes are usually classified together as "sensorineural"; these losses affect the cochlea, auditory nerve, or auditory cortex of the brain.

The most common cause of hearing loss in children is otitis media, or middle-ear infection, which causes fluid to build up behind the tympanic membrane. It is usually reversible with time and treatment. This is a type of conductive loss, as is hearing loss attributable to cerumen impaction (excessive buildup of earwax), which can occur in both children and adults. Sensorineural losses are caused by such things as excessive noise exposure, ototoxic drugs, exposure to toxins in

---

INFORMATION ON DEAFNESS

CAUSES: Aging; ear canal blockage (earwax, foreign body, fluid); ruptured or stiff eardrum; middle-ear infection; cochlea or auditory nerve damage (excessive noise exposure, ototoxic drugs, environmental toxins); genetic defect or predisposition

SYMPTOMS: Hearing loss ranging from moderate to total

DURATION: Acute, permanent, or progressive

TREATMENTS: Depends on cause; for permanent loss, hearing aids, cochlear implants, other assistive devices

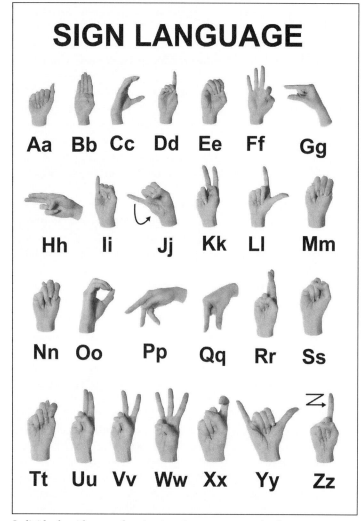

SIGN LANGUAGE

Aa Bb Cc Dd Ee Ff Gg

Hh Ii Jj Kk Ll Mm

Nn Oo Pp Qq Rr Ss

Tt Uu Vv Ww Xx Yy Zz

Individuals with severe hearing impairment may use sign language to communicate. (© Stephen Coburn/Dreamstime.com)

the environment, and diseases such as rubella (German measles). The type of sensorineural loss that many people experience as they get older is called presbycusis, which means "a condition of elder hearing." Many people with sensorineural losses have a genetic predisposition for hearing loss.

Congenital deafness is deafness that is present at the time a baby is born. Before the widespread availability of immunization against rubella, mothers who contracted German measles during pregnancy were at great risk of having a baby with congenital deafness. Congenital deafness may also be genetic. For example, if a child inherits a defective copy of the *GJB2* gene from each parent, then that child will be deaf even if both parents can hear.

Likewise, deafness that occurs after birth may be either acquired or genetic. Deafness associated with exposure to loud noises is acquired, for example, while many forms of deafness that occur in older age are genetic. About one-third of people between the ages of sixty-five and seventy-five years and 40 percent of those over seventy-five have hearing loss.

TREATMENT AND THERAPY

The best treatment for deafness is prevention. Immunizations against rubella, ear protection against noise exposure, and avoidance of too much aspirin are all examples of prevention against deafness.

Once hearing impairment has occurred, determination of the cause is essential. The primary care provider, an otorhinolaryngologist (ear, nose, and throat doctor), an audiologist (hearing specialist), and a neurologist may be involved in this assessment. Reversible causes of deafness or loss can be addressed medically or surgically, as in the removal of earwax. For nonreversible causes, hearing aids and other assistive hearing devices may be helpful. These devices have become increasingly sophisticated. Some allow the person to adjust the hearing aid to specific circumstances, while older versions amplified all sounds equally.

Cochlear implants are electronic devices that give profoundly deaf persons a sense of sound that helps them understand speech and other noises. A microphone picks up sounds, which are processed, converted to electric impulses, and sent to different areas of the auditory nerve.

In addition to these products, many new assistive devices are available to help persons with severe hearing impairment function independently. For example, special telephones, alarm clocks, and doorbells that flash a light or shake the bed in addition to ringing are readily available.

—Rebecca Lovell Scott, Ph.D., PA-C

See also Aging; Audiology; Ear infections and disorders; Ear surgery; Ears; Hearing; Hearing aids; Hearing loss; Hearing tests; Neuralgia, neuritis, and neuropathy; Otorhinolaryngology; Sense organs; Speech disorders.

FOR FURTHER INFORMATION:

American Medical Association. *American Medical Association Family Medical Guide*. 4th rev. ed. Hoboken, N.J.: John Wiley & Sons, 2004.

Carmen, Richard, ed. *The Consumer Handbook on Hearing Loss and Hearing Aids: A Bridge to Healing*. 3d rev. ed. Sedona, Ariz.: Auricle Ink, 2009.

Dillon, Harvey. *Hearing Aids*. New York: Thieme, 2001.

Komaroff, Anthony, ed. *Harvard Medical School Family Health Guide*. New York: Free Press, 2005.

Romoff, Arlene. *Hear Again: Back to Life with a Cochlear Implant*. New York: League for the Hard of Hearing, 1999.

Stoppard, Miriam. *Family Health Guide*. London: DK, 2006.

DEATH AND DYING

DISEASE/DISORDER

ANATOMY OR SYSTEM AFFECTED: Psychic-emotional system, all bodily systems

SPECIALTIES AND RELATED FIELDS: Family medicine, geriatrics and gerontology, psychology

KEY TERMS:

anticipatory depression: a depressive reaction to the awaited death of either oneself or a significant other; also called anticipatory grieving, preparatory grieving, or preparatory depression

bereavement: the general, overall process of mourning and grieving; considered to have progressive stages which include anticipation, grieving, mourning, postmourning, depression, loneliness, and reentry into society

depression: a general term covering mild states (sadness, inhibition, unhappiness, discouragement) to severe states (hopelessness, despair); typically part of normal, healthy grieving; considered the fourth stage of death and dying, between bargaining and acceptance

grief: the emotional and psychological response to loss; always painful, grieving is a type of psychological work and requires some significant duration of time

mourning: the acute phase of grief; characterized by distress, hopelessness, fear, acute loss, crying, insomnia, loss of appetite, anxiety, guilt, and restlessness

reactive depression: depression occurring as a result of overt events that have already taken place; it universally occurs in the bereaved

thanatology: the study and investigation of life-threatening actions, terminal illness, suicide, homicide, death, dying, grief, and bereavement

uncomplicated bereavement: a technical psychiatric label describing normal, average, and expectant grieving; despite an experience of great psychological pain, grieving is considered normal and healthy unless it continues much beyond one year

CAUSES AND SYMPTOMS

Medicine determines that death has occurred by assessing bodily functions in either of two areas. Persons with irreversible cessation of respiration and circulation are dead; persons with irreversible cessation of ascertainable brain functions are also dead. There are standard procedures used to diagnose death, including simple observation, brain-stem reflex studies, and the use of confirmatory testing such as electrocardiography (ECG or EKG), electroencephalography (EEG), and arterial blood gas analysis (ABG). The particular circumstances—anticipated or unanticipated, observed or unobserved, the patient's age, drug or metabolic intoxication, or suspicion of hypothermia—will favor some procedures over others, but in all cases both cessation of functions and their irreversibility are required before death can be declared.

Between 60 and 75 percent of all people die from chronic terminal conditions. Therefore, except in sudden death (as in a fatal accident) or when there is no evidence of consciousness (as in a head injury which destroys cerebral, thinking functions while leaving brain-stem, reflexive functions intact), dying is both a physical and a psychological process. In most cases, dying takes time, and the time allows patients to react to the reality of their own passing. Often, they react by becoming vigilant about bodily symptoms and any changes in them. They also anticipate changes that have yet to occur. For example, long before the terminal stages of illness become manifest, dying patients commonly fear physical pain, shortness of breath, invasive procedures, loneliness, becoming a burden to loved ones, losing decision-making authority, and facing the unknown of death itself.

As physical deterioration proceeds, all people cope by resorting to what has worked for them before: the unique means and mechanisms which have helped maintain a sense of self and personal stability. People seem to go through the process of dying much as they have gone through the process of living—with the more salient features of their personalities, whether good or bad, becoming sharper and more prominent. People seem to face death much as they have faced life.

Medicine has come to acknowledge that physicians should understand what it means to die. Indeed, while all persons should understand what their own deaths will mean, physicians must additionally understand how their dying patients find this meaning. Physicians who see death as the final calamity coming at the end of life, and thus primarily as something that only geriatric medicine has to face, are mistaken. Independent of beliefs about "life after life," the life process on this planet inexorably comes to an end for everyone, whether as a result of accident, injury, or progressive deterioration.

In 1969, psychiatrist Elisabeth Kübler-Ross published the landmark *On Death and Dying*, based on her work with two hundred terminally ill patients. Though the work of Kübler-Ross has been criticized for the nature of the stages described and whether or not every person experiences every stage, her model has retained enormous utility to those who work in the area of death and dying. Technologically driven, Western medicine had come to define its role as primarily dealing with extending life and thwarting death by defeating specific diseases. Too few physicians saw a role for themselves once the prognosis turned grave. In the decades that followed *On Death and Dying*, the profession has reaccepted that death and dying are part of life and that, while treating the dying may not mean extending the length of life, it can and should mean extending its quality.

Kübler-Ross provided a framework which explained how people cope with and adapt to the profound and terrible news that their illness is going to kill them. Although other physicians, psychologists, and thanatologists have shortened, expanded, and adapted her five stages of the dying process, neither the actual number of stages nor what they are specifically called is as important as the information and insight that any stage theory of dying yields. As with any human process, dying is complex, multifaceted, multidimensional, and polymorphic.

Well-intentioned, but misguided, professionals and family members may try to help move dying patients through each of the stages only to encounter active resentment or passive withdrawal. Patients, even dying patients, cannot be psychologically moved to where they are not ready to be. Rather than making the terminally ill die the "right" way, it is more respectful and helpful to understand any stage as a description of normal reactions to serious loss, and that these reactions normally vary among different individuals and also

within the same individual over time. The reactions appear, disappear, and reappear in any order and in any combination. What the living must do is respect the unfolding of an adaptational schema which is the dying person's own. No one should presume to know how someone else should die.

COMPLICATIONS AND DISORDERS

Denial is Kübler-Ross's first stage, but it is also linked to shock and isolation. Whether the news is told outright or gradual self-realization occurs, most people react to the knowledge of their impending death with existential shock: Their whole selves recoil at the idea, and they say, in some fashion, "This cannot be happening to me. I must be dreaming." Broadly considered, denial is a complex cognitive-emotional capacity which enables temporary postponement of active, acute, but in some way detrimental, recognition of reality. In the dying process, this putting off of the truth prevents a person from being overwhelmed while promoting psychological survival. Denial plays an important stabilizing role, holding back more than could be otherwise managed while allowing the individual to marshal psychological resources and reserves. It enables patients to consider the possibility, even the inevitability, of death and then to put the consideration away so that they can pursue life in the ways that are still available. In this way, denial is truly a mechanism of defense.

Many other researchers, along with Kübler-Ross, report anger as the second stage of dying. The stage is also linked to rage, fury, envy, resentment, and loathing. When "This cannot be happening to me" becomes, "This is happening to me. There was no mistake," patients are beginning to replace denial with attempts to understand what is happening to and inside them. When they do, they often ask, "Why me?" Though logically it is an unanswerable question, the logic of the question is clear. People, to remain human, must try to make intelligible their experiences and reality. The asking of this question is an important feature of the way in which all dying persons adapt to and cope with the reality of death.

People react with anger when they lose something of value; they react with greater anger when something of value is taken away from them by someone or something. Rage and fury, in fact, are often more accurate descriptions of people's reactions to the loss of their own life than is anger. Anger is a difficult stage for professionals and loved ones, more so when the anger and rage are displaced and projected randomly into any corner and crevice of the patient's world. An unfortunate result is that caregivers often experience the anger as personal, and the caregivers' own feelings of guilt, shame, grief, and rejection can contribute to lessening contact with the dying person, which increases his or her sense of isolation.

Bargaining is Kübler-Ross's third stage, but it is also the one about which she wrote the least and the one that other thanatologists are most likely to leave unrepresented in their own models and stages of how people cope with dying. Nevertheless, it is a common phenomenon wherein dying people fall back on their faith, belief systems, or sense of the transcendent and the spiritual and try to make a deal—with God, life, fate, a higher power, or the composite of all the randomly colliding atoms in the universe. They ask for more time to help family members reconcile or to achieve something of importance. They may ask if they can simply attend their child's wedding or graduation or if they can see their first grandchild born. Then they will be ready to die; they will go willingly. Often, they mean that they will die without fighting death, if death can only be delayed or will delay itself. Some get what they want; others do not.

At some point, when terminally ill individuals are faced with decisions about more procedures, tests, surgeries, or medications or when their thinness, weakness, or deterioration becomes impossible to ignore, the anger, rage, numbness, stoicism, and even humor will likely give way to depression, Kübler-Ross's fourth stage and the one reaction that all thanatologists include in their models of how people cope with dying.

The depression can take many forms, for indeed there are always many losses, and each loss individually or several losses collectively might need to be experienced and worked through. For example, dying parents might ask themselves who will take care of the children, get them through school, walk them down the aisle, or guide them through life. Children, even adult children who are parents themselves, may ask whether they can cope without their own parents. They wonder who will support and anchor them in times of distress, who will (or could) love, nurture, and nourish them the way that their parents did. Depression accompanies the realization that each role, each function, will never be performed again. Both the dying and those who love them mourn.

Much of the depression takes the form of anticipatory grieving, which often occurs both in the dying and in those who will be affected most by their death. It is a part of the dying process experienced by the living, both terminal and nonterminal. Patients, family, and friends can psychologically anticipate what it will be like when the death does occur and what life will, and will not, be like afterward. The grieving begins while there is still life left to live.

Bereavement specialists generally agree that anticipatory grieving, when it occurs, seems to help people cope with what is a terrible and frightening loss. It is an adaptive psychological mechanism wherein emotional, mental, and existential stability are painfully maintained. When depression develops, not only in reaction to death but also in preparation for it, it seems to be a necessary part of how those who are left behind cope to survive the loss themselves. Those who advocate or advise cheering up or looking on the bright side are either unrealistic or unable to tolerate the sadness in themselves or others. The dying are in the process of losing everything and everyone they love. Cheering up does not help them; the advice to "be strong" only helps the "helpers" deny the truth of the dying experience.

Both preparatory and reactive depression are frequently accompanied by unrealistic self-recrimination, shame, and guilt in the dying person. Those who are dying may judge themselves harshly and criticize themselves for the wrongs that they committed and for the good that they did not accomplish. They may judge themselves to be unattractive, unappealing, and repulsive because of how the illness and its treatment have made them appear. These feelings and states of minds, which have nothing to do with the reality of the situation, are often amenable to the interventions of understanding and caring people. Disfigured breasts do not make a woman less a woman; the removal of the testes does not make a man less a man. Financial and other obligations can be restructured and reassigned. Being forgiven and forgiving can help finish what was left undone.

Kübler-Ross's fifth stage, acceptance, is an intellectual and emotional coming to terms with death's reality, permanence, and inevitability. Ironically, it is manifested by diminished emotionality and interests and increased fatigue and inner (many would say spiritual) self-focus. It is a time without depression or anger. Envy of the healthy, the fear of losing all, and bargaining for another day or week are also absent. This final stage is often misunderstood. Some see it either as resignation and giving up or as achieving a happy serenity. Some think that acceptance is the goal of dying well and that all people are supposed to go through this stage. None of these viewpoints is accurate. Acceptance, when it does occur, comes from within the dying person. It is marked more by an emotional void and psychological detachment from people and things once held important and necessary and by an interest in some transcendental value (for the atheist) or his or her God (for the theist). It has little to do with what others believe is important or "should" be done. It is when dying people become more intimate with themselves and appreciate their separateness from others more than at any other time.

PERSPECTIVE AND PROSPECTS

Every person eventually dies, and the fact of death in each life is one that varies by culture in terms of its meaning. For some cultures, dying is seen as the ultimate difficulty for dying people and their loved ones. For other cultures, it is seen as not difficult at all, but more so like passing on to another realm of existence. In Western cultures, however, dying has very much become a medical process, and it is often a process filled with challenging questions. Patients ask questions that cannot be answered; families in despair and anger seek to find cause and sometimes lay blame. It takes courage to be with individuals as they face their deaths, struggling to find meaning in the time that they have left. Given this, in Western medicine, a profession that prides itself on how well it intervenes to avoid outcomes like death, it takes courage to witness the process and struggle involved in death. Working with death also reminds professionals of their own inevitable death. Facing that fact inwardly, spiritually, and existentially also requires courage.

Cure and treatment become care and management in the dying. They should live relatively pain-free, be supported in accomplishing their goals, be respected, be involved in decision making as appropriate, be encouraged to function as fully as their illness allows, and be provided with others to whom control can comfortably and confidently be passed. The lack of a cure and the certainty of the end can intimidate health care providers, family members, and close friends. They may dread genuine encounters with those whose days are knowingly numbered. Yet the dying have the same rights to be helped as any of the living, and how a society assists them bears directly on the meaning that its members are willing to attach to their own lives.

Today, largely in response to what dying patients have told researchers, medicine recognizes its role to assist these patients in working toward an appropriate death. Caretakers must determine the optimum treatments, interventions, and conditions which will enable such a death to occur. For each terminally ill person, these should be unique and specific. Caretakers should respond to the patient's needs and priorities, at the patient's own pace and as much as possible following the patient's lead. For some dying patients, the goal is to remain as pain-free as is feasible and to feel as well as possible. For others, finishing whatever unfinished business remains becomes the priority. Making amends, forgiving and being forgiven, resolving old conflicts, and reconciling with self and others may be the most therapeutic and healing of interventions. Those who are to be bereaved fear the death of those they love. The dying fear the separation from all they know and love, but they fear as well the loss of autonomy, letting family and friends down, the pain and invasion of further treatment, disfigurement, dementia, loneliness, the unknown, becoming a burden, and the loss of dignity.

The English writer C. S. Lewis said that bereavement is the universal and integral part of the experience of loss. It requires effort, authenticity, mental and emotional work, a willingness to be afraid, and an openness to what is happening and what is going to happen. It requires an attitude which accepts, tolerates suffering, takes respite from the reality, reinvests in whatever life remains, and moves on. The only way to cope with dying or witnessing the dying of loved ones is by grieving through the pain, fear, loneliness, and loss of meaning. This process, which researcher Stephen Levine has likened to opening the heart in hell, is a viscous morass for most, and all people need to learn their own way through it and to have that learning respected. Healing begins with the first halting, unsteady, and frightening steps of genuine grief, which sometimes occur years before the "time of death" can be recorded as a historical event and which may never completely end.

—Paul Moglia, Ph.D.

See also Acquired immunodeficiency syndrome (AIDS); Aging; Depression; Ethics; Euthanasia; Grief and guilt; Hospice; Living will; Midlife crisis; Palliative medicine; Phobias; Psychiatry; Psychiatry, child and adolescent; Psychiatry, geriatric; Stress; Sudden infant death syndrome (SIDS); Suicide; Terminally ill: Extended care.

FOR FURTHER INFORMATION:

Becker, Ernest. *The Denial of Death*. New York: Free Press, 1997. Written by an anthropologist and philosopher, this is an erudite and insightful analysis and synthesis of the role that the fear of death plays in motivating human activity, society, and individual actions. A profound work.

Cook, Alicia Skinner, and Daniel S. Dworkin. *Helping the Bereaved: Therapeutic Interventions for Children, Adolescents, and Adults.* New York: Basic Books, 1992. Although not a self-help book, this work is useful to professionals and nonprofessionals alike as a review of the state of the art in grief therapy. Practical and readable. Of special interest for those becoming involved in grief counseling.

Corr, Charles A., Clyde M. Nabe, and Donna M. Corr. *Death and Dying, Life and Living.* 6th ed. Belmont, Calif.: Wadsworth/Cengage Learning, 2009. This book provides perspective on common issues associated with death and dying for family members and others affected by life-threatening circumstances.

Forman, Walter B., et al., eds. *Hospice and Palliative Care: Concepts and Practice.* 2d ed. Sudbury, Mass.: Jones and Bartlett, 2003. A text that examines the theoretical perspectives and practical information about hospice care. Other topics include community medical care, geriatric care, nursing care, pain management, research, counseling, and hospice management.

Kübler-Ross, Elisabeth, ed. *Death: The Final Stage of Growth.* Reprint. New York: Simon & Schuster, 1997. A psychiatrist by training, Kübler-Ross brings together other researchers' views of how death provides the key to how human beings make meaning in their own personal worlds. Addresses practical concerns over how people express grief and accept the death of those close to them, and how they might prepare for their own inevitable ends.

Kushner, Harold. *When Bad Things Happen to Good People.* 20th anniversary ed. New York: Schocken Books, 2001. The first of Rabbi Kushner's works on finding meaning in one's life, it was originally his personal response to make intelligible the death of his own child. It has become a highly regarded reference for those who struggle with the meaning of pain, suffering, and death in their lives.

McFarlane, Rodger, and Philip Bashe. *The Complete Bedside Companion: No-Nonsense Advice on Caring for the Seriously Ill.* New York: Simon & Schuster, 1998. A comprehensive and practical guide to caregiving for patients with serious illnesses. The first section deals with the general needs of caring for the sick, while the second section covers specific illnesses in depth. Includes bibliographies and lists of support organizations.

DECONGESTANTS

TREATMENT

ANATOMY OR SYSTEM AFFECTED: Circulatory system, ears, nose, respiratory system, throat

SPECIALTIES AND RELATED FIELDS: Family medicine, otorhinolaryngology

DEFINITION: Oral and topical medications that are used to relieve nasal and sinus congestion and to promote the opening of collapsed Eustachian tubes.

KEY TERMS:

adjunctive: referring to the treatment of symptoms associated with a condition, not the condition itself

contraindication: a condition that makes a particular treatment not advisable; contraindications may be absolute (should never be used) or relative (should be used only with caution when the benefits outweigh the potential problems)

evidence-based medicine: a method of basing clinical medical practice decisions on systematic reviews of published medical studies

systemic: affecting the entire body; systemic treatments may be administered orally, directly into a vein, into the muscle, or through mucous membranes

topical: referring to treatments applied directly to the skin or mucous membranes that affect primarily the area in which they are applied

upper respiratory tract: the nose, sinuses, throat, ears, Eustachian tubes, and trachea

INDICATIONS AND PROCEDURES

Decongestants are used to shrink inflamed mucous membranes, promote drainage, or open collapsed Eustachian tubes. They are often used for the temporary relief of congestion caused by an upper respiratory tract infection (a cold), a sinus infection, or hay fever and other nasal allergies by promoting both nasal and sinus drainage. They are also often used as adjunctive therapy in the treatment of middle-ear infection (otitis media) to decrease congestion around the openings of the Eustachian tubes, and they may relieve the ear pressure, blockage, and pain experienced by some people during air travel. Careful scientific evaluation of the effectiveness of decongestants, however, has shown somewhat contradictory results.

The action of decongestants is accomplished primarily through stimulation of specific receptors in the smooth muscle of the upper respiratory tract, which in turn leads to constriction of the blood vessels and shrinkage of the mucous membranes. This improves air flow through the upper respiratory tract and relieves the sensation of stuffiness.

Uses and Complications

Decongestants may be applied topically, as sprays or drops, or taken by mouth. Commonly used decongestants include ephedrine, epinephrine, naphazoline, oxymetazoline, phenylephrine, pseudoephedrine, tetrahydrozoline, and xylometazoline. Some of these drugs are available over the counter and some by prescription only.

Oral preparations must be used with caution in elderly persons, children, and people with high blood pressure or other cardiac problems. If used as directed, decongestants do not usually cause excessive increases in blood pressure, overstimulate the heart, or change the distribution of blood in the circulatory system. The topical preparations are somewhat safer, because they are less likely to cause side effects, but they must also be used with caution.

The major advantage of oral decongestants is their long duration of action. Topical decongestants work more quickly but last a shorter period of time and are more likely to cause irritation of the tissues to which they are applied. If used too often or for too long a period of time (more than three to five days), nasal preparations may lead to a condition called rhinitis medicamentosa or rebound congestion, in which the congestion may be worse than before the person started using the medication.

People who take a certain type of antidepressant medication called a monoamine oxidase inhibitor (MAOI) and those with severe high blood pressure or heart disease should not take decongestants at all. People with thyroid disease, diabetes mellitus, glaucoma, or an enlarged prostate gland should take these drugs only after consulting a health care professional. Specific decongestants are contraindicated in infants and children.

People who take excessive doses of decongestants or who take them with other drugs that stimulate the central nervous system may experience insomnia, restlessness, dizziness, tremors, or nervousness. Overdose or long-term use of high doses may lead to hallucinations, convulsions, cardiovascular collapse, or even death.

Perspective and Prospects

Although decongestants have been widely used for decades, evidence-based medicine reveals few good studies indicating that decongestants do, in fact, treat illnesses. Systematic and careful reviews of the scientific studies available in the medical literature suggest that a single dose of a decongestant may relieve the stuffiness associated with the common cold in adults, but that no evidence exists for the usefulness of repeated doses. In people with a cough, a combination decongestant-antihistamine provides some relief in adults but not in children. In children with otitis media, there is a small statistical benefit from use of a combination decongestant-antihistamine, but it is not clear that the children benefit clinically. An evidence-based medicine review suggests that they not be used in children, especially given the increased risk of side effects from these medications in this age group.

—*Rebecca Lovell Scott, Ph.D., PA-C*

See also Allergies; Antihistamines; Anti-inflammatory drugs; Blood vessels; Common cold; Ear infections and disorders; Hay fever; Host-defense mechanisms; Immune system; Immunology; Inflammation; Multiple chemical sensitivity syndrome; Nasopharyngeal disorders; Otorhinolaryngology; Over-the-counter medications; Pharmacology; Pharmacy; Sinusitis; Smell.

For Further Information:

Flynn, C. A., G. Griffin, and F. Tudiver. "Decongestants and Antihistamines for Acute Otitis Media in Children." In *The Cochrane Library, Issue 4*. New York: John Wiley & Sons, 2003.

Komaroff, Anthony, ed. *Harvard Medical School Family Health Guide*. New York: Free Press, 2005.

Lacy, Charles F., et al. *The Drug Information Handbook*. 17th ed. Hudson, Ohio: Lexi-Comp, 2008.

Schiff, Donald, and Steven Shelov, eds. *American Academy of Pediatrics Guide to Your Child's Symptoms: The Official, Complete Home Reference, Birth Through Adolescence*. New York: Villard, 1999.

Schroeder, K., and T. Fahey. "Over-the-Counter Medications for Acute Cough in Children and Adults in Ambulatory Settings." In *The Cochrane Library, Issue 4*. New York: John Wiley & Sons, 2003.

Taverner, D., L. Bickford, and M. Draper. "Nasal Decongestants for the Common Cold." In *The Cochrane Library, Issue 4*. New York: John Wiley & Sons, 2003.

Deep vein thrombosis
Disease/disorder
Also known as: Blood clots, hypercoagulation

Anatomy or system affected: Blood, blood vessels, circulatory system, legs

Specialties and related fields: Family medicine, hematology

Definition: The formation of a blood clot (thrombus) in a deep vein that prevents blood circulation.

Key terms:

anticoagulant: a substance that hinders the clotting of blood

enzyme: a complex protein produced by living cells that catalyzes certain biochemical reactions at body temperature

fibrin: a fibrous insoluble protein formed from fibrinogen by the action of thrombin, especially in the clotting of blood

fibrinogen: a protein produced in the liver that is present in blood plasma and is converted to fibrin during the clotting of blood

platelet: a minute disk of vertebrate blood that assists in blood clotting

thrombin: an enzyme that facilitates the clotting of blood by catalyzing a conversion of fibrinogen to fibrin

Causes and Symptoms

Deep vein or venous thrombosis (DVT) is a blood clot (thrombus) in a deep vein. In vessels that transport blood toward the heart, various disorders including skin infections or phlebitis (inflammation of the vein) can occur; however, specific tests are required to diagnose the existence of DVT. While phlebitis afflicts superficial veins, DVT occurs in deep veins, usually the legs.

Because of the possibility of its breaking loose, lodging in the lungs, and creating a potentially fatal pulmonary embolism (blockage of blood to the lungs), a clot

---

INFORMATION ON DEEP VEIN THROMBOSIS

Causes: Prolonged inactivity, surgery, cancer, pregnancy, oral contraceptive use
Symptoms: Pain, redness, warmth; often none
Duration: Three to six months, possibly longer
Treatments: Anticoagulation drugs (heparin, coumadin)

---

in the leg is highly dangerous. Clots in veins in the legs generally follow inactivity, from surgery, long plane or car trips, pregnancy, obesity, smoking, estrogen therapy, oral contraceptive medication, or lengthy bed rest.

With DVT, the afflicted leg begins to swell, turn red, become warm, and throb. Occasionally, the area is tender to touch or movement. However, about one-half of the instances of DVT produce no symptoms, and it is frequently referred to as a silent killer.

Treatment and Therapy

Treatment for deep vein thrombosis begins with anticoagulants (blood thinners), specifically heparin, administered intravenously in the hospital, or through self-injections given at home. The anticoagulant warfarin (Coumadin), given as pills, are then prescribed daily to prevent clots from becoming larger. Frequent checkups with a physician are mandatory to maintain a certain level of medication effectiveness; depending upon the risk of further clotting, Coumadin can be required anywhere from three months to the remainder of the patient's life. Patients may also be advised to elevate the afflicted leg or apply a heating pad to the area. Walking is sometimes recommended, as is wearing tight-fitting stockings or compression stockings to reduce pain and swelling. In the event that Coumadin is unable to prevent blood clots, a filter may be surgically placed into the vena cava, the large vein carrying blood from the lower body to the heart, to prevent clots from entering the lungs. Also, a large clot may be removed through surgery or may be treated with powerful clot-destroying drugs.

Perspective and Prospects

Inquiries into the mysteries of blood coagulation have existed since 400 B.C.E., when Hippocrates observed that blood appeared to congeal as it cooled. By the nineteenth century, Pierre Andral, the founder of hematology (the branch of biology that deals with the blood and the blood-forming organs) and one of the first physicians to study the chemistry of the blood, formulated the classical hypothesis of blood coagulation. He found that the process of blood coagulation follows two pathways: the intrinsic, wherein, within seconds, platelets form a hemostatic plug at the site of the injury (primary hemostasis, or stoppage of bleeding); and the extrinsic, wherein fibrin molecules react in a complex cascade or network (secondary hemostasis) that ultimately moves into a third stage, wherein protein factors combine with the enzyme thrombin and contribute to the clotting of blood. Twentieth century research determined, however, that the tissue pathway (formerly known as the extrinsic) is a series of enzymes generated to participate with thrombin and catalyze fibrinogen into fibrin, which is essential to blood clotting. These factors, usually expressed in Roman numerals, are responsible for any abnormalities in the clotting of blood.

While the most commonly known blood clotting disorder is hemophilia, or uncontrolled bleeding, its opposite condition, hypercoagulation, specifically the formation of abnormal clots in veins, can also be life-threatening. In 1994, the clotting disorder factor V Leiden (named for the Dutch city in which it was discovered) was identified as a hereditary resistance to activated protein C. An estimated 30 percent of those individuals who suffer from hypercoagulation are afflicted by this enzyme mutation that encourages the overproduction of thrombin and, consequently, causes excessive clotting. Most of these persons are unaware of their condition or its dangers. Treatment and control of this disorder depends largely on antiplatelet medication, such as aspirin or clopidogrel (Plavix), that is designed to prevent platelets from sticking together.

Continued research into the complexities of coagulation account for new developments in medications, including thrombin inhibitors or molecular products that target enzymes controlling specific coagulation factors.

—Mary Hurd

See also Bleeding; Blood and blood disorders; Blood vessels; Circulation; Disseminated intravascular coagulation (DIC); Embolism; Hematology; Hematology, pediatric; Hemophilia; Lower extremities; Thrombus; Varicose vein removal; Vascular medicine; Vascular system.

FOR FURTHER INFORMATION:

Clayman, Charles B., ed. *American Medical Association Family Medical Guide.* Rev. 3d ed. New York: Random House, 1994.

Johnston, Bernard, ed. *Collier's Encyclopedia.* 24 vols. New York: Collier's, 1997.

Owen, Charles A. *History of Blood Coagulation.* Edited by William L. Nichols and E. J. Walter Bowie. Rochester, Minn.: Mayo Foundation for Medical Education and Research, 2001.

DEFIBRILLATION
PROCEDURE

ALSO KNOWN AS: Cardioversion, defib, shock

ANATOMY OR SYSTEM AFFECTED: Blood, blood vessels, brain, cells, chest, circulatory system, heart, nervous system, respiratory system

SPECIALTIES AND RELATED FIELDS: Anesthesiology, biotechnology, cardiology, critical care, emergency medicine, ethics, exercise physiology, family medicine, forensic medicine, general surgery, internal medicine, nursing, occupational health, pulmonary medicine, sports medicine, toxicology, vascular medicine

DEFINITION: A procedure that shocks the heart with therapeutic volts of electricity. Applied correctly and in the right circumstances, these shocks can change a life-threatening heart rhythm to a normal cardiac rhythm.

KEY TERMS:

automated external defibrillators (AEDs): portable and automated devices that deliver life-saving shocks

cardiac: referring to the heart

normal sinus rhythm: the heart's normal electrical activity

pulseless ventricular tachycardia (VT), ventricular fibrillation (VF): abnormal heart rhythms needing immediate defibrillation

INDICATIONS AND PROCEDURES

Defibrillation and cardioversion both deliver short bursts of direct electrical current across the chest to the heart. Heart tissue beats in a rhythmic manner as a result of electrical signals generated by the heart tissue. Sometimes, the normal heart rhythm, known as normal sinus rhythm, goes awry. Many different abnormal heart rhythms can develop from a variety of causes. These abnormal heart rhythms, known as arrhythmias, can be deadly since the heart cannot effectively pump blood when the heart is not in normal sinus rhythm.

Although cardioversion is used for a variety of abnormal and dangerous heart rhythms, defibrillation treats two very deadly arrhythmias, known as ventricular fibrillation (VF) and pulseless ventricular tachycardia (VT). The heart has four chambers: two atria and two ventricles. The ventricles pump blood to the lungs and body. In VF, the heart's electrical activity is chaotic and disorganized. This electrical chaos results in the ventricles quivering, like a bag of wiggling worms, and unable to pump blood. If blood is not pumped, the body will die in a manner of minutes. Therefore, defibrillation is of urgent and life-saving importance.

In VT, the ventricles are beating very fast. If the patient is unconscious and has no pulse (this can happen if the ventricles are beating too fast to fill up with enough blood to circulate), then VT treatment includes defibrillation.

A person with VF is unconscious because that person will have no cardiac output and no pulse. If the patient is placed on a cardiac monitor, a distinctive abnormal electrical pattern is displayed. The patient will shortly die if the fibrillation is not resolved quickly. The electrical current delivered during defibrillation shocks the heart tissue. This electrical shock stops all electrical heart activity, a process called depolarization, and resets the heart's electrical activity. Once the heart resets with defibrillation, normal sinus rhythm can take over.

Uses and Complications

Advanced cardiac life-support ambulance units and hospitals use devices equipped with electrical paddles and heart rhythm monitors for defibrillation. An unconscious patient with no pulse, showing the characteristic pattern of VF or VT on the cardiac monitor, will be urgently shocked with specified doses of electricity. The paddles are placed firmly on the patient's chest wall. Firm pressure, along with electrode paste, gel, or saline pads, helps ensure good electrical contact between the paddles and the chest wall.

Before discharging the electricity through the paddles, health care providers check the area surrounding the patient to ensure that no one is in physical contact with the patient or anything touching the patient. The electricity will shock anyone in direct contact with the patient or any metal touching the patient. This shock can change normal sinus rhythm into an abnormal rhythm. The health care person delivering the shock must quickly look around the area and shout "clear" and must avoid touching metal (like the stretcher frame) with any body part. Hands in the paddles are safely insulated from the delivered electricity.

Defibrillation protocols specify the sequencing and amount of electricity delivered during defibrillation. These protocols are quite detailed, involving cardiopulmonary resuscitation (CPR) and various medications.

Complications of defibrillation include damage to the heart muscle, which is rare unless repeated high energy shocks are used; blood clots dislodging from the heart and traveling to the body and lungs, causing problems when the clots block off blood supply; other abnormal heart rates emerging after defibrillation; fluid and blood backing up into the lungs, resulting in pulmonary edema; and low blood pressure that usually resolves in three to four hours.

Perspective and Prospects

Automated external defibrillators (AEDs) are life-saving devices that have gained in prominence and availability since the late twentieth century. AEDs are portable machines often found in public areas such as airports, sports arenas, shopping malls, or office buildings. They are different from the larger cart-based defibrillators found in health care facilities in several ways, so that they are easier and simpler to use. AED electrodes are attached to the patient with adhesive pads, rather than pressed down by hands and paddles, allowing hands-free operation. AEDs have microprocessors built into the system that detect ventricular fibrillation or ventricular tachycardia. If the device senses VF or VT, then the device advises the operator to deliver a shock.

The portable and automated nature of AEDs saves lives. Defibrillation is needed to reset the heart's electrical activity within minutes of the patient losing consciousness as the result of VF or VT. When defibrillation is indicated, earlier treatment is better. The increasing availability of AEDs, along with the ability of people trained to use the automated device in the right circumstances, promises to save even more lives in future.

—*Richard P. Capriccioso, M.D.*

See also Arrhythmias; Cardiac arrest; Cardiology; Cardiology, pediatric; Cardiopulmonary resuscitation (CPR); Emergency medicine; Emergency medicine, pediatric; Heart; Heart attack; Pacemaker implantation; Paramedics; Resuscitation.

For Further Information:

Chan, Paul S., et al. "Delayed Time to Defibrillation After In-Hospital Cardiac Arrest." *New England Journal of Medicine* 358, no. 1 (January 3, 2008): 9-17.

Picard, Andre. "School Defibrillators Could Be Lifesavers." *Globe and Mail*, March 31, 2009. Available at http://www.theglobeandmail.com/life/article756901.ece.

"2005 American Heart Association Guidelines for Cardiopulmonary Resuscitation and Emergency

Cardiovascular Care." *Circulation* 112, no. 24 Supplement (December 13, 2005): IV-1-IV-5. Available at http://circ.ahajournals.org/content/vol112/24_suppl.

DEHYDRATION
DISEASE/DISORDER
ANATOMY OR SYSTEM AFFECTED: Brain, cells, circulatory system

SPECIALTIES AND RELATED FIELDS: Exercise physiology, family medicine, sports medicine, vascular medicine

DEFINITION: Excessive loss of body water, which is often accompanied by disturbances in electrolyte balance.

KEY TERMS:

electrolytes: elements dissolved within body fluids that help regulate metabolism

plasma: the fluid portion of the blood

relative humidity: the percent moisture saturation of ambient air

CAUSES AND SYMPTOMS
The average adult's total body weight is approximately 60 percent water. Daily water requirements vary based on age, gender, level of physical activity, and climate. Dehydration, loss of 3 percent or more of body weight from the rapid loss of water, is often accompanied by the loss of essential electrolytes such as sodium, potassium, and chloride. Conditions that deplete body water faster than it is absorbed include fever-induced sweating, diarrhea, vomiting, acidosis, anorexia nervosa, bulimia, diabetes mellitus and insipidus, undernutrition,

---

INFORMATION ON DEHYDRATION

CAUSES: Fever-induced sweating, diarrhea, vomiting, acidosis, diabetes mellitus and insipidus, anorexia nervosa, bulimia, malnutrition, obesity, sedentary lifestyle, lack of acclimatization to heat stress

SYMPTOMS: Flushed skin, dark yellow urine, cramps, and heat exhaustion or stroke, causing cool and clammy skin, low blood pressure, rapid but weak heart rate, faintness, dizziness, headaches

DURATION: Acute

TREATMENTS: Rapid restoration of fluid volume and electrolyte balance

---

obesity, a sedentary lifestyle, and lack of acclimatization to heat stress. People exercising in hot, humid environments provide an excellent example of how dehydration develops and progresses. Symptoms of dehydration may include dry mouth, lips, and skin; decreased salivation; dizziness; weakness; constipation; and confusion.

Heat gain is higher and evaporative heat loss is lower during physical exertion in a hot environment in children as compared to adults, predisposing children to more rapid and severe dehydration. Both child and adult bodies attempt to reduce the buildup of metabolic heat through blood flow adjustments and sweat gland secretion. Flushed, red skin indicates that peripheral blood vessels have dilated, carrying blood and internal heat to the body surface for cooling. Once the heat is carried to the periphery by the bloodstream, dissipation occurs mainly by sweat evaporation. Large quantities of sweat may roll off the skin in a high humidity environment, but cooling only occurs when the sweat evaporates. Children exhibit a higher number of sweat glands per unit of body surface area than do adults, with each immature sweat gland producing about 40 percent as much sweat as an adult sweat gland. Children also gain heat from the environment faster than do adults because of their larger body surface area to body weight ratio; they dehydrate quicker as a result of lower overall fluid storage capacity. A large portion of the fluid released as sweat comes from the circulating blood plasma, making fluid consumption to rebuild blood plasma volume and to replenish lost water weight very important. Children acclimatize to a heat stress environment such as a sauna more slowly than do adults. They generally need at least six exposures before adjusting, whereas adults need only about three acclimation bouts.

The effects of dehydration are of particular concern in infants and young children, since their electrolyte balance can become precarious, leading to recommendations such as never allowing an infant to get a suntan.

TREATMENT AND THERAPY
Rapid restoration of fluid volume and electrolyte balance are primary treatment goals that may require intravenous infusion if sufficient fluid cannot be ingested orally.

"Prehydrating" the body by consuming liberal amounts of fluid before anticipated heat stress and "trickle hydrating" while losing body fluid are critical. Cool fluids of about 40 degrees Fahrenheit (about 5 degrees Celsius) empty from the gastrointestinal tract and supply the dehydrated cells quicker than warmer or colder temperature fluid. Studies of fluid absorption indicate that excessive sugar in electrolyte drinks slows water movement into the bloodstream. Children have been shown voluntarily to drink nearly twice as much when flavored fluids, as compared to plain water, are allowed.

Monitoring body weight before and after dehydration episodes and drinking enough water to regain lost weight is important. Nearly all body weight lost during exercise is attributable to water loss, not fat loss. Consuming 1 pint (473 milliliters) of fluid will replenish 1 pound (9.45 kilograms) of water weight loss. People should drink back all lost water weight even though they may not feel thirsty, as the human thirst mechanism is not a good indicator of actual need. Checking the urine is also recommended, as dark yellow urine indicates that more water consumption is needed and nearly colorless urine indicates that adequate rehydration has been achieved. Wearing light-colored, loose-fitting clothing in the heat is recommended, as rubberized or tight-weave clothing interferes with sweat evaporation and body cooling.

Other suggestions for countering dehydration include getting into good physical condition and acclimatizing to the heat. Conditioning increases the body's metabolic efficiency so that fewer of the calories burned accumulate as heat, enhances blood plasma volume to enable a larger sweat reserve, and reduces fat weight that insulates the body and retards heat dissipation. Eating a carbohydrate-enriched diet will retain water in muscle cells at a rate of nearly 3 grams of water per 1 gram of stored glycogen, whereas stored fat retains minimal water.

Perspective and Prospects

Many episodes of dehydration can be prevented from developing into heat cramps, heat exhaustion, and heatstroke during sporting events by adhering to the aforementioned guidelines. Heat cramps, especially muscle spasms in the calves and stomach, may occur during intense sweating, with the accompanying loss of electrolytes. Mineral loss, however, is always of secondary importance to fluid loss because water provides the medium in which all cellular processes occur.

Heat exhaustion occurs when increased sweating and peripheral blood flow reduce venous return of blood to the heart, resulting in cool and clammy skin, lower-than-normal blood pressure, and a rapid but weak heart rate. Less blood is pumped to the brain,

causing weakness, faintness, dizziness, headaches, and a grayish look to the face. Treatment includes lying down in a shaded, breezy place, drinking cool fluids, and removing excess clothing. Heatstroke occurs when the brain can no longer maintain thermal balance, as evidenced by the cessation of sweating, hot (sometimes white to gray) skin, rapid and full pulse, and a rise in body temperature over 104 degrees Fahrenheit leading to disorientation and unconsciousness. Heatstroke is rare but requires immediate medical attention to reduce body temperature. The body temperature should be lowered quickly by placing ice packs to the groin, neck, and under the arms. Cool sheets may be placed over and under the patient. The patient should not be allowed to shiver, which increases the body temperature. Others should be alert for seizures and the possible need to perform cardiopulmonary resuscitation (CPR). The most effective treatment is prevention through proper hydration.

—Daniel G. Graetzer, Ph.D.;
updated by Amy Webb Bull, D.S.N., A.P.N.

See also Anorexia nervosa; Appetite loss; Bulimia; Cardiovascular system; Constipation; Diabetes mellitus; Diarrhea and dysentery; Dizziness and fainting; Emergency medicine; Emergency medicine, pediatric; Enterocolitis; Exercise physiology; Fever; Headaches; Heat exhaustion and heatstroke; Malnutrition; Motion sickness; Nausea and vomiting; Nutrition; Obesity; Pyloric stenosis; Seizures; Sweating; Well-baby examinations.

For Further Information:

Brody, Jane E. "For Lifelong Gains, Just Add Water. Repeat." *The New York Times*, July 11, 2000, p. F8. The average American consumes slightly more than half the recommended amount of water per day. To avoid the symptoms of dehydration (headache, lethargy, dizziness, mental fuzziness, and loss of appetite), one should drink at least eight glasses of water per day.

McArdle, William, Frank I. Katch, and Victor L. Katch. *Exercise Physiology: Energy, Nutrition, and Human Performance.* 7th ed. Boston: Lippincott Williams & Wilkins, 2010. A wide-ranging text on exercise and the human body, covering topics such as nutrition, energy transfer, exercise training, systems of energy delivery and utilization, enhancement of energy capacity, the effect of environmental stress, and the effect of exercise on successful aging and disease prevention.

Sawka, Michael N., Samuel N. Cheuvront, and Robert Carter. "Human Water Needs." *Nutrition Reviews* 63, no. 6 (June, 2005): S30-S39. Provides information on daily water needs and the estimated amount of water intake required by an average adult male.

Sawka, Michael N., and Scott J. Montain. "Fluid and Electrolyte Supplementation for Exercise Heat Stress." *American Journal of Clinical Nutrition* 72, no. 2S (August, 2000): S564-S572. During exercise in the heat, sweat output often exceeds water intake, resulting in a body water deficit (hypohydration) and electrolyte losses. Because daily water losses can be substantial, persons need to emphasize drinking during exercise as well as at meals.

Scanlon, Valerie, and Tina Sanders. *Essentials of Anatomy and Physiology.* 5th ed. Philadelphia: F. A. Davis, 2007. A text designed around three themes: the relationship between physiology and anatomy, the interrelations among the organ systems, and the relationship of each organ system to homeostasis.

Sturt, Patty Ann. "Environmental Conditions." In *Mosby's Emergency Nursing Reference*, edited by Julia Fulz and Sturt. 3d ed. St. Louis, Mo.: Mosby/Elsevier, 2005. A helpful resource.

DELUSIONS

DISEASE/DISORDER

ANATOMY OR SYSTEM AFFECTED: Psychic-emotional system

SPECIALTIES AND RELATED FIELDS: Psychiatry, psychology

DEFINITION: False beliefs regarding the self or persons or objects outside the self that persist despite the facts and are common in paranoia, schizophrenia, and psychotic depressed states.

CAUSES AND SYMPTOMS

Clinical delusion is defined as the presence of one or more nonbizarre false beliefs, persisting for a period of at least one month. To avoid confusion, delusions are not typically linked to the direct physiological effects of a substance or a general medical condition. Determination of "nonbizarre false beliefs" may be difficult to determine. Usually "nonbizarre" refers to situations that could occur in real life; "bizarre" refers to situations that could not occur in real life.

Life management with delusions varies. Some individuals may appear relatively unimpaired in their interpersonal and occupational roles. In others, life management issues may be so severe that isolation and

---

INFORMATION ON DELUSIONS

CAUSES: Psychological disorders
SYMPTOMS: Isolation, withdrawal, impaired life management
DURATION: One month to chronic
TREATMENTS: Psychotherapy, counseling, drug therapy

---

withdrawal are common results. In general, however, life management functions are more likely to be adversely affected than cognitive or vocational activities.

TREATMENT AND THERAPY

Options for treatment and therapy vary depending on the severity of the delusions and the degrading effects on life management issues. Interventions vary depending on the theoretical orientation of the mental health professional combined with severity of the delusion. A thorough evaluation should begin the process. Clinical interviews should be combined with appropriate psychological testing and corroborative data collection. Therapy can vary from individual to group sessions, "talk" therapies to pharmacological therapy, and inpatient or outpatient venues. Delusions tend to wax and wane in intensity and degrees of severity. Maintaining good general physical health is an important part of managing delusions. Maintenance of neurochemical systems, especially neurotransmitters, with vitamin-B complex foods, is an important consideration.

PERSPECTIVE AND PROSPECTS

Delusions, in and of themselves, may not prevent successful life management functioning for most individuals. When the delusion represents a life management issue as a result of a loss of contact with reality, in the client's best interest, intervention and treatment is appropriate. Although popular media and common myths present otherwise, individuals with delusions are no more dangerous and no more aggressive than the general population. While they may be the targets of ridicule, challenge, and harassment, individuals with delusions may also reorient successfully with appropriate intervention.

—*Daniel L. Yazak, D.E.D.*

See also Antianxiety drugs; Anxiety; Hallucinations; Paranoia; Psychiatric disorders; Psychiatry; Psychiatry, child and adolescent; Psychiatry, geriatric; Psychosis; Schizophrenia.

FOR FURTHER INFORMATION:

American Psychiatric Association. *Diagnostic and Statistical Manual of Mental Disorders: DSM-IV-TR.* 4th ed. Arlington, Va.: Author, 2000.

Brems, Christiane. *Basic Skills in Psychotherapy and Counseling.* Belmont, Calif.: Brooks/Cole Thomson Learning, 2001.

Bruno, Frank J. *Psychological Symptoms.* New York: John Wiley & Sons, 1993.

Sadock, Benjamin James, and Virginia A. Sadock. *Kaplan and Sadock's Synopsis of Psychiatry: Behavioral Sciences/Clinical Psychiatry.* 10th ed. Philadelphia: Wolters Kluwer/Lippincott Williams & Wilkins, 2007.

Torrey, E. Fuller. *Surviving Schizophrenia: A Manual for Families, Consumers, and Providers.* 5th ed. New York: Collins, 2006.

DEMENTIAS

DISEASE/DISORDER

ANATOMY OR SYSTEM AFFECTED: Brain, nervous system, psychic-emotional system

SPECIALTIES AND RELATED FIELDS: Geriatrics and gerontology, neurology, psychiatry

DEFINITION: A group of disorders involving pervasive, progressive, and irreversible decline in cognitive functioning resulting from a variety of causes; differs from mental retardation, in which the affected person never reaches an expected level of mental growth.

KEY TERMS:

basal ganglia: a collection of nerve cells deep inside the brain, below the cortex, that controls muscle tone and automatic actions such as walking

cortical dementia: dementia resulting from damage to the brain cortex, the outer layer of the brain that contains the bodies of the nerve cells

delirium: an acute condition characterized by confusion, a fluctuating level of consciousness, and visual, auditory, and even tactile hallucinations; often caused by acute disease, such as infection or intoxication

hydrocephalus: a condition resulting from the accumulation of fluid inside the brain in cavities known as ventricles; as fluid accumulates, it exerts pressure on the neighboring brain cells, which may be destroyed

subcortical dementia: dementia resulting from damage to the area of the brain below the cortex; this area contains nerve fibers that connect various parts of the brain with one another and with the basal ganglia

vascular dementia: dementia caused by repeated strokes, resulting in interference with the blood supply to parts of the brain

CAUSES AND SYMPTOMS

Dementia affects between four and five million people in the United States and is a major cause of disability in individuals over sixty. Its prevalence increases with age. Dementia is characterized by a permanent memory deficit affecting recent memory in particular and of sufficient severity to interfere with the patient's ability to take part in professional and social activities. Dementia is not part of the normal aging process. It also is not synonymous with benign senescent forgetfulness, which is more common and affects recent memory. Although the latter is a source of frustration, it does not significantly interfere with the individual's professional and social activities because it tends to affect only trivial matters (or what the individual considers trivial). Furthermore, patients with benign forgetfulness usually can remember what was forgotten by utilizing a number of strategies, such as writing lists or notes to themselves and leaving them in conspicuous places. Individuals with benign forgetfulness also are acutely aware of their memory deficit, while those with dementia, except in the early stages of the disease or for specific types of dementia, generally have no insight into their memory deficit and often blame others for their problems.

In addition to the memory deficit interfering with the patient's daily activities, patients with dementia often show evidence of impaired abstract thinking, impaired judgment, or other disturbances of higher cortical functions such as aphasia (the inability to use or comprehend language), apraxia (the inability to execute complex, coordinated movements), or agnosia (the inability to recognize familiar objects).

INFORMATION ON DEMENTIAS

CAUSES: Aging, diseases (Alzheimer's, Pick's, Parkinson's), stroke, chronic infections, head trauma

SYMPTOMS: Impaired abstract thinking, impaired judgment, inability to use or comprehend language, inability to recognize familiar objects, inability to execute complex movements

DURATION: Chronic

TREATMENTS: None; alleviation of symptoms

Dementia may result from damage to the cerebral cortex (the outer layer of the brain), as in Alzheimer's disease, or from damage to the subcortical structures (the structures below the cortex), such as white matter, the thalamus, or the basal ganglia. Although memory is impaired in both cortical and subcortical dementias, the associated features are different. In cortical dementias, for example, cognitive functions such as the ability to understand speech and to talk and the ability to perform mathematical calculations are severely impaired. In subcortical dementias, on the other hand, there is evidence of disturbances of arousal, motivation, and mood, in addition to a significant slowing of cognition and of information processing.

Alzheimer's disease, the most common cause of presenile dementia, is characterized by progressive disorientation, memory loss, speech disturbances, and personality disorders. Pick's disease is another cortical dementia, but unlike Alzheimer's disease, it is rare, tends to affect younger patients, and is more common in women. In the early stages of Pick's disease, changes in personality, absence of inhibition, inappropriate social and sexual conduct, and lack of foresight may be evident—features that are not common in Alzheimer's disease. Patients also may become euphoric or apathetic. Poverty of speech is often present and gradually progresses to mutism, although speech comprehension is usually spared. Pick's disease is characterized by cortical atrophy localized to the frontal and temporal lobes.

Vascular dementia is the second most common cause of dementia in patients over the age of sixty-five and is responsible for 8 percent to 20 percent of all dementia cases. It is caused by interference with the blood flow to the brain. Although the overall prevalence of vascular dementia is decreasing, there are some geographical variations, with the prevalence being higher in countries with a high incidence of cardiovascular and cerebrovascular diseases, such as Finland and Japan. About 20 percent of patients with dementia have both Alzheimer's disease and vascular dementia. Several types of vascular dementia have been identified.

Multiple infarct dementia (MID) is the most common type of vascular dementia. As its name implies, it is the result of multiple, discrete cerebral infarcts (strokes) that have destroyed enough brain tissue to interfere with the patient's higher mental functions. The onset of MID is usually sudden and is associated with neurological deficit, such as the paralysis or weakness of an arm or leg or the inability to speak. The disease characteristically progresses in steps: With each stroke experienced, the patient's condition suddenly deteriorates and then stabilizes or even improves slightly until another stroke occurs. In about 20 percent of patients with MID, however, the disease displays an insidious onset and causes gradual deterioration. Most patients also show evidence of arteriosclerosis and other factors predisposing them to the development of strokes, such as hypertension, cigarette smoking, high blood cholesterol, diabetes mellitus, narrowing of one or both carotid arteries, or cardiac disorders, especially atrial fibrillation (an irregular heartbeat). Somatic complaints, mood changes, depression, and nocturnal confusion tend to be more common in vascular dementias, although there is relative preservation of the patient's personality. In such cases, magnetic resonance imaging (MRI) or a computed tomography (CT) scan of the brain often shows evidence of multiple strokes.

Strokes are not always associated with clinical evidence of neurological deficits, since the stroke may affect a "silent" area of the brain or may be so small that its immediate impact is not noticeable. Nevertheless, when several of these small strokes have occurred, the resulting loss of brain tissue may interfere with the patient's cognitive functions. This is, in fact, the basis of the lacunar dementias. The infarcted tissue is absorbed into the rest of the brain, leaving a small cavity or lacuna. Brain-imaging techniques and especially MRI are useful in detecting these lacunae.

A number of neurological disorders are associated with dementia. The combination of dementia, urinary incontinence, and muscle rigidity causing difficulties in walking should raise the suspicion of hydrocephalus. In this condition, fluid accumulates inside the ventricles (cavities within the brain) and results in increased pressure on the brain cells. A CT scan demonstrates enlargement of the ventricles. Although some patients may respond well to surgical shunting of the cerebrospinal fluid, it is often difficult to identify those who will benefit from surgery. Postoperative complications are significant and include strokes and subdural hematomas.

Dementia has been linked to Parkinson's disease, a chronic, progressive neurological disorder that usually manifests itself in middle or late life. It has an insidious onset and a very slow progression rate. Although intellectual deterioration is not part of the classical features of Parkinson's disease, dementia is being recognized as a late manifestation of the disease, with as many as one-third of the patients eventually being afflicted. The dementing process also has an insidious onset and slow progression rate. Some of the medication used to treat Parkinson's disease also may induce confusion, particularly in older patients.

Subdural hematomas (collections of blood inside the brain) may lead to mental impairment and are usually precipitated by trauma to the head. Usually, the trauma is slight and the patient neither loses consciousness nor experiences any immediate significant effects. A few days or even weeks later, however, the patient may develop evidence of mental impairment. By that time, the patient and caregivers may have forgotten about the slight trauma that the patient had experienced. A subdural hematoma should be suspected in the presence of a fairly sudden onset and progressing course. Headaches are common. A CT scan can reveal the presence of a hematoma. The surgical removal of the hematoma is usually associated with a good prognosis if the surgery is done in a timely manner, before irreversible brain damage occurs.

Brain tumors may lead to dementia, particularly if they are slow growing. Most tumors of this type can be diagnosed by CT scanning or MRI. Occasionally, cancer may induce dementia through an inflammation of the brain.

Many chronic infections affecting the brain can lead to dementia; they include conditions that, when treated, may reverse or prevent the progression of dementia, such as syphilis, tuberculosis, slow viruses, and some fungal and protozoal infections. Human immunodeficiency virus (HIV) infection is also a cause of dementia, and it may be suspected if the rate of progress is rapid and the patient has risk factors for the development of HIV infection. Although the dementia is part of the acquired immunodeficiency syndrome (AIDS) complex, it may occasionally be the first manifestation of the disease.

It is often difficult to differentiate depression from dementia. Nevertheless, sudden onset—especially if preceded by an emotional event, the presence of sleep disturbances, and a history of previous psychiatric illness—is suggestive of depression. The level of mental functioning of patients with depression is often inconsistent. They may, for example, be able to give clear accounts of topics that are of personal interest to them but be very vague about, and at times may not even attempt to answer, questions on topics that are of no interest to them. Variability in performance during testing is suggestive of depression, especially if it improves with positive reinforcement.

TREATMENT AND THERAPY

It is estimated that dementia affects about 1 percent of the population aged sixty to sixty-four years. By age eighty-five and higher, however, it affects anywhere from 30 to 50 percent of individuals. While different surveys may yield different results, depending on the criteria used to define dementia, it is clear that this is a significant problem.

For physicians, an important aspect of diagnosing patients with dementia is detecting potentially reversible causes that may be responsible for the impaired mental functions. A detailed history followed by a meticulous and thorough clinical examination and a few selected laboratory tests are usually sufficient to reach a diagnosis. Various investigators have estimated that reversible causes of dementia can be identified in 10 percent to 20 percent of patients with dementia. Recommended investigations include brain imaging (CT scanning or MRI), a complete blood count, and tests of erythrocyte sedimentation rate, blood glucose, serum electrolytes, serum calcium, liver function, thyroid function, and serum B_{12} and folate. Some investigators also recommend routine testing for syphilis. Other tests, such as those for the detection of HIV infection, cerebrospinal fluid examination, neuropsychological testing, drug and toxin screening, serum copper and ceruloplasmin analysis, carotid and cerebral angiography, and electroencephalography, are performed when appropriate.

It is of paramount importance for health care providers to adopt a positive attitude when managing patients with dementia. Although at present little can be done to treat and reverse dementia, it is important to identify the cause of the dementia. In some cases, it may be possible to prevent the disease from progressing. For example, if the dementia is the result of hypertension, adequate control of this condition may prevent further brain damage. Moreover, the prevalence of vascular dementia is decreasing in countries where efforts to reduce cardiovascular and cerebrovascular diseases have been successful. Similarly, if the dementia is the result of repeated emboli (blood clots reaching the brain) complicating atrial fibrillation, then anticoagulants or aspirin may be recommended.

Even after a diagnosis of dementia is made, it is important for the physician to detect the presence of other conditions that may worsen the patient's mental functions, such as the inadvertent intake of medications that may induce confusion and mental impairment. Medications with this potential are numerous and include not only those that act on the brain, such as sedatives and hypnotics, but also hypotensive agents (especially if given in large doses), diuretics, and antibiotics. Whenever the condition of a patient with dementia deteriorates, the physician meticulously reviews all the medications that the patient is taking, both medical prescriptions and medications that may have been purchased over the counter. Even if innocuous, some over-the-counter preparations may interact with other medications that the patient is taking and lead to a worsening of mental functions. Inquiries are also made into the patient's alcohol intake. The brain of an older person is much more sensitive to the effects of alcohol than that of a younger person, and some medications may interact with the alcohol to impair the patient's cognitive functions further.

Many other disease states also may worsen the patient's mental functions. For example, patients with diabetes mellitus are susceptible to developing a variety of metabolic abnormalities including a low or high blood glucose level, both of which may be associated with confusional states. Similarly, dehydration and acid-base or electrolyte disorders, which may result from prolonged vomiting or diarrhea, may also precipitate confusional states. Infections, particularly respiratory and urinary tract infections, often worsen the patient's cognitive deficit. Finally, patients with dementia may experience myocardial infarctions (heart attacks) that are not associated with any chest pain but that may manifest themselves with confusion.

The casual observer of the dementing process is often overwhelmed with concern for the patient, but it is the family that truly suffers. The patients themselves experience no physical pain or distress, and except in the very early stages of the disease, they are oblivious to their plight as a result of their loss of insight. Health care professionals therefore are alert to the stress imposed on the caregivers by dealing with loved ones with dementia. Adequate support from agencies available in the community is essential.

When a diagnosis of dementia is made, the physician discusses a number of ethical, financial, and legal issues with the family, and also the patient if it is believed that he or she can understand the implications of this discussion. Families are encouraged to make a list of all the patient's assets, including insurance policies, and to discuss this information with an attorney to protect the patient's and the family's assets. If the patient is still competent, it is recommended that he or she select a trusted person to have durable power of attorney. Un-

like the regular power of attorney, the former does not become invalidated when the patient becomes mentally incompetent and continues to be in effect regardless of the degree of mental impairment of the person who executed it. Because durable power of attorney cannot be easily reversed once the person is incompetent, great care should be taken when selecting a person, and the specific powers granted should be clearly specified. It is also important for the patient to make his or her desires known concerning advance directives and the use of life support systems.

Courts may appoint a guardian or conservator to have charge and custody of the patient's property (including real estate and money) when no responsible family members or friends are willing or available to serve as guardian. Courts supervise the actions of the guardian, who is expected to report all the patient's income and expenditures to the court once a year. The court may also charge the guardian to ensure that the patient is adequately housed, fed, and clothed and receiving appropriate medical care.

PERSPECTIVE AND PROSPECTS

Dementia is a very serious and common condition, especially among the older population. Dementia permanently robs patients of their minds and prevents them from functioning adequately in their environment by impairing memory and interfering with the ability to make rational decisions. It therefore deprives patients of their dignity and independence.

Because dementia is mostly irreversible, cannot be adequately treated at present, and is associated with a fairly long survival period, it has a significant impact not only on the patient's life but also on the patient's family and caregivers and on society in general. The expense of long-term care for patients with dementia, whether at home or in institutions, is staggering. Every effort, therefore, is made to reach an accurate diagnosis and especially to detect any other condition that may worsen the patient's underlying dementia. Finally, health care professionals do not treat the patient in isolation but also concern themselves with the impact of the illness on the patient's caregivers and family.

Much progress has been made in defining dementia and determining its cause. Terms such as "senile dementia" are no longer in use, and even the use of the term "dementia" to diagnose a patient's condition is frowned upon because there are so many types of dementia. The recognition of the type of dementia affecting a particular patient is important because of its practical implications, both for the patient and for research into the prevention, management, and treatment of dementia. The prevalence of vascular dementia, for example, is decreasing in many countries where the prevention of cardiovascular diseases such as hypertension and arteriosclerosis has been successful.

Unfortunately, there is little that can be done to cure dementia and no effective means to regenerate nerve cells. Researchers, however, are feverishly trying to identify factors that control the growth and regeneration of nerve cells. Although no single medication is expected to be of benefit to all types of dementia, it is hoped that effective therapy for many dementias will be developed.

—*Ronald C. Hamdy, M.D.,*
Louis A. Cancellaro, M.D.,
and Larry Hudgins, M.D.;
updated by Nancy A. Piotrowski, Ph.D.

See also Aging; Aging: Extended care; Alzheimer's disease; Amnesia; Brain; Brain disorders; Delusions; Frontotemporal dementia (FTD); Hallucinations; Hospice; Memory loss; Parkinson's disease; Pick's disease; Psychiatric disorders; Psychiatry; Psychiatry, geriatric; Strokes; Terminally ill: Extended care.

FOR FURTHER INFORMATION:

Ballard, Clive, et al. *Dementia: Management of Behavioural and Psychological Symptoms*. New York: Oxford University Press, 2001. Details the nature of dementia symptoms, assesses their severity, and recommends a structured and sequential approach to management.

Coons, Dorothy H., ed. *Specialized Dementia Care Units*. Baltimore: Johns Hopkins University Press, 1991. A collection of articles reviewing the benefits and disadvantages of caring for patients with dementia in specialized care units. Several problems encountered when running such units are addressed.

Dana.org. http://www.dana.org. A nonprofit organization of neuroscientists, which was formed to provide information about the personal and public benefits of brain research. The Web site is research oriented and gives excellent information and links on current brain studies, new diagnosis and treatment technology, and brain-related news stories.

Hamdy, Ronald C., J. M. Turnbull, and M. M. Lancaster, eds. *Alzheimer's Disease: A Handbook for Caregivers*. 3d ed. St. Louis, Mo.: Mosby Year Book, 1998. A comprehensive discussion of the symptoms and characteristic features of Alzheimer's disease and other dementias. Abnormal brain structure and function in these patients are discussed, and the normal effects of aging are reviewed.

Howe, M. L., M. J. Stones, and C. J. Brainerd, eds. *Cognitive and Behavioral Performance Factors in Atypical Aging*. New York: Springer, 1990. A review of the factors controlling behavior, test performance, and brain function in both young and older patients.

Kovach, Christine, ed. *Late-Stage Dementia Care: A Basic Guide*. Washington, D.C.: Taylor & Francis, 1997. Provides information on assessment and treatment management for individuals experiencing dementia. A valuable source for caregivers and family members of those affected.

Mace, Nancy L., and Peter V. Rabins. *The Thirty-six-Hour Day: A Family Guide to Caring for People with Alzheimer Disease, Other Dementias, and Memory Loss in Later Life*. 4th ed. Baltimore: Johns Hopkins University Press, 2006. Provides a wealth of information for families coping with Alzheimer's disease, including topics such as the evaluation of persons with dementia, hospice care, assisted living facilities and financing care, and the latest findings on eating and nutrition.

O'Brien, John, et al., eds. *Dementia*. 3d ed. New York: Oxford University Press, 2006. Text that covers advances in the research of degenerative disorders, current diagnostic criteria, rating scales, investigations, neurobiological mechanisms, therapeutic options and services, and all aspects of management, including psychosocial and psychological approaches, among other topics.

U.S. Congress. Office of Technology Assessment. *Confused Minds, Burdened Families: Finding Help for People with Alzheimer's and Other Dementias*. Washington, D.C.: Government Printing Office, 1990. A report from the Office of Technology Assessment analyzing the problems of locating and arranging services for people with dementia in the United States.

DENGUE FEVER

DISEASE/DISORDER

ALSO KNOWN AS: Break-bone fever

ANATOMY OR SYSTEM AFFECTED: Bones, eyes, glands, gums, head, mouth, musculoskeletal system, nose, skin

SPECIALTIES AND RELATED FIELDS: Family medicine, internal medicine, microbiology, public health, virology

DEFINITION: A flulike viral illness, contracted by humans through the bite of an infected *Aedes* mosquito.

KEY TERMS:

endemic: something commonly found in a specific geographic area or population

Flaviviridae: a family of single-strand RNA viruses that spread via mosquitoes and ticks

INFORMATION ON DENGUE FEVER

CAUSES: Viral infection transmitted by mosquitoes

SYMPTOMS: High fever, rash, joint and muscle pain, vomiting

DURATION: Subacute

TREATMENTS: Symptomatic treatment

CAUSES AND SYMPTOMS

Although dengue fever is primarily confined to the tropics, each year it causes more than 50 million infections worldwide. Dengue is caused by the dengue virus (DENV) that belongs to the Flaviviridae family. This viral family includes several other members, such as the yellow fever virus and the West Nile encephalitis virus, all of which have emerged as serious public health concerns over the years. All four serotypes of dengue virus (DENV-1 through DENV-4) are capable of causing the full spectrum of clinical manifestations, from asymptomatic presentation to dengue fever to the more severe dengue hemorrhagic fever or dengue shock syndrome. These forms are primarily found in hyperendemic areas that have all four serotypes of dengue virus.

Dengue virus enters the human host via the bite of an infected *Aedes* mosquito, primarily *A. aegypti* and occasionally *A. albopictus.* These vector populations are difficult to control because they are highly invasive and over time have accumulated adaptations that make them extremely resilient. The disease spreads from an infected individual to a healthy host through the bite of the *Aedes* mosquito. Once inside the mosquito, following a blood meal, the dengue virus needs to incubate for about eight to twelve days in the mosquito before it can initiate another round of infection in a healthy host. An *Aedes* mosquito that has acquired the dengue virus will forever act as a vector.

After being bitten by the infected *Aedes* mosquito, a human host will typically start showing symptoms anywhere between four to seven days; they last for as long as three to ten days. Once inside the human body, the dengue virus first replicates inside the dendritic cells. The replicated virus then infects macrophages and lymphocytes before entering the patient's bloodstream. Dengue fever patients can show a variety of symptoms, from mild feverishness to high fever of abrupt onset along with severe headache, pain behind the eyes (retro-orbital pain), flushing of the face, generalized joint and muscle pains, nausea, vomiting, and rash.

In dengue hemorrhagic and dengue shock syndrome, the more severe forms of dengue, clinical manifestations include fever, hemorrhage (diagnosed with a tourniquet test), low platelet count (thrombocytopenia), and increased vascular permeability. Some signs of hemorrhage seen in dengue hemorrhagic fever patients include pinpoint-sized red dots (petechiae), fragile capillaries that could lead to passage of blood from the ruptured blood vessels into subcutaneous tissue (purpura), and blood stains in vomit and stool (melena). The severity of dengue hemorrhagic fever is dependent on the extent of plasma leakage (detected by a rise in hematocrit level) from the capillaries that results in hypovolemia. As plasma continues to leak into the interstitial spaces, the patient can go into hypovolemic shock, a situation that can be fatal. These symptoms are typically accompanied by liver failure and hepatomegaly (increase in liver size). Concomitantly, as one would expect, viremia (the presence of virus in the bloodstream) titers are much more pronounced in cases of dengue hemorrhagic fever and dengue shock syndrome as compared to dengue fever.

Clinical diagnosis of dengue virus infection is based on signs of leukopenia (low white blood cell count), thrombocytopenia, and high serum transaminase levels in blood tests. Since rash is a common component of dengue fever, often the extent, nature, and location of the rash is used in the diagnostic process—for example, dengue rash is usually seen on the trunk and inner surfaces of the thighs and arms. With an increase in number of dengue cases, some unusual neurological complications such as convulsions, spasticity, and encephalopathy (resulting from water intoxication) have also been reported. To date, the exact molecular mechanism that underlies the pathogenesis seen in dengue hemorrhagic fever and dengue shock syndrome is not very well understood and is still under investigation.

TREATMENT AND THERAPY

Patients who have been diagnosed with dengue virus infection are required to maintain adequate hydration levels. Often the key to successful management of a patient with dengue hemorrhagic fever or dengue shock syndrome involves a careful monitoring of the patient's fluid level and replenishing any deficits with isotonic solution administered intravenously. Antipyretics such as acetaminophen are used for pain and fever management. Patients are advised to avoid using aspirin and nonsteroidal anti-inflammatory drugs (NSAIDs), since they may accentuate the bleeding problem associated with certain types of dengue infection.

The adaptive immune response of the patient plays an important role in clearing of the infection as well as providing immunity against reinfection. Infection with a DENV serotype (1-4) protects the individual only against reinfection by the same serotype. Since there are four serotypes of dengue virus, in theory a person can get dengue as many as four times during his or her lifetime. Efforts are underway to design a vaccine; the ideal vaccine would provide lifelong protection against all four DENV serotypes. Dengue vaccine candidates that are currently being investigated include live attenuated vaccines, inactivated virus vaccines, recombinant subunit vaccines, and deoxyribonucleic acid (DNA) vaccines.

PERSPECTIVE AND PROSPECTS

Dengue is considered an emerging infectious disease. As with the Ebola virus, the four serotypes are believed to have originated in monkeys and then mutated to move on to the human host several hundred years ago. Until the mid-twentieth century, dengue was largely a localized infection, primarily affecting populations in Africa and Southeast Asia. It is believed that the spread of the *Aedes* mosquito vector, and thus the dengue virus pathogen, via cargo ships to different parts of the world contributed to the global threat that the world is currently experiencing. A minimum of 2.5 billion people live in areas where dengue virus is endemic, and the number of dengue cases has gone up thirty-fold since the mid-twentieth century.

—Sibani Sengupta, Ph.D.

See also Bleeding; Ebola virus; Encephalitis; Epidemiology; Fever; Hemorrhage; Marburg virus; Tropical medicine; Viral hemorrhagic fevers; Viral infections; West Nile virus; Yellow fever; Zoonoses.

FOR FURTHER INFORMATION:

Halstead, S. B. "More Dengue, More Questions." *Emerging Infectious Diseases* 11, no. 5 (May, 2005): 740-741.

U.S. Department of Health and Human Services, Centers for Disease Control and Prevention, Division of Vector-Borne Infectious Diseases (DVBID). *Dengue and Dengue Hemorrhagic Fever: Information for Health Care Practitioners*. (2007). Available at http://www.cdc.gov/NCIDOD/dvbid/dengue/dengue-hcp.htm.

Whitehead, S. S., et al. "Prospects for a Dengue Virus Vaccine." *Nature Reviews Microbiology* 5 (July, 2007): 518-528.

DENTAL DISEASES
DISEASE/DISORDER

ANATOMY OR SYSTEM AFFECTED: Gums, mouth, teeth

SPECIALTIES AND RELATED FIELDS: Dentistry

DEFINITION: Diseases that affect the teeth, such as dental caries, and the gums, such as gingivitis, pyorrhea, or cancer.

KEY TERMS:

dental caries: tooth decay

dentin: a hard, bonelike tissue lying beneath the tooth enamel

enamel: the hard surface covering of teeth

gingivae: the soft tissue surrounding the teeth; the gums

gingivitis: an inflammation of the gums

periodontal diseases: diseases characterized by inflammation of the gingivae

pyorrhea: the second stage of gingivitis

tooth pulp: the tissue at the center of teeth, surrounded by dentin

Vincent's infection: a bacterial infection of the gingivae, also known as trench mouth

CAUSES AND SYMPTOMS

Dental diseases fall into four major categories: dental caries, or tooth decay; periodontal disease, including gingivitis and pyorrhea; Vincent's infection, or trench mouth; and oral cancer. The first of these diseases was the largest contributor to tooth loss among people under thirty-five in the United States before the widespread fluoridation of drinking water was begun; it remains a major cause of tooth loss in much of the world. Periodontal disease in its two stages, gingivitis and pyorrhea, is the most widespread dental problem for people over thirty-five. Most people who suffer the loss of all of their teeth are victims of this condition. Vincent's infection, which shares many characteristics with gingivitis, is bacterial. The infection flares up, is treated, and disappears, whereas gingivitis is more often a continuing condition that requires both persistent home treatment and specialized treatment. The most serious but least frequently occurring dental disease is oral cancer. It is the only dental disease commonly considered life-threatening, and there is a risk that it may spread to other parts of the body.

Dental caries occur because the food that one eats becomes trapped in the irregularities of the teeth, creating lactic acids that penetrate the enamel through holes (often microscopic) in it. Once lodged between the teeth or below the gum line, carbohydrates and starches combine with saliva to form acids that, over time, can penetrate a tooth's enamel, enter the dentin directly below it, and progressively destroy the dentin while spreading toward the tooth's center, the pulp.

This process often is not confined to a single tooth. As decay spreads, adjoining teeth may be affected. Some people have much harder tooth enamel than others. Therefore, some individuals may experience little or no decay, whereas others who follow similar diets and practice similar methods of dental hygiene may develop substantial decay.

Toothache occurs when decay eats through the dentin and enters the nerve-filled dental pulp, causing inflammation, infection, and pain. A dull, continuous ache, either mild or severe and often pulsating, may indicate that the infection has entered the jawbone beneath the tooth. An aching or sensitivity in the back teeth during chewing is sometimes a side effect of sinusitis.

One of dentistry's nagging problems is periodontal disease, which results from a buildup of calculus, or

INFORMATION ON DENTAL DISEASES

CAUSES: Tooth decay, periodontal disease (gingivitis, pyorrhea), Vincent's infection (trench mouth), oral cancer
SYMPTOMS: Vary; may include dull, continuous ache; gum soreness, swelling, and bleeding; receding gums forming pockets for infections; bone destruction and tooth loss; fever; persistent mouth sores
DURATION: Short-term to chronic
TREATMENTS: Dependent on condition; may include medications (dextrose, antibiotics), tooth implantation, gum surgery, laser treatment, radiation, chemotherapy, surgery

tartar, formed by hardened plaque. Plaque is formed when food, particularly carbohydrates and starches, interacts with the saliva that coats the teeth, creating a yellowish film. If this film is not removed, it inevitably lodges between the gums and the teeth, where, within twenty-four hours, it hardens into calculus. Dental hygienists can remove most of this calculus mechanically. If it is allowed to build up over extended periods, however, the calculus will irritate the gums, causing the soreness, swelling, and bleeding that signal gum infection. Eventually, this infection becomes entrenched and difficult to treat.

Periodontists can control but not cure most periodontal disease. In its early manifestations, periodontal disease results in gingivitis, marked by inflammation and bleeding. Untreated, it progresses to pyorrhea, which is characterized by gums that recede from the teeth and form pockets in which infections flourish. As pyorrhea advances, the bone that underlies the teeth and holds them in place is compromised and ultimately destroyed, causing looseness and eventual tooth loss.

Vincent's infection (trench mouth) is communicable through kissing or sharing eating utensils. Although it is sometimes mistaken for gingivitis, Vincent's infection has one distinguishing characteristic that gingivitis does not have: It is accompanied by a fever stemming from sustained bacterial infection, which also causes extremely foul breath. Vincent's infection is curable through proper treatment. It is unlikely to recur unless one is again exposed to the infection.

Oral cancer is the most serious of oral diseases. It often spreads quickly, destroying the tissues of the mouth during its ravaging advance. It not only threatens its original site but also can spread to other areas of the body and to vital organs. Fortunately, oral cancer is uncommon. Nevertheless, dentists look vigilantly for signs of it when they perform mouth examinations because early detection is vital to successful treatment, containment, and cure. People who have persistent mouth sores that do not heal may be experiencing the early manifestations of oral cancer and should see their dentists or physicians immediately.

Two other dental conditions afflict many people: malocclusion and toothache. Malocclusion occurs when, for a variety of reasons, the teeth are out of alignment. People with malocclusion are prime candidates for dental caries and periodontal disease, largely because their teeth are difficult to reach and hard to clean. Malocclusion may also cause one or more teeth to strike the teeth above or below them, causing injury to teeth and possibly fracturing them.

TREATMENT AND THERAPY

Modern dentistry has succeeded in controlling most dental diseases. In the United States, dental caries have been almost eliminated in the young by the addition of fluoride to most water systems. Used over time, fluoride strengthens the teeth by increasing the hardness of the enamel, making it resistant to the acids that form in the mouth and cause decay.

Since the 1950's, most American children have been reared on fluoridated water. Those whose water supply is not fluoridated have usually had their teeth treated with fluoride by their dentists. Many have brushed their teeth regularly with fluoridated toothpaste, which offers considerable protection from dental caries. From the 1950's to the 1990's, fluoride reduced dental decay in Americans under the age of twenty-one by more than 70 percent.

Current research into ways of preventing dental decay centers on several projects of the National Institute of Dental Research. Researchers for this organization discovered in the mid-1960's that a substance found in the mouth's streptococcal bacteria creates dextran. Dextran enables bacteria to cling to the surface of the teeth and invade them with the lactic acid that they generate. Researchers ultimately discovered dextrase, an enzyme effective in dissolving dextran. Strides are being made to use dextrase in toothpaste or mouthwash to reduce or eliminate the effects of dextran.

Some people's teeth seem to be impervious to tooth decay. It has been determined that such people have a common substance in their blood that protects their teeth from dental caries. Attempts are being made to identify and isolate this substance and to make it generally available to the public and to dentists in an applicable form. Some dentists coat the teeth with a durable plastic substance to make them resistant to penetration by the acids that cause dental decay, creating a hard protective coating above the enamel and making it difficult for food to lodge between the teeth or in irregularities in the teeth.

Because malocclusion, or poor spacing, can lead to tooth decay, dentists have become increasingly aware of the need to replace lost teeth so that the alignment of the remaining teeth will not be disturbed. Tooth implantation, a process by which a tooth, either artificial or natural, is anchored directly and permanently in the gum, solves many dental problems that in the past were

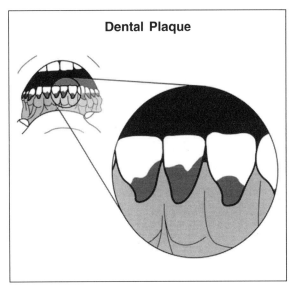

Dental Plaque

Plaque—a buildup of bacteria, mucus, and food debris— leads to dental caries (tooth decay) if not regularly removed by brushing, flossing, and professional tooth cleaning.

addressed by attaching artificial teeth to existing ones beside them. In situations where malocclusion is caused by malformations, the use of orthodontic braces results in a more regular alignment.

Nutrition has come to the forefront of recent research in dental health. A lack of calciferol, a form of vitamin D_2, may result in dental abnormalities, including malocclusion. Among substantial numbers of hospital patients who suffer from nutritional problems, the earliest symptoms occur in the soft tissue of the mouth.

Brushing the teeth after meals and before bed controls plaque, as does regular flossing. Such daily attention must be supplemented by twice-yearly cleaning, performed by a dentist or dental hygienist, and by annual or biennial whole-mouth X rays to reveal incipient decay. Various mouthwashes also contain substances that control decay.

People who cannot brush after every meal should use a mouthwash or rinse the mouth out with water after eating, then brush as soon as they can. Special attention must be given to the back surfaces of the lower front teeth because the salivary glands are located there. This area is a breeding ground for the bacteria that cause the formation of lactic acid. Routine home care of this kind, particularly daily flossing, will help prevent both tooth decay and periodontal disease, and can also reverse some of the inroads that periodontal disease has made. When gingivitis advances to pyorrhea, however, dental surgery may be indicated.

The major villain in both gingivitis and pyorrhea is tartar, or calculus, which is produced when plaque hardens. When tartar accumulates beneath the gums, it causes an irritation that can lead to infection. Sometimes, this infection moves to other parts of the body, causing joint problems and other difficulties.

People can control plaque by practicing daily dental hygiene at home. They must also have accumulated tartar regularly scraped away or removed by ultrasound in the dentist's office. Malocclusions and defects in the production of saliva can be corrected by dentists and can greatly reduce the progress of periodontal disease.

When gum surgery is advised for the removal of the deep gum pockets that occur with pyorrhea, further surgery can usually be avoided by regular home care. Meanwhile, researchers are trying to develop a vaccine to immunize its recipients against the bacteria that cause tooth decay. Other decay-inhibiting agents are being studied closely with the expectation that they may in time be added to common foods and beverages.

Vincent's infection is successfully treated with antibiotics, accompanied by a prescribed course of dental hygiene that is begun in the dentist's office and continues at home on a daily basis. Some patients have found a peroxide mouthwash helpful in treating this disease.

When dentists find evidence of oral cancer, they usually refer patients to their primary physicians, who coordinate referrals to oncologists. An oncologist will determine if the patient has cancer and will determine the best ways to treat it. Laser treatment and radiation are used in controlling oral cancer, as are chemotherapy and surgery. The most important element in cancer treatment is time. It is essential, therefore, that specialized treatment be initiated as soon as oral cancer is discovered or suspected. In cases of oral cancer, a delay of even days can affect outcomes negatively.

The most immediate treatments for toothache range from the application of cold compresses to the taking of aspirin or some other analgesic every few hours. If the decayed part of the tooth is visible and reachable, sometimes applying a mixture of oil of cloves and benzocaine to the decayed area with a small swab soothes the pain. These treatments, however, offer only temporary relief.

Dentists resist treating toothache by removing the tooth, although removal offers an immediate solution to the problem. In some cases, dentists can drill out the decay and fill the tooth with silver amalgam, gold, or plastic. Quite often, by the time a tooth begins to ache, the pulp and dentin have been ravaged by decay. The best solution is endodontistry, or root canal, which will preserve the tooth but may necessitate the attachment of a crown.

Perspective and Prospects

Great strides have been made in the United States in preventing and treating dental disease, as researchers have reached deeper understandings of the root causes of such disease. Dentistry has become increasingly less painful through the use of anesthetics and high-speed, water-cooled drills. The public at large has grown aware of the close relationship between dental health and general health. People are unwilling to accept tooth loss as a natural consequence of aging. They have also begun to realize that orthodontistry is more than a cosmetic procedure. Rather, it is a necessary procedure for correcting misalignments of the teeth that can result in difficulty if uncorrected.

National attention has been given to preventing tooth decay through the fluoridation of water supplies and, although some groups still fight fluoridation, it is for most Americans an accepted fact of modern life. Fluoridation, more than any other factor, has changed the emphasis in dentistry from preventing and treating dental caries to more sophisticated pursuits such as orthodontistry, endodontistry, and periodontistry. The establishment of the National Institute for Dental Research by Congress in 1948 has, more than any other single factor, stimulated dental research in the United States.

Advances in preventing and treating dental disease are constantly being made. Through genetic engineering, it is almost inevitable that substances will soon be available to increase an individual's resistance to tooth decay. Nevertheless, controlling the buildup of calculus, the major factor in periodontal disease, will probably remain the responsibility of individuals through daily home care and twice-yearly visits to their dentists.

—*R. Baird Shuman, Ph.D.*

See also Canker sores; Cavities; Crowns and bridges; Dentistry; Dentistry, pediatric; Dentures; Endodontic disease; Fluoride treatments; Fracture repair; Gingivitis; Gum disease; Jaw wiring; Oral and maxillofacial surgery; Orthodontics; Periodontal surgery; Periodontitis; Plaque, dental; Root canal treatment; Teeth; Teething; Tooth extraction; Toothache; Wisdom teeth.

For Further Information:

Anderson, Pauline C., and Alice E. Pendleton. *The Dental Assistant*. 7th ed. Albany, N.Y.: Delmar, 2001.

Designed as a textbook for dental hygienists, this popular volume is particularly clear in its discussion of periodontal disease and dental caries. Although it is not directed specifically to laypersons, the book is easily accessible to nonspecialized readers.

Diamond, Richard. *Dental First Aid for Families*. Ravensdale, Wash.: Idyll Arbor, 2000. Retired dentist Diamond discusses what to do when a dental problem arises and an immediate visit to the dentist is impossible. His practical, easy-to-understand advice is built on just enough basic science to put dental problems in context.

Fairpo, Jenifer E. H., and C. Gavin Fairpo. *Heinemann Dental Dictionary*. 4th ed. Boston: Butterworth-Heinemann, 1997. This is the fourth edition of a dictionary of dental and medical terms that includes several quick-reference charts on anatomy, abbreviations, and journals. The purpose is to provide a reference for dental students and other professional and nonprofessional people associated with the science and practice of dentistry.

Foster, Malcolm S. *Protecting Our Children's Teeth: A Guide to Quality Dental Care from Infancy Through Age Twelve*. New York: Insight Books, 1992. This book, written especially for parents, is clear and easy to understand. The illustrations, too, are useful. A good starting point.

Gluck, George M., and William M. Morganstein. *Jong's Community Dental Health*. 5th ed. St. Louis, Mo.: Mosby, 2003. Explores the role of dentistry in public health, examining such topics as dental care delivery, demographic shifts and dental health, distribution of dental disease and prevention, and research in dental public health.

Langlais, Robert P., and Craig S. Miller. *Color Atlas of Common Oral Diseases*. 4th ed. Philadelphia: Lippincott Williams & Wilkins, 2009. Provides six hundred color photographs of the most commonly seen oral problems accompanied by descriptive text for each condition.

Newman, Michael G., Henry H. Takei, and Perry R. Klokkevold, eds. *Carranza's Clinical Periodontology*. 10th ed. St. Louis, Mo.: Saunders/Elsevier, 2006. Explores the clinical aspects of modern periodontology and its relationships with anatomy, physiology, etiology, and pathology.

Ring, Malvin E. *Dentistry: An Illustrated History*. New York: Abradale, 1992. Ring's coverage of dentistry is broad and accurate. The illustrations are particularly useful in helping readers understand dental dis-

eases. An excellent starting point for those unfamiliar with the topic.

Woodall, Irene R., ed. *Comprehensive Dental Hygiene Care*. 4th ed. St. Louis, Mo.: Mosby, 1993. This illustrated text addresses topics in dental hygiene and prophylaxis.

Your Dental Health: A Guide for Patients and Families. Farmington: Connecticut Consumer Health Information Network, University of Connecticut Health Center, 2008. This is a user-friendly, practical Web resource for patients and the parents of younger patients, covering a wide range of information sources, including books and Web-based and printed pamphlets. http://library.uchc.edu/departm/hnet/dental health.html.

DENTISTRY

SPECIALTY

ANATOMY OR SYSTEM AFFECTED: Gums, mouth, teeth

SPECIALTIES AND RELATED FIELDS: Anesthesiology, orthodontics

DEFINITION: The field of health involving the diagnosis and treatment of diseases of the teeth and related tissues in the oral cavity.

KEY TERMS:

dental caries: the scientific term for tooth decay

dentist: a doctor with specialized training to diagnose and treat diseases of the teeth and oral tissues

endodontics: the dental specialty that treats diseases of infected pulp tissue

oral surgery: the dental specialty that surgically removes diseased teeth and oral tissues and treats fractures of the jawbone

orthodontics: the dental specialty that treats malocclusions or improperly aligned teeth by straightening the teeth in the jaws

pedodontics: the dental specialty that treats children

periodontics: the dental specialty that treats the diseases of the supporting tissues of the teeth

prosthodontics: the dental specialty that restores missing teeth with fixed or removable dentures

SCIENCE AND PROFESSION

The practice of dentistry is a highly specialized area of medicine that treats the diseases of the teeth and their surrounding tissues in the oral cavity. Dental education normally takes four years to complete, with predental training preceding it. Prior to entering a dental school, students are usually required to have a bachelor's degree from a college or university. This degree should have major emphasis in biology or chemistry. Predental courses are concentrated in both inorganic and organic chemistry. The biology courses can cover such subjects as comparative anatomy, histology, physiology, and microbiology. Other courses that can help students to prepare for both dental school and the future practice of dentistry are English, speech skills, economics, physics, computer technology, and subjects, such as sculpture, that teach spatial relationships. Upon entering dental school, students are faced with two distinct parts of their education: didactics and techniques.

The didactic courses offered in dental schools are required to achieve knowledge of the human body, most particularly the head and neck. Some of the courses required are human anatomy (including dissection of a human cadaver), physiology, biochemistry, microbiology, general and oral histology and pathology, dental anatomy, pharmacology, anesthesiology, and radiology. One course specific to dental school is occlusion, which emphasizes the structure of the temporomandibular joint and its accompanying neurology and musculature.

In addition, students must know the properties of the materials used in the practice of dentistry. The physical properties of metals, acrylic plastics, gypsum plasters, impression materials, porcelains, glass ionomers, dental composites, sealant resins, and other substances must be thoroughly understood to determine the proper restorations for diseased tissues in the mouth. Knowledge of resistance to wear by chewing forces, thermal conductivity, and corrosion and staining by mouth fluids and foods is important. Information concerning the materials used in dental treatment in terms of resistance to recurrent decay, possible toxicity, or irritation to the hard and soft tissues of the oral cavity is also necessary.

The technical phase of dental education addresses the practical use of this didactic knowledge in treating diseases of the mouth. Students are trained to operate on diseased teeth and to prepare the teeth to receive restorations that will function as biomechanical prostheses in, or adjacent to, living tissue. An understanding of anatomy, physiology, and pathology is necessary for successful restoration of the teeth. During this course of study, students are required to construct fillings, cast-gold crowns and inlays, fixed and removable dentures, porcelain crowns and inlays, and other restorations on mannequins, plastic models, or extracted teeth. These activities are undertaken prior to working on patients. Through practice and repetition of these techniques, dental students soon become aware of the importance of mastering this phase of the education prior to their application in a clinical environment.

The clinical phase of dental education integrates the didactic and technical instruction that has taken place throughout the first years of professional study. Students learn to treat patients under the close supervision of their instructors. The treatment of patients in all the specialties of dentistry is required of students before they receive the degree for general dentistry. Some students may opt for extra training in one of several specialties. To become a specialist, postgraduate education is required. This education commonly encompasses two years of study but is sometimes longer.

Upon graduation, students receive their professional degrees. Before they can legally practice dentistry in the United States, however, they must successfully pass an examination offered by the board of dental examiners in their chosen state. National exams in didactics are offered during dental school, and most states accept them as part of their state examination. The technical portion of the exam may only be taken after the student has received a doctorate. The emphasis regarding techniques may vary from state to state. Many states allow reciprocity, which means that a student who has passed the examination in one state may become licensed to practice in another. In states that do not accept reciprocity, the student must pass the practical examination of that state prior to obtaining a license. There have been attempts to make reciprocity universal among all states, but several states insist on governing the quality of their dental health care.

Dental education can be quite expensive. After a dentist receives a license to practice, the cost of equipping an office must also be borne. A dental office must have dental chairs, office and reception room furniture, a dental laboratory, a sterilizing room, X-ray units, instruments, and various supplies. Because of these expenses, new dentists often initially practice as an associate or partner of an established dentist, as an employee of a dental clinic, in the military or Public Health Service, or in state institutions. Some dentists enjoy the academic atmosphere of dental schools and return to become part-time or full-time educators.

DIAGNOSTIC AND TREATMENT TECHNIQUES

The practice of dentistry is quite different in modern times compared to the past. While some techniques and materials are still in use, there have been improvements in materials and instruments because of expanded knowledge in many scientific fields. This knowledge

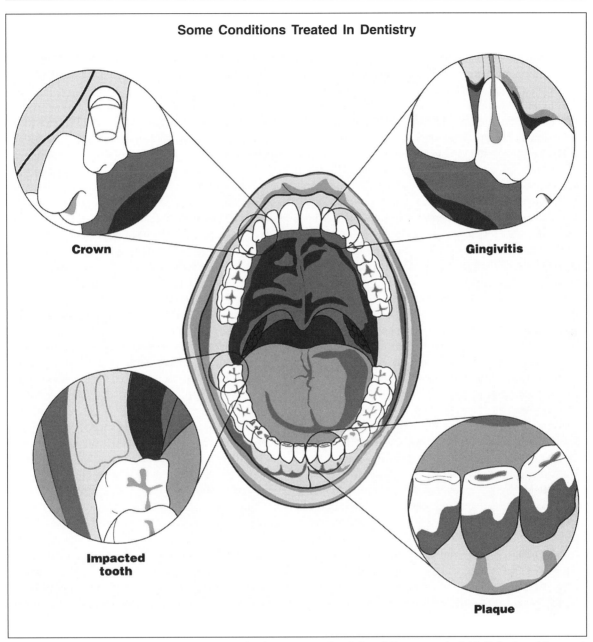

Some Conditions Treated In Dentistry

Crown

Gingivitis

Impacted tooth

Plaque

Care of the teeth and supporting structures may involve the treatment of such dental diseases as gingivitis (infection of the gums), the removal of dental plaque (hard deposits on the teeth), the surgical excision of impacted molars (teeth trapped beneath the gums), and the fitting of a crown (an artificial covering for a tooth) following root canal treatment.

has increased to such an extent that dentistry has divided into several specialties. While the general dentist uses all disciplines of dentistry to treat patients, complex problems often require referral and the expertise of a specialist.

The general dentist is involved primarily in the treatment of caries or tooth decay and the replacement of missing teeth. Bacterial acids that dissolve the enamel and dentin of teeth cause caries. A diseased or damaged tooth must be prepared mechanically by the removal of the decayed material using a dental drill and tough, sharp bits called burs. The amount of damage and the position of the tooth in the mouth determine the type of restoration. In the posterior or back teeth, initial cavities may be restored with silver amalgam or bonded composite resins. In addition to removing the decayed tooth structure, the dentist must take into consideration the closeness of the dental pulp, the chewing forces of the opposing teeth, and the aesthetics of the finished restoration. In the anterior or front teeth, aesthetic restorative materials are used to fill small cavities. In this case also, the size and position of the defect determine the choice of restorative material.

When the amount of tooth destruction caused by decay becomes too large for conservative filling materials, the remaining tooth structure must be reinforced by the use of cast metal or porcelain restorations. The tooth is prepared for the specific restoration, and accurate impressions are taken of the prepared teeth. The crown or inlay is fabricated on hard plaster models reproduced from the impressions and then cemented into place on the tooth. This process is also used for fixed partial dentures, or bridges, which are used to replace one or more missing teeth. Two or more teeth are prepared on either end of the space of missing teeth to support the span. The bridge is constructed with metal and porcelain as a single unit. It is then cemented on the prepared abutment teeth.

The health of the supporting tissues of the teeth, the periodontium, is necessary for the long-term retention of any mechanical restoration. When teeth become loose in the jaws because of periodontal disease, or pyorrhea, the restoration of these teeth often depends on the treatment by a periodontist, the specialist in this field. Periodontists treat the diseased tissues by scraping off harmful deposits on the roots of the teeth and by removing the diseased soft tissue and bone through curettage, surgery, or both techniques. At present, there is no means to regenerate or regrow bone lost by periodontal disease. Some newer techniques of grafting the patient's bone with sterile freeze-dried bone, implanting stainless steel pins, or using other artificial materials show great promise.

If the tooth decay reaches the dental pulp and infects it, there are two choices of treatment: removal of the tooth or endodontic therapy, commonly known as root canal treatment. If the tooth is well supported by a healthy periodontium, it is better to save the tooth by endodontics. The basic procedure of a root canal is to enter the tooth through the chewing surface on teeth toward the rear of the mouth or the inside surface or lingual aspect of teeth in the front of the mouth. Files, reamers, and broaches to the tip of the root remove diseased or decaying (necrotic) material of the dental pulp. The now-empty canal is filled by cementing a point that fits into it. Although the tooth is now nonvital, meaning that it has lost its blood supply and nerve, it can remain in the mouth for many years and provide good service.

The maintenance of the health of the primary dentition, or baby teeth, is very important. These deciduous teeth, although lost during childhood and adolescence, are important not only to the dental health of the child but to the permanent teeth as well. The deciduous teeth act as guides and spacers for the correct placement of adult teeth when they erupt. A pediodontist, who specializes in the practice of dentistry for children, must have a good knowledge of the specific mechanics of children's mouths in treating primary teeth. This specialist must also have a thorough foundation in the treatment of congenital diseases. The pediodontist prepares the way for dental treatment by an adult dentist and often assists an orthodontist by doing some preliminary straightening of teeth.

An orthodontist treats malocclusions, or ill-fitting teeth (so-called bad bites) with mechanical appliances that reposition the teeth into an occlusion that is closer to ideal. These appliances, known commonly as braces, move the teeth through the bone of the jaws until the opposing teeth occlude in a balanced bite. The side benefit of this treatment is that the teeth become properly positioned for an attractive smile.

Sometimes the teeth or their supporting tissues become so diseased that there is no alternative but to remove them. A general dentist often does routine extractions of these diseased teeth. If the patient has complications beyond the training of a general dentist or is medically compromised by systemic illness, an oral surgeon, with specialized training, is typically consulted. This specialist not only removes teeth under difficult conditions but also is trained to remove tumors of the oral cavity, treat fractures of the jaws, and perform the surgical placement of dental implants.

Although the total loss of teeth is becoming rarer, there are still many patients who are without teeth. Often, they have been wearing complete, removable dentures that, over a period of time, have caused the loss or resorption of underlying bone. Prosthodontists are specialists trained to construct fixed and removable dentures for difficult cases. The increased success of titanium implants in the jaws and the appliances connected to them have aided prosthodontists in treating the complex cases. They also construct appliances to replace tissues and structures lost from cancer surgery of the oral cavity and congenital deformities such as cleft palate.

PERSPECTIVE AND PROSPECTS

In the past, dentistry only treated pain caused by a diseased tooth; the usual mode of treatment was extraction. Today, the prevention of disease, the retention of teeth, and the restoration of the dentition are the treatment goals of dentists.

The development of composite resins has successfully addressed many aesthetic problems associated with restorations. Although metal fillings of silver amalgam (actually a mixture of silver, lead, and a small amount of mercury) and cast-gold restorations are often the treatments of choice, the display of metal is offensive to some patients. Plastic composite materials that are chemically bonded to the enamel and dentin of teeth are more aesthetically pleasing than metals. They have also shown great promise for longevity. There is still some concern about the resistance of these materials to chewing forces and leakage of the bonding to the tooth, but the techniques and materials are improving.

Dental porcelains improved greatly in the last half of the twentieth century. Although porcelain fused to metal crowns is often the material of choice, in certain cases crowns, inlays, and fixed bridges of a newer type of porcelain are being used. Thin veneers of porcelain are also used to restore front teeth that are congenitally or chemically stained. The result is cosmetically more appealing. Through a similar bonding process of composites, these veneers on the front surfaces of the teeth offer maximum aesthetics with minimum destruction of tooth structure.

While implantation of metals into the jawbones to support dentures and other prosthetic appliances is not new, the recent use of titanium implants and precision techniques promises long-term retention. Special drills are used to prepare the implant site, and titanium cylinders are either threaded into the bone or pushed into the jaw. The implant is covered by the gum tissue and allowed to heal for six to eight months, so that the process of osseointegration (joining of bone and metal) can occur. The bone will actually fuse to the pure metal, anchoring the implant for an eventual prosthetic appliance.

Laser technology is an exciting field that may have some applications in dentistry. Lasers have been used in gum surgery. Some theorists believe that if the enamel surface of the teeth were to be fused, it would be highly resistant to decay. The heat generated by lasers is a concern, but steps are being taken to control this problem. One of the most promising uses of lasers is in the specialty of endodontics. A thin laser fiber-optic probe advanced down the root canal, preparing and sterilizing the canal prior to filling, vaporizes diseased or degenerating pulp.

Computer science is also being integrated into the treatment phase of dentistry. For example, after scanning a patient's mouth, projected results of treatment can be displayed on a computer screen. In addition, restorations can be developed using the concept of computer-aided design/computer-aided manufacturing (CAD/CAM). A computer scans a prepared tooth for a crown or inlay. The restoration is then designed for a three-dimensional model on the screen. After the model restoration has been chosen, the computer transfers the data to a computer-activated milling machine in the dental laboratory, and a restoration is reproduced in a ceramic or composite resin material in the designed image. The restoration is then cemented into the prepared tooth.

Such improvements in techniques and materials have advanced dentistry into a new era in providing treatment for patients. The basic fundamentals of treatment of the teeth and their surrounding tissues must be maintained, however, in view of the peculiar anatomy and physiology of the teeth.

The above discussion reflects the state of dentistry in North America and Western Europe. In other parts of the world, resources are not available for such advanced techniques. In these countries, teeth are still more likely to be extracted than restored. Prosthetic devices are less common, and many chemical treatments are simply not available. The underlying reason is lack of money.

—William D. Stark, D.D.S.; updated by
L. Fleming Fallon, Jr., M.D., Ph.D., M.P.H.

See also Anesthesia; Anesthesiology; Braces, orthodontic; Canker sores; Cavities; Crowns and bridges; Dental diseases; Dentistry, pediatric; Dentures; Endodontic disease; Fluoride treatments; Fracture repair; Gastrointestinal system; Gingivitis; Gum disease; Halitosis; Head and neck disorders; Jaw wiring; Oral and maxillofacial surgery; Orthodontics; Periodontal surgery; Periodontitis; Plaque, dental; Root canal treatment; Teeth; Teething; Temporomandibular joint (TMJ) syndrome; Tooth extraction; Toothache; Wisdom teeth.

FOR FURTHER INFORMATION:

Foster, Malcolm S. *Protecting Our Children's Teeth: A Guide to Quality Dental Care from Infancy Through*

Age Twelve. New York: Insight Books, 1992. This book is written for parents and other interested readers. It gives insights and suggestions for promoting general dental health.

Gluck, George M., and William M. Morganstein. *Jong's Community Dental Health.* 5th ed. St. Louis, Mo.: Mosby, 2003. Explores the role of dentistry in public health, examining such topics as dental care delivery, demographic shifts and dental health, distribution of dental disease and prevention, and research in dental public health.

Kendall, Bonnie L. *Opportunities in Dental Care Careers.* Edited by Blythe Camenson. New York: McGraw-Hill, 2006. This text provides guidance for students interested in the field of dentistry. It provides information about careers in all allied dentistry fields. Admission requirements for different careers and the names of professional schools that can supply the training are listed.

Moss, Stephen J. *Growing Up Cavity Free: A Parent's Guide to Prevention.* New York: Edition Q, 1994. This rather brief book is written in easy-to-understand language. There are standard suggestions for preventing dental problems.

Parker, James N., and Philip M. Parker, eds. *The Official Patient's Sourcebook on Gingivitis.* San Diego, Calif.: Icon Health, 2002. Draws from public, academic, government, and peer-reviewed research to provide a wide-ranging handbook for patients with gingivitis.

_____. *The Official Patient's Sourcebook on Periodontitis.* San Diego, Calif.: Icon Health, 2002. Draws from public, academic, government, and peer-reviewed research to provide a wide-ranging handbook for patients with periodontitis.

Ring, Malvin E. *Dentistry: An Illustrated History.* New York: Abrams, 1985. Ring's coverage of dentistry is broad and accurate. The illustrations are particularly useful in helping readers understand dental diseases. An excellent starting point for those unfamiliar with the topic.

Smith, Rebecca W. *The Columbia University School of Dental and Oral Surgery's Guide to Family Dental Care.* New York: W. W. Norton, 1997. This classic text provides easy-to-understand explanations of all common dental problems and procedures and many less common procedures. The text is written for the general reader.

Your Dental Health: A Guide for Patients and Families. Farmington: Connecticut Consumer Health Information Network, University of Connecticut Health Center, 2008. This is a user-friendly, practical Web resource for patients and the parents of younger patients, covering a wide range of information sources, including books and Web-based and printed pamphlets. http://library.uchc.edu/departm/hnet/dentalhealth.html.

Dentistry, pediatric

Specialty

Anatomy or system affected: Gums, mouth, teeth

Specialties and related fields: Orthodontics

Definition: The specialty that addresses all aspects of dental treatment needed by children from infancy to age eighteen.

Key terms:

caries: tooth decay or cavities

deciduous teeth: the temporary teeth that normally appear between eight months and two years and that begin to fall out after the child turns six or seven; also called baby teeth

endodontist: a dentist whose specialty is the treatment of disorders of the dental pulp

orthodontist: a dentist whose specialty is straightening teeth

pedodontist: a dentist whose specialty is the treatment of children's teeth from infancy to late adolescence

permanent teeth: the teeth that appear between age seven and adolescence

sealant: a substance used to seal the chewing surfaces of teeth and prevent the development of caries

wisdom teeth: the permanent teeth that may appear between late adolescence and early adulthood

Science and Profession

Dental education normally takes four years to complete. Courses offered at dental schools teach knowledge of anatomy, particularly the head and neck. Students must also learn the properties of materials—such as metals, acrylic plastics, porcelains, and sealant resins—used in dentistry. Prior to working on patients, students are trained to operate on diseased teeth using mannequins, plastic models, or extracted teeth. Then they treat patients under the close supervision of instructors. Students must treat patients in all specialties of dentistry before they can receive a degree in general dentistry. Postgraduate education is required to become a specialist in pediatric dentistry.

General dental care for children may be given by a family dentist or by a pedodontist. Pedodontists are dentists specializing in the practice of dentistry for children. They must understand the specific mechanics of children's anatomy and have a thorough foundation in the treatment of congenital diseases. Many pedodontists also assist orthodontists by doing some preliminary straightening of teeth.

DIAGNOSTIC AND TREATMENT TECHNIQUES

In the second half of the twentieth century, dentists did an excellent job of educating parents and children about the importance of regular dental care. It is now generally understood that regular dental care from early childhood through adolescence is essential for the proper development of children. The dentist will also take advantage of each visit to discuss with parents and children proper techniques for brushing and flossing. If good habits are developed at an early age, serious dental problems can be reduced in the future.

Many parents do not understand the central importance of deciduous teeth, or baby teeth. These teeth appear in infants between eight months and two years and begin to fall out when children are about six or seven. By the age of two, most children have twenty deciduous teeth. If baby teeth are extracted too early, the other teeth will move, which will create orthodontic problems.

Dentists recommend that every child be examined by the age of three. If cavities or other problems are discovered, the affected teeth should be treated and saved. Fillings and even steel crowns are often required.

Since permanent teeth are located below baby teeth, abscesses in baby teeth can spread below the gums and damage permanent teeth. If X rays reveal that there are no permanent teeth to replace baby teeth, the dentist will make every effort to preserve baby teeth for as long as possible. Frequently, a dentist will have to explain to parents that paying for fillings or crowns now will save a much larger amount of money in the future by shortening the period of time required for orthodontics.

As the permanent teeth begin to break through and replace baby teeth, the dentist may discover that there are too many teeth or not enough teeth. Extra teeth,

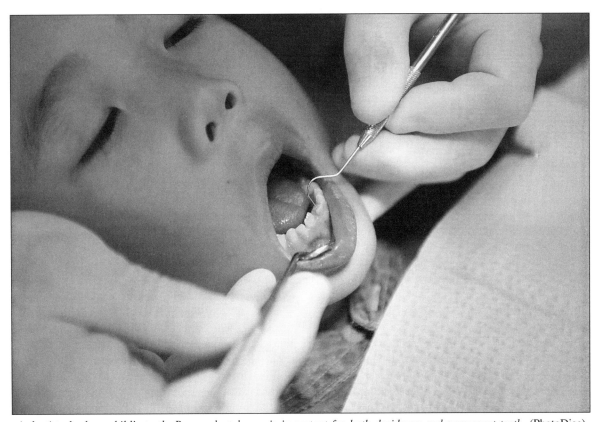

A dentist checks a child's teeth. Proper dental care is important for both deciduous and permanent teeth. (PhotoDisc)

called supernumerary teeth, must be extracted because they occupy space needed for the proper alignment of permanent teeth.

It is not uncommon for children's teeth to be injured as a result of accidents. In such cases, a dentist may refer the child to an endodontist, who will perform a root canal to repair damaged dental pulp. After the root canal has been completed, the family dentist or pedodontist will put a crown on the affected tooth.

A major expense for parents is orthodontics, but straightening teeth is not purely cosmetic. If there is a significant overbite, the child may develop speech problems that will not disappear until the malocclusion, or improper positioning of teeth, is eliminated. If a pedodontist or family dentist concludes that braces are needed to straighten a child's teeth, the child will be referred to an orthodontist, who will examine the child, take X rays, determine whether the child is ready for braces, and decide how to straighten the teeth and, if necessary, realign the jaws. Orthodontic treatment often lasts two to three years. Parents are usually asked to make a large initial payment and monthly payments thereafter. This expense can be significant if parents have two or more children in braces at the same time. Parents often consult several orthodontists to compare prices.

Orthodontists must motivate children to cooperate with their instructions in using bands as directed and brushing their teeth carefully. Both orthodontists and pedodontists or family dentists must remind children that it is easy for tooth decay to take place under braces.

As children become adolescents, other dental problems may occur, including tooth decay. Pedodontists often perform fluoride treatments, and they may apply sealants to the surface of the teeth. Frequently, oral surgery is performed on older adolescents or young adults to extract wisdom teeth that are impacted, or trapped within the gums.

PERSPECTIVE AND PROSPECTS

The quality of pediatric dental care available in economically advanced countries is excellent. Nevertheless, the cost of dental care concerns many parents, who wonder how they can afford to spend thousands of dollars for orthodontics and hundreds of dollars for a single crown or root canal. Dental insurance has become readily available in the United States, and most other countries have state-supported medical insurance programs that also cover dental treatment. Developing countries often have great difficulty paying for quality dental care. Efforts have been made to ensure that some of the international aid sent from developed to developing countries is used to improve dental care.

—*Edmund J. Campion, Ph.D.*

See also Braces, orthodontic; Dental diseases; Dentistry; Fluoride treatments; Orthodontics; Plaque, dental; Teeth; Teething; Thumb sucking; Wisdom teeth.

FOR FURTHER INFORMATION:

American Academy of Pediatric Dentistry. http://www.aapd.org/pediatricinformation.

Centers for Disease Control and Prevention. "Children's Oral Health." http://www.cdc.gov/oralhealth/topics/child.htm.

Foster, Malcolm S. *Protecting Our Children's Teeth: A Guide to Quality Dental Care from Infancy Through Age Twelve.* New York: Insight Books, 1992.

Moss, Stephen J. *Growing Up Cavity Free: A Parent's Guide to Prevention.* New York: Edition Q, 1994.

Nemours Foundation, The. KidsHealth. http://kidshealth.org/parent/general.

Schou, Lone, and Anthony S. Blinkhorn, eds. *Oral Health Promotion.* New York: Oxford University Press, 1993.

Taintor, Jerry F., and Mary Jane Taintor. *The Complete Guide to Better Dental Care.* New York: Checkmark Books, 1999.

DENTURES
TREATMENT

ANATOMY OR SYSTEM AFFECTED: Gums, mouth, teeth

SPECIALTIES AND RELATED FIELDS: Dentistry

DEFINITION: Removable artificial teeth worn to replace missing or diseased teeth, thus restoring both facial appearance and the ability to speak clearly and chew food by maintaining the shape of the jaw.

INDICATIONS AND PROCEDURES

With the aging process, disease of the teeth and surrounding tissues often increases, leading to the eventual loss of some or all the teeth. When teeth are missing, the remaining teeth can change position, drifting into the surrounding space. Teeth that are out of position can damage tissues in the mouth. It is also more difficult to clean thoroughly between crooked teeth, resulting in an increased risk of tooth decay, gum disease, and additional loss of teeth. The solution is to replace the missing teeth with a denture. In 1999, more than thirty-two million Americans were wearing some type of denture, and the majority were over fifty-five years of age.

When a large number of teeth are missing, and a sufficient number of adjacent teeth are not present to support a bridge, or fixed partial denture, a removable partial denture is the solution. It consists of replacement teeth attached to pink or gum-colored plastic bases, which are connected by a metal framework. This prosthetic device is usually secured by clasping it to several of the remaining teeth. The clasps are typically made out of gold or a cobalt-steel alloy. Although more costly, precision attachments are nearly invisible and generally more aesthetically pleasing than metal clasps. Crowns on the adjacent natural teeth may improve the fit of a removable partial denture, and they are usually required with precision attachments.

When all the teeth need replacement, a full denture is constructed. It is usually made of acrylic, occasionally reinforced with metal. Full dentures replace all the teeth in either jaw and are generally held in place by suction created between saliva and the soft tissues of the mouth. A temporary soft liner can be placed in a new or old denture to help improve the health of the gum tissues by absorbing some of the pressures of mastication and providing maximum retention by fitting around undercuts in the bone and gums.

USES AND COMPLICATIONS

A common misconception is that when all the teeth are extracted and replaced by full dentures, all teeth problems cease. In fact, properly fitted full dentures at best are only about 25 to 35 percent as efficient as natural teeth. Many elderly have little trouble adjusting, but some find it difficult to adapt to and learn to use dentures properly. Furthermore, the tissues of the mouth undergo constant changes, which may result in loose or bad-fitting dentures, which may cause damage to the mouth tissues. Consequently, a person who wears dentures should continue to see a dentist for regular annual checkups.

Full and partial dentures are removable and must be taken out frequently and cleansed. In addition, the supporting soft tissues of the mouth need thorough cleansing with a soft mouth brush two to three times daily. It typically takes a few weeks to get used to inserting, wearing, eating with, removing, and maintaining dentures. Careful attention to all the instructions given by the dentist is vital.

—*Alvin K. Benson, Ph.D.*

See also Aging; Bone disorders; Cavities; Crowns and bridges; Dental diseases; Dentistry; Otorhinolaryngology; Periodontitis; Teeth; Tooth extraction.

FOR FURTHER INFORMATION:

Connecticut Consumer Health Information Network. "Your Dental Health: A Guide for Patients and Families." http://library.uchc.edu/departm/hnet/dental health.html.

Devlin, Hugh. *Complete Dentures: A Clinical Manual for the General Dental Practitioner.* New York: Springer, 2002.

Schillingburg, Warren, et al. *Fundamentals of Fixed Prosthodontics.* 3d ed. Chicago: Quintessence, 1997.

Smith, Rebecca W. *The Columbia University School of Dental and Oral Surgery's Guide to Family Dental Care.* New York: W. W. Norton, 1997.

Woodforde, John. *The Strange Story of False Teeth.* New York: Universe Books, 1983.

DEPARTMENT OF HEALTH AND HUMAN SERVICES

ORGANIZATION

DEFINITION: A division of the executive branch of the U.S. government, with representation in the cabinet of the president, that is responsible for public health.

KEY TERMS:

Head Start: local preschool programs that help prepare children of economically disadvantaged or recent immigrant families for entry into regular primary school grades; encouraged by the Department of Health and Human Services through selective funding

Medicaid: a health care program, made available by the Department of Health and Human Services in conjunction with most states, to those with low-level income or those who are disabled and unable to pay health insurance premiums

Medicare: a governmental health insurance system for persons sixty-five years of age and older, supported by obligatory payroll withholding

HISTORY AND MISSION

Although several efforts were made in earlier decades to create a federal authority responsible for public health, it was not until Dwight D. Eisenhower's administration in the 1950's that a formal agency became part of the executive branch of government. Presidents Franklin D. Roosevelt and Harry S. Truman in particular had hoped, but failed, to create a federally administered health program as an added component of the Social Security Act put in place by Roosevelt in 1935. The Department of Health, Education, and Welfare (HEW)—restructured in 1979 as the Department of Health and Human Services (DHHS)—began operations in April, 1953. For a number of years, until 1995, the Social Security Administration remained under the DHHS. A number of legislative reorganization acts expanded and diversified responsibilities assigned to the DHHS. Among these was the major milestone when, as part of the Social Security Act of 1965 (a piece of President Johnson's Great Society legislation), two government-funded health care programs—Medicare and Medicaid—were placed under the administration of the secretary of HEW.

The shift in party control of the executive branch of government that came with Republican Richard M. Nixon's election in 1968 raised some question that there might be declining support for DHHS activities. This would not occur, however, mainly because public perceptions of the need for government responsibilities for health and social welfare had become a political given. In fact, there would be an expanding pattern of activities of, as well as budgetary allowances for, DHHS in the latter decades of the twentieth and first part of the twenty-first centuries.

The Department of Education Organization Act of 1979 provided for the creation of a separate Department of Education, while the DHHS retained responsibilities for operations relating to public health and welfare. In part, the evolving scope of DHHS operations reflected changing perceptions of the social definition of public health, as well as the impact on U.S. agencies of global health concerns, particularly those relating to HIV/AIDS and the avian and H1N1 influenza pandemics.

Since its inception as HEW and following restructuring as DHHS in 1980, as of 2009 there had been twenty-one secretaries appointed to head this executive branch of the U.S. government.

OVERVIEW

Overall responsibility for the activities of the DHSS rests with the secretary of Health and Human Services, assisted by the Office of Inspector General, whose task it is to report to the secretary and to Congress detailing both the budgetary soundness and managerial effectiveness of the activities assigned to more than ten subagencies of the department.

In general terms, work carried on by the DHHS falls into three categories: provision of direct services to specific groups within the overall population; gathering and disseminating technical information vital to the maintenance of optimal public health and safety standards within the United States; and support for scientific research that can contribute to the same health-related goals.

Closer examination of activities sponsored by several key DHHS subagencies suggests that many of their activities can be complementary. A first grouping, for example, consists of agencies providing direct assistance: Centers for Medicare and Medicaid (CMM), the Administration for Children and Families (ACF), the Administration on Aging, the Indian Health Service, and the Substance Abuse and Mental Health Services Administration (SAMHSA). In particular, SAMHSA is an example of complementary functions bridging several agencies.

Medicare and Medicaid clearly occupy the most public and politically sensitive position among all of DHHS's agencies. Unlike Medicare, which is fully funded by the federal government through withholding taxes on individual incomes, Medicaid programs involve budgetary and organizational cooperation between DHHS and each state. This fact of decentralization means that DHHS has the responsibility of monitoring a wide variety of state-run programs that set up eligibility standards (for example, low-income resources, disabilities, pregnancy) before providing free health care to Medicaid applicants. Some states include as much as half the cost of Medicaid services in their budgets, but others depend on DHHS for well over half of their expenditures. Nearly fifty million persons received Medicaid services across the country in 2008 at an estimated federal (DHHS) cost of more than $200 billion. Because many state programs face budgetary cuts that could decrease their ability to maintain Medicare services, measures had been underway by the end of 2008 to allow participating states to introduce minimal premiums and higher copayments for Medicaid recipients.

The ACF, organized with ten regional offices across the country, provides financial assistance to needy families, enforces child support obligations, and assists children held back by various economic or developmental disadvantages. Head Start is ACF's widely recognized program to help prepare children of qualifying economically disadvantaged families for entry into the regular school system. Grants are made available to local public and private nonprofit institutions to develop methods—ideally methods involving parent participation with their children—to develop necessary social and cognitive skills that may be lacking as a result of disadvantaged social and economic environments. Enrollments in Head Start since its inception in 1965 increased (although not steadily) from about 500,000 to more than 900,000 participants in 2007. Budgetary support also rose steadily, passing the billion dollar mark in 1985. By 2007, appropriations were close to $7 billion.

The activities of other important agencies of DHHS involve support for scientific research and dissemination of research findings to the general public. The National Institutes of Health (NIH) is the best known such agency focusing on "pure" scientific research. For its part, the Agency for Health Care Policy and Research, created in 1989 and reauthorized in 1999 as the Agency for Healthcare Research and Quality (AHRQ), supports research that gauges the effectiveness of existing or proposed health care programs around the country. These programs are studied, for example, in terms of costs, accessibility, and reduction of safety risks for patients. One should also note the social relevance of a number of AHRQ research projects, including studies of ethnic and racial disparities in access to health care. AHRQ also makes vital practical health care information available to the public. This is clear in the activities of one program in particular: the Office of Consumer Assessment of Healthcare Providers and Systems.

In the broader domain of informational services relating to public health, two agencies—the Food and Drug Administration (FDA) and Centers for Disease Control and Prevention (CDC)—stand out. The FDA is responsible for testing and approving (or rejecting) a broad spectrum of products proposed by manufacturers for the consumer market. These range from the obvious—vaccines and new pharmaceutical products or generic equivalents of brand-name drugs—through many categories of food additives and dietary supplements to cosmetics and tobacco products. FDA recommendations reach the public through a variety of media, most notably regular publications outlining the characteristics of individual drugs or providing advice on buying medicines online (including warnings on counterfeit products). Potentially the most direct protective impact of the FDA is the power to recall drugs or food items that, although they succeed in reaching the consumer market, later reveal dangerous health or safety risks. A number of FDA activities extend beyond

U.S. borders, both with the aim of sharing vital research information and encouraging cooperation when international public health safety questions (most notably in combating pandemic diseases) are involved. In these areas, the FDA coordinates its functions with the CDC, which has a program providing relevant disease risk information to travelers going abroad.

The CDC not only deals with common widespread infectious diseases such as influenza, hepatitis, and HIV/AIDS (as well as major debilitating chronic diseases such as diabetes and cancer) but also maintains specialized branches responsible for health and safety in the workplace as well as emergency preparedness in the event of bioterrorism, chemical and radiation disasters, and health hazards that stem from natural disasters.

SAMHSA has a wide range of programs that are either preventive or, when drug or alcohol abuse or mental health issues require treatment, provide referrals to appropriate public health institutions. It also maintains an online database, the National Registry of Evidence-Based Programs and Practices, that reviews modes of preventing or treating, or both, the most common mental disorders and cases of substance abuse. SAMHSA also provides funding to support qualified community programs involved in either substance abuse prevention or treatment. Grants in 2009, for example, included almost $2.5 million awarded to local juvenile court systems to help develop their ability to provide substance abuse treatment and some $15 million for the same need in geographically concentrated areas of particular need (mainly, but not solely, in large urban zones). A major sum (grants totaling $60 million) was earmarked in 2009 for local groups with existing or planned drug-free-community programs.

Other agencies of DHHS carry on programs whose importance to public health can be said to be visible in the very names they bear. For example, the Agency for Toxic Substances and Disease Registry (ATSDR) is responsible not only for monitoring dangerous substances that are easily recognizable by the general public (asbestos, lead, DDT, and mercury, for example) but for conducting research that can reveal new dangers in unsuspected places. Another responsibility of ATSDR is to monitor both public and specialized toxic waste sites across the country. The Indian Health Service and the Administration on Aging are two other agencies whose work within important subsectors of the U.S. population is easily recognized as a vital public service.

Perspective and Prospects

Because the budget for DHHS must be reviewed by Congress, a certain degree of uncertainty may surround the ongoing work of its several agencies. Some programs, like Medicare and Medicaid, are subject to close scrutiny not only because of their critical place within the total U.S. budget but also because of their importance as part of the health care reform debate, which came to center stage following the election of President Barack Obama in 2008. Other DHHS agencies, without being as politically "supercharged" as Medicare and Medicaid, are clearly identified in the public's mind because they represent easily visible dilemmas affecting everyday life. Within the brief period of two decades, questions of substance abuse and dysfunctional families, for example, have become the focus of major media attention. Because budgetary and political debates over the relative importance of the multidimensional activities of the DHHS can arise at any time, its administrators must be prepared for possible calls for prioritization.

—*Byron D. Cannon, Ph.D.*

See also Centers for Disease Control and Prevention (CDC); Environmental health; Epidemiology; Health care reform; Medicare; National Institutes of Health (NIH); Occupational health; Preventive medicine; World Health Organization.

For Further Information:

Daschle, Thomas, Scott Greenberger, and Jeanne Lambrew. *Critical: What We Can Do About the Health-Care Crisis.* New York: Thomas Dunne Books, 2008. Recommends several major and controversial reforms, including the creation of an independent federal health board and the incorporation into the Federal Employee Health Benefits Program of both Medicare and Medicaid, as well as a large number of private employers' plans.

Institute of Medicine. *An Assessment of the CDC Anthrax Vaccine Safety and Efficacy Research Program.* Washington, D.C.: National Academy Press, 2003. A representative example of independently contracted evaluations of the effectiveness of a DHHS agency project.

McCormick, Joseph B., Susan Fisher-Hoch, and Leslie Alan Horvitz. *Level 4: Virus Hunters of the CDC.* Atlanta: Turner, 1996. An extremely diversified collection of chapters dealing in human terms with the experiences of the CDC investigating potentially (and clearly established) infectious diseases around the world.

Moon, Marilyn, and Janemarie Mulvey. *Entitlements and the Elderly.* Washington, D.C.: Urban Institute Press, 1996. The authors review the three main support programs for the elderly (Social Security, Medicare, and Medicaid—the last two auspices of the DHHS). Attention on the possible consequences of budgetary cuts.

National Research Council, Committee on the Organizational Structure of the National Institutes of Health. *Enhancing the Vitality of the National Institutes of Health.* Washington, D.C.: National Academy Press, 2003. A seven-part review of the evolution of NIH programs also covers new challenges for `research given advances in the biomedical sciences.

Depression

Disease/disorder

Anatomy or system affected: Brain, heart, musculoskeletal system, psychic-emotional system

Specialties and related fields: Family medicine, geriatrics and gerontology, psychiatry, psychology

Definition: One of the most common psychiatric disorders to occur in most lifetimes, caused by biological, psychological, social, and/or environmental factors.

Key terms:

bipolar disorders: mood disorders characterized by symptoms of mania and symptoms of depression

cyclothymia: a mood disorder characterized by fewer and less intense symptoms of elevated mood and depressed mood than bipolar disorders

dysthymia: a mood disorder characterized by symptoms similar to depression that are fewer in number but last for a much longer period of time

electroconvulsive therapy (ECT): the use of electric shocks to induce seizure in depressed patients as a form of treatment

major depressive disorder: a pattern of major depressive episodes that form an identified psychiatric disorder

major depressive episode: a syndrome of symptoms characterized by depressed mood; required for the diagnosis of some mood disorders

manic episode: a syndrome of symptoms characterized by elevated, expansive, or irritable mood; required for the diagnosis of some mood disorders

psychopharmacology: the drug treatment of psychiatric disorders *psychosurgery:* the surgical removal or destruction of part of the brain of depressed patients as a form of treatment

psychotherapy: the "talk" therapies that target the emotional, social, and other contributors to and consequences of depression

seasonal affective disorder (SAD): a mood disorder associated with the winter season, when the amount of daylight hours is reduced

CAUSES AND SYMPTOMS

The word "depression" is used to describe many different things. For some, it defines a fleeting mood, for others an outward physical appearance of sadness, and for others a diagnosable clinical disorder. In any year, more than twenty million American adults suffer from a clinically diagnosed depression, a mood disorder that often affects personal, vocational, social, and health functioning. The *Diagnostic and Statistical Manual of Mental Disorders: DSM-IV-TR* (4th ed., 2000) of the American Psychiatric Association delineates a number of mood disorders that include clinical depression, known as major depression.

A major depressive episode is a syndrome of symptoms, present during a two-week period and representing a change from previous functioning. The symptoms include at least five of the following: depressed or irritable mood, diminished interest in previously pleasurable activities, significant weight loss or weight gain, insomnia or hypersomnia, physical excitation or slowness, loss of energy, feelings of worthlessness or guilt, indecisiveness or a diminished ability to concentrate, and recurrent thoughts of death. The clinical depression cannot be initiated or maintained by another illness or condition, and it cannot be a normal reaction to the death of a loved one (some symptoms of depression are a normal part of the grief reaction).

In major depressive disorder, the patient experiences a major depressive episode and does not have a history of mania or hypomania. Major depressive disorder is often first recognized in the patient's late twenties, while a major depressive episode can occur at any age, including infancy. Women are twice as likely to suffer from the disorder than are men.

There are several potential causes of major depressive disorder. Genetic studies suggest a familial link with higher rates of clinical depression in first-degree relatives. There also appears to be a relationship between clinical depression and levels of the brain's neurochemicals, specifically dopamine, norepineph-

INFORMATION ON DEPRESSION

CAUSES: Genetic factors, psychosocial stressors, neurochemical dysfunction, certain medications

SYMPTOMS: Irritable mood, diminished interest in previously pleasurable activities, significant weight loss or gain, insomnia or hypersomnia, physical excitation or slowness, loss of energy, feelings of worthlessness or guilt, indecisiveness, recurrent thoughts of death

DURATION: Ranges from short-term to chronic

TREATMENTS: Drug therapy, individual and group psychotherapy, light therapy, electroconvulsive therapy

rine, and serotonin, as well as hormones. It is important to keep in mind, however, that anywhere from 15 to 40 percent of adults will experience depression in their lifetimes. Furthermore, not everyone has a biological cause for this depression. Common causes of clinical depression also include psychosocial stressors such as the death of a loved one, financial stress, loss of a job, interpersonal problems, or world events. It is unclear, however, why some people respond to a specific psychosocial stressor with a clinical depression and others do not. Finally, certain prescription medications have been noted to cause or be related to clinical depression. These drugs include muscle relaxants, heart medications, hypertensive medications, ulcer medications, oral contraceptives, painkillers, narcotics, and steroids. Thus there are many causes of clinical depression, and no single cause is sufficient to explain all clinical depressions.

Another category of depressive disorder is bipolar disorders. Bipolar disorders occur in about 1 percent of the population as a whole. In persons over the age of eighteen, about two to three persons out of one hundred are diagnosed. Bipolar I disorder is characterized by one or more manic episodes along with persisting symptoms of depression. A manic episode is defined as a distinct period of abnormally and persistently elevated, expansive, or irritable mood. Three of the following symptoms must occur during the period of mood disturbance: inflated self-esteem, decreased need for sleep, unusual talkativeness or pressure to keep talking, racing thoughts, distractibility, excessive goal-oriented activities (especially in work, school, or social areas), and reckless activities with a high potential for negative consequences (such as buying sprees or risky business ventures). For a diagnosis of bipolar disorder, the symptoms must be sufficiently severe to cause impairment in functioning and/or concern regarding the person's danger to himself/herself or to others, must not be superimposed on another psychotic disorder, and must not be initiated or maintained by another illness or condition. Bipolar II disorder is characterized by symptoms of a history of a major depressive episode and symptoms of hypomania.

Cyclothymia is another cyclic mood disorder related to depression. It involves symptoms of both depression and mania. However, the manic symptoms are without marked social or occupational impairment and are known as hypomanic episodes. Similarly, the symptoms of major depressive episodes do not meet the clinical criteria (less than five of the nine symptoms described above), but the symptoms must be present for at least two years. Cyclothymia cannot be superimposed on another psychotic disorder and cannot be initiated or maintained by another illness or condition. This mood disorder is a particularly persistent and chronic disorder with an identified familial pattern.

Dysthymia is another chronic mood disorder affecting approximately 6 percent of the population in a lifetime. Dysthymia is characterized by at least a two-year history of depressed mood and at least two of the following symptoms: poor appetite, insomnia or hypersomnia, low energy or fatigue, low self-esteem, poor concentration or decision making, or feelings of hopelessness. There cannot be evidence of a major depressive episode during the first two years of the dysthymia or a history of manic episodes or hypomanic episodes. The individual cannot be without the symptoms for more than two months at a time, the disorder cannot be superimposed on another psychotic disorder, and it cannot be initiated or maintained by another illness or condition. Dysthymia is more common in adult females, equally common in both sexes of children, and with a greater prevalence in families. The causes of dysthymia are believed to be similar to those listed for major depressive disorder, but the disorder is less well understood than is depression.

A final variant of clinical depression is known as seasonal affective disorder. Patients with this illness demonstrate a pattern of clinical depression during the winter, when there is a reduction in the amount of daylight hours. For these patients, the reduction in available light is thought to be the cause of the depression.

Treatment and Therapy

Crucial to the choice of treatment for clinical depression is determining the variant of depression being experienced. Each of the diagnostic categories has associated treatment approaches that are more effective for a particular diagnosis. Multiple assessment techniques are available to the health care professional to determine the type of clinical depression. The most valid and reliable is the clinical interview. The health care provider may conduct either an informal interview or a structured, formal clinical interview assessing the symptoms that would confirm the diagnosis of clinical depression. If the patient meets the criteria set forth in the DSM-IV, then the patient is considered for depression treatments. Patients who meet many but not all diagnostic criteria are sometimes diagnosed with a "subclinical" depression. These patients might also be considered appropriate for the treatment of depression, at the discretion of their health care providers.

Another assessment technique is the "paper-and-pencil" measure, or depression questionnaire. A variety of questionnaires have proven useful in confirming the diagnosis of clinical depression. Questionnaires such as the Beck Depression Inventory, Hamilton Depression Rating Scale, Zung Self-Rating Depression Scale, and the Center for Epidemiologic Studies Depression Scale are used to identify persons with clinical depression and to document changes with treatment. This technique is often used as an adjunct to the clinical interview and rarely stands alone as the definitive assessment approach to diagnosing clinical depression.

Laboratory tests, most notably the dexamethasone suppression test, have also been used in the diagnosis of depression. The dexamethasone suppression test involves injecting a steroid (dexamethasone) into the patient and measuring the production levels of another steroid (cortisol) in response. Studies have demonstrated, however, that certain severely depressed patients do not reveal the suppression of cortisol production that would be expected following the administration of dexamethasone. The test has also failed to identify some patients who were depressed and has mistakenly identified others as depressed. Research continues to determine the efficacy of other measures of brain activity, including computed tomography (CT) scanning, positron emission tomography (PET) scanning, and magnetic resonance imaging (MRI). At this time, laboratory and imaging tests are not a reliable diagnostic strategy for depression.

Once a clinical depression (or a subclinical depression) is identified, several types of treatment options are available. These options are dependent on the subtype and severity of the depression. They include psychopharmacology (drug therapy), individual and group psychotherapy, light therapy, family therapy, electroconvulsive therapy (ECT), and other less traditional treatments. These treatment options can be provided to the patient as part of an outpatient program or, in certain severe cases of clinical depression in which the person is a danger to himself/herself or others, as part of a hospitalization.

Clinical depression often affects the patient physically, emotionally, and socially. Therefore, prior to beginning any treatment with a clinically depressed individual, the health care provider will attempt to develop an open and communicative relationship with the patient. This relationship will allow the health care provider to provide patient education on the illness and to solicit the collaboration of the patient in treatment. Supportiveness, understanding, and collaboration are all necessary components of any treatment approach.

Three primary types of medications are used in the treatment of clinical depression: cyclic antidepressants, monoamine oxidase inhibitors (MAOIs), and lithium salts. These medications are considered equally effective in decreasing the symptoms of depression, which begin to resolve in three to four weeks after initiating treatment. The health care professional will select an antidepressant based on side effects, dosing convenience (once daily versus three times a day), and cost.

The cyclic antidepressants are the largest class of antidepressant medications. As the name implies, the chemical makeup of the medication contains chemical rings, or "cycles." There are unicyclic (buproprion and fluoxetine, or Prozac), bicyclic (sertraline and trazodone), tricyclic (amitriptyline, desipramine, and nortriptyline), and tetracyclic (maprotiline) antidepressants. These antidepressants function to either block the reuptake of neurotransmitters by the neurons, allowing more of the neurotransmitter to be available at a receptor site, or increase the amount of neurotransmitter produced. The side effects associated with the cyclic antidepressants—dry mouth, blurred vision, constipation, urinary difficulties, palpitations, and sleep disturbance—vary and can be quite problematic. Some of these antidepressants have deadly toxic effects at high levels, so they are not prescribed to patients who are at risk of suicide. The newer drugs are more specific in terms of the drug action. For instance, fluoxetine is a selective serotonin reuptake inhibitor (SSRI) and works

specifically on the neurotransmitter serotonin. Similarly, buproprion is a norepinephrine and dopamine reuptake inhibitor (NDRI) and works specifically on the neurotransmitters norepinephrine and dopamine. More specific drugs generally create fewer side effects. Fewer side effects can be associated with greater medication compliance, potentially making these drugs a more effective treatment.

Monoamine oxidase inhibitors (isocarboxazid, phenelzine, and tranylcypromine) are the second class of antidepressants. They function by slowing the production of the enzyme monoamine oxidase. This enzyme is responsible for breaking down the neurotransmitters norepinephrine and serotonin, which are believed to be responsible for depression. By slowing the decomposition of these transmitters, more of them are available to the receptors for a longer period of time. Restlessness, dizziness, weight gain, insomnia, and sexual dysfunction are common side effects of the MAOIs. MAOIs are most notable because of the dangerous adverse reaction (severely high blood pressure) that can occur if the patient consumes large quantities of foods high in tyramine (such as aged cheeses, fermented sausages, red wine, foods with a heavy yeast content, and pickled fish). Because of this potentially dangerous reaction, MAOIs are not usually the first choice of medication and are more commonly reserved for depressed patients who do not respond to the cyclic antidepressants.

A third class of medication used in the treatment of mood disorders are mood stabilizers, the most notable being lithium carbonate, which is used primarily for bipolar disorder. Lithium is a chemical salt that is believed to effect mood stabilization by influencing the production, storage, release, and reuptake of certain neurotransmitters. It is particularly useful in stabilizing and preventing manic episodes and preventing depressive episodes in patients with bipolar disorder.

Psychotherapy refers to a number of different treatment techniques used to deal with the psychosocial contributors and consequences of clinical depression. Psychotherapy is a common supplement to drug therapy. In psychotherapy, the patients develop knowledge and insight into the causes and treatment for their clinical depression. In cognitive psychotherapy, symptom relief comes from assisting patients in modifying maladaptive, irrational, or automatic beliefs that can lead to clinical depression. In behavioral psychotherapy, patients modify their environment such that social or personal rewards are more forthcoming. This process might involve being more assertive, reducing isolation by becoming more socially active, increasing physical activities or exercise, or learning relaxation techniques. Research on the effectiveness of these and other psychotherapy techniques indicates that psychotherapy is as effective as certain antidepressants for many patients and, in combination with certain medications, is more effective than either treatment alone.

Electroconvulsive (or "shock") therapy is the single most effective treatment for severe and persistent depression. If the clinically depressed patient fails to respond to medications or psychotherapy and the depression is life-threatening, electroconvulsive therapy is considered. It is also considered if the patient cannot physically tolerate antidepressants, as with elders who have other medical conditions. This therapy involves inducing a seizure in the patient by administering an electrical current to specific parts of the brain. The therapy has become quite sophisticated and much safer than it was in the mid-twentieth century, and it involves fewer risks to the patient. Patients undergo several treatments over a period of time, such as a week, and show marked treatment benefit. Some temporary memory impairment is a common side effect of this treatment. In the past, however, more memory impairment, of lasting duration for some, was more common.

A special treatment used for individuals with seasonal affective disorder is light therapy, or phototherapy. Light therapy involves exposing patients to bright light for a period of time each day during seasons of the year when there is decreased light. This may be done as a preventive measure and also during depressive episodes. The manner in which this treatment approach modifies the depression is unclear and awaits further research, but some believe it affects the internal clock of the body, or circadian rhythm. Studies of the effectiveness of light therapy have been mixed, but interest in this promising treatment is strong, as it may prove useful for working with nonseasonal mood disorders as well. It should be noted, however, that light therapy does have some risks associated with it. Caution must be used to protect the eyes and use the light as directed. Additionally, the intensity of light must be correct so as to achieve therapeutic effects and not cause other problems. Finally, some individuals can experience manic episodes if they are exposed to too much light, so caution must be exercised in terms of the length of time for light exposure treatment sessions.

Psychosurgery, the final treatment option, is quite rare. It refers to surgical removal or destruction of certain portions of the brain believed to be responsible for causing severe depression. Psychosurgery is used only after all treatment options have failed and the clinical depression is life-threatening. Approximately 50 percent of patients who undergo psychosurgery benefit from the procedure.

PERSPECTIVE AND PROSPECTS

Depression, or the more historical term "melancholy," has had a history predating modern medicine. Writings from the time of the ancient Greek physician Hippocrates refer to patients with a symptom complex similar to the present-day definition of clinical depression.

The rates of clinical depression have increased since the early twentieth century, while the age of onset of clinical depression has decreased. Women appear to be at least twice as likely as men to suffer from clinical depression, and people who are happily married have a lower risk for clinical depression than those who are separated, divorced, or dissatisfied in their marital relationship. These data, along with recurrence rates of 50 to 70 percent, indicate the importance of this psychiatric disorder.

While most psychiatric disorders are nonfatal, clinical depression can lead to death. About 60 percent of individuals who commit suicide have a mood disorder such as depression at the time. In a lifetime, however, only about 7 percent of men and 1 percent of women with lifetime histories of depression will commit suicide. Though these numbers are very high, what this means is that not everyone who is depressed will commit suicide. In fact, many receive help and recover from this illness. There are, however, other costs of clinical depression. In the United States, billions of dollars are spent on clinical depression, divided among the following areas: treatment, suicide, and absenteeism (the largest). Clinical depression obviously has a significant economic impact on a society.

The future of clinical depression lies in early identification and treatment. Identification will involve two areas. The first is improving the social awareness of mental health issues to include clinical depression. By eliminating the negative social stigma associated with mental illness and mental health treatment, there will be an increased level of the reporting of depression symptoms and thereby an improved opportunity for early intervention, preventing the progression of the disorder to the point of suicide. The second approach to identification involves the development of reliable assessment strategies for clinical depression. Data suggest that the majority of those who commit suicide see a physician within thirty days of the suicide. The field will continue to strive to identify biological markers and other methods to predict and/or identify clinical depression more accurately. Treatment advances will focus on further development of pharmacological strategies and drugs with more specific actions and fewer side effects. Adjuncts to traditional drug therapies need continued development and refinement to maximize the success of integrated treatments.

> —*Oliver Oyama, Ph.D.;*
> *updated by Nancy A. Piotrowski, Ph.D.*

See also Antianxiety drugs; Antidepressants; Anxiety; Bipolar disorders; Brain; Death and dying; Dementias; Eating disorders; Emotions, biochemical causes and effects of; Geriatrics and gerontology; Grief and guilt; Hypochondriasis; Light therapy; Midlife crisis; Neurology; Neurology, pediatric; Neurosis; Neurosurgery; Obsessive-compulsive disorder; Palliative medicine; Panic attacks; Paranoia; Pharmacology; Phobias; Postpartum depression; Post-traumatic stress disorder; Psychiatric disorders; Psychiatry; Psychiatry, child and adolescent; Psychiatry, geriatric; Psychoanalysis; Psychosomatic disorders; Seasonal affective disorder; Shock therapy; Stress; Suicide; Terminally ill: Extended care.

FOR FURTHER INFORMATION:

American Psychiatric Association. *Diagnostic and Statistical Manual of Mental Disorders: DSM-IV-TR.* 4th ed. Arlington, Va.: Author, 2000. This reference book lists the clinical criteria for psychiatric disorders, including mood disorders.

DePaulo, J. Raymond, Jr., and Leslie Ann Horvitz. *Understanding Depression: What We Know and What You Can Do About It.* New York: Wiley, 2003. A leading expert on depression examines the disease's nature, causes, effects, and treatments.

Depression and Bipolar Support Alliance. http://www.dbsalliance.org. In addition to a comprehensive list of informative links, this site has information on mood disorders and support groups and offers lists of mental health professionals and discussion forums.

Jones, Steven. *Coping with Bipolar Disorder: A Guide to Living with Manic Depression.* Oxford, England: Oneworld, 2002. A handbook for living with bipolar disorder, outlining causes, symptoms, and treatments; giving case studies; and listing support organizations.

Koplewicz, Harold S. *More than Moody: Recognizing and Treating Adolescent Depression.* New York: Penguin, 2003. A leading clinician and researcher helps parents distinguish between normal teenage angst and depression, examining the warning signs, risk factors, and key behaviors, as well as treatment options.

National Institute of Mental Health. http://www.nimh.nih.gov.

DERMATITIS

DISEASE/DISORDER

ALSO KNOWN AS: Eczema

ANATOMY OR SYSTEM AFFECTED: Hair, skin

SPECIALTIES AND RELATED FIELDS: Dermatology

DEFINITION: A wide range of skin disorders, some the result of allergy, some caused by contact with a skin irritant, and some attributable to other causes.

KEY TERMS:

allergen: a substance that excites an immunologic response; also called an antigen

crusting: the appearance of slightly elevated skin lesions made up of dried serum, blood, or pus; they can be brown, red, black, tan, or yellowish

immunoglobulin E (IgE): ordinarily, a relatively rare antibody; in patients with atopic dermatitis, levels can be significantly higher than in the general population

lesion: any pathologic change in tissue

scaling: a buildup of hard, horny skin cells

secondary infection: a bacterial, viral, or other infection that results from or follows another disease

wheal: a small swelling in the skin

CAUSES AND SYMPTOMS

The term "dermatitis" does not refer to a single skin disease, but rather to a wide range of disorders. "Dermatitis" is often used interchangeably with "eczema." The two most common dermatitides are atopic (allergic) dermatitis, in which the individual appears to inherit a predilection for the disease, and contact dermatitis, in which the individual's skin reacts immediately on contact with a substance, or develops sensitivity to it.

Atopic dermatitis often occurs in individuals with a personal or family history of allergy, such as hay fever or asthma. Thirty to 50 percent of children with atopic dermatitis develop asthma or hay fever, a rate that is three to five times higher than for the general population. These people often have high serum levels of a certain antibody, immunoglobulin E (IgE), which may

---

INFORMATION ON DERMATITIS

CAUSES: Allergies, infection, contact irritation, altered immune system
SYMPTOMS: Dry and itchy skin, rashes, inflammation, pain
DURATION: Short-term to chronic
TREATMENTS: Topical corticosteroids or antihistamines, antibiotics, dietary changes, and specialized lotions, soaps, or shampoos

---

be associated with their skin's tendency to break out, although a specific antigen-antibody reaction has not been demonstrated.

There are many distinct characteristics of atopic dermatitis, some of which depend on the age of the patient. The disease usually starts early in childhood. It is often first discovered in infants in the first months of life when redness and weeping, crusted lesions appear mostly on the face, although the scalp, arms, and legs may also be affected. There is intense itching. Papules (pimples), vesicles (small, blisterlike lesions filled with fluid), edema (swelling), serous exudation (discharge of fluid), and scaly crusts may be seen. At one year of age, oval, scaly lesions appear on the arms, legs, face, and torso. In older children and adults, the lesions are usually localized in the crook of the elbow and the back of the knees, and the face and neck may be involved. The course of the disease is variable. It usually subsides by the third or fourth year of life, but periodic outbreaks may occur throughout childhood, adolescence, and adulthood. In 75 percent of cases, atopic dermatitis improves between the ages of ten and fourteen. Cases persisting past the patient's middle twenties, or beginning then, are the most difficult to treat.

Dryness and itching are always present in atopic dermatitis. People with atopic dermatitis seem to lose skin moisture more readily than average people: Rather than soft, pliable skin, they develop dry, rough, sensitive skin that is particularly prone to chapping and splitting. The skin becomes itchy, and the individual's tendency to scratch significantly aggravates the condition in what is called the "itch-scratch-itch" cycle or the "scratch-rash-itch" cycle: The individual scratches to relieve the itching, which causes a rash, which in turn causes increased itching, which invites increased scratching and increased irritation. After years of itching and scratching, the skin of older children and adults with atopic dermatitis develops red, lichenified (rough, thickened) patches in the crook of the arm and behind the knees, as well as on the eyelids, neck, and wrists.

Constant chafing of the affected area invites bacterial infection and lymphadenitis (inflammation of lymph nodes). Furthermore, patients with atopic dermatitis seem to have altered immune systems. They appear to be more susceptible than others to skin infections, warts, and contagious skin diseases. *Staphylococcus aureus* and certain streptococci are common infecting bacteria in these patients. Pyoderma is often seen as a result of bacterial infection in atopic dermatitis. This condition features redness, oozing, scaling, and crusting, as well as the formation of small pustules (pus-filled pimples).

Patients with atopic dermatitis are also particularly sensitive to herpes simplex and vaccinia viruses. Exposure to either could cause a severe skin disease called Kaposi's varicelliform eruption. Vaccinia virus (the agent that causes cowpox) is used in the preparation of smallpox vaccine. Therefore, patients with atopic dermatitis must not be vaccinated against smallpox. Furthermore, they must be isolated from patients with active herpes simplex and those recently vaccinated against smallpox.

Patients with atopic dermatitis may also develop contact dermatitis, which can greatly exacerbate their condition. They are also sensitive to a wide range of allergens, which can bring on outbreaks, as well as to low humidity (such as in centrally heated houses in winter), which would contribute to dry skin. They may not be able to tolerate woolen clothing.

A condition called keratosis pilaris often develops in the presence of atopic dermatitis. It is not seen in young infants, but it does appear in childhood. Hair follicles on the torso, buttocks, arms, and legs become plugged with horny matter and protrude above the skin, giving the appearance of goose bumps or "chicken skin." The palms of the hands of patients with atopic dermatitis have significantly more fine lines than those of average people. In many patients, there is a tiny "pleat" under the eyes. They are often prone to cold hands and may have pallor, seen as a blanching of the skin around the nose, mouth, and ears.

When ordinary skin is lightly rubbed with a pointed object, almost immediately there is a red line, followed by a red flare, and finally, a wheal or slight elevation of the skin along the line. In patients with atopic dermatitis, however, there is a completely different reaction: The red line appears, but almost instantly it becomes white. The flare and the wheal do not appear.

About 4 to 12 percent of patients with atopic dermatitis develop cataracts at an early age. Normally, cataracts do not appear until the fifties and sixties; those with atopic dermatitis may develop them in their twenties. These cataracts usually affect both eyes simultaneously and develop quickly.

Psychologically, children with atopic dermatitis often show distinct personality characteristics. They are reported to be bright, aggressive, energetic, and prone to fits of anger. Children with severe, unmanageable cases of atopic dermatitis may become selfish and domineering, and some go on to develop significant personality disorders.

It is not known exactly what happens to cause the itching and dry skin that are the fundamental signs of atopic dermatitis and the root of many of its complications. Theories suggest various origins. It is by definition an allergic disorder, but the allergens that are specifically involved and how they produce the signs of atopic dermatitis are unknown. One of the most interesting theories involves the antibody IgE. Theoretically, the union of IgE with an antigen causes certain cells to release pharmacologic mediators, such as histamine, bradykinin, and slow-reacting substance (SRS-A), that cause itching and thus begin the cycle of scratching and irritation characteristic of atopic dermatitis. The fact that patients with atopic dermatitis have higher than normal levels of IgE, and that there is a relationship between IgE levels and the severity of atopic dermatitis, seems to lend support to this theory.

Contact dermatitis could resemble atopic dermatitis at certain stages, but the dry skin of atopic dermatitis may not be seen. Contact dermatitis is usually characterized by a rash consisting of small bumps, itchiness, blisters, and general swelling. It occurs when the skin has been exposed to a substance to which the body is sensitive or allergic. If the contact dermatitis is caused by direct irritation by a caustic substance, it is called irritant contact dermatitis. The causative agents are primary irritants that cause inflammation at first contact. Some obvious irritants are acids, alkalis, and other harsh chemicals or substances. An example is fiberglass dermatitis, in which fine glass particles from fiberglass fabrics or insulation enter the skin and cause redness and inflammation.

If the dermatitis is caused by allergic sensitivity to a substance, it is called allergic contact dermatitis. In this case, it may take hours, days, weeks, or years for the patient to develop sensitivity to the point where exposure to these substances causes allergic contact dermatitis.

These agents include soaps, acetone, skin creams, cosmetics, poison ivy, and poison sumac.

Allergic contact dermatitis comprises the largest variety of contact dermatitides, many of them named for the allergens that cause them. Hence, there is pollen dermatitis; plant and flower dermatitis, such as poison ivy or poison oak; clothing dermatitis; shoe, and even sandal strap, dermatitis; metal and metal salt dermatitis; cosmetic dermatitis; and adhesive tape dermatitis, among others. They all have one thing in common: The skin is exposed to an allergen from any of these sources and becomes so sensitive to it that further exposure causes a rash, itching, and blistering.

The development of sensitivity to an allergen is an immunological response to exposure to that substance. With many allergens, the first contact elicits no immediate immunological reaction. Sensitivity develops after the allergen has been presented to the T lymphocytes that mediate the immune response.

Because it often takes a long time to develop sensitivity, patients are surprised to discover that they have become allergic to substances that they have been using for years. For example, a patient who has been applying a topical medication to treat a skin condition may one day find that the medication causes an outbreak of dermatitis. Ironically, some of the ingredients in medications commonly used to treat skin conditions are among the major allergens that cause allergic contact dermatitis. These include antibiotics, antihistamines, topical anesthetics, and antiseptics, as well as the inactive ingredients used in formulating the medications, such as stabilizers.

Other substances to which the patient may develop sensitivity include the chemicals used in making fabric for clothing, tanning chemicals used in making leather, dyes, and ingredients in cosmetics. Many patients develop sensitivity to allergens found in the workplace. The list of potential allergens in the industrial setting is virtually endless. It includes solvents, petroleum products, chemicals commonly used in manufacturing processes, and coal tar derivatives.

In some cases, the allergen requires sunlight or other forms of light to precipitate an outbreak of contact dermatitis. This is called photoallergic contact dermatitis, and it may be caused by such agents as aftershave lotions, sunscreens, topical sulfonamides, and other preparations applied to the skin. Another light reaction, termed phototoxic contact dermatitis, can be caused by exposure to sunlight after exposure to perfumes, coal tar, certain medications, and various chemicals.

A different form of dermatitis involves the sebaceous glands, which secrete sebum, a fatty substance that lubricates the skin and helps retain moisture. Sebaceous dermatitis is usually seen in areas of the body with high concentrations of sebaceous glands, such as on the scalp or face, behind the ears, on the chest, and in areas where skin rubs against skin, such as the buttocks and the groin. It is seen most often in infants and adolescents, although it may persist into adulthood or start at that time.

In infants, sebaceous dermatitis can begin within the first month of life and appears as a thick, yellow, crusted lesion on the scalp called cradle cap. There can be yellow scaling behind the ears and red pimples on the face. Diaper rash may be persistent in these infants. In older children, the lesion may appear as thick, yellow plaques in the scalp. When sebaceous dermatitis begins in adulthood, it starts slowly, and usually its only manifestation is scaling on the scalp (dandruff). In severe cases, yellowish-red scaling pimples develop along the hairline and on the face and chest. Its cause is unknown, but a yeast commonly found in the hair follicles, *Pityrosporum ovale*, may be involved.

There are many other kinds of dermatitis. Diaper dermatitis, or diaper rash, is a complex skin disorder that involves irritation of the skin by urine and feces, irritation by constant rubbing, and secondary infection by *Candida albicans*. Nummular dermatitis (from *nummus*, meaning coin) is characterized by crusting, scaly, disc-shaped papules and vesicles filled with fluid and often pus. Pityriasis alba is a common dermatitis with pale, scaly patches. In lichen simplex chronicus, there is intense itching, with lesions caused by, and perpetuated by, scratching and rubbing. Stasis dermatitis occurs at the ankles; brown discoloration, swelling, scaling, and varicose veins are common. Hyperimmunoglobulin E (Hyper IgE) syndrome is characterized by extremely high IgE levels, ten to one hundred times higher than normal, and a family history of allergy; the patient has frequent skin infections, suppurative (pus-forming) lymphadenitis, pustules, plaques, and abscesses. Pompholyx occurs on the hands and soles of the feet; there is excessive sweating, with eruptions of deep vesicles accompanied by burning or itching.

Friction can also cause dermatitis. In intertrigo, the friction of skin rubbing against skin causes inflammation that can become infected. In frictional lichenoid dermatitis, or sandbox dermatitis, it is thought that the abrasive action of sand or other gritty material on the skin causes the characteristic lesions. Winter eczema seems to be caused by the skin-drying effects of low humidity as well as by harsh soaps and overfrequent bathing; dry skin and itching are common. The acrodermatitis diseases (from *acro*, meaning the extremities) may be limited to the hands and feet, or, like acrodermatitis enteropathica, may erupt in other parts of the body, such as around the mouth and on the buttocks. In fixed-drug eruption, lesions appear in direct response to the administration of a drug; the lesions are generally in the same parts of the body, but they may spread. Swimmer's itch is a parasitic infection from an organism that lives in fresh water lakes and ponds, while seabather's eruption seems to be caused by a similar saltwater organism.

Treatment and Therapy

Many dermatitides resemble one another, and it is important for a physician to identify the patient's complaint precisely to treat it effectively. Therefore, the physician will confirm the identity of the condition through a process known as differential diagnosis. This method allows him or her to rule out all similar conditions, pinpoint the exact nature of the patient's problem, and develop a therapeutic regimen to treat it.

In treating atopic dermatitis, one of the first goals is to relieve dryness and itching. The patient is cautioned not to bathe excessively because this dries the skin. Lotions are used to lubricate the skin and retain moisture. The patient is advised not to scratch, because this could break the skin and invite infection. The patient is advised to avoid any known offending agents and not to apply any medication to the skin without the doctor's knowledge.

Wet compresses can bring relief to patients with atopic dermatitis. Topical corticosteroids are used to help resolve acute flare-ups, but only for short-term therapy, because their prolonged use might produce undesirable side effects. Oral antihistamines are often given to relieve itching and to help the patient sleep. Diet may play a role in atopic dermatitis in infants: Some pediatric dermatologists and other physicians recommend elimination of milk, eggs, tomatoes, citrus fruits, wheat products, chocolate, spices, fish, and nuts from the diets of these patients. Soft cotton clothing is recommended, as is the avoidance of pets or fuzzy toys that might be allergenic. For secondary infections that arise from atopic dermatitis, the physician prescribes appropriate antibiotic therapy.

In primary irritant contact dermatitis, the offending

agent is eliminated or avoided. In allergic contact dermatitis, one of the main goals is to discover the offending agent so that the patient can avoid contact with it. Sometimes this information can be elicited from the patient interview, and sometimes it is necessary to conduct a series of patch tests. In this procedure, known allergens are applied to the skin of the patient to find those that cause irritation. Avoidance of the offending agent can cause the patient some difficulty if the agent happens to be something that is found everywhere. An example is the metal nickel, which is in coins, jewelry, and hundreds of other objects. Patients who insist on wearing nickel-plated jewelry are advised to paint it with clear nail polish periodically to avoid contact of the metal with the skin. Similarly, many other allergens are in common use. Patients are advised to read cosmetics labels and food and medical ingredients lists to avoid contact with agents to which they are sensitive.

Because there is such a wide range of allergic contact dermatitides, treatment of the flare-ups varies considerably. Topical and oral steroids are used, as well as antihistamines. Sometimes the physician finds it necessary to drain large blisters and apply drying agents to weeping lesions. Sometimes the condition calls for wet compresses to relieve itching and soothe the patient. Specialized lotions, soaps, and shampoos are also used, some to treat dryness and others, as in the case of sebaceous dermatitis, to remove scales and to relieve oiliness.

Other treatments depend on the type of dermatitis from which the patient suffers. Patients with photoallergic or phototoxic dermatitis are advised to avoid light. Acrodermatitis enteropathica is caused by a zinc deficiency; in addition to palliative therapy to relieve the symptoms, these patients are given zinc sulfate, which results in complete remission of the disease. As with atopic dermatitis, bacterial infections occurring as a result of a flare-up of allergic contact dermatitis are treated with appropriate antibiotic therapy.

PERSPECTIVE AND PROSPECTS

The skin is the largest organ of the human body, and it is subject to an extraordinary range and number of diseases, with atopic dermatitis and contact dermatitis among the most common. They may afflict patients of all ages, but they are particularly prevalent in children. Many of the dermatitides start in the first weeks of life and continue through childhood. In many cases, the disease is resolved by the time that the child reaches adolescence, but in some it continues into adulthood.

In spite of the fact that disorders of the skin are readily apparent, an understanding of them has been imperfect throughout history. For example, the allergic nature of many of the dermatitides was not explained until the twentieth century. In addition, because their symptoms are similar to one another and to diseases that are not properly classified as dermatitides, there has been much confusion in identifying them. It has been suggested that many of the biblical lepers were in fact suffering only from a form of dermatitis. With prolonged exposure, however, they probably contracted leprosy in time.

The dermatitides are often highly complex diseases, involving genetic, allergic, metabolic, and immune and infective factors, among many others. They are not usually life-threatening, but they take an enormous toll in pain, discomfort, and disfigurement, with an equal toll in psychological distress that can be suffered by patients.

Understanding of these disorders improves constantly, and with understanding comes new methods of treating them. Nevertheless, progress will probably be limited. There is the possibility that patients can be desensitized to allow them to tolerate the allergens that bring about their eruptions, as many hay fever sufferers have been desensitized against the pollens and dusts that trigger their allergy. It is unlikely, however, that there will ever be vaccines to immunize against this group of diseases, nor can many of them be cured, except in the sense that the discomfort that they bring can be treated and the agents that cause them can be avoided.

—*C. Richard Falcon*

See also Acne; Allergies; Blisters; Dermatology; Dermatology, pediatric; Dermatopathology; Diaper rash; Eczema; Hives; Itching; Multiple chemical sensitivity syndrome; Poisonous plants; Psoriasis; Rashes; Rosacea; Scabies; Skin; Skin disorders.

FOR FURTHER INFORMATION:

Adelman, Daniel C., et al., eds. *Manual of Allergy and Immunology*. 4th ed. Philadelphia: Lippincott Williams & Wilkins, 2002. Examines research developments and the clinical diagnosis and treatment of allergies and immune disorders. Topics include asthma, disorders of the skin, diseases of the lung, anaphlaxism, insect allergies, drug allergies, rheumatic diseases, transplantation immunology, and immunization.

American Academy of Dermatology. http://www.aad

.org. The site's "Public Resources" section has good information about dermatitis, as well as coverage of other dermatological disorders.

Litin, Scott C., ed. *Mayo Clinic Family Health Book.* 4th ed. New York: HarperResource, 2009. An excellent general reference for the layperson, with good coverage of the dermatological diseases.

Middlemiss, Prisca. *What's That Rash? How to Identify and Treat Childhood Rashes.* London: Hamlyn, 2002. A comprehensive guide to the identification and treatment of childhood rashes.

Parker, James N., and Philip M. Parker, eds. *The Official Patient's Sourcebook on Atopic Dermatitis.* San Diego, Calif.: Icon Health, 2002. Draws from public, academic, government, and peer-reviewed research to provide a wide-ranging handbook for patients with dermatitis.

Rietschel, Robert L., and Joseph F. Fowler, eds. *Fisher's Contact Dermatitis.* 6th ed. Lewiston, N.Y.: Marcel Decker, 2008. An encyclopedic reference on contact dermatitis. Offers extensive lists of causative agents.

Titman, Penny. *Understanding Childhood Eczema.* New York: Wiley, 2003. Discusses the physical and emotional toll of eczema on young patients and provides practical advice for choosing and managing different treatments.

Weston, William L., et al. *Color Textbook of Pediatric Dermatology.* 4th ed. St. Louis, Mo.: Mosby/Elsevier, 2007. Clinical textbook that covers a range of disorders, including drug reactions, hair disorders, nail disorders, and sun sensitivity. Clinical features, differential diagnosis, pathogenesis, treatment, and patient education are discussed.

Williams, Hywel C., ed. *Atopic Dermatitis: The Epidemiology, Causes, and Prevention of Atopic Eczema.* New York: Cambridge University Press, 2000. Provides a comprehensive review of this increasingly common disorder. Discusses the distribution, frequency, and underlying causes of atopic dermatitis.

DERMATOLOGY
SPECIALTY
ANATOMY OR SYSTEM AFFECTED: Hair, immune system, nails, skin

SPECIALTIES AND RELATED FIELDS: Cytology, histology, immunology, oncology, public health

DEFINITION: The study of a variety of irritations or lesions affecting one of several layers of the skin.

KEY TERMS:
allergens: foreign substances in the surrounding environment that may cause an allergic response, such as a skin reaction

dermatitis: a general term for nonspecific skin irritations that may be caused by bacteria, viruses, or fungi

keratin: a fibrous molecule essential to the tissue structure of hair, nails, or the skin

melanin: a polymer made up of several compounds (including the amino acid tyrosine) that causes pigmentation in the skin, hair, and eyes

SCIENCE AND PROFESSION

Dermatology is the subfield of medicine that deals with diseases of the skin. Some disorders affecting the hair and fingernails may also fall under this category.

Dermatological study requires attention to three distinct layers of the skin, each of which can be affected differently by different disorders. The deepest layer is the subcutaneous tissue where fat is formed and stored. It is also here that the deeper hair follicles and sweat glands originate. Blood vessels and nerves pass from this layer to the dermis. The dermis is mainly connective tissue that contains the oil-producing, or sebaceous, glands and shorter hair follicles. On the surface of the skin is the epidermis, which is itself multilayered. The innermost basal layer is made up of specialized keratin- and melanin-forming cells, whereas the outermost, horny cell layer consists of keratinized dead cells.

The diagnosis of apparent skin disease requires dermatologists to determine whether symptomatic sores, or lesions, are primary (the original symptoms of suspected disease) or secondary (such as infection or irritation caused by scratching which may overshadow the original disorder). Dermatologists are trained to recognize categories of lesions and to determine whether they represent actual diseases or relatively common disorders characteristic of age, or even genetic predispositions. The most common categories of lesions include vesicles, bullae, and crusts; scaling; keratosis; lichenification; pustules; atrophy; and tumors.

Vesicles and bullae are bubblelike eruptions filled with clear serous fluid. As primary lesions, they are often the symptoms of diseases such as chickenpox and herpes zoster. Crusts are formed by tissue fluid that remains in a dried form after the rupture of microscopic vesicles.

Scaling is noticeably different from crusting. These

flakes on the surface of the skin may represent a subsiding stage of earlier inflammation. Scaling may be a secondary lesion associated with psoriasis. Keratoses are rough lesions that show strongly adherent (not loose) flaking. Lichenification involves a thickening of the epidermis, with a more pronounced visibility of lined patterns on the skin surface. Pustules are lesions filled with pus, which serves as a growth medium for microorganisms. Atrophy always involves shrinkage of skin tissues, creating in some cases visible depressions in the area of the lesion. The last category of primary lesions, tumors, may be found either on the surface of or underneath the skin. Tumorous growths can signal a condition as benign as seborrheic keratosis (the appearance of thick scales in isolated spots, particularly as age advances) or as serious as one of several forms of skin cancer.

Secondary lesions appear as the primary, or causal, skin disorder progresses, creating different symptoms in the secondary stage. Examples of secondary lesions include scales (dandruff and psoriasis), crusts (impetigo), ulcers (advanced syphilis), and scarring, the growth of connective tissue that actually replaces damaged tissues following burns or other traumatic injuries.

In addition to these general categories of lesions associated with dermatological diseases, a number of localized problems in blood flow—called vascular nevoid lesions, or birthmarks—may be visible at or soon after birth. Dermatologists assume that some of these lesions may be caused by genetic factors. The most common vascular nevi categories are nevus flammeus (port-wine stain), a purple discoloring of the skin resulting from dilated dermal vessels, and capillary hemangioma (strawberry mark), which begins as a bruiselike lesion but soon grows into a protruding mass. Unlike port-wine stains, which remain throughout the individual's lifetime unless they are removed through laser surgery, strawberry marks will usually subside and disappear on their own, leaving at most visible puckering of the skin. Unless there are complications (such as ulceration), treatment is usually simple, consisting of the application of elastic bandages to maintain constant pressure, thus reducing the distortion caused by the rapid expansion of skin tissue in a localized area.

Probably the most commonly recognized dermatological disorder, acne, usually occurs among adolescents and young adults. Although this problem is likely to occur as part of the normal process of maturation, lack of proper care of acne may cause complications

and lifelong scarring. Acne, as with equally common cases of seborrheic dermatitis (or dandruff, a subcategory of psoriasis), afflicts those areas of the body where oil gland secretions are plentiful and where many forms of bacteria are present on the skin (mainly the face, neck, and upper trunk). The points of lesion for acne are always specific: the hair follicles that are so numerous in these areas of the body. Two phenomena, so-called blackheads and the pimples associated with acne, occur when the normal draining of follicle secretions is blocked in a sac called a comedo. Blackheads occur when the residue trapped in the comedo—keratin, sebum, and various microorganisms—becomes chemically oxidized. When conditions associated with acne appear, an increase in bacterial growth within the comedones produces characteristic pimples which, if traumatized by scratching or picking, may burst, leading to the possibility of further infection. There is no way to prevent acne from appearing, but dermatological therapy to soothe the effects of advanced cases may be recommended.

Another relatively benign but persistently insoluble dermatological problem, the appearance of warts, occurs most often among the middle-aged or older segment of the adult population. Modern dermatological research dating from the 1960's has determined that warts are associated with particular viral strains (papillomaviruses). At least four subtypes have been associated with the appearance of warts on the human body. Warts may vary greatly in appearance—from plantar warts, which grow well below the skin surface and exhibit a drier consistency, to plane warts, which are even with the skin surface, to a very visible brownish and moist lump, which is often found on the face or hands. All warts are localized viral infections that destroy the normal skin tissue in the area of infection. Despite their common occurrence—dermatologists experience a high rate of patient demand for their removal—warts have always carried a certain social stigma. As viruses, they may be transferred to others through contact, particularly if the lesion is an open one.

The term "seborrheic dermatitis" can refer to the recurrent and common problem of dandruff (redness and scaling mainly in skin areas where body hair is present). Like acne, seborrheic dermatitis is more a condition resulting from secretion imbalances and chemical reactions affecting the skin than an actual disease. Dermatological complications arise when excessive scratching of sensitive areas causes secondary lesions to form.

Beyond these categories of common skin disorders are far more serious diseases that require professional dermatological treatment. For example, psoriasis, although varying in possible locations all over the body (including the hands and feet), seems to share symptoms with seborrheic dermatitis, specifically the flaking away of dry skin. What begins as limited patches of flaking, usually on elbows or in the armpits, however, may spread rapidly and have traumatic effects. Dermatologists usually associate psoriasis with stress and anxiety. When irritations are limited in scope, treatment through topical medications—most containing coal tar, sulfur, salicylic acid, or ammoniated mercury solutions—may be successful. Advanced cases may demand systemic treatment with more sophisticated drugs.

Herpes simplex is another common viral infection which leads directly to surface lesions that may be communicable, in this case cold sores. As with warts, folk knowledge has it that improper hygienic practices lead to the much more virulent eruptions associated with herpes simplex. Medical observations have shown, however, that various factors may unleash a dermatological reaction from latent viral sources in an individual. A herpes simplex reaction to increased levels of exposure to sunlight is a good example. On the other hand, many cases of herpes simplex occur in both the male and female genital areas. Although these eruptions are not necessarily connected with much more serious sexually transmitted diseases, their communicability is clearly associated with levels of hygiene in intimate sexual contact. Whatever the cause of herpes simplex, its highly contagious nature may demand dermatological attention to avoid more serious complications. Any occurrence of herpes simplex inflammation near a vital organ, for example, must be treated immediately to prevent the spread of viral infection, particularly in the area surrounding the eyes.

Herpes zoster, commonly referred to as shingles, is thought to be a recurrence in the adult years of a common viral infection that most people experience at an earlier age: chickenpox. The persistence of the symptoms of shingles among adults, however, is not comparable to the mild effect of the virus during childhood. The appearance of painful lesions, usually but not always in the trunk area, may come after a short period of tingling. Although inflammation may pass, many elderly patients, especially those suffering from systemic diseases such as diabetes mellitus, are plagued by continuous long-term discomfort. In addition to discom-

fort, there may be (as in herpes simplex) a danger of complications if the area of inflammation is close to vulnerable tissues or key organs, such as the eyes or ears. In cases where lesions may affect the eyes, dermatologists must go beyond topical treatment to enhance the healing process. Additional emergency therapy may include systemic steroid treatment, the intravenous administration of corticotropin, or oral doses of prednisone.

DIAGNOSTIC AND TREATMENT TECHNIQUES

The diagnosis of specific dermatoses, or potentially serious skin diseases, may or may not require cutaneous biopsies; because their symptoms are not shared by other diseases, a diagnosis can often be made by observation alone. Less easily recognized problems include lichen planus, an uncommon chronic pruritic disease; such potentially dangerous bullous diseases as pemphigus vulgaris, which is characterized by flat-topped papules on the wrists and legs that resemble poison ivy reactions; and skin cancer. Such conditions usually require biopsy to ensure that a mistaken diagnosis does not lead to the wrong treatment. Several methods of biopsy are employed, according to the nature of the lesion under examination. For example, the cutaneous punch technique, which utilizes a special surgical tool that penetrates to about 4 millimeters, may not be appropriate if the lesion is close to the surface. In this case, either curettage (scraping) or shave biopsy (cutting a layer corresponding to the thickness of the lesion) may be used in combination with the cutaneous punch method.

The total number of dermatoses that can be diagnosed is far too great for review here. The conditions that are most commonly treated, however, range from mildly serious but clearly irritating lesions such as acne or warts to much more serious phenomena such as psoriasis and lupus erythematosus. Several early and potentially dangerous conditions, especially basal cell carcinoma, may deteriorate into fatal skin cancers.

Dermatologists classify serious skin diseases under several key divisions. Pruritic dermatoses are characterized by itching. Vascular dermatoses, including several categories of urticaria, are all characterized by sudden outbreaks of papules—some temporary in their irritation and therefore merely disorders, as with hives as a reaction to poison ivy or medicines such as penicillin, and others more serious, such as swelling of the glottis, which may accompany angioneurotic edema. Papulosquamous dermatoses include psoriasis and lichen planus, both localized irritations that involve redness and flaking. In addition to these categories of dermatoses, a wide variety of common dermatologic viruses demand special medical attention because they are socially communicable. These include herpes simplex and herpes zoster. Other serious viruses affecting the skin, such as smallpox and measles, have been controlled by preventive vaccinations. Impetigo, once common during childhood in certain environments, is a bacterial infection, not a viral one. One formerly lethal sexually transmitted disease is syphilis, a form of spirochetal infection. Although far from eradicated, syphilis has been treatable through the use of benzathine penicillin since the mid-twentieth century.

The most serious challenge to dermatologists is the early diagnosis and treatment of skin cancer. The most common forms of skin cancer are basal cell epithelioma, which originates in the epidermis, often as a result of excessive exposure to the sun, and squamous cell carcinoma, which may affect the epidermis or mucosal surfaces (the inside of the mouth or throat). Early diagnosis of both types is essential to prevent metastasis (spreading). The most dangerous skin cancer is malignant melanoma, which may reveal itself through changes in size or color of a body mark such as a mole. This cancer can metastasize very rapidly and endanger the life of the patient.

Possible treatments for different types of skin disease vary considerably. Surgical operations, although certainly not unknown, tend to be associated with more extreme disorders, most notably skin cancer. In such cases, it is usually not the dermatologist but a specialized surgeon who performs the procedure.

The most common treatments used by dermatologists involve the application of various pharmaceutical preparations directly to the surface of the skin. For the treatment of common skin disorders, dermatologists may choose between a variety of medications.

The effect of antipruritic agents (menthol, phenol, camphor, or coal tar solutions) is to reduce itching. Keratoplastic agents (salicylic acid) and keratolytic agents (stronger doses of salicylic acid, resorcinol, or sulfur) affect the relative thickness or softness of the horny layer of the skin. They are associated with the treatment of diseases or disorders characterized by flaking.

Antieczematous agents, including coal tar solutions and hydrocortisone, halt oozing from vesicular lesions. By far the most commonly used drugs in dermatology are antiseptics which, according to their classification, control or kill bacteria, fungi, and viruses. Antibacterial agents that have been widely used for many years include iodochlorhydroxyquin and ammoniated mercury. Ointments to combat viral infections are much less common on the pharmaceutical market; however, several are available, mainly for the treatment of infection by herpes labialis (cold sores), herpes zoster (shingles), or varicella zoster (chickenpox).

These and many other topical applications may be only the first steps, however, in soothing the irritating side effects of more serious or chronically persistent dermatological diseases. Doctors may turn to more active therapies to treat specific ailments, beginning with the general category of electrosurgery, of which there are five specialized subtreatments: electrodesiccation, or the drying of tissues; electrocoagulation, which involves more intense heat; electrocautery, the actual burning of tissues; electrolysis, which produces the cauterization of lesions by chemical reaction; and electrosection, or the removal of tissues by cutting, achieved by the focus of electrical currents produced by various forms of vacuum tubes. By the 1990's, rapid progress in laser beam technology—particularly the carbon dioxide laser, which is a beam of infrared electromagnetic energy with an almost infinitesimal wavelength of 10,600 nanometers—began to replace some of these time-tested methods in cases in which electrosurgery had been commonplace for almost half a century.

Other modes of treatment that penetrate the subsurface layers of the skin include radiation therapy and cryosurgery, which is the immediate freezing of tissues by application of agents such as solid carbon dioxide (−78.5 degrees Celsius) or liquid nitrogen (−195.8 degrees Celsius). These methods are used to treat conditions ranging from psoriasis and pruritic dermatoses to skin cancer.

PERSPECTIVE AND PROSPECTS

One common feature—visible body surface symptoms—means that the medical identification and attempted treatment of human skin diseases can be traced to almost all cultures in all historical periods. An outstanding example of ancient peoples' concerns for eruptions on the skin can be found in the Old Testament or Talmud in Leviticus. In the Scripture, however, as well as in many medieval texts, one sees that a variety of skin diseases tended to be classified as leprosy. The physical location of skin lesions often determined the results of very general attempts at diagnosis.

It was not until the last quarter of the eighteenth century that Viennese physicians ushered in what could be called the first phase of scientific study of the skin and its disorders, or dermatology. This early Viennese school insisted on the study of the morphological nature of the lesions. Until this time, physicians had grouped skin diseases according to their appearance in different places on the body. By the mid-nineteenth century another Austrian, Ferdinand von Hebra, made considerable progress in classifying skin diseases.

Because so many lesions of the skin could potentially lead to diagnoses of sexually transmitted diseases, early generations of dermatologists concentrated most of their emphasis in this area. Discovery of a treatment for syphilis in the early twentieth century freed researchers to diversify their physiological investigations, opening the field to broader applications of biochemistry for treatment of different skin conditions, a field developed by the American doctor Stephen Rothman in the 1930's. Some categories, such as fungal diseases, were brought under control by treatments that were developed fairly quickly. By the second half of the century, dermatologists could alleviate most of the complications caused by psoriasis. Then, during the last quarter of the twentieth century, impressive advances in the discovery and patenting of sophisticated drugs brought most of the major dermatological diseases, including those caused in large part by nervous stress, under general control.

Although the treatment of life-threatening diseases, particularly skin cancers, continues to fall short of guaranteed cures, early recognition of their symptoms has steadily increased patients' chances for survival.

—*Byron D. Cannon, Ph.D.*

See also Abscess drainage; Abscesses; Acne; Age spots; Albinos; Athlete's foot; Bedsores; Biopsy; Birthmarks; Blisters; Boils; Bruises; Burns and scalds; Cancer; Carcinoma; Chickenpox; Collagen; Cryosurgery; Cyst removal; Cysts; Dermatitis; Dermatology, pediatric; Dermatopathology; Diaper rash; Eczema; Electrocauterization; Fifth disease; Fungal infections; Glands; Grafts and grafting; Hair; Hair loss and baldness; Hair transplantation; Hand-foot-and-mouth disease; Healing; Histology; Hives; Human papillomavirus (HPV); Itching; Impetigo; Lesions; Lice, mites, and ticks; Melanoma; Moles; Multiple chemical sensitivity syndrome; Nail removal; Necrotizing fasciitis; Neurofibromatosis; Pigmentation; Plastic surgery; Poisonous plants; Psori-

asis; Rashes; Ringworm; Rosacea; Scabies; Sense organs; Skin; Skin cancer; Skin disorders; Skin lesion removal; Styes; Sunburn; Systemic lupus erythematosus (SLE); Tattoo removal; Tattoos and body piercing; Touch; Warts; Wrinkles.

FOR FURTHER INFORMATION:

Braverman, Irwin M. *Skin Signs of Systemic Disease.* 3d ed. Philadelphia: W. B. Saunders, 1998. This book deals with the side effects of chronic diseases such as lymphomas and leukemia that may, at certain stages, be diagnosed through dermatological analysis.

Ceaser, Jennifer. *Everything You Need to Know About Acne.* Rev. ed. New York: Rosen, 2003. Covers the different forms of acne, their causes, and treatment forms in an approachable manner.

Hall, John C., and Gordon C. Sauer. *Sauer's Manual of Skin Diseases.* 10th ed. Philadelphia: Lippincott Williams & Wilkins, 2010. This detailed and frequently updated text is among the most widely used in medical schools. Part of its organization consists of "reminder boxes" to emphasize salient points for diagnosis and therapy.

Jacknin, Jeanette. *Smart Medicine for Your Skin.* New York: Putnam, 2001. An accessible guide to skin care, written in an A-to-Z format. Explores both alternative and conventional therapies for everything from common acne to diminishing wrinkles.

Monk, B. E., R. A. C. Graham-Brown, and I. Sarkany, eds. *Skin Disorders in the Elderly.* Boston: Blackwell Scientific, 1992. This collection of studies deals with typical skin problems among the elderly. Many of these skin problems stem from infections elsewhere in the body.

Turkington, Carol, and Jeffrey S. Dover. *The Encyclopedia of Skin and Skin Disorders.* 3d ed. New York: Facts On File, 2007. More than one thousand entries on skin-related topics, including diseases, treatments, resources and organizations, skin cancer, acne treatment, FDA approvals of new treatments, and remedies for wrinkled skin.

Weedon, David. *Skin Pathology.* 3d ed. New York: Churchill Livingstone/Elsevier, 2010. Text with extensive photographs, covering tissue reaction patterns; the epidermis, dermis, and subcutis; the skin in systemic and miscellaneous diseases; infections and infestations; and tumors, among other topics.

Dermatology, pediatric

Specialty

Anatomy or system affected: Skin

Specialties and related fields: Oncology, pediatrics, plastic surgery

Definition: The medical specialty that deals with the diagnosis and treatment of diseases and disorders of the skin that occur in infants and children.

Key terms:

congenital: existing or present at birth; usually also existing before birth

dermatitis: an inflammation of the skin

dermatosis: a condition of the skin; any skin disease not characterized by inflammation

skin biopsy: a small sample of skin removed for laboratory evaluation to help establish a diagnosis

systemic: affecting the entire body

topical treatment: a treatment that is placed on the skin itself

Science and Profession

A pediatric dermatologist is a skin doctor who has specialized training in the diagnosis and treatment of childhood skin disorders. The full course of training requires a medical degree followed by specialized residency training, usually at a large teaching hospital. Skin problems account for nearly one-third of all children's doctor visits. Most skin problems, however, are diagnosed in the primary care setting, by a pediatrician, family physician, physician assistant, or nurse practitioner. Primary care clinicians typically refer children with those conditions most difficult to diagnose or treat to the pediatric dermatologist. In addition, many general dermatologists also diagnose and treat children with skin problems.

The skin is the largest organ of the body and serves many functions. It is the body's first line of defense against infection, harmful substances, and radiation. It regulates body temperature. It conserves body fluids and also serves as a barrier to water. It helps in the production of vitamin D. The skin is also important in helping individuals sense the environment around them through special receptors for touch, heat, pain, and vibration. Any or all of these functions of the skin can be disrupted by the diseases and disorders that are diagnosed and treated by the pediatric dermatologist.

Children have some skin problems that are unique to childhood and share some skin problems with adults. For example, people of almost any age can have a condition called seborrheic dermatitis. Yet, each age group

from infancy through adolescence has its own characteristic skin conditions or problems. For example, newborns may have salmon patches (commonly known as stork bites), infants may have diaper rash, and adolescents may have acne. Some childhood diseases, such as chickenpox, are found mostly in toddlers and school-age children. Likewise, some skin conditions, such as seborrheic keratoses, are found primarily in adults.

Changes in the skin may represent diseases and disorders of the skin itself, as in diaper dermatitis (diaper rash) or sunburn. Skin changes may also reflect a systemic disease or disorder, as in the rash associated with scarlet fever. Some skin lesions are markers for serious underlying conditions, either congenital or acquired. For example, a condition called neurofibromatosis may be signaled by the presence of multiple café-au-lait spots on the trunk. Thus, the pediatric dermatologist must be knowledgeable not only about the skin but also about all systemic diseases that produce skin changes.

Diagnostic and Treatment Techniques

Most diagnoses relating to the skin are based on the appearance of the lesion itself. Lesions may be flat or raised, wet or dry, scattered or clustered, tender or nontender. They may have characteristic colors. They may be on the skin surface or extend beneath it. Typically, skin lesions are described according to their location on the body, their configuration, color, any changes that may have occurred as the result of secondary infection or scratching, and what the individual lesion itself looks like. In general, the pediatric dermatologist will inspect the skin of the entire body, even though only a small area may seem to be involved. In addition, the dermatologist will obtain a history related to the skin lesion: how long it has been there, whether it comes and goes, any changes that have taken place, what the patient or parents have used to treat the problem, allergies, and other symptoms such as pain or itching.

Usually, a thorough history and physical examination are sufficient to make the diagnosis of skin problems; however, the pediatric dermatologist may need to perform certain diagnostic or confirmatory tests. These tests may include a culture if a skin lesion is thought to be the result of an infection by a virus or bacterium. The dermatologist may gently scrape a lesion (particularly when a fungus is suspected) and examine the scrapings under a microscope. Certain dermatoses require the performance of a skin biopsy. In some cases, dermatologists punch out a small part of the skin lesion; in other cases, they cut out the entire lesion and a certain amount of surrounding tissue.

Treatments used by pediatric dermatologists may be topical, systemic, or surgical. Diaper dermatitis, for example, is usually treated with a topical cream or ointment aimed at killing the fungus that causes it. Impetigo, a bacterial infection of the skin, is usually treated with systemic antibiotics. Many kinds of skin lesions are treated with steroid creams, gels, or ointments. The dermatologist may surgically remove a mole with changes suspicious of skin cancer or use a laser to remove a birthmark.

PERSPECTIVE AND PROSPECTS

In the United States, many pediatric dermatologists (or general dermatologists with an interest in children's problems) belong to the Society for Pediatric Dermatology. The purpose of this group, formed in 1975, is to promote, develop, and advance education and research on skin conditions in children and to improve care. The group meets twice a year to present the latest advances in this field. The American Academy of Dermatology, while not specifically devoted to children's dermatology, also educates physicians about childhood problems. Another organization devoted specifically to children's skin problems is the International Society of Pediatric Dermatology.

—*Rebecca Lovell Scott, Ph.D., PA-C*

See also Acne; Albinos; Allergies; Birthmarks; Blisters; Boils; Bruises; Burns and scalds; Chickenpox; Childhood infectious diseases; Cradle cap; Dermatitis; Diaper rash; Fifth disease; Frostbite; Fungal infections; Hand-foot-and-mouth disease; Hives; Impetigo; Itching; Lesions; Lice, mites, and ticks; Measles; Moles; Neurofibromatosis; Pityriasis alba; Pityriasis rosea; Plastic surgery; Poisonous plants; Psoriasis; Rashes; Ringworm; Roseola; Rubella; Scabies; Scarlet fever; Skin; Skin disorders; Styes; Sunburn; Tattoo removal; Tattoos and body piercing; Warts.

FOR FURTHER INFORMATION:

American Medical Association. *American Medical Association Family Medical Guide.* 4th rev. ed. Hoboken, N.J.: John Wiley & Sons, 2004. An excellent reference for the beginner. The scientific accuracy of the text is not compromised by its accessibility.

Middlemiss, Prisca. *What's That Rash? How to Identify and Treat Childhood Rashes.* London: Hamlyn, 2002. A comprehensive guide to the identification and treatment of childhood rashes.

Porter, Robert S., et al., eds. *The Merck Manual Home Health Handbook.* Whitehouse Station, N.J.: Merck Research Laboratories, 2009. A team of nearly two hundred experts, consultants, and authors has assembled a body of information so vast that listing select items fails to do it justice.

Schmitt, Barton D. *Your Child's Health: The Parents' One-Stop Reference Guide to Symptoms, Emergencies, Common Illnesses, Behavior Problems, Healthy Development.* Rev. ed. New York: Bantam Books, 2005. Written for parents in a format that takes the guesswork out of when to call your health provider. This book covers almost any situation a parent could encounter. An essential resource.

Thompson, June. *Spots, Birthmarks, and Rashes: The Complete Guide to Caring for Your Child's Skin.* Toronto, Ont.: Firefly Books, 2003. Guide for identifying and treating skin disorders, with special attention to birthmarks and growths. Text accompanied by clear, color photographs.

Titman, Penny. *Understanding Childhood Eczema.* New York: Wiley, 2003. Discusses the physical and emotional toll of eczema on young patients and provides practical advice for choosing and managing different treatments.

Weston, William L., et al. *Color Textbook of Pediatric Dermatology.* 4th ed. St. Louis, Mo.: Mosby/Elsevier, 2007. Clinical textbook that covers a range of disorders, including drug reactions, hair disorders, nail disorders, and sun sensitivity. Clinical features, differential diagnosis, pathogenesis, treatment, and patient education are discussed.

Woolf, Alan D., et al., eds. *The Children's Hospital Guide to Your Child's Health and Development.* Cambridge, Mass.: Perseus, 2002. An authoritative and comprehensive guide to children's health, providing a guide to every common illness or condition that affects children and a carefully designed emergency section.

DERMATOPATHOLOGY
SPECIALTY

ANATOMY OR SYSTEM AFFECTED: Immune system, skin

SPECIALTIES AND RELATED FIELDS: Cytology, dermatology, forensic medicine, histology, immunology, oncology, pathology

DEFINITION: The study of the causes and characteristics of diseases or changes involving the skin.

KEY TERMS:

basal cells: cells at the base of the epidermis that migrate upward and become the principal source of epidermal tissue

dermatoses: disorders of the skin

dermis: the layer of skin just below the surface, in which is found blood and lymphatic vessels, sebaceous (oil) glands, and nerves; also called the corium

epidermis: the outer layer of the skin, consisting of a dead superficial layer and an underlying cellular section

SCIENCE AND PROFESSION

Dermatopathology is the medical specialty that utilizes external clinical features of the body's surface, as well as histological changes that are observed microscopically, to define diseases of the skin. The dermatopathologist is a physician who has specialized in pathology, the clinical study of disease, and/or in histology, the microscopic study of cells and tissues. Although the specific clinical field of this specialty involves the skin, the practitioner has also received broader training in pathology.

The skin is the tough, cutaneous layer that covers the entire surface of the body. In addition to the epidermal tissue of the surface, the skin contains an extensive network of underlying structures, including lymphatic vessels, nerves and nerve endings, and hair follicles. The dead cells on the surface of the epidermis continually slough off, to be replaced by dividing cells from the underlying basal layers. As these cells proceed to the surface, they mature and die, forming the outer layer of the skin.

When a disease or condition of the skin is being diagnosed, the initial observations are often carried out by a general practitioner or dermatologist. This person will make a gross observation; if warranted, biopsies or samples of the lesion may then be provided to the dermatopathologist for examination. The most common forms of skin lesions are those associated with allergies, such as contact dermatitis associated with exposure to plant oils (such as poison ivy) or chemicals (such as antibiotics). More serious dermatologic diseases may also require diagnosis. Specific types of disease are often represented by specific kinds of lesions; these may include a variety of forms of skin cancers, lesions associated with bacterial or viral infections (such as impetigo or herpes simplex), and autoimmune disorders (such as lupus). The dermatopathologist may also be concerned with diseases of underlying tissue, such as lymphoid cancers or lesions penetrating into mucous membranes.

The dermatopathologist is involved in the diagnosis of the problem but generally is not involved with specific forms of treatment. Nevertheless, his or her recommendations may certainly influence any decisions. The major role of the dermatopathologist is observation; this may then be followed by an interpretation of results, including a possible prognosis or outcome.

DIAGNOSTIC AND TREATMENT TECHNIQUES

The clinical examination of skin lesions initially falls within the realm of the dermatologist. If the gross observations are insufficient to warrant diagnosis, however, a sample of the lesion can be sent to the dermatopathologist for further examination. In addition to the tissue sample, information on the age, sex, and skin color of the patient should be included, along with any history of the suspected condition.

If the lesion is superficial, as in dermatoses such as warts or even certain types of cancer, a superficial shave biopsy is sufficient for examination. If the lesion involves an infiltrating tumor, inflammation, or possible metabolic problems, a deeper section of tissue is necessary. The specimen is immediately placed in a fixative solution, such as formalin, to prevent deterioration.

The dermatopathologist initially embeds the sample in paraffin, which can be sectioned into thin slices after hardening. The tissue is stained, most commonly with hematoxylin and eosin (H & E), and observed microscopically.

Anything about the cells that is out of the ordinary may be helpful in the diagnosis of the problem. For example, in the case of basal cell carcinoma, the cells may be abnormally shaped, with enlarged nuclei. They may also be observed infiltrating other layers of tissue. With contact dermatitis, the lesion is characterized by infiltration of large numbers of white blood cells, particularly lymphocytes, with their easily observed large nuclei. Edema, the abnormal accumulation of fluid, is also common with these types of lesions.

The presence of bacteria, as with boils or impetigo, warrants the use of antibiotics, unlike other inflammatory lesions. In this matter, the dermatopathology of the sample can determine the appropriate form of treatment.

While dermatopathology is primarily observational, recommendations regarding treatment may be made by its practitioners. For example, the study of a sample for the type and extent of cancer may lead to a recommendation concerning how extensive the surgical removal of the tumor should be.

Perspective and Prospects

The use of the physical appearance of the skin as a means of diagnosis represents one of the earliest attempts to understand disease. With the microscopic examination of tissue, first performed during the nineteenth century, it became possible to match the presence of histological lesions to specific diseases and to differentiate these diseases from one another.

The field of dermatopathology was greatly refined during the twentieth century. The development of differential and immunological staining methods allowed for a greater understanding of the roles played by the wide variety of cells in the body. For example, the dendritic cells of the skin were found to have a critical function in the immune responses that begin at that level.

In many Western countries, there was a significant shift during the twentieth century in the types of skin disease most commonly seen, mostly reflecting changes in lifestyle. The prevalence of malignant melanomas and basal cell carcinomas became much higher as a result of increased exposure to sun during leisure hours. The recognition of such problems has become an important aspect of the training of clinicians less specialized than dermatopathologists, such as family physicians.

—*Richard Adler, Ph.D.*

See also Autoimmune disorders; Bacterial infections; Biopsy; Cancer; Carcinoma; Cytopathology; Dermatitis; Dermatology; Diagnosis; Edema; Electrocauterization; Grafts and grafting; Herpes; Histology; Human papillomavirus (HPV); Lesions; Melanoma; Microscopy; Oncology; Pathology; Pigmentation; Plastic surgery; Skin; Skin cancer; Skin disorders; Skin lesion removal; Systemic lupus erythematosus (SLE); Viral infections; Warts.

For Further Information:

Caputo, Ruggero, and Carlo Gemetti. *Pediatric Dermatology and Dermatopathology: A Concise Atlas.* Washington, D.C.: Taylor & Francis, 2002. Reviews childhood dermatologic diseases in alphabetical order with a brief description and photos of clinical and pathological features.

McKee, Phillip. *A Concise Atlas of Dermatopathology.* New York: Gower Medical, 1993. This atlas of skin problems discusses histopathology, among other topics. Includes an index.

Mehregan, Amir H., et al. *Pinkus' Guide to Dermatohistopathology.* 6th ed. Norwalk, Conn.: Appleton & Lange, 1995. The sixth edition of a diagnostic reference to dermal pathology, for dermatology residents and practitioners. References extensively updated. Abundant halftone illustrations.

Tierney, Lawrence M., Stephen J. McPhee, and Maxine A. Papadakis, eds. *Current Medical Diagnosis and Treatment 2007.* New York: McGraw-Hill Medical, 2006. This text, updated yearly, is the point of reference for physicians and other health care practitioners. It incorporates each year's biomedical research discoveries that have immediate, relevant, and applicable use for the patient.

Weedon, David. *Skin Pathology.* 3d ed. New York: Churchill Livingstone/Elsevier, 2010. Text with extensive photographs, covering tissue reaction patterns; the epidermis, dermis, and subcutis; the skin in systemic and miscellaneous diseases; infections and infestations; and tumors, among other topics.

Developmental disorders

Disease/disorder

Also known as: Pervasive developmental disorders

Anatomy or system affected: Nervous system, psychic-emotional system

Specialties and related fields: Psychiatry, psychology

Definition: A group of conditions that indicate significant delays in or a lack of social skill development with deficiencies in adaptive behaviors, poor language skills, and a limited capacity to communicate effectively.

Key terms:

antipsychotic medication: a category of drugs helpful in the treatment of psychosis

Asperger's disorder: severe and sustained impairment in social interactions, often involving limited interests

disintegrative disorder: deterioration in functioning following a period of normal development

encephalopathy: disorder of the brain

infantile autism: the first term coined in 1943 for a diagnosis of autistic disorder

microcephaly: abnormal smallness of the head

regression: reverting to a pattern of behavior seen at an earlier age of development

CAUSES AND SYMPTOMS

The developmental disorders are categorized into five distinct disorders that all share the central feature of childhood development that is outside the norm in some manner. The five disorders are described in the *Diagnostic and Statistical Manual of Mental Disorders: DSM-IV-TR* (rev. 4th ed., 2000), which is published by the American Psychiatric Association. The DSM-IV-TR serves as the main resource for information concerning the diagnostic criteria for all psychiatric disorders and mental conditions. The developmental disorders are included under the heading of pervasive developmental disorders in the DSM-IV-TR. The term "pervasive" is used to indicate the extensive developmental deficits found among these disorders. The five developmental disorders in the DSM-IV-TR are autistic disorder, Rett's disorder, childhood disintegrative disorder, Asperger's disorder, and "pervasive developmental disorder not otherwise specified."

Autistic disorder is probably the best known of the disorders in the developmental disorders group, and reports indicate that it occurs in 2 to 20 cases per 10,000 births. Autistic disorder has an onset before age three years but may not be formally diagnosed until some years later. Children with autistic disorder do not commonly show any unusual physical characteristics, but they demonstrate a number of behavioral, social, and affective symptoms. There are usually major deficiencies in the capacity to show social relatedness to others, including parents. The social smile is absent during infancy, and autistic children continue to show deficits in play activities and social attachments throughout their lives. There is an inability to understand or infer the feelings and mental state of other people around them. Language development is usually limited, with difficulties in communicating ideas even when the vocabulary is present. Retardation occurs in a high percentage of children with autism, with greatest deficits in abstract reasoning and social understanding. Children from an early age do not show interactive play activity but rather engage in repetitive actions such as rocking and other unusual mannerisms. Children with autism usually form attachments to inanimate objects rather than to people. Their mood is usually marked with sudden changes and potentially aggressive outbursts. Although the exact cause in unknown, autistic disorder is considered to have a biological cause with a high genetic vulnerability. Research has indicated that two regions on chromosomes 2 and 7 contain genes involved with autistic disorder. Studies suggest that abnormal levels of serotonin and other neurotransmitters in the brain are found because there is a disruption of normal brain development early in fetal development caused by defects in the genes. The temporal lobe area of the brain has been implicated in the development of autism since this area is strongly associated with social development.

Rett's disorder features a period of normal development for approximately six months after birth that is followed with deterioration of functioning. Typical symptoms then occur, such as encephalopathy, seizures, breathing difficulties, loss of purposeful hand movements, loss of social engagement with others, poor coordination, and severely impaired language development. The growth of the head circumference slows and produces microcephaly. The child begins to show repetitive movements such as hand-wringing and problems in walking. The condition is progressive, and the skill level remains at the level of the first year of life. Children may live for ten years or more but must use a wheelchair as a result of muscle wasting. The cause of Rett's disorder has been identified as related to a genetic mutation. The gene is located at the Xq28 site on the X chromosome. Only one of the two X chromosomes need have the mutation in order for it to cause the disorder. This means that it is an X-linked dominant disorder. It is a rare condition usually found in females.

Childhood disintegrative disorder is diagnosed when there is marked regression or deterioration in a number of areas of functioning after age two. Children with this disorder begin to lose language and social skills previously developed in the first two years of life. Both bowel and bladder control can be lost as well as manual skills. It is common for these children to exhibit high levels of anxiety as the deterioration progresses. Children with this disorder also typically develop seizures. The cause of childhood disintegrative disorder is unknown, but it is considered to be related to some central nervous system pathology.

INFORMATION ON DEVELOPMENTAL DISORDERS

CAUSES: Genetic and biological causes
SYMPTOMS: Impairment in language, cognitive abilities, social skills, communication
DURATION: Chronic
TREATMENTS: Structured educational and behavioral interventions

Asperger's disorder is marked with symptoms of severe and sustained impairments in social interactions. Repetitive patterns of behavior are commonly seen. In contrast to autism, children with Asperger's disorder do not exhibit significant delays in language or cognitive development. Common characteristics that are used to describe Asperger's disorder include a lack of empathy toward the feelings of others, minimal social interactions, limited ability to form friendships, pedantic and monotonic speech, and intense fascination with trivial topics learned in rote fashion. The cause of Asperger's disorder is unknown but is believed to have a genetic base. Current research suggests that a tendency toward the condition may run in families. Children with Asperger's are also at risk for other psychiatric problems, including depression, attention-deficit disorder, schizophrenia, and obsessive-compulsive disorder. Persons with Asperger's have a variable prognosis depending upon their cognitive abilities and language skills, but all continue into adulthood showing an awkward manner toward other adults and lack of comfort in social settings. Asperger's disorder is usually first diagnosed in children between the ages of two and six.

"Pervasive developmental disorder not otherwise specified" is the fifth developmental disorder described in the DSM-IV-TR. It is viewed as a severe impairment in communication skills with deficiencies in social behavior. It differs from autistic disorder in terms of the severity of symptoms, and persons diagnosed with this disorder experience better functioning into adulthood than those with autistic disorder.

Treatment and Therapy

The goal for treatment of autistic disorder is to increase socially acceptable behaviors and decrease or extinguish unusual actions such as rocking and self-injurious behaviors. Therapy attempts to improve verbal and nonverbal communication skills to enhance interactions with other people. Therapy usually involves both educational and behavioral interventions with structured classroom training using behavioral techniques that employ rewards or positive reinforcements. Treatments for children with autistic disorder require a great deal of structure and repetition. Family members often participate in counseling sessions to help with the stressors of raising a child with autistic disorder. Medications are used as an adjunct to educational and behavioral treatments to diminish temper tantrums, self-injurious behaviors such as head banging, and hyperactivity. Antipsychotic medications such as risperidone and haloperidol are the most commonly used adjunctive treatments.

Rett's disorder has limited treatment options. The focus is on providing symptomatic relief whenever possible and structured behavioral techniques of positive rewards to concentrate on positive behaviors. Anticonvulsive medications are used to control seizures that can develop in this disorder and also diminish self-injurious behaviors. Physical therapy can assist with the distress associated with muscle deterioration.

Childhood disintegrative disorder is treated with similar methods as used in autistic disorder. Highly structured educational and behavioral programs are used to maintain the limited language and cognitive skills that had developed prior to the onset of the disorder.

Asperger's disorder treatments depend upon the level of functioning present among those with this disorder. Emphasis is usually placed upon improving social skills and adaptive functioning in social situations.

Treatment for "pervasive developmental disorder not otherwise specified" is basically the same as used with autistic disorder. Children with this disorder have a higher functioning of language skills than found with autistic disorder; consequently, the educational and behavioral treatments are supplemented with individual psychotherapy.

Perspective and Prospects

Autistic disorder was initially identified in 1867 by psychiatrist Henry Maudsley, but it was not until 1943 that Leo Kanner coined the term "infantile autism" and carefully described the associated signs and symptoms of the condition. Even with this description, many children with autism received the diagnosis of childhood schizophrenia. This tendency toward misdiagnosis continued into the 1980's. When considering the causes for the development of infantile autism, Kanner initially hypothesized that infantile autism was due to emotionally unresponsive or "refrigerator" mothers who were unable to provide nurturance and emotional warmth to their newborn infants. Some children reacted to this emotional coldness by turning inward as a defense mechanism. Due to this defense, the child with autism focused on his or her inner world and did not develop communication skills. The child with autism usually focuses on inanimate objects rather than people and exhibits repetitious or self-stimulating behaviors such as rocking to gain personal satisfaction. Additions to this theoretical idea focused on the unresponsiveness of both parents toward the child and feelings of rage directed toward the child. Theories focusing on parental factors have since been discarded with the current emphasis on identifying biological and genetic factors in the development of autism.

Rett's disorder was first identified by pediatrician Andreas Rett in 1966. Practicing in Austria, Rett based his descriptions on a pool of twenty-two girls who had developed normally until they were around six months of age. Rett published his findings in several German medical journals, but the information was largely ignored in the rest of the world. Awareness about the disorder increased when Rett published a description of the disease in English in 1977, but it was a 1983 article that appeared in the mainstream English-language journal *Annals of Neurology* that finally raised the recognition of this disorder and used the term "Rett's syndrome" for the disorder. Currently there is still limited information about this developmental disorder.

Childhood disintegrative disorder was first described in 1908 by Viennese remedial teacher Theodor Heller. He described six children who had unexpectedly developed a severe mental deterioration between their third and fourth years of life after previously normal development. Heller termed the condition "dementia infantilis," and it was subsequently called Heller's syndrome. The disorder is more often diagnosed in males than in females—at a ratio of 4:1—and occurs in approximately one birth out of 100,000. Although the DSM-IV-TR uses two years of age as the standard for its diagnosis, most cases emerge when a child is between three and four years of age.

Asperger's disorder was first described by Hans Asperger in 1944. Working in Austria, he used the term "autistic psychopathy" for the condition. Asperger described a number of children, and his descriptions were close to Kanner's idea of infantile autism. Asperger's portrayals differed from Kanner's, however, in that speech was less commonly delayed and the onset appeared to be somewhat later. The children that Asperger described were seen to have social behavior that was labeled as odd or unusual. Asperger called the children with this condition "little professors" because of their formal manner when talking about their favorite topics using great detail. Asperger also suggested that similar problems could be observed in family members, particularly fathers. Most of the scientific literature concerning Asperger's disorder initially appeared in the European professional journals until Asperger's syndrome was made official in 1994 when the diagnosis was added to the DSM-IV.

—Frank J. Prerost, Ph.D.

See also Antianxiety drugs; Anxiety; Asperger's syndrome; Autism; Bonding; Cognitive development; Developmental stages; Learning disabilities; Mental retardation; Neuroimaging; Psychiatric disorders; Psychiatry; Psychiatry, child and adolescent; Speech disorders.

For Further Information:

Aman, M., et al. "Medication and Parent Training in Children with Pervasive Developmental Disorders and Serious Behavior Problems: Results from a Randomized Clinical Trial." *Journal of the American Academy of Child and Adolescent Psychiatry* 23 (October, 2009): 1025-1038. This research article presents outcomes demonstrating the importance of family involvement in the education and treatment of children with autistic disorder.

Bopp, K., et al. "Behavior Predictors of Language Development over Two Years in Children with Autism Spectrum Disorders." *Journal of Speech, Language, and Hearing Research* 52 (October, 2009): 1106-1120. The authors examined the predictive relationships between such behaviors as repetitious actions and the future development of vocabulary and language skills in young children with autism.

Elder, J., et al. "Supporting Families of Children with Autism Spectrum Disorders: Questions Parents Ask and What Nurses Need to Know." *Pediatric Nursing* 35 (July/August, 2009): 240-245. The authors discuss the many questions that families of children with autistic disorders typically have and suggest how to help them provide meaningful lives for their children and themselves.

Noterdaeme, M., et al. "Asperger's Syndrome and High-Functioning Autism: Language, Motor, and Cognitive Profiles." *European Child and Adolescent Psychiatry* 8 (October, 2009): 875-925. This article provides a comparison of the cognitive profile, the motor and language functioning, and the psychosocial adaptation of children with Asperger's syndrome compared to children with high-functioning autism.

Developmental stages

Development

Anatomy or system affected: Brain, nervous system, psychic-emotional system

Specialties and related fields: Neurology, psychiatry, psychology

Definition: The growth and changes that occur over time in children's mental and physical processes as they develop from birth to adulthood.

Key terms:

attachment: special relationship of mutual closeness established between an infant and a caregiver; based on consistent caring, it confers an anticipation of security in relationships

concrete operations stage: Jean Piaget's cognitive stage in which concrete, easily visualized objects can be grouped together, combined, and transformed in equivalent ways; "concrete" contrasts with "formal" operations, which involve abstract and hypothetical transformations

initiative versus guilt: Erik Erikson's characterization for the young child's imaginative exploration of wishes and impulses in fantasy and dramatic play, restrained by emerging pangs of conscience

mental operations: comprehension of the reversibility of such events as regrouping objects into different categories or transferring a fixed quantity of a substance into containers of different shapes

preoperational stage: Piaget's transitional stage of young childhood in which absent objects can be remembered from mental representations but cannot be grouped or logically manipulated

sensorimotor stage: Piaget's stage in infancy in which objects can be recognized by appropriate habitual reactions to them

stage: a period in a progressive, invariant sequence of events when specified cognitive and motivational events are programmed to occur

Physical and Psychological Factors

The development of the human being from the infant to the child to the adolescent to the adult is a story of increasing physical, cognitive, social, and emotional adequacy in coping with environmental demands. Major observers of human development have added a key corollary concerning the nature and pace of this development: It occurs in stages.

Development in stages implies several features about the process. The first implication is that developmental changes are not simply quantitative but also qualitative, changes not only in degree but also in kind. With advancement to another stage, perceptions, thoughts, motives, and social interactions are fundamentally altered. A second implication is that development is uneven in its pace—sometimes flowing and sometimes ebbing, sometimes fast and sometimes slow and steady in apparent equilibrium. A third implication is that the order of the stages is invariant: One always moves from lower to higher stages. No individual skips stages; each subsequent stage is a necessary antecedent to the more mature or advanced stages to come. The invariant sequence is preordained by the biological maturation of neurological systems and by the necessary requirements of human societies.

Descriptions of development in terms of stages are found in the writings of many psychologists, especially cognitive psychologists, who are interested in age-related changes in thinking styles, and psychoanalytic psychologists, influenced by Sigmund Freud, who concern themselves with changes in the growing child's emotional involvements. The most significant, influential, and comprehensive of stage descriptions of development are those of two seminal scientists, Jean Piaget (1896-1980) and Erik Erikson (1902-1994).

Piaget, a cognitive developmental psychologist, outlined a series of shifts in children's cognition, their ways of thinking about and interpreting the world. They include the sensorimotor stage in infancy, the preoperational stage beginning in toddlerhood, the intuitive preoperational substage of the preschool child, the concrete operations stage of the school-age child, and the formal operations stage beginning in adolescence.

Erikson, who updated psychoanalytic theory, outlined a series of age-related shifts in motives and ways of relating to others, each one related to a psychosocial crisis. These psychosocial stages include an infancy stage of trust versus mistrust, a toddlerhood stage of autonomy versus shame and doubt, a preschool childhood stage of initiative versus guilt, a school-age stage of competence versus inferiority, and an adolescent stage of identity versus role diffusion.

The approaches of Piaget and Erikson originated independently, each emphasizing different aspects of development. The stages that they describe, however, should be viewed as complementary. Since the social changes result in large part from shifts in the child's thinking, the psychosocial stages of Erikson closely parallel the cognitive stages outlined by Piaget.

In infancy, a period lasting from birth to about eighteen months, sensorimotor cognitive development is initiated by rapid brain development. During the first six months of life, the nerve cells in the forebrain that control coordinated movements, refined sensory discriminations, speech, and intellect increase greatly in number and size and develop a rich network of connections. This neural growth makes possible dramatic progress in the child's ability to discriminate relevant objects and to coordinate precise movements of arms, legs, and fingers in relating to these objects. The infant who was capable of only a few reflexes at birth by six months can grasp a dangling object. The infant who was born with very poor visual acuity by six months can recognize detailed patterns in toys and faces. The infant shows recognition and knowledge of an object by relating to it repeatedly with the same pattern of movements. During the first few months of life, the infant has very limited ability to recall objects when they are not directly seen or heard and, in fact, will fail to look for a toy when it is not in view. Sensorimotor integrations, therefore, form the infant's principal method of representing reality. Only gradually does attention span increase and does the infant acquire the capacity to think about missing objects. The capacity to keep out-of-sight objects in mind, the gradual appreciation of object permanence, is a key achievement of the sensorimotor stage.

The corresponding psychosocial stage of infancy is built around the establishment of trust, some sort of sustaining faith in the stability of the world and the security of human relationships. Crucial to the establishing of this trust is the stability of the infant's relationship with a primary caregiver, most commonly a mother. Babies begin to pay special attention to the caregiver on a schedule determined by their cognitive development. The primary caregiving adult is among the first significant objects identified by the infant. Indeed, it appears that infants are wired to be especially responsive to a human caregiver. Infants of only two or three months of age find the human face the most interesting object and will focus on faces and facelike designs in preference to almost any other stimulus object. By the age of six months, infants clearly recognize the caregiver as special but for some time cannot appreciate that the caregiver continues to exist during absences. Thus, conspicuous anxiety sometimes occurs when the caregiver leaves.

It is little wonder that an infant perceives the caregiver as special. The human caregiver is wonderfully reinforcing to the infant. Relief from all kinds of pain, smiling responses to infantile smiles, vocal responses to infant babbling, soft and warm cuddling contact, and games all offer to the infant what is most craved. By six to nine months of age, the baby seems dependent on the caregiver for a basic feeling of security. Until the age of two or three, most infants seem more secure when their mother or primary caregiver is physically present. The relationship between the quality and warmth of infant-mother interactions and the infant's feelings of security has been supported by voluminous research on mother-infant attachment.

By about age two, neural and physical developments make possible the advance to more adaptive styles of cognitive interpretations. Piaget characterized the cognitive stage of toddlerhood as preoperational. Brain centers important for language and movement continue to develop rapidly. Now the child can deal cognitively with reality in a new way, by representing out-of-sight and distant objects and events by words, images, and symbols. The child can also imitate the actions of people not present. Thinking during this stage remains limited. The child cannot yet hold several thoughts simultaneously in mind and manipulate them—that is, perform mental operations. This stage is, therefore, "preoperational."

Erikson described the psychosocial crisis of toddlerhood as autonomy versus shame and doubt. This crisis results in part from the child's cognitive growth. The preoperational child has acquired an increasing ability to appreciate the temporary nature of a caregiver's absence and to move about independently. The toddler can now assert autonomy and often does so emphatically. Resistance to parental demands is possible, and the toddler seems to delight in such resistance. "No" becomes a favorite word. Since this period corresponds to the time when children are toilet trained, parent-child tugs-of-war often involve issues of bowel control and cleanliness. The beginning of shame, the humiliation that comes from overextending freedom foolishly and making mistakes, begins to serve as a self-imposed check on this autonomy.

Piaget characterized the thinking of three-, four-, and five-year-olds as "intuitive." This thinking is still preoperational. Children can represent to themselves all sorts of objects but cannot keep these objects in the focus of attention long enough to classify them or consider how these objects could be regrouped or transformed. If six tin soldiers are stretched into three groups of two, the preschool child assumes that there are now more than before. Thinking is egocentric because children lack the ability to put themselves in the perspective of others while keeping their own perspective. Yet preschool children make all sorts of intuitive attempts to fit remembered events and scenes into underlying plots or themes. Fanciful attempts to understand events often result in misconstruing the nature of things. Children at this stage are easily misled by appearances. A man in a tiger suit could become a tiger; a boy who wears a dress could become a girl and grow up to be a mother. Appearance becomes reality.

Erikson characterized the corresponding psychosocial stage of the preschool child as involving the crisis of initiative versus guilt. The child's new initiative is expressed in playful exploration of fanciful possibilities. Children can pretend and transform themselves in play as never before and never again. From dramatic play, the child's conceptions of the many possibilities of the world of bigger people are enacted. The earlier psychoanalyst, Freud, focused particularly on how children experience their first sexual urges at this time of life and sometimes weave into their ruminations fantastic themes of possession of the opposite-sex parent and jealous triumph over the same-sex parent. To Erikson, such themes are merely examples of the many playful fantasies essential to later, more realistic involvements.

Piaget characterized the cognitive stage of the school-age child as the concrete operations stage. The child is capable of mental operations. The school-age child can focus on several incidents, objects, or events simultaneously. Now it is obvious that six tin soldiers sorted into three pairs of two could easily be transformed back into a single group of six. Regardless of grouping, the total quantity is the same. The formerly egocentric child becomes cognitively capable of empathetic role taking, of assuming the perspective of another person while keeping the perspective of the self in mind. In making ethical choices, the child can now appreciate the impact of alternative possibilities on particular people in particular situations. The harshness of absolute dictates is softened by empathetic understanding of others.

Erikson characterized the psychosocial crisis of the school-age child as one of competence versus inferiority. Now is the time for children to acquire the many verbal, computational, and social skills that are required for adequate adulthood. Learning experiences are structured and planned, and performances are evaluated. Newly empathetic children are only too aware of how their skill levels are perceived by others. Adequacy is being assessed. The schoolchild must not only be good but also be good at something.

The cognitive stage of the adolescent was described by Piaget as formal operational. The dramatic physical changes that signal sexual maturity are accompanied by less obvious neural changes, especially a fine tuning of the frontal lobes of the brain, the brain's organizing, sequencing, executive center. Cognitively, the adolescent becomes capable of dealing with formal operations. Unlike concrete operations, which can be visualized, formal operations include abstract possibilities that are purely hypothetical, abstract strategies useful in ordering a sequence of investigations, and "as if" or "let us suppose" propositions.

Erikson's corresponding psychosocial crisis of adolescence was that of identity versus role diffusion. The many physical and mental changes and the impending necessity of finding occupational, social, marital, religious, and political roles in the adult world impel a concern with the question, "Who am I?" To interact as an adult, one must know what one likes and loathes, what one values and despises, and what one can do well, poorly, and not at all. Most adolescents succeed in finding themselves—some by adopting the identity of family and parents, some after a soul-searching struggle.

DISORDERS AND EFFECTS

Stage theories define success as advancement through the series of stages to maturity. Psychosocially, each successful advance yields a virtue that makes life endurable: hope, will, purpose, competence, and finally fidelity to one's own true self. As a final reward for normal developmental success, one can enjoy the benefits of adulthood: intimacy, or the sharing of one's identity with another, and generativity, or the contribution of one's own gifts to the benefit of the next generation and to the collective progress of humankind. Cognitively, maturity means the capacity for formal operational thought. Hypothetical thinking of this type is basic to most fields of higher learning, to the sciences, to philosophy, and even to the comprehension of such abstract moral principles as justice.

Advancement to each subsequent stage of cognitive development is dependent on both neurological maturation and a culture that presents appropriate problems. Adults who fail to attain concrete operational thought are considered mentally retarded. A failure in neurological maturation is a frequent cause. Failures to attain formal operational thought, on the other hand, are not unusual among normal adults. Cultural experience must nourish advancement to formal operational thinking within a domain of inquiry by the provision of moderately novel and challenging but not overwhelming tasks. When people are not confronted with such complex problems within some domain, then abstract, formal operational thought fails to occur. Abstract ethical reasoning is a case in point. Cross-cultural studies suggest that concepts of justice that involve the application of abstract rules are rare in cultures where people seldom confront questions of ethical complexity.

Psychosocial pathology is evidenced by development arrested in one of the immature stages of psychosocial development. It results from a social environment that fails to foster growth or exaggerates the particular apprehensions that are most acute in one of the developmental stages.

The development of trust in infancy requires a loving, available, and sensitive caretaker. If the infant's caretaker is unavailable, missing, neglectful, or abusive, the pathology of mistrust develops. The world is perceived as unstable. Close personal relationships are viewed as unreliable, fickle, and possibly malicious. Later, closeness in relationships may be rejected. Confident exploration of the possibilities of life may never be attempted.

Similarly, the apprehensions of each subsequent psychosocial stage can be exaggerated to the point of pathology. The toddler, shamed out of troublesome expressions of autonomy, may compensate for doubts with the rigidly excessive controls of the compulsive lifestyle. The preschool child can become so overwhelmed with guilt over playful fantasies, particularly sexual and aggressively tinged fantasies, that adult possibilities become severely restricted. The school-age child can become so wounded by humiliations in a harshly competitive school environment that the child becomes beaten down into enduring feelings of inferiority. An adolescent may so fear the risks of exploring the possibilities of life that future adulthood becomes a shallow diffusion of roles, a yielding to social pressures and whims unguided by any knowledge of who one really is.

The successful confrontation of the tasks of adulthood—finding a partner to share intimacy and caring for the next generation—are most easily attainable for adults who have overcome each of these earlier developmental hurdles.

Perspective and Prospects

Stage theories of development are found as early as 1900 in the work of American psychologist James Mark Baldwin and in Freud's psychoanalysis. Baldwin, much influenced by Charles Darwin's theory of evolution by natural selection, hypothesized that the infant emerges from a sensorimotor stage of infancy to a symbolic mode of thinking, an advancement yielding enormous evolutionary advantages. Freud, the Viennese psychoanalyst, based his conception of emotional development on what he called psychosexual stages. Progression occurs from an oral period of infancy, when sensory pleasure is concentrated on the mouth region, to an anal stage of toddlerhood, when anal pleasures and the control of such pleasures become of concern. When sexual pleasure shifts to the genital region in the three-year-old, the love of the opposite-sex parent becomes sexually tinged, and the child becomes jealous of the same-sex parent. Working through these so-called Oedipal fantasies was, to Freud, crucial to the formation of personality.

Neither Baldwin nor Freud and his followers were the sort of rigorous scientists most respected by scientific psychology in the mid-twentieth century. Far more influential in American psychology between 1920 to about 1960 were behavioral conceptions of the developmental process as steady, incremental growth. To behaviorists such as B. F. Skinner, becoming an adult was conceived as a process of continuously being reinforced for learning progressively more adequate responses.

The stage approaches of Piaget and Erikson were introduced to most American psychologists in 1950, the year that both Piaget's *Psychology of Intelligence* and Erikson's *Childhood and Society* were published in English. Piaget's description of cognitive stages was much more complete than Baldwin's earlier account and was much better supported by clever behavioral observations. Erikson's thesis of psychosocial stages incorporated most of Freud's observations about stages. Erikson treated the social environmental pressures intrinsic to each stage as events of primary importance and shifts in the locus of bodily pleasures as secondary.

By the 1970's, Piaget's and Erikson's accounts of stages were awarded an important place in most developmental texts. This influence occurred for several reasons. First, researchable hypotheses were derived, and most of this research was supportive. Cross-cultural comparisons suggested that these stages could be found in a similar sequence in differing cultures. Second, the theses of Piaget and Erikson were mutually supportive. The stage-related cognitive changes, in fact, would seem to explain the corresponding psychosocial concerns. Finally, these approaches generated productive spinoffs in related theory and research. In 1969, basing his work on the cognitive changes outlined by Piaget, Lawrence Kohlberg elaborated a stage sequence of progressively more adequate methods of moral reasoning. In 1978, basing her work on Erikson's hypotheses about trust, Mary Ainsworth began a productive research program on the antecedents and consequents of stable and unstable mother-infant attachment styles.

The most recent challenges to cognitive and psychosocial stage theory arise from the alternative perspectives of biopsychology and information-processing theory. Some psychologists argue that biologically rooted temperament, rather than the social environment, affects both styles of attachment and identity formation. Not only do babies respond to caregivers, but caregivers respond to babies as well. A baby who begins with a shy, passive temperament may be more susceptible to an avoidant attachment style and more likely to elicit detached, unresponsive caregiver behavior. Temperament, it is maintained, is more important than psychosocial environment.

Information processing theorists have challenged the discontinuity implied by stage concepts. They suggest that the appearance of global transformations in the structure of thought may be an illusion. Development is a continuous growth of efficiency in processing and problem solving. The growing child combines an expanding number of ideas, increases the level and speed of processing by increments, and learns more effective problem-solving strategies. To select particular points in this continuous development and call them "stages," they argue, is purely arbitrary.

The final research to settle the question of the ultimate nature of stages has not been performed. A psychosocial stage theorist can acknowledge the role of temperament but still maintain that loving, trust-creating environments are also significant in encouraging the child to apply temperamental potential in positive social directions rather than in angry antagonism or frightened withdrawal. At the very least, Piagetian and Eriksonian stage concepts have the practical usefulness of highlighting significant developmental events and interpersonal reactions to these events. The warmth of caregivers for infants, the later tolerance of children's struggles to become themselves, and environments that present challenging problems appropriate to the child's developmental level are vital to emotional and intellectual growth.

For some purposes, it may be instructive to break the achievement of cognitive and emotional growth into increments that can be seen as if under a microscope. For other purposes, it is instructive to go up for an aerial view to gain perspective on the nature and direction of such achievements. The aerial view is the contribution of stage theories of development.

—Thomas E. DeWolfe, Ph.D.

See also Bed-wetting; Bonding; Cognitive development; Developmental disorders; Motor skill development; Puberty and adolescence; Reflexes, primitive; Separation anxiety; Soiling; Speech disorders; Teething; Thumb sucking; Toilet training; Weaning.

FOR FURTHER INFORMATION:

Berk, Laura E. *Child Development.* 8th ed. Boston: Pearson/Allyn & Bacon, 2009. A text that reviews theory and research in child development, cognitive and language development, personality and social development, and the foundations and contexts of development.

Feldman, Robert S. *Development Across the Life Span.* 5th ed. Upper Saddle River, N.J.: Pearson/Prentice Hall, 2008. Traces the physical, cognitive, and social and personality development of one's life span, focusing on basic theories, research findings, and current applications of theory.

Ginsburg, Herbert, and Sylvia Opper. *Piaget's Theory of Intellectual Development.* 3d ed. Englewood Cliffs, N.J.: Prentice Hall, 1988. A detailed, book-length elaboration of Jean Piaget's stage theory of cognitive development.

Hall, Calvin S., Gardner Lindzey, and John B. Campbell. *Theories of Personality.* 4th ed. New York: John Wiley & Sons, 1998. Chapter 5, "Current Psychoanalytic Theory," describes Erikson's psychosocial stages and current research inspired by this theory. Chapter 2 describes Sigmund Freud's earlier psychosexual stages.

Karen, Robert. "Becoming Attached." *Atlantic Monthly* 265, no. 2 (February, 1990): 35-70. A thorough, fair, and readable account of the research on attachment and its relationship to trust in people.

Miller, Patricia H. *Theories of Developmental Psychology.* 5th ed. New York: Worth, 2010. A comparative analysis of developmental theories. Piaget's cognitive stage theory and Freud's and Erikson's psychoanalytic theories are described and compared with other developmental approaches.

Nathanson, Laura Walther. *The Portable Pediatrician:*

A Practicing Pediatrician's Guide to Your Child's Growth, Development, Health, and Behavior from Birth to Age Five. 2d ed. New York: HarperCollins, 2002. An engaging, easy-to-read guide for parents to assess their child's development, medical symptoms, and behavioral problems.

Parke, Ross D., et al., eds. *A Century of Developmental Psychology.* Washington, D.C.: American Psychological Association, 1994. Contains material on the early approaches of James Mark Baldwin and a review of attachment theory and research.

Sternberg, Robert J. *Psychology: In Search of the Human Mind.* 3d ed. Fort Worth, Tex.: Harcourt College, 2001. As in most other texts in introductory psychology, the stage theories of Erik Erikson and Jean Piaget are described in the chapter on human development. A good discussion of the concept of developmental stages.

DIABETES MELLITUS
DISEASE/DISORDER

ANATOMY OR SYSTEM AFFECTED: Abdomen, blood vessels, circulatory system, endocrine system, eyes, gastrointestinal system, glands, heart, kidneys, nervous system, pancreas

SPECIALTIES AND RELATED FIELDS: Endocrinology, family medicine, genetics, internal medicine, nephrology, neurology, pediatrics, vascular medicine

DEFINITION: A hormonal disorder in which proper blood sugar levels are not maintained; due either to insufficient production of insulin by the pancreas or to an inability of the body's cells to use insulin efficiently. If left untreated, diabetes mellitus leads to complications such as blindness, cardiovascular disease, dementia, kidney disease, and, eventually, death.

KEY TERMS:

beta cells: the insulin-producing cells located at the core of the islets of Langerhans in the pancreas; the alpha, or glucagon-producing, cells form an outer coat

cross-linking: a chemical reaction, triggered by the binding of glucose to tissue proteins, that results in the attachment of one protein to another and the loss of elasticity in aging tissues

glucosuria: a condition in which the concentration of blood glucose exceeds the ability of the kidney to reabsorb it; as a result, glucose spills into the urine, taking with it body water and electrolytes

hyperglycemia: excessive levels of glucose in the circulating blood

insulin-dependent diabetes mellitus (IDDM): type 1 diabetes, a state of absolute insulin deficiency in which the body does not produce sufficient insulin to move glucose into the cells

insulin resistance: a lack of insulin action; a reduction in the effectiveness of insulin to lower blood glucose concentrations; characteristic of type 2 diabetes

insulitis: the selective destruction of the insulin-producing beta cells in type 1 diabetes

islets of Langerhans: clusters of cells scattered throughout the pancreas; they produce three hormones involved in sugar metabolism: insulin, glucagon, and somatostatin

ketoacidosis: high levels of ketones in the blood that result from a lack of circulating insulin

non-insulin-dependent diabetes mellitus (NIDDM): type 2 diabetes, which is the state of a relative insulin deficiency; although insulin is released, its target cells do not adequately respond to it by taking up blood glucose

CAUSES AND SYMPTOMS

Diabetes mellitus is by far the most common of all endocrine (hormonal) disorders. The word "diabetes" is derived from the Greek word for "siphon" or "running through," a reference to the potentially large urine volume that can accompany the condition. *Mellitus,* the Latin word for "honey," was added when physicians began to make the diagnosis of diabetes mellitus based on the sweet taste of the patient's urine. The disease has been depicted as a state of starvation in the midst of plenty. Although there is plenty of sugar in the blood, without proper insulin action the sugar does not reach the cells that need it for energy. Glucose, the simplest form of sugar, is the primary source of energy for many vital functions. Deprived of glucose, cells starve and

---

INFORMATION ON DIABETES MELLITUS

CAUSES: Genetic and environmental factors

SYMPTOMS: Large urine output, excessive thirst, dehydration, low blood pressure, weight loss despite increased appetite, fatigue, nausea, vomiting, blurred vision

DURATION: Chronic

TREATMENTS: Insulin or oral hypoglycemic drugs, lifestyle changes (diet modification and exercise)

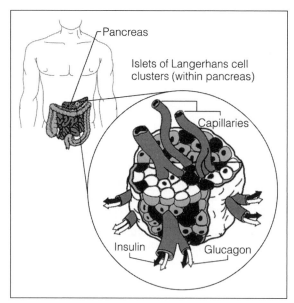

Location of the pancreas, with a section showing the specialized cells (islets of Langerhans) that produce the sugar-metabolizing hormones.

tissues begin to degenerate. The unused glucose builds up in the bloodstream, which leads to a series of secondary complications.

The most common symptoms of diabetes mellitus are related to hyperglycemia, glycosuria, and ketoacidosis. The acute symptoms of diabetes mellitus are all attributable to inadequate insulin action. The immediate consequence of an insulin insufficiency is a marked decrease in the ability of muscle, liver, and adipose (fat) tissue to remove glucose from the blood. In the presence of inadequate insulin action, a second problem manifests itself. People with diabetes continue to make the hormone glucagon. Glucagon, which raises the level of blood sugar, can be considered insulin's biological opposite. Like insulin, glucagon is released from the pancreatic islets. The release of glucagon is normally inhibited by insulin; therefore, in the absence of insulin, glucagon action elevates concentrations of glucose. For this reason, diabetes may be considered a "two-hormone disease." With a reduction in the conversion of glucose into its storage forms of glycogen in liver and muscle tissue and lipids in adipose cells, concentrations of glucose in the blood steadily increase (hyperglycemia). When the amount of glucose in the blood exceeds the capacity of the kidney to reabsorb this nutrient, glucose begins to spill into the urine (glucosuria). Glucose in the urine then drags additional body water along with it so that the volume of urine dra-

matically increases. In the absence of adequate fluid intake, the loss of body water and accompanying electrolytes (sodium) leads to dehydration and, ultimately, death caused by the failure of the peripheral circulatory system.

Insulin deficiency also results in a decrease in the synthesis of triglycerides (storage forms of fatty acids) and stimulates the breakdown of fats in adipose tissue. Although glucose cannot enter the cells and be used as an energy source, the body can use its supply of lipids from the fat cells as an alternate source of energy. Fatty acids increase in the blood, causing hyperlipidemia. With large amounts of circulating free fatty acids available for processing by the liver, the production and release of ketone bodies (breakdown products of fatty acids) into the circulation are accelerated, causing both ketonemia and an increase in the acidity of the blood. Since the ketone levels soon also exceed the capacity of the kidney to reabsorb them, ketone bodies soon appear in the urine (ketonuria).

Insulin deficiency and glucagon excess also cause pronounced effects on protein metabolism and result in an overall increase in the breakdown of proteins and a reduction in the uptake of amino acid precursors into muscle protein. This leads to the wasting and weakening of skeletal muscles and, in children who are diabetics, results in a reduction in overall growth. Unfortunately, the increased level of amino acids in the blood provides an additional source of material for glucose production (gluconeogenesis) by the liver. All these acute metabolic changes in carbohydrates, lipids, and protein metabolism can be prevented or reversed by the administration of insulin.

There are three distinct types of diabetes mellitus. type 1, or insulin-dependent diabetes mellitus (IDDM), is an absolute deficiency of insulin that accounts for approximately 10 percent of all cases of diabetes. Until the discovery of insulin, people stricken with type 1 diabetes faced certain death within about a year of diagnosis. In type 2 or non-insulin-dependent diabetes mellitus (NIDDM), insulin secretion may be normal or even increased, but the target cells for insulin are less responsive than normal (insulin resistance); therefore, insulin is not as effective in lowering blood glucose concentrations. Although either type can be manifested at any age, type 1 diabetes has a greater prevalence in children, whereas the incidence of type 2 diabetes increases markedly after the age of forty and is the most common type of diabetes. Genetic and environmental factors are important in the expression of both of these types of diabetes mellitus. The third type is gestational diabetes, which is characterized by high blood glucose during pregnancy in a person who did not previously have diabetes.

Type 1 diabetes is an autoimmune process that involves the selective destruction of the insulin-producing beta cells in the islets of Langerhans (insulitis). The triggering event that initiates this process in genetically susceptible persons is linked to environmental factors that result from an infection, a virus, or, more likely, the presence of toxins in the diet. The body's own T lymphocytes progressively attack the beta cells but leave the other hormone-producing cell types intact. T lymphocytes are white blood cells that normally attack virus-invaded cells and cancer cells. For up to ten years, there remains a sufficient number of insulin-producing cells to respond effectively to a glucose load, but when approximately 80 percent of the beta cells are destroyed, there is insufficient insulin release in response to a meal and the deadly spiral of the consequences of diabetes mellitus is triggered. Insulin injection can halt this lethal process and prevent it from recurring but cannot mimic the normal pattern of insulin release from the pancreas. It is interesting that not everyone who has insulitis actually progresses to experience overt symptoms of the disease, although it is known that the incidence of type 1 diabetes around the world is on the increase.

Type 2 diabetes is normally associated with obesity and lack of exercise as well as with genetic predisposition. Recently, with the reported increased rates of obesity and inactivity in children, there has also been an increase of type 2 diabetes at younger and younger ages. Family studies have shown that as many as 25 to 35 percent of persons with type 2 diabetes have a sibling or parent with the disease. The risk of diabetes doubles if both parents are affected. In the United States, the prevalence of type 2 diabetes in both adults and children is higher in some racial and ethnic groups—for example, African Americans, Native Americans, and Latinos—than it is among non-Latino Caucasians.

Because there is a reduction in the sensitivity of the target cells to insulin, people with type 2 diabetes must secrete more insulin to maintain blood glucose at nor-

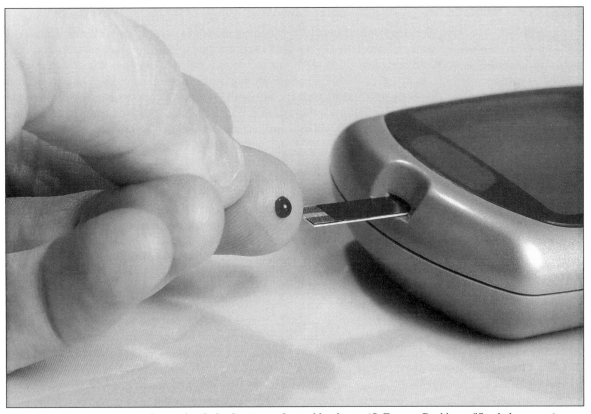

A diabetic performs a glucose level check using a finger blood test. (© Eugene Bochkarev/iStockphoto.com)

mal levels. Because insulin is a storage, or anabolic, hormone, this increased secretion further contributes to obesity. In response to the elevated insulin concentrations, the number of insulin receptors on the target cell gradually decreases, which triggers an even greater secretion of insulin. In this way, the excess glucose is stored despite the decreased availability of insulin binding sites on the cell. Over time, the demands for insulin eventually exceed even the reserve capacity of the "genetically weakened" beta cells, and symptoms of insulin deficiency develop as the plasma glucose concentrations remain high for increasingly longer periods of time. This phenomenon is known as beta-cell burn out. Because the symptoms of type 2 diabetes are usually less severe than those of type 1 diabetes, many persons have the disease but remain unaware of it. Unfortunately, once the diagnosis of diabetes is made in these individuals, they also exhibit symptoms of long-term complications that include atherosclerosis and nerve damage. Hence, type 2 diabetes has been called the silent killer.

Gestational diabetes develops during pregnancy in a person who did not have diabetes before becoming pregnant. It occurs in approximately 7 percent of all pregnancies. Women with gestational diabetes have an increased risk of developing diabetes after pregnancy. Children of women with gestational diabetes have a higher risk of obesity, glucose intolerance, and diabetes in adolescence.

Prediabetes is a condition in which individuals have blood glucose levels that are high, but not high enough to be diagnosed with type 2 diabetes. Persons with prediabetes are at higher risk to develop diabetes in the future.

Treatment and Therapy

Insulin is the only treatment available for type 1 diabetes, and in many cases it is used to treat individuals with type 2 diabetes. Insulin is available in many formulations, which differ in respect to the time of onset of action, activity, and duration of action. Insulin preparations are classified as fast-acting, intermediate-acting, and long-acting; the effects of fast-acting insulin last for thirty minutes to twenty-four hours, while those of long-acting preparations last from four to thirty-six hours. Some of the factors that affect the rate of insulin absorption include the site of injection, the patient's age and health status, and the patient's level of physical activity. For a person with diabetes, however, insulin is a reprieve, not a cure.

Because of the complications that arise from chronic exposure to glucose, it is recommended that glucose concentrations in the blood be maintained as close to physiologically normal levels as possible. For this reason, it is preferable to administer multiple doses of insulin during the day. By monitoring plasma glucose concentrations, the diabetic person can adjust the dosage of insulin administered and thus mimic normal concentrations of glucose relatively closely. Basal concentrations of plasma insulin can also be maintained throughout the day by means of electromechanical insulin delivery systems. Whether internal or external, such insulin pumps can be programmed to deliver a constant infusion of insulin at a rate designed to meet minimum requirements. The infusion can then be supplemented by a bolus injection prior to a meal. Increasingly sophisticated systems automatically monitor blood glucose concentrations and adjust the delivery rate of insulin accordingly. These alternative delivery systems are intended to prevent the development of long-term tissue complications.

There are a number of chronic complications that account for the shorter life expectancy of diabetic persons. These include atherosclerotic changes throughout the entire vascular system. The thickening of basement membranes that surround the capillaries can affect their ability to exchange nutrients. Cardiovascular lesions are the most common cause of premature death in diabetic persons. Kidney disease, which is commonly found in longtime diabetics, can ultimately lead to kidney failure. For these persons, expensive medical care, including dialysis and the possibility of a kidney transplant, overshadows their lives. Diabetes is the leading cause of new blindness in the United States. Delayed gastric emptying (gastroparesis) occurs when the stomach takes too long to empty its contents; it results from damage to the vagus nerve from long-term exposure to high glucose levels. In addition, diabetes leads to a gradual decline in the ability of nerves to conduct sensory information to the brain. For example, the feet of some diabetics feel more like stumps of wood than living tissue. Consequently, weight is not distributed properly; in concert with the reduction in blood flow, this problem can lead to pressure ulcers. If not properly cared for, areas of the foot can develop gangrene, which may then lead to amputation of the foot. Finally, in male patients, there are problems with reproductive function that generally result in impotence.

The mechanism responsible for the development of these long-term complications of diabetes is genetic in

In the News: Increase in Type 2 Diabetes in Adults and Children

There is no doubt that the United States, as well as many other countries around the world, is affected by an "obesity epidemic." Poor eating habits and sedentary lifestyles are causing higher rates of obesity across all age groups and ethnic backgrounds. Approximately 30 percent of adults in the United States are obese. The rate of obesity in children ages two to five and ages twelve to nineteen has tripled since the mid-1970's. In children ages six to eleven, this rate has quadrupled from 4 to an alarming 19 percent.

Type 2 diabetes is occurring with increasing frequency in children, adolescents, and adults. The number of people with diabetes has more than doubled in the United States, from 15 percent in 1980 to 34 percent in 2006. Type 2 diabetes accounts for 90 to 95 percent of these cases. In 2005-2006, 72 percent of adults ages twenty to seventy-four were overweight or obese.

The Centers for Disease Control and Prevention estimates that 8 to 43 percent of new cases of diabetes in children are type 2 diabetes. These young people are usually overweight or obese, have a family history of diabetes, have signs of insulin resistance such as acanthosis nigricans, are members of an ethnic group with a high risk of type 2 diabetes, and are more often girls than boys.

This increase has many causes. The serving sizes of foods sold in stores and restaurants have increased. In many neighborhoods, there are more fast food restaurants than grocery stores. Approximately 30 percent of all calories consumed by Americans are in the form of sodas and fruit-flavored drinks. Teenagers drink more soda than milk, and about half of children ages six to eleven drink soda daily. Less than 25 percent of Americans eat five or more servings of fruit and vegetables daily. To compound the problem, more than 30 percent of high school students do not exercise regularly, and more than half of adults do not get enough physical activity.

This epidemic can be stopped in a number of ways. Healthier eating habits and regular physical activity can decrease rates of obesity, diabetes, and many other chronic diseases. Breast-feeding is associated with lower rates of obesity in children. Parents can advocate for regular physical activity in schools and for healthy snacks and drinks in vending machines. Limiting television viewing and computer time, encouraging physical activity at home, and providing healthy meals and smaller portions can all contribute to controlling the "obesity epidemic" in children.

—*Julie M. Slocum, R.N., M.S., C.D.E.*

As an animal ages, most of its cells become less efficient in replacing damaged material, while its tissues lose their elasticity and gradually stiffen. For example, the lungs and heart muscle expand less successfully, blood vessels become increasingly rigid, and ligaments begin to tighten. These apparently diverse age-related changes are accelerated in diabetes, and the causative agent is glucose. Glucose becomes chemically attached to proteins and deoxyribonucleic acid (DNA) in the body without the aid of enzymes to speed the reaction along. What is important is the duration of exposure to the elevated glucose concentrations. Once glucose is bound to tissue proteins, a series of chemical reactions is triggered that, over the passage of months and years, can result in the formation and eventual accumulation of cross-links between adjacent proteins. The higher glucose concentrations in diabetics accelerate this process, and the effects become evident in specific tissues throughout the body.

Understanding the chemical basis of protein cross-linking in diabetes has permitted the development and study of compounds that can intervene in this process. Certain compounds, when added to the diet, can limit the glucose-induced cross-linking of proteins by preventing their formation. One of the best-studied compounds, aminoguanidine, can help prevent the cross-linking of collagen; this fact is shown in a decrease in the accumulation of trapped lipoproteins on artery walls. Aminoguanidine also prevents thickening of the capillary basement membrane in the kidney. Aminoguanidine acts by blocking glucose's ability to react with neighboring proteins. Vitamins C and B_6 are also effective in reducing cross-linking. Aminoguanidine and vitamins C and B_6 are thought to have anti-aging properties and may also improve the complications resulting from the high blood-glucose levels seen in diabetes mellitus;

origin and dependent on the amount of time the tissues are exposed to the elevated plasma glucose concentrations. What, then, is the link between glucose concentrations and diabetic complications?

however, aminoguanidine and vitamins C and B_6 are not currently approved by the Food and Drug Administration (FDA) as therapeutic treatments for diabetes.

Alternatively, transplantation of the entire pancreas is an effective means of achieving an insulin-independent state in persons with type 1 diabetes mellitus. Both the technical problems of pancreas transplantation and the possible rejection of the foreign tissue, however, have limited this procedure as a treatment for diabetes. Diabetes is usually manageable; therefore, a pancreas transplant is not necessarily lifesaving. Success in treating diabetes has been achieved by transplanting only the insulin-producing islet cells from the pancreas or grafts from fetal pancreas tissue. It may one day be possible to use genetic engineering to permit cells of the liver to self-regulate glucose concentrations by synthesizing and releasing their own insulin into the blood.

Some of the less severe forms of type 2 diabetes mellitus can be controlled by the use of oral hypoglycemic agents that bring about a reduction in blood glucose. These drugs can be taken orally to drive the beta cells to release even more insulin than usual. These drugs also increase the ability of insulin to act on the target cells, which ultimately reduces the insulin requirement. The use of these agents remains controversial, because they overwork the already strained beta cells. If a diabetic person is reliant on these drugs for extended periods of time, the insulin cells could "burn out" and completely lose their ability to synthesize insulin. In this situation, the previously non-insulin-dependent person would have to be placed on insulin therapy for life. Other hypoglycemic agents lower blood glucose by decreasing hepatic glucose output, reducing insulin resistance, and delaying the absorption of glucose from the gastrointestinal tract.

If obesity is a factor in the expression of type 2 diabetes, as it is in most cases, the best therapy is a combination of a reduction of calorie intake and an increase in activity. More than any other disease, type 2 diabetes is related to lifestyle. It is often the case that people

---

IN THE NEWS: ACCORD TRIAL

The Action to Control Cardiovascular Risk in Diabetes (Accord) trial, sponsored by the National Heart, Lung, and Blood Institute, was a large-scale clinical study of adults with type 2 diabetes who were at high risk for cardiovascular disease. More than ten thousand adults across the United States and Canada were enrolled in the study; participants were between the ages of forty and seventy, had diabetes for an average of ten years, and were at high risk for cardiovascular disease owing to at minimum two risk factors in addition to type 2 diabetes.

The Accord trial examined cardiovascular disease events in three treatment strategies compared to standard treatments: intensive lowering of blood glucose levels, treating cholesterol and triglycerides with a fibrate plus a statin, and intensive lowering of blood pressure.

In 2008, the intensive glucose control arm of the trial was stopped nearly eighteen months early because of safety concerns. After an average of 3.5 years of treatment, the intensive control group exhibited a 22 percent increased risk of death compared to the standard treatment group. The standard treatment group included 5,123 participants and aimed to lower blood-sugar levels to a hemoglobin A1C (HbA1C) of 7 to 7.9 percent. The intensive therapy group included 5,128 participants and aimed to lower HbA1C to less than 6 percent.

The causes of death were similar in both groups, and approximately half of the deaths were caused by cardiovascular events including heart attack, stroke, heart failure, or sudden cardiac death. The intensive treatment group had a 35 percent higher cardiovascular death rate than the standard treatment group. The death rates were consistent between the groups, regardless of baseline characteristics such as gender, age, race, or existing cardiovascular disease. The participants in the intensive treatment group were moved to the standard treatment arm of the study and followed to the study's planned conclusion.

Researchers have been unable to identify the exact cause of the increased risk of death, but believe it is due to a combination of factors and not a specific medication or treatment. The results underscore the importance of individualized treatment for type 2 diabetes. No changes to standard treatment guidelines are recommended. The results of the trial do not apply to people with type 1 diabetes.

The Accord trial began in 2003 and followed patients through 2009. The researchers published the final results of the study in 2010.

—*Jennifer L. Gibson, Pharm.D.*

prefer having an injection or taking a pill to improving their quality of life by changing their diet and level of activity. Attention to diet and exercise results in a dramatic decrease in the need for drug therapy in nine of ten diabetics. In some cases, the loss of only a small percentage of body weight results in an increased sensitivity to insulin. Exercise is particularly helpful in the management of both types of diabetes, because working muscle does not require insulin to metabolize glucose. Thus, exercising muscles take up and use some of the excess glucose in the blood, which reduces the overall need for insulin. Permanent weight reduction and exercise also help to prevent long-term complications and permit a healthier and more active lifestyle.

PERSPECTIVE AND PROSPECTS

Diabetes mellitus is a disease of ancient origin. The first written reference to diabetes, which was discovered in the tomb of Thebes in Egypt (1500 B.C.E.), described an illness associated with the passage of vast quantities of sweet urine and an excessive thirst.

The study of diabetes owes much to the Franco-Prussian War. In 1870, during the siege of Paris, it was noted by French physicians that the widespread famine in the besieged city had a curative influence on diabetic patients. Their glycosuria decreased or disappeared. These observations supported the view of clinicians at the time who had previously prescribed periods of fasting and increased muscular work for the treatment of the overweight diabetic individual.

It was Oscar Minkowski of Germany who, in 1889, accidentally traced the origin of diabetes to the pancreas. Following the complete removal of the pancreas from a dog, Minkowski's technician noted the animal's

---

IN THE NEWS:
BENEFITS AND RISKS OF DIABETES DRUGS

The benefits and risks of diabetes drugs have caused concern among patients and health care providers, and challenged traditional treatment options as safety concerns of new drugs mount and the effectiveness of older medications is confirmed.

Metformin is the most commonly used oral medication to treat type 2 diabetes. Metformin reduces triglycerides and LDL cholesterol and increases HDL cholesterol. According to the United Kingdom Prospective Diabetes Study, metformin reduces the risk of myocardial infarction and stroke, making it a first-choice treatment option for most patients with diabetes.

Thiazolidinediones can cause significant weight gain and fluid retention, leading to an increased risk of heart failure. Several studies suggest, but do not prove, that one agent, rosiglitazone, may increase the risk of heart attack and cardiovascular death. Conversely, another agent, pioglitazone, may reduce the risk of heart attack and stroke. Both thiazolidinediones have shown an increased risk of fractures in women. More research is needed to verify these findings.

Glucagon-like peptide-1 (GLP-1) agonists are incretin hormone-based therapies. Exenatide, a GLP-1 agonist, causes substantial gastrointestinal side effects, but these typically resolve after a few weeks of treatment. Of benefit in diabetes, exenatide leads to significant weight loss. Several cases of pancreatitis have been reported with the use of exenatide; most of the cases resolved with discontinuation of the drug. Also, several cases of kidney dysfunction have been reported with exenatide. The U.S. Food and Drug Administration (FDA) warns to use exenatide cautiously in patients with existing kidney or pancreatic disease.

Dipeptidyl peptidase-4 (DPP4) inhibitors are also incretin-based drugs. Rare cases of severe allergic reactions, including angioedema and Stevens-Johnson syndrome, have occurred with the use of DPP4 inhibitors. Sitagliptin, a DPP4 inhibitor, is also associated with several cases of severe pancreatitis; most of the cases resolved with discontinuation of the drug. In late 2009, the FDA ordered the manufacturer of sitagliptin to change the prescribing information to warn of the increased risk of pancreatitis with sitagliptin.

Many experts have questioned the urgency with which new diabetes medications have emerged, and clinicians now advocate weighing the benefits of blood glucose control with the undesirable risks associated with many diabetes drugs.

—*Jennifer L. Gibson, Pharm.D.*

---

subsequent copious urine production. Acting on the basis of a hunch, Minkowski tested the urine and determined that its sugar content was greater than 10 percent.

In 1921, Frederick Banting and Charles Best, at the University of Toronto in Canada, successfully extracted the antidiabetic substance "insulin" using a cold alcohol-hydrochloric acid mixture to inactivate the harsh digestive enzymes of the pancreas. Using this substance, they first controlled the disease in a depancreatized dog and then, a few months later, successfully treated the first human diabetic patient. The clinical application of a discovery normally takes a long time, but in this case a mere twenty weeks had passed between the first injection of insulin into the diabetic dog and the first trial with a diabetic human. Three years later, in 1923, Banting and Best were awarded the Nobel Prize in Physiology or Medicine for their remarkable achievement.

Although insulin, when combined with an appropriate diet and exercise, alleviates the symptoms of diabetes to such an extent that a diabetic can lead an essentially normal life, insulin therapy is not a cure. The complications that arise in diabetics are typical of those found in the general population except that they happen much earlier in the diabetic. With regard to these glucose-induced complications, it was first postulated in 1908 that sugars could react with proteins. In 1912, Louis Camille Maillard further characterized this reaction at the Sorbonne and realized that the consequences of this reaction were relevant to diabetics. Maillard suggested that sugars were destroying the body's amino acids, which then led to increased excretion in diabetics. It was not until the mid-1970's, however, that Anthony Cerami in New York introduced the concept of the nonenzymatic attachment of glucose to protein and recognized its potential role in diabetic complications. A decade later, this development led to the discovery of aminoguanidine, the first compound to limit the cross-linking of tissue proteins and thus delay the development of certain diabetic complications.

In 1974, Josiah Brown published the first report showing that diabetes could be reversed by transplanting fetal pancreatic tissue. By the mid-1980's, procedures had been devised for the isolation of massive numbers of human islets that could then be transplanted into diabetics. For persons with diabetes, both procedures represent more than a treatment; they may offer a cure for the disease.

By the turn of the twenty-first century, there was a noticeable rise in the prevalence of type 2 diabetes in both developing and developed countries. In the United States, an estimated 24 million people have diabetes, a number expected to rise. It is believed that 57 million people have prediabetes, meaning that they could develop diabetes if they do not take preventive measures to lower their blood glucose levels. Although the incidence of type 2 diabetes typically increases with age, the first decade of the twenty-first has seen a dramatic rise in the number of cases in younger people.

Obesity is clearly linked to the increase of type 2 diabetes. The growing sedentary lifestyle and increase in energy-dense food intake in the United States are significant risk factors. The Centers for Disease Control reported that obesity more than doubled in the United States from 15 percent in 1980 to 34 percent in 2006. In 2005-2006, 72 percent of adults ages twenty to seventy-four were overweight or obese.

—Hillar Klandorf, Ph.D.;
updated by Sharon W. Stark, R.N., A.P.R.N., D.N.Sc.

See also Blindness; Endocrine disorders; Endocrine glands; Endocrinology; Endocrinology, pediatric; Eye infections and disorders; Gangrene; Gastroenterology; Gastroenterology, pediatric; Gastrointestinal system; Gestational diabetes; Glands; Heart attack; Hormones; Hyperadiposis; Hypoglycemia; Internal medicine; Metabolic disorders; Metabolic syndrome; Obesity; Obesity, childhood; Pancreas; Pancreatitis.

For Further Information:

American Diabetes Association. "Gestational Diabetes." *Diabetes Care* 26 (2003): S103-S105. Discussion of gestational diabetes risk factors, diagnosis, and treatment.

_____. http://www.diabetes.org. Comprehensive information on both type 1 and type 2 diabetes and current research and scientific findings, provides community forums and news stories, and helps decipher health insurance issues, among other features.

American Diabetes Association Complete Guide to Diabetes. 4th rev. ed. Alexandria, Va.: American Diabetes Association, 2006. A comprehensive consumer guide for all issues surrounding diabetes.

Becker, Gretchen. *The First Year—Type 2 Diabetes: An Essential Guide for the Newly Diagnosed.* 2d ed. New York: Marlowe, 2007. A unique guide for persons with type 2 diabetes, setting expectations and answering questions related to the first week of diagnosis, the first months, and the first year. Topics include treatment options, dietary choices, and holistic alternatives.

Centers for Disease Control and Prevention. http://www.cdc.gov/diabetes/consumer. A concise overview of diabetes—its diagnosis, treatment, and prevention.

Children with Diabetes. http://www.childrenwith diabetes.com. Site provides information that helps children with diabetes and their families learn about the disease, meet people with diabetes, and help others with diabetes.

Jovanovic-Peterson, Lois, Charles M. Peterson, and Morton B. Stori. *A Touch of Diabetes*. 3d ed. Minneapolis, Minn.: Chronimed, 1998. A straightforward guide for people with type 2 diabetes. Provides useful information on the disease and suggestions of how to change eating habits and monitor one's lifestyle.

Kronenberg, Henry M., et al., eds. *Williams Textbook of Endocrinology*. 11th ed. Philadelphia: Saunders/ Elsevier, 2008. Comprehensive information regarding endocrine diseases, pathophysiology, diagnoses, treatment, and prognoses.

McCulloch, David. *The Diabetes Answer Book: Practical Answers to More than Three Hundred Top Questions*. Naperville, Ill.: Sourcebooks, 2008. Answers to three hundred questions about diabetes, including lifestyle changes, diet and nutrition, and therapy.

Magee, Elaine. *Tell Me What to Eat If I Have Diabetes: Nutrition You Can Live With*. 3d ed. Franklin Lakes, N.J.: Career Press, 2008. This guide gives a nontechnical overview of diabetes combined with the latest nutritional advice for diabetics.

National Diabetes Information Clearinghouse. National Institute of Diabetes and Digestive and Kidney Diseases. http://diabetes.niddk.nih.gov/dm/ pubs/overview. A good discussion of diabetes, diagnosis, treatment, future directions in treatment, and other points to remember.

DIAGNOSIS

PROCEDURE

ANATOMY OR SYSTEM AFFECTED: All

SPECIALTIES AND RELATED FIELDS: All

DEFINITION: A methodical evaluation of symptoms and complaints through interview, observation, testing instruments, or procedures, including biological tests, to determine if an illness is present.

KEY TERMS:

criteria: specific items, denoting symptoms, which are part of diagnostic decision making and rules

differential diagnosis: the process used to discern between conditions with similar or overlapping symptoms

epidemiology: the science of studying the distributions of illness across populations of people

false negative: when a specific diagnosis was ruled absent, when in fact it is actually present

false positive: when a specific diagnosis is identified as being present, when in reality it is actually absent

INDICATIONS AND PROCEDURES

When individuals see health care professionals for treatment, they are evaluated to determine the nature of their concerns. The process of evaluation usually involves a combination of assessment, screening, reassessment, and then formal diagnosis. They typically initially describe their experience, concerns, and history, and then the professional asks more questions and may follow up with screening questions.

Screening questions identify risk for any more serious conditions and for which additional assessment is needed. Screening is inexpensive and involves a small amount of time on questions that are easy to ask and answer, providing a determination of whether the person is at risk for a specific problem. If the screening result is positive, then the risk is there and further evaluation is needed; if it is negative, then the risk is deemed absent and no further evaluation is needed. Unfortunately, no screening process is perfect, and so sometimes there are false negatives. This is why it is important that if problems continue, individuals seeking care get second opinions or return for evaluation.

If a screening result is positive, then additional assessment is conducted to determine if a diagnosable condition is present. This usually involves a complete symptom history, comparing the symptoms described to known disorders, and doing differential diagnosis. If the information collected does not yield anything, then the screening process resulted in a false positive. If, on the other hand, the collection of information yields enough information to show that the criteria for a condition are satisfied, then a diagnosis is confirmed. The most common diagnostic systems in use are the *Diagnostic and Statistical Manual of Mental Disorders: DSM-IV-TR* (rev. 4th ed., 2000), and the *International Classification of Diseases* (2000).

An example of how diagnosis may work is as follows. A person comes to an emergency room, has alcohol on the breath and no other medical problems, and is screened positive for alcohol problems by a nurse asking a few questions. Additional assessment is done by a psychologist, and they determine that the individual meets the criteria for alcohol dependence. Alcohol dependence is a condition with seven criteria, and an individual who demonstrates three or more in any twelve-month period qualifies for the diagnosis. The patient might report having tolerance (using more to get the same effect), withdrawal (insomnia when stopping using), and a persistent desire to quit, all in the past year. The psychologist then diagnoses the patient with alcohol dependence, and treatment will address that problem.

USES AND COMPLICATIONS

Diagnoses are useful in facilitating effective and quick communications among treatment professionals and other stakeholders in the care of the client. These stakeholders include other treatment providers, insurance companies, researchers in epidemiology and other areas of science, and the clients and their families.

One complication related to diagnoses, however, is that some diagnoses have symptoms that overlap and methods of differential diagnoses are always developing. As such, it is possible for misdiagnoses to occur. When this occurs, individuals may be treated for the wrong problem, or even overdiagnosed or underdiagnosed, and thus not properly treated. As such, it is often advised for more serious conditions that are costly to treat for patients to use multiple methods of diagnosis and even seek secondary opinions to confirm the diagnosis.

PERSPECTIVE AND PROSPECTS

All forms of healers and health care providers have been involved, since the beginning human societies, in the process of diagnosis in one form or another. As science has advanced in its understanding of causes of death and illness, procedures for diagnosis have also evolved. The procedures and rules for making diagnoses in many areas of health care continue to evolve as new technology and research develop. New technologies take many forms, ranging from improved questionnaires, to new interview procedures, to automated tests and screening online, to the use of new magnetic resonance imaging (MRI), and to even the use of virtual reality-assisted robots entering the body and allowing diagnosticians to see what is happening inside specific organs. All these methods aid in quicker diagnoses and faster paths to effective treatment.

One challenge to evolving diagnostic methods is that the world has become more interconnected over the last century. As a result, it is important for diagnosticians of all types to recognize cultural differences in terms of how symptoms are experienced, expressed, and understood. This is true for both physical and mental health

problems. Therefore, relevant screening, assessment, and other diagnostic technologies may need to adjust both in terms of how early symptoms are identified and in how information about diagnoses is conveyed to individuals of different backgrounds. This is the case as well because while diagnosis does involve technology, it is also a procedure involving human communication. As definitions and understandings of illness and health vary by culture, so too will communications about diagnosis need to adjust as cultures and health care providers interact more and more.

—*Nancy A. Piotrowski, Ph.D.*

See also Apgar score; Biopsy; Blood testing; Disease; Epidemiology; Hearing tests; Invasive tests; Laboratory tests; Mammography; Noninvasive tests; Pap test; Physical examination; Prognosis; Screening; Well-baby examinations.

FOR FURTHER INFORMATION:

American Psychiatric Association. *Diagnostic and Statistical Manual of Mental Disorders: DSM-IV-TR*. Rev. 4th ed. Washington, D.C.: Author, 2000. The technical manual outlines the major mental health disorders diagnosed in the United States.

Helman, Cecil G., ed. *Culture, Health, and Illness*. 5th ed. London: Hodder Education, 2007. Presents a useful discussion on how different cultures define and respond to illness, as well as how they define health.

World Health Organization. *International Statistical Classification of Diseases and Related Health Problems: 10th Revision–ICD-10*. 2d ed. Geneva, Switzerland: Author, 2000. This technical source is used internationally by professionals as a manual for classifying diseases, including both psychiatric and medical conditions.

DIALYSIS

PROCEDURE

ANATOMY OR SYSTEM AFFECTED: Abdomen, blood, circulatory system, kidneys, urinary system

SPECIALTIES AND RELATED FIELDS: Biotechnology, hematology, internal medicine, nephrology, serology, urology

DEFINITION: The artificial replacement of renal (kidney) function, which involves the removal of toxins in the blood by selective diffusion through a semipermeable membrane.

KEY TERMS:

hemodialysis: the removal of toxins from blood through the process of dialysis *osmosis:* the diffusion of molecules through a semi-permeable membrane until there is an equal concentration on either side of the membrane

peritoneal dialysis: the removal of toxins from blood by dialysis in the peritoneal cavity

peritoneum: the membrane lining the walls of the abdominal cavity and enclosing the viscera

INDICATIONS AND PROCEDURES

The two major functions of the kidneys are to produce urine, thereby excreting toxic substances and maintaining an optimal concentration of solutes in the blood, and to produce and secrete hormones that regulate blood flow, blood production, calcium and bone metabolism, and vascular tone. These functions can be impaired or even completely halted by kidney failure that may or may not be related to diseases such as hepatitis and diabetes. The kidney is the only human organ with a function—that is, the excretion of toxic substances from the blood—that can be artificially replaced on a reliable and chronic basis. Although dialysis cannot duplicate the intricate processes of normal renal function, it is possible to provide patients with a tolerable level of life.

If a solute is added to a container of water, it will be distributed at uniform concentration through the water. This process is called diffusion and results from random movement of the solute molecules in the solvent; it can be seen as a chemical mixing of the solution. The mixing will ensure an even distribution of solute molecules throughout the solution. The time required for complete mixing depends on factors such as the nature of the solute, its molecular size, the temperature of the solution, and the size of the container. The process of dialysis is based on the diffusion of solute molecules (urea and other substances) from the blood or fluids of a patient to a sterile solution called dialysate. The artificial kidney or dialysis system is designed to provide controllable osmosis, or the transfer of solutes and water across a semipermeable membrane separating streams of blood (contaminated as a result of renal failure) and dialysate (a sterile solution). For solutes such as urea, the outflowing blood concentration is high, while the concentration in the inflowing dialysate is usually zero. The result is a concentration gradient that guarantees osmosis of urea molecules from the blood to the dialysate solution. The same process will take place for other toxins present in the blood but absent from the dialysate solution.

There are two types of clinical dialysis, hemodialysis and peritoneal dialysis. In hemodialysis, the device utilized is called a dialyzer. The three basic structural elements of all dialyzers are the blood compartment, the membrane, and the dialysate compartment. In a perfect dialyzer, diffusion equilibrium would result in the blood and dialysate streams during passage through the device, and virtually all the urea and toxins contained in the inflowing blood stream would be transferred to the dialysate stream. This level of efficiency is not achieved, however, and for maximum efficiency, dialysate flow rate should be from two to two and one-half times the actual blood flow rate.

Several fundamental material and design requirements must be met in the construction of efficient dialyzers suitable for clinical use. First, the surfaces in contact with blood and the flow geometry must not induce the formation of blood clots. The materials used must be nontoxic and free of leachable toxic substances. The ratio of membrane surface area to contained volume must be high to ensure maximum transference of substances, and the resistance to blood flow must be low and predictable.

There are three basic designs for a dialyzer: the coil, parallel plate, and hollow fiber configurations. The coil dialyzer was the earliest design. In it, the blood compartment consisted of one or two membrane tubes placed between support screens and then wound with the screens around a plastic core. This resulted in a coiled tubular membrane laminated between support screens, which was then enclosed in a rigid cylindrical case. This design had serious performance limitations, such as a high hydraulic resistance to blood flow and an increase in contained blood volume as blood flow through the device was increased.

The coil design has all but been replaced by more efficient devices. In the parallel plate dialyzer, sheets of membrane are mounted on a plastic support screen and then stacked in multiple layers, allowing for multiple parallel blood and dialysate flow channels. The original design had problems with membrane stretching and nonuniform channel performance. To minimize these problems, smaller plates and better membrane supports have been developed. The hollow fiber dialyzer is the most effective design for providing low volume and high efficiency together with modest resistance to flow. Developed in the 1970's, the membrane is composed of tiny cellulose or synthetic hollow fibers about the size of a human hair. Between seven thousand and twenty-five thousand of those fibers are enclosed in a cylindrical jacket, with the blood inlet and outlet at the top and

The Administration of Hemodialysis

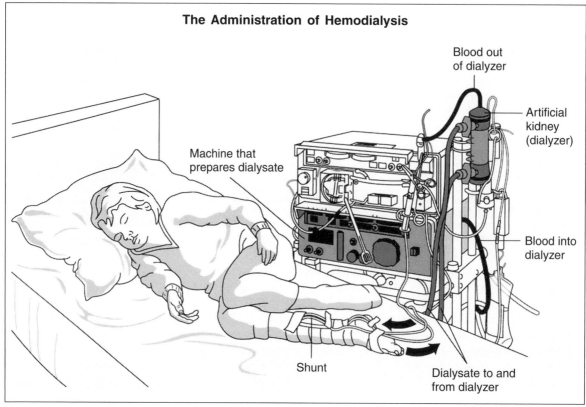

Dialysis is a method of removing wastes from the blood when the kidneys have failed to do so. Hemodialysis, which employs a machine that acts as an artificial kidney, is performed in a hospital or a local dialysis center in a session lasting two to six hours in which the blood is filtered to eliminate wastes, toxins, and excess fluid.

bottom of the cylinder and the dialysate inlet and outlet being simply expanded sections of the jacket itself. This is the most commonly used geometry for hemodialysis. Extreme care must be taken to ensure that all the extra fluids that might have entered the blood during dialysis are removed. Ultrafiltration refers to the removal of water from the blood after dialysis and is a critical component of the dialysis process.

The delivery system of a dialyzer provides on-line proportioning of water with dialysate concentrate and monitors the dialysate for temperature, composition, and blood leaks. It also controls the ultrafiltration rate and regulates the dialysate flow. Normally included in the system are a blood pump, blood pressure and air monitors, and an anticoagulant pump.

The composition of the dialysate is designed to approximate the normal electrolyte concentration found in plasma and extracellular water; it contains calcium, magnesium, sodium and potassium chloride, sodium acetate, sodium carbonate, and lactic acid, kept at a pH of 7.4. The water used in this preparation is purified,

heated to between 35 and 37 degrees Celsius, and deaerated to prevent air embolism. An anticoagulant must be added in the process to prevent the formation of blood clots. Heparin is the most commonly used anticoagulant, mainly because its effect is immediate, is easily measured, and can be almost immediately terminated by adding protamine. In addition, because of its high molecular weight and substantial protein binding, it is not dialyzable and will not be lost from the blood in the process.

Several types of polymers are commonly employed for the manufacture of the membranes utilized in hemodialysis. Cellulosic membranes, or membranes generated from the plant product cellulose, are the most commonly used polymers. (Cellophane was originally used, and later cuprophan and hemophan were introduced.) Noncellulosic artificial membranes made from synthetic polymers such as polycarbonate and polyamide are also used.

The development of efficient and more permeable synthetic membranes and ultrafiltration control delivery systems has reduced treatment time to two or three hours. Dialysis remains a potentially lethal procedure, and careful monitoring of equipment and solutions is necessary. For example, the dialysate must be monitored for hypertonic or hypotonic conditions that can result in hemolysis and death, and the flow from the dialyzer outlet back to the patient must have, among other things, an air bubble detector and filters to remove clots.

Peritoneal dialysis involves the transfer of solutes and water from the peritoneal capillary blood to the dialysate in the peritoneal cavity and the absorption of glucose and other solutes from the peritoneal fluid into the blood. The physiology of this process is less understood than that of hemodialysis. The process involves the introduction in the peritoneal cavity of a certain volume of dialysate and its removal after the dialysis process is complete. The main type of procedure is chronic intermittent peritoneal dialysis (CIPD). This process is performed three to seven times per week and takes from eight to twelve hours. It is mostly done overnight, when a pump introduces the dialysate to the peritoneal cavity and gravity removes it. Two systems are commonly used for this purpose: One is the reverse osmosis machine, which provides continuous flow through the night in a fast manner, while the other system utilizes a cycler for the cycling of the dialysate during the night. Cyclers are semiautomated systems with simple operation and a low initial expense that provide basically trouble-free performance but are expensive in the long run because they use premixed dialysates and many disposable components. Chronic ambulatory peritoneal dialysis (CAPD) is the most versatile and manageable of the techniques. In this case, the inflow and outflow of dialysate is done manually by gravity. With about 2 liters of dialysate used per exchange, it normally takes ten minutes for inflow and fifteen to twenty minutes for outflow. There are an average of four exchanges per day and one overnight. This is an easy, safe, and effective method of dialysis. A variation of CAPD is continuous cycling peritoneal dialysis (CCPD), introduced in 1980. It basically reverses the CAPD cycle: Cyclers are used during the night to achieve three to four exchanges, and there is a long period without exchange during the day. This minimizes the inconvenience of scheduling exchanges during the day, and many patients can alternate between the two methods without experiencing problems.

For peritoneal dialysis, the dialysate includes dextrose, lactate, sodium, calcium, and magnesium salts.

An anticoagulant such as heparin can be added when needed, such as if blood is seen in the peritoneal fluid. Other substances—such as insulin for both diabetic and nondiabetic patients, antibiotics if there is peritonitis, and bicarbonate to prevent abdominal discomfort—can also be added without major complications.

Peritoneal dialysis may be a better choice than hemodialysis for certain patients when factors such as coronary artery disease, diabetes mellitus, age, or severe hemodialysis-related symptoms are present. It is also the choice for patients whose residence is remote from a dialysis center, who wish to travel frequently, or who live alone.

Uses and Complications

Hemodialysis is used in acute and chronic renal failure patients. Some individuals, however, do not tolerate hemodialysis well, such as children, infants, geriatric patients, diabetics, and victims of traumatic injuries. Therefore, the selection of patients for this procedure must be closely monitored. The process also can be used for treatment of drug overdose (since drugs can be removed from the blood during the dialysis procedure) and hypercalcemia, an excess of calcium.

For many years, peritoneal dialysis was reserved for the treatment of acute renal failure (ARF) or for those patients awaiting transplantation or the availability of hemodialysis. Although it is used principally for the treatment of patients with end-stage renal disease, it remains a valuable tool in the management of ARF because of its simplicity and widespread availability. Essentially, it can be provided in any hospital by most internists or surgeons without the need for specially trained nephrology personnel. It also avoids the need for systematic anticoagulation, making it a good choice for patients in the immediate postoperative period with severe trauma, intracerebral hemorrhage, or hypocoagulable states. It is most suitable for the treatment of patients with an unstable cardiovascular system and for pediatric or elderly patients. It could be impossible to use, however, in postsurgical patients with many abdominal drains, with hernias, or with severe gastroesophageal reflux.

For many years, peritoneal dialysis was not used for patients with CRF (chronic renal failure) because of the problems involved in the maintenance of permanent peritoneal access, the inconvenience of manual dialysate exchanges, the high rate of peritonitis observed in these patients, and the rapid progress made in hemodialysis in the early 1960's. The advent of a safe, permanent peritoneal catheter in the late 1960's and the simultaneous development of automated reverse osmosis peritoneal delivery systems created new interest in the technique and resulted in safer, more effective systems. Peritoneal dialysis can also be used or is recommended in the following cases: for diabetic patients, since it provides a continuous source of insulin and also has the advantage of providing blood pressure control; for edema patients, since the process is useful in the treatment of intractable edema states such as congestive heart failure; and for pancreatitis patients or individuals who suffer from the release of pancreatic enzymes into the abdominal cavity and their subsequent absorption into the circulation. For the latter, the removal of the enzymes through peritoneal dialysis may prevent the necrotic process. Individuals exhibiting hypothermia as a consequence of accidental exposure, cold water immersion, central nervous system disorders, intoxication, or burns can be treated by performing peritoneal dialysis with dialysate solutions between 40 and 45 degrees Celsius. This will bring the body back to 34 degrees Celsius (a stable temperature) in a few hours, and, if the cause of the hypothermia is intoxication, the drugs causing the condition can be removed at the same time.

Perspective and Prospects

As early as the seventeenth century, the relationship between blood and various diseases was known. At that time, however, great difficulties existed in the transport and study of blood. By the nineteenth century, the techniques for entering the blood vessels had been refined. The dangers of air embolization (air entering the patient) and clotting were well recognized. Prior to 1850, there was no treatment for patients with renal failure, but crude methods such as applying heat, immersing in warm baths, bloodletting, or administering diaphoretic (perspiration-inducing) mixtures of nitric acid in alcohol and wine were commonly used. (In fact, diaphoretic mixtures and bloodletting for renal failure were used as late as the 1950's.)

In 1854, Thomas Graham, a Scottish chemist, presented a paper on osmotic force, which was the first reference to the process of separating a substance using a semipermeable membrane. His definitions and experimental proofs of the laws of diffusion and osmosis form the foundation upon which dialysis is based. Between 1872 and 1900, the control of membrane manufacture and the dialysis of animal blood were critical developments. One of the key turning points in the

development of dialysis occurred in 1913, when John Jacob Abel, using anticoagulants, created the first extracorporeal device that could be used to diffuse a substance from blood and developed methods to quantify this diffusion. World War I brought the development of the first plate dialyzer, by Heinrich Necheles, a German-born physician. It included an air bubble trap, continuous blood flow, and an entry port for a saline solution to be used as dialysate; it was only used for animals. George Haas must be credited as the first to perform dialysis on a uremic human, in October, 1924. He used heparin, an anticoagulant discovered by William H. Howell and Luther E. Holt, two Americans. Haas had all the pieces together: a dialyzer with a large surface area, a workable membrane, a blood pump, and an anticoagulant.

The emergence of manufactured membranes in the 1930's (such as cellophane, which allows small molecules to pass through it) was crucial in the development of the technique. The lifesaving potential of an artificial kidney was shown by Willem Kolff, a physician from the Netherlands, who saved a patient from coma. His classic work *New Ways of Treating Uraemia*, published in 1947, laid out the principles that are still used and was the first manual for the treatment of patients undergoing hemodialysis. In the United States, the first clinical dialysis was performed on January 26, 1948, at Mt. Sinai Hospital in New York City, by physicians Irving Kroop and Alfred Fishman. The number of groups developing artificial kidney devices and programs between 1945 and 1950 was large. The first complete artificial kidney system commercially available came into existence in 1956, and the first home patient was treated in 1964 by Belding Scribner, from the University of Washington.

Soon the dialyzing fluid delivery systems became smaller and easier to use, the designs were simplified and made more compact, and a better understanding of the physiology of the patient was obtained. Calcium depletion, bone disease, neuropathy, dietary management, and anemia were being looked at closely in order to determine better how much dialysis was required for effective treatment. The late 1960's brought the miniaturization of the systems, in-home care, and lower prices. In fact, in 1973, legislation was enacted in the United States that provided payment through the Social Security system for the care of dialysis patients.

In the latter part of the 1970's, a shift to totally automated systems and an emphasis on negative-pressure dialysis had major impacts, resulting in a move from coil to hollow-fiber dialyzers. Some patients, however, such as diabetics, children, and older patients, did not tolerate hemodialysis well. Therefore, a closer look was taken at peritoneal and automated peritoneal dialysis delivery systems. The earliest reference to peritoneal diffusion was in 1876, and in 1895 it was formally presented as an alternative to remove toxins from the bloodstream. Nevertheless, peritoneal dialysis lay dormant until the 1940's. The basic procedure of using solutions and instilling them into the peritoneal cavity in order to reduce the toxin levels in the blood was first used in 1945 by a group of physicians in Beth Israel Hospital in Boston. The full implications of its use came in the late 1970's, with the development of reverse osmosis technology and the introduction of continuous ambulatory peritoneal dialysis. In the 1980's, the introduction of continuous intermittent peritoneal dialysis gave patients yet another treatment option.

One of the main goals of the medical community and industry is to provide the quality of care that will minimize the burden of those afflicted with renal disease. The main goal, however, remains to obtain the necessary knowledge to understand the causes of progressive renal failure and then prevent, control, or eliminate the consequences of renal disease.

—Maria Pacheco, Ph.D.

See also Blood and blood disorders; Circulation; Diabetes mellitus; Edema; Heart failure; Hematology; Hematology, pediatric; Hemolytic uremic syndrome; Hepatitis; Hyperthermia and hypothermia; Kidney cancer; Kidney disorders; Kidney transplantation; Kidneys; Nephrectomy; Nephritis; Nephrology; Nephrology, pediatric; Pancreatitis; Polycystic kidney disease; Renal failure; Uremia.

FOR FURTHER INFORMATION:

Cameron, J. Stewart. *History of the Treatment of Renal Failure by Dialysis*. New York: Oxford University Press, 2002. Traces the history of dialysis, including discussions of the concepts of diffusion and anticoagulation, early attempts of dialysis in animals and humans, and recent developments in the field.

Cogan, Martin G., and Patricia Schoenfeld, eds. *Introduction to Dialysis*. 2d ed. New York: Churchill Livingstone, 1991. An excellent and thorough presentation of the topic. Somewhat technical, however, since it includes derivations for the equations governing the different parts of the process. A good reference work for those interested in the theoretical and practical aspects of the dialysis process.

Fine, Leonard W., Herbert Beall, and John Stuehr. *Chemistry for Engineers and Scientists*. Fort Worth, Tex.: Saunders College, 2000. A good chemistry book that explains the chemical and physical bases of diffusion and dialysis in a nontechnical presentation.

Nissenson, Allen R., and Richard N. Fine, eds. *Clinical Dialysis*. 4th ed. New York: McGraw-Hill Medical, 2005. A compilation of works by various authorities in the field of dialysis. Contains an excellent presentation of the development of the technique and of its many aspects and applications.

_____. *Dialysis Therapy*. 3d ed. Philadelphia: Hanley and Belfus, 2002. A compilation of works dealing with the theory, applications, advantages, and complications of dialysis. The reader will need some background in the area to make the best use of the book.

Voet, Donald, and Judith G. Voet. *Biochemistry*. 3d ed. Hoboken, N.J.: John Wiley & Sons, 2004. A good book to use for the description and explanation of the chemical processes taking place in the kidney and other areas of the body.

DIAPER RASH
DISEASE/DISORDER
ANATOMY OR SYSTEM AFFECTED: Anus, skin

SPECIALTIES AND RELATED FIELDS: Family medicine, pediatrics

DEFINITION: A skin condition characterized by irritation in the diaper area which can vary from slight redness to severe inflammation with sores or blisters.

KEY TERMS:

rash: the breaking out of spots or patches on the skin

sensitive skin: skin that is easily irritated

CAUSES AND SYMPTOMS

Nearly all babies have diaper rash at some time during their infancy. Whether cloth diapers or disposable diapers are used does not affect whether the baby will have this rash. Diaper rash is less likely to occur, however, in very young infants who are fed breast milk than it is in babies who are bottle-fed. Breast milk is more completely digested by the baby than is formula or cow's milk. Thus, babies who are breast-fed produce less waste material than do babies who are bottle-fed, providing fewer opportunities for fecal material to irritate the baby's diaper area.

When a baby starts on solids or juices, occasional diaper rash is likely to occur. Sometimes when new foods are fed to the baby, the baby's body may not be able to digest the food completely; enzymes in the food can cause diaper rash. These enzymes can break down a baby's skin, causing irritation and even sores. Acid in foods and juices can also cause irritation; a bright red scald around the urethral opening or on the buttocks can result when the baby cannot digest the acid in such foods as tomatoes or orange juice.

Interaction between the baby's urine and bacteria on the baby's skin produces ammonia. Ammonia can be caustic to the diaper area, causing burns. Prolonged wetness can cause the rash to form bumps, which then become white-headed pimples and even weeping areas. These white-headed, weeping pimples are likely to appear if a baby sleeps in a wet diaper for ten to twelve hours or if a baby has a cold, sore throat, or ear infection.

Another cause of diaper rash is yeast infections, such as candidiasis. A rash from a yeast infection is fiery red and bumpy; it may have scaly edges. The rash caused by candidiasis may appear when a baby has been ill, since some antibiotics taken for certain illnesses may destroy the bacteria that control the growth of yeast in the body.

Babies are likely to get diaper rash when they have had diarrhea or an illness. Diarrhea burn is indicated by a bright red burn encircling the baby's anus after a bout with diarrhea. Streptococcal bacteria may also produce diaper rash; often, diaper rash caused by strep infection will appear after other members of the family have been infected. This rash will be bright red, with swollen areas near the rectum. There may also be slits in the skin.

There are also inorganic causes of diaper rash. A diaper that fits too snugly may cause a rash. Usually, such a rash is shiny and red but not sore. Sensitive skin may also develop a rash when exposed to fabric softeners, detergents, and various toiletries. Such rashes are often tiny red blisters. If the baby wears cloth diapers, a rash can occur if the diaper has been washed in a detergent that contains an enzyme or bleach. The plastic in some disposable diapers can also cause red patches.

Treatment and Therapy

When diaper rash develops, particularly a rash that appears to be a burn, the baby's diet should be examined to determine if certain foods are contributing to the rash. Highly acidic foods such as orange juice and tomatoes can cause scalding burns. Mixing water with acidic juices will help reduce the likelihood of rash formation.

The best way to eliminate diaper rash is to keep a baby clean and dry. Caregivers should remove wet or soiled diapers as soon as they are aware of them. The baby should be washed with warm water and dried off at each diaper change. If there is a rash, the baby should be allowed, whenever possible, to lie for an hour with the diaper area uncovered. If air is allowed to move around the diaper area, it is less likely that a rash will form, and if one does occur, it is more likely that the rash will heal. Therefore, the baby's diapers should not be fastened too tightly to the skin.

If the baby's diaper rash is caused by a yeast infection, then a prescription medication such as nystatin will be needed to clear up the problem. Severe diaper rash caused by prolonged wetness can sometimes be controlled by using extra-absorbency disposable diapers. A doctor may recommend 1 percent hydrocortisone ointment for such a rash, but caregivers should be careful when using hydrocortisone creams, since they can affect the baby's own production of cortisone.

If the diaper rash appears to be a result of irritation from detergents used in washing cloth diapers, then the diapers should be washed in milder detergents. Drying diapers in a very hot dryer or in the sunshine will kill organisms that can cause rashes. If all else fails, boiling diapers for a half hour or more will destroy most bacteria.

Diaper rash can be prevented by coating the diaper area with a protective ointment such as petroleum jelly. If a diaper rash does develop, the ointment can prevent further spread of the rash. Care must be taken, however, because medicated ointments can prevent the stay-dry liner of disposable diapers from drawing moisture away from the body, making the rash worse.

A physician should be consulted for a diaper rash that resembles a chemical burn, develops blisters, or becomes infected. Impetigo, which must be treated by a doctor, is a fairly common complication of diaper rash. This communicable infection is characterized by blisters that itch, break, ooze, and crust over.

PERSPECTIVE AND PROSPECTS
Undoubtedly, diaper rash has been around since babies began to wear diapers. It can be largely prevented through vigilant caregivers who make sure that diapers are changed as soon as they become soiled or wet. Nevertheless, when new foods are introduced, a baby is sick, or sensitive skin comes in contact with irritants such as detergents, it is likely that diaper rash will occur.

—*Annita Marie Ward, Ed.D.*

See also Allergies; Bacterial infections; Breastfeeding; Burns and scalds; Dermatology, pediatric; Fungal infections; Impetigo; Lesions; Nutrition; Pediatrics; Rashes; Skin; Skin disorders.

FOR FURTHER INFORMATION:

Illingworth, Ronald S. *The Normal Child: Some Problems of the Early Years and Their Treatment.* 10th ed. New York: Churchill Livingstone, 1991. Although intended as a text for pediatric students, the approach and style make this book equally useful for parents who are unafraid of occasional medical terminology.

Jones, Sandy. *Crying Baby, Sleepless Nights: Why Your Baby Is Crying and What You Can Do About It.* Rev. ed. Boston: Harvard Common Press, 1992. Writing with empathy for parents and infants alike, Jones helps parents identify the source of their baby's distress. She covers basic soothing techniques, infants' sleep-wake patterns, feeding problems, the colic-allergy connection, and colic drugs.

Kemper, Kathi J. *The Holistic Pediatrician: A Pediatrician's Comprehensive Guide to Safe and Effective Therapies for the Twenty-five Most Common Ailments of Infants, Children, and Adolescents.* Rev. ed. New York: Quill, 2002. Integrates mainstream and alternative medicine to aid parents in dealing with the most common childhood health problems such as diaper rash, ear infections, and allergies.

Leach, Penelope. *Your Baby and Child: From Birth to Age Five.* London: Dorling Kindersley, 2003. Each developmental stage—newborn, settled baby, older baby, toddler, and young child—is discussed in terms of feeding, teeth and teething, growing, excreting, crying, sleeping, playing, and everyday care.

Sullivan, Michele G. "Diaper Rash: Common, Yet Poorly Understood." *Pediatric News* 38, no. 9 (September 1, 2004): 43. Discusses the etiology of and treatment options for diaper rash.

Woolf, Alan D., et al., eds. *The Children's Hospital Guide to Your Child's Health and Development.* Cambridge, Mass.: Perseus, 2002. An authoritative and comprehensive guide to children's health, providing a guide to every common illness or condition that affects children and a carefully designed emergency section.

DIAPHRAGM
ANATOMY

ANATOMY OR SYSTEM AFFECTED: Chest, lungs, muscles, musculoskeletal system, respiratory system, spine

SPECIALTIES AND RELATED FIELDS: Internal medicine, pulmonary medicine

DEFINITION: The diaphragm, a dome-shaped muscle that is unique to mammals, is the major muscle of respiration and separates the thoracic and abdominal cavities. When the diaphragm contracts, it decreases the pressure within the lungs by expanding the rib cage and increasing the volume of the lungs as it flattens.

STRUCTURE AND FUNCTIONS
The diaphragm is attached to the spine, the ribs, and the sternum. It is pierced by the esophagus, the phrenic nerve, the aorta, and the vena cava. The human body has three types of muscles: cardiac, which is striated and under involuntary control; smooth, which is not striated and is under involuntary control; and skeletal, which is striated and under voluntary control. The diaphragm is composed of skeletal muscle and is under both voluntary and involuntary control. That is, one is able to hold the breath, take deeper breaths, or take faster breaths (panting), examples of voluntary control. However, a person normally breathes, allowing the diaphragm to contract and relax as skeletal muscle does, involuntarily—that is, without the conscious effort that is required with holding one's breath.

As skeletal muscle, the diaphragm must be innervated; that is, it must receive a nerve impulse before it will contract. The impulses that are sent to the diaphragm originate in the higher brain centers when one voluntarily controls breathing but originate in the lower brain when low oxygen concentrations or high carbon dioxide concentrations are present. The diaphragm relies on the phrenic nerve for its innervations.

When innervated, the diaphragm contracts, as all skeletal muscle does, and flattens or pulls downward. This movement serves to cause the ribs to pull outward, increasing the volume within the lungs. Air pressure inside the lungs is now lower than air pressure outside the lungs (the environment), so air rushes in. As the diaphragm muscle relaxes, it once again domes upward, allowing the ribs to move back to a resting position. The lung volume decreases, but since the lungs are filled with air, the pressure inside the lungs is now greater than the pressure outside the lungs. Air moves outward, as one exhales. (This simple expansion and contraction of the lung volume is the premise behind the original iron lung machine.) This cycle of contraction and relaxation is repeated approximately twelve to fourteen times per minute; with heavy exercise, it may be repeated forty times per minute.

The diaphragm has a role in laughing, singing, crying, yawning, hiccupping, vomiting, coughing, sneezing, whistling, defecating, and urinating, as well as in childbirth.

Disorders and Diseases

The diaphragm may be affected by both neurological and anatomical processes. Common neurological problems are disorders of innervation as a result of trauma to the head or brain stem; nerve impulses to the diaphragm are disrupted and the diaphragm cannot contract and relax. These injuries are often fatal. Poliomyelitis, demyelinating diseases, and other disease may also impair the innervation of the diaphragm. Anatomical problems may include hernias (protrusion of the stomach through the diaphragm and into the thoracic cavity). Blunt trauma from car accidents and the like may rupture the diaphragm.

—*M. A. Foote, Ph.D.*

See also Abdomen; Chest; Muscles; Pulmonary medicine; Respiration.

For Further Information:

Koch, Wijnand F. R. M., and Enrico Marani. *Early Development of the Human Pelvic Diaphragm.* New York: Springer, 2007.

Marieb, Elaine N. *Essentials of Human Anatomy and Physiology.* 9th ed. San Francisco: Pearson/Benjamin Cummings, 2009.

Diarrhea and dysentery
Disease/disorder

Anatomy or system affected: Abdomen, gastrointestinal system, intestines

Specialties and related fields: Family medicine, gastroenterology, internal medicine, pediatrics, public health

Definition: Intestinal disorders that may indicate minor emotional distress or a variety of diseases, some serious; diarrhea is loose, watery, copious bowel movements, whereas dysentery is a process, usually infectious and characterized by severe diarrhea, sometimes with passage of blood, mucus, and pus.

Key terms:

electrolytes: inorganic ions dissolved in body water, including sodium, potassium, calcium, magnesium, chloride, phosphate, bicarbonate, and sulphate

functional disease: a derangement in the way that normal anatomy operates

gastroenterology: the medical subspecialty devoted to care of the digestive tract and related organs

intestines: the tube connecting the stomach and anus in which nutrients are absorbed from food; divided into the small intestine and the colon, or large intestine

mucosa: the semipermeable layers of cells lining the gut, through which fluid and nutrients are absorbed

organic disease: disease resulting from an identifiable cause, such as an enzyme deficiency, growth, hole, or organism

pathogen: an organism that causes disease

peristalsis: the wavelike muscular contractions that move food and waste products through the intestines; problems with peristalsis are called motility disorders

stool: the waste products expelled from the anus during defecation

Causes and Symptoms

A symptom of various diseases rather than a disease in itself, diarrhea is so difficult to define and can result from so many disparate causes that it is sometimes called the gastroenterologist's nightmare. Dysentery (bloody diarrhea), a more threatening symptom, presents even further complexity.

Uncontrolled, some forms of diarrhea result in dehydration, weakness, and malnutrition and quickly turn deadly. Diarrhea is implicated in more infant deaths worldwide than any other affliction. Even in mild forms, it produces so much distress in victims and has inspired so many remedies that its psychological and economic toll is monumental.

Common medical definitions of diarrhea seek to bring diagnostic precision to a nebulous complaint and to distinguish between acute and chronic forms and between organic and functional causes. For example, *The Merck Manual of Diagnosis and Therapy* (18th ed., 2006), a widely respected reference for physicians, associates diarrhea with increased amount and fluidity of fecal matter and frequent defecation relative to a person's usual pattern, emphasizing the importance of volume (more than 300 grams of stool daily, of which 60 to 90 percent is water) in the definition. The key phrase here is "relative to a usual pattern": Because quantity, frequency, and firmness of bowel movements vary greatly among healthy people, a more precise generalization is difficult to make. Yet some specialists demand greater specificity from the definition. For example, W. Grant Thompson, a professor of medicine and popular author on the digestive tract, proposed the operational definition of "loose or watery stools more than 75 percent of the time" in *Gut Reactions* (1989). Acute diarrhea seldom lasts more than five days, although acute dysentery may continue up to ten days; most causes are infections, that is, resulting from the presence of microorganisms (viruses, bacteria, or parasites). Physicians differ over how long the symptoms must persist before a condition is identified as chronic diarrhea, proposing from two weeks to three months; impaired functioning of the intestinal tract (functional diarrhea) is usually responsible, although persistent malfunctions may originate from pathogens that in most cases provoke only acute diarrhea.

In a single day, water intake, saliva, gastric juice, bile, pancreatic juices, and electrolyte secretions in the upper small intestine produce about 9 to 10 liters of fluid in the average person. About 1 to 2 liters of this amount empty into the colon, and 100 to 150 milligrams are excreted in the stool; the rest is absorbed through the intestinal mucosa. If for any reason more fluid enters the colon than it can absorb, diarrhea results. Schemes classifying diarrhea according to the biochemical mechanisms causing it vary considerably, although all authorities agree on three broad types of malfunction.

The first is secretory diarrhea. The intestines, especially the small intestine, normally add water and electrolytes—principally sodium, potassium, chloride, and bicarbonate—into the nutrient load during the biochemical reactions of digestion. In a healthy person, more fluid is absorbed than is secreted. Many agents and conditions can reverse this ratio and stimulate the mucosa to exude more water than can be absorbed: toxin-producing bacteria; various organic chemicals, including caffeine and some laxatives; acids; hormones; some cancers; and inflammatory diseases of the bowel. Large stool volume (more than 1 liter a day), with little or no decrease during fasting and with normal sodium and potassium content in the body fluid, characterizes secretory diarrhea.

Second, the nutrient load in the gut may include substances that exert osmotic force but cannot be absorbed, causing osmotic diarrhea. Some laxatives (especially those containing magnesium), an inability to absorb the lactose in dairy products or the artificial fats and sweeteners in diet foods, and enzyme deficiencies are the principal causes. Stool volume tends to be less than 1 liter a day and decreases during fasting, and the sodium and potassium content of stool water is low.

Third, motility disorders occur when peristalsis, the natural wavelike contractions of the bowel wall that move waste matter toward the rectum for defecation, becomes deranged. Some drugs, irritable bowel syndrome (IBS), hyperthyroidism, and gut nerve damage (as from diabetes mellitus) may have this effect. Fluid passes through the intestines too quickly or in an uncoordinated fashion, and too little is removed from the waste matter.

These mechanisms do not conform exactly with popular names for diarrhea. For example, travelers' diarrhea, the most infamous, comprises a diverse group of microorganism infections that come from drinking polluted water or eating tainted foods. When a person is not a native to an area, and so has little or no resistance to locally abundant pathogens, these pathogens can radically alter the balance of intestinal flora or attack the mucosa, increasing secretion and disrupting absorption and motility. Similarly, terms such as "Monte-

---

INFORMATION ON DIARRHEA AND DYSENTERY

Causes: Bacterial, viral, or parasitic infection; laxative abuse; hormones; inflammatory bowel disease

Symptoms: Dehydration, weakness, malnutrition, nausea, bleeding, fever, bloating, persistent intestinal pain

Duration: Acute to chronic

Treatments: Oral rehydration, antibiotics if needed

zuma's revenge," "the backdoor trots," and "beaver fever" can refer to a variety of organic diseases, although the last commonly refers to *Giardia lamblia* infection.

Dysentery may occur with infectious diarrhea due to certain organisms, most commonly amoebas and other unicellular or multicellular parasites, or to bacterial organisms such as *Shigella*, *Campylobacter*, and some strains of *Escherichia coli*, or *E. coli*. Any pathogen or process that injures and inflames the bowel wall—ulcerating the mucosa—may cause blood and pus to ooze into the feces. Dysentery is also seen in inflammatory diseases of the bowel, such as ulcerative colitis and Crohn's disease. Severe diarrhea, with or without dysentery, may be associated with fever, chills, nausea, and in extreme cases, delirium, convulsions, coma, and death. Dehydration is the most common complication, but systemic infection may occur. Dysentery also may be associated with significant blood loss.

Although most diarrheas result from physiological mechanisms, one relatively rare form of chronic diarrhea ultimately has a psychological origin: laxative abuse. Physicians consider this curious phenomenon a specialized manifestation of Münchausen syndrome, named after the German soldier Baron Münchausen (1720-1797), who was famous for his wild tales of military exploits and injuries in battles. To be admitted to hospitals, patients mutilate themselves in such a way that the injuries mimic acute, dramatic, and convincing symptoms of serious physiological diseases. Laxative abusers secretly dose themselves with nonprescription laxatives and suffer continual diarrhea, weight loss, and weakness. When they present themselves to physicians, they lie about taking laxatives, which makes a correct diagnosis extremely difficult; even when confronted with irrefutable evidence of the abuse, they deny it and persist in taking the laxatives.

TREATMENT AND THERAPY

Almost everyone, at one time or another, produces stools that seem somehow unusual; if the bowel movement comes swiftly and is preceded by intestinal cramps and if the stool has anything from a watery to an

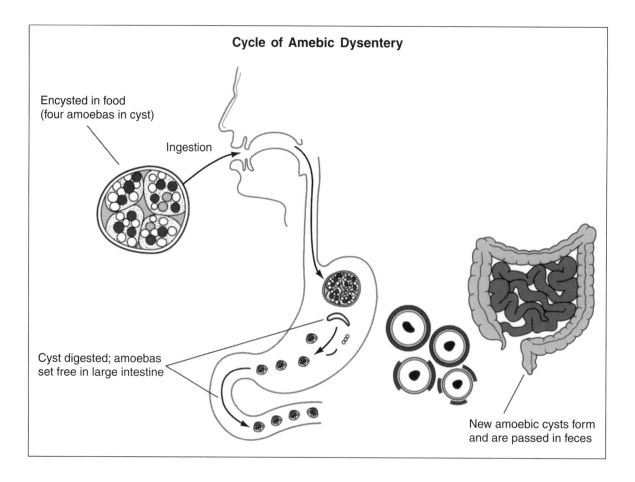

Cycle of Amebic Dysentery

Encysted in food
(four amoebas in cyst)

Ingestion

Cyst digested; amoebas
set free in large intestine

New amoebic cysts form
and are passed in feces

oatmeal-like consistency, victims are likely to believe that they have diarrhea. Such episodes seldom indicate anything except perhaps a dietary excess or a temporary motility disturbance. Normal bowel movement returns on its own, and no medical treatment is called for. When loose feces are uncontrollable, even explosive, however, and other symptoms coexist, such as nausea, bleeding, fever, bloating, and persistent intestinal pain, the distress may indicate serious illness.

Because so many organic and functional diseases can lead to diarrhea, physicians follow carefully designed algorithms when treating patients. Essentially, such an algorithm seeks to eliminate possibilities systematically. Step by step, physicians interview patients, conduct physical examinations, and, when called for, perform tests that gradually narrow the range of possible causes until one seems most likely. Only then can the physician decide upon an effective therapy. This painstaking approach is necessary because treatments for some mechanisms of diarrhea prove useless against or worsen other mechanisms. If the underlying disease is complex or uncommon, the process can be long and frustrating.

One treatment, however, always precedes a complete investigation. Because dehydration is the most immediately serious effect of diarrhea, the physician first tries to prevent or reduce dehydration in a patient through oral rehydration; that is, the patient is given fluids with electrolytes to drink. Often, mineral water or clear fruit juice with soda crackers is sufficient to restore fluid balance.

If the diarrhea lasts fewer than three days and no other serious symptoms accompany it, the physician is unlikely to recommend treatment other than oral rehydration because whatever caused the upset is already resolving itself. If the diarrhea is persistent, however, the physician queries the patient about his or her recent experience, which is called "taking a history." Fever, tenesmus (the urgent need to defecate without the ability to do so satisfactorily), blood in the stool, and abdominal pain will suggest that a pathogen has infected the patient. If the patient has recently eaten seafood, traveled abroad, suffered an immune system disorder, or engaged in sexual activity without the protection of condoms, the physician has reason to suspect that viruses, bacteria, or parasites are responsible.

At that point, a stool sample is taken. If few or no white cells turn up in the stool, then the diarrhea has not caused inflammation. Several common bacteria and parasites, usually contracted during travel, induce diar-

rhea without inflammation, most notably some types of *E. coli*, cryptosporidium, rotavirus, Norwalk virus, and *Giardia lamblia*. Further tests, such as the culturing and staining of stool samples and electron microscopy of stool or bowel wall tissue, will distinguish between bacterial and parasite infection. Most noninflammatory bacterial diarrheas are allowed to run their course without drug therapy; only the effects of the diarrhea (especially dehydration) are treated. If the agent responsible is a parasite, the patient is given specific antiparasite medications.

The presence of white cells in the stool is evidence of inflammatory diarrhea, and the physician considers a completely separate group of microorganisms, especially *Shigella*, *Salmonella*, amoebas, and various forms of *E. coli*. Because the inflammation may cause bleeding and pockets of pus, which in turn can lead to anemia and fever, inflammatory diarrhea often requires aggressive treatment. Cultures help identify the specific microorganism involved, and that identification enables the physician to select the proper antibiotic to kill the infecting agents.

If cultures, microscopic examination of stool samples, biopsies, or staining fails to identify a microorganism (and some, like the parasite *Giardia lamblia*, are difficult to spot), the physician suspects that the diarrhea derives from a source other than an infectious agent. IBS, a chronic and relapsing disorder, may be making its first appearance. Overuse of antibiotics, antacids, or laxatives is frequently the cause, in which case the cure is simple: Elimination of the drugs clears up the symptom.

When neither drugs nor IBS is responsible, the physician looks for other diseases, organic or functional; these can range from the readily identifiable to the obscure, and they are often chronic. Chemical tests, for example, can show that a patient has enzyme deficiencies that produce intolerance to types of food, such as dairy products, or conditions resulting from malfunctioning organs, such as hyperthyroidism and pancreatic insufficiency. Looking through an endoscope, a long flexible fiber-optic tube, the physician can locate diarrhea-causing tumors or the abrasions and inflammation typical of colitis and Crohn's disease. Yet neither tests nor direct examination may pin down the dysfunction. For example, diarrhea figures prominently among a group of symptoms, probably derived from assorted dysfunctions, that characterize IBS; this mild functional disease is estimated to afflict between 10 and 20 percent of Americans.

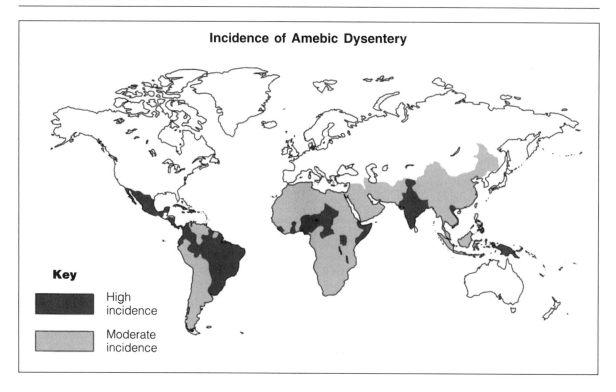

Incidence of Amebic Dysentery

Key

High incidence

Moderate incidence

Cancers, Crohn's disease, and some forms of colitis can be alleviated with surgery, although in the case of Crohn's disease the relief from diarrhea may be only temporary. The surgery itself, however, may impair bowel function, worsening diarrhea rather than stopping it. Food intolerances are managed by removing the offending food from the patient's diet; similarly, some types of colitis and IBS sometimes improve after the physician and patient experiment with altering the patient's diet. Medications are available that supplement or counteract the biochemical imbalances created by malfunctioning organs, such as treatment for hyperthyroidism. Yet, in many cases, the disease must simply be endured and the diarrhea can only be palliated with bulking agents, which often contain aluminum and bismuth, or opiates, such as morphine and codeine, which slow peristalsis.

The surest protection from diarrhea of all types is a balanced, moderate, pathogen-free diet, although diet alone seldom prevents organic diseases. When dietary control is difficult, such as when a person travels and especially when the itinerary includes underdeveloped countries, other measures may help. Bacterial infection accounts for 80 percent of cases of travelers' diarrhea, so some physicians recommend regular doses of antibiotics or a bismuth subsalicylate preparation (such as Pepto Bismol) to kill off the pathogens before they can cause trouble. Such prophylactic treatment is controversial because the drugs, taken over long periods, can have serious side effects, including rashes, tinnitus (ringing in the ear), sensitivity to sunlight, and shock. Also, preventive doses of drugs may give travelers a false sense of security so that they fail to exercise caution in eating foreign foods. Also, widespread use of antibiotics for this purpose fosters the emergence of bacteria that are resistant to them, ultimately making the treatment of disease more difficult.

PERSPECTIVE AND PROSPECTS

In effect, diarrhea is an urgent message from the body that something is wrong. Although it is often difficult for a physician to interpret, persistent diarrhea sends a signal that cannot be ignored without endangering the patient. Similarly, when significant numbers of people in an area suffer diarrhea, the disease is an urgent social and political message to local governments: Public health is endangered and steps must be taken to improve living conditions.

Although some endemic diarrheal diseases do exist in wealthy industrialized countries such as the United States, most severe, long-lasting plagues of diarrhea occur in impoverished nations that have inadequate sanitation systems and poor standards for food handling. Most viral, bacterial, and parasitic diarrheas are transmitted by food and water. Any food can harbor bacteria after being grown in or washed with infected water. Meat is especially vulnerable during slaughtering, but refrigerating, drying, salting, fermenting, freezing, or irradiating it prevents the bacteria from proliferating to numbers that cause illness. If the food is stored in a warm place, as is often the case in countries lacking the resources for refrigeration or other safe storage techniques, the diarrhea-causing organisms can spoil the food in hours. Spoiled food becomes a particular nuisance when served at restaurants or by street vendors, because great numbers and varieties of people are infected.

Organisms that cause many forms of diarrhea travel in human excrement. When an infected person defecates, the organism-rich stool enters the sewer system, and if that system is not well designed, the infected excrement may leak into the local water supply, spreading the infection when the water is drunk or used to wash food. Furthermore, infected persons, if they fail to wash themselves well, may have traces of excrement on their hands, and when they touch food during its preparation or touch other people directly, the organism can find a new host.

In 1989, the World Health Organization (WHO) issued ten rules for safe food preparation in an attempt to improve food handling practices worldwide and combat diarrheal diseases. The effort, it was hoped, would reduce infant mortality in developing countries, since diarrheal dehydration kills children younger than two years of age at rates disproportionate to other age groups. WHO advises food handlers to choose foods that are already processed, to cook foods thoroughly, to serve cooked foods immediately, to store foods carefully, to reheat foods thoroughly, to prevent raw and cooked foods from touching, to wash their hands repeatedly, to clean all kitchen surfaces meticulously, to protect foods from insects and rodents, and to use pure water.

Eliminating endemic infectious diarrheal diseases would improve general health significantly throughout the world, since diarrhea is one of the most incapacitating of afflictions even in its mild forms. International travel would also become safer; of the estimated 300 million people who cross national borders yearly, 20 to 50 percent contract diarrheal illnesses. Noninfectious diarrhea from chronic functional diseases will remain a knotty problem, but it is rare in comparison to acute infectious diarrhea and cannot be transmitted, so has little or no effect on public health.

—*Roger Smith, Ph.D.*

See also Abdominal disorders; Amebiasis; Bacterial infections; Bile; *Campylobacter* infections; *Clostridium difficile* infections; Colitis; Colon; Colorectal cancer; Crohn's disease; Digestion; *E. coli* infection; Food poisoning; Gastroenteritis; Gastroenterology; Gastroenterology, pediatric; Gastrointestinal disorders; Gastrointestinal system; Giardiasis; Incontinence; Indigestion; Intestinal disorders; Intestines; Irritable bowel syndrome (IBS); Lactose intolerance; Noroviruses; Over-the-counter medications; Rotavirus; Shigellosis; Viral infections.

FOR FURTHER INFORMATION:

Biddle, Wayne. *A Field Guide to Germs*. 2d ed. New York: Anchor Books, 2002. This comprehensive book is easily accessible to the nonspecialist and includes a discussion of nearly every virus, bacterium, and fungus known to cause human and nonhuman animal disease. The history of the microbe and the treatment of diseases are included.

DuPont, Herbert L., and Charles D. Ericsson. "Drug Therapy: Prevention and Treatment of Traveler's Diarrhea." *New England Journal of Medicine* 328 (June 24, 1993): 1821-1826. This article, a periodic update on the subject from the Center for Infectious Diseases, is a review of existing knowledge. It should be basic reading for international travelers, or anyone who wants an accurate overview of travelers' diarrhea.

Gracey, Michael, ed. *Diarrhea*. Boca Raton, Fla.: CRC Press, 1991. The fourteen essays in this collection cover major types of acute and chronic diarrhea in depth. Although written by academic physicians, the essays are accessible to readers with a basic knowledge of physiology, and the clarity and wealth of information make the book a valuable resource.

Janowitz, Henry D. *Your Gut Feelings: A Complete Guide to Living Better with Intestinal Problems*. Rev. ed. New York: Oxford University Press, 1995. An eminent gastroenterologist and popular writer on intestinal subjects, Janowitz writes plainly and offers much helpful advice. His section on travelers' diarrhea is particularly valuable.

Parker, James N., and Philip M. Parker, eds. *The Official Patient's Sourcebook on Diarrhea*. San Diego, Calif.: Icon Health, 2002. Draws from public, academic, government, and peer-reviewed research to provide a wide-ranging handbook for patients with diarrhea.

Peikin, Steven R. *Gastrointestinal Health*. Rev. ed.

New York: Quill, 2001. Examines a range of gastro-intestinal ailments in depth, including diarrhea and colitis, and offers tips for managing them via diet, stress management, and drugs.

Saibil, Fred. *Crohn's Disease and Ulcerative Colitis: Everything You Need to Know.* Rev. ed. Toronto, Ont.: Firefly Books, 2009. A leading expert on in-flammatory bowel disease (IBD), Saibil covers top-ics such as signs and symptoms, how the gastrointes-tinal system works normally and how IBD affects it, procedures and instruments used to diagnose IBD, effects of diet, and children and IBD.

Scarpignato, Carmelo, and P. Rampal, eds. *Traveler's Diarrhea: Recent Advances.* New York: S. Karger, 1995. The authors discuss the latest methods in the prevention, control, and treatment of diarrhea.

Thompson, W. Grant. *Gut Reactions: Understanding Symptoms of the Digestive Tract.* New York: Plenum Press, 1989. With much charm, Grant writes for the general reader, laying out the essential information that patients need in order to comprehend most gas-trointestinal ailments. His chapter on diarrhea ad-dresses only the functional diseases.

DIET. *See* NUTRITION.

DIETARY DEFICIENCIES. *See* MALNUTRITION; NUTRITION; VITAMINS AND MINERALS.

DIETARY REFERENCE INTAKES (DRIs)
BIOLOGY

ANATOMY OR SYSTEM AFFECTED: All
SPECIALTIES AND RELATED FIELDS: Nutrition
DEFINITION: The official U.S. guidelines for nutrient intakes in order to maintain health.

DEVELOPMENT

The dietary reference intakes (DRIs) include four ref-erence values that can be used in assessing and plan-ning a healthy diet throughout the life span: estimated average requirement (EAR), recommended dietary al-lowance (RDA), adequate intake (AI), and tolerable upper intake limit (UL). The RDA is the amount of a nutrient needed to meet the needs of nearly all healthy individuals. In setting the RDA, an EAR is first deter-mined. The EAR is the amount of a specific nutrient that is believed to meet the needs of half of the popula-tion. Using the assumption of a normal distribution of nutrient needs, the RDA is calculated from the EAR

and the standard deviation of requirements. When data are insufficient to calculate an EAR, the available data are used to estimate an AI. The AI is similar to the RDA but acknowledges that additional research concerning nutrient requirements is needed in that area. The UL represents the highest daily intake of a nutrient that is known to pose no health risks.

The EAR, RDA, and AI cannot be used to address the needs of those with chronic or acute disease. It can be assumed that intakes below the EAR probably need to be improved, since at this level 50 percent of the pop-ulation would have inadequate intake. Intakes between the EAR for a specific nutrient and the RDA also may be improved. Intakes at or above the RDA probably are adequate, although many days of intake should be eval-uated because of day-to-day variation. It is more diffi-cult to be certain of the adequacy of intake when using AIs. However, in general, intakes below the AIs should probably be improved. Intakes at or above the UL should be lowered.

Nutrients for which EARs and RDAs have been es-tablished include phosphorus, magnesium, thiamine, riboflavin, niacin, vitamin B_6, folate, vitamin B_{12}, vita-min C, vitamin E, and selenium for adults and children over one year of age. Those for which an AI has been set include calcium, vitamin D, fluoride, pantothenic acid, biotin, and choline.

PERSPECTIVE AND PROSPECTS

Although these reference values could be used for la-beling and fortification guidelines, they are not yet be-ing implemented as such. The current daily value (DV percent) on the nutrition facts labels rely on the 1968 version of the nutrient reference values. The major dif-ficulty in applying the newer reference values for label-ing purposes rests on how to choose a "reference" age group or gender. Currently the DV reflect needs for a male adult.

The first nutrient-based guidelines for healthy intake were released in 1941 in the United States, with similar guidelines released in Canada in 1938. Much research has occurred since that time concerning recording and assessing nutrient intake and in determining human re-quirements. However, the use of these guidelines has always been to assist in planning meals for individuals and groups, including federal assistance programs.

—*Karen Chapman-Novakofski, R.D., L.D.N., Ph.D.*

See also Antioxidants; Beriberi; Carbohydrates; Cholesterol; Digestion; Fiber; Food biochemistry; Food Guide Pyramid; Kwashiorkor; Malnutrition; Nutrition; Obesity; Obesity, childhood; Phytonutrients; Protein; Supplements; Vitamins and minerals.

FOR FURTHER INFORMATION:

Institute of Medicine, Food and Nutrition Board, Committee on the Use of Dietary Reference Intakes in Nutrition Labeling. Dietary Reference Intakes. *Guiding Principles for Nutrition Labeling and Fortification.* Washington, D.C.: National Academy Press, 2003.

Institute of Medicine, Food and Nutrition Board, Subcommittee on Interpretation and Uses of Dietary Reference Intakes and the Standing Committee on the Scientific Evaluation of Dietary Reference Intakes. *Dietary Reference Intakes: Applications in Dietary Assessment.* Washington, D.C.: National Academy Press, 2000.

_____. *Dietary Reference Intakes: Applications in Dietary Planning.* Washington, D.C.: National Academy Press, 2003.

DiGeorge syndrome
DISEASE/DISORDER

ALSO KNOWN AS: Chromosome 22 interstitial deletion, 22q11.2 deletion syndrome

ANATOMY OR SYSTEM AFFECTED: Glands, heart, immune system, lymphatic system, mouth

SPECIALTIES AND RELATED FIELDS: Cardiology, genetics, immunology, pediatrics, plastic surgery

DEFINITION: A pediatric syndrome caused by a missing piece of chromosome 22 and characterized by congenital heart defects, the absence or hypoplasia of the thymus and parathyroid glands, cleft palate, and dysmorphic facial features.

CAUSES AND SYMPTOMS

Chromosomes possess two parts. The upper arms are called "p" arms and the lower arms are called "q" arms. Patients with DiGeorge syndrome are missing a tiny interstitial piece inside the long arm of chromosome 22. The specific region inside the long "q" arm is labeled 11.2. Thus, DiGeorge syndrome is also referred to as 22q11.2 deletion syndrome or chromosome 22 interstitial deletion.

Most microdeletions such as these cannot be observed under a microscope because they are so tiny. A molecular cytogenetic test known as fluorescence in situ hybridization (FISH) is used. It includes the use of deoxyribonucleic acid (DNA) probes made from the DiGeorge chromosomal region (DGCR). A green fluo-

---

INFORMATION ON DiGEORGE SYNDROME

CAUSES: Chromosomal abnormality resulting in absence of thymus and parathyroid glands

SYMPTOMS: Recurrent viral infections, reduced or absent T lymphocytes, defects in antibody production, congenital heart disease, cleft palate, learning difficulties

DURATION: Lifelong

TREATMENTS: Growth hormone, speech therapy, surgery to correct heart defects and cleft palate

---

rescent probe is used to identify chromosome 22, while a red probe is specific to the DGCR. In DiGeorge syndrome, one of the chromosomes will lack the red fluorescence.

About 93 percent of patients have a spontaneous (de novo) deletion of a 22q11.2, and 7 percent have inherited the deletion from a parent. The very high de novo rate indicates that the deletion recurs with a high frequency as a result of new mutations occurring in the population. This deletion is inherited in an autosomal dominant manner. The offspring of persons with the deletion have a 50 percent chance of inheriting it. This interstitial deletion encompasses about 3 million base pairs of DNA in the majority of patients. About 90 percent of patients have the same 3 million base pair deletion, while 10 percent have a 1.5 million base pair deletion. Therefore, the deletion is large enough to contain nearly one hundred genes.

DiGeorge syndrome is initiated by defective embryonic development of the third and fourth pharyngeal pouches during the fifth week of development. These pouches normally become the thymus and the parathyroid glands. In the absence of a thymus, T lymphocyte maturation is stopped at the pre-cell stage. DiGeorge syndrome is one of the most severe forms of deficient T-cell immunity. Children with DiGeorge syndrome develop recurrent viral infections and have abnormal cellular immunity, as characterized by severely reduced or absent T lymphocytes. They also have defects in T cell-dependent antibody production. A spectrum of abnormal phenotypes may develop. These defects arise from the absence of key genes that are not available for normal development when a 22q microdeletion is present. Infants with this disease may suffer from congenital heart disease of various types, palatal abnormalities (such as cleft palate), and learning difficulties.

TREATMENT AND THERAPY

Children with a 22q11.2 deletion may exhibit a wide spectrum of problems and much variation in the severity of symptoms. A patient with DiGeorge syndrome may have several organs or systems affected. DiGeorge syndrome may result in problems in different body systems, such as the heart or palate, and in cognition, such as learning style. Consequently, a multidisciplinary approach is needed for management of a specific patient.

In the neonatal period, the following clinical and laboratory studies are pursued. The serum is tested for calcium; a low concentration points to the need for supplementation. The lymphocytes are measured; a low absolute count means referral to an immunologist, who will look at T and B cell subsets. A renal ultrasound examination should be performed because of the high incidence of structural renal abnormalities. A chest X ray is needed to identify thoracic vertebral anomalies. A cardiac evaluation is recommended for all patients with DiGeorge syndrome because possible malformations may include tetralogy of Fallot, ventricular septal defect, interrupted aortic arch, or truncus arteriosus. Pediatric cardiologists are necessary for the treatment and therapy that is needed. An endocrinologist could follow up possible growth hormone deficiencies. Since there is a high incidence of speech and language delay, speech therapy and early educational intervention are highly recommended. All children with the 22q deletion should be seen by a cleft palate team to diagnose problems and schedule surgery if necessary.

Other medical needs of children are met through evaluation by a feeding specialist, especially in the newborn period; a neurologist, for possible seizure disorders or problems with balance; a urologist, for possible kidney problems; and an otorhinolaryngologist (ear, nose, and throat doctor) for problems in this region.

PERSPECTIVE AND PROSPECTS

DiGeorge syndrome is relatively frequent, occurring with a frequency of 1 in 4,000 live births. Therefore, this disorder is a significant health concern in the general population. Since the phenotype associated with it is broad and variable, many types of clinical and laboratory specialists are needed. The medical geneticist is the most likely person to have an overview of the diagnosis. A yearly genetics evaluation is beneficial in answering questions. Parents should be tested to determine their chromosomal status. Genetic counseling could provide individuals and families with information on the nature, inheritance, and implications of DiGeorge syndrome to help them make informed medical and personal decisions. Current and future research using model organisms may help to explain the problems of phenotypic variability in DiGeorge syndrome.

—Phillip A. Farber, Ph.D.

See also Birth defects; Cleft lip and palate; Congenital disorders; Congenital heart disease; Genetic counseling; Genetic diseases; Genetics and inheritance; Immune system; Immunodeficiency disorders; Lymphatic system.

FOR FURTHER INFORMATION:

Emanuel, Beverly S., et al. "The 22q11.2 Deletion Syndrome." *Advances in Pediatrics* 48 (2001): 33-73.

King, Richard A., Jerome I. Rotter, and Arno G. Motulsky, eds. *The Genetic Basis of Common Diseases.* 2d ed. New York: Oxford University Press, 2002.

Maroni, Gustavo. *Molecular and Genetic Analysis of Human Traits.* Malden, Mass.: Blackwell Scientific, 2001.

Rimoin, David L., et al., eds. *Emery and Rimoin's Principles and Practice of Medical Genetics.* 5th ed. Philadelphia: Churchill Livingstone/Elsevier, 2007.

Stocker, J. Thomas, and Louis P. Dehner, eds. *Pediatric Pathology.* 2d ed. Philadelphia: Lippincott Williams & Wilkins, 2001.

Turnpenny, Peter, and Sian Ellard. *Emery's Elements of Medical Genetics.* 13th ed. New York: Churchill Livingstone/Elsevier, 2007.

DIGESTION

BIOLOGY

ANATOMY OR SYSTEM AFFECTED: Abdomen, gastrointestinal system, intestines, pancreas, stomach

SPECIALTIES AND RELATED FIELDS: Biochemistry, family medicine, gastroenterology, internal medicine, nutrition, pharmacology

DEFINITION: The chemical breakdown of food materials in the stomach and small intestine and the absorption into the bloodstream of essential nutrients through the intestinal walls.

KEY TERMS:

amino acids: the product of proteins broken down by digestive enzymes; essential for the building of tissue throughout the body *cecum:* the dividing passageway between the small intestine and the large intestine, or colon

chyme: partially broken-down food materials that pass from the stomach into the small intestine

dyspepsia: a general term applied to several forms of indigestion

villi: fingerlike projections on the intestinal lining that absorb essential body nutrients after enzymes break down chyme

STRUCTURE AND FUNCTIONS

In the most general terms, digestion is a multiple-stage process that begins by breaking down foodstuffs taken in by an organism. Some specialists consider that the actual process of digestion occurs after this breaking-down stage, when essential nutritional elements are absorbed into the body. Even after division of the digestive process into two main functions, there remains a third, by-product stage: disposal by the body of waste material in the form of urine and feces.

Several different vital organs, all contained in the abdominal cavity, contribute either directly or indirectly to the digestive process at each successive stage. Certain imbalances in the functioning of any one of these organs, or a combination, can lead to what is commonly called indigestion. Chronic imbalances in the functioning of any of the key digestive organs—the stomach, small intestine, large intestine (or colon), liver, gallbladder, and pancreas—may indicate symptoms of diseases that are far more serious than mere indigestion.

In a very broad sense, the process of digestion begins even before food that has been chewed and swallowed passes into the stomach. In fact, while chewing is underway, a first stage of glandular activity—the release of saliva by the salivary glands into the food being chewed (a process referred to as intraluminal digestion)—provides a natural lubricant to help propel masticated material down the esophagus. Although the esophagus does not perform a digestive function, its muscular contractions, which are necessary for swallowing, are like a preliminary stage to the muscular operation that begins in the stomach.

The human stomach has two main sections: the baglike upper portion, or fundus, and the lower part, which is twice as large as the fundus, called the antrum. The function of the fundus is essentially to receive and hold foods that reach the stomach via the esophagus, allowing intermittent delivery into the antrum. Here two dynamic elements of the breaking-down process occur, one physical, the other chemical. The muscular tissue surrounding the antrum acts to churn the partially liquefied food in the lower stomach, while a series of what are commonly called gastric juices flow into the mixture held by the stomach.

The most active element that is secreted from special parietal cells in the mucous membranes lining the stomach is hydrochloric acid. The possibility of damage to the stomach lining is minimized (but not removed entirely) first by the chemical reaction between the acid and the mildly alkaline chewed food and second by the presence of other gastric juices in the antrum. Primary among these is the enzyme pepsin, which is secreted by a different set of specialized cells in the gastric lining. Secretions of both hydrochloric acid and pepsin become mixed and interact chemically with food materials, while the antrum itself moves in rhythmic pulses caused by muscular contractions (peristalsis). One of the key functions of pepsin during this stage is to break down protein molecules into shorter molecular strings of less complicated amino acids, which eventually serve as building material for many body tissues.

At a certain point, food materials are sufficiently reduced to pass beyond the antrum into the duodenum, the first section of the small intestine, where a different stage in the digestive process takes place. At this juncture, the partially broken-down food material is referred to as chyme. The transfer of food from one digestive organ to another is actually monitored by a special autonomic nerve, called the vagus nerve, which originates in the medulla at the head of the spinal cord. Although the vagus nerve innervates a number of vital zones in the abdominal cavity, its function here is quite specific: It adjusts the intensity of muscular movement in the stomach wall and thus limits the amount of food passing into the small intestine.

The exact amount of food that is allowed to enter the intestinal tract represents only part of the essential question of balance between agents contributing to the digestive process. The presence of a now slightly acidic food-gastric juice mixture in the duodenum sparks what is called an enterogastric reflex. Two hormones, secretin and cholecystokinin, begin to flow from the mucous membranes of the duodenum. These hormones serve to limit the acidic strength of stomach secretions and trigger reactions in the liver, gallbladder, and pancreas—other key organs that contribute to digestion as the chyme passes through the intestines.

While in the compact, coiled mass of the small intestine (compared to the thicker, but much shorter, colon, or large intestine), food materials, especially proteins, are broken down into one of twenty possible amino acid components by the chemical action of two pancreatic enzymes, trypsinogen and chymotrypsinogen, and two enzymes produced in the intestinal walls themselves, aminopeptidase and dipeptidase. It is interesting to note that the body, which is itself in large part constructed of protein material, has its own mechanism to prevent protein-splitting enzymes from devouring the very organs that produce them. Thus, when they leave the pancreas, both trypsinogen and chymotrypsinogen are inactive compounds. They become active "protein-breakers" only when joined by another enzyme—enterokinase—which is secreted from cells in the wall of the small intestine itself.

Other nutritional components contained in chyme interact chemically with other specialized enzymes that are secreted into the small intestine. Carbohydrate molecules, especially starch, begin to break down when exposed to the enzyme amylase in saliva. This process is intensified greatly when pancreatic amylase flows into the small intestine and mixes with the chyme. The products created when carbohydrates break down are simple sugars, including disaccharides and monosaccharides, especially maltose. As these sugars are all broken down into monosaccharides, a final process that occurs in the wall of the small intestine itself (which contains more specialized enzymes such as maltase, sucrase, and lactase), they become the most rapidly assimilated body nutrients.

The process needed to break down fats is more complicated, since fats are water insoluble and enter the intestine in the form of enzyme-resistant globules. Before the fat-splitting enzyme lipase can be chemically active, bile, a fluid produced by the liver and stored in the gallbladder, must be present. Bile serves to dissolve fat globules into tiny droplets that can be broken down for absorption, like all other nutritive elements, into the body via the epithelial lining of the intestinal wall. Such absorption is locally specialized. Iron and calcium pass through the epithelial lining of the duodenum. Protein, fat, sugars, and vitamins pass through the lining of the jejunum, or middle small intestine. Finally, salt, vitamin B_{12}, and bile salts pass through the lining of the lower small intestine, or ileum.

It is this stage that many scientists consider to be the true process of digestion. Absorption occurs through enterocytes, which are specialized cells located on the surface of the epithelium. The surface of the epithelium is increased substantially by the existence of fingerlike projections called villi. These tiny protrusions are surrounded by the fluid elements of chemically altered food. Specialized enterocyte cells selectively absorb these elements into the capillaries that are inside each of the hundreds of thousands of villi. From the capillaries, the nutrients enter the blood and are carried by the portal vein to the liver. This organ carries out the essential chemical processes that prepare fats, carbohydrates, and proteins for their eventual delivery, through the main bloodstream, to various parts of the body.

Elements that are left after the enzymes in the small intestine have done their work are essentially waste material, or feces. These pass from the small intestine to the large intestine, or colon, through a dividing passageway called the cecum. The disposal of waste materials may or may not be considered to be technically part of the main digestive process.

After essential amounts of water and certain salts are absorbed into the body through the walls of the colon, the remaining waste material is expulsed from the bowels through the rectum and anus. If any prior stage in the digestive process is incomplete or if chemical imbalances have occurred, the first symptoms of indigestion may manifest themselves as bowel movement irregularities.

DISORDERS AND DISEASES

Malfunctions in any of the delicate processes that make up digestion can produce symptoms that range from what is commonly called simple indigestion to potentially serious diseases of the gastrointestinal tract. Functional indigestion, or dyspepsia, is one of the most common sources of physical discomfort experienced not only by human beings but by most animals as well. Generally speaking, dyspepsias are not the result of organic disease, but rather of a temporary imbalance in one of the functions described above. There are many possible causes of such an imbalance, including nervous stress and changes in the nature and content of foods eaten.

The most common causes of dyspepsia and their symptoms, although serious enough in chronic cases to require expert medical attention, are far less dangerous than diseases afflicting one of the digestive organs. Such diseases include gallstones, pancreatitis, peptic ulcers (in which excessive acid causes lesions in the stomach wall), and, most serious of all, cancers afflicting any of the abdominal organs.

Dyspepsia may stem from either physical or chemical causes. On the physical side, it is clear that an important part of the digestive process depends on muscular or nerve-related impulses that move partially digested food through the gastrointestinal tract. When, for reasons that are not yet fully understood, the organism fails to coordinate such physical reactions, spasms may occur at several points from the esophagus through to the colon. If extensive, such muscular contractions can create abdominal pains that are symptomatic of at least one category of functional indigestion.

Problems of motility, or physical movement of food materials through the digestive tract, may also cause one common discomfort associated with indigestion: heartburn. This condition occurs when the system fails to move adequate quantities of the mixture of food and gastric juices, including hydrochloric acid, from the stomach into the duodenum. The resultant backup of food forces part of the acidic liquid mass into the esophagus, causing instant discomfort.

Insufficient motility may also cause delays in the movement of feces through the colon, resulting in constipation. Just as the vagus nerve monitors the muscular movements that are necessary to move food from the stomach to the small intestine, an essential gastrocolic reflex, tied to the organism's nervous system, is needed to ensure a constant rhythm in the movement of feces into the rectum for elimination. If this function is delayed (as a result of nervous stress in some individuals, or because of the dilated physical state of the colon in aged persons), food residues become too tightly compressed in the bowels. As the colon continues to carry out its normal last-stage digestive function of reabsorbing essential water from waste material before it is eliminated, the feces become drier and even more compacted, making defecation difficult and sometimes painful.

Most other imbalances in digestive functions are chemical in nature. Highly spiced or unfamiliar foods frequently upset the balance in the body's chemical digestion. Symptoms may appear either in the abdomen itself (in particular, a bloated stomach accompanied by what is commonly called gas, a symptom of chemical disharmony in the digestive process) or in the stool. If the chemical breakdown of chyme is incomplete because of an imbalance in the proportion (either excessive or inadequate) of enzymes secreted into the stomach or intestines, the normal process of absorption will not take place, creating one of a number of symptoms of indigestion.

The most common symptom of indigestion is diarrhea, which can result from a variety of causes. Because movement in the bowels is affected by different nerve signals, some diarrhea attacks may be linked to nonchemical reactions, such as extreme nervousness. Relaxation of the sphincter, however, as well as the rise in the contractile pressure of the lower colon that precedes defecation (the gastroileal reflex), is also affected by the presence of gastrointestinal hormones, particularly gastrin itself. An imbalance in the amount of concentration of such components in the gastrointestinal tract (attributable to incomplete digestive chemistry) tends to relax the bowels to such a degree that elimination cannot be prevented except through determined mental resistance. It is important to note that if diarrhea continues for an extended time, its effect on the body is not simply the loss of essential body nutrients that pass through the bowels without being fully digested; the inability of the colon to reabsorb into the body an adequate proportion of the water content from the feces can lead to dehydration of the organism, especially in infants.

In most areas of the world, there is widespread consensus that treatment of indigestion is a matter of taking over-the-counter drugs whose function is to right the imbalance in some of the chemical processes described above. In theory as well as in practice, such treatments do work, since the basic chemical imbalance, if it is has not extended beyond the point of indigestion (in the case of peptic ulcers, for example), is fairly easily diagnosed, even by pharmacists. Increasingly, however, the public is becoming aware that digestion can be aided, and indigestion avoided, by paying closer attention to dietary habits, particularly the importance of increasing fiber intake to facilitate the digestive process. Critical advances are also being made in knowledge of the potentially harmful effects on digestion of chemical additives to processed foods.

PERSPECTIVE AND PROSPECTS

Historical traces of the medical observation of indigestion, as well as the prescription of remedies, can be found as far back as ancient Egypt. A famous medical text from about 1600 B.C.E. known as the Ebers Papyrus contains suggested remedies (mainly herbal drugs) for digestive ailments, as well as instructions for the use of suppositories to loosen the lower bowel. For centuries, however, such practical advice for treating indigestion was never accompanied by an adequate theoretical conception of the digestion function itself.

In the medieval Western world, many erroneous guidelines for understanding the digestive process were handed down from the works of Galen of Pergamum (129-c. 199 C.E.). Galen taught that food material passed from the intestines to the liver, where it was transformed into blood. At this point, a vital life-giving spirit, or "pneuma," gave the blood power to drive the body. Similar misconceptions would continue until, following the work of William Harvey (1578-1657), medical science gained more accurate knowledge of the circulatory function of the bloodstream. By the eighteenth century, rapid advances had been made in studies of the function of the stomach and intestines, notably by the French naturalist René de Réaumur (1683-1757), who demonstrated that food is broken down by gastric juices in the stomach, and by the Italian physiologist Lazzaro Spallanzani (1729-1799), who discovered that the stomach itself is the source of gastric juices.

It was an American army surgeon, William Beaumont (1785-1853), who wrote what became, until well into the twentieth century, the most complete medical guide to digestive functions. Beaumont carried out direct clinical observations of the actions of gastric juices in humans. He also observed the way in which the anticipation of eating can spark not only the secretion of such fluids but also the muscular stimuli that promote motility in the digestive process. Soon after Beaumont's findings were published, the German physiologist Theodor Schwann (1810-1882) first isolated pepsin. Others would show that a variety of enzymes in the gastrointestinal tract are secreted by different organs in the abdomen, notably the pancreas.

—*Byron D. Cannon, Ph.D.*

See also Acid-base chemistry; Acid reflux disease; Bile; Celiac sprue; Chyme; Colitis; Constipation; Crohn's disease; Diarrhea and dysentery; Enzymes; Esophagus; Fiber; Food biochemistry; Food poisoning; Gastroenteritis; Gastroenterology; Gastroenterology, pediatric; Gastrointestinal disorders; Gastrointestinal system; Heartburn; Hirschsprung's disease; Indigestion; Intestines; Irritable bowel syndrome (IBS); Malabsorption; Metabolism; Nutrition; Over-the-counter medications; Peristalsis; Supplements; Ulcer surgery; Ulcers; Vagotomy; Vitamins and minerals.

For Further Information:

Bonci, Leslie. *American Dietetic Association Guide to Better Digestion*. New York: Wiley, 2003. A user-friendly guide to help analyze one's eating habits, map out a dietary plan to manage and reduce the uncomfortable symptoms of digestive disorders, and find practical recommendations for implementing lifestyle changes.

Jackson, Gordon, and Philip Whitfield. *Digestion: Fueling the System*. New York: Torstar Books, 1984. This compact and excellently illustrated volume is designed for the informed layperson.

Janowitz, Henry D. *Indigestion: Living Better with Upper Intestinal Problems, from Heartburn to Ulcers and Gallstones*. New York: Oxford University Press, 1994. Deals with common problems of indigestion and includes medical approaches to the treatment of chronic cases.

Johnson, Leonard R., ed. *Gastrointestinal Physiology*. 7th ed. Philadelphia: Mosby/Elsevier, 2007. This book contains a variety of different "self-contained" specialized topics dealt with by experts. Offers the excellent chapters "Gastric Motility" and "Pancreatic Secretion."

Magee, Donal F., and Arthur F. Dalley. *Digestion and the Structure and Function of the Gut*. Basel, Switzerland: S. Karger, 1986. This textbook is part of a continuing education publication series. Although it covers all topics with full technical detail, it is easily understood by a well-informed reader.

Mayo Clinic. *Mayo Clinic on Digestive Health: Enjoy Better Digestion with Answers to More than Twelve Common Conditions*. 2d ed. Rochester, Minn.: Author, 2004. Reviews the causes and treatments of common digestive conditions.

Scanlon, Valerie, and Tina Sanders. *Essentials of Anatomy and Physiology*. 5th ed. Philadelphia: F. A. Davis, 2007. A text designed around three themes: the relationship between physiology and anatomy, the interrelations among the organ systems, and the relationship of each organ system to homeostasis.

Diphtheria

Disease/disorder

Anatomy or system affected: Heart, nervous system, throat

Specialties and related fields: Bacteriology, cardiology, epidemiology, family medicine, microbiology, pediatrics, toxicology

Definition: An acute, contagious disease found primarily in children, associated with toxin production by the bacterium *Corynebacterium diphtheriae*.

Causes and Symptoms

The etiological agent of diphtheria, *Corynebacterium diphtheriae*, is found in some individuals as an inhabitant of the nasopharynx (nose and throat). Its symptoms

INFORMATION ON DIPHTHERIA

CAUSES: Toxin production by bacteria
SYMPTOMS: Sore throat, malaise, mild fever, pseudomembrane formation in throat; when systemic, damage to heart, nervous system, or other organs
DURATION: Acute
TREATMENTS: Antibiotics (penicillin, erythromycin), antitoxin

are associated with the production of a toxin. Only those strains of the organism carrying a bacteriophage in a lysogenic state produce the toxin. Spread of diphtheria is generally person to person through respiratory secretions or through contaminated environmental surfaces.

Following an incubation period of several days to a week, symptoms often have a sudden onset and typically include a sore throat, malaise, and a mild fever. The disease is further characterized by an exudative, pseudomembrane formation on the mucous surface of the throat, which results from replication of the organism in the pharynx or surrounding areas. The pseudomembrane can become quite thick and may cause respiratory stress through obstruction of the breathing passages. Toxin is secreted into the bloodstream, where its presence can result in damage to the heart, nervous system, or other organs. Diagnosis is based upon a combination of symptoms, as well as isolation of the organism in a throat culture.

A less common form of diphtheria may be observed on skin surfaces. It contains bacteria that can be spread through contaminated environmental surfaces. Infection generally occurs through small cuts in the skin. Cutaneous diphtheria is characterized by an ulcer that heals slowly. If the organism is a strain that produces toxin, then systemic damage may result.

TREATMENT AND THERAPY

Most diphtheria infections respond to antibiotics, either a single dose of penicillin or a seven-day or ten-day course of erythromycin. Since symptoms are associated with toxin production, the administration of antitoxin is critical to early treatment. Once toxin has been incorporated into the target, cell death is irreversible. Antibiotic treatment, however, does result in the elimination of the organism and the termination of further toxin production.

Vaccination with diphtheria toxoid, an inactivated form of the toxin, has proven effective in immunization against the disease. Prophylaxis is generally started early in childhood as part of the trivalent DPT (diphtheria, pertussis, tetanus) series. Boosters are recommended at ten-year intervals.

PERSPECTIVE AND PROSPECTS

Introduction of the diphtheria vaccine in the first decades of the twentieth century served to reduce significantly the incidence of the disease in the West. The use of antibiotic therapy further reduced the fatality rate associated with this disease, which ranged from 30 to 50 percent at its peak. On average, fewer than ten cases per year are now observed in the United States, generally associated with asymptomatic carriers. Diphtheria still exists as a childhood scourge, however, in much of the developing world.

—*Richard Adler, Ph.D.*

See also Antibiotics; Bacterial infections; Bacteriology; Childhood infectious diseases; Immunization and vaccination; Sore throat.

FOR FURTHER INFORMATION:

Forbes, Betty, Daniel F. Sahm, and Alice S. Weissfeld. *Bailey and Scott's Diagnostic Microbiology.* 12th ed. St. Louis, Mo.: Mosby/Elsevier, 2007.

Grob, Gerald N. *The Deadly Truth: A History of Disease in America.* Cambridge, Mass.: Harvard University Press, 2002.

Parker, James N., and Philip M. Parker, eds. *The Official Patient's Sourcebook on Diphtheria.* San Diego, Calif.: Icon Health, 2002.

DISEASE

DISEASE/DISORDER
ANATOMY OR SYSTEM AFFECTED: All
SPECIALTIES AND RELATED FIELDS: All
DEFINITION: A morbid (pathological) process with a characteristic set of symptoms that may affect the entire body or any of its parts; the cause, pathology, and course of a disease may be known or unknown.

KEY TERMS:

diagnosis: the art of distinguishing one disease from another

lesion: any pathologic or traumatic discontinuity of tissue or loss of function of a body part

pathology: the study of the essential nature of disease, especially as it relates to the structural and functional changes that are caused by that disease *prognosis:* a forecast regarding the probable cause and result of an attack of disease

syndrome: a congregation of a set of signs and symptoms that characterize a particular disease process, but without a specific etiology or a constant lesion

TYPES OF DISEASE

It is difficult to answer the question "What is disease?" To the patient, disease means discomfort and disharmony with the environment. To the treating physician or surgeon, it means a set of signs and symptoms. To the pathologist, it means one or more structural changes in body tissues, called lesions, which may be viewed with or without the aid of magnifying lenses.

The study of lesions, which are the essential expression of disease, forms part of the modern science of pathology. Pathology had its beginnings in the morgue and the autopsy room, where investigations into the cause of death led to the appreciation of "morbid anatomy"—at first by gross (naked-eye) examination and later microscopically. Much later, the investigation of disease moved from the cold autopsy room to the patient's bedside, from the dead body to the living body, on which laboratory tests and biopsies are performed for the purpose of establishing a diagnosis and addressing proper treatment.

Diagnosis is the art of determining not only the character of the lesion but also its etiology, or cause. Because so much of this diagnostic work is done in laboratories, the term "laboratory medicine" has gained in popularity. The explosion in high technology has expanded the field of laboratory medicine tremendously. The diagnostic laboratory today is highly automated and sophisticated, containing a team of laboratory technologists and scientific researchers rather than a single pathologist.

The lesions laid bare by the pathologist usually bear an obvious relation to the symptoms, as in the gross lesions of acute appendicitis, the microscopic lesions in poliomyelitis, or even the chromosomal lesions in genetically inherited conditions such as Down syndrome. Yet there may be lesions without symptoms, as in early cancer or "silent" diseases such as tuberculosis. There may also be symptoms without obvious lesions, as in the so-called psychosomatic diseases, functional disorders, and psychiatric illnesses. It is likely that future research will reveal the presence of "biochemical lesions" in these cases. The presence of lesions distinguishes organic disease, in which there are gross or microscopic pathologic changes in an organ, from

functional disease, in which there is a disturbance of function without a corresponding obvious organic lesion. Although most diagnoses consist largely of naming the lesion (such as cancer of the lung or a tooth abscess), diseases should truly be considered in the light of disordered function rather than altered structure. Scientists are searching beyond the presence of obvious lesions in tissues and cells to the submicroscopic, molecular, and biochemical alterations affecting the chemistry of cells.

Not every disease has a specific etiology. A syndrome is a complex of signs and symptoms with no specific etiology or constant lesion. It results from interference at some point with a chain of body processes, causing impairment of body function in one or more systems. With a syndrome, a specific biochemical molecular derangement caused by yet undiscovered agents is usually found. An example is acquired immunodeficiency syndrome (AIDS), for which a specific human immunodeficiency virus (HIV) agent is now accepted as the etiologic agent.

Some diseases have an acute (sudden) onset and run a relatively short course, as with acute tonsillitis (strep throat) or the common cold. Others run a long, protracted course, as with tuberculosis and rheumatoid arthritis; these are called chronic illnesses. The healthy body is in a natural state of readiness to combat disease, and thus there is a natural tendency to recover from disease. This is especially true in acute illness, in which inflammation tends to heal with full resolution of structure and function. Sometimes, however, healing does not occur and the disease overwhelms the body and leads to death. Therefore, a patient with acute pneumonia may have a full recovery, with complete healing and resolution of structure and function, or may die. The outcome of disease can vary between the extremes of full recovery or death and can run a chronic, protracted course eventually leading to severe loss of function. This outcome is the prognosis, a forecast of what may be expected to happen. The accurate diagnosis of disease is essential for its treatment and prognosis.

There are four aspects to the study of disease. The first is etiology or cause; for example, the common cold virus causes the common cold. The second is pathogenesis, or course; it refers to the sequence of events in the body that occurs in response to injury and the method of the lesion's production and development. The relation of an etiologic agent to disease, of cause to effect, is not always as simple a matter as it is in most acute illnesses; for example, a herpesvirus causes the development of fever blisters. In many illnesses, indeed in most chronic illnesses, the concept of one agent causing one disease is an oversimplification. In tuberculosis, for example, the causative agent is a characteristic slender microbe called tubercle bacillus (*Mycobacterium tuberculosis*). Many people may be exposed to and inhale the tuberculosis bacteria, but only a few will get the disease; also, the bacteria may lurk in the body for years and become clinically active only as a result of an unrelated, stressful situation that alters the body's immunity, such as prolonged strain, malnutrition, or another infection. In investigating the causation and pathogenesis of disease, several factors—such as heredity, sex, environment, nutrition, immunity, and age—must be considered. That is why there is no simple answer to the questions, "Does cigarette smoking cause cancer?" or "Does a cholesterol-rich diet cause hardening of the blood vessels (atherosclerosis)?" The third aspect to the study of disease relates to morphologic and structural changes associated with the functional alterations in cells and tissues that are characteristic of the disease. These are the gross and microscopic findings that allow the pathologist to establish a diagnosis. The fourth aspect to disease study is the evaluation of functional abnormalities and their clinical significance; the nature of the morphologic changes and their distribution in different organs or tissues influence normal function and determine the clinical features, signs and symptoms, and course and outcome (prognosis) of disease.

All forms of tissue injury start with molecular and structural changes in cells. Cells are the smallest living units of tissues and organs. Along with their substructural components, they are the seat of disease. Cellular pathology is the study of disease as it relates to the origins, molecular mechanisms, and structural changes of cell injury.

The normal cell is similar to a factory. It is confined to a fairly narrow range of function and structure, dictated by its genetic code, the constraints of neighboring cells, the availability of and access to nutrition, and the disposal of its waste products. It is said to be in a "steady state," able to handle normal physiologic demands and to respond by adapting to other excessive or strenuous demands (such as the muscle enlargement seen in bodybuilders) to achieve a new equilibrium with a sustained workload. This type of adaptive response is called hypertrophy. Conversely, atrophy is an adaptive response to decreased demand, with a resulting diminished size and function.

If the limits of these adaptive responses are exceeded, or if no adaptive response is possible, a sequence of events follows that results in cell injury. Cell injury is reversible up to a certain point, but if the stimulus persists or is severe, then the cell suffers irreversible injury and eventual death. For example, if the blood supply to the heart muscle is cut off for only a few minutes and then restored, the heart muscle cells will experience injury but can recover and function normally. If the blood flow is not restored until one hour later, however, the cells will die.

Whether specific types of stress induce an adaptive response, a reversible injury, or cell death depends on the nature and severity of the stress and on other inherent, variable qualities of the cell itself. The causes of cell injury are many and range from obvious physical trauma, as in automobile accidents, to a subtle, genetic lack of enzymes or hormones, as in diabetes mellitus. Broadly speaking, the causes of cell injury and death can be grouped into the following categories: hypoxia, or a decrease in the delivery of available oxygen; physical agents, as with mechanical and thermal injuries; chemical poisons, such as carbon monoxide and alcohol, tobacco, and other addictive drugs; infectious agents, such as viruses and bacteria; immunological and allergic reactions, as in patients with certain sensitivities; genetic defects, as with sickle cell disease; and nutritional imbalances, such as severe malnutrition and vitamin deficiencies or nutritional excesses predisposing a patient to heart disease and atherosclerosis.

CAUSES OF DISEASE
By far the most common cause of disease is infection, especially by bacteria. Certain lowly forms of animal life known as animal parasites may also live in the body and produce disease; parasitic diseases are common in poor societies and countries. Finally, there are viruses, forms of living matter so minute that they cannot be seen with the most powerful light microscope; they are visible, however, with the electron microscope. Viruses, as agents of disease, have attracted much attention for their role in many diseases, including cancer.

Bacteria, or germs, can be divided into three morphologic groups: cocci, which are round; bacilli, which are rod-shaped; and spirilla or spirochetes, which are spiral-shaped, like a corkscrew. Bacteria produce disease either by their presence in tissues or by their production of toxins (poisons). They cause inflammation and either act on surrounding tissues, as in an abscess, or are carried by the bloodstream to other distant organs. Strep throat is an example of a local infection by cocci—in this case, streptococci. Some dysenteries and travelers' diarrheas are caused by coliform bacilli. Syphilis is an example of a disease caused by a spirochete. The great epidemics of history, such as bubonic plague and cholera, have been caused by bacteria, as are tuberculosis, leprosy, typhoid, gas gangrene, and many others. Bacterial infections are treatable with antibiotics, such as penicillin.

Viruses, on the other hand, are not affected by antibiotics; they infect the cell itself and live within it, and are therefore protected. Viruses cause a wide variety of diseases. Some are short-lived and run a few days' course, such as many childhood diseases, the measles, and the common cold. Others can cause serious body impairment, such as poliomyelitis and AIDS. Still others are probably involved in causing cancer and such diseases as multiple sclerosis.

Of the many physical agents causing injury, trauma is the most obvious; others relate to external temperatures, ones that are either too high or too low. A high temperature may produce local injury, such as a burn, or general disease, such as heatstroke. Heatstroke results from prolonged direct exposure to the sun (sunstroke) or from very high temperatures, so that the heat-regulating mechanism of the body becomes paralyzed. The internal body temperature shoots up to alarming heights; collapse, coma, and even death may result. Low temperatures can cause local frostbite or general hypothermia, which can also lead to death.

Other forms of physical agents causing injury are radiation and atmospheric pressure. Increased atmospheric pressure is best illustrated by the "bends," a decompression sickness that can affect deep sea divers. The pressure of the water causes inert gases, such as nitrogen, to be dissolved in the blood plasma. If the diver passes too rapidly from a high to a normal atmospheric pressure, the excessive nitrogen is released, forming gas bubbles in the blood. These tiny bubbles can cause the blockage of small vessels of the brain and result in brain damage. The same problem can occur in high-altitude aviators unless the airplane is pressurized.

The study of chemical poisoning, or toxicology, as a cause of disease is a large and specialized field. Poisons may be introduced into the body by accident (especially in young children), in the course of suicide or homicide, and, most important, as industrial pollution. Lead poisoning is a danger because of the use of lead in paints and soldering. Acids and carbon monoxide are

emitted into the atmosphere by industry, and various chemicals are dumped into the ground and water. Such environmental damage will eventually affect plants, livestock, and humans.

Hypoxia (lack of oxygen) is probably the most common cause of cell injury, and it may also be the ultimate mechanism of cell death by a wide variety of physical, biological, and chemical agents. Loss of adequate blood and oxygen supply to a body part, such as a leg, is called ischemia. (This is a local loss of blood, in contrast to anemia, which is a general condition of poor oxygen-carrying capacity affecting the entire body.) If the blood loss is very severe, the result is hypoxia or anoxia. This condition may also result from narrowing of the blood vessels, called atherosclerosis. If this narrowing occurs in the artery of the leg, as may be seen in patients with advanced diabetes, then the tissues of the foot will eventually die, a condition known as gangrene. An even more critical example of ischemia is blockage of the coronary arteries of the heart, resulting in a myocardial infarction (heart attack), with damage to the heart muscle. Similarly, severe blockage of arteries to the brain can cause a stroke.

Nutritional diseases can be caused either by an excessive intake and storage of foodstuffs, as in extreme obesity, or by a deficiency. Obesity is a complex condition, often associated with hereditary tendencies and hormonal imbalances. The deficiency conditions are many. Starvation and malnutrition can occur because of intestinal illnesses that prevent the delivery of food to the blood (malabsorption) or because of debilitating diseases such as advanced cancer. Even more important than general malnutrition as a cause of disease is a deficiency of essential nutrients such as minerals, vitamins, and other trace elements. Iron deficiency causes anemia, and calcium deficiency causes osteoporosis (bone fragility). Vitamin deficiencies are also numerous, and deficiency of the trace element iodine causes a thyroid condition called goiter.

Genetic defects as a cause of cellular injury and disease are of major interest to many biologists. The genetic injury may be as gross as the congenital malformations seen in patients with Down syndrome or as subtle as molecular alterations in the coding of the hemoglobin molecule that causes sickle cell disease.

Cellular injuries and diseases can be induced by immune mechanisms. The anaphylactic reaction to a foreign protein, such as a bee sting or drug, can actually cause death. In the so-called autoimmune diseases, such as lupus erythematosus, the immune system turns against the cellular components of the very body that it is supposed to protect.

Finally, neoplastic diseases, or cancer, are presently of unknown etiology. Some are innocuous growths, while others are highly lethal. Diagnosing cancer and determining its precise nature can be an elaborate, and elusive, process. The methods involve clinical observations and laboratory tests; a biopsy of the involved organ may be taken and analyzed.

PERSPECTIVE AND PROSPECTS

It is sometimes said that the nature of disease is changing, that one hears more often of people dying of heart failure and cancer than was once the case. This does not mean that these diseases have actually become more common, although more people do die from them. This increase is attributable to a longer life span and vastly improved diagnostic methods.

For primitive humans, there were no diseases, only patients stricken by evil; therefore, magic was the plausible recourse. Magic entails recognition of the principle of causality—that, given the same predisposing conditions, the same results will follow. In a profound sense, magic is early science. In ancient Egypt, the priests assumed the role of healers. Unlike magic, religion springs from a different source. Here the system is based on the achievement of results against, or in spite of, a regular sequence of events. Religion heals with miracles and antinaturals that require the violation of causality. The purely religious concept of disease, as an expression of the wrath of gods, became embodied in many religious traditions.

The ancient Greeks are credited with attempts at introducing reason to the study of disease by asking questions about the nature of things and considering the notion of health as a harmony, as the adjustment of such opposites as high and low, hot and cold, dry and moist. Disease, therefore, was a disharmony of the four elements that make up life: earth, air, fire, and water. This concept was refined by Galen in the second century and became dogma throughout the Dark Ages until the Renaissance, when the seat of disease was finally assigned to organs within the body itself through autopsy studies. Much later, in the nineteenth century, the principles espoused by French physiologist Claude Bernard were introduced, whereby disease was considered not a thing but a process that distorts normal physiologic and anatomic features. The nineteenth century German pathologist Rudolf Virchow emphasized the same principle—that disease is an alteration of life's processes—

by championing the concept of cellular pathology, identifying the cell as the smallest unit of life and as the seat of disease.

As new diseases are discovered and old medical mysteries are deciphered, as promising new medicinal drugs and vaccines are tested and public health programs implemented, the age-old goal of medicine as a healing art seems to be closer at hand.

—*Victor H. Nassar, M.D.*

See also Centers for Disease Control and Prevention (CDC); Childhood infectious diseases; Dental diseases; Diagnosis; Environmental diseases; Gallbladder diseases; Genetic diseases; Infection; Insect-borne diseases; Motor neuron diseases; National Institutes of Health (NIH); Parasitic diseases; Pathology; Prion diseases; Prognosis; Protozoan diseases; Pulmonary diseases; Sexually transmitted diseases (STDs); Signs and symptoms; Syndrome; Zoonoses; *specific diseases.*

FOR FURTHER INFORMATION:

Biddle, Wayne. *A Field Guide to Germs.* 2d ed. New York: Anchor Books, 2002. This comprehensive book is easily accessible to the nonspecialist and includes a discussion of nearly every virus, bacterium, and fungus known to cause human and nonhuman animal disease. The history of the microbe and the treatment of diseases are included.

Boyd, William. *Boyd's Introduction to the Study of Disease.* 11th ed. Philadelphia: Lea & Febiger, 1992. A textbook for students in the medical and allied health sciences. The text and illustrations emphasize the view of disease as a disturbed functional alteration.

Frank, Steven A. *Immunology and Evolution of Infectious Disease.* Princeton, N.J.: Princeton University Press, 2002. Blends research from molecular biology, immunology, pathogen biology, and population dynamics to discuss how and why parasites vary to escape recognition by the immune system, vaccine design, and the control of epidemics.

Grist, Norman R., et al. *Diseases of Infection: An Illustrated Textbook.* 2d ed. New York: Oxford University Press, 1992. An informative survey of communicable diseases. Contains copious illustrations.

Kumar, Vinay, Abul K. Abbas, and Nelson Fausto, eds. *Robbins and Cotran Pathologic Basis of Disease.* 8th ed. Philadelphia: Saunders/Elsevier, 2010. The standard textbook on disease for medical students.

McCance, Kathryn L., and Sue M. Huether. *Pathophysiology: The Biologic Basis for Disease in Adults and Children.* 6th ed. St. Louis, Mo.: Mosby/Elsevier, 2010. A text that explores the myriad cellular and genetic causes of disease. Topics include cell injury, immunity, inflammation and wound healing, coping and illness, and ontogenesis.

Shaw, Michael, ed. *Everything You Need to Know About Diseases*. Springhouse, Pa.: Springhouse Press, 1996. This well-illustrated consumer reference, compiled by more than one hundred doctors and medical experts, describes five hundred illnesses and conditions, their causes, symptoms, diagnosis, treatment, and prevention. A valuable reference book for everyone interested in health and disease.

Strauss, James, and Ellen Strauss. *Viruses and Human Disease*. 2d ed. Boston: Academic Press/Elsevier, 2008. An undergraduate text that examines virology from a human disease perspective.

DISK REMOVAL

PROCEDURE

ANATOMY OR SYSTEM AFFECTED: Back, bones, nervous system, spine

SPECIALTIES AND RELATED FIELDS: General surgery, neurology, orthopedics, physical therapy

DEFINITION: A surgical procedure used to remove intervertebral disks that are compressing nerves that enter and exit the spinal cord.

KEY TERMS:

cervical vertebrae: the first seven bones of the spinal column, located in the neck

disk prolapse: the protrusion (herniation) of intervertebral disk material, which may press on spinal nerves

intervertebral disks: flattened disks of fibrocartilage that separate the vertebrae and allow cushioned flexibility of the spinal column

lumbar vertebrae: the five bones of the spinal column in the lower back, which experience the greatest stress in the spine

spinal cord: a column of nervous tissue housed in the vertebral column that carries messages to and from the brain

INDICATIONS AND PROCEDURES

A relatively common disorder that causes lower back and sometimes leg pain is the herniation or prolapse of an intervertebral disk in the lower back. These disks are made of cartilage and serve to separate the bones that make up the vertebral column. The spinal cord is located within the bony structure of the vertebrae and has nerves which enter and exit between these bones.

These sensory and motor nerves must pass alongside the intervertebral disks. When a disk's jellylike center bulges out through a weakened area of the firmer outer core, the disk is said to be herniated or prolapsed. This may compress the spinal cord or the nerve roots and yield such symptoms as interference with muscle strength or pain and numbness of the lower back and leg.

More than 90 percent of disk prolapses occur in the lumbar region of the back, but they may also occur in the cervical vertebrae. Occasionally, disk herniation is caused by improper lifting of heavy objects, sudden twisting of the spinal column, or trauma to the back or neck. More typically, however, a prolapsed disk develops gradually as the patient ages and the intervertebral disks degenerate.

To diagnose a prolapsed disk, a physician will likely want to visualize the vertebrae and spinal cord using X rays, computed tomography (CT) scans, or magnetic resonance imaging (MRI). Once diagnosed, most cases can be treated with analgesics, muscle relaxants (such as cyclobenzaprine and methocarbamol), and physical therapy. If the symptoms recur, however, it may be necessary to have the protruding portion of the disk or the whole disk surgically removed. This procedure usually requires that the patient have general anesthesia and remain hospitalized for several days.

For a lumbar procedure, the patient is anesthetized and placed on the operating room table in a modified kneeling position, with the abdomen suspended and the legs placed over the end of the table. The lower back is then prepared for a sterile procedure, and the surgeon makes an incision in the middle of the back along the spine. The surrounding tissues are retracted, and the vertebrae are exposed. At this time, the surgeon must make a careful dissection of the tissues in order to identify the affected nerves and intervertebral disk. Once the prolapsed disk is found, the physician will cut away the fragment of the disk impinging on the nerve. It is important that all free fragments be removed, as these could cause symptoms at a later time. Often, the surgeon must remove some of the vertebrae to gain access to the disk. This is known as a laminectomy.

USES AND COMPLICATIONS

Because the vertebral column houses the spinal cord, any surgical manipulation of this area must be approached with extreme caution. Very large arteries (the aorta) and veins (the vena cava) lie adjacent to the spinal column, and accidental cuts can lead to rapid blood loss. The spinal cord is surrounded by a covering called the meninges, which helps to protect the cord and which contains the cerebral spinal fluid. Trauma to the meninges may cause the fluid to leak out or lead to meningitis (inflammation of the meninges). One surgical approach to reduce the adverse affects of a lesion on the meninges is to use some of the patient's fat to pack the leak and help prevent scarring. Patients with operative trauma to the meninges may complain of headache, which usually decreases in severity as the lesion heals.

Other complications that may arise include infections in approximately 3 percent of patients, thromboembolism in less than 1 percent, and death in about one patient per 1,000. One study reports an overall complication rate of 4 percent. Unfortunately, one of the major long-term complications reported in the study involved a worsening of symptoms after surgery.

PERSPECTIVE AND PROSPECTS

Even with some potential complications, disk removal typically has a favorable outcome, although this varies somewhat depending on the patient, the treatment method, and what the patient and physician consider to be a good result. Typically, favorable outcomes range from 50 to 95 percent. The number of patients who need a second operation ranges from 4 to 25 percent.

Health care professionals are beginning to emphasize the importance of prevention of back pain. Educating patients on proper lifting techniques, such as bending the legs rather than the back and avoiding twisting, will reduce the potential for damage to the intervertebral disks. Individuals who are overweight are also at risk for developing lower back pain because of the added stress to the lumbar spine, as well as because of their relatively weak abdominal muscles. The abdominal muscles are important in stabilizing and supporting the lower back. Exercises that help strengthen these muscles are recommended for a weight-reducing exercise and diet program. Patients who must sit for long periods of time are also at risk for lower back pain. These people should take several quick breaks to stand and stretch, which reduces the constant stress on the lumbar spine.

—*Matthew Berria, Ph.D., and Douglas Reinhart, M.D.*

See also Back pain; Bone disorders; Bones and the skeleton; Braces, orthopedic; Laminectomy and spinal fusion; Meningitis; Orthopedic surgery; Orthopedics; Slipped disk; Spinal cord disorders; Spine, vertebrae, and disks.

FOR FURTHER INFORMATION:

Aminoff, Michael J. "Nervous System." In *Current Medical Diagnosis and Treatment 2007*, edited by Lawrence M. Tierney, Jr., Stephen J. McPhee, and Maxine A. Papadakis. New York: McGraw-Hill Medical, 2006. A chapter in a text that is the point of reference for physicians and other health care practitioners. Incorporates each year's biomedical research discoveries that have immediate, relevant, and applicable use for the patient.

Bradford, David S., and Thomas A. Zdeblick, eds. *The Spine*. 2d ed. Philadelphia: Lippincott Williams & Wilkins, 2004. Discusses surgical methods and options for the treatment of the spine. Includes bibliographical references and an index.

Canale, S. Terry, ed. *Campbell's Operative Orthopaedics*. 11th ed. 4 vols. St. Louis, Mo.: Mosby/Elsevier, 2008. The section "The Spine" contains an essay, "Lower Back Pain and Disorders of Intervertebral Discs," which discusses such topics as microsurgery, nontraumatic bone and joint disorders, arthrodesis, arthroplasty, and congenital anomalies.

Filler, Aaron G. *Do You Really Need Back Surgery? A Surgeon's Guide to Back and Neck Pain and How to Choose Your Treatment*. Rev. ed. New York: Oxford University Press, 2007. A good review of diagnosis and treatment options.

Haldeman, Scott, William H. Kirkaldy-Willis, and Thomas N. Bernard, Jr. *Atlas of Back Pain*. Boca Raton, Fla.: Parthenon, 2002. A clinical text that explains how to determine the underlying causes of back conditions and describes the various treatment options available.

Leikin, Jerrold B., and Martin S. Lipsky, eds. *American Medical Association Complete Medical Encyclopedia*. New York: Random House Reference, 2003. A concise presentation of numerous medical terms and illnesses. A good general reference.

DISLOCATION. *See* FRACTURE AND DISLOCATION.

DISSEMINATED INTRAVASCULAR COAGULATION (DIC)
DISEASE/DISORDER
ALSO KNOWN AS: Consumption coagulopathy
ANATOMY OR SYSTEM AFFECTED: Blood, blood vessels, circulatory system, immune system
SPECIALTIES AND RELATED FIELDS: Hematology, internal medicine, neonatology, obstetrics, oncology

DEFINITION: A hemorrhagic disorder that occurs as a complication of several different disease states and results from abnormally initiated and accelerated blood clotting.

KEY TERMS:

acute DIC: a disorder of the blood-clotting mechanism that develops within hours of an initial attack on an underlying body system

chronic DIC: a disorder of the blood-clotting mechanism that persists in a suppressed state until a coagulation disorder worsens

coagulation: the process of blood clot formation

coagulation cascade: the series of steps starting with the activation of the intrinsic or extrinsic pathways of coagulation and proceeding through the common pathway of coagulation leading to the formation of fibrin clots

ecchymosis: bleeding into the skin, subcutaneous tissue, or mucous membranes, resulting in bruising

hemostasis: the stopping of blood flow through the blood vessels, usually as a result of blood clotting

petechiae: round pinpoint hemorrhages in the skin

platelets: cells, found in the blood of all mammals, that are involved in the coagulation of blood and the contraction of blood clots

thrombocytopenia: a markedly decreased number of platelets in the blood

thromboembolism: the obstruction of a blood vessel with a clot that has broken loose from its site of origin

CAUSES AND SYMPTOMS

Disseminated intravascular coagulation (DIC) is a disorder that occurs as a life-threatening complication of many different conditions. It is most commonly seen as a complication of bacterial, fungal, parasitic, or viral infections; inflammatory bowel disease; pregnancy; cancer; surgery; major trauma; burns; heatstroke; shock; transplant rejection; toxicity resulting from recreational drug use; or snakebite. It can occur as either an acute or a chronic condition, depending on the underlying cause.

In both forms, DIC involves the systemic activation of the hemostasis system. In its acute form, DIC involves hemorrhaging, the development of ecchymoses, bleeding of the mucosa, and depletion or absence of platelets and clotting factors in the blood. In the most severe cases, it is accompanied by extensive consumption of the proteins involved in coagulation, sig-

nificant deposits of fibrin in the vasculature and organs, and bleeding that may lead to organ failure and death. In its chronic form, it is more subtle and usually includes thromboembolism along with activation of the coagulation system.

In acute DIC, the introduction of tissue factors into the circulation (from injury, surgery, or tissue necrosis), stagnant blood flow (from shock or cardiac arrest), or the presence of infectious agents leads to systemic activation of the coagulation system. A massive clotting cascade is triggered and leads to the formation of blood clots, possibly compromising the blood supply to major organs, and simultaneously to the exhaustion of platelets and coagulation factors, resulting in hemorrhaging.

Thus, DIC occurs when endothelial cells or monocytes are damaged by toxic substances. When these cells are injured, they release tissue factor on the surface of the cell, which in turn triggers the hemostasis system, activating a coagulation cascade. Thrombin accumulates rapidly, and fibrin is produced in large quantities and is deposited in the microvasculature, leading to blood clots throughout the capillary system. This clot formation leads rapidly to the depletion of platelets and coagulation factors throughout the body. Simultaneously, thrombin activates fibrinolytic pathways that release anticoagulants and dissolve the clots by turning them into fibrin split products, further contributing to uncontrollable bleeding. In chronic DIC, these events occur more slowly, allowing compensation to take place.

INFORMATION ON DISSEMINATED INTRAVASCULAR COAGULATION (DIC)

CAUSES: Accelerated blood clotting that may be a complication of bacterial, fungal, parasitic, or viral infections; inflammatory bowel disease; pregnancy; cancer; surgery; major trauma; burns; heatstroke; shock; transplant rejection; drug use; snakebite

SYMPTOMS: Hemorrhaging, bruising, bleeding of mucosa, depletion or absence of platelets and clotting factors in blood

DURATION: Acute or chronic, depending on cause

TREATMENTS: Dependent on underlying condition; anticoagulants (heparin, antithrombin III), antifibrinolytics (Amicar, Cykokapron), blood products (fresh frozen plasma, cryoprecipitate, red blood cells, platelets)

The diagnosis of DIC is based on clinical signs and laboratory findings. In acute DIC, the symptoms include multiple bleeding sites, the development of petechiae on the skin, ecchymoses of the skin and mucous membranes, visceral hemorrhaging, and the development of ischemic tissue. In chronic DIC, symptoms will include deep vein or arterial thrombosis or embolism, superficial venous thrombosis (especially in the absence of varicose veins), multiple and simultaneous thrombus sites, or serial thrombotic episodes. Laboratory findings indicative of DIC are decreased platelet count, prolonged prothrombin time (PT), activated partial thromboplastin time (APTT), and thrombin time along with decreased fibrinogen levels and increased fibrin-fibrinogen degradation product (FDP) levels. Peripheral smears will show the presence of schistocytes (fragments of red blood cells).

TREATMENT AND THERAPY

The treatment of either the acute or the chronic form of DIC is based on the etiology and pathophysiology of the underlying clinical condition. Aside from the treatment of the underlying disorder, acute DIC requires aggressive treatment of the bleeding through the use of anticoagulants (such as heparin or antithrombin III) and antifibrinolytics (Amicar or Cykokapron), as well as the administration of blood products, including fresh frozen plasma, cryoprecipitate, red blood cells, and platelets. The prognosis is determined by the underlying condition that led to DIC, as well as the severity of the DIC. Follow-up care for those who survive is provided by a primary physician, for the underlying disorder, and by a hematologist.

PERSPECTIVE AND PROSPECTS

It is unclear when disseminated intravascular coagulation was first mentioned in the medical literature. Historically, it has always been considered a secondary disease (resulting as a consequence of some underlying disorder). Thus, DIC has always referred to the secondary activation of the coagulation system as a result of an underlying problem. It occurs with equal frequency in males and females and does not appear to be age-related. Approximately 20,000 cases per year were diagnosed in the United States during the mid-1990's.

While DIC is generally categorized, treated, and evaluated based on the pathophysiology of the underlying disorder, Rodger L. Bick has proposed a DIC scoring system to assess the severity of the coagulation disorder, as well as the effectiveness of the treatment modalities. New treatment modalities, such as the use of recombinant activated protein C, are being investigated in large multicenter clinical trials.

—*Robin Kamienny Montvilo, R.N., Ph.D.*

See also Bleeding; Blood and blood disorders; Circulation; Hematology; Hematology, pediatric; Hemorrhage; Ischemia; Thrombosis and thrombus.

FOR FURTHER INFORMATION:

Bick, Roger L. "Disseminated Intravascular Coagulation: Objective Criteria for Diagnosis and Management." *Medical Clinics of North America* 78 (1994): 511-543.

Kasper, Dennis L., et al., eds. *Harrison's Principles of Internal Medicine.* 16th ed. New York: McGraw-Hill, 2005.

Lichtman, Marshall A., et al., eds. *Williams Hematology.* 7th ed. New York: McGraw-Hill, 2006.

DIURETICS

TREATMENT

ALSO KNOWN AS: Water pill

ANATOMY OR SYSTEM AFFECTED: Bladder, blood, blood vessels, cells, circulatory system, heart, kidneys, urinary system

SPECIALTIES AND RELATED FIELDS: Cardiology, critical care, internal medicine, nephrology, nursing, pharmacology, urology

DEFINITION: Prescription medications used to prevent passive reabsorption of water in the kidney unit (nephron), resulting in an increased urinary output.

KEY TERMS:

acid-base balance: the balance between acids (proton donors) and bases (proton acceptors) in the blood that normally maintains the blood pH (hydrogen ion concentration) between 7.35 and 7.45; components of the acid-base system include the lungs, blood buffer system, and kidneys

aldosterone: a hormone produced by the adrenal gland that helps regulate the salt (sodium) and water balance in the body by increasing both sodium and water retention

diuresis: increased formation and excretion of urine

electrolyte: minerals (sodium, potassium, calcium, magnesium, chloride, bicarbonate) that carry an electrical charge and assist in body functions (metabolic processes, nerve conduction, heart rhythm and contraction, and muscle contraction)

filtrate: water and small solute molecules filtered from the blood by the glomerulus of the nephron

nephron: the functional unit of the kidney consisting of the glomerulus, the proximal convoluted tubule, the loop of Henle, and the distal convoluted tubule; the nephron produces urine

osmotic: an agent resulting in osmosis, the movement of a solvent (such as water) through a semipermeable membrane (such as a cell wall) from an area of lower solute concentration to an area of higher solute concentration; aim is to equalize the solvent-solute ratio (concentration) on both sides of the membrane

ototoxic: creating damage resulting in hearing loss; the loss may or may not be reversible when the damaging agent is removed

reabsorption: in the kidney, the process of reabsorbing water and electrolytes from the filtrate and returning them to the bloodstream (circulation)

solute: the dissolved particles in a solution; common solutes in humans are the electrolytes

INDICATIONS AND PROCEDURES

The basic functional unit of the kidney is the nephron. It consists of four regions: glomerulus, proximal convoluted tubule, loop of Henle, and distal convoluted tubule. The purpose of the nephron is to filter waste products from the blood and excrete these products as urine. Blood filtering occurs in the glomerulus. In the adult, approximately 180 liters of filtrate is produced daily. The purpose of the other three segments of the nephron are to reabsorb the majority of water and electrolytes from the filtrate and return these items to circulation, leaving approximately 1.8 liters to be discarded as urine.

In certain disease states it becomes necessary to enhance urine production to relieve symptoms and prevent morbidity (illness) or mortality (death). Increased urine production can be accomplished by the administration of a category of drugs known as diuretics. Diuretics are prescription medications that work by blocking the reabsorption of solutes, especially salt (sodium) and water, which passively follows sodium. Thus, solutes and water are excreted from the body rather than being returned to circulation. Diuretics are prescribed for conditions such as high blood pressure (hypertension), heart failure, pulmonary edema, kidney (renal) failure, and liver (hepatic) failure or cirrhosis with accompanying fluid in the abdominal cavity (ascites). Diuresis results in a lower blood volume and reduces blood pressure and the work of the heart. By removing fluid from the lungs breathing is less labored. Diuretics also maintain urine production in shock states. This prevents acute renal failure. Removing abdominal fluid makes it easier to breathe and comfort of the individual is increased.

The care provider will prescribe diuretic therapy after examining a patient and obtaining supporting information such as blood pressure, radiological examinations, and laboratory tests. The patient's lifestyle, preferences, and the cost of medications are considered in the decision to prescribe diuretics and which type of diuretics to prescribe.

USES AND COMPLICATIONS

There are four major types of diuretics: high-ceiling, thiazide, potassium-sparing, and osmotic diuretics. The most potent are high-ceiling agents (for example, furosemide). These drugs are commonly referred to as loop diuretics because they exert effects on the loop of Henle portion of the nephron. Administration of loop diuretics may result in profound fluid and electrolyte loss. This can lead to serious side effects such as low blood volume (hypovolemia), low blood pressure (hypotension), and electrolyte and acid-base disturbances requiring treatment. Loop diuretics are ototoxic and can lead to hearing loss. Hearing loss may be reversed if reported to the care provider and the medication is stopped. An advantage of loop diuretics is that they continue to work even if renal blood flow is decreased. This is not true with other types of diuretics.

Another class of diuretic agents is the thiazides (for example, hydrochlorothiazide). Thiazides exert their effects on the proximal portion of the distal convoluted tubule. Although not as potent as high-ceiling diuretics they produce losses of electrolytes and water. Thiazide diuretics do not cause as much calcium excretion as loop diuretics and are useful in patients prone to calcium kidney stones. They suppress insulin production and glycogen storage resulting in higher blood glucose levels. This requires diabetic patients receiving thiazide diuretics to monitor blood glucose closely. Thiazides also decrease the excretion of uric acid. As uric acid blood levels rise, gout may develop. This class of diuretics is relatively inexpensive and well tolerated and is often used as first-line therapy for hypertension.

Potassium-sparing diuretics exert only a modest increase in urine output. There are two types of potassium-sparing agents: aldosterone antagonists (for example, spironalactone) and non-aldosterone antagonists (for example, amiloride). Aldosterone, a hormone secreted by the adrenal gland, increases sodium and water reabsorption in the nephron. By blocking aldosterone the reuptake of sodium and water is prohibited. Aldosterone antagonists require approximately forty-eight hours to demonstrate an effect. Non-aldosterone antagonists directly inhibit sodium and water reabsorption and effects begin without delay. Potassium-sparing diuretics cause minimal amounts of potassium to be lost in the urine. This class of diuretics is frequently used with loop or thiazide diuretics, not for diuresis, but to prevent potassium depletion. Side effects include too much potassium in the body (hyperkalemia) resulting in fatal heart rhythms, and endocrine effects. Because aldosterone antagonists are steroid hormones gynecomastia, menstrual irregularities, impotence, hirsutism, and deepening of the voice may occur. Potassium-sparing diuretics should not be taken with other drugs which are potassium sparing (angiotensin-converting enzyme inhibitors, angiotensin receptor blockers, or direct renin inhibitors), potassium supplements, or salt substitutes containing potassium.

Osmotic diuretics are the final class of diuretic agents (for example, mannitol). Osmotic agents differ from other diuretic groups in their mechanism of action and indications for use. Osmotic drugs work by creating an osmotic force. When utilized to maintain urine production and prevent renal failure in patients suffering from shock, the drug is administered intravenously. In the kidney, the osmotic agent is freely filtered from the blood into the filtrate. It remains in the filtrate and holds water close to it in an attempt to maintain a normal solute-solvent ratio. The degree of diuresis is directly proportional to the concentration of osmotic agent in the filtrate. In treating increased pressure within the eye (intraocular pressure) as in glaucoma, osmotic eye drops work the same way—they create an osmotic force thus reducing pressure within the eye.

Diuretic drugs should be used with caution in patients with diabetes, gout, or renal impairment; during pregnancy; and when taking other drugs such as

In the News: Antihypertensive and Lipid-Lowering Treatment to Prevent Heart Attack Trial (ALLHAT)

This five-year study involving forty thousand subjects was funded by the National Institutes of Health: National Heart, Lung, and Blood Institute and demonstrated reduced illness (morbidity) including heart attack and stroke, and deaths (mortality) when high blood pressure (hypertension) was controlled. The original study found that an older, and cheaper, thiazide diuretic worked just as well or better to control blood pressure than three newer and more expensive types of antihypertensive medications. This finding led to changes in recommendations on the management of hypertension. *The Seventh Report of the Joint National Committee on Prevention, Detection, Evaluation, and Treatment of High Blood Pressure* (JNC 7), published in 2003, recommended thiazide diuretics, usually in conjunction with another antihypertensive drug to treat hypertension. Diuretics remove fluid from the body by increasing urinary output thus reducing blood pressure and the work of the heart. Patients can breathe easier with less fluid in the lungs. The work of the heart is reduced when the volume of blood is lowered through urinary losses (diuresis).

A ten-year follow-up analysis of ALLHAT study subjects' morbidity and mortality outcomes was presented in the late fall of 2009 by the ALLHAT Collaborative Research Group at the American Heart Association's 2009 Scientific Session. The follow-up data continued to demonstrate improved outcomes when hypertension is controlled regardless of the type of medication used to lower blood pressure. These data reinforce the need for the public to have blood pressure monitored and to be treated when hypertension is detected.

—*Wanda Todd Bradshaw, M.S.N., N.N.P., P.N.P., C.C.R.N.*

digoxin, lithium, ototoxic medications, nonsteroidal anti-inflammatory drugs (NSAIDs), or additional antihypertensive agents. Individuals should weigh daily in the morning before eating or drinking and keep a weight record that should be shared with the care provider. Also, they should check and record the blood pressure as instructed and remain alert to side effects of dehydration (dry mouth, thirst, low urine output), low potassium levels (irregular heartbeat, muscle weakness, cramping), or high potassium levels (slow or irregular heartbeat, high muscle tone, tingling).

Perspective and Prospects

Control of fluid and electrolytes to treat pathologic conditions such as hypertension, heart failure, pulmonary edema, and ascites is not new. Historical references go back to ancient Egypt. Throughout the centuries various medications to control these pathologies have been utilized including plants and herbs, and in the 1940's, mercury compounds. Thiazide diuretics were introduced in 1958 followed by the loop diuretic, furosemide in 1966. Since that time additional diuretics have been invented. As the rate of obesity, type 2 diabetes mellitus, and hypertension continue to rise in the United States the need for diuretic agents will increase. Pharmaceutical companies consider new compounds that may show benefit as the next diuretic agent.

—Wanda Todd Bradshaw,
M.S.N., N.N.P., P.N.P., C.C.R.N.

See also Hypertension; Kidney disorders; Kidneys; Nephrectomy; Nephritis; Nephrology; Pharmacy; Renal failure; Urinalysis; Urinary system; Urology.

FOR FURTHER INFORMATION:

Adams, Michael, and Robert Koch. "Diuretic Therapy and the Pharmacotherapy of Renal Failure." In *Pharmacology: Connections to Nursing Practice.* Upper Saddle River, N.J.: Pearson, 2010.

Broyles, Bonita, Barry Reiss, and Mary Evans, eds. *Pharmacological Aspects of Nursing Care.* 7th ed. Clifton Park, N.Y.: Thomson-Delmar, 2007.

Herbert-Ashton, Marilyn, and Nancy Clarkson, eds. *Pharmacology.* 2d ed. Sudbury, Mass.: Jones and Bartlett, 2008.

Will, Julie. "Diuretic Therapy and Drugs for Renal Failure." In *Pharmacology for Nurses: A Pathophysiologic Approach*, edited by Michael Adams, Leland Holland, Jr., and Paula Bostwick. Upper Saddle River, N.J.: Pearson-Prentice Hall, 2008.

DIVERTICULITIS AND DIVERTICULOSIS
DISEASE/DISORDER

ANATOMY OR SYSTEM AFFECTED: Abdomen, gastrointestinal system, intestines

SPECIALTIES AND RELATED FIELDS: Gastroenterology, internal medicine, proctology

DEFINITION: Diverticulosis is a disease involving multiple outpouchings, or diverticuli, of the wall of the colon; these diverticuli may become inflamed, leading to the painful condition called diverticulitis.

KEY TERMS:

colon: the portion of the large intestine excluding the cecum and rectum; it includes the ascending, transverse, descending, and sigmoid colon

dietary fiber: indigestible plant substances that humans eat; fiber may be soluble, meaning that it dissolves in water, or insoluble, meaning that it does not dissolve in water

hernia: the bulging out of part or all of an organ through the wall of the cavity that usually contains it

infection: multiplication of disease-causing microorganisms in the body; the body normally also contains microorganisms that do not cause disease

inflammation: a tissue response to injury involving local reactions that attempt to destroy the injurious material and begin healing

lumen: the channel within a hollow or tubular organ

mucosa: the inner lining of the digestive tract; in the colon, the major function of the mucosal cells is to reabsorb liquid from feces, creating a semisolid material

perforation: an abnormal opening, such as a hole in the wall of the colon

peritoneal cavity: the cavity in the abdomen and pelvis that contains the internal organs

prevalence: the frequency of disease cases in a population, often expressed as a fraction (such as cases per 100,000)

CAUSES AND SYMPTOMS

Diverticulosis is an acquired condition of the colon that involves a few to hundreds of blueberry-sized outpouchings of its wall, called diverticuli. Diverticular disease is usually manifested by the presence of multiple diverticuli that are at risk of causing abdominal pain, inflammation, or bleeding.

Although the wall of the colon is thin, microscopically it has four layers. The innermost layer is called the mucosa. Its main function is to absorb fluids from the substance entering the colon, turning it into a semisolid material called feces. Outside the mucosa is the submucosa, a layer which contains blood vessels as well as nerve cells that control the functions of mucosal cells. Outside the submucosa is the muscularis, which contains muscle cells that are able to contract, pushing feces along the colon and eventually out through the rectum. Outside the muscularis is the serosa, which forms a wrap around the colon and helps prevent infections in this organ from spreading beyond its walls.

The definition of a diverticulum, taken from *Stedman's Medical Dictionary* (27th ed., 2000), is "a pouch or sac opening from a tubular or saccular organ, such as the gut or bladder." The diverticuli that form in the colon are not true diverticuli, in that the entire wall is not present in the outpouching. If examined microscopically, only the mucosal and submucosal layers pouch out through weakened areas in the muscularis layer. If examined by the naked eye, however, it appears as if the entire wall of the colon is involved in the tiny outpouching. The mucosa bulges out in the part of the colonic wall that is weakened: This is where arteries penetrate through clefts in the muscularis.

The large intestine begins with the cecum, which is connected to the small intestine. The cecum is a pouch leading to the colon, whose components are the ascending, transverse, descending, and sigmoid colon. The sigmoid colon leads to the rectum, which is connected to the outside of the body by the anal canal. Although diverticuli can appear at a variety of locations in the gastrointestinal (GI) tract, they are usually located in the colon, most commonly in the sigmoid colon.

The most common form of diverticulosis is called spastic colon diverticulosis, which is a condition involving diverticuli in the sigmoid colon whose lumen is abnormally narrowed. Since the circumference of the colon normally alternately narrows and widens along its length, muscle contractions may result in local occlusions of the lumen at the narrowed sections. Occlusion may cause the lumen of the colon to become multiple, separate chambers. When this happens, the pressure within the chambers can increase to the point where the mucosa herniates out through small clefts in the muscularis, creating diverticuli.

Most people with diverticulosis never notice it. When abdominal pain related to painful diverticular disease develops, it is felt in the lower abdomen and may last for hours or days. Eating usually makes it worse, whereas passing gas or having a bowel movement may relieve it.

Besides causing abdominal pain, diverticuli may cause rectal bleeding, which may vary from mild to life-threatening. Usually, there is a sudden urge to defecate followed by passage of red blood, clots, or maroon-colored stool. If the stool is black, the bleeding is probably from the upper GI tract.

Since the colon may be studded with multiple diverticuli, and the bleeding may stop by the time of evaluation, it is often difficult to tell which one bled. Diverticulosis is most common in elderly people, who may have other conditions of the colon that are associated with bleeding. Therefore, it is often impossible to confirm that the cause of bleeding was diverticular disease—even if the colon is lined with hundreds of diverticuli.

What is most important is to establish what part of the GI tract is bleeding. To find out if the bleeding could have come from the upper GI tract, a tube is passed through the nose into the stomach, and the contents are aspirated. If blood is not present, this suggests lower GI bleeding. In addition, the esophagus, stomach, and upper small intestine can be visualized with a flexible,

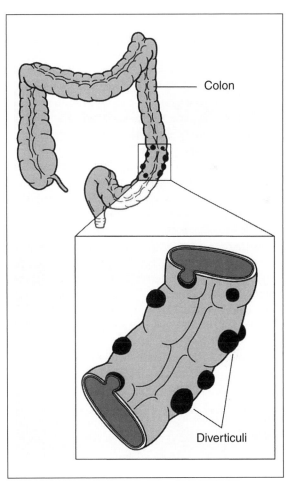

Diverticulosis occurs when multiple diverticuli (outpouchings) appear on the colon wall.

snakelike instrument called an endoscope to exclude a source such as a bleeding ulcer.

It is more difficult to examine the lower GI tract. The simplest procedure is anoscopy, by which the physician can examine the inside of the anal canal for hemorrhoids. Proctosigmoidoscopy, a procedure similar to endoscopy, offers a view of the rectum and part of the sigmoid colon. It may reveal diverticuli or other lesions such as a bleeding growth called a polyp. Colonoscopy is most easily performed after bleeding has stopped. It requires cleaning out the contents of the colon and then inserting a long, flexible instrument called a colonoscope all the way to the cecum. The entire lining of the colon can be visualized while withdrawing the colonoscope.

Angiography is a test done in the radiology department; it involves injecting dye into the vessels that lead to the colon. If there is active bleeding, it can help localize the source. Even if the bleeding has stopped, this procedure can sometimes identify abnormal blood vessel formations suggestive of cancer or a blood vessel abnormality called angiodysplasia.

About 15 percent of people with diverticulosis suffer from one or more episodes of diverticulitis, which is an inflammatory condition that may progress to an infection. Initially, feces may become trapped and inspissated (thickened) in a diverticulum, irritating it and leading to inflammation. Inflammation is a tissue response to injury which involves local reactions that attempt to destroy the injurious material and begin the healing process. It is usually the first step in the body's attempt to prevent infection and involves the migration of white blood cells out of blood vessels and into tissues, where they begin to fight off bacteria. The white blood cells release enzymes that cause tissue destruction. Because it is thin, the wall of the diverticulum may develop a tiny perforation.

Feces are made up of waste material and bacteria that normally do not cause problems when confined within the lumen of the colon. When a diverticulum perforates, however, they travel outside the colon and into other regions such as the peritoneal cavity, causing an infection. This infection along the outside of the colon is often limited, because many adjacent structures are able to wall off the bacteria, limiting their ability to extend through the peritoneal cavity. Although they become sealed off, they often form a pus-filled lesion called an abscess.

Fever and abdominal pain are the most common symptoms of diverticulitis. The fever may be high and

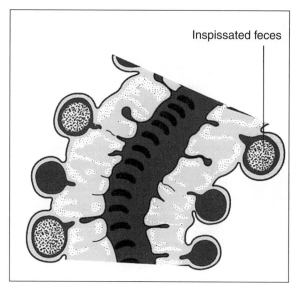

Diverticulitis begins when fecal material invades diverticuli and thickens (inspissated feces); when a diverticulum perforates, bacteria travel outside the colon into other regions and cause serious symptoms, including lower abdominal pain, fever, chills, and abscesses.

associated with shaking chills. The pain is often sudden in onset, is often continuous, and may radiate from the left lower abdomen to the back. Laboratory findings usually include an elevated white blood cell count, a nonspecific finding that occurs with a variety of infections.

Radiographic studies are helpful for diagnosing and assessing the severity of diverticulitis. For example, a computed tomography (CT) scan can detect diverticuli or a thickening of the bowel wall associated with diverticulitis and can help assess whether abscesses are present.

TREATMENT AND THERAPY

There are two treatment goals in treating uncomplicated, painful diverticular disease: prevention of further development of diverticuli and pain relief. It is important to understand that the pressure that is able to develop inside the lumen of the colon is inversely related to the radius of the lumen. Therefore, if the lumen's radius can be increased, the pressures within the lumen will lessen, theoretically decreasing the chance of diverticuli formation. One key to increasing the radius of the lumen of the colon is to increase the bulk of the stool by the addition of dietary fiber.

A Western diet tends to be high in fiber-free animal foods and to lose much of its fiber during processing.

This low-fiber diet may contribute to diverticulosis, which is prevalent in countries that have low-fiber diets. The typical American diet contains an average of 12 grams of fiber per day, whereas diets from Africa and India contain from 40 to 150 grams of fiber per day. A high-fiber diet can increase stool bulk by 40 to 100 percent. Fiber adds bulk to the stool because it acts like a sponge, retaining water that would normally be reabsorbed by the colonic mucosa. Fiber also increases stool bulk because 50 to 70 percent of the fiber is degraded by the bacteria in the colon and the products of degradation attract water by a process called osmosis.

The main fibers that increase stool bulk are the water-insoluble fibers, such as cellulose, hemicellulose, and lignin; they are derived from plants such as vegetables and whole grain cereals. Diets high in these fibers have been shown to decrease the intraluminal pressure in the sigmoid colon, as well as to relieve the pain associated with uncomplicated diverticular disease. The best results have been with the addition of 10 to 25 grams per day of coarse, unprocessed wheat bran to various liquid and semisolid foods. The sudden addition of large amounts of bran to one's diet, however, may cause bloating. Commercial preparations such as methylcellulose may be better tolerated during the first few weeks of therapy; their use may then be tapered off as bran is added to the diet. There are also various antispasmodic drugs available for inhibiting the muscle spasms of the colon, but many of those used in the United States are not very effective for decreasing symptoms.

For diverticular bleeding, the most effective therapy is patience. Most episodes stop on their own, and conservative treatments such as maintaining the patient's blood volume with intravenous fluids and possibly performing blood transfusions are all that is necessary. In those patients with continued active bleeding and in whom the source of the bleeding can be identified with angiography, a drug called vasopressin may be administered into the artery over several hours. This causes constriction of the vessel and stops bleeding most of the time. Once the vasopressin is stopped, however, patients may resume bleeding.

If vasopressin fails, surgery may be necessary. Surgery is most often successful if the bleeding site has been well localized before the operation. In that case, only the involved segment of the colon needs to be removed. If the bleeding site cannot be identified, it may be necessary to remove a majority of the colon; this procedure is associated with a higher rate of postoperative complications.

Diverticulitis that warrants hospitalization is initially treated with intravenous antibiotics for seven to ten days. Antibiotics help prevent 70 to 85 percent of patients from needing surgery. Most of those who respond to antibiotics will not have future attacks severe enough to warrant hospitalization.

Other measures may be necessary for the care of someone with diverticulitis, because the inflammation around the colon may be associated with problems such as narrowing of the bowel lumen to the point where it causes a partial or complete colonic obstruction. In this case, nothing should be given by mouth, and a tube should be passed through the nose into the stomach in order to suck out air and the stomach contents. This suction helps to reduce the amount of material that can pass through the colon and worsen the dilation of the colon that occurs proximal to the obstruction.

If the fever persists for more than a few days, the diverticulitis may be associated with complications. One complication is the formation of a large abscess outside the colon, which may be detected by a CT scan. An abscess has a rim around it that makes it difficult for antibiotics to penetrate the liquid center. If it does not go away despite antibiotic therapy, surgery may be necessary. If the abscess is small, it is possible to remove the involved segment of bowel and reattach the two free ends. If the abscess is very large, it may be necessary first to drain the abscess and then to cut across the colon proximal to the diseased segment, attaching the free end of the proximal segment to the abdominal wall, a procedure called a diverting colostomy. Later, the diseased segment of colon can be removed, and the remaining two free ends of colon can be joined. Another option is to drain the abscess with the aid of visual guidance by the CT scan and then operate on the colon. Draining the abscess in this manner helps get the infection under control before surgery is performed. Other indications for surgery in diverticulitis include complications such as a persistent bowel obstruction. In this case, it is often necessary to use a two-stage approach rather than to cure the problem in one operation.

Another complication of diverticulitis is a generalized infection of the peritoneal cavity, called peritonitis. Surgery for peritonitis involves removing the leaking segment of bowel and attaching the remaining two free ends of the colon to the abdominal wall. In addition, the peritoneal cavity is rinsed with a sterile solution in an attempt to clean out the contaminating materials.

Diverticulitis may also be complicated by the presence of a perforation of a diverticulum leading to a fistula, an abnormally existing channel connecting two hollow organs. When there is a fistula between the colon and the bladder, stool can travel into the bladder. The bacteria in the stool can cause severe, recurrent urinary tract infections. Another symptom is that bowel gas gets into the bladder; when the patient urinates, there is an intermittent stream because of colonic gas being passed along with the urine. When a fistula exists, it is necessary to remove the diseased segment of colon, the fistula tract, and a small portion of the bladder where the tract entered it.

Even if a patient with diverticulitis seems to improve and is able to return home from the hospital without needing surgery, there is still a chance that surgery will be necessary in the future. Surgery may be needed if the patient continues to have repeated, severe attacks of diverticulitis, or when a fistula between the colon and bladder causes recurring urinary tract infections. Another reason for surgery is persistent partial colonic obstruction and no possibility of inspecting the narrowed region of colon to exclude a constricting cancerous lesion as the cause of the obstruction.

PERSPECTIVE AND PROSPECTS

Diverticuli are quite common in the United States and other developed countries that tend to eat processed, low-fiber foods. In the United States, for example, diverticulosis is uncommon before the age of forty but is seen in 30 to 50 percent of elderly people at autopsy. Of those with diverticuli, only about one-fifth suffer any symptoms. Although members of ethnic groups who live in underdeveloped countries and eat a high-fiber diet tend to have a low prevalence of diverticulosis, their risk of developing this disease increases within ten years of moving to more developed countries.

Before 1900, the presence of colonic diverticuli in the United States was considered a curiosity, whereas now it is found in one-third to one-half of all autopsies of people over the age of sixty. There are a few possible explanations for why this increasing prevalence is seen.

First, the change in the American diet probably plays a large part in the pathogenesis of diverticular disease. Fiber consumption may have fallen off by as much as 30 percent during the twentieth century. Many people in the United States eat foods such as quick-cooking rice, highly processed cereals, and processed flour, all of which contain less fiber than their unprocessed counterparts. In addition, the population tends to eat more fats and proteins and less carbohydrates. Many fibers are from food sources rich in carbohydrates and are carbohydrates themselves.

The increasing prevalence of diverticular disease may also be attributable to the changing survival pattern. In 1900, the average life expectancy in the United States was forty-nine; in 1983, it was seventy-one years for men and seventy-eight years for women. The proportion of people over sixty-five has risen: It was 4.1 percent in 1900 and increased to 11.6 percent in 1986. Thus, the American population is not only growing but also getting older. Since diverticulosis is seen in increasing frequencies with aging, it is understandable that more of it was seen in the late twentieth century than during the early twentieth century.

Most poor people in the world live largely on plant foods rich in fiber, being largely dependent on cereal grains such as wheat, rice, and corn for both their calorie and their protein sources. Although one can look at the amount of fiber in the diet of rural societies and compare it to that in the United States, there may be other differences in lifestyles that contribute to the higher prevalence of diverticular disease in the United States. Living in rural societies, without traffic jams and the fast pace of developed countries, may cause people to have less stressful lives, and the lower stress is associated with fewer muscle spasms in the colon. Since it has been documented that stress can increase colonic contractions, and stress may worsen another disorder of the colon involving muscle spasm called irritable bowel syndrome (IBS), one might postulate that the stress of Western society contributes to the spasms in the sigmoid colon that may lead to diverticular disease.

Another reason for the increase in the prevalence of diverticular disease could be improvements in detection. Now it is detected not only at autopsy but also by barium enema, during sigmoidoscopy, and during surgery. Thus, there are more opportunities for discovering diverticulosis.

—Marc H. Walters, M.D.

See also Colon; Colon therapy; Colonoscopy and sigmoidoscopy; Colorectal cancer; Colorectal polyp removal; Colorectal surgery; Constipation; Digestion; Gastroenterology; Gastroenterology, pediatric; Gastrointestinal disorders; Gastrointestinal system; Intestinal disorders; Intestines; Irritable bowel syndrome (IBS); Nutrition; Peritonitis.

For Further Information:

Achkar, Edgar, Richard G. Farmer, and Bertram Fleshler, eds. *Clinical Gastroenterology.* 2d ed. Philadelphia: Lea & Febiger, 1992. This book is written by gastroenterologists from the Cleveland Clinic. Contains excellent chapters on abdominal pain, gastrointestinal bleeding, and diverticular disease. Less detailed but more readable than Marvin Sleisenger and John Fordtran's textbook.

Feldman, Mark, Lawrence S. Friedman, and Lawrence J. Brandt, eds. *Sleisenger and Fordtran's Gastrointestinal and Liver Disease: Pathophysiology, Diagnosis, Management.* New ed. 2 vols. Philadelphia: Saunders/Elsevier, 2010. This text is the best comprehensive textbook on gastrointestinal diseases and physiology. Contains excellent information on diverticular disease.

Ganong, William F. *Review of Medical Physiology.* 23d ed. New York: Lange Medical Books/McGraw-Hill Medical, 2009. This classic book has an excellent section emphasizing normal gastrointestinal physiology that provides a solid background for understanding diverticulosis.

Kapadia, Cyrus R., James M. Crawford, and Caroline Taylor. *An Atlas of Gastroenterology: A Guide to Diagnosis and Differential Diagnosis.* Boca Raton, Fla.: Pantheon, 2003. Provides a fully illustrated, nonspecialist understanding of myriad gastrointestinal diseases, including heartburn, dyspepsia, diarrhea, irritable bowel syndrome, and pancreatitis. Includes bibliographic references and an index.

Kumar, Vinay, et al., eds. *Robbins Basic Pathology.* 8th ed. Philadelphia: Saunders/Elsevier, 2007. An introductory pathology textbook. Less detailed than texts used by physicians, but still contains useful information on diverticular disease.

Peikin, Steven R. *Gastrointestinal Health.* Rev. ed. New York: Quill, 2001. Discusses a range of gastrointestinal disorders, including diverticulosis, IBS, and ulcers.

Tortora, Gerard J., and Bryan Derrickson. *Principles of Anatomy and Physiology.* 12th ed. Hoboken, N.J.: John Wiley & Sons, 2009. An outstanding textbook of human anatomy and physiology, and a good first text to consult before reading more advanced gastroenterology texts and journal articles.

Dizziness and fainting

Disease/disorder

Anatomy or system affected: Blood vessels, brain, circulatory system, head, nervous system, psychic-emotional system

Specialties and related fields: Cardiology, emergency medicine, family medicine, internal medicine, neurology

Definition: Dizziness is a feeling of light-headedness and unsteadiness, sometimes accompanied by a feeling of spinning or other spatial motion; fainting is a loss of consciousness as a result of insufficient amounts of blood reaching the brain. Both are symptoms of many conditions, which may be harmless or serious.

Key terms:

cardiac output: the amount of blood that the heart can pump per unit of time (usually per minute); if the brain does not receive enough of the cardiac output, the person becomes dizzy and may faint

dizziness: a sensation of whirling, with difficulty balancing·

fainting: a weak feeling followed by a loss of consciousness, usually due to a lack of blood flow to the brain; also called syncope

hypertension: a condition in which the patient's blood pressure is higher than that demanded by the body

hypotension: decrease in blood pressure to the point that insufficient blood flow causes symptoms

vasoconstriction: a reduction in the diameter of arteries, which increases the amount of work required for the heart to move blood

vasodilation: an increase in the diameter of arteries, which decreases the amount of work required for the heart to move blood

venous return: the amount of blood returning to the heart; one factor that determines the amount of blood the heart can pump out

vertigo: a sensation of moving in space or having objects move about when the patient is stationary, the most common symptom of which is dizziness; vertigo results from a disturbance in the organs of equilibrium

Causes and Symptoms

In humans, several mechanisms have evolved by which adequate blood flow to organs is maintained. Without a constant blood supply, the body's tissues would die from a lack of essential nutrients and oxygen. In particular, the brain and heart are very sensitive to changes

INFORMATION ON DIZZINESS AND FAINTING

CAUSES: Environmental factors, dehydration, postural hypotension, inner ear infection, brain stem disorders, brain tumors, blood flow deficiency disorders
SYMPTOMS: Light-headedness, unsteadiness, feeling of spinning or other spatial motion, nausea, vomiting
DURATION: Usually temporary
TREATMENTS: Deep breathing, rest, adequate blood flow to brain, drug therapy, rehydration

in their blood supply as they, more than any other organs, must receive oxygen and nutrients at all times. If they do not, their cells will die and cannot be replaced.

While the heart supplies most of the force needed to propel the blood throughout the body, tissues rely on changes in the size of arteries to redirect blood flow to where it is needed most. For example, after a large meal the blood vessels that lead to the gastrointestinal tract enlarge (vasodilate) so that more blood can be present to collect the nutrients from the meal. At the same time, the blood vessels that supply muscles decrease in diameter (vasoconstrict) and effectively shunt the blood toward the stomach and intestines. During exercise, the blood vessels that supply the muscles dilate and the ones leading to the intestinal tract vasoconstrict. This mechanism allows the cardiovascular system to supply the most blood to the most active tissues.

The brain is somewhat special in that the body tries to maintain a nearly constant blood flow to it. Located in the walls of the carotid arteries, which carry blood to the brain, are specialized sensory cells that have the ability to detect changes in blood pressure. These cells are known as baroreceptors. If the blood pressure going to the brain is too low, the baroreceptors send an impulse to the brain, which in turn speeds up the heart rate and causes a generalized vasoconstriction. This reflex response raises the body's blood pressure, reestablishing adequate blood flow to the brain. If the baroreceptors detect too high a blood pressure, they send a signal to the brain, which in turn slows the heart rate and causes the arteries of the body to dilate. These reflexes prevent large fluctuations in blood flow to the brain and other tissues.

Most people have experienced a dizzy feeling or maybe even a fainting response when they have stood up too quickly from a prone position. The ability of the baroreceptors to maintain relatively constant arterial pressure is extremely important when a person stands after having been lying down. Immediately upon standing, the pressure in the carotid arteries falls, and a reduction of this pressure can cause dizziness or even fainting. Fortunately, the falling pressure at the baroreceptors elicits an immediate reflex, resulting in a more rapid heart rate and vasoconstriction, minimizing the decrease in blood flow to the brain.

Blood pressure is not the only factor that is essential in maintaining tissue viability. The accumulation of waste products and a lack of essential nutrients and gases can also have a profound effect on how much blood flows through a particular tissue and how quickly. In a region of the carotid arteries near the baroreceptors are chemoreceptors. Chemoreceptors detect the concentration of the essential gas oxygen and the concentration of the gaseous waste product carbon dioxide. When carbon dioxide concentrations increase and oxygen concentrations decrease, the chemoreceptors stimulate regions in the brain to increase the heart rate and blood pressure in an attempt to supply the tissues with more oxygen and flush away the excess carbon dioxide. If the chemoreceptors detect high levels of oxygen and low levels of carbon dioxide, an impulse is transmitted to the brain, which in turn slows the heart rate and decreases the blood pressure.

Normally, most of the blood flow to the brain is controlled by the baroreceptor and chemoreceptor reflexes. However, the brain has a backup system. If blood flow decreases enough to cause a deficiency of nutrients and oxygen and an accumulation of waste products, special nerve cells respond directly to the lack of adequate energy sources and become strongly excited. When this occurs, the heart is stimulated and blood pressure rises.

Dizziness is a sensation of light-headedness often accompanied by a sensation of spinning (vertigo). Occasionally, a person experiencing dizziness will feel nauseated and may even vomit. Most attacks of dizziness are harmless, resulting from a brief reduction in blood flow to the brain. There are several causes of dizziness, and each alters blood flow to the brain for a slightly different reason.

A person rising rapidly from a sitting or lying position may become dizzy. This is known as postural hypotension, which is caused by a relatively slow reflexive response to the reduced blood pressure in the arteries providing blood to the brain. Rising requires increased blood pressure to supply the brain with adequate amounts of blood. Postural hypotension is more common in the elderly and in individuals prescribed antihypertensive medicines (drugs used to lower high blood pressure).

If the patient experiences vertigo with dizziness, the condition is usually caused by a disorder of the inner ear equilibrium system. Two disorders of the inner ear that can cause dizziness are labyrinthitis and Ménière's disease. Labyrinthitis, inflammation of the fluid-filled canals of the inner ear, is usually caused by a virus. Since these canals are involved in maintaining equilibrium, when they become infected and inflamed, one experiences the symptom of dizziness. Ménière's disease is a degenerative disorder of the ear in which the patient experiences not only dizziness but also progressive hearing loss.

Some brain-stem disorders also cause dizziness. The brain stem houses the vestibulocochlear nerve, which transmits messages from the ear to several other parts of the nervous system. Any disorder that alters the functions of this nerve will result in dizziness and vertigo. Meningitis (inflammation of the coverings of the brain and spinal cord), brain tumors, and blood-flow deficiency disorders such as atherosclerosis may affect the function of the vestibulocochlear nerve.

Syncope (fainting) is often preceded by dizziness. Syncope is the temporary loss of consciousness as a result of an inadequate blood flow to the brain. In addition to losing consciousness, the patient may be pale and sweaty. The most common cause of syncope is a vasovagal attack, in which an overstimulation of the vagus nerve slows the heart. Often vasovagal syncope results from severe pain, stress, or fear. For example, people may faint when hearing bad news or at the sight of blood. More commonly, individuals who have received a painful injury will faint. Rarely, vasovagal syncope may be caused by prolonged coughing, straining to defecate or urinate, pregnancy, or forcing expiration. Standing still for long periods of time or standing up rapidly after lying or sitting can cause fainting. With the exception of vasovagal syncope, all the causes of syncope are attributable to inadequate blood returning to the heart. If blood pools in the lower extremities, there is a reduced amount available for the heart to pump to the brain. In vasovagal syncope and some disorders of heart rhythm such as Adams-Stokes syndrome, it is the heart itself that does not force enough blood toward the brain.

TREATMENT AND THERAPY

Short periods of dizziness usually subside after a few minutes. Deep breathing and rest will usually help relieve the symptom. Prolonged episodes of dizziness and vertigo should be brought to the attention of a physician.

Recovery from fainting likewise will occur when adequate blood flow to the brain is reestablished. This happens within minutes because falling to the ground places the head at the same level as the heart and helps return the blood from the legs. If a person does not regain consciousness within a few minutes, a physician or emergency medical team should be notified.

The most common cause of syncope is decreased cerebral blood flow resulting from limitation of cardiac output. When the heart rate falls below its normal seventy-five beats per minute to approximately thirty-five beats per minute, the patient usually becomes dizzy and faints. Although slow heart rates can occur in any age group, they are most often found in elderly people who have other heart conditions. Drug-induced syncope can also occur. Drugs for congestive heart failure (digoxin) or antihypertensive medications that slow the heart rate (propranolol, metoprolol) may reduce blood flow to the brain sufficiently to cause dizziness and fainting.

Exertional syncope occurs when individuals perform some physical activity to which they are not accustomed. These physical efforts demand more work from the cardiovascular system, and in patients with some obstruction of the arteries which leave the heart, the cardiovascular system is overstressed. This defect, combined with the vasodilation in the blood vessels that provide blood to the working muscles, reduces the amount of blood available for use by the brain. If the person also hyperventilates during exercise, he or she will effectively reduce the amount of carbon dioxide in the blood and rid the cardiovascular system of this normal stimulus for increasing heart rate and blood flow to the brain. Some persons also hold their breath during periods of high exertion. For example, people attempting to lift something very heavy often take a deep breath just prior to exerting and then hold their breath when they lift the object. This practice, known as the Valsalva maneuver, increases the pressure within the chest cavity, which in turn reduces the amount of blood returning to the heart. A decrease in blood returning to the heart (venous return) causes a decrease in the availability of blood to be pumped out of the heart and reduces cardiac output. The reduction in cardiac output decreases the amount of blood flowing to the brain and initiates a fainting response. It is interesting to note that humans also use the Valsalva maneuver when defecating or urinating, particularly when they strain. These acts can also lead to exertional syncope.

For a physician to diagnose and treat dizziness and fainting accurately, he or she must take an accurate medical history, paying particular attention to cardiovascular and neurological problems. In addition to experiencing episodes of dizziness and fainting, patients often have a weak pulse, low blood pressure (hypotension), sweating, and shallow breathing. Heart rate and blood pressure are monitored while the patient assumes different positions. The clinician also listens to the heart and carotid arteries to determine whether there are any problems with these tissues, such as a heart valve problem or atherosclerosis of the carotid arteries. An electrocardiogram (ECG or EKG) can detect abnormal heart rates and rhythms that may reduce cardiac output. Laboratory tests are used to determine whether the patient has low blood sugar (hypoglycemia), too little blood volume (hypovolemia), too few red blood cells (anemia), or abnormal blood gases suggesting a lung disorder. Finally, if the physician suspects a neurological problem such as a seizure disorder, he or she may run an electroencephalogram (EEG) to record brain activity.

Treatment for any of these underlying disorders may cure the dizziness and fainting episodes. In patients with postural hypotension, merely being aware of the condition will allow them to change their behavior to lessen the chances of becoming dizzy and fainting. These patients should not make any sudden changes in posture that could precipitate an attack. Often, this means simply slowing down their movements and learning to assume a horizontal position if they feel dizzy. Patients also can learn to contract their leg muscles and not hold their breath when rising. This increases the amount of blood available for the heart to pump toward the brain. If these techniques do not provide an adequate solution for postural hypotension, then a physician can prescribe drugs, such as ephedrine, which increase blood pressure.

Heart rhythm disturbances that cause an abnormally fast or slow heart rate can be corrected with drug therapy such as quinidine or disopyramide (if the rate is too rapid) or a pacemaker (if the rate is too slow). It is interesting to note that even too fast a heart rate can cause dizziness and fainting. In patients with this type of arrhythmia, the heart beats at such a rapid rate that it cannot efficiently fill with blood before the next contraction. Therefore, less blood is pumped with each beat.

Other treatments for dizziness and fainting may include correcting the levels of certain blood elements. Patients with hypoglycemia often feel dizzy. The brain and spinal cord require glucose as their energy source. In fact, the brain and spinal cord have a very limited ability to utilize other substrates such as fat or protein for energy. Because of this, patients often feel lightheaded when there are inadequate levels of glucose in the blood. Patients can correct this condition by eating more frequent meals, and if necessary, physicians can administer drugs such as epinephrine or glucagon. These agents liberate glucose from storage sites in the liver.

Individuals with a low blood volume are often dehydrated and upon becoming rehydrated no longer have dizziness or fainting episodes. If dehydration is not corrected and becomes worse, the patient can go into shock, a state of inadequate blood flow to tissues that will result in death if left untreated. In addition to being dizzy or fainting, the patient is often cold to the touch and has a rapid heart rate, low blood pressure, bluish skin, and rapid breathing. These patients are treated by emergency medical personnel, who keep the individual warm, elevate the legs, and infuse fluid into a vein. Drugs may be used to help bring blood pressure back to normal. The cause of the shock should be identified and corrected.

Perspective and Prospects

As humans evolved, they assumed an upright posture. This was advantageous because it allows for the use of the front limbs for other things besides locomotion. Unlike most four-legged animals, however, humans have their brains above their hearts and must continually force blood uphill to reach this vital tissue. This adaptation to the upright posture is a continuing physiological problem because the cardiovascular system must counteract the forces of gravity to provide the brain with blood. If this does not occur, the individual becomes dizzy and faints.

Another significant problem that humans face is adaptation to brain blood flow during exercise. The amount of blood flowing to a tissue is usually proportional to the metabolic demand of the tissue. At rest, various organs throughout the body receive a certain amount of the cardiac output. For example, blood flow to abdominal organs such as the spleen and the kidneys requires about 43 percent of the total blood volume.

The total flow to the brain is estimated to be only 13 percent, and the skin and skeletal muscles require 21 percent and 9 percent, respectively. Other areas such as the gastrointestinal tract and heart receive the remaining 14 percent. During exercise, the skeletal muscles may receive up to 80 percent of the cardiac output while the rest of the organs are perfused at a much reduced rate.

Most data indicate that the brain receives only 3 percent of the total cardiac output during heavy exercise. Even though there is a large change in the redistribution of cardiac output, physiologists do not know the absolute amount of blood reaching the brain or the mechanism for the change in the perfusion rate.

With strenuous aerobic exercise such as jogging, there is an increase in cardiac output. During strenuous anaerobic exercise such as weight lifting, however, there may be a decrease in cardiac output, attributable to the Valsalva maneuver. Therefore, it has been difficult to predict accurately, using available techniques, the volume of blood reaching this critical tissue.

—Matthew Berria, Ph.D.

See also Anxiety; Balance disorders; Blood vessels; Brain; Brain disorders; Circulation; Ear infections and disorders; Ears; Exercise physiology; Headaches; Huntington's disease; Hypotension; Ménière's disease; Meningitis; Migraine headaches; Multiple chemical sensitivity syndrome; Narcolepsy; Nausea and vomiting; Nervous system; Neuralgia, neuritis, and neuropathy; Neurology; Neurology, pediatric; Palpitations; Unconsciousness.

FOR FURTHER INFORMATION:

Babikian, Viken K., and Lawrence R. Wechsler, eds. *Transcranial Doppler Ultrasonography.* 2d ed. Boston: Butterworth-Heinemann, 1999. Describes a noninvasive way to measure blood flow to the brain using ultrasound techniques. The authors provide information on how drugs such as anesthetics alter this blood flow.

Brandt, Thomas. *Vertigo: Its Multisensory Syndromes.* 2d ed. New York: Springer, 2003. Uses an interdisciplinary approach in its discussion of clinical symptoms; central vestibular, nerve, and labyrinthine disorders; hereditary factors; and epilepsy, among other topics.

Furman, Joseph M., and Stephen P. Cass. *Vestibular Disorders: A Case-Study Approach.* New York: Oxford University Press, 2003. A text that examines case studies to elucidate the causes of vestibular disorders. History, physical examination, laboratory testing, differential diagnosis, and treatment are discussed.

Geelen, G., and J. E. Greenleaf. "Orthostasis: Exercise and Exercise Training." *Exercise and Sport Sciences Reviews* 21 (1993): 201-230. Provides an excellent, complete discussion of the relationship between exercise and dizziness and fainting. These authors describe the current theories on blood flow regulation to the brain in athletes.

Guyton, Arthur C. *Human Physiology and Mechanisms of Disease.* 6th ed. Philadelphia: W. B. Saunders, 1997. This textbook introduces human physiology and basic pathology for individuals without an extensive background in medicine. Guyton offers several chapters on blood pressure regulation in humans and gives brief explanations as to what happens when blood pressure is not adequately regulated.

Leikin, Jerrold B., and Martin S. Lipsky, eds. *American Medical Association Complete Medical Encyclopedia.* New York: Random House Reference, 2003. This encyclopedia lists in alphabetical order medical terms, diseases, and medical procedures. It does an excellent job of explaining rather complex medical subjects for the nonprofessional audience. In the sections on dizziness and fainting, flow charts detail the appropriate first aid treatments.

DNA AND RNA

BIOLOGY

ANATOMY OR SYSTEM AFFECTED: Cells

SPECIALTIES AND RELATED FIELDS: Genetics

DEFINITION: Molecules that store coded genetic information and express this information as functional proteins; deoxyribonucleic acid (DNA) is a long, thin, double-stranded fibrous molecule which holds coded information that determines the type, amount, and timing of protein production, while ribonucleic acid (RNA) is a long, single-stranded molecule that amplifies, transports, and expresses this coded information.

KEY TERMS:

genetic disease: a disease state that exists because of a decrease in or the absence of normal protein activity as the result of an alteration in the information carried in the DNA

mutation: an alteration in the information stored in DNA that may lead to an alteration in the structure of proteins produced from this information *replication:* the process by which the DNA of a cell is duplicated so that the information stored there can be passed on to new cells after cell division

transcription: the process by which the information stored in DNA is copied into the structure of RNA for transport to the cytoplasm

translation: the process by which the copied information in RNA is utilized in the production of a protein

STRUCTURE AND FUNCTIONS

Each human being is a biologically unique individual. That uniqueness has its basis in one's cellular makeup. Appearance derives from the arrangement of cells during fetal development, size depends on the cells' ability to grow and divide, and the function of organs depends on the biochemical function of the individual cells that constitute each organ. The functions of cells depend on the types and amounts of the different proteins that they synthesize. The substance that holds the information that determines the structure of proteins, when they should be produced, and in what amounts is deoxyribonucleic acid (DNA).

DNA is the molecule of heredity, and as a child receives half of his or her DNA from each biological parent, each individual is the product of a mixture of information. Therefore, while children resemble their parents, they are unique. Each cell in an individual's body (except for the sex cells) has a complete set of genetic information contained in the chromosomes of the cell's nucleus. Human cells have forty-six chromosomes (twenty-three pairs). Each chromosome is a single piece of DNA associated with many types of proteins. The major function of DNA is to store, in a stable manner, the information that is the "blueprint" for all physiological aspects of an individual. Stability is one of the key attributes of DNA. An information storage molecule is of little use if it can be altered or damaged easily. Another key characteristic of DNA is its ability to be replicated. When a cell divides, the information in the DNA must be replicated so that each of the two new cells can have a complete set.

Stability, the ability to be replicated, and the ability to store vast amounts of coded information have their basis in the structure of DNA. DNA is a long, incredibly thin fiber. The chromosomes in some cells would be as long as a foot or more if they were fully extended. The shape of the DNA molecule can be imagined as a long ladder whose rails are chains of two alternating molecules: deoxyribose (a sugar) and phosphate (an acid containing phosphorus and oxygen). The steps of

the ladder are made of pairs of organic bases, of which there are four types: adenine (A), guanine (G), thymine (T), and cytosine (C). Adenine always pairs up with thymine to form a step in the ladder (A-T), and guanine always pairs with cytosine (C-G). This complementarity of base-pairing is the basis for DNA replication and for transferring information from DNA out of the nucleus and into the cytoplasm. Finally, the whole DNA molecule is twisted into a stable right-handed spiral, or helix. Because there is no restriction on the sequence in which the base pairs appear along the molecule, the bases have the potential to be used as a four-letter alphabet that can encode information into "words" of varying lengths, called genes. Each information sequence, or gene, holds the information needed to synthesize a linear chain of amino acids, which are the building blocks of proteins. The information encoded in the base sequences of DNA determines the quantities and composition of all proteins made in the cell.

Under certain conditions, DNA can be separated lengthwise into two halves, or denatured, by breaking the base pairs so that one of each pair remains attached to one sugar-phosphate chain and the other base remains attached to the other sugar-phosphate chain. Because this forms two strands of DNA, whole DNA is usually referred to as being double-stranded. Such separation rarely happens by accident because of the extreme length of DNA. If any area becomes denatured, the rest of the base pairs hold the molecule together. In addition, an area of denaturation will automatically try to renature, since complementary bases have a natural attraction for each other. As stable as these traits make it, DNA must be capable of being duplicated so that each newly divided cell has a complete copy of the stored information. DNA is replicated by breaking the base pairs, separating the DNA into two halves, and building a new half onto each of the old halves. This is possible because the complementarity rule (A pairs with T, and C pairs with G) allows each half of a denatured DNA molecule to hold the information needed to construct a new second half. This is accomplished by special sets of proteins that separate the old DNA as they move along the molecule and build new DNA in their wake.

All the information needed to produce proteins is located in the DNA within the nucleus of the cell, but all protein synthesis occurs outside the nucleus in the cytoplasm. An information transfer molecule is required to copy or transcribe information from the genes of the DNA and carry it to the cytoplasm, where large globular protein complexes called ribosomes take the information and translate it into the amino acid structure of specific proteins. This information transfer molecule is ribonucleic acid (RNA). Many RNA copies can be made for any single piece of information on the DNA and used as a template to synthesize many proteins. In this way, the information in DNA is also amplified by RNA. RNA also participates in the synthesis of proteins from the genetic information. RNA resembles one half of a DNA molecule and is usually referred to as being single stranded. It consists of a single chain of alternating sugars and phosphates with a single organic base attached to each sugar. The sugar in this case is ribose, similar to deoxyribose, and the bases are identical to those in DNA with the exception of

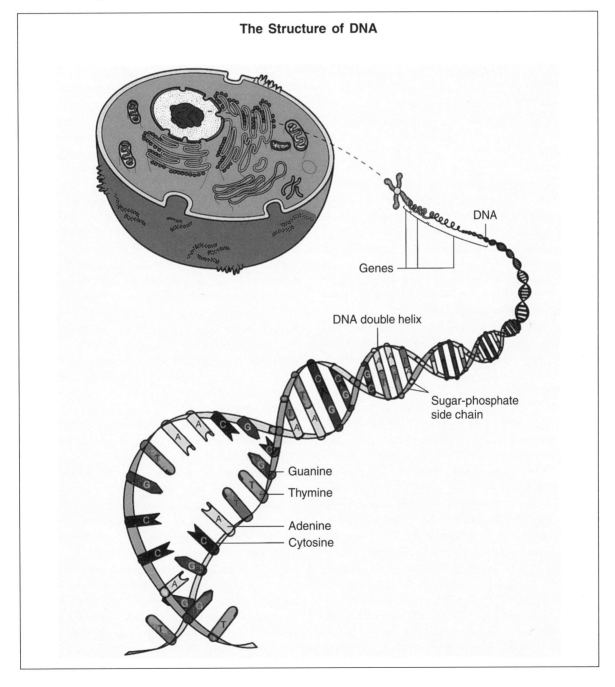

The Structure of DNA

DNA

Genes

DNA double helix

Sugar-phosphate side chain

Guanine
Thymine

Adenine
Cytosine

thymine, which is replaced by a very similar base called uracil (U).

There are four major types of RNA. Messenger RNA (mRNA) is responsible for the transfer of information from the DNA sequences in the nucleus to the ribosomes in the cytoplasm. Ribosomal RNA (rRNA) interacts with dozens of proteins to form the ribosome. It aids in the interaction between mRNA and the ribosome. Transfer RNA (tRNA) is a group of small RNAs that helps translate the information coded in the mRNA into the structure of specific proteins. They carry the amino acids to the ribosome and match the correct amino acid to its corresponding sequence of bases in the mRNA.

The first step in producing a specific protein is the accurate copying or transcription of information in a gene into information on a piece of mRNA. There are specific sets of proteins that separate the double-stranded DNA in the immediate vicinity of a gene into two single-stranded portions and then, using the DNA as a template, build a piece of mRNA that is a complementary copy of the information in the gene. This is possible because RNA also uses organic bases in its structure. The A, C, G, and T of the single-stranded portion of DNA form base pairs with the U, G, C, and A of the mRNA, respectively. The complementary copy of mRNA, when complete, falls away from the DNA and moves to the cytoplasm of the cell.

In the cytoplasm, the mRNA binds to a ribosome. As the ribosome moves down the length of the mRNA, the tRNAs interact with both the ribosome and the mRNA in order to match the proper amino acid (carried by the tRNAs) to the proper sequence of bases in the mRNA. The order of amino acids in the protein is thus determined by the order of bases in the DNA. Achieving the correct order of amino acids is critical for the correct functioning of the protein. The order of amino acids in the chain determines the way in which it interacts with itself and folds into a three-dimensional structure. The function of all proteins depends on their assuming the correct shape for interaction with other molecules. Therefore, the sequence of bases in the DNA ultimately determines the shape and function of proteins.

Another class of RNA is involved in translation regulation, by a process called RNA interference, or RNAi. The two types of RNA in this class are short interfering RNA (siRNA) and micro RNA (miRNA). SiRNA is a double-stranded molecule of twenty to twenty-five base-pairs in length, whereas miRNA is single stranded and consists of nineteen to twenty-three nucleotides.

SiRNA and miRNA become incorporated in a protein complex known as the RNA-induced silencing complex (RISC). The RISC-associated siRNA targets a specific sequence in its target mRNA, and when bound to the mRNA causes destruction. MiRNA bound RISC binds to the mRNA and inhibits translation of that mRNA; in this case, however, the mRNA is not destroyed. RNAi plays a role in diverse cellular functions such as cell differentiation, fetal development, cell proliferation, and cell death. It is also involved in pathogenic events such as viral infection and certain cancers.

DISORDERS AND DISEASES

When the normal structure of DNA is altered (a process called a mutation), the number of proteins produced and/or the functions of proteins may be affected. At one extreme, a mutation may cause no problem at all to the person involved. At the other extreme, it may cause devastating damage to the person and result in genetic disease or cancer.

Mutations are changes in the normal sequence of bases in the DNA that carry the information to build a protein or that regulate the amount of protein to be produced. There are different types of mutations, such as the alteration of one base into another, the deletion of one or many bases, or the insertion of bases that were not in the sequence previously. Mutations can have many different causes, such as ultraviolet rays, X rays, mutagenic chemicals, invading viruses, or even heat. Sometimes mutations are caused by mistakes made during the process of DNA replication or cell division. Cells have several systems that constantly repair mutations, but occasionally some of these alterations slip by and become permanent.

Mutations may affect protein structure in several ways. The protein may be too short or too long, with amino acids missing or new ones added. It might have new amino acids substituting for the correct ones. Sometimes as small a change as one amino acid can have noticeable effects. In any of these cases, changes in the amino acid sequence of a protein may drastically affect the way the protein interacts with itself and folds itself into a three-dimensional structure. If a protein does not assume the correct three-dimensional structure, its function may be impaired. It is important to note that how severely a protein's function is affected by a mutation depends on which amino acids are involved. Some amino acids are more important than others in maintaining a protein's shape and function. A change in amino acid sequence may have virtually no effect on a protein or it may destroy that protein's ability to function.

If a mutation occurs that affects the regulation of a particular protein, that gene may be perfectly normal and the protein may be fully functional, but it may exist in the cell in an improper amount—too much, too little, or even none at all. It is important to note that the overproduction of a protein, as well as its underproduction or absence, can be harmful to the cell or to the person in general. The genetic disease known as Down syndrome, for example, is the result of the overproduction of many proteins at the same time.

The term "genetic disease" is used for a heritable disease that can be passed from parent to child. The mutation responsible for the disease is contributed by the parents to the affected child via the sperm or the egg or (as is usually the case) both. The parents are, for the most part, quite unaffected. Because all creatures more complex than bacteria have at least two copies of all their genes, a person may carry a mutated gene and be perfectly healthy because the other normal gene compensates by producing adequate amounts of normal protein. If two individuals carrying the same mutated gene produce a child, that child has a chance of obtaining two mutant genes—one from each parent. Every

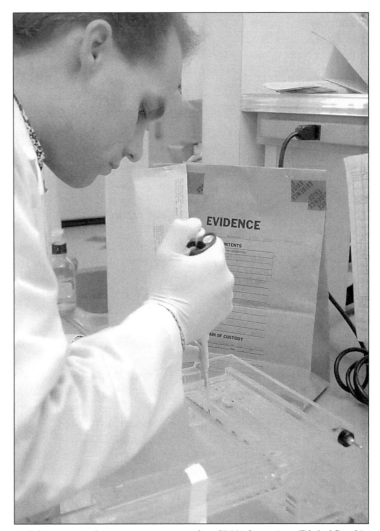

A laboratory technician prepares samples of DNA for testing. (Digital Stock)

cell in that child's body carries the error with no normal genes to compensate, and every cell that would normally use that gene must produce an abnormal protein or abnormal amounts of that protein. The medical consequences vary, depending on which gene is affected and which protein is altered. The following are two specific examples of genetic diseases in which the connection between specific mutations and the disease states are well documented.

Sickle cell disease is a genetic disease that results from an error in the gene that carries the information for the protein beta globin. Beta globin is one of the building blocks of hemoglobin, the molecule that binds to and carries oxygen in the red blood cells. The error or mutation is a surprisingly small one and serves to illustrate the fact that the replacement of even a single

amino acid can change the chemical nature and function of a protein. Normal beta globin has a glutamic acid as the sixth amino acid in the protein chain. The mutation of a single base in the DNA changes the coded information such that the amino acid valine replaces glutamic acid as the sixth position in the protein chain. This single alteration causes the hemoglobin in the red blood cell to crystallize under conditions of low oxygen concentration. As the crystals grow, they twist and deform the normally flexible and disk-shaped red blood cells into rigid sickle shapes. These affected cells lose their capacity to bind and hold oxygen, thereby causing anemia, and their new structure can cause blockages in small capillaries of the circulatory system, causing pain and widespread organ damage. There is no safe and effective treatment or cure for this condition.

Phenylketonuria (PKU) is caused by a mutation in the gene that controls the synthesis of the protein phenylalanine hydroxylase (PAH). There are several mutations of the *PAH* gene that can lead to a drastic decrease in PAH activity (by greater than 1 percent of normal activity). Some are changes in one base that lead to the replacement of a single amino acid for another. For example, one of the most common mutations in the *PAH* gene is the alteration of a C to a T that results in amino acid number 408 changing from an arginine to a tryptophan. Some mutations are deletions of whole sequences of bases in the gene. One such deletion removes the tail end of the gene. In any case, the amino acid structure of *PAH* is altered significantly enough to remove its ability to function. Without this protein, the amino acid phenylalanine cannot be converted into tyrosine, another useful amino acid. The problem is not a shortage of tyrosine, since there is plenty in most foods, but rather an accumulation of undesirable products that form as the unused phenylalanine begins to break down. Since developing brain cells are particularly sensitive to these products, the condition can cause mental retardation unless treated immediately after birth. While there is no cure, the disease is easily diagnosed and treatment is simple. The patient must stay on a diet in which phenylalanine is restricted. Food products that contain the artificial sweetener aspartame (NutraSweet) must have warnings to PKU patients printed on them since phenylalanine is a major component of aspartame.

PERSPECTIVE AND PROSPECTS

Genetics is a young science whose starting point is traditionally considered to be 1866, the year in which Gregor Mendel published his work on hereditary patterns in pea plants. While he knew nothing of DNA or its structure, Mendel showed mathematically that discrete units of inheritance, which are now called genes, existed as pairs in an organism and that different combinations of these units determined that organism's characteristics. Unfortunately, Mendel's work was ahead of its time and thus ignored until rediscovered by several researchers simultaneously in 1900.

DNA itself was discovered in 1869 by Friedrich Miescher, who extracted it from cell nuclei but did not realize its importance as the carrier of hereditary information. Chromosomes were first seen in the 1870's as threadlike structures in the nucleus, and because of the precise way they are replicated and equally parceled out to newly divided cells, August Weismann and The-

odor Boveri, in the 1880's, postulated that chromosomes were the carriers of inheritance.

In 1900, Hugo de Vries, Karl Correns, and Erich Tschermak von Seysenegg—all plant biologists who were working on patterns of inheritance—independently rediscovered Mendel's work. De Vries had in the meantime discovered mutation around 1890 as a source of hereditary variation, but he did not postulate a mechanism. Mendel's theories and the then-current knowledge of chromosomes merged perfectly. Mendel's units of inheritance were thought somehow to be carried on the chromosomes. Pairs of chromosomes would carry Mendel's pairs of hereditary units, which, in 1909, were dubbed "genes."

At that point, genes were still a theoretical concept and had not been proved to be carried on the chromosomes. In 1909, Thomas Hunt Morgan began the work that would provide that proof and allow the mapping of specific genes to specific areas of a chromosome. The nature of a gene, or how it expressed itself, was still a mystery. In 1941, George Beadle and Edward Tatum proved that genes regulated the production of proteins, but the nature of genes was still in debate. There were two candidates for the chemical substance of genes; one was protein and the other was the deceptively simple DNA. In 1944, Oswald Avery proved in experiments with pure DNA that DNA was indeed the molecule of inheritance. In 1953, James D. Watson and Francis Crick, using the work of Rosalind Franklin, elucidated the chemical structure of the double helix, and soon after, Matthew Meselson and Franklin Stahl proved that DNA replicated itself. By the end of the 1950's, RNA was being implicated in protein synthesis, and much of the mechanism of translation was postulated by Marshall Nirenberg and Johann Matthaei in 1961.

Craig Mello and Andrew Fire were awarded the 2006 Nobel Prize in Physiology or Medicine for their discovery of siRNA and for their research on the RNAi system. In 1993, Victor Ambros was the first person to describe miRNA. Both siRNA and micro RNA have possible therapeutic use. Clinical trials involving siRNA and miRNA are in progress. Examples are the use of siRNA in the treatment of macular degeneration, an age-related eye disorder, and the use of miRNA in the treatment of chronic hepatitis C. The major barriers to the use of these molecules are inefficient delivery to target cells and off-target effects.

The concept of heritable genetic disease is also a relatively recent one. The first direct evidence that a mutation can result in the production of an altered protein came in 1949 with studies on sickle cell disease. Since then, thousands of genetic diseases have been characterized. The advent in the 1970's of recombinant DNA technology, which allows the direct manipulation of DNA, has greatly increased the knowledge of these diseases, as well as demonstrated the genetic influences in maladies such as cancer and behavioral disorders. This technology has led to vastly improved diagnostic methods and therapies while pointing the way toward potential cures.

—*Robert D. Meyer, Ph.D.*

See also Bioinformatics; Cells; Gene therapy; Genetic counseling; Genetic diseases; Genetic engineering; Genetics and inheritance; Genomics; Karyotyping; Mutation; Proteomics.

FOR FURTHER INFORMATION:

Campbell, Neil A., et al. *Biology: Concepts and Connections*. 6th ed. San Francisco: Pearson/Benjamin Cummings, 2008. This classic introductory textbook provides an excellent discussion of essential biological structures and mechanisms. Its extensive and detailed illustrations help to make even difficult concepts accessible to the nonspecialist. Of particular interest are the chapters constituting the unit titled "The Gene."

Drlica, Karl. *Understanding DNA and Gene Cloning: A Guide for the Curious*. 4th ed. Hoboken, N.J.: Wiley, 2004. This book for the uninitiated explains the basic principles of genetic mechanisms without requiring knowledge of chemistry. The first third is especially good on the fundamentals, but the remainder may be too deep for some readers.

Frank-Kamenetskii, Maxim D. *Unraveling DNA: The Most Important Molecule of Life*. Translated by Lev Liapin. Rev. ed. Reading, Mass.: Addison-Wesley, 1997. This very readable book provides an excellent history of the discovery of DNA. Also describes the nature of DNA and discusses genetic engineering and the ethical questions that surround its use.

Glick, Bernard, Jack J. Pasternak, and Cheryl L. Patten. *Molecular Biotechnology: Principles and Applications of Recombinant DNA*. 4th ed. Washington, D.C.: ASM Press, 2010. Explores the scientific principles of recombinant DNA technology and its wide-ranging use in industry, agriculture, and the pharmaceutical and biomedical sectors.

Gonick, Larry, and Mark Wheelis. *The Cartoon Guide to Genetics*. Rev. ed. New York: Collins Reference, 2007. An effective mixture of humor and fact makes this book a nonthreatening reference on genetics. Presented using historical context, it covers DNA and RNA structure and function and much more.

Gribbin, John. *In Search of the Double Helix*. New York: Bantam Books, 1985. Gribbin is a renowned science writer who is capable of explaining complex subjects in a way that anyone can understand. In this book, he goes from Charles Darwin's theories to quantum mechanics in his rendition of the history of the discovery of DNA. Very readable.

Hofstadter, Douglas R. "The Genetic Code: Arbitrary?" In *Metamagical Themas: Questing for the Essence of Mind and Pattern*. New York: Basic Books, 1985. While only a thirty-page chapter in a large book, this piece by Hofstadter is an excellent and thought-provoking explanation of transcription and translation written for the nonscientist.

Micklos, David A., Greg A. Freyer, and David A. Crotty. *DNA Science: A First Course*. 2d ed. Cold Springs Harbor, N.Y.: Cold Springs Harbor Press, 2003. Text that combines an introductory discussion of the principles of genetics, DNA structure and function, and methods for analyzing DNA with twelve laboratory experiments that illustrate the basic techniques of DNA restriction, transformation, isolation, and analysis.

Nicholl, Desmond S. T. *Introduction to Genetic Engineering*. 3d ed. New York: Cambridge University Press, 2008. A valuable textbook for the nonspecialist and anyone interested in genetic engineering. It provides an excellent foundation in molecular biology and builds on that foundation to show how organisms can be genetically engineered.

Paddison, Patrick J., and Peter J. Voght. *RNA Interference*. New York: Springer, 2008. A comprehensive book about the field of RNA interference that includes detailed and updated mechanistic descriptions of the RNAi process.

Watson, James D., and Andrew Berry. *DNA: The Secret of Life*. New York: Knopf, 2004. Nobel Prize-winning scientist Watson guides readers through the rapid advances in genetic technology and what these advances mean for modern life. Covers all aspects of the genome in a readable fashion.

DOMESTIC VIOLENCE
DISEASE/DISORDER

ANATOMY OR SYSTEM AFFECTED: Psychic-emotional system, all bodily systems

SPECIALTIES AND RELATED FIELDS: Emergency medicine, family medicine, geriatrics and gerontology, internal medicine, pediatrics, psychiatry, psychology, public health

DEFINITION: Assaultive behavior intended to punish, dominate, or control another person in an intimate family relationship; health care providers are often best able to identify situations of domestic violence and to assist victims to implement preventive interventions.

KEY TERMS:

cycle of violence: a repeating pattern of violence characterized by increasing tension, culminating in violent action, and followed by remorse

family violence: violence against a family member, typically to assert domination, control actions, or punish, which occurs as a pattern of behavior, not as a single, isolated act; also called battering, marital violence, domestic violence, relationship violence, spousal abuse, child abuse, or elder abuse

funneling: an interviewing technique for assessing violence in a patient's relationship, beginning with broad questions of relationship conflict and gradually narrowing to focus on specific violent actions

hands-off violence: indirect attacks meant to terrorize or control a victim; may include property or pet destruction, threats, intimidating behavior, verbal abuse, stalking, and monitoring

hands-on violence: direct attacks upon the victim's body, including physical and sexual violence; comprises a continuum of acts ranging from seemingly minor to obviously severe

lethality: the potential, given the particular dynamics of violence in a relationship, for one or both partners to be killed

safety planning: the development of a specific set of actions and strategies to enable a victim either to avoid violence altogether or, once violence has begun, to escape and minimize damage and injury

CAUSES AND SYMPTOMS

Domestic or family violence is the intentional use of violence against a family member. The purpose of the violence is to assert domination, to control the victim's actions, or to punish the victim for some actions. Family violence generally occurs as a pattern of behavior over time rather than as a single, isolated act.

Forms of family violence include child physical abuse, child sexual abuse, spousal or partner abuse, and elder abuse. These forms of violence are related, in that they occur within the context of the family unit. Therefore, the victims and perpetrators know one another, are related to one another, may live together, and may love one another. These various forms of violence also differ insofar as victims may be children, adults, or frail, elderly adults. The needs of victims differ with age and independence, but there are also many similarities between the different types of violence. One such similarity is the relationship between the offender and the victim. Specifically, victims of abuse are always less powerful than abusers. Power includes the ability to exert physical and psychological control over situations. For example, a child abuser has the ability to lock a child in a bathroom or to abandon him or her in a remote area in order to control access to authorities. A spouse abuser has the ability to physically injure a spouse, disconnect the phone, and keep the victim from leaving for help. An elder abuser can exert similar control. Such differences in power between victims and offenders are seen as a primary cause of abuse; that is, people batter others because they can.

Families that are violent are often socially isolated, meaning they are not well connected to others outside the family or home. The members usually keep to themselves and have few or no friends or relatives with whom they are involved, even if they live in a city. This social isolation prevents victims from seeking help from others and allows the abuser to establish rules for the relationship without answering to anyone for these actions. Abuse continues and worsens because the violence occurs in private, with few consequences for the abuser.

Victims of all forms of family violence share common experiences. In addition to physical violence, victims are also attacked psychologically, being told they are worthless and responsible for the abuse that they receive. Because they are socially isolated, victims do not have an opportunity to take social roles where they can experience success, recognition, or love. As a result, victims often have low self-esteem and truly believe that they cause the violence. Without the experience of being worthwhile, victims often become severely depressed and anxious, and they experience more stress-related illnesses such as headaches, fatigue, or gastrointestinal problems.

Child and partner abuse are linked in several ways. About half of the men who batter their wives also batter their children. Furthermore, women who are battered are more likely to abuse their children than are nonbattered women. Even if a child of a spouse-abusing father is not battered, living in a violent home and observing the father's violence has negative effects. Such children often experience low self-esteem, aggression toward other children, and school problems. Moreover, abused children are more likely to commit violent offenses as adults. Children, especially males, who have observed violence between parents are at increased risk of assaulting their partners as adults. Adult sexual offenders have an increased likelihood of having been sexually abused as children. Yet, while these and other problems are reported more frequently by adults who were abused as children than by adults who were not, many former victims do not become violent. The most common outcomes of childhood abuse in adults are emotional problems. Although much less is known about the relationship between child abuse and future elder abuse, many elder abusers did suffer abuse as children. While most people who have been abused do not themselves become abusers, this intergenerational effect remains a cause for concern.

In its various forms, family violence is a public health epidemic in the United States. Once thought to be rare, family violence occurs with high frequency in the general population. Although exact figures are lacking and domestic violence tends to be under-reported, it is estimated that each year 1.9 million children are physically abused, 250,000 children are sexually molested, 1.6 million women are assaulted by their male partners, and between 500,000 and 2.5 million elders are abused. Rates of violence directed toward unmarried heterosexual women, married heterosexual women, and members of homosexual male and female couples tend to be similar. No one is immune: Victims come from all social classes, races, and religions. Partner violence directed toward heterosexual men, however, is rare and usually occurs in relationships in which the male hits first.

Because family violence is so pervasive, physicians encounter many victims. One out of every three to five women visiting emergency rooms is seeking medical care for injuries related to partner violence. In primary care clinics, including family medicine, internal medicine, and obstetrics and gynecology, one out of every four female patients reports violence in the past year, and two out of five report violence at some time in their lives. It is therefore reasonable to expect all physicians

and other health care professionals working in primary care and emergency rooms to provide services for victims of family violence.

Family violence typically consists of a pattern of behavior occurring over time and involving both hands-on and hands-off violence. Hands-on violence consists of direct attacks against the victim's body. Such acts range from pushing, shoving, and restraining to slapping, punching, kicking, clubbing, choking, burning, stabbing, or shooting. Hands-on violence also includes sexual assault, ranging from forced fondling of breasts, buttocks, and genitals; to forced touching of the abuser; to forced intercourse with the abuser or with other people.

Hands-off violence includes physical violence that is not directed at the victim's body but is intended to display destructive power and assert domination and control. Examples include breaking through windows or locked doors, punching holes through walls, smashing objects, destroying personal property, and harming or killing pet animals. The victim is often blamed for this destruction and forced to clean up the mess. Hands-off violence also includes psychological control, coercion, and terror. This includes name calling, threats of violence or abandonment, gestures suggesting the possibility of violence, monitoring of the victim's whereabouts, controlling of resources (such as money, transportation, and property), forced viewing of pornography, sexual exposure, or threatening to contest child custody. These psychological tactics may occur simultaneously with physical assaults or may occur separately. Whatever the pattern of psychological and physical tactics, abusers exert extreme control over their partners.

Neglect—the failure of one person to provide for the basic needs of another dependent person—is another form of hands-off abuse. Neglect may involve failure to provide food, clothing, health care, or shelter. Children, older adults, and developmentally delayed or physically disabled people are particularly vulnerable to neglect.

Family violence differs in two respects from violence directed at strangers. First, the offender and victim are related and may love each other, live together, share property, have children, and share friends and relatives. Hence, unlike victims of stranger violence, victims of family violence cannot quickly or easily sever ties with or avoid seeing their assailants. Second, family violence often increases slowly in intensity, progressing until victims feel immobilized, unworthy, and responsible for the violence that is directed toward them. Victims may also feel substantial and well-grounded fear about leaving their abusers or seeking legal help, because they have been threatened or assaulted in the past and may encounter significant difficulty obtaining help to escape. In the case of children, the frail and elderly, or people with disabilities, dependency upon the caregiver and cognitive limitations make escape from an abuser difficult. Remaining in the relationship increases the risk of continued victimization. Understanding this unique context of the violent family can help physicians and other health care providers understand why battered victims often have difficulty admitting abuse or leaving the abuser.

Family violence follows a characteristic cycle. This cycle of violence begins with escalating tension and anger in the abuser. Victims describe a feeling of "walking on eggs." Next comes an outburst of violence. Outbursts of violence sometimes coincide with episodes of alcohol and drug abuse. Following the outburst, the abuser may feel remorse and expect forgiveness. The abuser often demands reconciliation, including sexual interaction. After a period of calm, the abuser again becomes increasingly tense and angry. This cycle generally repeats, with violence becoming increasingly severe. In partner abuse, victims are at greatest risk when there is a transition in the relationship such as pregnancy, divorce, or separation. In the case of elder abuse, risk increases as the elder becomes increasingly dependent on the primary caregiver, who may be inexperienced or unwilling to provide needed assistance. Without active intervention, the abuser rarely stops spontaneously and often becomes more violent.

TREATMENT AND THERAPY

Physicians play an important role in stopping family violence by first identifying people who are victims of violence, then taking steps to intervene and help. Physicians use different techniques with each age group because children, adults, and older adults each have special needs and varying abilities to help themselves. This section will first consider the physician's role with children and will then examine the physician's role with adults and older adults.

Because children do not usually tell a physician directly if they are being abused physically or sexually, physicians use several strategies to identify child and adolescent victims. Physicians screen for abuse during regular checkups by asking children if anyone has hurt them, touched them in private places, or scared them.

To accomplish this screening with five-year-old patients having routine checkups, physicians may teach their young patients about private areas of the body; let them know that they can tell a parent, teacher, or doctor if anyone ever touches them in private places; and ask the patients if anyone has ever touched them in a way that they did not like. For fifteen-year-old patients, physicians may screen potential victims by providing information on sexual abuse and date rape, then asking the patients whether they have ever experienced either.

A second strategy that physicians use to identify children who are victims of family violence is to remain alert for general signs of distress that may indicate a child or youth lives in a violent situation. General signs of distress in children, which may be caused by family violence or by other stressors, include depression, anxiety, low self-esteem, hyperactivity, disruptive behaviors, aggressiveness toward other children, and lack of friends.

In addition to general signs of distress, there are certain specific signs and symptoms of physical and sexual abuse in children which indicate that the child has probably been exposed to violence. For example, a bruise that looks like a handprint, belt mark, or rope burn would indicate abuse. X rays can show a history of broken bones that are suspicious. Intentional burns from hot water, fire, or cigarettes often have a characteristic pattern. Sexually transmitted diseases in the genital, anal, or oral cavity of a child who is aged fourteen or under would suggest sexual abuse.

A physician observing specific signs of abuse or violence in a child, or even suspecting physical or sexual abuse, has an ethical and legal obligation to provide this information to state child protective services. Every state has laws that require physicians to report suspected child abuse. Physicians do not need to find proof of abuse before filing a report. In fact, the physician should never attempt to prove abuse or interview the child in detail because this can interfere with interviews conducted by experts in law, psychology, and the medicine of child abuse. When children are in immediate danger, they may be hospitalized so that they may receive a thorough medical and psychological evaluation while also being removed from the dangerous situation. In addition to filing a report, the physician records all observations in the child's medical file. This record includes anything that the child or parents said, drawings or photographs of the injury, the physician's professional opinion regarding exposure to violence, and a description of the child abuse report.

The physician's final step is to offer support to the child's family. Families of child victims often have multiple problems, including violence between adults, drug and alcohol abuse, economic problems, and social isolation. Appropriate interventions for promoting safety include foster care for children, court-ordered counseling for one or both parents, and in-home education in parenting skills. The physician's goal, however, is to maintain a nonjudgmental manner while encouraging parental involvement.

Physicians also play a key role in helping victims of partner violence. Like children and adolescents, adult victims will usually not disclose violence; therefore, physicians should screen for partner violence and ask about partner violence whenever they notice specific signs of abuse or general signs of distress. Physicians screen for current and past violence during routine patient visits, such as during initial appointments; school, athletic, and work physicals; premarital exams; obstetrical visits; and regular checkups. General signs of distress include depression, anxiety disorders, low self-esteem, suicidal ideation, drug and alcohol abuse, stress illnesses (headache, stomach problems, chronic pain), or patient comments about a partner being jealous, angry, controlling, or irritable. Specific signs of violence include physical injury consistent with assault, including that requiring emergency treatment.

When a victim reports partner violence, there are several steps that a physician can take to help. Communicating belief and support is the first step. Sometimes abuse is extreme and patient reports may seem incredible. The physician validates the victim's experience by expressing belief in the story and exonerating the patient of blame. The physician can begin this process by making eye contact and telling the victim, "You have a right to be safe and respected" and "No one should be treated this way."

Another step is helping the patient assess danger. This is done by asking about types and severity of violent acts, duration and frequency of violence, and injuries received. Specific factors that seem to increase the risk of death in violent relationships include the abuser's use of drugs and alcohol, threats to kill the victim, and the victim's suicidal ideation or attempts. Finally, the physician should ask if the victim feels safe returning home. With this information, the physician can help the patient assess lethal potential and begin to make appropriate safety plans.

Another step is helping the patient identify resources and make a safety plan. The physician begins this process by simply expressing concern for the victim's safety and providing information about local resources such as mandatory arrest laws, legal advocacy services, and shelters. For patients planning to return to an abusive relationship, the physician should encourage a detailed safety plan by helping the patient identify safe havens with family members, friends, or a shelter; assess escape routes from the residence; make specific plans for dangerous situations or when violence recurs; and gather copies of important papers, money, and extra clothing in a safe place in or out of the home against the event of a quick exit. Before the patient leaves, the physician should give the patient a follow-up appointment within two weeks. This provides the victim with a specific, known resource. Follow-up visits should continue until the victim has developed other supportive resources.

The physician's final step is documentation in the patient's medical file. This written note includes the victim's report of violence, the physician's own observations of injuries and behavior, assessment of danger, safety planning, and follow-up. This record can be helpful in the event of criminal or civil action taken by the victim against the offender. The medical file and all communications with the patient are kept strictly confidential. Confronting the offender about the abuse can place the victim at risk of further, more severe violence. Improper disclosure can also result in loss of the patient's trust, precluding further opportunities for help.

There are several things that a physician should never do when working with a patient-victim. The physician should not encourage a patient to leave a violent relationship as a first or primary choice. Leaving an abuser is the most dangerous time for victims and should be attempted only with adequate planning and resources. The physician should not recommend couples counseling. Couples counseling endangers victims by raising the victim's expectation that issues can be discussed safely. The abuser often batters the victim after disclosure of sensitive information. Finally, the physician should not overlook violence if the violence appears to be "minor." Seemingly minor acts of aggression can be highly injurious.

Physicians also play an important role in helping adults who are older, developmentally delayed, or physically disabled. People in all three groups experience a high rate of family violence. Each group presents unique challenges for the physician. One common element among all three groups is that the victims may be somewhat dependent upon other adults to meet their basic needs. Because of this dependence, abuse may sometimes take the form of failing to provide basic needs such as adequate food or medical care. In many states, adults who are developmentally delayed are covered by mandatory child abuse reporting laws.

The signs and symptoms of the abuse of elders are similar to those of the other forms of family violence. These include physical injuries consistent with assault, signs of distress, and neglect, including self-neglect. Elder abuse victims are often reluctant to reveal abuse because of fear of retaliation, abandonment, or institutionalization. Therefore, a key to intervention is coordinating with appropriate social service and allied health agencies to support an elder adequately, either at home or in a care center. Such agencies include aging councils, visiting nurses, home health aides, and respite or adult day care centers. Counseling and assistance for caregivers are also important parts of intervention.

Many states require physicians to report suspected elder abuse. Because many elder abuse victims are mentally competent, however, it is important that they be made part of the decision-making and reporting process. Such collaboration puts needed control in the elder's hands and therefore facilitates healing. Many other aspects of intervention described for partner abuse apply to working with elders, including providing emotional support, assessing danger, safety planning, and documentation.

In addition to helping the victims of acute, ongoing family violence, physicians have an important role to play in helping survivors of past family violence. People who have survived family violence may continue to experience negative effects similar to those experienced by acute victims. Physicians can identify survivors of family violence by screening for past violence during routine exams. A careful history can determine whether the patient has been suffering medical or psychological problems related to the violence. Finally, the physician should identify local resources for the patient, including a mutual help group and a therapist.

Physicians can also help prevent family violence. One avenue of prevention is through education of patients by discussing partner violence with patients at key life transitions, such as during adolescence when youths begin dating, prior to marriage, during pregnancy, and during divorce or separation. A second avenue of prevention is making medical clinic waiting rooms and examination rooms into education centers by displaying educational posters and providing pamphlets.

PERSPECTIVE AND PROSPECTS

Despite its frequency, family violence has not always been viewed as a problem. In the nineteenth century, it was legal in the United States for a husband to beat his wife, or for parents to use brutal physical punishment with their children. Although the formation of the New York Society for the Prevention of Cruelty to Children in 1874 signaled rising concern about child maltreatment, the extent of the problem was underestimated. As recently as 1960, family violence was viewed as a rare, aberrant phenomenon, and women who were victims of violence were often seen as partially responsible because of "masochistic tendencies." Several factors combined to turn the tide during the next thirty years. Medical research published in the early 1960's began documenting the severity of the problem of child abuse. By 1968, every state in the United States had passed a law requiring that physicians report suspected child abuse, and many states had established child protective services to investigate and protect vulnerable children.

Progress in the battle against partner violence was slower. The battered women's movement brought new attention and a feminist understanding to the widespread and serious nature of partner violence. This growing awareness provided the impetus, during the 1970's and 1980's, for reform in the criminal justice system, scientific research, continued growth of women's shelters, and the development of treatment programs for offenders.

The medical profession's response to partner abuse followed these changes. In 1986, Surgeon General C. Everett Koop declared family violence to be a public health problem and called upon physicians to learn to identify and intervene with victims. In 1992, the American Medical Association (AMA) echoed the surgeon general and stated that physicians have an ethical obligation to identify and assist victims of partner violence, and it established standards and protocols for identifying and helping victims of family violence. Because partner and elder abuse have been recognized only recently by the medical community, many physicians are just beginning to learn about their essential role.

Family violence has at various times been considered as a social problem, a legal problem, a political problem, and a medical problem. Because of this shifting understanding and because of the grassroots political origins of the child and partner violence movements, some may question why physicians should be involved. There are three compelling reasons.

First, there is a medical need: Family violence is one

of the most common causes of injury, illness, and death for women and children. Victims seeking treatment for acute injuries make up a sizable portion of emergency room visits. Even in outpatient clinics, women report high rates of recent and ongoing violence and injury from partners. In addition to physical injuries, many victims experience stress-related medical problems for which they seek medical care. Among obstetrical patients who are battered, there is a risk of injury to both the woman and her unborn child. Hence, physicians working in clinics and emergency rooms will see many people who are victims.

Second, physicians have a stake in breaking the cycle of violence because they are interested in injury prevention and health promotion. When a physician treats a child or adult victim for physical or psychological injury but does not identify root causes, the victim will return to a dangerous situation. Prevention of future injury requires proper diagnosis of root causes, rather than mere treatment of symptoms.

Third, physicians have a stake in treatment of partner violence because it is a professional and ethical obligation. Two principles of medical ethics apply. First, a physician's actions should benefit the patient. Physicians can benefit patients who are suffering the effects of family violence only if they correctly recognize the root cause and intervene in a sensitive and professional manner. Physicians should also "do no harm." A physician who fails to recognize and treat partner violence will harm the patient by providing inappropriate advice and treatment.

—L. Kevin Hamberger, Ph.D.,
and Bruce Ambuel, Ph.D.

See also Addiction; Alcoholism; Bipolar disorders; Depression; Ethics; Intoxication; Münchausen syndrome by proxy; Paranoia; Psychiatric disorders; Psychiatry; Psychiatry, child and adolescent; Psychiatry, geriatric; Psychoanalysis; Psychosis; Rape and sexual assault; Schizophrenia; Stress.

For Further Information:

Bancroft, Lundy, and Jay G. Silverman. *The Batterer as Parent: Addressing the Impact of Domestic Violence on Family Dynamics.* Thousand Oaks, Calif.: Sage, 2002. Examines how partner abuse affects each relationship in a family and explains how children's emotional recovery is inextricably linked to the healing and empowerment of their mothers.

Barnett, Ola, Cindy L. Miller-Perrin, and Robin D. Perrin. *Family Violence Across the Lifespan: An In-troduction.* 2d ed. Thousand Oaks, Calif.: Sage, 2005. Provides information about the different ways that domestic violence, and the warning signs associated with it, may be recognized at various stages in the life spans of individuals and families.

Dutton, Donald G. *The Abusive Personality: Violence and Control in Intimate Relationships.* 2d ed. New York: Guilford Press, 2007. Dutton, a psychologist, began as a disciple of social learning theory and eventually came to understand that theory alone was inadequate to explain the multifaceted origins of spousal abuse.

Island, David, and Patrick Letellier. *Men Who Beat the Men Who Love Them: Battered Gay Men and Domestic Violence.* New York: Haworth Press, 1991. The first published book that addresses the issue of violence between gay partners. The authors write in a lively, straightforward manner that is easy to understand. Proposes novel ways of thinking about partner violence.

Kakar, Suman. *Domestic Abuse: Public Policy/Criminal Justice Approaches Towards Child, Spousal, and Elderly Abuse.* San Francisco: Austin & Winfield, 2002. Offers theoretical and analytical explanations for domestic violence and includes detailed discussion of violence against children, spouses, and the elderly.

Levine, Murray, and Adeline Levine. *Helping Children: A Social History.* 2d ed. New York: Oxford University Press, 1992. The Levines provide an excellent history of child maltreatment in the United States, as well as the various legal, social, and medical strategies that have been used to help abused children.

National Coalition Against Domestic Violence. http://www.ncadv.org. A site that helps to define domestic violence and that offers information on community responses, getting help, and public policy.

Raphael, Jody. *Saving Bernice: Battered Women, Welfare, and Poverty.* Boston: Northeastern University Press, 2000. Raphael uses the case study of one welfare mother and survivor of domestic violence to exemplify the broader issues connecting domestic violence and poverty. In interviews taped during 1995-1999, Bernice, a mother of two and on welfare for eight years, recounts the trauma of abuse, harassment, and stalking by her former partner.

Wilson, K. J. *When Violence Begins at Home: A Comprehensive Guide to Understanding and Ending Domestic Violence.* Alameda, Calif.: Hunter House,

1997. Wilson seeks to share her wealth of knowledge stemming from experience as a training director at the Austin Center for Battered Women, as an educator, and as a survivor of domestic abuse.

DOWN SYNDROME
DISEASE/DISORDER

ANATOMY OR SYSTEM AFFECTED: Brain, nervous system, psychic-emotional system

SPECIALTIES AND RELATED FIELDS: Embryology, genetics, obstetrics, pediatrics

DEFINITION: A congenital abnormality characterized by moderate to severe mental retardation and a distinctive physical appearance caused by a chromosomal aberration, the result of either an error during embryonic cell division or the inheritance of defective chromosomal material.

KEY TERMS:

chromosomes: small, threadlike bodies containing the genes that are microscopically visible during cell division

gametes: the egg and sperm cells that unite to form the fertilized egg (zygote) in reproduction

gene: a segment of the DNA strand containing instructions for the production of a protein

homologous chromosomes: chromosome pairs of the same size and centromere position that possess genes for the same traits; one homologous chromosome is inherited from the father and the other from the mother

meiosis: the type of cell division that produces the cells of reproduction, which contain one-half of the chromosome number found in the original cell before division

mitosis: the type of cell division that occurs in nonsex cells, which conserves chromosome number by equal allocation to each of the newly formed cells

translocation: an aberration in chromosome structure resulting from the attachment of chromosomal material to a nonhomologous chromosome

CAUSES AND SYMPTOMS

Down syndrome is an example of a genetic disorder, that is, a disorder arising from an abnormality in an individual's genetic material. Down syndrome results from an incorrect transfer of genetic material in the formation of cells. Genetic information is contained in large "library" molecules of deoxyribonucleic acid (DNA). DNA molecules are formed by joining together units called nucleotides which come in four different varieties: adenosine, thymine, cytosine, and guanine (identified by their initials A, T, C, and G). These nucleotides store hereditary information by forming "words" with this four-letter alphabet. In a gene, a section of DNA which contains the chemical message controlling an inherited trait, three consecutive nucleotides combine to specify a particular amino acid. This word order forms the "sentences" of a recipe telling cells how to construct proteins, such as those coloring the hair and eyes, from amino acids.

In living systems, tissue growth occurs through cell division processes in which an original cell divides to form two cells containing duplicate genetic material. Just before a cell divides, the DNA organizes itself into distinct, compact bundles called chromosomes. Normal human cells, diploid cells, contain twenty-three pairs (or a total of forty-six) of these chromosomes. Each pair is a set of homologues containing genes for the same traits. These chromosomes are composed of two DNA strands, chromatids, joined at a constricted region known as the centromere. The bundle is similar in shape to the letter X. The arms are the parts above and below the constriction, which may be centered or offset toward one end (giving arms of equal or different lengths, respectively). During mitosis, the division of nonsex cells, the chromatids separate at the centromere, forming two sets of single-stranded chromosomes, which migrate to opposite ends of the cell. The cell then splits into two genetically equivalent cells, each containing twenty-three single-stranded chromosomes that will duplicate to form the original number of forty-six chromosomes.

In sexual reproduction, haploid egg and sperm cells, each containing twenty-three single-stranded chromosomes, unite in fertilization to produce a zygote cell with forty-six chromosomes. Haploid cells are created through a different, two-step cell division process termed meiosis. Meiosis begins when the homologues in a diploid cell pair up at the equator of the cell. The at-

---

INFORMATION ON DOWN SYNDROME

CAUSES: Genetic defect

SYMPTOMS: Mental retardation, characteristic facial appearance, lack of muscle tone, increased risk for heart malformations, increased disease susceptibility

DURATION: Lifelong

TREATMENTS: None

tractions between the members of each pair then break, allowing the homologues to migrate to opposite ends of the cell, each twin to a different pole, without splitting at the centromere. The parent cell then divides once to give two cells containing twenty-three double-stranded chromosomes, and then divides again through the process of mitosis to form cells that contain only twenty-three single-stranded chromosomes. Thus, each cell contains half of the original chromosomes.

Although cell division is normally a precise process, occasionally an error called nondisjunction occurs when a chromosome either fails to separate or fails to migrate to the proper pole. In meiosis, the failure to move to the proper pole results in the formation of one gamete having twenty-four chromosomes and one having twenty-two chromosomes. Upon fertilization, zygotes of forty-seven or forty-five chromosomes are produced, and the developing embryo must function with either extra or missing genes. Since every chromosome contains a multitude of genes, problems result from the absence or excess of proteins produced. In fact, the embryos formed from most nondisjunctional fertilizations die at an early stage in development and are spontaneously aborted. Occasionally, nondisjunction occurs in mitosis, when a chromosome migrates before the chromatids separate, yielding one cell with an extra copy of the chromosome and no copy in the other cell.

Down syndrome is also termed trisomy 21 because it most commonly results from the presence of an extra copy of the smallest human chromosome, chromosome 21. Actually, it is not the entire extra chromosome 21 that is responsible, but rather a small segment of the long arm of this chromosome. Only two other trisomies occur with any significant frequency: trisomy 13 (Patau's syndrome) and trisomy 18 (Edwards' syndrome). Both of these disorders are accompanied by multiple severe malformations, resulting in death within a few months of birth. Most incidences of Down syndrome are a consequence of a nondisjunction during meiosis. In about 75 percent of these cases, the extra chromosome is present in the egg. About 1 percent of Down syndrome cases occur after the fertilization of normal gametes from a mitosis nondisjunction, producing a mosaic in which some of the embryo's cells are normal and some exhibit trisomy. The degree of mosaicism and its location will determine the physiological consequences of the nondisjunction. Although mosaic individuals range from apparent normality to completely affected, typically the disorder is less severe.

In about 4 percent of all Down syndrome cases, the individual possesses not an entire third copy of chromosome 21 but rather extra chromosome 21 material, which has been incorporated via a translocation into a nonhomologous chromosome. In translocation, pieces of arms are swapped between two nonrelated chromosomes, forming "hybrid" chromosomes. The most common translocation associated with Down syndrome is that between the long arm (Down gene area) of chromosome 21 and an end of chromosome 14. The individual in whom the translocation has occurred shows no evidence of the aberration, since the normal complement of genetic material is still present, only at different chromosomal locations. The difficulty arises when this individual forms gametes. A mother who possesses the 21/14 translocation, for example, has one normal 21, one normal 14, and the hybrid chromosomes. She is a genetic carrier for the disorder, because she can pass it on to her offspring even though she is clinically normal. This mother could produce three types of viable gametes: one containing the normal 14 and 21; one containing both translocations, which would result in clinical normality; and one containing the normal 21 and the translocated 14 having the long arm of 21. If each gamete were fertilized by normal sperm, two apparently normal embryos and one partial trisomy 21 Down syndrome embryo would result. Down syndrome that results from the passing on of translocations is termed familial Down syndrome and is an inherited disorder.

The presence of an extra copy of the long arm of chromosome 21 causes defects in many tissues and organs. One major effect of Down syndrome is mental retardation. The intelligence quotients (IQs) of affected individuals are typically in the range of 40-50. The IQ varies with age, being higher in childhood than in adolescence and adult life. The disorder is often accompanied by physical traits such as short stature, stubby fingers and toes, protruding tongue, and an unusual pattern of hand creases. Perhaps the most recognized physical feature is the distinctive slanting of the eyes, caused by a vertical fold (epicanthal fold) of skin near the nasal bridge which pulls and tilts the eyes slightly toward the nostrils. For normal Caucasians, the eye runs parallel to the skin fold below the eyebrow; for Asians, this skin fold covers a major portion of the upper eyelid. In contrast, the epicanthal fold in trisomy 21 does not cover a major part of the upper eyelid.

It should be noted that not all defects associated with Down syndrome are found in every affected individual. About 40 percent of Down syndrome patients have

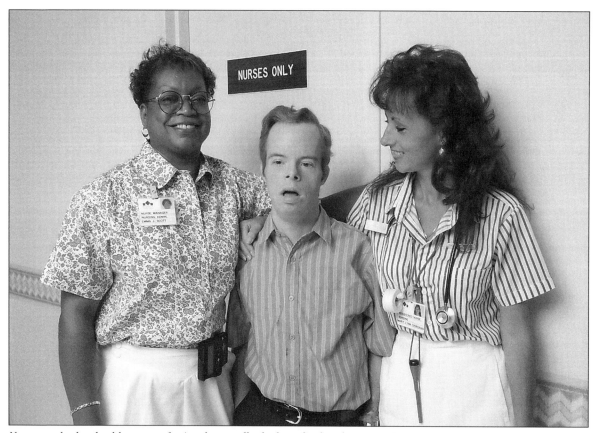

Nurses and other health care professionals can offer both medical and emotional support to people with Down syndrome. (PhotoDisc)

congenital heart defects, while about 10 percent have intestinal blockages. Affected individuals are prone to respiratory infections and contract leukemia at a rate twenty times that of the general population. Although Down syndrome children develop the same types of leukemia in the same proportions as other children, the survival rates of the two groups are markedly different. While the survival rate for patients without Down syndrome after ten years is about 30 percent, survival beyond five years is negligible in those with Down syndrome. It appears that the extra copy of chromosome 21 not only increases the risk of contracting the cancer but also exerts a decisive influence on the disease's outcome. Reproductively, males are sterile while some females are fertile. Although many Down syndrome infants die in the first year of life, the average life expectancy is about fifty years. This reduced life expectancy results from defects in the immune system, causing a high susceptibility to infectious disease. Many individuals with Down syndrome develop an Alzheimer's-like condition later in life.

TREATMENT AND THERAPY

Trisomy 21 is one of the most common human chromosomal aberrations, occurring in about 0.5 percent of all conceptions and in one out of every seven hundred to eight hundred live births. About 15 percent of the patients institutionalized for mental deficiency suffer from Down syndrome.

Even before the chromosomal basis for the disorder was determined, the frequency of Down syndrome births was correlated with increased maternal age. For mothers at age twenty, the incidence of Down syndrome is about 0.05 percent, which increases to 0.9 percent by age thirty-five and 3 percent at age forty-five. Studies comparing the chromosomes of the affected offspring with those of both parents have shown that the nondisjunction event is maternal about 75 percent of the time. This maternal age effect is thought to result from the different manner in which the male and female gametes are produced. Gamete production in the male is a continual, lifelong process, while it is a one-time event in females.

Formation of the female's gametes begins early in embryonic life, somewhere between the eighth and twentieth weeks. During this time, cells in the developing ovary divide rapidly by mitosis, forming cells called primary oocytes. These cells then begin meiosis by pairing up the homologues. The process is interrupted at this point, and the cells are held in a state of suspended animation until needed in reproduction, when they are triggered to complete their division and form eggs. It appears that the frequency of nondisjunction events increases with the length of the storage period. Studies have demonstrated that cells in a state of meiosis are particularly sensitive to environmental influences such as viruses, X rays, and cytotoxic chemicals. It is possible that environmental influences may play a role in nondisjunction events. Up to age thirty-two, males contribute an extra chromosome 21 as often as do females. Beyond this age, there is a rapid increase in nondisjunctional eggs, while the number of nondisjunctional sperm remains constant. Where the maternal age effect is minimal, mosaicism may be an important source of the trisomy. An apparently normal mother who possesses undetected mosaicism can produce trisomy offspring if gametes with an extra chromosome are produced. In some instances, characteristics such as abnormal fingerprint patterns have been observed in the mothers and their Down syndrome offspring.

Techniques such as amniocentesis, chorionic villus sampling, and alpha-fetoprotein screening are available for prenatal diagnosis of Down syndrome in fetuses. Amniocentesis, the most widely used technique for prenatal diagnosis, is generally performed between the fourteenth and sixteenth weeks of pregnancy. In this technique, about one ounce of fluid is removed from the amniotic cavity surrounding the fetus by a needle inserted through the mother's abdomen. Although some testing can be done directly on the fluid (such as the assay for spina bifida), more information is obtained from the cells

IN THE NEWS: NEW SCREENING TESTS FOR DOWN SYNDROME

Down syndrome is the most common chromosome condition, occurring in 1 of every 750 live births. Individuals who have Down syndrome usually have an extra copy of chromosome number 21 (trisomy 21). The extra chromosome leads to a distinctive appearance, mild-to-moderate mental retardation, and sometimes additional medical complications such as a heart defect or digestive system problems.

The risk to have a pregnancy with Down syndrome increases with a women's age, but all women have a risk to have an affected pregnancy. Therefore, all pregnant women are offered screening tests for Down syndrome. These screening tests can be performed as early as the first trimester of pregnancy. The accumulation of fluid behind the fetal neck—called a nuchal translucency, or NT—can be measured on ultrasound between ten and thirteen weeks of gestation. This measurement tends to be larger in fetuses that have Down syndrome. The NT measurement can be combined with a measurement of hormones found in the maternal blood that are produced by the pregnancy as well as a woman's age, weight, and ethnicity to give a personalized risk estimate for the fetus to have Down syndrome. There are many variations of this testing, and some versions of this screening test involve an additional maternal blood sample in the second trimester.

Although these tests can detect more than 90 percent of fetuses with Down syndrome, they do not give a definitive diagnosis. Women found to be in the high-risk category on screening, also called a screen positive, are offered additional testing, such as a detailed level II ultrasound at approximately 18 weeks gestation. Half of fetuses with Down syndrome will display a marker, or soft sign on ultrasound, such as thickened skin behind the neck, short bones, or a bright spot in the heart. The presence or absence of a soft marker can be used to further refine the risk for the pregnancy to have Down syndrome, but is not diagnostic.

The only diagnostic testing for Down syndrome in the pregnancy is chorionic villus sampling (CVS) or amniocentesis. Both tests are invasive and carry a small risk of miscarriage and many women forgo this testing due to the procedure-related risk. The technology to detect fetal cells in the maternal bloodstream is rapidly evolving, and soon pregnant woman may be able to learn if their fetus has Down syndrome with a simple blood draw. This technology could certainly revolutionize the field of prenatal diagnosis for Down syndrome.

—*Lauren Lichten, M.S., C.G.C.*

shed from the fetus that accompany the fluid. The mixture obtained in the amniocentesis is spun in a centrifuge to separate the fluid from the fetal cells. Unfortunately, the chromosome analysis for Down syndrome cannot be conducted directly on the amount of cellular material obtained. Although the majority of the cells collected are nonviable, some will grow in culture. These cells are allowed to grow and multiply in culture for two to four weeks, and then the chromosomes undergo karyotyping, which will detect both trisomy 21 and translocational aberration.

In karyotyping, the chromosomes are spread on a microscope slide, stained, and photographed. Each type of chromosome gives a unique, observable banding pattern when stained, which allows it to be identified. The chromosomes are then cut out of the photograph and arranged in homologous pairs, in numerical order. Trisomy 21 is easily observed, since three copies of chromosome 21 are present, while the translocation shows up as an abnormal banding pattern. Termination of the pregnancy in the wake of an unfavorable amniocentesis diagnosis is complicated, because the fetus at this point is usually about eighteen to twenty weeks old, and elective abortions are normally performed between the sixth and twelfth weeks of pregnancy. Earlier sampling of the amniotic fluid is not possible because of the small amount of fluid present.

An alternate testing procedure called chorionic villus sampling became available in the mid-1980's. In this procedure, a chromosomal analysis is conducted on a piece of placental tissue that is obtained either vaginally or through the abdomen during the eighth to eleventh week of pregnancy. The advantages of this procedure are that it can be done much earlier in the pregnancy and that enough tissue can be collected to conduct the chromosome analysis immediately, without the cell culture step. Consequently, diagnosis can be completed during the first trimester of the pregnancy, making therapeutic abortion an option for the parents. Chorionic villus sampling does have some negative aspects. One disadvantage is the slightly higher incidence of test-induced miscarriage as compared to amniocentesis—around 1 percent (versus less than 0.5 percent). Also, because tissue of both the mother and the fetus are obtained in the sampling process, they must be carefully separated, complicating the analysis. Occasionally, chromosomal abnormalities are observed in the tested tissue that are not present in the fetus itself.

Prenatal maternal alpha-fetoprotein testing has also been used to diagnose Down syndrome. Abnormal levels of a substance called maternal alpha-fetoprotein are often associated with chromosomal disorders. Several research studies have described a high correlation between low levels of maternal alpha-fetoprotein and the occurrence of trisomy 21 in the fetus. By correlating alpha-fetoprotein levels, the age of the mother, and specific female hormone levels, between 60 percent and 80 percent of fetuses with Down syndrome can be detected. Although techniques allow Down syndrome to be detected readily in a fetus, there is no effective intrauterine therapy available to correct the abnormality.

The care of a Down syndrome child presents many challenges for the family unit. Until the 1970's, most of these children spent their lives in institutions. With the increased support services available, however, it is now common for such children to remain in the family environment. Although many Down syndrome children have happy dispositions, a significant number have behavioral problems that can consume the energies of the parents, to the detriment of other children. Rearing a Down syndrome child often places a large financial burden on the family: Such children are, for example, susceptible to illness; they also have special educational needs. Since Down syndrome children are often conceived late in the parents' reproductive period, the parents may not be able to continue to care for these children throughout their offspring's adult years. This is problematic because many Down syndrome individuals do not possess sufficient mental skills to earn a living or to manage their affairs without supervision.

All women in their mid-thirties have an increased risk of producing a Down syndrome infant. Since the resultant trisomy 21 is not of a hereditary nature, the abnormality can be detected only by the prenatal screening, which is recommended for all pregnancies of women older than age thirty-four.

For parents who have produced a Down syndrome child, genetic counseling can be beneficial in determining their risk factor for future pregnancies. The genetic counselor determines the specific chromosomal aberration that occurred utilizing chromosome studies of the parents and affected child, along with additional information provided by the family history. If the cause was nondisjunction and the mother is young, the recurrence risk is much less than 1 percent; for mothers over the age of thirty-four, it is about 5 percent. If the cause was translocational, the Down syndrome is hereditary and risk is greater—statistically, a one-in-three chance. In addition, there is a one-in-three chance that clinically normal offspring will be carriers of the syndrome, producing it in the next generation. It is suggested that couples who come from families having a history of spontaneous abortions, which often result from lethal chromosomal aberrations, and/or incidence of Down syndrome, undergo chromosomal screening to detect the presence of a Down syndrome translocation.

PERSPECTIVE AND PROSPECTS

English physician John L. H. Down is credited with the first clinical description of Down syndrome, in 1886. Since the distinctive epicanthic fold gave Down children an appearance that John Down associated with Asians, he called the condition "mongolism"—an unfortunate term implying that those affected with the condition are throwbacks to a more "primitive" racial group. Today, the inappropriate term has been replaced with the name Down syndrome.

A French physician, Jérôme Lejeune, suspected that Down syndrome had a genetic basis and began to study the condition in 1953. A comparison of the fingerprints and palm prints of affected individuals with those of unaffected individuals showed a high frequency of abnormalities in the prints of those with Down syndrome. These prints appear very early in development and serve as a record of events that take place early in embryogenesis. The extent of the changes in print patterns led Lejeune to the conclusion that the condition was not a result of the action of one or two genes but rather of many genes or even an entire chromosome. Upon microscopic examination, he observed that Down syndrome children possess forty-seven chromosomes instead of the forty-six chromosomes found in normal children. In 1959, Lejeune published his findings, showing that Down syndrome is caused by the presence of the extra chromosome which was later identified as a copy of chromosome 21. This first observation of a human chromosomal abnormality marked a turning point in the study of human genetics. It demonstrated that genetic defects not only were caused by mutations of single genes but also could be associated with changes in chromosome number. Although the presence of an extra chromosome allows varying degrees of development to occur, most of these abnormalities result in fetal death, with only a few resulting in live birth. Down syndrome is unusual in that the affected individual often survives into adulthood.

—*Arlene R. Courtney, Ph.D.*

See also Amniocentesis; Birth defects; Chorionic villus sampling; Congenital disorders; DNA and RNA; Genetic diseases; Genetics and inheritance; Leukemia; Mental retardation; Mutation.

FOR FURTHER INFORMATION:

Cohen, William, Lynn Nadel, and Myra E. Madnick, eds. *Down Syndrome: Visions for the Twenty-first Century.* New York: Wiley-Liss, 2002. Reviews the medical and research advances in the clinical, educational, developmental, psychosocial, and vocational aspects of Down syndrome.

Hassold, Terry J., and David Patterson, eds. *Down Syndrome: A Promising Future, Together.* New York: Wiley-Liss, 1999. Discusses clinical, educational, developmental, psychosocial, and vocational issues relevant to people with Down syndrome.

Miller, Jon F., Mark Leddy, and Lewis A. Leavitt, eds. *Improving the Communication of People with Down Syndrome.* 2d ed. Baltimore: Paul H. Brookes, 2003. Discusses how to assess and treat speech, language, and communication problems in children and adults with Down syndrome.

Moore, Keith L., and T. V. N. Persaud. *The Developing Human.* 8th ed. Philadelphia: Saunders/Elsevier, 2008. An outstanding textbook on human embryonic development, with specific information about the causes of congenital malformations and common defects occurring in each of the body's systems.

National Down Syndrome Society. http://www.ndss.org. An excellent organization that focuses on research, advocacy, and education. The Web site promotes virtual communities and provides updated information about coming events.

Pueschel, Siegfried M. *A Parent's Guide to Down Syndrome.* Rev. ed. Baltimore: Paul H. Brookes, 2001. An informative guide highlighting the important developmental stages in the life of a child with Down syndrome.

_____, ed. *Adults with Down Syndrome.* Baltimore: Paul H. Brookes, 2006. Discusses health care and medical issues, psychiatric disorders, sexuality, education and employment, and community involvement.

Rondal, Jean A., et al., eds. *Down's Syndrome: Psychological, Psychobiological, and Socioeducational Perspectives.* San Diego, Calif.: Singular, 1996. An academic text on issues surrounding Down syndrome. Includes references and an index.

DROWNING

DISEASE/DISORDER

ANATOMY OR SYSTEM AFFECTED: Brain, circulatory system, heart, kidneys, lungs, nervous system, respiratory system, stomach, throat

SPECIALTIES AND RELATED FIELDS: Critical care, emergency medicine, environmental health, nursing, pulmonary medicine

DEFINITION: A drowning victim dies by suffocation from submersion in a liquid medium, usually water.

KEY TERMS:

alveolar ventilation: the volume of air that ventilates all the perfused alveoli; the normal average is four to five liters per minute

asphyxia: cessation of breathing

bradycardia: a heart rate below sixty beats per minute

glottis: the opening to the larynx

hypertonic fluid: a solution that increases the degree of osmotic pressure on a semipermeable membrane

hypothermia: an abnormal and dangerous condition in which the temperature of the body is below 95 degrees Fahrenheit; usually caused by prolonged exposure to cold

hypoxia: inadequate oxygen at the cellular level

intrapulmonary shunting: a condition of perfusion without ventilation

laryngospasm: spasm of the larynx

CAUSES AND SYMPTOMS

Drowning is the leading cause of accidental death in the United States. The victim dies by suffocation from submersion in a liquid medium. Although suffocation most commonly results from aspiration of fresh or salt water into the lungs, about 10 percent to 20 percent of victims experience laryngospasm with subsequent glottic closure followed by asphyxiation. Near-drowning is defined as recovery after submersion. Victims are typically children or adolescents. Males more often engage in risk-taking behavior and have a significantly greater incidence of drowning and near-drowning than do females.

Victims of near-drowning, if rescued and resuscitated quickly enough, may fully recover. In many instances, however, near-drowning victims are left with mild to severe neurologic effects. Even if the victim has been submerged in water for some time, vigorous attempts at resuscitation are indicated because of documented recovery following such incidents.

Boating and swimming accidents account for the largest number of drownings in the adult population,

and many are alcohol-related. Factors that influence the extent of damage in near-drowning include the length of time submerged, the temperature of the water, and the victim's resistance to asphyxia and anoxia (oxygen deprivation). Recovery may be more successful if the victim drowns in cold water, because the induced hypothermia lowers the body's metabolic demands and, therefore, oxygen needs. Extremely cold water may decrease the victim's core body temperature so rapidly that death from hypothermia may actually occur before drowning.

Generally, there is an inverse relation between the victim's age and the victim's resistance to asphyxia and anoxia. The younger the victim, the greater the resistance. The resistance is especially strong in very young victims, usually under two or three years of age, because of the diving reflex triggered in young children when the face is immersed in very cold water. Blood is shunted to the vital organs, especially the brain and heart. Hypothermia offers some protection to the hypoxic brain by reducing the cerebral metabolic rate. Although the victim suffers severe bradycardia, the remaining oxygen supply is concentrated in the heart and brain. The diving reflex is generally not a factor in adult drownings.

Approximately 10 percent of drowning victims develop laryngospasm concurrently with the first gulp of water and thus do not aspirate (swallow) fluid. Even in the majority of victims who do aspirate, the amount of fluid aspirated is small. In the past, salt water and freshwater drowning were differentiated. These differences are of little clinical significance in humans, primarily because so little fluid is aspirated. In both cases, drown-

---

INFORMATION ON DROWNING

CAUSES: Submersion in a liquid medium, resulting in aspiration or asphyxiation

SYMPTOMS: Slow heart rate, hypoxemia, ineffective circulation, cardiac arrest, brain injury, brain death; following near-drowning, may include acute respiratory failure, cerebral and pulmonary edema, shock acidosis, electrolyte imbalance, stupor, coma, cardiac arrest

DURATION: Acute and often fatal; possible permanent effects for near-drowning

TREATMENTS: For near-drowning, cardiopulmonary resuscitation (CPR), intubation, mechanical ventilation, stomach decompression, sometimes induced coma and hypothermia

ing quickly diminishes perfusion to the alveoli, interfering with ventilation and soon leading to hypoxemia, ineffective circulation, cardiac arrest, brain injury, and brain death.

When water is aspirated into the lungs, the composition of the water is a key factor in the pathophysiology of the near-drowning event. Aspiration of freshwater causes surfactant to wash out of the lungs. Surfactant reduces surface tension within the alveoli, increases lung compliance and alveolar radius, and decreases the work of breathing. Loss of surfactant from freshwater aspiration destabilizes the alveoli and leads to increased airway resistance. Conversely, salt water—a hypertonic fluid—creates an osmotic gradient that draws protein-rich fluid from the vascular space into the alveoli. The consequences of both types of aspiration include impaired alveolar ventilation and resultant intrapulmonary shunting, which further compound the hypoxic state.

When submersion is brief, the near-drowning victim may spontaneously regain consciousness or may recover quickly following rescue. Even when victims have not aspirated fluid, they should be hospitalized for observation because respiratory symptoms may not develop for twelve to twenty-four hours. Victims who have been submerged for longer periods may show varying degrees of recovery following resuscitation. Manifestations may include acute respiratory failure, pulmonary edema, shock acidosis, electrolyte imbalance, stupor, coma, and cardiac arrest. Damage causes cerebral edema (brain swelling) and may lead to increased intracranial pressure. Care for the patient who has suffered brain damage involves careful and frequent assessment of the patient's neurologic status, including vital signs, pupil reaction, and reflexes.

TREATMENT AND THERAPY

Immediate care should focus on a safe rescue of the victim. Once rescuers gain access to the victim, priorities include safe removal from the water, while maintaining spine stabilization with a board or flotation device, and initiating airway clearance and ventilatory support measures. If hypothermia is a concern, then gentle handling of the victim is essential to prevent ventricular fibrillation. Abdominal thrusts should only be delivered if airway obstruction is suspected. Once the victim is safely removed from the water, airway and cardiopulmonary support interventions begin. Emergency care involves cardiopulmonary resuscitation (CPR), intubation, and mechanical ventilation with 100 percent oxygen.

In the clinical setting, stomach decompression using a tube down the nose or mouth is indicated to prevent the aspiration of gastric contents and to improve breathing.

Patients who experience near-drowning require complex care to support their body systems. The full spectrum of critical care technology may be needed to manage the physiological problems and effects associated with near-drowning, including lung infection, acute respiratory distress syndrome, and central nervous system impairment. Metabolic acidosis results from severe hypoxia. Arterial blood gases must be monitored frequently, and sodium bicarbonate is usually administered to correct the acidosis. Coma may be induced with barbiturates and a state of hypothermia maintained for several days following the near-drowning. These interventions reduce the metabolic and oxygen demands of the brain. Diuretics are prescribed to treat pulmonary and cerebral edema. Fluid therapy must be monitored carefully to prevent fluid overload and promote adequate renal function.

PERSPECTIVE AND PROSPECTS

Drowning is the second leading cause of preventable death in children according to the American Academy of Pediatrics. New drowning prevention recommendations warn parents to be certain that everyone caring for a child understands the need for constant supervision around water and other liquids.

—*Jane C. Norman, Ph.D., R.N., C.N.E.*

See also Accidents; Asphyxiation; Brain damage; Cardiopulmonary resuscitation (CPR); Choking; Critical care; Critical care, pediatric; Emergency medicine; Emergency medicine, pediatric; First aid; Hyperbaric oxygen therapy; Lungs; Pulmonary medicine; Pulmonary medicine, pediatric; Respiration; Resuscitation; Unconsciousness.

FOR FURTHER INFORMATION:

Black, Joyce M., and Jane H. Hawks, eds. *Medical-Surgical Nursing: Clinical Management for Positive Outcomes.* 8th ed. St. Louis, Mo.: Saunders/Elsevier, 2009.

Lewis, Sharon M., et al., eds. *Medical-Surgical Nursing: Assessment and Management of Clinical Problems.* 7th ed. St. Louis, Mo.: Mosby/Elsevier, 2007.

Smeltzer, Suzanne C., and Brenda G. Bare, eds. *Brunner and Suddarth's Textbook of Medical-Surgical Nursing.* 12th ed. Philadelphia: Wolters Kluwer/Lippincott Williams & Wilkins, 2010.

886 • Drug resistance

DRUG ADDICTION. *See* **ADDICTION.**

DRUG RESISTANCE
DISEASE/DISORDER

ANATOMY OR SYSTEM AFFECTED: All

SPECIALTIES AND RELATED FIELDS: Bacteriology, microbiology, pharmacology, public health, virology

DEFINITION: The ability of a microorganism, formerly susceptible to a particular medication, to change in such a way that it is no longer affected by that medication.

KEY TERMS:

antibiotic: a substance that kills or prevents the growth of a pathogen

bacteria: microscopic single-celled organisms

bacterial chromosome: a circular cell component in bacteria that contains deoxyribonucleic acid (DNA)

bacteriophage: a virus that attaches itself to bacteria

conjugation: the direct exchange of genetic material between bacteria

nosocomial infection: an infection that is acquired in a hospital

pathogen: a living organism that causes disease

plasmids: circular pieces of DNA within bacteria; these are much smaller than bacterial chromosomes

transduction: the indirect transfer of genetic material between bacteria by a bacteriophage

transposons: pieces of DNA that can be transferred between plasmids and chromosomes

virus: a microscopic organism consisting of DNA or ribonucleic acid (RNA) within a protein coating

CAUSES AND SYMPTOMS

Drug resistance occurs whenever microorganisms such as bacteria, viruses, or fungi—that have been exposed to a chemical agent—develop the ability to resist that agent. The most clinically important form of drug resistance is the ability of bacteria to develop resistance to antibiotics.

An antibiotic attacks a bacterial cell by interfering with a vital biochemical process needed by the organism. Antibiotics generally are engineered to kill bacteria, while leaving body cells unharmed. This bacteria-specific approach creates a safe way of killing pathogens, while keeping the affected person safe from harm.

Bacteria can develop resistance to an antibiotic in several ways, and that resistance may be propagated through the evolutionary process of natural selection. Selection is the "weeding out" of those individuals in a population who fail to adapt to changing conditions, leaving a smaller number of "tougher" individuals. If environmental pressure (such as an antibiotic treatment) is placed on any population of organisms, the only individuals who will survive and reproduce are those resistant to that pressure.

Resistance to a particular antibiotic arises in a bacterial cell by random genetic mutation. Because a particular cell is genetically altered and survives the antibiotic treatment that destroys other bacteria of the same kind, it is able to survive, unlike its susceptible relatives. The small, resistant population that is left can perpetuate infection despite the presence of antibiotics. Nonpathogenic bacteria, too, are affected by this selective pressure, and the development of antibiotic resistance in organisms that do not ordinarily cause infection can still have a powerful impact on disease processes.

The human body contains billions of bacteria of many different kinds. These bacteria fill large and small environmental niches in the microflora that human beings carry in and on their bodies. When one or more of these susceptible bacteria types are eliminated by an antibiotic, their niches are left empty. This leaves room for the resistant bacteria that are left to multiply in greater numbers. When these surviving organisms grow to such large numbers, the mix of "normal (nonpathogenic) flora" is disturbed, and normally harmless organisms can cause disease in those circumstances. Additionally, some of these organisms may have the ability to transfer resistance genes to pathogenic bacteria.

The ability to resist a particular antibiotic is encoded as genetic information in deoxyribonucleic acid (DNA) molecules. Bacterial DNA is located in a special bacterial chromosome found in the cytoplasm of a bacterial cell. Additionally, bacterial DNA may be found on small, circular fragments of DNA called plasmids. These plasmids are separate from the bacterial chromosome and carry special information needed for the bacteria to survive under adverse environmental conditions. Plasmids carry "mating" genes, which allow the bacteria to transfer a plasmid from one bacteria to another. They also carry genes that make a bacteria resistant to a particular antibiotic. Consequently, plasmids are of particular importance because they allow antibiotic resistance to be transferred between bacteria.

Two bacterial cells may exchange plasmids by direct contact in a process known as conjugation. Not all plasmids can be exchanged in this way, but the genetic information that encodes for resistance may be transferred from a plasmid that cannot be exchanged to one that can. This occurs when a small piece of DNA known as a transposon breaks away from one plasmid and attaches itself to another. A transposon may also break away from a bacterial chromosome and attach itself elsewhere on the chromosome or onto a plasmid.

Antibiotic resistance may also be transferred between bacteria indirectly by a bacteriophage in transduction. A bacteriophage is a virus that attaches itself to a bacterial cell. The virus sometimes incorporates DNA from the invaded bacterial cell into its own DNA. The virus may then transfer this DNA to the next bacterial cell to which it attaches. In this way, it can transfer drug resistance between bacteria that are unable to undergo conjugation.

The various ways in which genetic information can be exchanged between bacteria may result in organisms with resistance to multiple drugs. Some bacteria are known to be resistant to at least ten different antibiotics. They carry a series of genes on their plasmids able to make enzymes that can degrade and destroy antibiotics. For example, bacteria able to resist penicillin treatments carry an enzyme called penicillinase that destroys penicillin, thus protecting the bacteria. Other genes may code for a change in the structure of bacterial sites to which an antibiotic binds, reducing or eliminating its effect.

Frequent exposure to antibiotics increases the evolutionary pressure in bacterial populations and increases the likelihood that resistance will develop. An important factor in the emergence of antibiotic resistance is the misuse of antibiotics. For example, antibiotics have no effect on viruses but are often used against viral illnesses. A study published in 1997 revealed that at least half of all patients in the United States who visited doctors' offices with colds, upper respiratory tract infections, and bronchitis received antibiotics, even though 90 percent of these illnesses are caused by viruses. The same study showed that almost one-third of all antibiotic prescriptions were used for these kinds of illnesses. It is also important to remember that misuse can include underutilizing prescribed drugs, such as may stem from poor patient compliance with medical directions. Failure to take as directed, typically until the whole course of antibiotics has been consumed, may encourage the development of drug resistance, as the antibiotics will not have the opportunity to exert their full effect on the bacteria causing the problem. The bacteria that survive the partial course may be more likely to be resistant to that drug, making future administrations less effective.

This misuse of antibiotics has been one of the strongest forces pushing selection of antibiotic-resistant bacteria—but this is not only because of its use in humans. Specifically, even if doctors stop overprescribing antibiotics, other factors are at work. In 2000, an estimated fifty million pounds of antibiotics were used in the United States; half that amount was used for veterinary and agricultural purposes. Antibiotics are administered in huge doses to farm animals to keep them healthy and allow them to grow larger. These drugs are even being used in the petroleum industry for cleaning pipelines. The World Health Organization (WHO) noted a sharp decrease in the incidence of antibiotic-resistant bacterial strains in Denmark after antibiotic use in livestock was all but eliminated in 1998.

A final factor in the increase in antibiotic resistance is the use and overuse of substandard and counterfeit antimicrobial agents in developing countries. In Nigeria, for example, WHO estimates that there are twenty thousand unlicensed medical stands scattered throughout the country. These street vendors do not require prescriptions to dose patients. Additionally, the common use of antibiotics in developing nations to "sterilize" households risks the development of cross-resistant bacterial strains.

Several public health concerns have arisen as a result of drug resistance. Since the mid-twentieth century, multiple antibiotic resistance has emerged in bacteria, causing pneumonia, gonorrhea, meningitis, and other serious illnesses.

In the 1980's, drug-resistant tuberculosis emerged as a public health concern. In 1991, in New York City, for example, 33 percent of all tuberculosis infections were resistant to at least one drug, and 19 percent were resistant to both of the most effective drugs used to treat the disease. Because of resistance, many tuberculosis patients now require treatment with four drugs for several months. Some patients are required to be directly observed by a health care worker every time they take a dose of medication to ensure compliance. The use of multiple drugs and the need for increased numbers of health care workers greatly increase the cost of treating tuberculosis.

A new challenge appeared in 1997, when patients in Japan and the United States developed infections caused by a highly resistant strain of the bacteria known as *Staphylococcus aureus*. This bacteria is an organism often found on human skin, and it can cause potentially fatal infections when it enters the bloodstream. Shortly after the development of penicillin in the 1940's, it was reported that some strains of this organism, initially highly susceptible to penicillin, had developed resistance to it by producing an enzyme that inactivated it (penicillinase). In response, scientists developed a new generation of penicillins (including methicillin) that could withstand penicillinase. Within a few years, many strains of *staphylococci* developed resistance to methicillin and to all classes of penicillins and related drugs through a different mechanism, an alteration in the bacterial cell wall component to which these drugs bind. Few drugs remained active against these strains of methicillin-resistant *S. aureus* (MRSA); the most reliable and the mainstay of treatment for these infections was vancomycin. In 1997, vancomycin-resistant *Staphylococcus aureus* (VRSA) emerged, threatening to cause major public health problems. Fortunately, in part owing to strict practices of isolation and to heightened awareness of the potential for life-threatening, untreatable infections, VRSA has not yet become a frequent cause of infection. MRSA, however, once found primarily in hospitals and nursing homes, is now frequently found to cause community-acquired infections, including some fatal infections in high school athletes (infected through minor traumatic wounds) and children with complications of influenza.

Another problem bacteria is pneumococcus. This bacterial species was once completely sensitive to penicillin, but now, according to bacteriologist Perry Dickinson, up to 55 percent of the pneumococcal strains are penicillin-resistant. The group most at risk for infection with the drug-resistant *Streptococcus pneumoniae* (DRSP) is children age six or younger. The resistant strains are becoming quite a serious threat among children, but pneumococcus is still vancomycin-sensitive, and some derivatives of penicillin remain effective.

As might be expected, hospitals and nursing homes, where antibiotic usage is highest, are the sites where antibiotic resistance is most common and most complex. The last few decades of the twentieth century saw the development of high levels of resistance among gram-negative bacilli in addition to the gram-positive organisms previously discussed. These organisms frequently cause nosocomial (hospital-acquired) pneumonia, urinary tract infections, surgical wound infections, and other complications. MRSA continues to be a problem in hospitals as well as in the community. It is a major cause of surgical wound infections and infections related to intravenous devices, including hemodialysis accesses. Although VRSA has not yet emerged as a common pathogen, another gram-positive organism, the enterococcus, has acquired resistance to penicillins and vancomycin; vancomycin-resistant enterococci (VRE) are now an important cause of nosocomial infections. These bacteria often give rise to infections in the urinary tracts of patients, but they are also the cause of meningitis, septicemia, and endocarditis. Most frequently, *Enterococcus* is found in children, the elderly, HIV-infected individuals, or the immunologically compromised, whose immune systems are not fully functioning.

TREATMENT AND THERAPY

In the context of emerging drug resistance, treatment of most infections requires culture of the pathogen as well as laboratory testing to establish the antibiotics to which the cultured strain is susceptible, a process that lasts several days. A physician may prescribe an antibiotic in the meantime, using knowledge of prevalent antibiotic susceptibility patterns. Laboratory results may subsequently confirm the effectiveness of that choice or guide selection of a replacement.

The rapidity with which microorganisms develop resistance to antibiotics has been a challenge to pharmaceutical companies, which are working to create a widening array of safe and effective new therapies. Some efforts aim at expanding previously developed lines of antibiotics. For example, a number of drug classes have been derived from penicillins. These "beta-lacatam" antibiotics have a common mechanism of action on bacterial cell walls; modifications have extended their spectrum of activity against an ever-widening variety of organisms and have stabilized them against the activity of penicillinase-like inactivating enzymes. Some of these newer agents include carbapenems and monobactams.

The expanding classes of previously developed drugs include the quinolone antibiotics, derived from nalidixic acid, an early drug for urinary tract infections. Likewise, teicoplanin is chemically related to the glycopeptide vancomycin.

A number of entirely new antibiotics have been developed. One of the most promising new superdrugs, linezolid (Zyvox), developed to combat antibiotic resistance, falls into a new category of antibiotics called oxazolidinones. These drugs act at an early stage in the synthesis of protein by bacteria. Without protein production, bacteria cannot multiply, and they die. The antibiotic linezolid is effective against many gram-positive bacteria, including MRSA, VRSA, VRE, and penicillin-resistant pneumococci. In hospital trials involving patients with MRSA infections, linezolid produced clinical success in more than 83 percent of the patients. The drug can be taken orally or injected, making it quite versatile. Robert Moellering of Harvard University Medical School suggests that this versatility is convenient for patients because they can complete their therapy at home. This drug has also been shown to have few side effects. The streptogramins (qunupristin/dalfopristin) and lipopeptides (daptomycin) are other newly developed classes active against gram-positive bacteria.

While much of the experience and knowledge of drug resistance centers on bacteria, similar problems occur in viruses, fungi, and parasites. Human immunodeficiency virus (HIV) rapidly developed resistance to the early antiretroviral drugs. Despite enormous research and development efforts, drug resistance continues to pose significant challenges in the treatment of HIV infection. Likewise, malaria and tuberculosis are two highly adaptable organisms responsible for a huge proportion of deaths worldwide. Both have developed resistance to many of the available drugs, compounding the difficulties in treating and preventing these infections, particularly in underdeveloped countries with limited resources.

Perspective and Prospects

Several different strategies have been suggested for handling the problem of drug resistance. In general, these strategies involve educating the public and health care workers; monitoring antibiotic, antiviral, and antifungal use; and promoting research into methods to deal with resistant pathogens.

The general public should be aware of the proper use of these medicines as well. Many patients expect to be given antibiotics for illnesses that do not respond to them, such as viral infections. Similarly, they may pressure physicians into prescribing antiviral or antifungal medications even when physicians are aware that these drugs are useless. Patients must learn to understand the difference between a bacterial and a viral infection and how each is treated. Patients must also be educated not to use another person's medicines or an old supply of medicines that they have saved from previous illnesses. Finally, patients must learn to take the entire course of medicines. Often, patients who begin to feel better may fail to take the entire amount

prescribed. This leads to an increased risk of drug-resistant infection if they do not completely eliminate the original infection.

All health care workers should be aware of the importance of avoiding the spread of resistant pathogens from one patient to another. In the late 1990's, about two million Americans per year acquired nosocomial infections. These infections were responsible for about eighty thousand deaths per year. The most important factors in reducing the rate of nosocomial infections are frequent and thorough hand washing, glove changes, and disinfectant applications.

Children should be immunized at a young age against pneumococcal infections. Children who are immunized do not get the infections; hence, no antibiotics are needed, and no extra antibiotics enter into the general population. Additionally, children who are ill should be kept home from day care centers. Day care centers are becoming dangerous incubators, where disease may potentially run rampant. In these places, children spread bacterial infections among themselves, often amplifying pathogenicity and drug resistance. This can be avoided by isolating sick children at home.

Physicians need to be aware of the proper ways to use antibiotics. Microbiologists have suggested better instruction in antibiotic use in medical schools, more continuing education on the subject for practicing physicians, and the development of computer programs to aid physicians in selecting antibiotics. Some have suggested that all physicians prescribing antibiotics in hospitals be required to consult with physicians who specialize in infectious diseases. Standardized order forms that include guidelines for proper use of each antibiotic have also been proposed. Additionally, doctors who have been thoroughly educated must learn not to accede to patient demands for antibiotics, and they must defer antibiotic use in self-limiting infections that will heal on their own. They must also avoid prescribing antibiotics over the phone.

Unfortunately, overall antibiotic prescription rates still seem to be rising, despite warnings of increased antimicrobial resistance. Since 1992, yearly prescriptions have increased by more than thirty million. The most commonly prescribed antibiotic has been amoxicillin, which represents more than 25 percent of the total prescriptions. Erythromycin use has fallen to less than 7 percent, while penicillin and tetracycline use have fallen as well. The new broad-spectrum antibiotics have replaced these drugs and make up more than 10 percent of antibiotic use. Despite the overall increases, the proportion of antibiotic prescriptions for the common cold has decreased to 40 percent from a high of 52 percent in 1994.

Researchers agree that monitoring antibiotic use is critical in fighting drug resistance. A study published in 1997 demonstrated the effectiveness of education and monitoring in reducing resistance. Physicians in Finland were educated in the proper use of the antibiotic erythromycin, and use of the drug was monitored. In 1992, 16.5 percent of bacteria known as group A *Streptococci* were resistant to erythromycin. In 1996, only 8.6 percent were resistant. Some experts have proposed using computers to share information about antibiotic use and resistance among as many health care facilities as possible.

Faster development of new antibiotics for use on multiply resistant bacteria is another improvement. Researchers stress, however, that these new antibiotics must be used only when necessary, in order to avoid promoting resistance to them. Consequently, linezolid and other new antibiotics are being used sparingly.

Other methods have been proposed for minimizing antibiotic resistance. Because patients often expect or demand prescriptions when they visit physicians, some experts have suggested that the physician write a lifestyle prescription when drug use is not appropriate. Such a prescription would explain why antibiotics should not be used in a particular situation and would give the patient specific instructions on how to treat the illness without them.

Eliminating the routine use of antibiotics in farm animals would be of great help. As the Danish study suggests, the risk of resistant bacterial strains in livestock could be reduced, making human lives safer as well.

International concerns over antibiotic resistance are at such a height that in 2000, eight international medical societies gathered to spend a full day discussing the problem. They called this event Global Resistance Day, and the medical professionals discussed the dilemma and solutions for global antibiotic resistance.

—*Rose Secrest; James J. Campanella, Ph.D.;*
Nancy A. Piotrowski, Ph.D.;
updated by Margaret Trexler Hessen, M.D.

See also Antibiotics; Bacterial infections; Bacteriology; Epidemiology; Fungal infections; Hospitals; Iatrogenic disorders; Infection; Microbiology; Mutation; Pharmacology; Pharmacy; Viral infections.

FOR FURTHER INFORMATION:

Brooks, G. F., et al., eds. *Jawetz, Melnick, and Adelberg's Medical Microbiology.* 24th ed. New York: McGraw-Hill, 2007. A comprehensive text with chapters on bacterial cell functions, antibiotics and modes of action, mechanisms of antibiotic resistance and transfer of resistance genes.

Fischback, M. A., and C. T. Walsh. "Antibiotics for Emerging Pathogens." *Science* 325, no. 5944 (August 28, 2009): 1089-1093. Discusses options for developing new antibiotics to circumvent existing bacterial resistance mechanisms.

Levy, Stuart B. *The Antibiotic Paradox: How the Misuse of Antibiotics Destroys Their Curative Powers.* Cambridge, Mass.: Perseus, 2002. A leading researcher in molecular biology explores a modern-day massive evolutionary change in bacteria due to misuse of antibiotics. He argues that a buildup of new antibiotic-resistant bacteria in individuals and in the environment is leading medicine into a dangerous territory where "miracle" drugs may be obsolete.

Science 321, no. 5887 (July 18, 2008). The entire issue of this magazine is devoted to problems of antibiotic resistance, highlighting some particularly difficult infections and discussing some issues pertaining to the genetics of antibiotic resistance.

Shnayerson, Michael, and Mark J. Plotkin. *The Killers Within: The Deadly Rise of Drug Resistant Bacteria.* Boston: Little, Brown, 2003. Traces the evolution of drug-resistant bacteria and how physicians are trying to combat them.

Walsh, Christopher. *Antibiotics: Actions, Origins, Resistance.* Washington, D.C.: ASM Press, 2003. Examines such topics as how antibiotics block specific proteins, how the molecular structure of drugs enables such activity, the development of bacterial resistance, and the molecular logic of antibiotic biosynthesis.

DRUG THERAPY. *See* **ANTIANXIETY DRUGS; ANTIBIOTICS; ANTIDEPRESSANTS; ANTIHISTAMINES; ANTI-INFLAMMATORY DRUGS; CHEMOTHERAPY; DECONGESTANTS; DIURETICS; NARCOTICS; OVER-THE-COUNTER MEDICATIONS; STEROIDS.**

Dwarfism

Disease/disorder

Anatomy or system affected: Back, bones, brain, endocrine system, glands, hips, legs, musculoskeletal system, nervous system, respiratory system

Specialties and related fields: Endocrinology, genetics, orthopedics, pediatrics

Definition: Underdevelopment of the body, most often caused by a variety of genetic or endocrinological dysfunctions and resulting in either proportionate or disproportionate development, sometimes accompanied by other physical abnormalities and/or mental deficiencies.

Key terms:

amino acid: the building blocks of protein

autosomal: refers to all chromosomes except the X and Y chromosomes (sex chromosomes) that determine body traits

cleft palate: a gap in the roof of the mouth, sometimes present at birth and frequently combined with harelip

collagen: protein material of which the white fibers of the connective tissue of the body are composed

hypoglycemia: low blood sugar

laminae: arches of the vertebral bones

spondylosis: a condition characterized by restriction of movement of the vertebral bones; occurs naturally as a child grows

stenosis: any narrowing of a passage or orifice of the body

Causes and Symptoms

A person of unusually small stature is generally termed a "dwarf." Dwarfism in humans may be caused by a number of conditions that occur either before birth or in early childhood. When short stature is the only observable feature, growth—though abnormal relative to height—is proportionate. Short stature is nearly always blamed on endocrinological dysfunction, but few cases are actually the result of endocrinopathy. If shortness is caused by endocrinopathy, it is often attributable to a deficiency in one or two glands: the pituitary gland (which produces growth hormone) and the thyroid gland. Those who are unusually short but have no other obvious disease are divided into two categories: those who were afflicted prenatally and those who were afflicted postnatally. Many of those born "growth-retarded" are actually the result of chromosomal aberrations and skeletal abnormalities; other events that

may cause prenatal growth retardation might include magnesium deficiency (which would prohibit ribosome synthesis and, in turn, halt protein synthesis) or a uterus that is too small. Postnatal growth retardation may be caused by heredity if both parents are short; there is no skeletal abnormality at fault. Other short-statured children may simply mature at a much slower rate, yet grow normally. Typically, one of the parents may have had a late onset of puberty; such children may reach normal height in their late teens.

Unusually short-statured males are those who are shorter than five feet tall; in females, fifty-eight inches and below is short-statured. Children are classified as dwarfs if their height is below the third percentile for their age. When this is the case, doctors will look primarily to four major causes of dwarfism: an underactive or inactive pituitary gland, achondroplasia (failure of normal development in cartilage), emotional or nutritional deprivation, or Turner syndrome (the possession of a single, X, chromosome). If the answer is not found in one of these alternatives, then it may be found in rarer causes, either genetically based or disease-induced.

Growth hormone, also called somatotropin, determines a person's height. Growth hormone does not affect brain growth but may influence the brain's functions. In addition, it may enhance the growth of nerves radiating from the brain so that they can reach their targets. Growth hormone elevates the appetite, increases metabolic rate, maintains the immune system, and works in coordination with other hormones to regulate carbohydrate, protein, lipid, nucleic acid, water, and electrolyte metabolism. Target areas for growth hormone include cell membranes, as well as other cell organelles, in bone, cartilage, bone marrow, adipose tissue, and the liver, kidney, heart, pancreas, mammary glands, ovaries, testes, thymus gland, and hypothalamus. Fetuses not producing growth hormone still grow normally until birth; they may even weigh more than average at birth. These babies may thrive at first, but if no growth hormone is administered, they will be "miniature" adults with a maximum height of two and a half feet. Other telltale physical attributes include higher-than-average body fat, a high forehead, wrinkled skin, and a high-pitched voice. During childhood, there may be episodic hypoglycemia attacks. If the endocrine system is functioning properly, puberty may be delayed but still will occur. Complete reproductive maturity will be reached, and there is great likelihood that the afflicted person will develop his or her complete intellec-

INFORMATION ON DWARFISM

CAUSES: Genetic or endocrinological dysfunctions

SYMPTOMS: Short stature, higher-than-average body fat, high forehead, wrinkled skin, high-pitched voice, episodic hypoglycemia during childhood, late onset of puberty

DURATION: Lifelong

TREATMENTS: Growth hormone

tual potential. When it is inherited, growth hormone deficiency occurs as an autosomal recessive trait. Yet the genetic basis for growth hormone deficiency may not simply be caused by a gene. The condition could, in theory, be the result of a structural defect in the pituitary gland or the hypothalamus, or in the secretory mechanisms of growth hormone itself. Prenatal factors that contribute to growth retardation include toxemia, kidney and heart disease, rubella, maternal malnutrition, maternal age, small uterus, and environmental influences such as alcohol and drug use.

Prenatal thyroid dysfunction that goes untreated results in congenital hypothyroidism, commonly known as cretinism. Child with this disorder do not undergo nervous, skeletal, or reproductive maturation; they may not grow over thirty inches tall. Before two months of age, treatment can cause a complete reversal of symptoms. Delayed treatment, however, cannot reverse brain damage, although growth and reproductive organs can be dramatically affected.

Achondroplasia is the most common form of short-limb dwarfism. It is inherited as an autosomal dominant form of dwarfism. Only when one dominant gene is inherited is achondroplasia expressed; when an offspring inherits the dominant gene from both parents, the condition is lethal. Incidence of achondroplasia increases with parental age and is more closely related to the father's age. Mutations may account for a majority of cases of achondroplasia, since in only 15 to 20 percent of cases is there an afflicted parent. Achondroplasia results from abnormal embryonic development that affects bone growth; metaphyseal development is prevented, which means that cartilaginous bone growth is impaired. This impairment is accompanied by unusually small laminae of the spine, resulting in spinal stenosis. The spinal cord may become compressed during the normal process of spondylosis. These individuals may experience slowly progressing spastic weakness

of the legs as a result of the spinal cord compression. The torso may be normal, but the head will be disproportionately large and the limbs may be dwarfed and curved. In addition, there will be a prominent forehead and a depressed nasal bridge. A shallow thoracic cage and pelvic tilt may cause a protuberant abdomen. Bowlegs are caused by overly long fibulae. Many infants so affected are stillborn. Those surviving to adulthood are typically three feet to five feet tall and have unusual muscular strength; reproductive and mental development are not affected, and neither is longevity.

Marasmus, severe emaciation resulting from malnutrition prenatally or in early infancy, may be considered a form of dwarfism. It is caused by extremely low caloric and protein intake, which causes a wasting of body tissues. Usually marasmus is found in babies either weaned very early or never breast-fed. All growth is retarded, including head circumference. If the area housing the brain fails to grow, then it cannot house a normal-sized brain, and some degree of retardation will occur. Not only is growth stunted, but such infants will be apathetic and hyperirritable as well. As they lie in bed, they are completely unresponsive to their environment and are irritable when moved or handled. Although the symptoms are treatable and may disappear, the growth failure is permanent.

Occasionally, dwarfism may be induced by emotional starvation. This type of child abuse causes extreme growth retardation, inhibition of skeletal growth, and delayed psychomotor development. Fortunately, it can be reversed by social and dietary changes. These children are extremely small but perfectly proportioned; however, they have distended abdomens.

The height achieved in females with Turner syndrome is typically between four and a half and five feet. Turner syndrome results when an egg has no X chromosome and is fertilized by an X-bearing sperm. The offspring are females with only one X; their ovaries never develop and are unable to function. These individuals cannot undergo puberty; physical manifestations of Turner syndrome include short stature, stocky build, and a webbed neck.

Another cause of short stature may be as a consequence of chronic disease. Children suffering from chronic renal (kidney) failure nearly always experience growth retardation because of hormonal, metabolic, and nutritional abnormalities, effects seen in 35 to 65 percent of children with renal failure. The failure to grow occurs more often in children with congenital renal disease than in those with acquired renal disease.

With congenital heart disease, several factors may prohibit growth. Growth failure may be a direct result of the disease or an indirect result of other problems associated with heart disease. These babies experience stress, with periods of cardiac failure, and either caloric or protein deficiency. These inadequacies grossly slow the multiplication of cells and hence growth. If surgery corrects the condition, some catching up can be expected, but normal growth is dependent on how much time has elapsed without treatment.

TREATMENT AND THERAPY

In the United States population in 1992, there were roughly five million people of short stature, with 40 percent of this number under the age of twenty-one. The more a child is below the average stature, the greater is the likelihood of determining the cause. A child who is short-statured should be evaluated so that if an endocrine disorder is the root, the child can be treated. Time is an important consideration with hypothyroidism especially, since the longer it goes untreated, the more likely it is that mental development will be arrested.

Children born with congenital growth hormone deficiency are sometimes small for their gestational age; however, the majority of growth hormone-deficient children acquire the disorder after birth. The first year or two, the children grow normally; then growth dramatically decreases. Diagnosis of growth hormone deficiency requires numerous tests and sampling. If bone age appears the same as the child's age, then growth hormone deficiency can be eliminated. A test for normal growth hormone secretion is done by measuring a blood sample for growth hormone twenty minutes after exercise in a fasting child. If this test shows a hormone deficiency, then growth hormone therapy may help the child overcome the obstacles of being labeled "short."

At first, growth hormone was harvested from human pituitary glands after persons' deaths. This process was so expensive, however, that few children with hormone deficiency could be treated. Even worse, some of those who did get this treatment were inadvertently infected

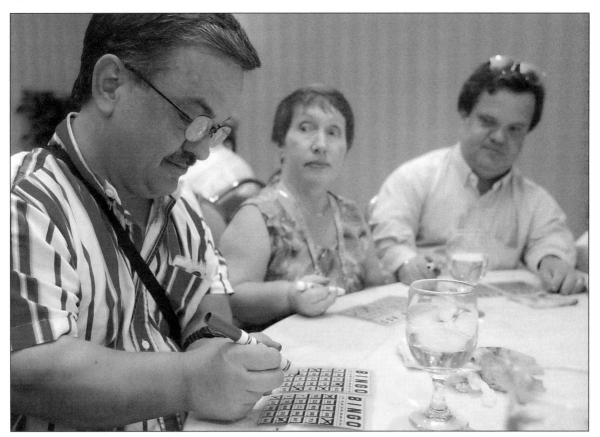

Participants at a convention of Little People of America, an organization for people with dwarfism, play bingo. (AP/Wide World Photos)

with a slow-acting virus that proved fatal. In the mid-1980's, it was found that some men who had received human growth hormone died at an early age of a neurological disorder called Creutzfeldt-Jakob disease (CJD). These men were found to have been given the disease via a growth hormone that had been obtained from pituitary glands during autopsies. Once the relationship was determined, more victims were traced. CJD is a nervous disorder caused by a slow-acting, viruslike particle. Its symptoms include difficulty in balance while walking, loss of muscular control, slurred speech, impairment of vision, and other muscular disorders including spasticity and rigidity. Behavioral changes and mental incapacities may also occur (memory loss, confusion, dementia). The symptoms appear, progress rapidly over the next months, and usually cause death in less than a year. There is no treatment or cure.

These unfortunate circumstances led to the development of a synthetic growth hormone. It is made by encoding bacterial deoxyribonucleic acid (DNA) with the sequence of human growth hormone; the bacteria used are those that grow normally in the human intestinal tract. The bacteria synthesize human growth hormone using the preprogrammed human sequence of DNA; it is then purified so that no bacteria remain in the hormone that is used for treatment. The Food and Drug Administration (FDA) approved the biosynthetic hormone in 1985. The sole difference between the synthetic and the naturally produced growth hormone was one amino acid; in 1987, a new synthetic form without the extra amino acid became available. This synthetic hormone works exactly as natural growth hormone does. Moreover, it does not carry the danger of contamination attributed to human growth hormone. In most cases, the patient's immune system fails to interfere with the synthetic growth hormone's effectiveness. In fact, no major health-threatening side effects have surfaced in using artificial growth hormone. In 1992, more than 150,000 growth hormone-deficient children in the United States were receiving growth hormone therapy.

Those children suffering from various forms of chondrodystrophies (cartilage disorders), such as achondroplasia, are diagnosed by using skeletal measurements, clinical manifestations, X rays, laboratory study and analysis of cartilage, and observed abnormalities of the body's proteins, such as collagen and cell membranes. In chondrodystrophies, skeletal growth is disproportionate, with shortened limbs more common than a shortened trunk. If visual examination is not confirmation enough, the diagnosis may be assured through X rays. Although histological studies do not necessarily enhance diagnosis, making an analysis of the patient's cartilage may lead to a better understanding of the disease. Biochemical studies of abnormal proteins in chondrodystrophies actually have little diagnostic value, but they too may lead to better understanding. Because achondroplasia is genetically inherited, prevention of the affliction involves genetic counseling before conception.

A child so affected may be treated symptomatically; surgery on the fibulae to correct bowlegs may be desirable, either for cosmetic reasons or for functional reasons. Laminectomies or skull surgery may be indicated for neurological problems. Orthodontic surgery may be necessary to correct malocclusions and other dental deformities. If hearing loss occurs because of recurrent ear infections, then corrective surgery may be necessary. Achondroplasiacs generally enjoy a normal life span, barring complications.

Other chondrodystrophies that cause dwarfism may have more severe symptoms than achondroplasia. Cockayne syndrome, a type of progeria, is the sudden onset of premature old age in extremely young children. It is the result of inheritance of an autosomal recessive gene. Physical signs of the disease begin after a normal first year of life. In the second year, growth begins to falter, and psychomotor development becomes abnormal. As time passes, dwarfism, and sometimes mental retardation, becomes evident. Other observable characteristics that develop are a shrunken face with sunken eyes and a thin nose, optic degeneration, cavities of the teeth, a photosensitive skin rash that produces scarring, disproportionately long limbs with large hands and feet, and hair loss. The life span for children with this disease is very short.

Another chondrodystrophy inherited through autosomal recessive genes is thanotophoric dwarfism. All known cases have died during the first four weeks of life as a result of respiratory distress; most are stillborn. Postnatal death occurs as a result of an extremely small thoracic cage with only eleven pairs of ribs present. Other physical characteristics of the disease are that the infant has a large skull relative to its face, which is often elongated with a prominent forehead. The eyes are widely spaced, and there is a broad, flat nasal bridge. Frequently, cleft palate is present. The ears are low-set and poorly formed, and the neck is short and fleshy. The limbs, particularly the legs, are bowed; clubfoot is common, as are dislocated hip joints.

A small percentage of short-statured individuals may be unusually short because of social and psychological factors. This condition is called psychosocial dwarfism. This type of nongrowth is secondary to emotional deprivation and is representative of a type of child abuse. The behavior of such children is characterized by apathy and inadequate interpersonal relationships, with retarded motor and language development. They generally do not gain weight in spite of their extraordinary appetite and excessive thirst; such a child may steal and hoard food yet have the distended abdomen of a starving child. Diagnosis generally identifies a growth hormone deficiency, and when these children are moved to stimulating and accepting environments, their behavior becomes more normal. Their caloric intake decreases as their growth hormone secretion becomes normal, and their growth undergoes a dramatic catch-up.

PERSPECTIVE AND PROSPECTS

Dwarfism is certainly not a new phenomenon. Two well-known Egyptian deities, Bes and Ptah, are represented as dwarfs. At one time, short-statured individuals were attractions in the royal courts. Jeffery Hudson, a favorite of Charles I of England, is said to have been only eighteen inches high at the age of thirty, and Bébé, the celebrated dwarf in the court of Stanisław I of Poland, was thirty-three inches tall. More recently, perfectly proportioned dwarfs have made a living by working in circuses and sideshows. It is likely that the best known of these individuals was P. T. Barnum's General Tom Thumb (Charles Stratton), who at age twenty-five was thirty-one inches tall.

Today, because of the negative consequences of being short-statured, counseling should begin early. Counseling would be preceded by a physical examination to determine the nature of the affliction. If it is ascertained that the short stature cannot be treated, both patient and parents should be informed of the nature of the disease. The patient should be assured that intelligence will not be affected, even if the head is somewhat large. Ear infections are common, and the child should be closely watched to avoid hearing loss. Normal fertility is the rule, but giving birth will necessitate a cesarean section. These characteristics of a majority of dwarfism cases should assure families that, as the child matures, he or she will not be limited physically or mentally. The problems that the patients may face usually deal with social and emotional consequences. Short-statured children will usually be thought younger than their age; finding appropriate clothes and shoes may be difficult. Children are often cruel, and as afflicted individuals are highly noticeable, they may be the butt of jokes and teasing and will experience discrimination on many fronts. Seeking affiliation with support groups may aid in coping with the difficulties that a short-statured person will undoubtedly meet. Additionally, counseling for children and parents of dwarf children should be provided to assist in coping with their anomalies and to facilitate positive outcomes.

The rate at which those diagnosed with dwarfism develop psychologically is directly related to two components: if their parents treat them according to their age rather than their size, and if they can cope with the notoriety that their size brings them. It is common for such children to lag in development; personality traits often exhibited with delayed maturation are withdrawal, inhibition, dissociation, and learning problems. There have been no observed tendencies toward aggression or acting out. Inhibition and withdrawal are likely if affected children are appalled by their notoriety; if they use it to measure popularity, they may act the clown to minimize their size difference.

—Iona C. Baldridge;
updated by Sharon W. Stark, R.N., A.P.R.N., D.N.Sc.

See also Congenital disorders; Congenital heart disease; Congenital hypothyroidism; Cornelia de Lange syndrome; Endocrine disorders; Endocrinology; Endocrinology, pediatric; Gigantism; Growth; Hormones; Metabolic disorders; Rubinstein-Taybi syndrome.

FOR FURTHER INFORMATION:

Adelson, B., and J. Hall. *Dwarfism: Medical and Psychological Aspects of Profound Short Stature.* Baltimore: Johns Hopkins University Press, 2005. Overview of problems related to dwarfism and medical progress in treatment.

Brooks, S. J., and Robert S. Bar. *Early Diagnosis and Treatment of Endocrine Disorders.* Totowa, N.J.: Humana Press, 2003. Reviews the early signs and symptoms of common endocrine diseases, surveys the clinical testing needed for a diagnosis, and presents recommendations for therapy.

Healthline. "Dwarfism." http://www.healthline.com/search?q1=dwarfism. Compilation of articles examining various types of dwarfism and including definitions, causes, and treatments.

Juul, Anders, and Jens O. L. Jorgensen, eds. *Growth Hormone in Adults: Physiological and Clinical Aspects.* 2d ed. New York: Cambridge University Press, 2000. This book examines the use of somatotropin on adults to treat dwarfism.

Kelly, Thaddeus E. *Clinical Genetics and Genetic Counseling.* 2d ed. Chicago: Year Book Medical, 1986. This text of genetic disorders and their treatment was written to aid medical students and physicians. Aside from the sometimes difficult medical terminology, the case illustrations and discussions of genetic counseling are interesting.

Kronenberg, Henry M., et al., eds. *Williams Textbook of Endocrinology.* 11th ed. Philadelphia: Saunders/Elsevier, 2008. Comprehensive information regarding endocrine diseases, pathophysiology, diagnoses, treatment, and prognoses.

Little People of America. http://www.lpaonline.org. A nonprofit organization that provides support and information to people of short stature and their families. Web site offers a research library, FAQs, information on local chapters, and more.

MedlinePlus. "Dwarfism." http://www.nlm.nih.gov/medlineplus/dwarfism.html. This Web site offers an overview of dwarfism and resources from which to obtain additional information.

Morgan, Brian L. G., and Roberta Morgan. *Hormones: How They Affect Behavior, Metabolism, Growth, Development, and Relationships.* Los Angeles: Price, Stern, Sloan, 1989. A book written for use by the general reader as a resource on hormones and their roles in the human body. Very readable, it also contains sections about hormonal diseases and includes a bibliography.

Shaw, Michael, ed. *Everything You Need to Know About Diseases.* Springhouse, Pa.: Springhouse Press, 1996. This well-illustrated consumer reference, compiled by more than one hundred doctors and medical experts, describes five hundred illnesses and conditions, as well as their causes, symptoms, diagnosis, treatment, and prevention. Of particular interest is chapter 21, "Genetic Disorders."

DYSENTERY. *See* DIARRHEA AND DYSENTERY.

DYSKINESIA
DISEASE/DISORDER

ALSO KNOWN AS: Hyperkinesia, levodopa-induced dyskinesia, paroxysmal dyskinesia, tardive dyskinesia

ANATOMY OR SYSTEM AFFECTED: Arms, brain, feet, hands, head, legs, mouth, neck, nerves, nervous system, psychic-emotional system

SPECIALTIES AND RELATED FIELDS: Geriatrics and gerontology, neurology, pharmacology, physical therapy, psychiatry

DEFINITION: Abnormal involuntary movements with different causes and clinical presentations.

KEY TERMS:

anticholinergic: an agent that blocks the neurotransmitter acetylcholine

anticonvulsant: an agent that prevents or relieves seizures

antiemetic: an agent that prevents or relieves nausea and vomiting

basal ganglia: a group of interconnected deep brain nuclei that includes striatum, pallidum, subthalamic nucleus, and substantia nigra

benzodiazepine: any of a group of drugs with strong sedative and hypnotic action

brain stem: a part of the brain that connects the cerebral hemispheres with the spinal cord

dopaminergic: related to the neurotransmitter dopamine; nerve terminals releasing the neurotransmitter dopamine

levodopa: a precursor to the neurotransmitter dopamine, used in treating Parkinson's disease

neuroleptic: an agent that modifies psychotic behavior; in general, synonymous with "antipsychotic"

CAUSES AND SYMPTOMS

There are many types of dyskinesia, with different clinical appearances, pathogenetic mechanisms, and treatment modalities. The most common manifestations are akathisia (restlessness), athetosis (slow, writhing movements), ballism (arm or leg flinging), chorea (jerky, dancelike movements), dystonia (increased muscle tone with repetitive patterned movements and distorted posturing), myoclonus (lightning-fast movements), stereotypy (repetitive, patterned, coordinated ritualistic movements), restless legs, tic, and tremor. These abnormal movements may involve the head, face, mouth, limbs, or trunk. Depending on the specific clinical type, the disease mechanism includes damage to cerebral cortex or subcortical structures such as basal ganglia, brain stem and cerebellum. In adults, multiple neurodegenerative diseases, inherited conditions, vascular disorders (stroke), tumors, infections, malformations, and drug treatments can lead to dyskinesia. In children, abnormal involuntary movements can be caused by genetic conditions, hypoxia, and excessive bilirubin in the nervous system (kernicterus).

Huntington's disease, an autosomal dominant neu-

INFORMATION ON DYSKINESIA

CAUSES: Neurologic, vascular, genetic, or metabolic disorders; pharmacotherapy
SYMPTOMS: Abnormal involuntary movements
DURATION: Acute, chronic
TREATMENTS: Pharmacotherapy, drug treatment modification, deep brain stimulation

rodegenerative disorder, is a common genetic cause of chorea and ballism. Cerebral palsy, overactive thyroid, pregnancy, metabolic abnormalities, and drug-induced disorders are some of the nongenetic causes of choreic motions.

Combinations of various involuntary movements occur in a group of conditions called paroxysmal dyskinesias, characterized by the sudden occurrence of dyskinetic movements (dystonia, chorea, athetosis, ballism), either spontaneous or triggered by an unexpected stimulus.

Neuroleptic-induced tardive dyskinesia and levodopa-induced dyskinesia are the two most common drug-induced abnormal movement syndromes. Tardive dyskinesia manifests with grimacing, masticatory motions of the mouth and tongue, and choreo-athetoid movements of the trunk and limbs. Most often it develops after months or years of neuroleptic treatment, especially with typical antipsychotic drugs (such as haloperidol). Nevertheless, it was observed in schizophrenic patients long before the advent of antipsychotic dopaminergic antagonists, which suggests that these individuals might be susceptible to involuntary movements. It is also known to occur after antiemetic treatment (metoclopramide). The pathophysiology of tardive dyskinesia is not completely understood, but dopaminergic hypersensitivity and oxidative stress are believed to be involved.

Dyskinesia can occur after years of levodopa, or L-dopa, therapy for Parkinson's disease. Some movements appear at the peak blood levels of medication (peak-dose dyskinesia), others when the drug level is peaking and falling (biphasic dyskinesia) and even at low drug levels. Young age, longer disease duration, and high levodopa dosage are known risk factors for these complications. The intricate mechanism generating levodopa-induced dyskinesia involves an interplay between the loss of dopaminergic nerve terminals and long-term drug treatment with pulsatile stimulation of receptors.

TREATMENT AND THERAPY

Therapeutic approaches vary, depending on the type of movement and etiology of dyskinesia. Recommended pharmacologic treatments include benzodiazepines (myoclonus, tremor, dystonia), tetrabenazine (chorea, stereotypy, tremor), anticholinergic agents (dystonia), dopaminergic drugs (restless legs), anticonvulsants (tremor, myoclonus), botulinum toxin (tremors, tics, dystonia), antipsychotics, and brain metabolism enhancers. Deep brain stimulation and repetitive transcranial magnetic stimulation are effective procedures. Stress and activity often aggravate dyskinesia, while relaxation and sleep alleviate it. Physical therapy and self-help groups should be employed as necessary.

In drug-induced dyskinesia, prevention is crucial. Once the levodopa-induced dyskinesia occurs, modification of the Parkinson's disease treatment regimen becomes necessary. Deep brain stimulation and pharmacotherapy (dopaminergic agents, amantadine) are beneficial in certain categories of patients.

Patients treated with neuroleptics should be examined for involuntary movements before commencing therapy and subsequently maintained on the lowest effective dose. If symptoms develop, then dosage reduction is advised. No agent is truly effective in treating tardive dyskinesia, but vitamin E, tetrabenazine and botulinum toxin have been shown to alleviate the symptoms. Mild tardive dyskinesia may improve with benzodiazepines and cholinergic agents. Atypical antipsychotic drugs (clozapine, olanzapine, risperidone) are less prone to inducing dyskinesia and may even be beneficial in patients who develop the symptoms.

PERSPECTIVE AND PROSPECTS

In the sixteenth century, Andrea Vesalius and Francisco Piccolomini distinguished subcortical nuclei from cerebral cortex and white matter. Paracelsus introduced the concept of chorea. The nineteenth century brought the recognition of striatal lesions as causes of chorea and athetosis. Classifications and descriptions for myoclonic movements were introduced. In the late nineteenth century, Gilles de la Tourette and Jean M. Charcot presented cases of tic disorders. A relationship between subthalamic nucleus lesions and ballism was demonstrated in the first half of the twentieth century. Since then, the important role played by this nucleus in hyperkinetic disorders has become evident. In the late twentieth century, genetic mutations were identified in families with dystonia. Therapeutic strategies for levodopa-induced dyskinesia were implemented. Physicians and neuroscientists continue to make significant progress in elucidating the physiology of basal ganglia and the pathogenesis of hyperkinetic movement disorders. Brain imaging, animal models, and molecular techniques are widely used. New modalities of delivering levodopa are being explored. Tardive dyskinesia remains a source of concern as a result of its drug-induced nature. The available data suggest a lower risk of dyskinesia with newer medications. However, more studies of relative risk and appropriate doses are needed.

While attempting to find pathogenesis-targeted therapies, it is imperative to achieve a good understanding of the clinical syndromes and to use comprehensive rating systems. This will allow for more effective patient management, with the goal of improving the quality of life by reducing disability and reliance on caregivers.

—*Mihaela Avramut, M.D., Ph.D.*

See also Cerebral palsy; Huntington's disease; Muscle sprains, spasms, and disorders; Muscles; Nervous system; Neuroimaging; Neurology; Palsy; Parkinson's disease; Seizures; Tics; Tourette's syndrome; Trembling and shaking.

FOR FURTHER INFORMATION:

Bradley, Walter G., et al., eds. *Neurology in Clinical Practice*. 5th ed. Philadelphia: Butterworth Heinemann/Elsevier, 2007.

Jankovic, Joseph. "Treatment of Hyperkinetic Movement Disorders." *Lancet Neurology* 8, no. 9 (September, 2009): 844-856.

Parker, James N., and Philip M. Parker, eds. *The Official Patient's Sourcebook on Tardive Dyskinesia: A Revised and Updated Directory for the Internet Age*. San Diego, Calif.: Icon Health, 2002.

DYSLEXIA

DISEASE/DISORDER

ANATOMY OR SYSTEM AFFECTED: Brain, ears, eyes, nervous system, psychic-emotional system

SPECIALTIES AND RELATED FIELDS: Audiology, neurology, psychology, speech pathology

DEFINITION: Severe reading disability in children with average to above-average intelligence.

KEY TERMS:

auditory dyslexia: the inability to perceive individual sounds that are associated with written language

cognitive: relating to the mental process by which knowledge is acquired

computed tomography (CT) scan: a detailed X-ray picture that identifies abnormalities of fine tissue structure

dysgraphia: illegible handwriting resulting from impaired hand-eye coordination

electroencephalogram: a graphic record of the brain's electrical activity

imprinting: training that overcomes reading problems by use of repeated, exaggerated language drills

kinesthetic: related to sensation of body position, presence, or movement, resulting mostly from the stimulation of sensory nerves in muscles, tendons, and joints

phonetics: the science of speech sounds; also called phonology

visual dyslexia: the inability to translate observed written or printed language into meaningful terms

CAUSES AND SYMPTOMS

Nearly 25 percent of the individuals in the United States and in many other industrialized societies who otherwise possess at least average intelligence cannot read well. Many such people are viewed as suffering from a neurological disorder called dyslexia. This term was first introduced by the German ophthalmologist Rudolf Berlin in the nineteenth century. Berlin defined it as designating all those individuals who possessed average or above-average intelligence quotients (IQs) but who could not read adequately because of their inability to process language symbols. At the same time as Berlin and later, others reported on dyslexic children. These children saw everything perfectly well but acted as if they were blind to all written language. For example, they could see a bird flying but were unable to identify the written word "bird" seen in a sentence.

The problem involved in dyslexia has been defined and redefined many times since its introduction. The modern definition of the disorder, which is close to Berlin's definition, is based on long-term, extensive studies of dyslexic children. These studies have identified dyslexia as a complex syndrome composed of a large number of associated behavioral dysfunctions that are related to visual-motor brain immaturity and/or brain dysfunction. These problems include a poor memory for details, easy distractibility, poor motor skills, visual letter and word reversal, and the inability to distinguish between important elements of the spoken language.

Understanding dyslexia in order to correct this reading disability is crucial and difficult. To learn to read well, an individual must acquire many basic cognitive and linguistic skills. First, it is necessary to pay close attention, to concentrate, to follow directions, and to understand the language spoken in daily life. Next, one must develop an auditory and visual memory, strong sequencing ability, solid word decoding skills, the ability to carry out structural-contextual language analysis, the capability to interpret the written language, a solid vocabulary that expands as quickly as is needed, and speed in scanning and interpreting written language. These skills are taught in good developmental reading programs, but some or all are found to be deficient in dyslexic individuals.

Two basic explanations have evolved for dyslexia. Many physicians propose that it is caused by brain damage or brain dysfunction. Evolution of the problem is attributed to accident, disease, and/or hereditary faults in body biochemistry. Here, the diagnosis of dyslexia is made by the use of electroencephalograms (EEGs), computed tomography (CT) scans, and related neurological technology. After such evaluation is complete, medication is often used to diminish hyperactivity and nervousness, and a group of physical training procedures called patterning is used to counter the neurological defects in the dyslexic individual.

In contrast, many special educators and other researchers believe that the problem of dyslexia is one of dormant, immature, or undeveloped learning centers in the brain. Many proponents of this concept strongly encourage the correction of dyslexic problems by the teaching of specific reading skills. While such experts agree that the use of medication can be of great value, they attempt to cure dyslexia mostly through a process called imprinting. This technique essentially trains dyslexic individuals and corrects their problems via the use of exaggerated, repeated language drills.

Another interesting point of view, expressed by some experts, is the idea that dyslexia may be the fault of the written languages of the Western world. For example, Rudolf F. Wagner notes that Japanese children exhibit an incidence of dyslexia that is less than 1 percent. The explanation for this, say Wagner and others, is that unlike Japanese, the languages of Western countries require both reading from left to right and phonetic word attack. These characteristics—absent in Japanese—may make the Western languages either much harder to learn or much less suitable for learning.

A number of experts propose three types of dyslexia. The most common type and the one most often identified as dyslexia is called visual dyslexia, the lack of

---

INFORMATION ON DYSLEXIA

CAUSES: Unknown; possibly neurological disorder from accident, disease, or hereditary faults in body biochemistry; dormant, immature, or undeveloped learning centers in the brain
SYMPTOMS: Poor written schoolwork, easy distractibility, clumsiness, poor coordination, poor spatial orientation, confused writing and/or spelling, poor left-right orientation
DURATION: Often long term
TREATMENTS: Medication, patterning, teaching of specific reading skills and repeated language drills (imprinting)

---

ability to translate the observed written or printed language into meaningful terms. The major difficulty is that afflicted people see certain words or letters backward or upside down. The resultant problem is that—to the visual dyslexic—any written sentence is a jumble of many letters whose accurate translation may require five or more times as much effort as is needed by an unafflicted person. The other two problems viewed as dyslexia are auditory dyslexia and dysgraphia. Auditory dyslexia is the inability to perceive individual sounds of spoken language. Despite having normal hearing, auditory dyslexics are deaf to the differences between certain vowel and/or consonant sounds, and what they cannot hear they cannot write. Dysgraphia is the inability to write legibly. The basis for this problem is a lack of the hand-eye coordination that is required to write clearly.

Many children who suffer from visual dyslexia also exhibit elements of auditory dyslexia. This complicates the issue of teaching many dyslexic students because only one type of dyslexic symptom can be treated at a time. Also, dyslexia appears to be a sex-linked disorder, being much more common in boys than in girls. Estimates vary between three and seven times as many boys having dyslexia as girls.

TREATMENT AND THERAPY

The early diagnosis and treatment of dyslexia is essential to its eventual correction. Many experts agree that if a treatment begins before the third grade, there is an 80 percent probability that the dyslexia can be corrected. If the disorder remains undetected until the fifth grade, however, success at treating dyslexia is cut in half. If treatment does not begin until the seventh grade, the probability of successful treatment drops below 5 percent.

The preliminary identification of a dyslexic child can be made from symptoms that include poor written schoolwork, easy distractibility, clumsiness, poor coordination, poor spatial orientation, confused writing and/or spelling, and poor left-right orientation. Because numerous nondyslexic children also show many of these symptoms, a second step is required for such identification: the use of written tests designed to identify dyslexics. These tests include the Peabody Individual Achievement Test, the Halstead-Reitan Neuropsychological Test Battery, and the SOYBAR Criterion Tests.

Electroencephalograms and CT scans are often performed in the hope of pinning down concrete brain abnormalities in dyslexic patients. There is considerable disagreement, however, over the value of these techniques, beyond finding evidence of tumors or severe brain damage—both of which may indicate that the condition observed is not dyslexia. Most researchers agree that children who seem to be dyslexic but who lack tumors or damage are no more likely to have EEG or CT scan abnormalities than nondyslexics. An interesting adjunct to EEG use is a technique called brain electrical activity mapping (BEAM). BEAM converts an EEG into a brain map. Viewed by some workers in the area as a valuable technique, BEAM is contested by many others.

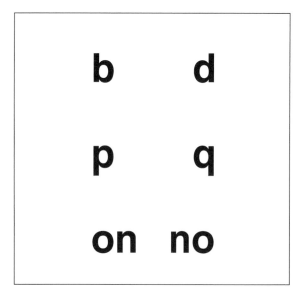

Dyslexia may make it difficult to distinguish letters and words that are mirror images of each other, thus making it difficult for an otherwise intelligent child to learn to read.

Once conclusive identification of a dyslexic child has been made, it becomes possible to begin corrective treatment. Such treatment is usually the preserve of special education programs. These programs are carried out by the special education teacher in school resource rooms. They also involve special classes limited to children with reading disabilities and schools that specialize in treating learning disabilities.

An often-cited method used is that of Grace Fernald, which utilizes kinesthetic imprinting, based on combined language experience and tactile stimulation. In this popular method or adaptations of it, a dyslexic child learns to read in the following way. First, the child tells a spontaneous story to the teacher, who transcribes it. Next, each word that is unrecognizable to the child is written down by the teacher, and the child traces its letters repeatedly until he or she can write the word without using the model. Each word learned becomes part of the child's word file. A large number of stories are handled this way. Though the method is quite slow, many reports praise its results. Nevertheless, no formal studies of its effectiveness have been made.

A second common teaching technique used by special educators is the Orton-Gillingham-Stillman method, which was developed in a collaboration between two teachers and a pediatric neurologist, Samuel T. Orton. The method evolved from Orton's conceptualization of language as developing from a sequence of processes in the nervous system that ends in its unilateral control by the left cerebral hemisphere. He proposed that dyslexia arises from conflicts between this cerebral hemisphere and the right cerebral hemisphere, which is usually involved in the handling of nonverbal, pictorial, and spatial stimuli.

Consequently, the corrective method that is used is a multisensory and kinesthetic approach, like that of Fernald. It begins, however, with the teaching of individual letters and phonemes. Then, it progresses to dealing with syllables, words, and sentences. Children taught by this method are drilled systematically, to imprint them with a mastery of phonics and the sounding out of unknown written words. They are encouraged to learn how the elements of written language look, how they sound, how it feels to pronounce them, and how it feels to write them down. Although the Orton-Gillingham-Stillman method is as laborious as that of Fernald, it is widely used and appears to be successful.

Another treatment aspect that merits discussion is the use of therapeutic drugs in the handling of dyslexia. Most physicians and educators propose the use of these drugs as a useful adjunct to the special education training of those dyslexic children who are restless and easily distracted and who have low morale because of continued embarrassment in school in front of their peers. The drugs that are utilized most often are amphetamine, Dexedrine, and methylphenidate (Ritalin).

These stimulants, given at appropriate dose levels, will lengthen the time period during which certain dyslexic children function well in the classroom and can also produce feelings of self-confidence. Side effects of their overuse, however, include loss of appetite, nausea, nervousness, and sleeplessness. Furthermore, there is also the potential problem of drug abuse. When they are administered carefully and under close medical supervision, however, the benefits of these drugs far outweigh any possible risks.

A proponent of an entirely medical treatment of dyslexia is psychiatrist Harold N. Levinson. He proposes that the root of dyslexia is in inner ear dysfunction and that it can be treated with the judicious application of proper medications. Levinson's treatment includes amphetamines, antihistamines, drugs used against motion sickness, vitamins, health food components, and nutrients mixed in the proper combination for each patient. He asserts that he has cured more than ten thousand dyslexics and documents many cases. Critics of Levinson's work pose several questions, including whether the studies reported were well controlled and whether the patients treated were actually dyslexics. A major basis for the latter criticism is Levinson's statement that many of his cured patients were described to him as outstanding students. The contention is that dyslexic students are never outstanding students and cannot work at expected age levels.

An important aspect of dyslexia treatment is parental support of these children. Such emotional support helps dyslexics to cope with their problems and with the judgment of their peers. Useful aspects of this support include a positive attitude toward an afflicted child, appropriate home help that complements efforts at school, encouragement and praise for achievements, lack of recrimination when repeated mistakes are made, and positive interaction with special education teachers.

Perspective and Prospects

The identification of dyslexia by German physician Rudolf Berlin and England's W. A. Morgan began the efforts to solve this unfortunate disorder. In 1917, Scottish eye surgeon James Hinshelwood published a book on dyslexia, which he viewed as being a hereditary problem, and the phenomenon became much better known to many physicians.

Attempts at educating dyslexics were highly individualized until the endeavors of Orton and his coworkers and of Fernald led to more standardized and widely used methods. These procedures, their adaptations, and several others not mentioned here had become the standard treatments for dyslexia by the late twentieth century.

Many famous people—including Hans Christian Andersen, Winston Churchill, Albert Einstein, George Patton, and Woodrow Wilson—had symptoms of dyslexia, which they subsequently overcame. This was fortunate for them, because adults who remain dyslexic are very often at a great disadvantage. In many cases in modern society, such people are among the functionally illiterate and the poor. Job opportunities open to dyslexics of otherwise adequate intelligence are quite limited.

Furthermore, with the development of a more complete understanding of the brain and its many functions, better counseling facilities, and the conceptualization and actualization of both parent-child and parent-counselor interactions, the probability of success in dyslexic training has improved greatly. Moreover, while environmental and socioeconomic factors contribute relatively little to the occurrence of dyslexia, they strongly affect the outcome of its treatment.

The endeavors of special education have so far made the greatest inroads in the treatment of dyslexia. It is hoped that many more advances in the area will be made as the science of the mind grows and diversifies, and the contributions of psychologists, physicians, physiologists, and special educators mesh even more effectively. Perhaps BEAM or the therapeutic methodology suggested by Levinson may provide or contribute to definitive understanding of and treatment of dyslexia.

—Sanford S. Singer, Ph.D.

See also Brain; Brain disorders; Developmental disorders; Developmental stages; Learning disabilities.

For Further Information:

Huston, Anne Marshall. *Understanding Dyslexia: A Practical Approach for Parents and Teachers.* Rev. ed. Lanham, Md.: Madison Books, 1992. Explains dyslexia, describes its three main types, identifies causes and treatments, and covers useful teaching techniques. A bibliography, a useful glossary, appendixes, and teaching materials are valuable additions.

International Dyslexia Association. http://www.inter dys.org. Association Web site includes a bookstore and information on new assistive technologies. Site is divided into sections for children, teens, college students, adults, educators, and parents.

Jordan, Dale R. *Overcoming Dyslexia in Children, Adolescents, and Adults.* 3d ed. Austin, Tex.: Pro-Ed, 2002. Examines the role of genetics and brain development in relation to learning disabilities and explains the perceptual and emotional nature of dyslexia. Eight "success stories," strategies for improving academic performance and social skills, and assessment checklists are included.

Levinson, Harold N. *Smart but Feeling Dumb: The Challenging New Research on Dyslexia—and How It May Help You.* Rev. ed. New York: Warner Books, 2003. Argues that the basis of dyslexia and other disorders is an inner ear dysfunction that can be cured with judicious application of the correct medications. Also discusses adults and families with dyslexia, speech disorders, and attention deficit disorders.

Reid, Gavin, and Jane Kirk. *Dyslexia in Adults: Education and Employment.* New York: John Wiley & Sons, 2001. Offers a comprehensive guide for professionals to working with adults with dyslexia in the learning and working environment.

Snowling, Margaret. *Dyslexia: A Cognitive Developmental Perspective.* 2d ed. Malden, Mass.: Blackwell, 2002. Covers aspects of dyslexia, including its identification, associated cognitive defects, the basis for language skill development, and the importance of phonetics.

Wolraich, Mark L., ed. *Disorders of Development and Learning: A Practical Guide to Assessment and Management.* 3d ed. Hamilton, Ont.: B. C. Decker, 2003. Summarizes salient facts about learning disorders, including etiology, assessment, management, and outcome.

DYSMENORRHEA
DISEASE/DISORDER

ANATOMY OR SYSTEM AFFECTED: Reproductive system, uterus

SPECIALTIES AND RELATED FIELDS: Gynecology

DEFINITION: A common menstrual disorder characterized by painful menstrual flow that is more severe than the usual cramps experienced by women with menstruation.

CAUSES AND SYMPTOMS

Dysmenorrhea is classified into primary and secondary dysmenorrhea. In primary dysmenorrhea, no organic cause of the menstrual pain is found, although multiple theories exist in the medical literature as to why pain occurs. Dysmenorrhea is associated with a number of psychological symptoms, including depression, irritability, and insomnia, although it is not clear whether these psychological symptoms are causes or effects.

Secondary dysmenorrhea is painful menstruation that occurs in the setting of known pelvic disease, such as endometriosis, adenomyosis, infection such as endometritis or pelvic inflammatory disease (PID), or anatomic abnormalities such as uterine fibroids or developmental abnormalities of the uterus, cervix, or vagina.

The symptoms of dysmenorrhea involve dull lower abdominal pain or cramping at the midline. The discomfort may radiate to the lower back or thighs. It can be associated with a number of other symptoms, most commonly nausea and vomiting or fatigue. Dysmenorrhea can occur up to one to two days before the onset of menstrual flow and usually lasts for forty-eight to seventy-two hours. The most severe pain usually occurs on the first day of menstrual flow.

TREATMENT AND THERAPY

Treatment is recommended if dysmenorrhea interferes with the activities of daily living. The two most common treatments are hormones and nonsteroidal anti-inflammatory drugs (NSAIDs). Ibuprofen is particularly effective and commonly prescribed in doses of 600 and even 800 milligrams every six hours, which exceeds the over-the-counter limits of 400 milligrams every six hours. Ibuprofen should never be taken on an empty stomach or by women with gastric conditions that are contraindications to the drug. In women who do not desire pregnancy, combined hormonal contraception, either in the form of birth control pills, the Ortho Evra patch, or NuvaRing are an effective method of controlling dysmenorrhea, as they can reduce the volume of blood flow. An intrauterine device (IUD) such as Mirena may also be effective. If combined hormonal contraception is utilized, dosing in a continuous or extended fashion can help to reduce symptoms. Application of heat, such as through a heating pad, and exercise provide relief to some women.

In women nearing menopause, hormones that artificially induce menopause can serve as a bridge until natural menopause occurs. In women with primary dys-

INFORMATION ON DYSMENORRHEA

CAUSES: Primary type unknown but associated with psychological symptoms (depression, irritability, insomnia); secondary type caused by pelvic disease (endometriosis or adenomyosis), infection (endometritis or pelvic inflammatory disease), or anatomic abnormalities (uterine fibroids or developmental abnormalities of uterus, cervix, or vagina)

SYMPTOMS: Dull lower abdominal pain or cramping radiating to lower back or thighs; associated with nausea, vomiting, fatigue

DURATION: Two or three days

TREATMENTS: Hormones, prostaglandin synthetase inhibitors, treatment of underlying condition

menorrhea whose symptoms do not improve after six to twelve months of medical treatment, laparoscopy may be considered to search for organic causes of pain.

In secondary dysmenorrhea, the treatment of any underlying pelvic disease may ameliorate the symptoms. For instance, any anatomic abnormalities may be amenable to surgery. Endometriosis may be treated with hormones or removal procedures.

Pain from either primary or secondary amenorrhea is often responsive to prostaglandin synthetase inhibitors, such as ibuprofen. These drugs decrease the levels of prostaglandins (which cause uterine cramping) in the menstrual blood. Patients with psychological symptoms accompanying their dysmenorrhea may benefit from psychological counseling and therapy. In cases of dysmenorrhea that resist standard treatment, a number of alternate treatments have been tried, with varying levels of success. They include nonspecific analgesics (such as opioids), acupuncture, and even surgical procedures such as presacral neurectomy, the interruption of the nerves going to the uterus.

—*Anne Lynn S. Chang, M.D.*

See also Contraception; Endometriosis; Genital disorders, female; Gynecology; Hormones; Menstruation; Pain; Pain management; Pelvic inflammatory disease (PID); Premenstrual syndrome (PMS); Reproductive system; Uterus; Women's health.

FOR FURTHER INFORMATION:

Golub, Sharon. *Periods: From Menarche to Menopause.* Newbury Park, Calif.: Sage, 1992.

Kasper, Dennis L., et al., eds. *Harrison's Principles of Internal Medicine.* 16th ed. New York: McGraw-Hill, 2005.

Minkin, Mary Jane, and Carol V. Wright. *The Yale Guide to Women's Reproductive Health: From Menarche to Menopause.* New Haven, Conn.: Yale University Press, 2003.

Stenchever, Morton A., et al. *Comprehensive Gynecology.* 5th ed. St. Louis, Mo.: Mosby/Elsevier, 2007.

Tierney, Lawrence M., Stephen J. McPhee, and Maxine A. Papadakis, eds. *Current Medical Diagnosis and Treatment 2007.* New York: McGraw-Hill Medical, 2006.

DYSPHASIA. *See* **APHASIA AND DYSPHASIA.**

E. COLI INFECTION

DISEASE/DISORDER

ANATOMY OR SYSTEM AFFECTED: Blood, gastrointestinal system, intestines, nervous system, urinary system

SPECIALTIES AND RELATED FIELDS: Bacteriology, epidemiology, family medicine, gastroenterology, internal medicine, microbiology, neonatology, nephrology, pediatrics, public health, urology

DEFINITION: Infection by a gram-negative bacillus that normally colonizes the gastrointestinal tract of humans and other mammals.

KEY TERMS

conjugation: a process in which two bacteria come together and the donor transfers genetic material (plasmid) to the recipient via tubular bridges called fimbriae

facultative anaerobe: a bacterium that prefers to live and grow in oxygen-rich conditions but can also grow in reduced-oxygen concentration

fimbriae: small hairlike projections on the outside of *E. coli* that enable attachment to human or animal cells; also called pili

plasmids: small, double-stranded loops of deoxyribonucleic acid (DNA) inside bacteria that are independent of the chromosome and capable of autonomous replication

CAUSES AND SYMPTOMS

Escherichia coli (*E. coli*) is a rod-shaped, gram-negative bacterium and a member of the Enterobacteriaceae family. Its cytoplasm is enclosed by an inner membrane, a periplasmic space, a peptidoglycan layer, an outer membrane, and, finally, a capsule. Most strains produce two types of projections, flagellae for motility and fimbriae (pili) for cellular adhesion and genetic transfer. There is no nucleus. The genome consists of a single circular chromosome that is usually complemented by multiple plasmids. There are no intracellular organelles, and respiratory processes occur at the cellular membrane.

E. coli are found as normal flora in the gastrointestinal tracts of mammals and are the most common facultative anaerobes in the human intestinal tract. The traits that transform these benign inhabitants into disease-causing pathogens are called virulence factors. The virulence factors of *E. coli* may be divided into adhesins, toxins, and capsules. Adhesins consist of fimbriae or outer membrane proteins that allow the bacteria to bind to host cells and exert their disease-causing effects.

Toxins are proteins made by *E. coli* that can be released to damage, or even kill, host cells. Capsules can enable the bacteria to elude the immune system and invade host tissues.

Plasmids can be transmitted between various strains of *E. coli* and other bacteria by a process called conjugation. Conjugation might be thought of as "bacterial sex." In order for a bacterium to conjugate, it must possess F (fertility) factor, which is a specific type of plasmid that contains genes for plasmid DNA replication and pili construction. A bacterium with F factor can use its F factor-generated pili to hold onto another bacterium and inject selected portions of genetic material into the bacterial partner. This genetic material can add new virulence factors or antibiotic resistance attributes to the recipient bacterium.

The diseases caused by *E. coli* may be divided into intestinal and extraintestinal. The *E. coli* strains causing intestinal diseases are of several different types. Enteropathogenic *E. coli* (EPEC) cause disease by adhering to intestinal epithelial cells with an outer membrane adhesin (intimin) and special pili, both of which are plasmid-mediated. The exact mechanism by which these virulence factors alter the intestine—resulting in watery diarrhea, low-grade fever, and vomiting—is unclear. Enterotoxigenic *E. coli* (ETEC) cause illness using a combination of mucosal adherence and toxin production. The enterotoxin is similar to cholera toxin and alters ionic transfer in the intestinal cells, producing copious amounts of watery diarrhea. The illness can vary greatly, from a lack of symptoms to severe diarrhea with cramps, nausea, and dehydration. The adhesins and toxins appear to be mediated by both chromosomal and plasmid genes. Some *E. coli* have acquired genes from *Shigella dysenteriae* via conjugation, and these strains can produce Shiga toxins (STEC). The toxins permit intestinal invasion resulting in painful, bloody di-

---

INFORMATION ON
E. COLI INFECTION

CAUSES: Bacterial infection

SYMPTOMS: Stomach cramping, fever, watery or bloody diarrhea, bowel wall inflammation, difficulty urinating, platelet and red blood cell destruction, organ damage

DURATION: Acute

TREATMENTS: None; symptom management and supportive therapy

arrhea indistinguishable from shigellosis; such strains are referred to as enterohemorrhagic (EHEC). In about 5 percent of cases, Shiga toxins enter the bloodstream, causing damage to red blood cells, endothelial cells, and kidney cells; this is called the hemolytic-uremic syndrome (HUS). The life-threatening HUS is usually associated with the O157:H7 strain of *E. coli* and is seen more often in children than in adults. The O157:H7 strain often colonizes cattle, and humans may then acquire the infection from eating beef or fresh vegetables contaminated by cattle manure.

The extraintestinal diseases caused by *E. coli* vary widely. *E. coli* is the most common cause of urinary tract infections (UTIs). The strains that cause UTIs are different from those strains that colonize healthy individuals. These uropathogenic *E. coli* possess fimbriae the bind to cells lining the urinary tract. They are also encapsulated and produce a toxin (hemolysin). The *E. coli* may ascend the urinary tract through the urethra to the bladder and kidney. The route is more common in women because of a shorter urethra and can be facilitated in both men and women by the use of a urinary catheter. Infection of the kidney can also occur via the bloodstream. *E. coli* infection can follow surgery, especially when the intestinal tract is violated. Surgical wound infection, abscesses, and peritonitis are possible. Because ducts connect the gallbladder and pancreas directly with the intestinal lumen, *E. coli* often play a prominent role in cholecystitis and pancreatitis. Newborns with undeveloped immune systems may experience ear infections, bacteremia, or meningitis caused by *E. coli*. The strains producing neonatal meningitis have a K1 capsule, which may facilitate passage into the brain. Because *E. coli* are so common and possess many virulence factors, they can produce many additional types of infection.

TREATMENT AND THERAPY

Mild cases of diarrhea caused by EPEC strains usually can be managed with fluids and other supportive therapies, but the duration of illness may be made shorter with the use of antibiotic therapy. ETEC diarrhea is treated with loperamide and oral antibiotics. STEC and HUS are treated with supportive care. HUS may require renal dialysis.

Extraintestinal infection is treated by antibiotic therapy. Since *E. coli* are becoming increasingly resistant to antibiotics, susceptibility testing on the particular strain of *E. coli* causing the infection isolated from diagnostic cultures must be utilized.

PERSPECTIVE AND PROSPECTS

Escherichia coli is named after Theodore Escherich, who described the bacterium in a paper published in 1885. Frederick Blattner of the University of Wisconsin completed the sequencing of the 4,288 genes of the *E. coli* genome in 1997. Nearly half of these genes were newly identified. In an effort to further understand the genome and biochemical machinery of *E. coli*, a constantly evolving informatics database is available on the Internet at http://ecocyc.org.

Epidemiological studies have assisted in the understanding of the origins of *E. coli* infections. Intestinal illness can be prevented with improved farming methods, better food processing and handling, expanded sewage and sanitation facilities, clean drinking water, and handwashing. Hospital-acquired infection, such as UTIs, can be reduced by limiting the use of urinary catheters and the employment of closed drainage systems when catheters are necessary.

The treatment of extraintestinal *E. coli* infection, and some intestinal infections, depends upon the use of one or more effective antibiotics. Resistance is a rapidly growing problem and can be controlled only thorough reduction of the inappropriate use of antibiotics and the development of new agents.

H. Bradford Hawley, M.D.

See also Antibiotics; Bacterial infections; Bacteriology; Centers for Disease Control and Prevention (CDC); Colitis; Diarrhea and dysentery; Drug resistance; Food poisoning; Gastroenteritis; Gastroenterology; Gastroenterology, pediatric; Gastrointestinal disorders; Gastrointestinal system; Hemolytic uremic syndrome; Infection; Intestinal disorders; Intestines; Meningitis; Microbiology; Mutation; Renal failure.

FOR FURTHER INFORMATION:

Alcamo, I. Edward. *Fundamentals of Microbiology.* 6th ed. Sudbury, Mass.: Jones and Bartlett, 2001. This is an outstanding textbook of basic microbiology by a now deceased author.

Forbes, Betty A., Daniel F. Sahm, and Alice S. Weissfeld. *Bailey & Scott's Diagnostic Microbiology.* 12th ed. St. Louis: Mosby Elsevier, 2007. This microbiology text describes the bacteria and their diseases.

Koneman, Elmer W. *The Other End of the Microscope: The Bacteria Tell Their Own Story.* Washington, D.C.: ASM Press, 2002. An entertaining book that tells the story of bacteria and infections as told by bacteria meeting at a fantasy conference by a small pond.

Mandell, Gerald L., John E. Bennett, and Raphael Dolin, eds. *Principles and Practice of Infectious Diseases*. 7th ed. 2 vols. Philadelphia: Churchill Livingstone Elsevier, 2010. The standard reference text on infectious diseases. Contains a chapter covering the Enterobacteriaceae.

EAR INFECTIONS AND DISORDERS

DISEASE/DISORDER

ANATOMY OR SYSTEM AFFECTED: Ears

SPECIALTIES AND RELATED FIELDS: Audiology, neurology, otorhinolaryngology

DEFINITION: Infections or disorders of the outer, middle, or inner ear, which may result in hearing impairment or loss.

KEY TERMS:

conductive loss: a hearing loss caused by an outer-ear or middle-ear problem which results in reduced transmission of sound

frequency: the number of vibrations per second of a source of sound, measured in hertz; correlates with perceived pitch

intensity of sound: the physical phenomenon that correlates approximately with perceived loudness; measured in decibels

otitis: any inflammation of the outer or middle ear

sensorineural loss: a hearing loss caused by a problem in the inner ear; this impairment is caused by a hair cell or nerve problem and is usually not amenable to surgical correction

CAUSES AND SYMPTOMS

The hearing mechanism, one of the most intricate and delicate structures of the human body, consists of three sections: the outer ear, the middle ear, and the inner ear. The outer ear converts sound waves into the mechanical motion of the eardrum (tympanic membrane), and the middle ear transmits this mechanical motion to the inner ear, where it is transformed into nerve impulses sent to the brain.

The outer ear consists of the visible portion, the ear canal, and the eardrum. The middle ear is a small chamber containing three tiny bones—the auditory ossicles, termed malleus (hammer), incus (anvil), and stapes (stirrup)—which transmit the vibrations of the eardrum (attached to the hammer) into the inner ear. The chamber is connected to the back of the throat by the Eustachian tube, which allows equalization with the external air pressure. The inner ear, or cochlea, is a fluid-filled cavity containing the complex structure necessary to

---

> ### INFORMATION ON EAR INFECTIONS AND DISORDERS
>
> **CAUSES:** Infection, buildup of earwax, fluid retention, injury, fungal growth, allergies, exposure to loud noise, sudden change in air pressure, certain drugs
>
> **SYMPTOMS:** Hearing impairment or loss, itchiness, pain, inflammation, discharge, tinnitus
>
> **DURATION:** Temporary to chronic
>
> **TREATMENTS:** Wide ranging; can include flushing ear with a warm solution under pressure, antibiotics, surgery

---

convert the mechanical vibrations of the cochlear fluid into nerve pulses. The cochlea, shaped something like a snail's shell, is divided lengthwise by a slightly flexible partition into upper and lower chambers. The upper chamber begins at the oval window, to which the stirrup is attached. When the oval window is pushed or pulled by the stirrup, vibrations of the eardrum are transformed into cochlear fluid vibrations.

The lower surface of the cochlear partition, the basilar membrane, is set into vibration by the pressure difference between the fluids of the upper and lower ducts. Lying on the basilar membrane is the organ of Corti, containing tens of thousands of hair cells attached to the nerve transmission lines leading to the brain. When the basilar membrane vibrates, the cilia of these cells are bent, stimulating them to produce electrochemical impulses. These impulses travel along the auditory nerve to the brain, where they are interpreted as sound.

Although well protected against normal environmental exposure, the ear, because of its delicate nature, is subject to various infections and disorders. These disorders, which usually lead to some hearing loss, can occur in any of the three parts of the ear.

The ear canal can be blocked by a buildup of waxy secretions or by infection. Although earwax serves the useful purpose of trapping foreign particles that might otherwise be deposited on the eardrum, if the canal becomes clogged with an excess of wax, less sound will reach the eardrum, and hearing will be impaired.

Swimmer's ear, or otitis externa, is an inflammation caused by contaminated water which has not been completely drained from the ear canal. A moist condition in a region with little light favors fungal growth. Symptoms of swimmer's ear include an itchy and tender ear canal and a small amount of foul-smelling drainage. If the canal is allowed to become clogged by the concomitant swelling, hearing will be noticeably impaired.

A perforated eardrum may result from a sharp blow to the side of the head, an infection, the insertion of objects into the ear, or a sudden change in air pressure (such as a nearby explosion). Small perforations are usually self-healing, but larger tears require medical treatment.

Inflammation of the middle ear, acute otitis media, is one of the most common ear infections, especially among children. Infection usually spreads from the throat to the middle ear through the Eustachian tube. Children are particularly susceptible to this problem because their short Eustachian tubes afford bacteria in the throat easy access to the middle ear. When the middle ear becomes infected, pus begins to accumulate, forcing the eardrum outward. This pressure stretches the auditory ossicles to their limit and tenses the ligaments so that vibration conduction is severely impaired. Untreated, this condition may eventually rupture the eardrum or permanently damage the ossicular chain. Furthermore, the pus from the infection may invade nearby structures, including the facial nerve, mastoid bones, the inner ear, or even the brain. The most common symptom of otitis is a sudden severe pain and an impairment of hearing resulting from the reduced mobility of the eardrum and the ossicles.

Secretory otitis media is caused by occlusion of the Eustachian tube as a result of conditions such as a head cold, diseased tonsils and adenoids, sinusitis, improper blowing of the nose, or riding in unpressurized airplanes. People with allergic nasal blockage are particularly prone to this condition. The blocked Eustachian tube causes the middle-ear cavity to fill with a pale yellow, noninfected discharge which exerts pressure on the eardrum, causing pain and impairment of hearing. Eventually, the middle-ear cavity is completely filled with fluid instead of air, impeding the movement of the ossicles and causing hearing impairment.

A mild, temporary hearing impairment resulting from airplane flights is termed aero-otitis media. This disorder results when a head cold or allergic reaction does not permit the Eustachian tube to equalize the air pressure in the middle ear with atmospheric pressure when a rapid change in altitude occurs. As the pressure outside the eardrum becomes greater than the pressure within, the membrane is forced inward, while the opening of the tube into the upper part of the throat is closed by the increased pressure. Symptoms are a severe sense of pressure in the ear, pain, and hearing impairment.

Although the pressure difference may cause the eardrum to rupture, more often the pain continues until the middle ear fills with fluid or the tube opens to equalize pressure.

Chronic otitis media may result from inadequate drainage of pus during the acute form of this disease or from a permanent eardrum perforation that allows dust, water, and bacteria easy access to the middle-ear cavity. The main symptoms of this disease are fluids discharging from the outer ear and hearing loss. Perforations of the eardrum result in hearing loss because of the reduced vibrating surface and a buildup of fibrous tissue that further induces conductive losses. In some cases, an infection may heal but still cause hearing loss by immobilizing the ossicles. There are two distinct types of chronic otitis, one relatively harmless and the other quite dangerous. An odorless, stringy discharge from the mucous membrane lining the middle ear characterizes the harmless type. The dangerous type is characterized by a foul-smelling discharge coming from a bone-invading process beneath the mucous lining. If neglected, this process can lead to serious complications, such as meningitis, paralysis of the facial nerve, or complete sensorineural deafness.

The ossicles may be disrupted by infection or by a jarring blow to the head. Most often, a separation of the

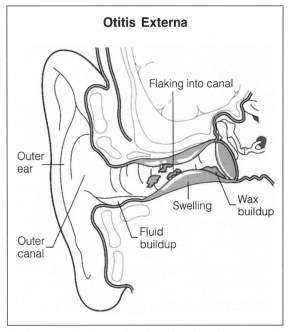

Otitis externa (swimmers' ear) results when the outer ear is inflamed by contaminated water that has not been completely drained from the ear canal.

linkage occurs at the weakest point, where the anvil joins the stirrup. A partial separation results in a mild hearing loss, while complete separation causes severe hearing impairment.

Disablement of the mechanical linkage of the middle ear may also occur if the stirrup becomes calcified, a condition termed otosclerosis. The normal bone is resorbed and replaced by very irregular, often richly vascularized bone. The increased stiffness of the stirrup produces conductive hearing loss. In extreme cases, the stirrup becomes completely immobile and must be surgically removed. Although the exact cause of this disease is unknown, it seems to be hereditary. About half of the cases occur in families in which one or more relatives have the same condition, and it occurs more frequently in females than in males. There is also some evidence that the condition may be triggered by a lack of fluoride in drinking water and that increasing the intake of fluoride may retard the calcification process.

Tinnitus is characterized by ringing, hissing, or clicking noises in the ear that seem to come and go spontaneously without any sound stimulus. While technically tinnitus is not a disease of the ear, it is a common symptom of various ear problems. Possible causes of tinnitus are earwax lodged against the eardrum, a perforated or inflamed eardrum, otosclerosis, high aspirin dosage, or excessive use of the telephone. Tinnitus is most serious when caused by an inner-ear problem or by exposure to very intense sounds, and it often accompanies hearing loss at high frequencies.

Ménière's disease is caused by production of excess cochlear fluid, which increases the pressure in the cochlea. This condition may be precipitated by allergy, infection, kidney disease, or any number of other causes, including severe stress. The increased pressure is exerted on the walls of the semicircular canals, as well as on the cochlear partition. The excess pressure in the semicircular canals (the organs of balance) is interpreted by the brain as a rapid spinning motion, and the victim experiences abrupt attacks of vertigo and nausea. The excess pressure in the cochlear partition has the same effect as a very loud sound and rapidly destroys hair cells. A single attack causes a noticeable hearing loss and could result in total deafness without prompt treatment.

Of all ear diseases, damage to the hair cells in the cochlea causes the most serious impairment. Cilia may be destroyed by high fevers or from a sudden or prolonged exposure to intensely loud sounds. Problems include

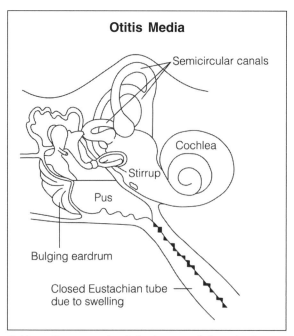

Otitis media occurs when infection spreads from the throat to the middle ear via the Eustachian tube; it is a serious condition which, left untreated, may lead to permanent ear damage and even infection of the brain.

destroyed or missing hair cells, hair cells that fire spontaneously, and damaged hair cells that require unusually strong stimuli to excite them. At the present time, there is no means of repairing damaged cilia or of replacing those which have been lost.

Viral nerve deafness is a result of a viral infection in one or both ears. The mumps virus is one of the most common causes of severe nerve damage, with the measles and influenza viruses as secondary causes.

Ototoxic (ear-poisoning) drugs can cause temporary or permanent hearing impairment by damaging auditory nerve tissues, although susceptibility is highly individualistic. A temporary decrease of hearing (in addition to tinnitus) accompanies the ingestion of large quantities of aspirin or quinine. Certain antibiotics, such as those of the mycin family, may also create permanent damage to the auditory nerves.

Repeated exposure to loud noise (in excess of 90 decibels) will cause a gradual deterioration of hearing by destroying cilia. The extent of damage, however, depends on the loudness and the duration of the sound. Rock bands often exceed 110 decibels; farm machinery averages 100 decibels.

Presbycusis (hearing loss with age) is the inability to hear high-frequency sounds because of the increasing deterioration of the hair cells. By age thirty, a perceptible high-frequency hearing loss is present. This deterioration progresses into old age, often resulting in severe impairment. The problem is accelerated by frequent unprotected exposure to noisy environments. The extent of damage depends on the frequency, intensity, and duration of exposure, as well as on the individual's predisposition to hearing loss.

TREATMENT AND THERAPY

The simplest ear problems to treat are a buildup of earwax, swimmer's ear, and a perforated eardrum. A large accumulation of wax in the ear canal is best removed by having a medical professional flush the ear with a warm solution under pressure. One should never attempt to remove wax plugs with a sharp instrument. A small accumulation of earwax may be softened by a few drops of baby oil left in the ear overnight, then washed out with warm water and a soft rubber ear syringe. Swimmer's ear can usually be prevented by thoroughly draining the ears after swimming. The disease can be treated by an application of antibiotic eardrops after the ear canal has been thoroughly cleaned. A small perforation of the eardrum will usually heal itself. Larger tears, however, require an operation, tympanoplasty, that grafts a piece of skin over the perforation.

Fortunately, the bacteria that usually cause acute otitis respond quickly to antibiotics. Although antibiotics may relieve the symptoms, complications can arise unless the pus is thoroughly drained. The two-part treatment—draining the fluid from the middle ear and antibiotic therapy—resolves the acute otitis infection within a week. Secretory otitis is cured by finding and removing the cause of the occluded Eustachian tube. The serous fluid is then removed by means of an aspirating needle or by an incision in the eardrum so as to inflate the tube by forcing air through it. In some cases, a tiny polyethylene tube is inserted through the eardrum to aid in reestablishing normal ventilation. If the Eustachian tube remains inadequate, a small plastic grommet may be inserted. The improvement in hearing is often immediate and dramatic. The pain and hearing loss of aero-otitis is usually temporary and disappears of its own accord. If, during or immediately after flight, yawning or swallowing does not allow the Eustachian tube to open and equalize the pressure, medicine or surgical puncture of the eardrum may be required. The harmless form of chronic otitis is treated with applied medications to kill the bacteria and to dry the chronic drainage. The eardrum perforation may then be closed

to restore the functioning of the ear and to recover hearing. The more dangerous chronic form of this disease does not respond well to antibacterial agents, but careful X-ray examination allows diagnosis and surgical removal of the bone-eroding cyst.

Ossicular interruption can be surgically treated to restore the conductive link by repositioning the separated bones. This relatively simple operation has a very high success rate. Otosclerosis is treated by operating on the stirrup in one of several ways. The stirrup can be mechanically freed by fracturing the calcified foot plate, or by fracturing the foot plate and one of the arms. Although this operation is usually successful, recalcification often occurs. Alternatively, the stirrup can be completely removed and replaced by a prosthesis of wire or silicon, yielding excellent and permanent results.

Since tinnitus has many possible, and often not readily identifiable, causes, only about 10 percent of the cases are treated successfully. The tinnitus masker has been invented to help sufferers live with this annoyance. The masker, a noise generator similar in appearance to a hearing aid, produces a constant, gentle humming sound which masks the tinnitus.

Ménière's disease, usually treated by drugs and a restricted diet, may also require surgical correction to relieve the excess pressure in severe cases. If this procedure is unsuccessful, the nerves of the inner ear may be cut. In drastic cases, the entire inner ear may be removed.

Presently there is no cure for damaged hair cells; the only treatment is to use a hearing aid. It is more advantageous to take preventive measures, such as reducing noise at the source, replacing noisy equipment with quieter models, or using ear protection devices. Recreational exposure to loud music should be severely curtailed, if not completely eliminated.

PERSPECTIVE AND PROSPECTS

For many centuries, treatment of the ear was associated with that of the eye. In the nineteenth century, the development of the laryngoscope (to examine the larynx) and the otoscope (to examine the ears) enabled doctors to examine and treat disorders such as croup, sore throat, and draining ears, which eventually led to the control of these diseases. As an offshoot of the medical advances made possible by these technological devices, the connection between the ear and throat became known, and otologists became associated with laryngologists.

The study of ear diseases did not develop scientifically until the early nineteenth century, when Jean-Marc-Gaspard Itard and Prosper Ménière made systematic investigations of ear physiology and disease. In 1853, William R. Wilde of Dublin published the first scientific treatise on ear diseases and treatments, setting the field on a firm scientific foundation. Meanwhile, the scientific investigation of the diseased larynx was aided by the laryngoscope, invented in 1855 by Manuel Garcia, a Spanish singing teacher who used his invention as a teaching aid. During the late nineteenth century, this instrument was adopted for detailed studies of larynx pathology by Ludwig Türck and Jan Czermak, who also adapted this instrument to investigate the nasal cavity, which established the link between laryngology and rhinology. Friedrich Voltolini, one of Czermak's assistants, further modified the instrument so that it could be used in conjunction with the otoscope. In 1921, Carl Nylen pioneered the use of a high-powered binocular microscope to perform ear surgery. The operating microscope opened the way for delicate operations on the tiny bones of the middle ear. With the founding of the American Board of Otology in 1924, otology (later otolaryngology) became the second medical specialty to be formally established in North America.

Prior to World War II, the leading cause of deafness was the various forms of ear infection. Advances in technology and medicine have now brought ear infections under control. Today the leading type of hearing loss in industrialized countries is conductive loss, which occurs in those who are genetically predisposed to such loss and who have had lifetime exposure to noise and excessively loud sounds. In the future, ear protection devices and reasonable precautions against extensive exposure to loud sounds should reduce the incidence of hearing loss to even lower levels.

—*George R. Plitnik, Ph.D.*

See also Altitude sickness; Audiology; Balance disorders; Deafness; Decongestants; Ear surgery; Ears; Earwax; Hearing; Hearing aids; Hearing loss; Hearing tests; Ménière's disease; Motion sickness; Myringotomy; Nasopharyngeal disorders; Neurology; Neurology, pediatric; Otoplasty; Otorhinolaryngology; Sense organs; Sinusitis; Speech disorders; Tinnitus; Tonsillitis.

For Further Information:

Canalis, Rinaldo, and Paul R. Lambert, eds. *The Ear: Comprehensive Otology*. Philadelphia: Lippincott Williams & Wilkins, 2000. A text covering all aspects of otology.

Dugan, Marcia B. *Living with Hearing Loss*. Washington, D.C.: Gallaudet University Press, 2003. Offers a range of practical advice for those with hearing loss, including strategies for dealing with everyday situations and emergencies, speech reading (lipreading), oral interpreters, and assertive communication.

Ferrari, Mario. *PDxMD Ear, Nose, and Throat Disorders*. Philadelphia: PDxMD, 2003. A clinical yet accessible reference text that provides a comprehensive list of disorders, with a summary of the condition, background, diagnosis, treatment, outcomes, prevention, and resources.

Friedman, Ellen M., and James M. Barassi. *My Ear Hurts! A Complete Guide to Understanding and Treating Your Child's Ear Infections*. Darby, Pa.: Diane, 2004. Reviews current research on ear infections and reviews a range of treatment approaches from both conventional and alternative medicine.

Greene, Alan R. *The Parent's Complete Guide to Ear Infections*. Reprint. Allentown, Pa.: People's Medical Society, 2004. Every parent who has ever had a child with recurrent otitis will appreciate this book. It explains the anatomy of normal ears, causes of infections, prevention, symptoms, evaluation, initial and ongoing treatment, antibiotics, the pros and cons of surgical intervention, hearing loss, tubes, and complications.

Jerger, James, ed. *Hearing Disorders in Adults: Current Trends*. San Diego, Calif.: College-Hill Press, 1984. A reliable and readable introductory treatise on common hearing disorders.

Kemper, Kathi J. *The Holistic Pediatrician: A Pediatrician's Comprehensive Guide to Safe and Effective Therapies for the Twenty-five Most Common Ailments of Infants, Children, and Adolescents*. Rev. ed. New York: Quill, 2002. Integrates mainstream and alternative medicine to aid parents in dealing with the most common childhood health problems such as diaper rash, ear infections, and allergies.

"Lack of Consensus About Surgery for Ear Infections." *Health News* 18, no. 3 (June/July, 2000): 11. Children who suffer from recurrent otitis media, or ear infections, may be candidates for a surgical procedure called "myringotomy," which involves the insertion of tiny tubes into the eardrums. The goal of the surgery is to prevent future infections and reduce the chances of hearing loss.

Pender, Daniel J. *Practical Otology*. Philadelphia: J. B.

Lippincott, 1992. A well-illustrated text on diseases of the ear and their surgical correction.

Roland, Peter S., Bradley F. Marple, and William L. Meyerhoff, eds. *Hearing Loss*. New York: Thieme, 1997. Provides information on hearing disorders and discusses the anatomy and physiology of the ear.

EAR, NOSE, AND THROAT MEDICINE. *See* OTORHINOLARYNGOLOGY.

EAR SURGERY

PROCEDURE

ANATOMY OR SYSTEM AFFECTED: Bones, ears, musculoskeletal system, nervous system

SPECIALTIES AND RELATED FIELDS: Audiology, general surgery, otorhinolaryngology, speech pathology

DEFINITION: An invasive procedure to correct structural problems of the ear that produce some degree of hearing loss.

KEY TERMS:

cochlea: a structure in the inner ear that receives sound vibrations from the ossicles and transmits them to the auditory nerve

myringotomy: incision of the tympanic membrane used to drain fluid and reduce middle-ear pressure

ossicles: tiny bones located between the eardrum and the cochlea

otosclerosis: a condition in which the stapes becomes progressively more rigid, and hearing loss results

stapedectomy: a surgical procedure in which the stapes is replaced with an artificial substitute

stapes: the ossicle that makes contact with the cochlea

tympanic membrane: the eardrum, which separates the external ear canal from the middle ear and ossicles and which transmits sound vibration to the ossicles

tympanoplasty: a surgical procedure to repair the tympanic membrane

INDICATIONS AND PROCEDURES

Humans are able to detect sound because of the interaction between the ears and the brain. When sound waves strike the tympanic membrane (eardrum), it vibrates. The movement of the tympanic membrane then causes the movement of the ossicles, the three tiny bones within the middle ear (malleus, incus, and stapes). These moving bones transfer the vibrations to the cochlea of the inner ear, which stimulates the auditory nerve and eventually the brain.

Hearing problems may result when any part of the ear is damaged. Hearing difficulties can be categorized into two main areas: conductive and sensorineural hearing loss. In conductive hearing loss, the ear loses its ability to transmit sound from the external ear to the cochlea. Common causes include earwax buildup in the outer ear canal; otosclerosis, in which the stapes loses mobility and cannot stimulate the cochlea effectively; and otitis media, in which the middle ear becomes infected and a sticky fluid is produced which causes the ossicles to become inflexible. Otitis media is the most common cause of conductive hearing loss and typically occurs in children. If antibiotics such as amoxicillin or ampicillin fail to clear the ear of infection, surgery may be required. Sensorineural hearing loss results from damage to the cochlea or auditory nerve. Common causes include loud noises, rubella (a type of viral infection) during embryonic development, and certain drugs such as gentamicin and streptomycin. Occasionally, a tumor (neuroma) of the auditory nerve may cause sensorineural hearing loss.

Myringotomy is a surgical procedure in which an incision is made in the tympanic membrane to allow drainage of fluid (effusion) from the middle ear to the external ear canal. The surgeon usually performs this operation to treat recurrent otitis media, a condition in which pressure builds in the middle ear and pushes outward on the tympanic membrane. The patient, usually a child, is given general anesthesia. An incision is made in the eardrum so that a small tube can be inserted to allow continuous drainage of the pus. The tube usually falls out in a few months, and the tympanic membrane heals rapidly.

Otosclerosis, the overgrowth of bone that impedes the movement of the stapes, can be treated by stapedectomy (surgical removal of the stapes). General anesthesia is used to prevent pain or movement when an incision is made in the ear canal and the tympanic membrane is folded to access the ossicles. The stapes can then be removed and a metal or plastic prosthesis inserted in its place. The eardrum is then repaired.

Tympanoplasty is an operation to repair the tympanic membrane or ossicles. Sudden pressure changes in an airplane or during deep-sea diving may perforate the tympanic membrane (barotrauma) and require tympanoplasty. The procedure is similar to stapedectomy. With the patient under general anesthesia, an incision is made next to the eardrum to provide access to the tympanic membrane and ossicles. The tympanic membrane may need to be repaired if the perforated eardrum does not heal on its own. An operating microscope is employed for optimal visualization of the middle ear. If the tympanoplasty involves the ossicles, microsurgical instruments are used to reposition, repair, or replace the damaged bones. They are then reset in their natural positions, and the eardrum is repaired.

Auditory neuromas are benign tumors of the supporting cells surrounding the auditory nerve. Although rare, these tumors can cause deafness. Once neuromas are confirmed by computed tomography (CT) scanning, surgical removal is necessary. With the patient under general anesthesia, the surgeon must make a hole in the skull and attempt to remove the tumor carefully without damaging the auditory nerve or adjacent nerves.

USES AND COMPLICATIONS

More than 90 percent of the patients undergoing stapedectomy experience improved hearing. Approximately 1 percent, however, show deterioration of hearing or total hearing loss postoperatively. For this reason, most surgeons perform stapedectomy on one ear at a time.

Occasionally, the surgical removal of auditory neuromas causes total deafness because of damage to the auditory nerve itself. In rare cases, damage to nearby nerves may cause weakness and/or numbness in that part of the face. Depending on the extent of nerve damage, the symptoms may or may not lessen with time.

PERSPECTIVE AND PROSPECTS

Improvements in technology promise new methods of treating hearing loss. For example, cochlear implants have been developed for the treatment of total sensorineural hearing loss. These implants are surgically inserted into the inner ear. Electrodes in the cochlea receive sound signals transmitted to them from a miniature receiver implanted behind the skin of the ear. Directly over the implant, the patient wears an external transmitter which is connected to a sound processor and microphone. As the microphone picks up sound, the sound is eventually conducted to the electrodes within the cochlea.

—*Matthew Berria, Ph.D.,*
and Douglas Reinhart, M.D.

See also Audiology; Deafness; Ear infections and disorders; Ears; Hearing; Hearing loss; Ménière's disease; Myringotomy; Neurology; Neurology, pediatric; Otoplasty; Otorhinolaryngology; Plastic surgery; Sense organs.

FOR FURTHER INFORMATION:

Brunicardi, F. Charles, et al., eds. *Schwartz's Principles of Surgery.* 9th ed. New York: McGraw-Hill, 2010. A standard textbook on the topic. Intended for practicing surgeons, but valuable to general readers for its details.

Ferrari, Mario. *PDxMD Ear, Nose, and Throat Disorders.* Philadelphia: PDxMD, 2003. A clinical yet accessible reference text that provides a comprehensive list of disorders, with a summary of the condition, background, diagnosis, treatment, outcomes, prevention, and resources.

Leikin, Jerrold B., and Martin S. Lipsky, eds. *American Medical Association Complete Medical Encyclopedia.* New York: Random House Reference, 2003. A concise presentation of numerous medical terms and illnesses. A good general reference.

Nadol, Joseph B., Jr., and Michael J. McKenna. *Surgery of the Ear and Temporal Bone.* 2d ed. Philadelphia: Lippincott Williams & Wilkins, 2005. Written by specialists at the Massachusetts Eye and Ear Infirmary, details surgical techniques that have been found reproducible and effective, as well as surgical decision making, including discussions of indications, contraindications, complications, and therapeutic alternatives.

Pender, Daniel J. *Practical Otology.* Philadelphia: J. B. Lippincott, 1992. A well-illustrated text on diseases of the ear and their surgical correction.

Tierney, Lawrence M., Stephen J. McPhee, and Maxine A. Papadakis, eds. *Current Medical Diagnosis and Treatment 2007.* New York: McGraw-Hill Medical, 2006. The point of reference for physicians and other health care practitioners. It incorporates each year's biomedical research discoveries that have immediate, relevant, and applicable use for the patient.

EARS

ANATOMY

ANATOMY OR SYSTEM AFFECTED: Bones, musculoskeletal system, nervous system

SPECIALTIES AND RELATED FIELDS: Audiology, neurology, otorhinolaryngology, speech pathology

DEFINITION: The organs responsible for both hearing and balance.

KEY TERMS:

auditory nerve: the nerve that conducts impulses originating in hair cells of cochlea to the brain for processing as the sensation of sound

cochlea: the fluid-filled coil of the inner ear containing hair cells that change vibrations in the fluid into nerve impulses

eardrum: the membrane separating the outer ear canal

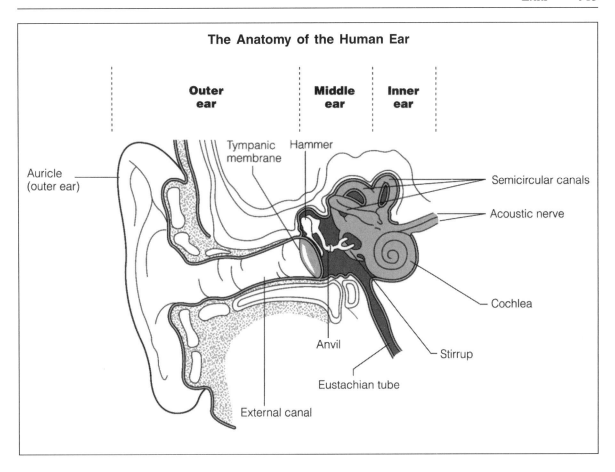

The Anatomy of the Human Ear

from the middle ear that changes sound waves into movements of the ossicles; also called the tympanic membrane

Eustachian tube: the tube connecting the middle ear to the back of the throat; air exchange through this tube equalizes air pressure in the middle ear with the outside air pressure

inner ear: an organ that includes the cochlea (for detection of sound) and the labyrinth (for detection of movement)

labyrinth: a structure consisting of three fluid-filled, semicircular canals at right angles to one another in the inner ear; they monitor the position and movement of the head

middle ear: the air-filled cavity in which vibrations are transmitted from the eardrum to the inner ear via the ossicles

ossicles: three small bones in the middle ear that transmit vibrations from the eardrum to the fluid of the inner ear

otoscope: an instrument for viewing the ear canal and the eardrum

outer ear: the visible, fleshy part of the ear and the ear canal; transmits sound waves to the eardrum

tympanic membrane: another term for the eardrum

STRUCTURE AND FUNCTIONS

The ear is composed of three parts: the outer ear, the middle ear, and the inner ear. All three parts are involved in hearing, while only the inner ear is involved in balance.

Sound can be thought of as pressure waves that travel through the air. These waves are collected by the fleshy part of the outer ear and are funneled down the ear canal to the eardrum. The eardrum, being a thin membrane, vibrates as it is hit by the sound waves. Attached to the eardrum is the first of the ossicles (the hammer or malleus), which moves when the eardrum moves. The second ossicle (the anvil or incus) is attached to the first, and the third to the second. Therefore, as the first bone moves, the others move also. The base of the third bone (the stirrup or stapes) is in contact with the oval window at the beginning of the inner ear. Movement of the oval window sets up vibrations in the fluid of the cochlea. These vibrations are detected by hair cells. Depending on their position in the cochlea, the hair cells are sensitive to being moved by vibrations of different frequencies. When the hair of a hair cell is bent by the fluid, an impulse is generated. The impulses are transmitted to the brain via the auditory nerve. The nerve impulses are processed in the brain, and the result is the sensation of sound, in particular the sense of pitch. Thus the three parts of the ear turn sound waves into "sound" by changing air vibrations into eardrum vibrations, then ossicle movement, then fluid vibrations, and finally nerve impulses.

DISORDERS AND DISEASES

Each of the three parts of the ear can be affected by diseases that can lead to temporary or, in some cases, permanent hearing loss. Damage to the eardrum, ossicles, or any part of the ear before the cochlea results in conductive hearing loss, as these structures conduct the sound or vibrations. Damage to the hair cells or to the auditory nerve results in sensorineural hearing loss. Sound may be conducted normally but cannot be detected by the hair cells or transmitted as nerve impulses to the brain.

Disorders of the outer ear include cauliflower ear, blockage by earwax, otitis externa, and tumors. Cauliflower ear is a severe hematoma (bruise) to the outer ear. In some cases, the blood trapped beneath the skin does not resorb and instead turns into fibrous tissue that may become cartilaginous or even bonelike.

Earwax is secreted by the cells in the lining of the ear canal. Its function is to protect the eardrum from dust and dirt, and it normally works its way to the outer opening of the ear. The amount secreted varies from person to person. In some people, or in people who are continually exposed to dusty environments, excessive amounts of wax may be secreted and may block the ear canal sufficiently to interfere with its transmission of sound waves to the eardrum.

Otitis externa can take two forms, either localized or generalized. The localized form, a boil or abscess, is a bacterial infection that results from breaks in the lining of the ear canal and is often caused by attempts to scratch an itch in the ear or to remove wax. The generalized form can be a bacterial or fungal infection, known as otomycosis. Generalized otitis externa is also called swimmer's ear because it often results from swimming in polluted waters or from chronic moisture in the ear canal.

Tumors of the ear can be benign (noncancerous) or malignant (cancerous) growths of either the soft tissues

or the underlying bone. Bony growths, or osteomas, can cause sufficient blockage, by themselves or by leading to the buildup of earwax, to result in hearing loss.

The middle ear consists of the eardrum, three small bones called the ossicles, and the Eustachian tube. The bones of the middle ear move in an air-filled cavity. Air pressure within this cavity is normally the same as the outside air pressure because air is exchanged between the middle ear and the outside world via the Eustachian tube. When this tube swells and closes, as it often does with a head cold, one experiences a stuffy feeling, decreased hearing, mild pain, and sometimes ringing in the ears (tinnitus) or dizziness. The middle ear is susceptible to infection, such as otitis media, because bacteria and viruses can sometimes enter via the Eustachian tube. Young children are especially prone to middle-ear infections because a child's Eustachian tubes are shorter and more directly in line with the back of the throat than those of adults. Untreated ear infections can sometimes spread into the surrounding bone (mastoiditis) or into the brain (meningitis).

Fluid in the middle ear during an ear infection interferes with the free movement of the ossicles, causing hearing loss that, although significant while it lasts, is temporary. In other instances, there is the prolonged presence of clear fluid in the middle ear, resulting from a combination of infection or allergy and Eustachian tube dysfunction, which itself can result from swelling caused by allergy. This condition, known as glue ear or persistent middle-ear effusion, can last long enough to cause detrimental effects on speech, particularly in young children. Middle-ear infections can sometimes become chronic, as in chronic otitis media; permanent damage to the hearing can result from the ossicles being dissolved away by the pus from these chronic infections.

During a middle-ear infection, fluid can build up and increase pressure within the middle-ear cavity sufficiently to rupture (perforate) the eardrum. Very loud noises are another form of increased pressure, in this case from the outside. If a loud noise is very sudden, such as an explosion or gunshot, then pressure cannot be equalized fast enough and the eardrum can rupture. Scuba diving without clearing one's ears (that is, getting the Eustachian tube to open and allow airflow) can also result in ruptured eardrums. Other causes of ruptured eardrums include puncture by a sharp object inserted into the ear canal to remove wax or relieve itching, a blow to the ear, or a fractured skull. Some hearing is lost when the eardrum is ruptured, but if the damage is not too severe, the eardrum heals itself and hearing returns.

The middle ear does not always fill with fluid if the Eustachian tube is blocked. In some instances, the middle-ear cavity remains filled with trapped air. This trapped air is taken up by the cells lining the middle-ear cavity, decreasing the air pressure inside the middle ear and allowing the eardrum to push inward. Cells that are constantly shed from the eardrum collect in this pocket and form a ball that can become infected. This infected ball, or cholesteatoma, produces pus, which can erode the ossicles. If left untreated, the erosion can continue through the roof of the middle-ear cavity (causing brain abscesses or meningitis) or through the walls (causing abscesses behind the ear). The symptoms of a cholesteatoma go beyond the symptoms of an earache to include headache, dizziness, and weakness of the facial muscles.

Permanent conductive hearing loss can also result from calcification of the ossicles, a condition called osteosclerosis. Abnormal spongy bone can form at the base of the stirrup bone, interfering with its normal movement against the oval window. Hearing loss caused by osteosclerosis occurs gradually over ten to fifteen years, although it may be accelerated in women by pregnancy. There is a hereditary component.

The inner ear begins at the oval window, which separates the air-filled cavity at the middle ear from the fluid-filled cavities of the inner ear. The inner ear consists of the cochlea, which is involved in hearing, and the labyrinth, which maintains balance.

Disorders of the cochlea result in permanent sensorineural hearing loss. Hair cells can be damaged by the high fever accompanying some diseases such as meningitis. They may also be damaged by some drugs. The largest, and most preventable, sources of damage to the hair cells are occupational and recreational exposure to loud sounds, particularly if they are prolonged. In some occupations, the hearing loss from working without ear protection may be confined to certain frequencies of sounds, while other occupations lead to general loss at all sound frequencies. Prolonged exposure to over-amplified music will likewise cause permanent hearing loss at all frequencies. This is more severe and has much earlier onset than presbycusis—the progressive loss of hearing, particularly in the high frequencies, that occurs with normal aging.

The labyrinth is the part of the ear that maintains one's balance; therefore the major system of disorders of the labyrinth is vertigo (dizziness). Labyrinthitis is an infection, generally viral, of the labyrinth. The vertigo can be severe but is temporary.

With Ménière's disease, there is an increase in the volume of fluid in the labyrinth and a corresponding increase in internal pressure, which distorts or ruptures the membrane lining. The symptoms, which include vertigo, noises in the ear, and muffled or distorted hearing especially of low tones, flare up in attacks that may last from a few hours to several days. The frequency of these attacks varies from one individual to another, with some people having episodes every few weeks and others having them every few years. This condition, which may be accompanied by migraine headaches, usually clears spontaneously but in some people may result in deafness.

DIAGNOSTIC AND TREATMENT TECHNIQUES
The most common ear disorders, outer-ear or middle-ear infections, are diagnosed visually with an otoscope. This handheld instrument is a very bright light with a removable tip. Tips of different sizes can be attached so that the doctor can look into ear canals of various sizes. Infections or obstructions in the outer ear are readily visible. Middle-ear infections can often be discerned by the appearance of the eardrum, which may appear red and inflamed. Fluid in the middle ear can sometimes be seen through the eardrum, or its presence can be surmised if the eardrum is bulging toward the ear canal. In other cases, the eardrum will be seen to be retracted or bulging inward toward the middle-ear cavity. Holes in the eardrum can also be seen, as can scars from previous ruptures that have since healed.

Impedance testing may be used in addition to the otoscope for diagnosis of middle-ear problems. Impedance testing is based on the fact that, when sound waves hit the eardrum, some of the energy is transmitted as vibrations of the drum, while some of the energy is reflected. If the eardrum is stretched tight by fluid pushing against it or by being retracted, it will be less mobile and will reflect more sound waves than a normal eardrum. In the simplest form, the mobility of the eardrum is tested with a small air tube and bulb attached to an otoscope. The doctor gently squeezes a puff of air into the ear canal while watching through the otoscope to see how well the eardrum moves.

A far more quantitative version of impedance testing can be done in cases of suspected hearing loss. This type of impedance testing is generally administered by an audiologist, a professional trained in administering and interpreting hearing tests. The ear canal is blocked with an earplug containing a transmitter and receiver. The transmitter releases sound of known frequency and intensity into the ear canal while also changing the pressure in the ear canal by pumping air into it. The receiver then measures the amount of energy reflected back. The machine analyzes the efficiency of reflection at various pressures and prints out a graph. By comparison of the graph to that from an eardrum with normal mobility, conclusions can be drawn about the degree of immobility and, consequently, about the stage of the middle-ear infection. Many pediatricians or family physicians have handheld versions of this instrument, which resembles an otoscope but is capable of transmitting sound and measuring reflected sound intensity.

When an ear infection has been diagnosed, the treatment is generally with antibiotics. For outer-ear infections, drops containing antibiotic or antifungal agents are prescribed. For middle-ear infections, antibiotics are prescribed that can be taken by mouth. The patient is rechecked in about three weeks to ensure that the ear has healed.

In some cases, the ear does not heal, or the fluid in the middle ear does not go away. This can occur if a new infection starts before the ear is fully recovered or if the infecting microorganisms are resistant to the antibiotic used for treatment. In cases of chronic or repeated otitis media, a surgical procedure called a myringotomy can be performed in which a small slit is made in the eardrum to release fluid from the middle ear. Often, a small tube is inserted into the slit. These ear tubes, or tympanostomy tubes, keep the middle ear ventilated, allowing it to dry and heal. In most cases, these tubes are spontaneously pushed out by the eardrum as healing takes place, usually within three to six months. Patients must be cautious to keep water out of their ears while the tubes are in place.

A permanently damaged eardrum—from an explosion, for example—can be replaced by a graft. This procedure is called tympanoplasty, and the tissue used for the graft is generally taken from a vein from the same person. If the ossicles are damaged, they too can be replaced, in this case by metal copies of the bones. For example, when otosclerosis has damaged the stapes (stirrup) bone, hearing can often be restored by replacing it with a metal substitute.

Tumors, osteomas in the ear canal, or cholesteatomas on the eardrum may need to be removed surgically. Surgery may also be needed if infections have spread into the surrounding bone. Bone infections or abnormalities of the inner ear are diagnosed by X rays or by computed tomography (CT) scans.

For some persons who have complete sensorineural hearing loss, some awareness of sound can be restored with a cochlear implant. This electronic device is surgically implanted and takes the place of the nonexistent hair cells in detecting sound and generating nerve impulses.

Problems of balance may sometimes be treated successfully with drugs to limit the swelling in the labyrinth. Ringing in the ears (tinnitus) is usually resolved when the underlying condition is resolved. In some cases, tinnitus is caused by drugs (large doses of aspirin, for example) and will cease when the drugs are stopped.

Doctors who specialize in diagnosis and treatment of disorders of the ear and who do these surgeries are called otorhinolaryngologists (ear, nose, and throat doctors). They are medical doctors who have several years of training beyond medical school in surgery and in problems of the ear, nose, and throat.

PERSPECTIVE AND PROSPECTS

The basic anatomy of the ear has been known for some time. Bartolommeo Eustachio (1520-1574), an Italian anatomist, first described the Eustachian tube as well as a number of the nerves and muscles involved in the functioning of the ear. An understanding of how the ear functions to discriminate the pitch of sounds, however, was not arrived at until the twentieth century. Georg von Békésy won the Nobel Prize in Physiology or Medicine in 1961 for his work on the acoustics of the ear and how it functions to analyze sounds of varying frequencies (pitch).

Treatment of diseases of the ear has been radically changed by the advent of antibiotics. Older texts describe rupture of the eardrum by middle-ear fluid as a desired outcome of middle-ear infection, one which would ensure that the infection drained and healed, rather than becoming chronic.

Chronic ear infections used to be associated with diseases such as tuberculosis, measles, and syphilis, which themselves became far less common with the widespread use of antibiotics or vaccines. In the past, chronic ear infections were much more likely to result in mastoiditis, or infection of the air spaces of the mastoid bone, requiring surgical removal of the infected portions of the mastoid bone.

Adenoids and tonsils were frequently removed from patients with recurrent ear infections, as these were thought to be the source of the reinfection. It is now known that these tissues are involved in the formation of immunity to infectious bacteria and viruses. Their removal is not advocated in most circumstances—except, for example, when they are large enough to block the opening of the Eustachian tube.

Reconstructive surgery began in the 1950's with the development by Samuel Rosen and others of the operation to free up the calcified stapes bone in cases of otosclerosis. Today virtually all the components of the middle ear can be replaced.

While ear infections used to be much more dangerous, perhaps there is an equal danger today of taking threats to the ears too lightly. Chronic ear infections can still cause permanent hearing loss and even become life-threatening infections if left untreated. Damage involving the inner ear remains untreatable, as do many cases of tinnitus and loss of balance. Because the largest source of inner ear damage is prolonged exposure to noise, the prevention of damage is far more effective than treatment.

—Pamela J. Baker, Ph.D.

See also Altitude sickness; Anatomy; Audiology; Balance disorders; Biophysics; Deafness; Dyslexia; Ear infections and disorders; Ear surgery; Earwax; Hearing; Hearing loss; Hearing tests; Ménière's disease; Motion sickness; Myringotomy; Nervous system; Neurology; Neurology, pediatric; Otoplasty; Otorhinolaryngology; Plastic surgery; Sense organs; Speech disorders; Systems and organs; Tinnitus.

For Further Information:

Gelfand, Stanley A. *Essentials of Audiology.* 3d ed. New York: Thieme, 2009. Undergraduate text covering a wide range of relevant topics, including acoustics, anatomy and physiology, sound perception, auditory disorders, and the nature of hearing impairment.

Katz, Jack, ed. *Handbook of Clinical Audiology.* 6th ed. Philadelphia: Wolters Kluwer/Lippincott Williams & Wilkins, 2009. Text that examines advances in the scientific, clinical, and philosophical understanding of audiology. Sections of the book cover behavioral tests, physiologic tests, special populations, and the management of hearing disorders.

Leikin, Jerrold B., and Martin S. Lipsky, eds. *American Medical Association Complete Medical Encyclopedia.* New York: Random House Reference, 2003. Includes a nondetailed, readable description of the anatomy of the ear and a complete listing of common ailments, each with a section on treatment that includes "self-help" and "professional help." Good illustrations and some photographs are provided.

Mendel, Lisa Lucks, Jeffrey L. Danhauer, and Sadanand Singh. *Singular's Illustrated Dictionary of Audiology.* San Diego, Calif.: Singular, 1999. A comprehensive reference guide to the field that includes numerous photographs, charts, and diagrams. Appendixes cover acronyms, illustrations, topic categories, and physical quantities.

Nettina, Sandra M., ed. *The Lippincott Manual of Nursing Practice.* 8th ed. Philadelphia: Lippincott Williams & Wilkins, 2006. Presents hearing problems and other problems of the ear, each in outline form, with sections including clinical manifestations, management, and patient education. Contains an extensive bibliography.

Pender, Daniel J. *Practical Otology.* Philadelphia: J. B. Lippincott, 1992. A well-illustrated text on diseases of the ear and their surgical correction.

Zuckerman, Barry S., and Pamela A. M. Zuckerman. *Child Health: A Pediatrician's Guide for Parents.* New York: Hearst Books, 1986. A very readable description of the ear ailments and treatments most common to children. Includes sections on swimmer's ear, otitis media, glue ear, ear tubes, hearing tests, and other topics.

Earwax

Anatomy

Also known as: Cerumen

Anatomy or system affected: Ears

Specialties and related fields: Audiology, family medicine, otorhinolaryngology

Definition: A normal, waxy product with antibacterial properties that forms in the outer third of the ear canal. It protects the ear from water and helps to prevent infection.

Structure and Functions

Earwax is made of a combination of dead skin cells, sebum (an oily substance produced by sebaceous glands), and a wax that is secreted by special glands in the outer third of the ear canal. There are two basic types of earwax, described as wet or dry; a gene has been identified that determines this characteristic: Wet earwax contains more fat.

The function of earwax is to protect the ear by trapping dust, bacteria, and foreign particles. Earwax moves out of the ear canal to the ear opening, where it becomes dry and falls out. This action is assisted by the motion of the jaw during chewing and speaking.

DISORDERS AND DISEASES

Too much or too little earwax can both increase the possibility of infection. Too little earwax compromises the protection of the ear from bacteria and foreign particles. Too much earwax can trap bacteria in the ear and cause infection, plug the ear and cause some loss in hearing, or cause a blockage that does not allow a doctor to adequately see the outer and middle ear canal during examination.

Symptoms of a wax blockage, called cerumen impaction, can be a decrease in hearing, an earache, a feeling of fullness in the ear, or a feeling that the ear is plugged. When individuals probe or try to clean out their own ears using a cotton swab or other device, such as a hairpin, this often pushes the wax deeper into the ear and can cause wax blockage against the eardrum and possible perforation of the eardrum.

The best method for earwax removal is by a doctor using a device, a microscope or an otoscope, to see a lighted and magnified view of the outer and middle ear; earwax can then be removed using a cerumen spoon or with forceps or mild suction. Other methods of earwax removal by a doctor include use of a cerumenolytic agent (a wax softener) or by irrigation of the ear with water. Over-the-counter irrigation products for individuals to use at home are available, but some studies have shown that water is as effective as these products. Other do-it-yourself products for earwax removal, including vacuum kits and "candling," where a cone-shaped device is put in the ear canal and lighted at the outside end to draw wax and impurities from the ear, are strongly discouraged.

—*Vicki J. Miskovsky*

See also Audiology; Ear infections and disorders; Ears; Hearing; Hearing loss; Host-defense mechanisms; Otorhinolaryngology; Sense organs.

FOR FURTHER INFORMATION:

Harkin, H. "A Nurse-Led Ear Care Clinic: Sharing Knowledge and Improving Patient Care." *British Journal of Nursing* 14, no. 5 (March 10-23, 2005): 250-254.

Kraszewski, Sarah. "Safe and Effective Ear Irrigation." *Nursing Standard* 22, no. 43 (July, 2008): 45-48.

Roland, P. S., et al. "Clinical Practice Guideline: Cerumen Impaction." *Archives of Otolaryngology—Head and Neck Surgery* 139, no. 3, supp. 2 (September, 2008): S1-S21.

EATING DISORDERS
DISEASE/DISORDER

ANATOMY OR SYSTEM AFFECTED: Abdomen, bones, gastrointestinal system, intestines, mouth, psychic-emotional system, reproductive system, stomach, teeth, throat

SPECIALTIES AND RELATED FIELDS: Dentistry, family medicine, pediatrics, psychiatry, psychology

DEFINITION: A group of conditions characterized by disordered eating patterns, preoccupation with body size and weight, and distorted body image. Eating disorders can cause serious medical complications and even death. The causes of eating disorders are complex and involve biological, psychological, and societal factors.

KEY TERMS:

amenorrhea: the absence of menstruation

antidepressant: medication used to treat depression

cardiomyopathy: disease of the heart muscle

diuretic: an agent that promotes the secretion of urine

fast: to abstain from food

laxative: an agent that promotes evacuation of the bowel

neurotransmitters: chemicals in the brain that stimulate activity

osteopenia: reduced bone mass

osteoporosis: demineralization of the bone

pharmacotherapy: the treatment of disease with medication

satiety: the state of feeling full or fed and free from hunger

serotonin: the neurotransmitter associated with pain perception, sleep, impulsivity, and aggression; implicated in disorders associated with anxiety, depression, and migraines

CAUSES AND SYMPTOMS

Identified eating disorders include anorexia nervosa, bulimia nervosa, and binge-eating disorder. These disorders are not always distinct, and many individuals exhibit symptoms of more than one. Their prevalence has increased during the past several decades. Anorexia nervosa and bulimia nervosa predominantly affect adolescent and young adult females. However, they can also occur in males and the elderly, and binge-eating disorder occurs more frequently in males. Approximately 4 percent of females have eating disorders, although the number of those who do not meet the full criteria for diagnosing any specific disorder is much higher. There is an approximately 9 to 1 ratio of females to males with eating disorders. The incidence of eating disorders in males is rising, however, and they are most commonly associated with sports (such as wrestling), bodybuilding, and the performing arts (such as dance). The disorders can be chronic and recur across the life span of an individual. Recognition of eating disorders in the elderly has increased, as have the negative health affects of the conditions on this population.

Anorexia nervosa is characterized by refusal to maintain normal body weight (less than 85 percent of expected weight), extreme fear of becoming fat, and relentless pursuit of thinness. Individuals with anorexia nervosa have a distorted perception of body weight and size and consider themselves to be overweight even when the opposite is true. Their view of themselves is heavily dependent on factors such as their level of adherence to a restrictive diet or the fit of their clothes. They often deny the negative aspects of low weight even in the face of serious health problems.

Two types of anorexia nervosa have been identified: the restricting type, involving dieting, fasting, or skipping meals, but not bingeing/purging; and the binge-eating/purging type, involving binge eating and purging (self-induced vomiting or misusing laxatives, enemas, or diuretics). The latter type is primarily distinguished from bulimia nervosa by refusal to maintain 85 percent of normal body weight. Dieting regimens may be severe, with intake reduced to between 300 and 600 kilocalories (Calories) per day and strict habits regarding food selection and eating.

Individuals with anorexia nervosa commonly display a set of personality and behavioral characteristics including being goal driven, perfectionistic, and overtly competent at school or work. Underlying these tendencies is often a lack of confidence and low sense of self-worth. As dieting increases, individuals may become depressed and fatigued, causing school or work to suffer and further eroding self-perception. Rigid "all or nothing" thinking influences the severity of dieting. Thus, anorexic people might believe that if they permit themselves even one lapse in dieting, then they will become obese. As starvation develops, focus on food and weight increases, and behaviors such as hoarding food, gazing in mirrors, or seeking reassurance about appearance may be observed. Significant energy is expended

to keep secret the severity of weight loss efforts. Consequently, exercise may be conducted privately, family meals and public eating avoided, or food disposed of surreptitiously. In some cases, anorexia nervosa is not discovered until after a health problem has developed consequent to malnutrition.

A number of serious health problems stemming from starvation and malnutrition are seen in people with anorexia nervosa. Among the most serious are those associated with cardiac functioning, including cardiomyopathy, arrhythmias, and altered heart rates. In rare cases, sudden death can occur as a result of irregular heart muscle contractions. Other health problems caused by anorexia nervosa involve the gastrointestinal system (bloating and constipation), the reproductive system (amenorrhea, hormonal abnormalities, and infertility), and the skeletal system (osteoporosis and osteopenia). Additional complications include lowered metabolism, cold intolerance, weakness, loss of muscle mass, low body temperature, and growth suppression. While elderly individuals with anorexia nervosa may not exhibit a drive for thinness, behaviors such as food refusal, the hoarding or hiding of food, and distorted body image are often observed. The health effects of anorexia nervosa in this population are significant and worsen coexisting illnesses, sometimes hastening death. A very serious condition known as the "female athlete triad" is a combination of factors involving athletic training: disordered eating, amenorrhea, and osteoporosis. Permanent damage to bone strength can result from this condition. Despite the numerous medical problems caused by anorexia nervosa, many with the disorder appear superficially healthy even after significant weight loss.

INFORMATION ON EATING DISORDERS

CAUSES: Psychological disorder
SYMPTOMS: Intense preoccupation with food and weight, disordered eating; may include ingestion of laxatives, depression and suicidal feelings, nutritional deficiencies, dehydration, hormonal changes, gastrointestinal problems, changes in metabolism, heart disorders, persistent sore throat, teeth and gum damage
DURATION: Chronic
TREATMENTS: Psychotherapy, nutritional counseling, medication

Bulimia nervosa is characterized by recurrent episodes of binge eating followed by purging or other inappropriate efforts to avoid weight gain. The episodes are accompanied by feelings of being out of control and subsequent self-disgust, guilt, and depression. Bingeing involves eating over a limited period of time an amount of food that is markedly larger than most people would under similar circumstances. Caloric intake during binges may range from 2,000 to 10,000. Social interruption, fear of discovery, or physical discomfort (nausea or abdominal pain) typically terminates the binge episode. The binge-purge cycle may occur several times per day, with considerable effort directed toward keeping the episodes secret. Typically, bulimics recognize that their behavior is abnormal and desire to change (as opposed to those with anorexia nervosa). The disorder is divided into two types. The purging type involves self-induced vomiting or laxative, diuretic, or enema misuse as methods to avoid weight gain. The nonpurging type involves fasting or excessive exercise to prevent weight gain.

Self-induced vomiting is the most frequent method of purging and is typically accomplished by initiating the gag reflex by placing fingers down the throat. Over time, many bulimics are able to vomit reflexively without the need to use their fingers. Though employed less frequently as the sole methods of purging, laxatives, enemas, and rarely diuretics may be used in conjunction with vomiting. Abuse of laxatives is more common among the elderly.

Individuals with nonpurging bulimia nervosa, especially males, engage in hours of exercise every day or fast following bingeing. Typically, the fast is broken by another binge episode and the cycle continues.

Those with bulimia nervosa place strong emphasis on appearance, and their mood and view of themselves are highly dependent on their weight and body shape. Most are at a normal weight, but some are underweight or overweight. Often bulimia nervosa is initiated by a restrictive diet that appears to cause many of the unusual behaviors and thinking patterns associated with anorexia nervosa, such as secretive behavior, food hoarding, and extreme focus on food and eating. There may be signs of depression and anxiety as well as compulsive behavior. As opposed to anorexia nervosa, those with bulimia nervosa are more likely to be interested in social relations and to worry more about how others perceive them. Some engage in impulsive behaviors such as substance abuse or shoplifting.

Serious medical complications can result from bulimia nervosa. Chronic vomiting or laxative abuse and consequent loss of body fluids may cause dizziness, cardiac abnormalities, dehydration, and weakness. Tooth decay caused by repeated exposure to gastric acids from vomiting may occur. Erosion or tearing of the esophagus can result from chronic vomiting. Bingeing is associated with a variety of gastrointestinal disturbances including bloating, diarrhea, and constipation.

Binge-eating disorder is a relatively newly identified condition, and less is known about it. The disorder is similar to bulimia nervosa but does not involve efforts to avoid weight gain (such as purging). Individuals with the disorder regularly engage in binges lasting up to several hours, during which from 2,000 to 10,000 Calories may be consumed. Eating during binges is typically at a rapid pace and continues in spite of feeling discomfort or pain. Bingeing may occur when an individual is not very hungry, after attempting to keep a strict diet, or as a means to reduce stress. It is usually done in private and kept secret. Feeling out of control during binges is common, followed by feelings of self-disgust and shame. Preoccupation with food and unusual food-related behaviors (such as hiding food) are common. Individuals with binge-eating disorder are typically overweight and unhappy with their body shape and size. General mood and self-perception may be dependent on their weight and size. Depression and anxiety are common coexisting conditions. Distorted body image is less likely than with anorexia nervosa and bulimia nervosa. The health problems related to obesity are seen in those with binge-eating disorder. They include high blood pressure, diabetes, high cholesterol, and heart disease. Gastrointestinal problems may also result from bingeing.

The precise causes of eating disorders are unknown; however, a number of factors involving biological, psychological, and social variables have been identified as contributing to the conditions. The primary biological influences on all eating disorders are related to hunger and starvation. Research indicates that in healthy individuals, severe dieting produces moodiness, irritability, depression, food obsessions, social isolation, and apathy. These symptoms are also found in eating disorders and become more pronounced as starvation emerges. Thus, anorexia nervosa, bulimia nervosa, or binge-eating disorder may develop after food deprivation has occurred as a result of purposeful dieting in order to lose weight or enhance athletic performance, or consequent to food restriction resulting from illness (especially in the elderly) or stress. Hunger resulting from restrictive dieting is the major stimulus for bingeing. Because a majority of those who diet do not develop eating disorders, there is likely some as yet unidentified biological or genetic predisposition in some individuals. Biological abnormalities associated with the hypothalamus and thyroid gland have been identified in some individuals with anorexia nervosa, while other research points to neurochemical or hormonal imbalances. In the elderly, medications, coexisting health problems, and even poorly fitting dentures may initiate restricted eating, leading to anorexia nervosa. Irregular levels of the neurotransmitter serotonin may influence bingeing in bulimia nervosa and binge-eating disorder since it is associated with triggering signals of satiety to the brain. Knowledge of the causes of binge-eating disorder is limited; however, as with bulimia nervosa, there often is a history of being overweight or obese prior to developing the disorder.

A number of psychological factors have been identified as causing eating disorders. Most of these are not mutually exclusive, and none has been universally accepted as the primary causative factor for the conditions. Factors proposed to account for anorexia nervosa include phobic responses to food and weight gain, conflicted feelings over adolescent development and sexual maturity,

---

IN THE NEWS: GENETIC LINKS TO EATING DISORDERS

A study published in the April, 2003, volume of the *International Journal of Eating Disorders* revealed substantial heritability for obesity and moderate heritability for binge eating among 2,163 female twins. The study also showed that obesity and binge eating share a moderate genetic correlation. Another study published in the same volume demonstrated that some genetic influences may be activated during puberty, suggesting that age-related development may be an important factor to consider in the study of eating disorders. This study used 530 twins who were eleven years of age and 602 twins who were seventeen years of age from the Minnesota Twins Family Study. The genetic contribution was zero in the eleven-year-olds but 55 percent in the seventeen-year-olds. The correlation of developmental stage with eating disorders was also highlighted in *Aging and Mental Health* (2001), which reported on anorexia and the elderly.

In February, 2003, *Clinical Psychology Review* presented a review of relevant literature suggesting that disorders such as anorexia nervosa and bulimia nervosa may also share relationships with other conditions that have genetic contributions. For instance, both disorders may be associated with depression, and anorexia has been associated with obsessive-compulsive disorder.

Similarly, a study of 256 female twins reported in the *Journal of Abnormal Psychology* (2002) suggested that eating disorders might be related to inherited personality characteristics. In this study, the results indicated that phenotypic associations between the Multidimensional Personality Questionnaire and the Eating Disorders Inventory were more likely to be genetic; however, their shared genetic variance was limited. Thus, personality may play a role in the expression of eating disorders, but this role may be limited.

Together, these studies suggest that genetics and environment play roles in the development of various eating disorders. They also suggest that more than one mechanism may account for these contributions related to factors such as psychiatric conditions (depression or anxiety), personality factors, and even age-related development.

—Nancy A. Piotrowski, Ph.D.

---

and reactions to feelings of personal ineffectiveness by "controlling" hunger and the body. Faulty thinking, known as cognitive distortions, may cause misperceptions in body image and undue emphasis on the importance of appearance. Powerful needs to demonstrate self-discipline and to develop feelings of uniqueness and independence may also contribute to anorexia nervosa. Individuals with bulimia nervosa often exhibit mood fluctuations as well as impulsive behaviors. Bulimia nervosa is thought by some to be a variant of

obsessive-compulsive disorder (OCD) in which bingeing results from irresistible urges to eat and purging is engaged in to alleviate overwhelming anxiety. Fewer psychological causes have been identified in binge-eating disorder. Some research suggests that characteristics seen in bulimia nervosa such as impulsivity and mood changes are also associated with this disorder. Depression, especially in the elderly population, appears to play a role in all eating disorders. Middle-aged and elderly individuals may employ behaviors such as extreme dieting, bingeing, and purging to reduce anxiety or to exert control in their lives.

Societal factors appear to also contribute to eating disorders. Popular media increasingly promotes physical appearance, and thinness is held up as the ideal body type. Since the 1950's, there have been steady decreases in the weights of influential persons such as actors, fashion models, and musicians. Many popular role models for females and males are underweight. Significant social approval is often associated with weight loss and disapproval with weight gain. Thus, females and males may feel pressured to attain an unhealthy weight or unrealistic body shape. A number of Web sites are devoted to promoting anorexia nervosa and bulimia nervosa as a means of personal choice and self-expression and minimizing the medical and psychological damage caused by these disorders. No reliable family characteristics have been conclusively associated with eating disorders; however, some families appear to have higher than usual levels of depression, difficulties in communication, conflict, and focus on weight and appearance.

Treatment and Therapy

Treatment of eating disorders incorporates medical, behavioral, and psychological interventions. Typically, those with anorexia nervosa believe that their diet is justified, and resistance to treatment is the norm. Males may be especially resistant. Weight restoration is the central focus of initial treatment. Hospitalization is recommended for persons with more serious medical complications or who have less than 75 percent of expected weight. During hospitalization, daily monitoring of weight and caloric intake occurs, as well as any other necessary medical management. Behavioral therapy is employed to facilitate eating habits, and privileges such as social activity or family visits are made dependent upon increased eating and daily weight gains. Individual and family therapy are introduced as malnutrition eases and irritability, depression, and preoccupation with diet diminishes. Lengths of hospital stays vary from weeks to months depending on severity of illness and treatment progress.

Outpatient treatment may be recommended with individuals who have less severe medical complications, who are motivated to cooperate with treatment, and who have families that can independently monitor diet and health status. Weight restoration is facilitated by supervision of caloric intake and regular measurements as well as behavioral therapy techniques. Individual

therapy focuses on altering cognitive distortions and assumptions about diet, weight, and body image and developing more effective means of dealing with stress. Family therapy aims to improve communication patterns, eating habits, and supportive behaviors.

No medications have been identified as effective agents in treating the core symptoms of anorexia nervosa. Medications that promote hunger may be used during the initial stages of treatment to facilitate eating. Also, medications to treat coexisting conditions such as depression and anxiety are often employed in the treatment regimen.

Most patients with bulimia nervosa do not require hospitalization unless medical complications are severe. Outpatient treatment involves individual psychotherapy, family therapy, and pharmacotherapy. Individual psychotherapy addresses cognitive distortions involving appearance and body image as well as behaviors, thoughts, and emotions that lead to binge episodes. Skills for problem solving and stress reduction are also taught. Treatment methods used for obsessive-compulsive disorder may also be employed, involving exposure to stimuli that usually trigger binge-purge behaviors while preventing them from occurring. Family therapy for bulimia nervosa aims at strengthening support and communication and developing healthy eating habits. With adolescents, impulsive behaviors associated with bulimia nervosa may be addressed by helping parents develop more effective methods of discipline and behavior management.

Antidepressant medications that regulate the neurotransmitter serotonin have been found to reduce bingeing, improve mood, and lesson preoccupation with weight and size. These same medications are useful in treating depression and anxiety, which are also commonly seen in those with bulimia nervosa.

Treatment of binge-eating disorder is similar to that of bulimia nervosa. Psychotherapy aims toward identifying and altering behaviors and feelings that lead to bingeing and developing effective methods of dealing with stress. Group therapy and weight loss programs with medical management may also be utilized. Antidepressants have also been found effective with binge-eating disorder.

Perspective and Prospects

Behaviors associated with eating disorders have been identified in the earliest writings of Western civilization, including those by the ancient Greeks and early Christians. Formal identification of eating disorders as medical illnesses occurred in the nineteenth century when case studies were first recorded. Treatment methods at that time were limited and often involved "mental hygiene" measures such as rest, fresh air, and cold or hot baths.

In the early to mid-twentieth century, psychological theories influenced by Sigmund Freud, an Austrian psychiatrist, dominated treatment methods for eating disorders. These conditions were viewed as resulting from early childhood experiences that caused problems with psychological and sexual development. Treatment involved psychoanalysis, a form of psychotherapy, often lasting several years. Limited evidence for the success of this approach caused its decline in use.

More recent and successful treatment approaches involve cognitive and behavioral therapy that aims to alter thinking and behavior contributing to eating disorders. Medications have increasingly been used in treating eating disorders since the 1980's. Identifying biological causes of the conditions and refining pharmacotherapy may offer the best hope for improving treatment in the future.

Eating disorders were once thought to occur exclusively among young Caucasian females from middle- and upper-class families. Consequently, research into the disorders has historically focused on this population. Increased awareness of the illnesses has revealed that they occur in all socioeconomic classes and races, as well as in males and the elderly. Additional research into these groups is needed.

Awareness of eating disorders and their dangers has expanded among the general public since the 1970's. Nevertheless, rates of these disorders are rising. The media publicizes celebrities' struggles with these conditions, which may glamorize the illnesses even when negative aspects are reported. Establishing healthy eating habits and identifying potential problems early constitute the current focus of prevention efforts in medicine and education.

—Paul F. Bell, Ph.D.

See also Addiction; Amenorrhea; Anorexia nervosa; Anxiety; Appetite loss; Bariatric surgery; Bulimia; Depression; Diuretics; Enemas; Hyperadiposis; Malnutrition; Nausea and vomiting; Nutrition; Obesity; Obesity, childhood; Obsessive-compulsive disorder; Psychiatric disorders; Psychiatry; Psychiatry, child and adolescent; Puberty and adolescence; Sports medicine; Stress; Vitamins and minerals; Weight loss and gain; Weight loss medications; Women's health.

FOR FURTHER INFORMATION:

American Psychiatric Association. *Diagnostic and Statistical Manual of Mental Disorders: DSM-IV-TR.* 4th ed. Arlington, Va.: Author, 2000. A manual used by most mental health professionals to diagnose patients. It details the diagnostic criteria for mental health disorders, including eating disorders, identified by the American Psychiatric Association.

Duyff, Roberta Larson, ed. *365 Days of Healthy Eating from the American Dietetic Association.* Hoboken, N.J.: John Wiley & Sons, 2006. A guide for developing healthy eating habits. Provides practical recommendations for making good food choices, as well as preparation suggestions and recipes that promote healthy nutrition. Offers strategies for incorporating exercise and health-promoting activity into daily living.

National Association of Anorexia Nervosa and Associated Disorders. http://www.anad.org. A site that provides hotline counseling, a national network of free support groups, referrals to health care professionals, and education and prevention programs to promote self-acceptance and healthy lifestyles.

Parker, James M., and Philip M. Parker, eds. *The 2002 Official Patient's Sourcebook on Binge Eating Disorder.* San Diego, Calif.: Icon Health, 2002. Draws from public, academic, government, and peer-reviewed research to provide a wide-ranging handbook for patients with this eating disorder.

Paterson, Anna. *Fit to Die: Men and Eating Disorders.* Thousand Oaks, Calif.: Sage, 2004. This book examines the causes and effects of eating disorders in men. Issues are explored such as how depression, self-esteem, and the drive for fitness contribute to disordered eating and disturbed body image. It offers advice and hope for those experiencing the illnesses.

Sackler, Ira M., and Marc A. Zimmer. *Dying to Be Thin: Understanding and Defeating Anorexia Nervosa and Bulimia—A Practical, Lifesaving Guide.* New York: Warner Books, 2001. Includes case histories of individuals suffering from eating disorders, with accounts from patients, family members, and treatment professionals. Reviews the causes and symptoms of eating disorders, and presents treatment options and resources. Information included can be helpful to those who are concerned about eating disorders for themselves or loved ones.

Thompson, Ron A., and Roberta Trattner Sherman. *Helping Athletes with Eating Disorders.* Champaign, Ill.: Human Kinetics, 1993. This book examines the connection between sports and eating disorders and the characteristics of athletes that put them at risk. The effects of eating disorders on performance and methods for coaches to approach athletes with eating disorders are detailed.

EBOLA VIRUS
DISEASE/DISORDER

ANATOMY OR SYSTEM AFFECTED: Blood, circulatory system, gastrointestinal system, muscles, skin

SPECIALTIES AND RELATED FIELDS: Epidemiology, public health, virology

DEFINITION: A virus responsible for a severe and often fatal hemorrhagic fever.

KEY TERMS:

Filoviridae: the family to which the Ebola virus belongs

maculopapular rash: a discolored skin rash observed in patients with Ebola fever

CAUSES AND SYMPTOMS

The Ebola virus is named after the Ebola River in northern Zaire, Africa, where it was first detected in 1976, when hundreds of deaths were recorded there as well as in neighboring Sudan. Three subtypes of the virus

---

INFORMATION ON EBOLA VIRUS

CAUSES: Viral infection

SYMPTOMS: Severe blood clotting and hemorrhaging, fever, lethargy, appetite loss, headaches, muscle aches, skin rash

DURATION: Acute

TREATMENTS: None

---

cause human disease: Ebola-Zaire, Ebola-Sudan, and Ebola-Ivory Coast. A fatal disease among cynomolgus laboratory monkeys that were imported from the Philippines to Texas in 1996 was caused by Ebola-Reston, a fourth subtype of the virus that causes disease in nonhuman primates, but not in humans. An equally devastating outbreak among humans took place again in early 1995 in Kirkwit, 500 kilometers east of Kinshasha, Zaire; the disease claimed the lives of 244 patients out of 315 reported cases, a 77 percent fatality rate. It is interesting to note that the epidemic ended within a few months, as suddenly as it began; this puzzled scientists, who are still unaware of the causes and nature of this so-called hot virus. Despite the dreadful speed with which the disease killed its victims, scien-

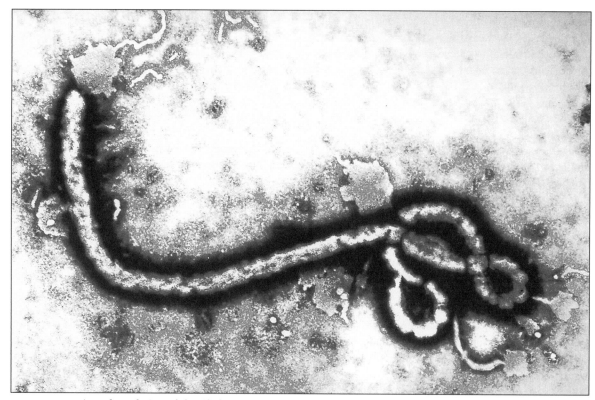

An enlarged view of the Ebola virus that causes African hemorrhagic fever. (Digital Stock)

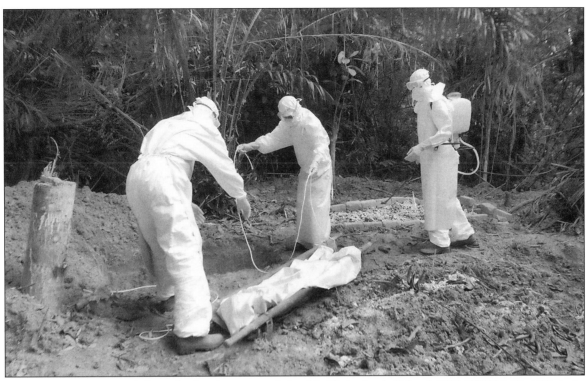

Workers wear protective clothing when burying a young victim of the Ebola virus in Gabon in 2001. (AP/Wide World Photos)

tists were happy that they contained it with a relatively small number of fatalities. Outbreaks in Africa have continued to occur; a recent outbreak in Sudan resulted in twenty cases with five deaths. Recently obtained historical documentation suggests the possibility that the Athenian plague at the beginning of the Peloponnesian War around 430 B.C.E. could be attributed to the Ebola virus.

The Ebola virus appears to have an incubation period of two to twenty-one days, after which time the impact is devastating. The patient develops appetite loss, increasing fever, headaches, and muscle aches. The next stage involves disseminated intravascular coagulation (DIC), a condition characterized by both blood clots and hemorrhaging. The clots usually form in vital internal organs such as the liver, spleen, and brain, with subsequent collapse of the neighboring capillaries. Other symptoms include vomiting, diarrhea with blood and mucus, and conjunctivitis. An unusual type of skin irritation known as maculopapular rash first appears in the trunk and quickly covers the rest of the body. The final stages of the disease involve a spontaneous hemorrhaging from all body outlets, coupled with shock and kidney failure and often death within eight to seventeen days.

TREATMENT AND THERAPY

The Ebola virus is classified as a ribonucleic acid (RNA) virus and is closely related to the Marburg virus, first discovered in 1967. The Marburg and the Ebola viruses are the only two members of the Filoviridae family, which was first established in 1987. Electron microscope studies show the Ebola virus as long filaments, 650 to 14,000 nanometers in length, that are often either branched or intertwined. Its virus part, known as the virion, contains one single noninfectious minus-strand RNA molecule and an endogenous RNA polymerase. The lipoprotein envelope contains a single glycoprotein, which behaves as the type-specific antigen. Spikes are approximately 7 nanometers in length, are spaced at approximately 10-nanometer intervals, and are visible on the virion surface. It is believed that once in the body, the virus produces proteins that suppress the organism's immune system, thus allowing its uninhibited reproduction. In 2002, researchers announced a new discovery about how Ebola makes entry into and subverts human cells. Findings show that the virus targets a "lipid raft," tiny fat platforms that float atop the membranes of human cells. These rafts act as gateways for the virus, the assembly platform for making new virus particles, and the exit point where new

In the News:
Congo Outbreak of Ebola in 2003

In December, 2002, reports that gorillas and chimpanzees were dying in remote forests within the northern region of the Republic of Congo alarmed Congolese authorities. The following month, word spread of a possible outbreak of Ebola virus in the country's Cuvette-Ouest district. At that point in time, twelve people had died of apparent hemorrhagic fever in the town of Kelle, and four more persons had died at Mbomo. The previous year, in the same area, a similar episode led to the deaths of forty-three people in the Republic of Congo and fifty-three residents of neighboring Gabon.

At the peak of the epidemic, most of the population of Kelle fled into the forest in the attempt to hide from the deadly virus. Volunteers from the Congolese Red Cross, clad in protective suits, cared for the sick and the elderly who were left behind. Few villagers believed that the epidemic was a natural disease brought about by eating infected primate meat—rather, they suspected witchcraft. Four teachers, accused of causing the outbreak, were reportedly killed by a mob.

Medical teams from the United Nations World Health Organization (WHO), the Red Cross, and Médecins Sans Frontières set up makeshift hospital wards in the affected area. The U.S. Centers for Disease Control and Prevention (CDC) sent an expert epidemiologist. The European Commission's Humanitarian Aid Office appropriated 500,000 euros to support the relief work.

Aid workers began a public awareness campaign to halt the spread of the disease. WHO held meetings with local leaders to assure them they could limit the outbreak by avoiding primate meat and by not touching the bodies of those sick with the disease. People were urged to refrain from washing deceased family members, a ritual required by traditional burial practices.

By late April, the epidemic appeared to be under control, and people began to return to their homes. Fears that the returning villagers might start a new series of infections after eating the meat of dead gorillas while hiding in the forest proved unfounded. Out of 144 reported cases, the disease claimed 126 lives, a death rate approaching 90 percent.

—*Milton Berman, Ph.D.*

ble at room temperature. Its inactivation is accomplished via ultraviolet or gamma irradiation, 1 percent formalin, beta propiolactone, and an exposure to phenolic disinfectants and lipid solvents, such as deoxycholase and ether. The virus isolation is usually achieved from acute-phase serum of appropriate cell cultures, such as the Ebola-Sudan virus MA-104 cells from a fetal rhesus monkey kidney cell line. Satisfactory results have been accomplished using tissues obtained from the liver, spleen, lymph nodes, kidneys, and heart during autopsy. The virus isolation from brain and other nervous tissues, however, has been rather unsuccessful so far. Neutralization tests have been inconsistent for all filoviruses. Ebola strains, however, show cross-reactions in tests of immunofluorescence assays.

There appears to be no known or standard treatment for Ebola fever. No chemotherapeutic or immunization strategies are available, and no antiviral drug has been shown to provide positive results, even under in vitro conditions. Human interferon, human convalescent plasma, and anticoagulation therapy have been used with unconvincing results.

At this stage, therapy involves sustaining the desired fluid and electrolyte balance by the frequent administration of fluids. Bleeding may be fought off with blood and plasma transfusion. Sanitary conditions to avoid further contact with the disease are required. Proper decontamination of medical equipment, isolation of the patients from the rest of the community, and prompt disposal of infected tissues, blood, and even corpses limit the spread of the disease.

particles bud. This research is a significant step toward one day creating drugs that would stop viruses from replicating.

The Ebola virus can be transmitted through contact with body fluids, such as blood, semen, mucus, saliva, and even urine and feces. It is thought that the first person in an outbreak acquires the virus through contact with an infected animal, including carcasses of dead animals.

The level of infectivity of the Ebola virus is quite sta-

Perspective and Prospects

The puzzling characteristics of the Ebola virus are the location of its primary natural reservoir, its sudden eruption and the unknown reason for its quick end, and the unusual discovery of the virus in the organs of people who have survived it.

In the past, experimental work on the virus has been slow because of its high pathogenicity. The progress of recombinant deoxyribonucleic acid (DNA) technology has shed the first light on the molecular structure of this virus. It is hoped that further work using this technique as well as the results of viruses of lower pathogenicity (such as the Reston virus) will provide the desired information on replication and virus-host interactions. Finally, the improvement of the various diagnostic tools will allow more accurate virus identification and assessment of transmission modes.

In 1995, the World Health Organization (WHO) investigators and epidemiologists captured about three thousand birds, rodents, and other animals and insects that are suspected of spreading the disease in order to investigate the source of the virus. The results, however, were obscure and inconclusive, and the main facts about the disease are still a mystery, with the exception of the established link between primates and Ebola virus infection in humans. This conclusion was reached after the fatal infection of a French researcher in Ivory Coast who performed an autopsy on a chimpanzee that had died from a disease with the same symptoms as Ebola fever. Yet, the human outbreaks in Zaire and the Sudan have not been traced to primates. As long as these puzzling questions linger, the disease should be contained, with particular emphasis on the improvement of sanitary conditions and the control of body fluid contact.

—*Soraya Ghayourmanesh, Ph.D.;*
updated by H. Bradford Hawley, M.D.

See also Bleeding; Centers for Disease Control and Prevention (CDC); Dengue fever; Epidemiology; Hemorrhage; Marburg virus; Tropical medicine; Viral hemorrhagic fevers; Viral infections; Zoonoses.

For Further Information:

Balter, Michael. "On the Trail of Ebola and Marburg Viruses." *Science* 290, no. 5493 (November 3, 2000): 923-925. Researchers are making headway on understanding hemorrhagic fever viruses. Perplexing to researchers is how Marburg and Ebola viruses cause such devastating symptoms as shock and massive bleeding.

Biddle, Wayne. *A Field Guide to Germs.* 2d ed. New York: Anchor Books, 2002. This comprehensive book is easily accessible to the nonspecialist and includes a discussion of nearly every virus, bacterium, and fungus known to cause human and nonhuman animal disease. The history of the microbe and the treatment of diseases are included.

Dyer, Nicole. "Killers Without Cures." *Science World* 57, no. 3 (October 2, 2000): 8-12. In the last thirty years, more than fifty lethal viruses once found only in animals have infected humans. A look at how virus hunters on a 1995 mission worked to stop a deadly outbreak of the Ebola virus in the Congo.

Jaax, Nancy. *Lethal Viruses, Ebola, and the Hot Zone: Worldwide Transmission of Fatal Viruses.* Lincoln: University of Nebraska Foundation, 1996. This text is based on a forum on world issues sponsored by the Cooper Foundation and the University of Nebraska at Lincoln. Illustrated.

Jahrling, Peter B., et al. "Filoviruses and Arenaviruses." In *Manual of Clinical Microbiology*, edited by Patrick R. Murray et al. 8th ed. Washington, D.C.: ASM Press, 2007. A chapter in a text devoted to medical and diagnostic microbiology. Includes bibliographical references and an index.

McGraw-Hill Encyclopedia of Science and Technology. 10th ed. 20 vols. New York: McGraw-Hill, 2007. A complete reference for the nonspecialist that offers thousands of articles written by world-renowned scientists and engineers. It includes many new and revised articles and extensive cross-references and bibliographies and is fully illustrated.

Peters, C. J., and J. W. LeDuc. "An Introduction to Ebola: The Virus and the Disease." *Journal of Infectious Diseases* 179, supp. 1 (1999): ix-xvi. This paper is sponsored by the World Health Organization and the Centers for Disease Control and Prevention. Includes bibliographical references.

Strauss, James, and Ellen Strauss. *Viruses and Human Disease.* 2d ed. Boston: Academic Press/Elsevier, 2008. An undergraduate text that examines virology from a human disease perspective.

ECG or EKG. *See*
Electrocardiography (ECG or EKG).

Echocardiography
Procedure

Also known as: Cardiac ultrasound, 2-D echo, stress echo

Anatomy or system affected: Circulatory system, heart

Specialties and related fields: Cardiology, critical care, emergency medicine, family medicine, internal medicine

Definition: A diagnostic technique that uses ultrasound to display anatomical and physiological characteristics of the heart and related structures.

Key terms:

stress echocardiography: echocardiography procedure performed while the heart is stressed, either with medications or by exercising on a treadmill

transducer: the tip of the ultrasound probe

transesophageal echocardiography: the method of performing echocardiography with the ultrasound probe inserted via the esophagus (food pipe)

transthoracic echocardiography: the routine method of performing echocardiography by placing the ultrasound probe on the chest

Indications and Procedures

Echocardiography is a technique that uses ultrasound waves to detect the structures of the heart. The most common indication for echocardiography is to evaluate chamber size, thickness of the heart muscle, valve abnormalities, and the flow of blood through the heart. The procedure is usually performed to evaluate the functioning of the heart in a patient with heart failure and can detect any damage to the heart muscles after a heart attack. In addition, valvular abnormalities of any of the four heart valves, such as thickening or leakage, can be detected. Other indications include evaluation of congenital or birth defects of the heart and fluid collection in the sac covering the heart (pericardial effusion). The use of a color Doppler further helps in assessing the velocity of blood flow through the heart.

Transthoracic echocardiography (TTE) is a simple outpatient, noninvasive procedure. While undergoing echocardiography, the patient lies down on his or her back and turns a little toward to the left so that the heart can be better visualized. The area on the left side of chest is wiped dry (no shaving is necessary), and a gel is applied over the skin for better conduction of the ultrasound waves. The operator then applies the transducer or the ultrasound probe over the chest, and two-dimensional images of the heart are seen on the attached monitor. Multiple still and motion pictures of the heart are recorded, which are then read by a cardiologist. The procedure takes about thirty minutes, and the patient is able to go home immediately after the procedure.

Special types of echocardiography include transesophageal echocardiography (TEE) and stress echocardiography. In TEE, the ultrasound probe is mounted on an endoscope and introduced into the esophagus. The structures at the back of the heart and valves are better visualized with this procedure. Stress echocardiography includes performing echocardiography while the patient is undergoing a stress test (while exercising on a treadmill or after medications such as dobutamine have been given). Both these procedures take a longer time and require experienced operators. Patients may be observed for a few hours after the procedure.

Uses and Complications

Echocardiography helps in identifying congenital heart defects such as tetralogy of Fallot, atrial and ventricular septal defects, valvular abnormalities such as stenosis (narrowing) or regurgitation (leaking) of the four heart valves, the functioning of the heart muscle after a heart attack, the collection of fluid in the sac covering the heart, the rupture of heart muscle, and the progression of heart failure.

Different modes of echocardiography are used in clinical practice. The most common is two-dimensional echocardiography (2-D echo), as described above, which detects cardiac structure and function and displays results in two dimensions. A newer, more expensive three-dimensional echocardiography is gaining popularity, as it displays the findings in a three-dimensional form and localizes specific lesions more accurately. Stress echocardiography is used to detect areas in the heart that have a reduced blood flow, especially during exercise or stress. This enables cardiologists to locate the diseased artery and correct it by stenting or by surgery. TEE specifically looks for blood clots in one of the heart chambers called the left atrium and also looks closely at infections of the valves (endocarditis).

TTE is a safe procedure without any known complications. Patients undergoing TEE or stress echocardiography are carefully screened before undergoing the procedure. Rare complications of stress echocardiography are chest pain and heart attack in patients with very poor circulation to the heart, and this procedure should not be performed in persons with ongoing heart attack symptoms. TEE rarely can cause rupture of the esophagus because of the invasive nature of the procedure. Occasionally, aspiration of food contents into the lungs can occur, and hence patients are required to have an empty stomach before the procedure. If complications do occur, then patients are hospitalized and treated appropriately.

Perspectives and Prospects

The term "echo" was first coined by the Roman architect Vesuvius during the rule of the Roman Empire.

Karl Dussik first used ultrasound in medicine to outline the ventricles of the brain. The first use of ultrasound to examine the heart was by W. D. Keidel in the 1940's. Clinical echocardiography was initiated by Helmut Hertz and Inge Edler of Sweden using a commercial ultrasonoscope to examine the heart. Though echocardiography was introduced in the United States by John J. Wild, H. D. Crawford, and John Reid in the 1960's, most of the credit for its further development and popularity goes to Harvey Feigenbaum at Indiana University.

Echocardiography is a great tool for assessing cardiac function. Recent echocardiography machines are portable and allow physicians to do bedside evaluation of the heart. Newer models are handheld, further enhancing ease of use. A role for echocardiography has been proposed in other systemic diseases such as diabetes, hypertension, pregnancy, kidney disease, and thyroid disease and also in the screening of athletes. Echocardiography is a cost-effective, versatile procedure that has a significant role in clinical medicine.

—*Venkat Raghavan Tirumala, M.D., M.H.A.*

See also Angiography; Arrhythmias; Arteriosclerosis; Cardiac rehabilitation; Cardiology; Cardiology, pediatric; Circulation; Congenital heart disease; Diagnosis; Electrocardiography (ECG or EKG); Endocarditis; Exercise physiology; Heart; Heart attack; Heart disease; Heart failure; Hypertension; Imaging and radiology; Magnetic resonance imaging (MRI); Mitral valve prolapse; Noninvasive tests; Pacemaker implantation; Palpitations; Sports medicine; Ultrasonography; Vascular medicine; Vascular system.

For Further Information:

Feigenbaum, Harvey, William F. Armstrong, and Thomas Ryan. *Feigenbaum's Echocardiography.* 7th ed. Philadelphia: Lippincott Williams & Wilkins, 2010. An interesting read authored by the founder of echocardiography in the United States.

Kasper, Dennis L., et al., eds. *Harrison's Principles of Internal Medicine.* 16th ed. New York: McGraw-Hill, 2005. A textbook of medicine that includes a detailed description of echocardiography.

Tierney, Lawrence M., Stephen J. McPhee, and Maxine A. Papadakis, eds. *Current Medical Diagnosis and Treatment 2007.* New York: McGraw-Hill Medical, 2006. An annually updated resource for medical topics.

ECLAMPSIA. *See* PREECLAMPSIA AND ECLAMPSIA.

ECTOPIC PREGNANCY
DISEASE/DISORDER

ALSO KNOWN AS: Tubal pregnancy

ANATOMY OR SYSTEM AFFECTED: Reproductive system

SPECIALTIES AND RELATED FIELDS: Embryology, gynecology

DEFINITION: The implantation of an embryo outside the uterine endometrium, most commonly in the Fallopian tube.

CAUSES AND SYMPTOMS

Although ectopic pregnancies can occur without any known cause, several factors increase a woman's risk. Studies have shown an increase in ectopic pregnancies in women with previous pelvic inflammatory disease (PID). Intrauterine devices (IUDs), so effective at preventing pregnancies, do not increase the risk of ectopic pregnancy. However, when a woman with an IUD does get pregnant, the risk for an ectopic pregnancy is increased, especially for women using an IUD containing progestin at the time of conception. There is also an increased risk in women who have had tubal ligations and other surgeries of the Fallopian tubes.

Endometriosis, multiple induced abortions, and pelvic adhesions also may increase a woman's chance of ectopic pregnancy. In general, women whose Fallopian tubes are damaged for any reason have a higher risk. The risk is heightened because damage slows the progress of the developing embryo through the tube, allow-

---

INFORMATION ON ECTOPIC PREGNANCY

CAUSES: Unknown; factors may include previous pelvic inflammatory disease, IUD use, tubal ligation, endometriosis, multiple abortions, pelvic adhesions

SYMPTOMS: Similar to those of early pregnancy, followed by spotting, cramping, abdominal pain (especially on one side); if Fallopian tube ruptures, bleeding and severe pain

DURATION: Acute

TREATMENTS: Only in early cases, methotrexate to end pregnancy; usually surgical removal of embryo and Fallopian tube

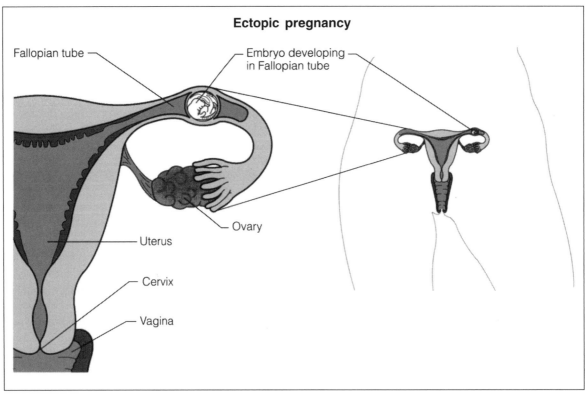

Ectopic pregnancy

Fallopian tube

Embryo developing
in Fallopian tube

Ovary

Uterus

Cervix

Vagina

Ectopic pregnancy results when the fertilized egg implants itself outside the uterus and begins to develop; surgical intervention is usually required.

ing the embryo to be mature enough to implant itself before reaching the uterus. Another factor that may increase the chances of ectopic pregnancy is smoking. Nicotine slows the movement of cilia in the Fallopian tubes, thus slowing the progress of the embryo.

The symptoms of an early ectopic pregnancy are similar to those of any early pregnancy, except that spotting, cramping, and pain, especially on only one side of the abdomen, may occur as the embryo grows. Hormone levels mimic early pregnancy but usually do not rise as high as in a normal intrauterine implantation. If the tube ruptures, then bleeding and severe pain may occur.

TREATMENT AND THERAPY

If a tubal ectopic pregnancy is diagnosed early enough, methotrexate, a chemical that attacks quickly growing cells, may be administered, and surgery may be avoided. The drug causes the death of the embryo. Surgical removal is now less common than is management with methotrexate; when surgery is performed, however, it is usually done through laparoscopy. Following

surgery, methotrexate may be administered to help remove any remaining tissues from the pregnancy. Because there is no known way to implant the removed embryo in the uterus, surgical removal also results in the death of the embryo.

—*Richard W. Cheney, Jr., Ph.D.*

See also Conception; Contraception; Genital disorders, female; Miscarriage; Obstetrics; Pregnancy and gestation; Women's health.

FOR FURTHER INFORMATION:

Carson, Sandra Ann, ed. *Ectopic Pregnancy*. Philadelphia: Lippincott-Raven, 1999.

Hey, Valerie, et al., eds. *Hidden Loss: Miscarriage and Ectopic Pregnancy*. 2d ed. London: Women's Press, 1997.

Leach, Richard E., and Steven J. Ory, eds. *Management of Ectopic Pregnancy*. Malden, Mass.: Blackwell Science, 2000.

Stabile, Isabel. *Ectopic Pregnancy: Diagnosis and Management*. New York: Cambridge University Press, 1996.

ECZEMA

DISEASE/DISORDER
ALSO KNOWN AS: Dermatitis
ANATOMY OR SYSTEM AFFECTED: Skin
SPECIALTIES AND RELATED FIELDS: Dermatology, pediatrics
DEFINITION: An inflammation of the skin.

CAUSES AND SYMPTOMS

The term "eczema" refers to a noncontagious inflammation of the skin. Several types of eczema exist, resulting in a range of symptoms that vary in appearance, duration, and severity. The common characteristic, however, is red, dry, and itchy skin. Other symptoms may include scaling, thickening, or cracking of the skin, leading to infections and severe discomfort.

Atopic dermatitis, the most common form of eczema, is characterized by itchy and cracked skin of the cheeks, arms, and legs. The onset of this chronic type of eczema occurs most often during infancy or childhood, although symptoms may continue into adulthood. The cause of atopic dermatitis is thought to be a hereditary predisposition to skin sensitivities to various environmental factors. These factors include irritants such as soaps, detergents, and rough clothes; allergens such as certain foods, pollen, or animal dander; and changes in climate or temperature. Other forms of eczema, such as contact dermatitis, have similar environmental causes. Seborrheic eczema, nummular eczema, and dishydrotic eczema may result from a combination of several possible causes. Emotional factors, such as stress or frustration, may aggravate the symptoms.

The diagnosis of eczema requires a careful and detailed observation of symptoms. Family and personal medical histories are often useful to determine the presence of allergies or exposure to allergens or irritants. Dermatologists may also use skin biopsies or blood tests to determine a tendency toward elevated allergic or immune response.

TREATMENT AND THERAPY

The treatment of eczema involves minimizing exposure to possible causes while at the same time managing symptoms to maintain a high quality of life. Identifying known allergens and irritants specific to the individual is an important first step. Lifestyle changes aimed at avoiding exposure to these possible causes can lower the frequency and duration of symptoms dramatically. Proper skin care to avoid excessive drying of the skin, including the use of moisturizers or creams and minimizing exposure to water, may also help reduce skin irritation. Avoiding scratching of existing irritations and eliminating sources of emotional stress are other ways that patients can lessen the severity of their symptoms. Dermatologists may prescribe additional treatments, such as corticosteroid creams and ointments, antihistamines, or antibiotics. In more severe cases, systemic corticosteroid treatments or phototherapy, the use of ultraviolet (UV) light, may be tried.

The approval of a new type of treatment for eczema called topical immunomodulators has changed the way eczema is treated in recent years. This new class of drug counteracts the inflammation of the skin without interfering in the body's normal immune response. This treatment has been successful in preventing and even eliminating symptoms of eczema.

—*Paul J. Frisch*

See also Allergies; Dermatitis; Dermatology; Dermatology, pediatric; Itching; Lesions; Rashes; Skin; Skin disorders; Wiskott-Aldrich syndrome.

INFORMATION ON ECZEMA

CAUSES: Genetic sensitivity to irritants (soaps, detergents, rough clothes), allergens (certain foods, pollen, animal dander), and climate or temperature changes
SYMPTOMS: Red, dry, and itchy skin; scaling, thickening, or cracking of skin
DURATION: Often chronic
TREATMENTS: Minimal exposure to irritants, drugs (corticosteroid creams and ointments, antihistamines, antibiotics); in severe cases, oral corticosteroids or phototherapy

---

FOR FURTHER INFORMATION:
Fry, Lionel. *An Atlas of Atopic Eczema.* New York: Parthenon, 2004.
National Eczema Society. http://www.eczema.org.
Rakel, Robert E., and Edward T. Bope, eds. *Conn's Current Therapy.* Philadelphia: Saunders/Elsevier, 2007.
Ring, J., B. Przybilla, and T. Ruzicka, eds. *Handbook of Atopic Eczema.* 2d ed. New York: Springer, 2006.
Turkington, Carol A., and Jeffrey S. Dover. *Skin Deep: An A-Z of Skin Disorders, Treatments, and Health.* 3d ed. New York: Checkmark Books, 2007.
Westcott, Patsy. *Eczema: Recipes and Advice to Provide Relief.* New York: Welcome Rain, 2000.

EDEMA

DISEASE/DISORDER

ANATOMY OR SYSTEM AFFECTED: Blood vessels, circulatory system, liver, lungs, lymphatic system, respiratory system, skin

SPECIALTIES AND RELATED FIELDS: Internal medicine, nephrology, pulmonary medicine

DEFINITION: Accumulation of fluid in body tissues that may indicate a variety of diseases, including cardiovascular, kidney, liver, and medication problems.

KEY TERMS:

extracellular fluid: the fluid outside cells; includes the fluid within the vascular system and the lymphatic system and the fluid surrounding individual cells

hydrostatic pressure: the physical pressure on a fluid, such as blood; it tends to push fluids across membranes toward areas of lower pressure

interstitial fluid: the fluid between the vascular system and cells; nutrients from the vascular compartment must diffuse across the interstitial compartment to enter the cells

intracellular fluid: the fluid within cells

intravascular fluid: the fluid carried within the blood vessels; it is in a constant state of motion because of the pumping action of the heart

osmotic pressure: the ability of a concentrated fluid on one side of a membrane to draw water away from a less concentrated fluid on the other side

PROCESS AND EFFECTS

Edema is not a disease, but a condition that may be caused by a number of diseases. It signals a breakdown in the body's fluid-regulating mechanisms. The body's water can be envisioned as divided into three compartments: the intracellular compartment, the interstitial compartment, and the vascular compartment. The intracellular compartment consists of the fluid contained within the individual cells. The vascular compartment consists of all the water that is contained within the heart, the arteries, the capillaries, and the veins. The last compartment, and in many ways the most important for a discussion of edema, is called the interstitial compartment. This compartment includes all the water not contained in either the cells or the blood vessels. The interstitial compartment contains all the fluids between the intracellular compartment and the vascular compartment and the fluid in the lymphatic system. The sizes of these compartments are approximately as follows: intracellular fluid at 66 percent, interstitial fluid at 25 percent, and the vascular fluid at only 8 percent of the total body water.

When the interstitial compartment becomes overloaded with fluid, edema develops. To understand the physiology of edema formation, it may be helpful to follow a molecule of water as it travels through the various compartments, beginning when the molecule enters the aorta soon after leaving the heart. The blood has just been ejected from the heart under high pressure, and it speedily begins its trip through the body. It passes from the great vessel, the aorta, into smaller and smaller arteries that divide and spread throughout the body. At each branching, the pressure and speed of the water molecule decrease. Finally, the molecule enters a capillary, a vessel so small that red blood cells must flow in a single file. The wall of this vessel is composed only of the membrane of a single capillary cell. There are small passages between adjacent capillary cells leading to the interstitial compartment, but they are normally closed.

The hydrostatic pressure on the water molecule is much lower than when it was racing through the aorta, but it is still higher than that of the surrounding interstitial compartment. At the arterial end of the capillary, the blood pressure is sufficient to overcome the barrier of the capillary cell's membrane. A fair number of water and other molecules are pushed through the membrane into the interstitial compartment.

In the interstitial compartment, the water molecule is essentially under no pressure, and it floats amid glucose molecules, oxygen molecules, and many other compounds. Glucose and oxygen molecules enter the cells, and when the water molecule is close to a glucose molecule it is taken inside a cell with that molecule. The water molecule is eventually expelled by the cell, which has produced extra water from the metabolic process.

Back in the interstitial compartment, the molecule floats with a very subtle flow toward the venous end of the capillary. This occurs because, as the arterial end of the capillary pushes out water molecules, it loses hydrostatic pressure, eventually equaling the pressure of the interstitial compartment. Once the pressure equalizes, another phenomenon that has been thus far overshadowed by the hydrostatic pressure takes over—osmotic pressure. Osmotic pressure is the force exercised by a concentrated fluid that is separated by a membrane from a less concentrated fluid. It draws water molecules across the membrane from the less concentrated side. The more concentrated the fluid, the greater is the drawing power. The ratio of nonwater molecules to water molecules determines concentration.

The fluid that stays within the capillary remains more concentrated than the interstitial fluid for two reasons. First, the plasma proteins in the vascular compartment are too large to be forced across the capillary membrane; albumin is one such protein. These proteins stay within the vascular compartment and maintain a relatively concentrated state, compared to the interstitial compartment. At the same time, the concentration of the fluid in the interstitial compartment is being lowered constantly by the cellular compartment's actions. Cells remove molecules of substances such as glucose to metabolize, and afterward they release water—a by-product of the metabolic process. Both processes conspire to lower the total concentration of the interstitial compartment. The net result of this process is that water molecules return to the capillaries at the venous end because of osmotic pressure.

The water molecule is caught by this force and is returned to the vascular compartment. Back in the capillary, the molecule's journey is not yet complete. Now in a tiny vein, it moves along with blood. On the venous side of the circulatory system, the process of branching is reversed, and small veins join to form increasingly larger ones. The water molecule rides along in these progressively larger veins. The pressure surrounding the molecule is still low, but it is now higher than the pressure at the venous end of the capillary. One may wonder how this is possible if the venous pressure at the beginning of the venous system is essentially zero, and there is only one pump, the heart, in the body. As the molecule flows through the various veins, it occasionally passes one-way valves that allow blood to flow only toward the heart. The action of these valves, combined with muscular contractions from activities such as walking or tapping the foot, force blood toward the heart. Without these valves, it would be impossible for the venous blood to flow against gravity and return to the heart; the blood would simply sit at the lowest point in the body. Fortunately, these valves and contractions move the molecule against gravity, returning it to the heart to begin a new cycle.

In certain disease states, there is marked capillary dilation and excessive capillary permeability, and excessive amounts of fluid are allowed to leave the intravascular compartment. The fluid accumulates in the interstitial space. When capillary permeability is increased, plasma proteins also

tend to leave the vascular space, reducing the intravascular compartment's osmotic pressure while increasing the interstitial compartment's osmotic pressure. As a result, the rate of return of fluid from the interstitial compartment to the vascular compartment is lowered, thus increasing the interstitial fluid levels.

Another route of return of interstitial fluid to the circulation is via the lymphatic system. The lymphatic system is similar to the venous system, but it carries no red blood cells. It runs through the lymph nodes, carrying some of the interstitial fluid that has not been able to return to the vascular compartment at the capillary level. If lymphatic vessels become obstructed, water in the interstitial compartment accumulates, and edema may result.

CAUSES AND SYMPTOMS

Heart failure is a major cause of edema. When the right ventricle of the heart fails, it cannot cope with all the venous blood returning to the heart. As a consequence, the veins become distended, the interstitial compartment is overloaded, and edema occurs. If the patient with heart failure is mostly upright, the edema collects in the legs; if the patient has been lying in bed for some time, the edema tends to accumulate in the lower back. Other clinical signs of right heart failure include distended neck veins, an enlarged and tender liver, and a "galloping" sound on listening to the heart with a stethoscope.

When the left ventricle of the heart fails, the congestion affects the pulmonary veins instead of the neck and leg veins. Fluid accumulates in the same fashion within the interstitial compartment of the lungs; this condition is termed pulmonary edema. Patients develop shortness of breath with minimal activity, upon lying down,

---

INFORMATION ON EDEMA

CAUSES: Wide ranging; includes disease, heart failure, deep vein thrombosis, inadequate blood levels of albumin

SYMPTOMS: Varies; may include accumulated fluid, shortness of breath, pain and tenderness, impacted mobility

DURATION: Acute to chronic

TREATMENTS: Dependent on cause; may include frequent elevation of feet to heart level, support stockings, avoidance of prolonged standing or sitting, dietary changes, medications (e.g., diuretics)

and periodically through the night. They may need to sleep on several pillows to minimize this symptom. This condition can usually be diagnosed by listening to the lungs and heart through a stethoscope and by taking an X ray of the chest.

Deep vein thrombosis is another common cause of edema of the lower limbs. When a thrombus (a blood clot inside a blood vessel) develops in a large vein of the legs, the patient usually complains of pain and tenderness of the affected leg. There is usually redness and edema as well. If the thrombus affects a small vein, it may not be noticed. The diagnosis can be made by several specialized tests, such as ultrasound testing and/or impedance plethysmography. Other tests may be needed to make the diagnosis, such as injecting radiographic dye in a vein in the foot and then taking X rays to determine whether the flow in the veins has been obstructed, or using radioactive agents that bind to the clot. Risks for developing venous thrombosis include immobility (even for relatively short periods of time such as a long car or plane ride), injury, a personal or family history of venous thrombosis, the use of birth control pills, and certain types of cancer. Elderly patients are at particular risk because of relative immobility and an increased frequency of minor trauma to the legs.

When repeated or large thrombi develop, the veins deep inside the thigh (the deep venous system) become blocked, and blood flow shifts toward the superficial veins. The deep veins are surrounded by muscular tissue, and venous flow is assisted by muscular contractions of the leg (the muscular pump), but the superficial veins are surrounded only by skin and subcutaneous tissue and cannot take advantage of the muscular pump. As a consequence, the superficial veins become distended and visible as varicose veins.

When vein blockage occurs, the valves inside become damaged. Hydrostatic pressure of the venous system below the blockage then rises. The venous end of the capillary is normally where the osmotic pressure of the vascular compartment pulls water from the interstitial compartment back into the vascular compartment. In a situation of increased hydrostatic pressure, however, this process is slowed or stopped. As a result, fluid accumulates in the interstitial space, leading to the formation of edema.

A dangerous complication of deep vein thrombosis occurs when part of a thrombus breaks off, enters the circulation, and reaches the lung; this is called a pulmonary embolus. It blocks the flow of blood to the lung,

impairing oxygenation. Small emboli may have little or no effect on the patient, while larger emboli may cause severe shortness of breath, chest pain, or even death.

Another potential cause of edema is the presence of a mass in the pelvis or abdomen compressing the large veins passing through the area and interfering with the venous return from the lower limbs to the heart. The resulting venous congestion leads to edema of the lower limbs. The edema may affect either one or both legs, depending on the size and location of the mass. This diagnosis can usually be established by a thorough clinical examination, including rectal and vaginal examinations and X-ray studies.

Postural (or gravitational) edema of the lower limbs is the most common type of edema affecting older people; it is more pronounced toward the end of the day. It can be differentiated from the edema resulting from heart failure by the lack of signs associated with heart failure and by the presence of diseases restricting the patient's degree of mobility. These diseases include Parkinson's disease, osteoarthritis, strokes, and muscle weakness. Postural edema of the lower limbs results from a combination of factors, the most important being diminished mobility. If a person stands or sits for prolonged periods of time without moving, the muscular pump becomes ineffective. Venous compression also plays an important role in the development of this type of edema. It will occur when the veins in the thigh are compressed between the weight of the body and the surface on which the patient sits, or when the edge of a reclining chair compresses the veins in the calves. Other factors that aggravate postural edema include varicose veins, venous thrombi, heart failure, some types of medication, and low blood albumin levels.

Albumin is formed in the liver from dietary protein. It is essential to maintaining adequate osmotic pressure inside the blood vessels and ensuring the return of fluid from the interstitial space to the vascular compartment. When edema is caused by inadequate blood levels of albumin, it tends to be quite extensive. The patient's entire body and even face are often affected. There are several reasons that the liver may be unable to produce the necessary amount of albumin, including malnutrition, liver impairment, the aging process, and excessive protein loss.

In cases of malnutrition, the liver does not receive a sufficient quantity of raw material from the diet to produce albumin; this occurs when the patient does not ingest enough protein. Healthy adults need at least 0.5 gram of protein for each pound of their body weight.

Two groups of people are particularly susceptible to becoming malnourished: the poor and the elderly. Infants and children of poor families who cannot afford to prepare nutritious meals often suffer from malnutrition. The elderly, especially men living on their own, are also vulnerable, regardless of their income.

A liver damaged by excessive and prolonged consumption of alcohol, diseases, or the intake of some types of medication or other chemical toxins will be unable to manufacture albumin at the rate necessary to maintain a normal concentration in the blood. Clinically, the patient shows other evidence of liver impairment in addition to edema. For example, fluid may also accumulate in the abdominal cavity, a condition known as ascites. The diagnosis of liver damage is made by clinical examination and supporting laboratory investigations. The livers of older people, even in the absence of disease, are often less efficient at producing albumin.

The albumin also can be deficient if an excessive amount of albumin is lost from the body. This condition may occur in certain types of diseases affecting the kidneys or the gastrointestinal tract. An excessive amount of protein also may be lost if a patient has large, oozing pressure ulcers, extensive burns, or chronic lung conditions that produce large amounts of sputum.

Patients with strokes and paralysis sometimes develop edema of the paralyzed limb. The mechanism of edema formation in these patients is not entirely understood. It probably results from a combination of an impairment of the nerves controlling the dilation and a constriction of the blood vessels in the affected limb, along with postural and gravitational factors.

Severe allergic states, toxic states, or local inflammation are associated with increased capillary permeability that results in edema. The amount of fluid flowing out to the capillaries far exceeds the amount that can be returned to the capillaries at the venous end. A number of medications, including steroids, estrogens, some arthritis medications, a few blood pressure medications, and certain antibiotics, can induce edema by promoting the retention of fluid. Salt intake tends to cause retention of fluid as well. Obstruction of the lymphatic system often leads to accumulation of fluid in the interstitial compartment. Obstruction can occur in certain types of cancer, after radiation treatment, and in certain parasitic infestations.

TREATMENT AND THERAPY

The management of edema depends on the specific reason for its presence. To determine the cause of edema, a thorough history, including current medications, dietary habits, and activity level, is of prime importance. Performing a detailed physical examination is also a vital step. It is frequently necessary to obtain laboratory, ultrasound, and/or X-ray studies before a final diagnosis is made. Once a treatable cause is found, then therapy aimed at the cause should be instituted.

If no treatable, specific disease is responsible for the edema, conservative treatment aimed at reducing the edema to manageable levels without inducing side effects should be initiated. Frequent elevation of the feet to the level of the heart, support stockings, and an avoidance of prolonged standing or sitting are the first steps. If support stockings are ineffective or are too uncomfortable, then custom-made, fitted stockings are available. A low-salt diet is important in the management of edema because a high salt intake worsens the fluid retention. If all these measures fail, then diuretics in small doses may be useful.

Diuretics work by increasing the amount of urine produced. Urine is made of fluids removed from the vascular compartment by the kidneys. The vascular compartment then replenishes itself by drawing water from the interstitial compartment. This reduction in the amount of interstitial fluid improves the edema. There are various types of diuretics, which differ in their potency, duration of action, and side effects. Potential side effects include dizziness, fatigue, sodium and potassium deficiency, excessively low blood pressure, dehydration, sexual dysfunction, the worsening of a diabetic's blood sugar control, increased uric acid levels, and increased blood cholesterol levels. Although diuretics are a convenient and effective means of treating simple edema, it is important to keep in mind that the cure should not be worse than the disease. When the potential side effects of diuretic therapy are compared to the almost total lack of complications of conservative treatment, one can see that mild edema which is not secondary to significant disease is best managed conservatively. Edema caused by more serious diseases, however, calls for more intensive measures.

PERSPECTIVE AND PROSPECTS

The prevalence of edema could decrease as people become more health-conscious and medical progress is made. Nutritious diets, avoidance of excessive salt, and an increased awareness of the dangers of excessive alcohol intake and of the benefits of regular physical exercise all contribute to decreasing the incidence of edema. Improved methods for the early detection, prevention, and management of diseases that may ultimately result in edema could also significantly reduce the scope of the problem. It is also expected that safer and more convenient methods of treating edema will become available.

—*Ronald C. Hamdy, M.D., Mark R. Doman, M.D.,*
and Katherine Hoffman Doman

See also Arteriosclerosis; Circulation; Diuretics; Elephantiasis; Embolism; Heart; Heart disease; Heart failure; Kidney disorders; Kidneys; Kwashiorkor; Liver; Liver disorders; Lungs; Malnutrition; Nutrition; Phlebitis; Protein; Pulmonary diseases; Pulmonary medicine; Pulmonary medicine, pediatric; Respiration; Signs and symptoms; Thrombosis and thrombus; Varicose vein removal; Varicose veins; Vascular medicine; Vascular system; Venous insufficiency.

FOR FURTHER INFORMATION:

Andreoli, Thomas E., et al., eds. *Andreoli and Carpenter's Cecil Essentials of Medicine.* 8th ed. Philadelphia: Saunders/Elsevier, 2010. A good introductory text to internal medicine that is appropriate and helpful for nonscientists as well.

Guyton, Arthur C., and John E. Hall. *Human Physiology and Mechanisms of Disease.* 6th ed. Philadelphia: W. B. Saunders, 1997. The standard reference text in human physiology. A background in basic physiology is helpful in understanding this work.

Hosenpud, Jeffrey D., and Barry H. Greenberg, eds. *Congestive Heart Failure.* 3d ed. Philadelphia: Lippincott Williams & Wilkins, 2007. A thorough treatise on the subject of heart failure. The authors discuss the circulatory system in states of both health and disease and the drug treatment for heart failure.

Marieb, Elaine N., and Katja Hoehn. *Human Anatomy and Physiology.* 9th ed. San Francisco: Pearson/Benjamin Cummings, 2010. Details the interrelationships of body organ systems, homeostasis, and how structure and function complement one another.

EDUCATION, MEDICAL
HEALTH CARE SYSTEM

DEFINITION: In the United States, the educational process that leads to obtaining and maintaining a state license to practice medicine, a process which generally involves obtaining two academic degrees and one or more medical certifications; the entire medical education takes a minimum of eleven years beyond high school.

KEY TERMS:

continuing medical education (CME): medical lectures given by hospitals, medical societies, specialists, and conferences that, in the United States, must be approved to meet the requirements for CME credits

generalist: a medical practitioner who belongs to one of the three largest specialties of medicine—family medicine, internal medicine, and pediatrics; sometimes, practitioners of obstetrics/gynecology (OB/GYN) and general surgery are considered to be generalists

internship: the first year of supervised, postgraduate training after receiving a doctor of medicine (M.D.) or doctor of osteopathy (D.O.) degree, which allows individuals to practice clinical medicine with a limited license; for M.D.'s, this is called year one of residency, and for D.O.'s this is called year one of internship

residency: a course of postgraduate medical education undertaken after receiving an M.D. or D.O. degree and leading to certification in a generalist or specialist branch of medicine

specialist: referring to specialties of medicine not categorized as generalist

STRUCTURE AND CURRICULUM

During the course of the twentieth century, the medical education system in the United States developed from a one-year or two-year program to the present requirement of eleven or more years of formal education and training after completion of secondary school.

College or university. A person who wishes to be licensed as a physician by one of the fifty states usually begins by completing a bachelor's degree at an accredited college or university. This is, by far, the norm, although it is not an absolute requirement. Some colleges and universities offer a premedical undergraduate program that emphasizes biology, chemistry, and other courses in scientific disciplines. In the past, medical schools preferred graduates of these premedical programs over those with liberal arts or science degrees. Today, many medical schools seek more well rounded students who have degrees in liberal arts disciplines. This change has been made in response to societal pressures to graduate more physicians who have a humanistic approach to medical practice. An effort has also been made to provide educational opportunities for members of disadvantaged and minority groups. Therefore, any person with a good grade point average may consider applying to medical school regard-

THE REQUIREMENTS FOR FULLY LICENSED PHYSICIANS

Place or Event	Degree or Program	Years
College or University	B.A. or B.S.	4
Medical School	Preclinical	2
Medical School	Clinical	2
Graduation	D.O. or M.D.	-
Internship or Residency	D.O. or M.D. Limited License	1
Residency (1st)	Generalist or Specialist	2-5
Residency (2d/3d)	Subspecialist (Optional)	0-5
Continuing Education	CME (150 credits)	every 3
	TOTAL	11-19+

less of the type or the nature of the bachelor-level education.

Preparation. The first choice that an individual must make when considering a career as a physician is, "What type of medical school do I wish to attend?" In the United States, two medical degrees are granted: doctor of medicine (M.D.) and doctor of osteopathy (D.O.). M.D.'s are occasionally referred to as allopathic physicians to distinguish them from osteopathic physicians. Historically, allopathic education stressed the importance of disease in causing illness. Laboratory tests and the prescription of medications are generally used in diagnosis and treatment. Osteopathic education historically looked to the musculoskeletal system with respect to health and illness. This distinction is largely a historical remnant. The curricula of both M.D. and D.O. schools are nearly identical. Both types of physicians train in the same residencies, and both receive the same license to practice medicine and surgery.

Medical school (preclinical). The first two years of medical school are generally devoted to the study of academic medicine. This period is known as preclinical education. These years stress the need to master material from basic sciences and to understand the scientific method of research. Courses such as anatomy, biochemistry, histology, immunology, microbiology, neurology, pathology, and physiology are taught. Achievement is marked by success in test taking through memorization, the analysis of detailed information, and the integration of new material. Actual contact with practicing physicians and their patients is not stressed.

As a result, this phase is sometimes criticized for teaching medical knowledge that is separated from medical practice. Some medical schools are adjusting the curriculum in the preclinical years to reduce this dichotomy. At the end of the second year, students must pass the first component of the examination to obtain licensure.

Medical school (clinical). The second two years of medical education stress the clinical knowledge needed to become a physician. Classroom education is concerned with physical diagnosis, the identification of diseases, treatments, and associated procedures and techniques. Medical schools require students to observe physicians practicing medicine with patients in both hospital and office settings. Opportunities are available for students to spend time away from their medical school learning about various specialties. The standard curriculum requires all students to study internal medicine, surgery, pediatrics, obstetrics and gynecology, and psychiatry. Other specialties are studied on an elective basis. For example, a medical student may spend a month observing family physicians working in hospitals and their offices and receive a grade for that month. In this manner, students gain some experience by direct exposure to several medical specialties. At the end of the fourth year, students must pass the second component of the examination to obtain licensure.

It has been suggested that general medical education should include as part of the core curriculum courses in bioethics, communication, and the legal issues that affect the practice of medicine. Components of such courses would include informed consent and refusal of treatment; the ethical limits of paternalism, truth-telling, trust, confidentiality, and communication; medical research; human reproduction and the status of the embryo; issues regarding children; issues surrounding genetics, mental health, and reproduction; special duties involving death and dying; and prolonging life. Medical education in Great Britain includes such courses. In the United States, however, those courses are not a mandatory part of the curriculum with the exception of a very few medical schools. It is only through continuing education and individual cases that physicians and other health care providers are exposed to these problems. Humanities courses are also part of the undergraduate medical curriculum in Great Britain because it is believed that art, drama, and literature, for example, are means by which people express their joy and sorrow through human creativity. These subjects are not required in the United States curriculum.

Internship. In the past, many generalist physicians, after one year of internship, entered private practice. Today, the year of internship is completed under close medical supervision. This prepares a new physician for more independent practice. All new physicians complete their first year of internship in a residency program before receiving a full medical license in the second year of residency. Physicians who receive their medical education outside the United States must pass the same test as American medical students before being eligible to complete residency training. Some internships are spent rotating through the areas of medicine, surgery, pediatrics, and obstetrics before entering specialized training in areas such as radiology, dermatology, and some surgical specialties. During the first year of residency, a physician has a limited license to practice medicine. Upon completion of the internship or first-year residency and successful passage of the third portion of the standard licensure examination, a physician is granted a full license to practice medicine and surgery.

Residency. The three generalist areas in which resident physicians learn clinical medicine, also known as primary care specialties, are family medicine, internal medicine, and pediatrics. Family medicine treats the whole family throughout life, internal medicine treats adults, and pediatrics treats children and teenagers. The end of childhood and the beginning of adulthood are not clearly defined, and there is some overlap. Most pediatricians will treat patients up to the age of twenty-two, when they typically complete college. The lowest age for patients of internists is usually sixteen. The many specialist areas of medicine are concerned with specific organ systems, disease processes, or prevention. For example, a psychiatrist has a residency in the area of mental illness, while an emergency room (ER) physician has a residency in the practice of medicine in the ER.

Residency education is the time when a physician who has graduated from medical school first becomes responsible for patient care, under both direct and indirect supervision. Resident physicians are often referred to as "house officers" or "house staff." Residency teaches and evaluates the skill of a new physician

in applying the knowledge gained in medical school to clinical practice. Residency programs are usually three to five years in length. After each year, the resident is given more independence of practice and more responsibility to supervise newer physicians. Upon completion of a residency program, a physician becomes eligible for certification by one of the generalist or specialist boards of medicine. Most boards require one or two years of independent practice before allowing candidates to seek board certification. A physician must take and pass yet another examination concerning knowledge related to the specialty area for which certification is desired. Many board certifications must be renewed periodically (every five to seven years) as a condition of retaining board-certified status.

Second residency (subspecialization). Some physicians choose to complete additional training in their medical specialties. This subspecialty medical education is usually called a fellowship. For example, a general surgeon may complete a multiyear residency in cardiac surgery, or a psychiatrist may complete a subspecialty residency in children's mental illness. Some highly subspecialized physicians need seven to ten years after medical school to complete their subspecialty training. An example of this level of specialization is forensic pathology, which requires residency training in pathology and fellowships in forensic and chemical pathology. Pediatric neurosurgery is another example.

Continuing medical education. All states require that physicians complete a certain number of continuing medical education (CME) credits in order to maintain their medical licensure. A common requirement is 150 CME credits over three years. Some specialties also require national examinations for recertification in the specialty. For physicians in the United States, medical education is an exercise in lifelong learning.

ISSUES AND PHILOSOPHIES

American medical education is undergoing one of the greatest challenges in its history. Medical schools are being asked to teach physicians how to be effective and efficient caregivers to all persons. The corporate system of medical care demands medical care that is effective, cost-conscious or economically efficient, and delivered in a positive and caring manner. Health maintenance organizations (HMOs), preferred provider organizations (PPOs), and other organizational alliances of physicians expect the medical educational system to teach these values and skills.

The national government adds one more criterion: Physicians must be able to do the above for all citizens. In a pluralistic and democratic society, a physician must acknowledge various social, ethnic, cultural, and regional needs. Medical educators must train socially conscious physicians. Physicians must be available to practice in either rural or inner-city areas. They must be able to treat various populations, such as African Americans and Native Americans, for their specific needs. Physicians are being asked to be cognizant of and caring toward all Americans.

The medical philosophy that allows for an increase of psychological skills and social awareness in medical education is called the biopsychosocial model. As the label indicates, it conceptualizes a medical education system which teaches physicians solid medical knowledge ("bio"), an improved ability to relate to patients ("psycho"), and an awareness of different social systems and cultural attitudes as they affect medical care ("social"). The biopsychosocial model of care is a proposed revision of what the medical education system should teach physicians. It may be the medical school curriculum of the future.

PERSPECTIVE AND PROSPECTS

The history of American medical education can be understood as falling into five periods of development. Each period stressed a certain philosophy and direction unique to its times. The current philosophy of medical education has aspects of all five periods, affecting how and what physicians are taught.

The British period (1750-1815). American medical education was established on the British model. The emphasis in British medical education was on developing a physician's medical knowledge through direct observation of patient care in clinical settings. There were few formal centers for medical training. They functioned to instruct teaching physicians and to transmit new medical knowledge. In America, there were only six medical schools. Most medical education was clinical and taught by older physicians to younger physicians in office settings. There were no formal educational requirements. Most physicians could read and write, possessing the equivalent of only two or three years of formal education.

The French period (1815-1865). French physicians, who developed the skills of classification, influenced American medical education through methods of diagnosis and the use of hospitals. In the United States, many hospitals were built, and there was a significant expansion in the number of medical schools. Large groups of patients were admitted to hospitals and grouped on wards by diagnosis. The hospital-office model of medical education began to develop.

The German period (1865-1915). Laboratory methods and germ theory were introduced into medical education from Germany. Some medical schools began to educate physicians in the laboratory approach to medicine. Office practice was less important in medical education. The period of formal education was still relatively brief, often less than two years in total length. At the end of the German period, many medical schools that were not teaching laboratory methods were closed.

The American period (1915-1965). American medical education embraced a scientific approach, first detailed by Abraham Flexner in *Medical Education in the United States and Canada*, published in 1910 in a report on reforming American medical education. Physician-scientists were to be educated by quality medical schools to provide clinical medicine according to the scientific method. This model was successfully introduced into American medical education. It was considered the norm until the concerns of corporate interests and government interests became vital.

The corporate period (1965-   ). Medicare and Medicaid programs were created and supported by the national government in order to provide quality medical care to all Americans. Corporate interests require that medical education be effective in controlling health costs to industry. Many of the current challenges facing medical education revolve around teaching physicians the two concerns of access and cost-effectiveness.

In the early 1990's, the Council on Graduate Medical Education (COGME) suggested that certain humanistic and corporate medical education goals be reached by the year 2000. At least 50 percent of residency graduates should enter practice as generalist physicians. The number of underrepresented minority students should be doubled. Shortages of physicians in rural and urban areas should be eliminated. The purpose of these goals was to avoid a severe physician shortage for some populations, areas of specialty, and geographic centers. With a system of managed medical care in place, COGME projected a shortage of 35,000 generalist physicians and a surplus of 115,000 specialist physicians by the year 2000. COGME released a report in 1999 that noted the rate of growth in the physician supply had moderated slightly but still was likely to lead to a surplus of physicians, and that the number of generalist physicians was increasing.

In 1990, fewer than one-third of all American physicians practiced primary care. It appears that in the future, the trend toward specialization will be reversed. Those who plan, those who pay, and those who organize the various systems to deliver medical care in the United States no longer believe that so many specialty-trained physicians will be needed. Yet, the demand by Americans for specialized health care services has not diminished. A clash between recipients and providers appears to be inevitable. The next decades in American medicine are likely to be turbulent, as various stakeholders struggle to redefine the American system of health care.

There is an acknowledged maldistribution of physicians. Most prefer to practice in suburban and medical center settings, leaving significant numbers of Americans without easy access to adequate health care. Many planners also believe that the promised efficiency of managed care will result in a decreased need for physicians. In the mid-1990's, state legislatures began to reduce the amounts of support for medical education, effectively forcing medical schools to reduce the number of physicians that they graduate. The final outcomes of these policy changes are unclear. The results of this trend, however, will be felt by American society for decades.

Women in medicine. Despite a long history of discrimination against women in medicine, women have actually practiced the profession for many centuries. In ancient Egypt, in the time of Moses, and throughout the nineteenth century and the reign of King Henry V of England, female physicians were active. Opportunities for female physicians were scarce, however, and admissions to "regular" medical schools were an anomaly.

In the United States, three medical schools were opened specifically for female applicants in 1864: in Boston, Cincinnati, and Philadelphia. Medical societies refused admission to women, however, and it was difficult for women to obtain academic positions outside a women's medical school. By 1870, women represented only 0.8 percent of physicians in the United States. By 1900, 6 percent of all physicians were women. By 1940, the percentage of women in medicine declined to 4.4 percent, and it did not reach 6 per-

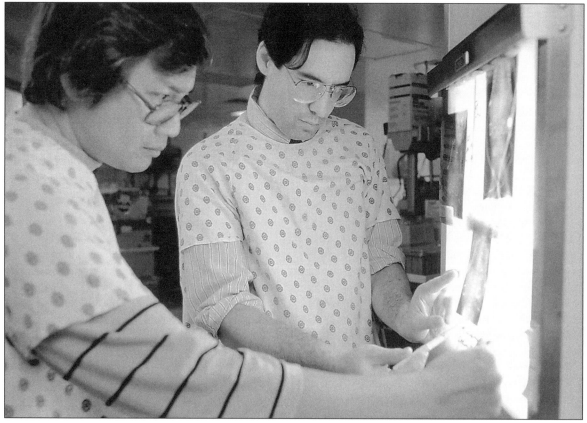

Interns gain experience by reviewing X rays. (Digital Stock)

cent again until 1950. A major surge in female admissions occurred in the 1970's, when the percentage of women in medicine reached 8.9 percent. Overall, by 1997 women represented 22 percent of physicians. They are, however, an increasing proportion of the profession, constituting close to half of all medical students in the early twenty-first century. Despite the relative paucity of their numbers as physicians, women occupy the majority position as workers in the health care sector generally (85 percent).

Discrimination is present in medical schools and workplaces, and sexual harassment exists within the medical sector, a disproportionate amount of which is directed toward women. Some patients also discriminate, preferring not to deal with female physicians. Research during the 1970's revealed that patients often felt that women physicians lacked competency and experience, but as more women entered the profession, patients' attitudes toward female physicians became more positive. Overall, female physicians have a greater percentage of female patients than do male physicians. They are more likely to discuss psychological and sexual issues with their patients and to bring a sense of participation to the physician-patient relationship, relative to male physicians. Data suggest that there is greater disclosure in the same-sex doctor-patient relationship.

Women in medicine have also had to combat sexual stereotyping. The characteristics of leaders—assertion, capability, and decisiveness—when applied to women become negative attributes—pushiness, lack of femininity, and aggression. Sociologists have reported that women and men think differently and approach situations from different perspectives. Consequently, many people believe that women bring the positive traits of humanism and caring to the practice of medicine. In 2000, it was predicted that in the future male physicians will use high-tech medicine while female physicians will practice hands-on medicine.

Female physicians also experience many stresses in their professional lives. They advance more slowly in their careers and earn less money than do male physicians. One study reported that almost 65 percent of female family practitioners felt overwhelmed at least once a week. Women reportedly complain of less support from their employers and their families than do their male counterparts, and they rely more heavily on their spouses for support. A common solution to stress management has been avoidance; that is, some female physicians back off from ambition. Others, in contrast, play a domestic role while simultaneously pursuing a career. The latter group experiences extreme strain, fatigue, anxiety, and resentment about work overload with little time to accomplish their tasks. Statistics in 1999 demonstrated that about 90 percent of married female physicians have a spouse who also is a professional, and half of these marry another physician.

Techniques for reducing strain when combining roles of marriage and motherhood with medicine include role cycling (prioritizing one or another role at different times); changed expectations (developing a flexible attitude toward daily problems); decreased confrontations with social norms (reducing conflict by seeking out friends with similar backgrounds, thus reaching one's own comfort level); hiring help for child care, housework, and other chores; and concentrating one's life within a small geographic area. Relaxation techniques such as meditation and biofeedback, support groups, coaches, and professional counseling are helpful means to assist female physicians in stress reduction and in coping.

—Gerald T. Terlep, Ph.D.;
L. Fleming Fallon, Jr., M.D., Ph.D., M.P.H.;
updated by Marcia J. Weiss, M.A., J.D.

See also American Medical Association (AMA); Ethics; Hippocratic oath; Medical College Admission Test (MCAT); Nursing; Osteopathic medicine; *specific specialties.*

FOR FURTHER INFORMATION:

Birenbaum, Aaron. *Wounded Profession: American Medicine Enters the Age of Managed Care.* Westport, Conn.: Greenwood Press, 2002. Traces the evolution of health care in the United States during the 1990's and examines the rising costs, consumer backlash, and new legislation.

Bowman, Marjorie A., and Deborah I. Allen. *Stress and Women Physicians.* 2d ed. New York: Springer, 1990. Discusses professional qualities of practicing women physicians.

Bowman, Marjorie A., Erica Frank, and Deborah I. Allen. *Women in Medicine: Career and Life Management.* New York: Springer, 2002. An honest discussion of the challenges facing women physicians. Includes cases, appendixes, resource lists, organizations, and Web site addresses. An updated version of *Stress and Women Physicians.*

Brown, Stanford J. *Getting into Medical School.* 9th ed. Hauppauge, N.Y.: Barron's, 2001. Advice on recommended undergraduate courses, taking the Medical College Admission Test (MCAT), applying to medical school, getting through the personal interview, and alternatives for students who have been rejected. Directory of American medical schools included.

Ludmerer, Kenneth M. *Time to Heal: American Medical Education from the Turn of the Century to the Managed Care Era*. New York: Oxford University Press, 2005. Ludmerer looks at the future of medicine in America and reveals some very disturbing trends in managed care, education, and research funding. Contains a wealth of factual details and insightful questions.

Rivo, Marc L., et al. "Defining the Generalist Physician's Training." *Journal of the American Medical Association* 271 (May 18, 1994): 1499-1504. Rivo presents a clear, fact-filled article on major current issues in medical education. The article is accessible to the general reader. It also contains charts and references for further research.

Starr, Paul. "The Framework of Health Care Reform." *New England Journal of Medicine* 330, no. 15 (April 14, 1994): 1086-1088. This article reviews several proposals for health care reform. The author has provided commentary on the American health care system for many years.

Zebala, John A., Daniel B. Jones, and Stephanie B. Jones. *Medical School Admissions: The Insider's Guide*. 5th rev. ed. Memphis, Tenn.: Mustang, 2000. Written by medical students for medical students, this book gives practical advice on admission tasks such as the preparation of an effective application, improving scores on the MCAT, and writing a compelling personal essay.

EEG. *See* ELECTROENCEPHALOGRAPHY (EEG).

EHRLICHIOSIS
DISEASE/DISORDER

ANATOMY OR SYSTEM AFFECTED: Immune system, musculoskeletal system, nervous system

SPECIALTIES AND RELATED FIELDS: Family medicine, pediatrics

DEFINITION: Infection by one of a group of intracellular bacteria transmitted to humans through tick bites.

CAUSES AND SYMPTOMS

Human ehrlichiosis is a group of tick-borne bacterial infections caused by *Anaplasma phagocytophilum* (formerly *Ehrlichia phagocytophilum*), *Ehrlichia chaf-*

INFORMATION ON EHRLICHIOSIS

CAUSES: Bite of an infected tick
SYMPTOMS: Fever, chills, headache, muscle aches and weakness, joint pain, nausea
DURATION: Acute
TREATMENTS: Antibiotics

feensis, and *Ehrlichia ewingii*. These bacteria are transmitted by the bite of *Ixodes spp.* or *Amblyomma americanum* ticks, which subsequently infect circulating white blood cells (leukocytes).

After an incubation period of five to ten days, the disease is typically characterized by fever, chills, and other nonspecific symptoms. A percentage of asymptomatic infections have also been documented. Confirmation of ehrlichiosis infection is accomplished via laboratory methods including blood smear examination, polymerase chain reaction, culture, and serologic analysis for the presence of anti-ehrlichia antibodies.

TREATMENT AND THERAPY

Ehrlichiosis is effectively treated with a tetracycline antibiotic, most commonly doxycycline. With the increased number of diagnoses, more significant cases requiring hospitalization and condition appropriate treatment have been documented. Significant complications include respiratory distress, myocarditis, neurological complications, hepatitis, septicemia, and opportunistic infections. Despite clinical similarities between the causative agents, a higher percentage of opportunistic infection has been documented with human granulocytic anaplasmosis (HGA), caused by *A. phagocytophila*, whereas increased disease severity and higher mortality has been associated with human monocytic ehrlichiosis (HME), caused by *E. chaffeensis*. Death resulting from complications may occur in up to 3 percent of cases.

PERSPECTIVE AND PROSPECTS

The reported prevalence and incidence of human ehrlichiosis has been on the rise in regions where specified tick vectors are found. Although historically considered an acute infection conferring long-term immunity, one study found a percentage of HME patients experienced a significantly higher than expected rate of fever, chills, sweats, and fatigue one to three years after the initial illness. Because these symptoms did not correlate with the severity or duration of the initial episode, nor did serological tests confirm the presence of ehrlichia, determination of whether these findings are attributed to a persistent/recurrent infection or a type of post-infection syndrome is still under investigation.

—*Pam Conboy*

See also Bacterial infections; Bacteriology; Bites and stings; Insect-borne diseases; Lice, mites, and ticks; Lyme disease; Parasitic diseases.

FOR FURTHER INFORMATION:

Dumler, J. S. "Anaplasma and Ehrlichia Infection." *Annals of the New York Academy of Sciences* 1063 (December, 2005): 361-373.

_____, et al. "Ehrlichioses in Humans: Epidemiology, Clinical Presentation, Diagnosis, and Treatment." *Clinical Infectious Diseases* 45, suppl. 1 (July 15, 2007): S45-S51.

Dumler, J. S, R. J. Thomas, and J. A. Carlyon. "Current Management of Human Granulocytic Anaplasmosis, Human Monocytic Ehrlichiosis, and Ehrlichia Ewingii Ehrlichiosis." *Expert Review of Anti-Infective Therapy* 7, no. 6 (August, 2009): 709-722.

Ganguly, S., and S. K. Mukhopadhayay. "Tick-Borne Ehrlichiosis Infection in Human Beings." *Journal of Vector Borne Diseases* 45, no. 4 (December, 2008): 273-280.

ELECTRICAL SHOCK

DISEASE/DISORDER

ANATOMY OR SYSTEM AFFECTED: Heart, nervous system, skin

SPECIALTIES AND RELATED FIELDS: Critical care, emergency medicine, neurology

DEFINITION: The physical effect of an electrical current entering the body and the resulting damage.

CAUSES AND SYMPTOMS

Electrical shock ranges from a harmless jolt of static electricity to a power line's lethal discharge. The severity of the shock depends on the current flowing through the body, and the current is determined by the skin's electrical resistance. Dry skin has a very high resistance; thus, 110 volts produces a small, harmless current. The resistance for perspiring hands, however, is lower by a factor of 100, resulting in potentially fatal currents. Currents traveling between bodily extremities are particularly dangerous because of their proximity to the heart.

Electrical shock causes injury or death in one of

> ### INFORMATION ON ELECTRICAL SHOCK
>
> **CAUSES:** Electrical current entering the body
> **SYMPTOMS:** Unconsciousness, moderate to severe pain, ventricular fibrillation, burning or charring of skin
> **DURATION:** Acute
> **TREATMENTS:** Resuscitation, emergency care

---

three ways: paralysis of the breathing center in the brain, paralysis of the heart, or ventricular fibrillation (extremely rapid and uncontrolled twitching of the heart muscle).

The threshold of feeling (the minimum current detectable) ranges from 0.5 to 1.0 milliamperes. Currents up to 5.0 milliamperes, the maximum harmless current, are not hazardous, unless they trigger an accident by involuntary reaction. Currents in this range create a tingling sensation. The minimum current that causes muscular paralysis occurs between 10 and 15 milliamperes. Currents of this magnitude cause a painful jolt. Above 18 milliamperes, the current contracts chest muscles, and breathing ceases. Unconsciousness and death follow within minutes unless the current is interrupted and respiration resumed. A short exposure to currents of 50 milliamperes causes severe pain, possible fainting, and complete exhaustion, while currents in the 100- to 300-milliampere range produce ventricular fibrillation, which is fatal unless quickly corrected. During ventricular fibrillation, the heart stops its rhythmic pumping and flutters uselessly. Since blood stops flowing, the victim dies from oxygen deprivation in the brain in a matter of minutes. This is the most common cause of death for victims of electrical shock.

Relatively high currents (above 300 milliamperes) may produce ventricular paralysis, deep burns in the body's tissue, or irreversible damage to the central nervous system. Victims are more likely to survive a large but brief current, even though smaller, sustained currents are usually lethal. Burning or charring of the skin at the point of contact may be a contributing factor to the delayed death that often follows severe electrical shock. Very high voltage discharges of short duration, such as a lightning strike, tend to disrupt the body's nervous impulses, but victims may survive. On the other hand, any electric current large enough to raise body temperature significantly produces immediate death.

TREATMENT AND THERAPY

Before medical treatment can be applied, the current must be stopped or the shock victim must be separated from the current source without being touched. Nonconducting materials such as dry, heavy blankets or pieces of wood can be used for this purpose. If the victim is not breathing, artificial respiration immediately applied provides adequate short-term life support, though the victim may become stiff or rigid in reaction to the shock. Victims of electrical shock may suffer from severe burns and permanent aftereffects, including eye cataracts, angina, or disorders of the nervous system.

Electrical shock can usually be prevented by strictly adhering to safety guidelines and using common-sense precautions. Careful inspection of appliances and tools, compliance with manufacturers' safety standards, and the avoidance of unnecessary risks greatly reduce the chance of an electrical shock. Electrical appliances or tools should never be used when standing in water or on damp ground, and dry gloves, shoes, and floors provide considerable protection against dangerous shocks from 110-volt circuits.

Electrical safety is also provided by isolation, guarding, insulation, grounding, and ground-fault interrupters. Isolation means that high-voltage wires strung overhead are not within reach, while guarding provides a barrier around high voltage devices, such as those found in television sets.

Old wire insulation may become brittle with age and develop small cracks. Defective wires are hazardous and should be replaced immediately. Most modern power tools are double-insulated; the motor is insulated from the plastic insulating frame. These devices do not require grounding, as no exposed metal parts become electrically live if the wire insulation fails.

In a home, grounding is accomplished by a third wire in outlets, connected through a grounding circuit to a water pipe. If an appliance plug has a third prong, it will ground the frame to the grounding circuit. In the event of a short circuit, the grounding circuit provides a low resistance path, resulting in a current surge which trips the circuit breaker.

In some instances the current may be inadequate to trip a circuit breaker (which usually requires 15 or 20 amperes), but current in excess of 10 milliamperes could still be lethal to humans. A ground-fault inter-rupter ensures nearly complete protection by detecting leakage currents as small as 5 milliamperes and breaking the circuit. This relatively inexpensive device operates very rapidly and provides an extremely high degree of safety against electrocution in the household. Many localities now have codes which require the installation of ground-fault interrupters in bathrooms, kitchens, and other areas where water is used.

—George R. Plitnik, Ph.D.

See also Burns and scalds; Cardiac arrest; Critical care; Critical care, pediatric; Emergency medicine; First aid; Intensive care unit (ICU); Resuscitation; Shock; Unconsciousness.

FOR FURTHER INFORMATION:

Atkinson, William. "Electric Injuries Can Be Worse than They Seem." *Electric World* 214, no. 1 (January/February, 2000): 33-36. Whether an electrical shock initially seems serious or mild, it is always a cause for concern. Aspects of electrical shock injuries are explored.

Bridges, J. E., et al., eds. *International Symposium on Electrical Shock Safety Criteria.* New York: Pergamon Press, 1985. The summary of a symposium covering the physiological effects of shock, bioelectrical conditions, and safety measures.

Hewitt, Paul G. *Conceptual Physics.* 11th ed. San Francisco: Pearson Addison Wesley, 2010. Comprehensive coverage of physics for the layperson, which includes detailed discussions of the laws of electricity and electrical devices.

Hogan, David E., and Jonathan L. Burstein. *Disaster Medicine.* 2d ed. Philadelphia: Lippincott Williams & Wilkins, 2007. Examines a wide range of relevant topics including natural, industrial, transportation, and conflict-related disasters; and infectious diseases, winter storms, fires, and mass burns.

Liu, Lynda. "Pullout Emergency Guide: Electric Shock." *Parents* 75, no. 1 (January, 2000): 65-66. A pull-out emergency guide for the prevention and treatment of electrical shock in children. Household hazards and electricity dos and don'ts are among the tips offered.

U.S. Department of Labor. Occupational Safety and Health Administration. *Controlling Electrical Hazards.* Rev. ed. Washington, D.C.: Author, 2002. A report which identifies common electrical hazards and discusses their prevention.

ELECTROCARDIOGRAPHY (ECG OR EKG)

PROCEDURE

ANATOMY OR SYSTEM AFFECTED: Chest, circulatory system, heart

SPECIALTIES AND RELATED FIELDS: Biotechnology, cardiology, critical care, emergency medicine, exercise physiology, preventive medicine

DEFINITION: A noninvasive procedure that provides insight into the rate, rhythm, and general health of the heart.

KEY TERMS:

ECG waves: the repeated deflections of an electrocardiogram; one complete wave consists of a P wave, followed by a QRS complex, and then a T wave and represents one complete cardiac cycle, or heartbeat

electrocardiogram (ECG or EKG): a record of the waves produced by the rhythmically changing electrical conduction within the heart; often recorded by a strip chart recorder

INDICATIONS AND PROCEDURES

Electrocardiography is a useful medical diagnostic and evaluative procedure that reveals much information about the function or malfunction of a person's heart. ECG is a noninvasive, easy-to-use, and economical tool that is an essential part of diagnosing chest pain. It serves an important role in both cardiology and emergency medicine. ECG is also commonly used in preventive medicine to monitor heart health. For this purpose, ECG is frequently used in a format known as a stress test. Athletes often have ECG analysis performed as a part of their training and cardiovascular conditioning.

In a stress test, a person is studied for regularity of rhythm, rate, and unimpeded flow of electrical conduction within the heart. ECG recordings are first made while the person is at rest, then during light exercise, and, finally, if healthy enough, during rigorous exercise. Such exercise causes the heart to work harder and allows a physician to determine whether a person has a

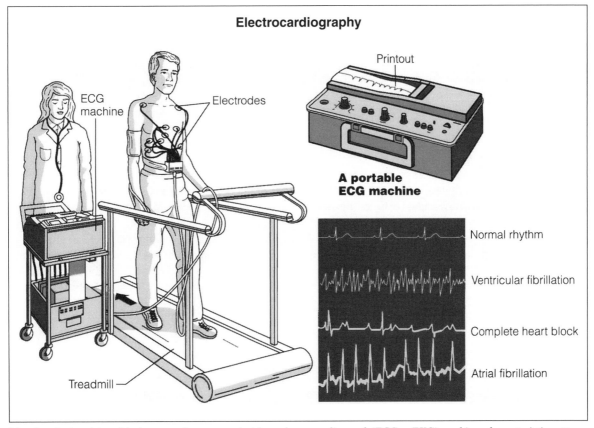

Electrocardiography

Printout

Electrodes

ECG machine

A portable ECG machine

Normal rhythm

Ventricular fibrillation

Complete heart block

Atrial fibrillation

Treadmill

The electrical activity of the heart can be measured with an electrocardiograph (ECG or EKG) machine; characteristic patterns can be used to diagnose arrhythmias (irregular heartbeats). The patient may also be asked to walk on a treadmill while the heart is monitored in order to gauge its function during exercise.

heart that beats with a regular, repetitive rhythm and at an appropriate pace for the level of rest or exercise. The stress of exercise can also help in assessing whether the heart muscle masses contract in the proper sequence: atrial contraction followed by ventricular contraction. An irregularity of electrical conduction, poor muscle contraction, dead regions of heart tissue (from a recent or old heart attack), and other maladies can be revealed.

To obtain an electrocardiogram, small metallic contact points are taped to the patient's skin via an electrically conductive adhesive or gel. The electric impulses travel across the skin to these contact points; from there, leads (plastic-coated wires) are attached to the recording device so that a complete circuit is made. Either a monitor screen or a strip chart recorder traces the electrical impulses. The waves are plotted in units of millivolts (on the y-axis) versus time in units of seconds (on the x-axis).

A twelve-lead ECG has replaced the original four-lead type. A twelve-lead ECG allows the physician to explore the performance of the heart from twelve different orientations, or angles, so that much more of the heart mass can be evaluated. Ten electrodes are placed on the body as follows: one on the right leg, which serves as the ground electrode; one on each of the other extremities; and six on the precordium, which is the area around the sternum and on the left chest wall (over the heart). The leads are explored in different combinations.

Uses and Complications

Healthy people, including athletes or certain members of the armed services, may take stress tests in order to have their health and cardiovascular conditioning monitored during training. Some professionals are required to take stress tests on a regular basis, such as commercial airline pilots and astronauts. In addition, people who have a family history of cardiovascular disease, or who are concerned about their heart health for other reasons, may have a stress test performed to find early warning signs and allow intervention before a crisis occurs. Finally, it should be noted that some insurance companies require stress tests of their applicants in order to determine insurability before issuing or rejecting a policy.

Treatment for chest pain is highly dependent on the electrical patterns seen on the ECG. Drugs may be administered or withheld depending on the shape or duration reported for the P-wave, QRS-complex, and T-wave patterns. Left-sided versus right-sided heart disease can

be discerned from the traces, and infarction (heart attack) can be distinguished from angina. Although the waves in the electrocardiogram for an infarcted or anginal heart are abnormal, the patterns become abnormal in a predictable, and therefore diagnostic, manner.

Diagnostic patterns can also be seen for arrhythmias (unusual and abnormal beating patterns), such as ectopic foci, in which some part of the heart other than the sinoatrial (S-A) node (the natural pacemaker) is abnormally in control of determining when the heart contracts, or heart block, whereby electrical conduction is interrupted.

ECG is routinely used to keep close tabs on heart patients and in the postsurgery monitoring of patients who have had open heart or thoracic surgery. Certain kinds of neonatal or infant malformations or malfunctions may also be evaluated with ECG.

Because ECG is a superficial and noninvasive technique, there are no real risks associated with having this procedure performed.

Perspective and Prospects

Electrocardiography was once a wet, messy, and awkward procedure to perform: A patient dangled one arm in a huge jar filled with a conducting salt solution and placed the left leg in another saline-filled container. Changing the leads to include other limbs required the patient to take a good amount of soaking. Although it was a clumsy procedure, the basic premise of ECG remains unchanged: The heart exhibits regular patterns of electrical activity that can be useful diagnostically.

Advances in electrocardiography have involved the use of multiple electrode systems along with computers and recorders that allow rapid and simultaneous multiple-lead input and output. In addition, modern electronic instrumentation allows continuous ECG monitoring so that patients in intensive care units, coronary care units, or emergency rooms can be assessed on a second-by-second basis when seconds count. Undoubtedly, modern ECG systems, coupled with thoughtful and informed interpretation by medical doctors and emergency medical technicians (EMTs), save many lives.

—Mary C. Fields, M.D.

See also Angina; Arrhythmias; Biofeedback; Cardiac arrest; Cardiology; Cardiology, pediatric; Cardiopulmonary resuscitation (CPR); Critical care; Critical care, pediatric; Diagnosis; Echocardiography; Emergency medicine; Emergency medicine, pediatric; Exercise physiology; Heart; Heart attack; Paramedics; Stress; Stress reduction.

FOR FURTHER INFORMATION:

Brady, William, John Camm, and June Edhouse. *ABC of Clinical Electrocardiography.* Malden, Mass.: Blackwell Science, 2002. A quick-reference text showing a wide range of electrocardiogram patterns seen in clinical practice.

Conover, Mary Boudreau. *Understanding Electrocardiography.* 8th ed. St. Louis, Mo.: Mosby, 2003. This standard text is divided into four sections: introduction to the 12-lead electrocardiogram, arrhythmia recognition, abnormal 12-lead electrocardiograms, and special diagnostic and therapeutic procedures.

Phibbs, Brendan. *The Human Heart: A Complete Text on Function and Disease.* 5th ed. St. Louis, Mo.: G. W. Manning, 1992. Designed for the general reader, this resource discusses cardiology. Includes bibliographical references and an index.

Surawicz, Borys, and Timothy K. Knilans. *Chou's Electrocardiography in Clinical Practice: Adult and Pediatric.* 6th ed. Philadelphia: Saunders/Elsevier, 2008. Explores the values and limitations of the electrocardiogram and covers such topics as pericarditis and cardiac surgery, atrial and atrioventricular rhythms, ventricular arrhythmias, and effects of drugs on the ECG.

Thaler, Malcom S. *The Only EKG Book You'll Ever Need.* 6th ed. Philadelphia: Lippincott Williams & Wilkins, 2010. Many EKG texts delve heavily into the physics and myocardial electrophysiology associated with EKGs and overwhelm and confuse the early learner. This book avoids lengthy discussions of theory and uses wide spacing, open pages, simple text, and diagrams to allow for speedier mastery of the basics.

Wellens, Hein J. J., and Mary Conover. *The ECG in Emergency Decision Making.* 2d ed. St. Louis, Mo.: Saunders/Elsevier, 2006. This resource offers guidance for the professional regarding the diagnosis of heart disease in an emergency setting.

Wiederhold, Richard. *Electrocardiography: The Monitoring and Diagnostic Leads.* Philadelphia: W. B. Saunders, 1999. This textbook is intended to be a primary or introductory text to the field of electrocardiography (ECG) for students in the health care professions or clinicians who are not cardiologists.

ELECTROCAUTERIZATION

PROCEDURE

ANATOMY OR SYSTEM AFFECTED: Blood vessels, cells, circulatory system, joints, ligaments, muscles, skin, uterus

SPECIALTIES AND RELATED FIELDS: Cardiology, critical care, dermatology, emergency medicine, family medicine, general surgery, gynecology, internal medicine, vascular medicine

DEFINITION: The surgical control of bleeding from small blood vessels or the removal of unwanted tissue using a controlled electric current.

INDICATIONS AND PROCEDURES

Electrocauterization is a procedure used in many surgical operations. As a surgeon's scalpel penetrates layers of skin and tissue, numerous tiny blood vessels are cut open. To stop the associated bleeding, an assisting surgeon can seal these vessels immediately using an electrical instrument to burn just enough of the tissue to produce a tiny scar. Electrocauterization is also used to destroy unwanted tissue, such as skin lesions.

Prior to any surgery involving electrocautery, local anesthesia is applied by injection. Electrocauterization is carried out with a small needle probe that is heated with an electrical current. Enough current is applied to heat the probe to temperatures at which blood will coagulate. To prevent electrical shock, a grounding pad is placed on the patient and a small electrode is attached to the skin near the surgery site to direct any excess current away from the body. Depending on the surgery site and the size and shape of unwanted tissue, the cautery pattern may be circular, dotted, or linear. In some applications, a temperature sensor near the electrical probe allows a microprocessor-based control unit to regulate the delivered electrical power as a function of tissue temperature.

USES AND COMPLICATIONS

Electrocauterization is commonly used to destroy unwanted tissue. It has been applied to remove growths in the nasal passage, noncancerous polyps in the colon, canker sores, and lesions on or around the skin, muscles, ligaments, blood vessels, joints, and bones. It is used to stop bleeding during surgery and also when biopsies are performed. It has been used in women to remove abnormal tissue from the cervix and to stop abnormal bleeding from the uterus that is not caused by menstruation.

The healing time after electrocauterization procedures is usually two to three weeks. After electrocautery, a patient may experience pain, swelling, redness, drainage, bleeding, bruising, scarring, or itching at or around the surgery site. Headache, muscle aches, dizziness, fever, tiredness, and a general ill feeling may also occur following electrocauterization. The most serious complication can be the onset of infection. Antibiotics are typically administered if this occurs. Acetaminophen is used to diminish pain.

Excessive electrocautery can produce superficial to deep burns, which can be treated with cold packs. Electrocauterization of the cervix may lead to the misinterpretation of future Pap tests. When electrocauterization is performed multiple times to stop the occurrence of frequent nosebleeds, scar tissue can build up in the nose, leading to increased nosebleeds because of the lack of elasticity of scar tissue.

—*Alvin K. Benson, Ph.D.*

See also Biopsy; Bleeding; Blood vessels; Canker sores; Cervical procedures; Colorectal polyp removal; Cryosurgery; Dermatology; Dermatopathology; Genital disorders, female; Healing; Laser use in surgery; Lesions; Nosebleeds; Skin; Skin disorders; Skin lesion removal; Surgery, general; Surgical procedures; Tumor removal; Tumors.

FOR FURTHER INFORMATION:
Bland, Kirby I., ed. *The Practice of General Surgery.* Philadelphia: W. B. Saunders, 2002.

Brunicardi, F. Charles, et al., eds. *Schwartz's Manual of Surgery.* 8th ed. New York: McGraw-Hill Medical, 2006.

Morreale, Barbara, David L. Roseman, and Albert K. Straus. *Inside General Surgery: An Illustrated Guide.* New Brunswick, N.J.: Johnson & Johnson, 1991.

Pollack, Sheldon V. *Electrosurgery of the Skin.* New York: Churchill Livingstone, 1991.

ELECTROENCEPHALOGRAPHY (EEG)
PROCEDURE

ANATOMY OR SYSTEM AFFECTED: Brain, head, nervous system, psychic-emotional system

SPECIALTIES AND RELATED FIELDS: Biotechnology, critical care, emergency medicine, neurology, pathology, psychiatry, psychology, speech pathology

DEFINITION: The tracing of the electrical potentials produced by brain cells on a graphic chart, as detected by electrodes placed on the scalp.

KEY TERMS:

brain stem: the medulla oblongata, pons, and mesencephalon portions of the brain, which perform motor, sensory, and reflex functions and contain the corticospinal and reticulospinal tracts

cerebrum: the largest and uppermost section of the brain, which integrates memory, speech, writing, and emotional responses

epilepsy: uncontrollable excessive activity in either all or part of the central nervous system

lesion: a visible local tissue abnormality such as a wound, sore, rash, or boil which can be benign, cancerous, gross, occult, or primary

neurological: dealing with the nervous system and its disorders

seizure: a sudden, violent, and involuntary contraction of a group of muscles; may be paroxysmal and episodic

INDICATIONS AND PROCEDURES

Clinical electroencephalography (EEG) uses from eight to sixteen pairs of electrodes called derivations. The "international 10-20" system of electrode placement provides coverage of the scalp at standard locations denoted by the letters F (frontal), C (central), P (parietal), T (temporal), and O (occipital). Subscripts of odd for left-sided placement, even for right-sided placements, and z for midline placement further define electrode location. During the procedure, the patient remains quiet, with eyes closed, and refrains from talking or moving. In some circumstances, however, prescribed activities such as hyperventilation may be requested. An EEG test is used to diagnose seizure disorders, brain-stem disorders, focal lesions, and impaired consciousness.

Electrical potentials caused by normal brain activity have atypical amplitudes of 30 to 100 millivolts and irregular, wavelike variations in time. The main generators of the EEG are probably postsynaptic potentials, with the largest contribution arising from pyramidal cells in the third cortical layer. The ongoing rhythms on an EEG background recording are classified according to the frequencies that they produce as delta (less than 3.5 hertz), theta (4.0 to 7.5 hertz), alpha (8.0 to 13.0 hertz), and beta (greater than 13.5 hertz). In awake but relaxed normal adults, the background consists primarily of alpha activity in occipital and parietal areas and beta activity in central and frontal areas. Variations in this activity can occur as a function of behavioral state and aging. Alpha waves disappear during sleep and are replaced by synchronous beta waves of higher frequency but lower voltage. Theta waves can occur during emotional stress, particularly during extreme disappointment and frustration. Delta waves occur in deep sleep and infancy and with serious organic brain disease.

USES AND COMPLICATIONS

During neurosurgery, electrodes can be applied directly to the surface of the brain (intracranial EEG) or placed within brain tissue (depth EEG) to detect lesions or tumors. Electrical activity of the cerebrum is detected through the skull in the same way that the electrical activity originating in the heart is detected by an electrocardiogram (ECG or EKG) through the chest wall. The amplitude of the EEG, however, is much smaller than that of the ECG because the EEG is generated by cells that are not synchronously activated and are not geometrically aligned, whereas the ECG is generated by cells that are synchronously activated and aligned. Variations in brain wave activity correlate with neurological conditions such as epilepsy, abnormal psychopathological states, and level of consciousness such as during different stages of sleep.

The two general categories of EEG abnormalities are alterations in background activity and paroxysmal activity. An EEG background with global abnormalities indicates diffuse brain dysfunction associated with developmental delay, metabolic disturbances, infections, and degenerative diseases. EEG background abnormalities are generally not specific enough to establish a diagnosis—for example, the "burst-suppression" pattern may indicate severe anoxic brain injury as well as a coma induced by barbiturates. Some disorders do have characteristic EEG features: An excess of beta activity suggests intoxication, whereas triphasic slow waves are typical of metabolic encephalopathies, particularly as a result of hepatic or renal dysfunction. Psychiatric illness is generally not associated with prominent EEG changes. Therefore, a normal EEG helps to distinguish psychogenic unresponsiveness from neurologic disease. EEG silence is an adjunctive test in the determination of brain death, but it is not a definitive one because it may be produced by reversible conditions such as hypothermia. Focal or lateralized EEG abnormalities in the background imply similarly localized disturbances in brain function and thus suggest the presence of lesions.

Paroxysmal EEG activity consisting of spikes and sharp waves reflects the pathologic synchronization of neurons. The location and character of paroxysmal activity in epileptic patients help clarify the disorder, guide rational anticonvulsant therapy, and assist in de-

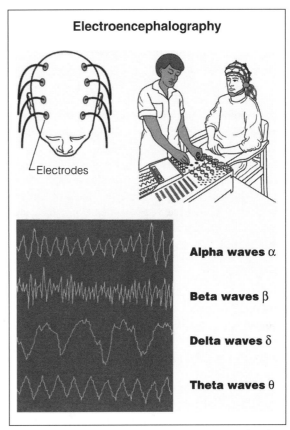

The electrical activity of the brain can be measured with an electroencephalograph (EEG) machine; characteristic patterns can be used to diagnose some brain disorders and to determine levels of consciousness.

termining a prognosis. The diagnostic value of an EEG is often enhanced by activation procedures, such as hyperventilation, photic (light) stimulation, and prolonged ambulatory monitoring, or by using special recording sites, such as nasopharyngeal leads, anterior temporal leads, and surgically placed subdural and depth electrodes. During a seizure, paroxysmal EEG activity replaces normal background activity and becomes continuous and rhythmic. In partial seizures, paroxysmal activity begins in one brain region and spreads to uninvolved regions.

PERSPECTIVE AND PROSPECTS

One of the most important uses of EEGs has been to diagnose certain types of epilepsy and to pinpoint the area in the brain causing the disturbance. Epilepsy is characterized by uncontrollable excessive activity in either all or part of the central nervous system and is classified into three types: grand mal epilepsy, petit mal epilepsy, and focal epilepsy. Additionally, EEGs are often used to localize tumors or other space-occupying lesions in the brain. Such abnormalities may be so large as to cause a complete or partial block in electrical activity in a certain portion of the cerebral cortex, resulting in reduced voltage. More frequently, however, a tumor compresses the surrounding nervous tissue and thereby causes abnormal electrical excitation in these areas.

Some researchers predict new uses of EEG technology in the future, although many of these applications appear dubious. Attempts to interpret thought patterns so that an EEG could serve as a lie detector or measurement of intellectual ability, for example, have proven unsuccessful.

—Daniel G. Graetzer, Ph.D.

See also Brain; Brain damage; Brain disorders; Brain tumors; Critical care; Critical care, pediatric; Diagnosis; Emergency medicine; Epilepsy; Headaches; Neuroimaging; Neurology; Neurology, pediatric; Neurosurgery; Positron emission tomography (PET) scanning; Seizures; Tumor removal; Tumors.

FOR FURTHER INFORMATION:

Daube, Jasper R., ed. *Clinical Neurophysiology.* 3d ed. New York: Oxford University Press, 2009. Covers the basics of clinical neurophysiology, considers the assessment of disease by anatomical system, and explains how clinical neurophysiologic techniques are used in the clinical assessment of diseases of the nervous system. Electroencephalography is covered extensively.

Ebersole, John S., and Timothy A. Pedley, eds. *Current Practice of Clinical Electroencephalography.* 3d ed. Philadelphia: Lippincott Williams & Wilkins, 2003. The thoroughly revised and greatly expanded third edition of this classic work covers the full range of applications of EEG and evoked potentials in current clinical practice. The most advanced instrumentation and techniques and their use in evaluating various disorders are discussed by more than twenty of the foremost authorities in the field.

Evans, James R., and Andrew Abarbanel, eds. *Introduction to Quantitative EEG and Neurofeedback.* San Diego, Calif.: Academic Press, 2004. The stated purpose of this text is to provide "an overview of the basics of QEEG and neurofeedback in one source."

Hayakawa, Fumio, et al. "Determination of Timing of Brain Injury in Preterm Infants with Periventricular Leukomalacia with Serial Neonatal Electroencephalography." *Pediatrics* 104, no. 5 (November, 1999): 1077-1081. The authors determine the timing of brain injury in infants with periventricular leukomalacia with serial encephalography recordings during the neonatal period.

Powledge, Tabitha M. "Unlocking the Secrets of the Brain: Part II." *Bioscience* 47, no. 7 (July/August, 1997): 403-408. In the second article in a two-part series, Powledge discusses positron emission tomography (PET) scanning, electroencephalography, magnetoencephalography, and other imaging techniques that help provide an understanding of the brain.

Ricker, Joseph H., and Ross D. Zafonte. "Functional Neuroimaging and Quantitative Electroencephalography in Adult Traumatic Head Injury: Clinical Applications and Interpretive Cautions." *Journal of Head Trauma Rehabilitation* 15, no. 2 (April, 2000): 859. This article provides an overview of the use of procedures such as positron emission tomography, single photon emission computed tomography, and quantitative electroencephalography in adults.

ELECTROLYTES. *See* FLUIDS AND ELECTROLYTES.

ELECTROMYOGRAPHY
PROCEDURE

ANATOMY OR SYSTEM AFFECTED: Muscles, nerves, nervous system

SPECIALTIES AND RELATED FIELDS: Neurology, physical therapy

DEFINITION: A procedure used to evaluate the electrical activity of nerves when muscles are both contracting and at rest.

KEY TERMS:

carpal tunnel syndrome: excessive compression of the median nerve located in the wrist that leads to irritation and eventually nerve damage

muscle: tissue that provides power to help the body function

myasthenia gravis: a disorder in which the nicotinic acetylcholine receptors located in junctions between nerve cells and muscles are attacked by the immune system, causing exhaustion of the muscles

nerve: a bundle of fibers that can transmit sensory and motor information among body parts

nerve compression: excessive pressure causing a nerve to be pinched *sciatica:* pain related to the sciatic nerve; a herniated disc in the lower back can cause this pain, as well as several other types of inflammation

INDICATIONS AND PROCEDURES

The term "electromyography" originated in 1890, but the process of measuring and recording the electrical signals conducted by nerves as muscles move was first studied as early as the seventeenth century by such scientists as Francesco Redi, Luigi Galvani, and Emil duBois-Reymond. It was not until 1922 that an oscilloscope, which looks like a small television set, was used to show these electrical signals on a screen, making visual monitoring possible. In the 1960's, electromyography (EMG) began to be used in medical clinics and doctors' offices to diagnose muscular and nerve injuries and disorders, such as carpal tunnel syndrome.

Today, the electrical activity measured by EMG is displayed on a computer monitor and can also be printed out or recorded as an electromyogram. The results can also be heard through an audio speaker. This electrical activity can be recorded because an electrode detects any electrical activity of the muscles. When a patient does not move the muscle, no signal is detected, but when a patient contracts a muscle by raising a leg or finger, then the nerve cells produce a smooth, wavy line. The exact size and shape of this wave form shown on the computer monitor gives information about the specific muscle's response to the nerve cells. This wave form is called the action potential. The EMG technician may also use a small electrical stimulus to cause a specific muscle to twitch, and this twitching produces an action potential that can be measured and recorded using electromyography as well.

USES AND COMPLICATIONS

The EMG is very safe, and most patients find that only the insertion of the needles or pins and the mild electrical voltage are somewhat uncomfortable. Any bruises heal within a few days. Very little preparation is required, but a patient does need to follow some guidelines to prevent complications. Cream and lotion should not be used before the EMG test, and smoking as well as caffeine-containing drinks and foods should be avoided for at least three hours prior to the test to avoid inaccurate results. A patient should also avoid taking any muscle relaxant medications such as anticholinergics for at least three to six days prior to the EMG testing. A pacemaker could also cause complications.

IN THE NEWS:
WIRELESS EMG APPLIED TO STUDIES INVOLVING BACKPACKS AND TEXT MESSAGES

A portable surface electromyography (EMG) device has been developed by researchers at Johns Hopkins University and also by Portuguese investigator Joao Eduardo Castro Ribeiro. According to the September, 2004, issue of *Engineering in Medicine and Biology*, this portable EMG uses a wireless acquisition module to measure electric potentials of the muscles in the vertebral column. These muscles are subjected to a large amount of stress from heavy backpacks. Children carrying these heavy backpacks can develop scoliosis and lordosis because the weight of these backpacks can cause muscles to be affected by an altered center of gravity for the body, thus exerting unnecessary pressure on the vertebrae. The wireless acquisition module of the EMG uses two 1.5 volt class AA batteries to monitor the impact of heavy backpacks on children.

Another application of this EMG technology is the measurement of hand-applied forces important for training and rehabilitation. Muscle contractions in the upper arm and forearm when gripping an object by using the hands produce biopotentials that generate voltage. These voltage readings of a patient are then compared to the normal pull and clenching force readings of a person in a variety of movements.

Ergonomist Ewa Gustafsson at the Sahlgrenska Academy has applied this EMG technology to study the thumb movements of fifty-six young adults while typing messages on cell phones. The results of her study, reported in June, 2009, indicate that nearly 50 percent of the young people studied experienced pain in the neck, arm, and hand after typing messages on the keypads of their mobile phones because of the use of one thumb instead of both thumbs. Subjects who used both thumbs did not experience pain in these areas. Additional differences were also measured by the EMG, thus confirming Gustafsson's hypothesis regarding the improper use of just one thumb to type text messages.

—*Jeanne L. Kuhler, Ph.D.*

Other tests performed along with EMG include the nerve conduction velocity test, often abbreviated as the nerve conduction test. It can also be completed by the same EMG technician in the same location but does not require any needles or small pins. Instead, small electrodes can be taped to the skin, and as the name implies, the nerve conduction velocity test can measure the speed of electrical signals, thus allowing additional disorders that affect the peripheral nervous system to be diagnosed, such as post-polio syndrome, which can develop even years after a human has suffered from polio. An EMG cannot evaluate brain or spinal cord diseases. Thus an EMG and a nerve conduction test are often completed together to more completely diagnose a range of disorders, such as carpal tunnel syndrome, sciatica (nerve root injury), muscular dystrophy, myasthenia gravis, ruptured spinal disks, spinal cord injuries, and various other nerve disorders.

PERSPECTIVE AND PROSPECTS

EMG has evolved extensively since the observation by Redi in the year 1666 that the muscle of an electric ray fish could produce electricity. It only takes thirty to sixty minutes for an EMG to record the data. Because the waves can be transmitted through a loudspeaker as well, a patient's physician can instantly hear them broadcast from a speaker, or recorded on a video that the physician can see instantly.

There is no risk of infection from an EMG because the needles used are sterile and the electrical pulse is of very low voltage and is used for less than a second. Once the testing has been completed, the EMG technician removes the electrodes and cleans the patient's skin. Some patients may experience bruising or tenderness of the muscles for a few days, but this minor discomfort should disappear within a week.

Research continues to expand the useful scope of conditions that can be diagnosed using EMG. Urination problems can now be diagnosed by recording the electrical signals of the external urinary sphincter, which is a group of muscles that surround the urethra. Also, myasthenia gravis can be diagnosed by using a special type of single fiber EMG that is able to monitor the contraction of a single fiber contraction.

—*Jeanne L. Kuhler, Ph.D.*

See also Carpal tunnel syndrome; Electroencephalography (EEG); Motor neuron diseases; Muscle sprains, spasms, and disorders; Muscles; Nervous system; Neuralgia, neuritis, and neuropathy; Neurology; Neurology, pediatric; Poliomyelitis.

FOR FURTHER INFORMATION:

Chernecky, C., and B. Berger. *Laboratory Tests and Diagnostic Procedures.* 4th ed. Philadelphia: Saunders, 2004.

Fischbach, F., and M. Dunning. *Manual of Laboratory and Diagnostic Tests.* 7th ed. Philadelphia: Lippincott Williams & Wilkins, 2004.

Pagana, K., and T. Pagana. *Mosby's Manual of Diagnostic and Laboratory Tests.* 3d ed. St. Louis: Mosby/Elsevier, 2006.

ELEPHANTIASIS

DISEASE/DISORDER

ALSO KNOWN AS: Bancroft's filariasis

ANATOMY OR SYSTEM AFFECTED: Lymphatic system

SPECIALTIES AND RELATED FIELDS: Environmental health, epidemiology, public health

DEFINITION: A grossly disfiguring disease caused by a roundworm parasite; it is the advanced stage of the disease Bancroft's filariasis, contracted through roundworms.

KEY TERMS:

acute disease: a disease in which symptoms develop rapidly and which runs its course quickly

chronic disease: a disease that develops more slowly than an acute disease and persists for a long time

host: any organism on or in which another organism (called a parasite) lives, usually for the purpose of nourishment or protection

inflammation: a response of the body to tissue damage caused by injury or infection and characterized by redness, pain, heat, and swelling

lymph nodes: globular structures located along the routes of the lymphatic vessels that filter microorganisms from the lymph

lymphatic system: a body system consisting of lymphatic vessels and lymph nodes that transports lymph through body tissues and organs; closely associated with the cardiovascular system

lymphatic vessels: vessels that form a system for returning lymph to the bloodstream

parasite: an organism that lives on or within another organism, called the host, from which it derives sustenance or protection at the host's expense

CAUSES AND SYMPTOMS

Elephantiasis is characterized by gross enlargement of a body part caused by the accumulation of fluid and connective tissue. It most frequently affects the legs, but may also occur in the arms, breasts, scrotum, vulva, or any other body part. The disease starts with the slight enlargement of one leg or arm (or other body part). The limb increases in size with recurrent attacks of fever. Gradually, the affected part swells, and the swelling, which is soft at first, becomes hard following the growth of connective tissue in the area. In addition, the skin over the swollen area changes so that it becomes coarse and thickened, looking almost like elephant hide. The elephant-like skin, along with the enlarged body parts, gave the disease the name elephantiasis.

Elephantiasis is found worldwide, mostly in the tropics and subtropics. Most cases of elephantiasis are a result of infection with a parasitic worm called *Wuchereria bancrofti* (*W. bancrofti*). *W. bancrofti* belongs to a group of worms called filaria, or roundworms, and infection with a filarial worm is called filariasis. Filariasis caused by *W. bancrofti* is the most common and widespread type of human filarial infection and is often called Bancroft's filariasis. Elephantiasis is the advanced, chronic stage of Bancroft's filariasis, and only a small percentage of persons with Bancroft's filariasis will develop elephantiasis. During Bancroft's filariasis, adult forms of *W. bancrofti* live inside the human lymphatic system, and it is the person's reaction to the presence of the worm that causes the symptoms of the disease. The worm's life cycle is important in understanding how the disease is transmitted from one person to another, how the symptoms develop, and how to prevent and reduce the incidence of the disease.

The adult worms live in human lymphatic vessels and lymph nodes and measure about 4 centimeters in length for the male and 9 centimeters in length for the female. Both are threadlike and about 0.3 millimeter in diameter. After mating, the female releases large numbers of embryos or microfilariae (microscopic roundworms), which are more than one hundred times smaller in length and ten times thinner than their parents. They make their way from the lymphatic system into the bloodstream, where they can circulate for two years or longer. Interestingly, most strains of microfilariae (all except those found in the South Pacific Islands) exhibit a nocturnal periodicity, in which they appear in the peripheral blood system (the outer blood vessels, such as those in the arms, legs, and skin) only at night, mostly between the hours of 10 P.M. and 2 A.M., and the remainder of the time they spend in the blood vessels of the lungs and other internal organs. This nighttime cycling into the peripheral blood is somehow related to the pa-

tient's sleeping habits, and although it is unknown exactly how or why the microfilariae do this, it is necessary for the survival of the worms. The microfilariae must develop through at least three different stages (called the first, second, and third larval stages) before they are ready to mature into adults; these stages take place not within humans, but within certain types of mosquitoes, which bite at night. Thus, the microfilariae appear in the peripheral blood just in time for the mosquitoes to bite an infected human and extract them so that they can continue their life cycle. It is important to note, therefore, that both humans and the proper type of mosquito are needed to keep a filariasis infection going in a particular area.

Female night-feeding mosquitoes of the genera *Culex*, *Aedes*, and *Anopheles* serve as intermediate hosts for *Wuchereria bancrofti*. The mosquitoes bite an infected person and ingest microfilariae from the peripheral blood. The microfilariae pass into the intestines of the mosquito, invade the intestinal wall, and within a day find their way to the thoracic muscles (the muscles in the middle part of the mosquito's body). There they develop from first-stage to third-stage larvae in about two weeks, and the new third-stage larvae move from the thoracic muscles to the head and mouth of the mosquito. Only the third-stage larvae are able to infect humans successfully, and the third stage can mature only inside humans. When the mosquito takes a blood meal, infective larvae make their way through the proboscis (the tubular sucking organ with which a mosquito bites a person) and enter the skin through the puncture wound. After they enter the skin, the larvae move by an unknown route to the lymphatic system, where they develop into adult worms. It takes about one year or longer for the larvae to grow into adults, mate, and produce more microfilariae.

A person contracts Bancroft's filariasis by being bitten by an infected mosquito. Various forms of the dis-

---

INFORMATION ON ELEPHANTIASIS

CAUSES: Infection from roundworm parasite
SYMPTOMS: Recurrent fever, inflammation of lymph vessels, swollen and painful lymph nodes, possible gross enlargement of body part
DURATION: Acute to chronic
TREATMENTS: Bed rest, supportive measures (e.g., hot and cold compresses to reduce swelling), drug diethylcarbamazine (DEC)

ease can occur, depending on the person's immune response and the number of times the person is bitten. The period of time from when a person is first infected with larvae to the time microfilariae appear in the blood can be between one and two years. Even after this time some persons, especially young people, show no symptoms at all, yet they may have numerous microfilariae in their blood. This period of being a carrier of microfilariae without showing any signs of disease may last several years, and such carriers act as reservoirs for infecting the mosquito population.

In those patients showing symptoms from the infection, there are two stages of the disease: acute and chronic. In acute disease, the most common symptoms are a recurrent fever and lymphangitis and/or lymphadenitis in the arms, legs, or genitals. These symptoms are caused by an inflammatory response to the adult worms trapped inside the lymphatic system. Lymphangitis, an inflammation of the lymph vessels, is characterized by a hard, cordlike swelling or a red superficial streak that is tender and painful. Lymphadenitis is characterized by swollen and painful lymph nodes. The attacks of fever and lymphangitis or lymphadenitis recur at irregular intervals and may last from three weeks up to three months. The attacks usually become less frequent as the disease becomes more chronic. In the absence of reinfection, there is usually a steady improvement in the victim, each relapse being milder. Thus, without specific therapy, this condition is self-limiting and presumably will not become chronic in those acquiring the infection during a brief visit to an area where the disease is endemic.

The most obvious symptoms caused as a result of *W. bancrofti* infection, such as elephantiasis, are noted in the chronic stage. Chronic disease occurs only after years of repeated infection with the worms. It is seen only in areas where the disease is endemic and only occurs in a small percentage of the infected population. The symptoms are the result of an accumulation of damage caused by inflammatory reactions to the adult worms. The inflammation causes tissue death and a buildup of scar tissue that eventually results in the blockage of the lymphatic vessels in which the worms live. One of the functions of lymphatic vessels is to carry excess fluid away from tissues and bring it back to the blood, where it enters the circulation again as the fluid portion of the blood. If the lymphatic vessels are blocked, the excess fluid stays in the tissues, and swelling occurs. When this swelling is extensive, grotesque enlargement of that part of the body occurs.

TREATMENT AND THERAPY

One way in which doctors can tell whether a person has Bancroft's filariasis is by taking a sample of peripheral blood between 10 P.M. and 2 A.M. and looking at the blood under a microscope to try to find microfilariae. Sometimes, the ability to find microfilariae is enhanced by filtering the blood to concentrate the possible microfilariae in a smaller volume of liquid. Many persons infected with *W. bancrofti* have no detectable microfilariae in their blood, so other methods are available. In the absence of microfilariae, a diagnosis can be made on the basis of a history of exposure, symptoms of the disease, positive antibody or skin tests, or the presence of worms in a sample of lymph tissue. It is important to note that occasionally a few other filarial worms and at least one bacteria can also cause elephantiasis; therefore, if symptoms of elephantiasis are observed, it is important to discover the correct cause so that the proper treatment can be given. Since chronic infection occurs after prolonged residence in areas where the disease occurs, patients with acute disease should be removed from those areas. They also should be reassured that elephantiasis is a rare complication that is limited to persons who have had constant exposure to infected mosquitoes for years.

The best way to avoid contracting filariasis when traveling to an affected area is to avoid being bitten by mosquitoes. Insect repellent, mosquito netting, and other methods are helpful in this regard. No drugs or vaccines are available to prevent infection once a person is bitten.

A problem in the treatment of all parasitic diseases is finding a drug that will kill the parasite without harming the human host. The drug diethylcarbamazine (DEC) is the drug of choice in treating Bancroft's filariasis. Its advantages are that it can be taken orally, patients have a relatively high tolerance to the drug, and it has relatively rapid, beneficial clinical effects. Generally, in the treatment of acute disease, excellent results are obtained when the proper dosage of the drug is given. There are only two relatively mild side effects of DEC. The first is nausea or vomiting. This symptom depends on the amount of the drug given; therefore, lower doses help alleviate this side effect. The second is fever and dizziness, the severity of which depends on the number of microfilariae a person has in his or her blood; the more microfilariae, the more severe the reaction. It is important to warn patients ahead of time about the fever reaction and encourage them to continue taking their doses anyway. The fever reaction is a sign that the patient is being cured, but the cure will not completely work if the patient does not finish the whole regimen of drug doses. Other drugs have been used in the treatment of filariasis (suramin, metrifonate, levamisole) but are generally less effective or more toxic than DEC. Additional treatment measures include bed rest and supportive measures, such as using hot and cold compresses to reduce swelling. The administration of antibiotics for patients with secondary bacterial infections and painkillers as well as anti-inflammatory agents during the painful, acute stage is helpful. Sometimes, swollen limbs can be wrapped in pressure bandages to force the lymph from them. If the distortion is not too great, this method is successful. It should also be noted that, although drugs such as DEC might be effective in killing *W. bancrofti*, the chronic lesions resulting from the infection are mostly incurable. Signs of chronic filariasis, such as elephantiasis of the limbs or the scrotum, are usually unaffected or only incompletely cured by medication, and it sometimes becomes necessary to apply surgical or other symptomatic treatments to relieve the suffering of the patients. Chronic obstruction in less advanced stages is sometimes improved by surgery. The surgical removal of an elephantoid breast, vulva, or scrotum is sometimes necessary.

Theoretically, it should be possible first to control and eventually to eliminate Bancroft's filariasis. Conditions that are highly favorable for continued propagation of the infection include a pool of microfilariae carriers in the human population and the right species of mosquitoes breeding near human habitations. Thus, control can be effected by treating all microfilariae carriers in an affected area and eliminating the necessary mosquitoes. Microfilariae carriers can be effectively treated with DEC. The decision usually is between giving mass drug treatment to the entire population in an affected area or only treating those persons who are microfilariae positive. Usually, if the infection is at a high rate and very widespread in an area, it is best to treat the entire population, since it would be very time-consuming, difficult, and expensive to find all the microfilariae carriers. In other areas that are smaller or in which the pockets of infection are well defined, it is better to identify all the microfilariae-positive persons and treat only those persons until they are cured.

The second control measure is to eliminate the mosquito population. It is important to note that eliminating the mosquitoes alone will not control the disease, especially in tropical areas, since the breeding period and season in which the disease can be transmitted is so ex-

tensive. In some temperate areas, where Bancroft's filariasis used to be endemic, measures that removed the mosquitoes alone aided in the elimination of the disease from that area, since in temperate areas the breeding period and thus the season for transmission is so short. In tropical areas, both DEC therapy and mosquito control must be applied in order to control the disease.

The mosquito population can be controlled in four ways. First, general sanitation measures can be carried out in order to reduce the areas where the mosquitoes are breeding; for example, draining swamps. Second, insecticides can be used to kill the adult mosquitoes. Third, larvacides can be applied to sources of water where mosquitoes breed in order to kill the mosquito larvae. Finally, natural mosquito predators, such as certain species of fish, can be introduced into waters where mosquitoes breed to eat the mosquito larvae. Numerous problems stand in the way of eradication, such as

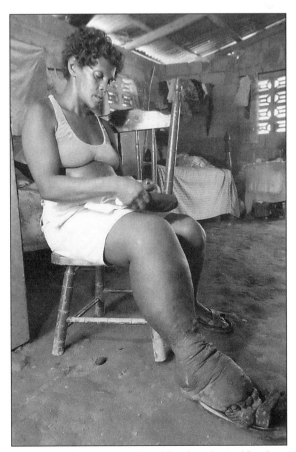

A woman in the Dominican Republic whose leg and foot have become crippled with elephantiasis, which affects many people in developing countries. (AP/Wide World Photos)

poor sanitation, persons who do not cooperate with medical intervention, mosquitoes that become resistant to all known insecticides, increasing technology that yields increasing water supplies and therefore places for mosquitoes to breed, large populations, ignorance of the cause of the disease, and lack of medicine and a way of distributing that medicine.

PERSPECTIVE AND PROSPECTS

Dramatic symptoms of elephantiasis, especially the enormous swelling of legs or scrotum, were recorded in much of the ancient medical literature of India, Persia, and the Far East. The embryonic form of microfilariae was first discovered and described by a Frenchman in Paris in 1863. The organism was named for O. Wucherer, who also discovered microfilariae in 1866, and Joseph Bancroft, who discovered the adult worm in 1876. Two important facts about *W. bancrofti*—namely, its development in mosquitoes and the nocturnal periodicity of the microfilariae—were discovered by Patrick Manson between 1877 and 1879. This was the first example of a disease being transmitted by a mosquito, and its discovery earned for Manson the title of founder of tropical medicine. These and most of the other essential facts of the disease were discovered before the end of the nineteenth century. Progress in the epidemiology and control of filariasis came after World War II. In 1947, DEC was shown to kill filariae in animals, and this result was followed by the successful use of DEC in the treatment of humans. The first promising results in the control of Bancroft's filariasis by mass administration of DEC were reported in 1957 on a small island in the South Pacific. Through subsequent studies, it has become clear that effective control of the infection can be achieved if sufficient dosages of DEC are administered to infected populations.

Filariasis is a serious health hazard and public health problem in many tropical countries. Infection with *W. bancrofti* has been recorded in nearly all countries or territories in the tropical and subtropical zones of the world. The infection occurs primarily in coastal areas and islands that experience long periods of high humidity and heat. Infections have also been noted from some temperate zone districts, such as mainland Japan, central China, and some European countries. There is more Bancroft's filariasis now than there was a hundred years ago, principally because of increases in population in affected areas and in increased resistance of mosquitoes to insecticides. In 1947, it was estimated that 189 million people were infected with *W. ban-*

crofti. More recently, the World Health Organization estimated that 250 million people are infected and 400 million are at risk.

Bancroft's filariasis was introduced into and became endemic to Charleston, South Carolina, until 1920. It disappeared in the United States before World War II, presumably because of a reduction of mosquitoes resulting from improved sanitation. Servicemen in the Pacific in World War II were concerned about contracting elephantiasis; although several thousand showed signs of acute filariasis, only twenty had microfilariae in their blood, and no one developed elephantiasis. In the United States today, the infection is most frequently seen in immigrants, military veterans, and missionaries. It is important for physicians to be aware of this and other tropical diseases so that they can treat the occasional patient who is suffering from one of them, since most of these diseases are more successfully treated in the early stages of the disease.

—*Vicki J. Isola, Ph.D.*

See also Bites and stings; Edema; Inflammation; Insect-borne diseases; Lymphadenopathy and lymphoma; Lymphatic system; Parasitic diseases; Roundworms; Tropical medicine; Worms; Zoonoses.

FOR FURTHER INFORMATION:

Beaver, Paul C., and Rodney C. Jung. *Animal Agents and Vectors of Human Disease*. 5th ed. Philadelphia: Lea & Febiger, 1985. Discusses all major parasitic diseases. Chapter 12, "Filariae," which describes those diseases caused by filarial worms, contains helpful photographs and diagrams.

Biddle, Wayne. *A Field Guide to Germs*. 2d ed. New York: Anchor Books, 2002. This comprehensive book is easily accessible to the nonspecialist and includes a discussion of nearly every virus, bacterium, and fungus known to cause human and nonhuman animal disease. The history of the microbe and the treatment of diseases are included.

Frank, Steven A. *Immunology and Evolution of Infectious Disease*. Princeton, N.J.: Princeton University Press, 2002. Blends research from molecular biology, immunology, pathogen biology, and population dynamics to discuss how and why parasites vary to escape recognition by the immune system, vaccine design, and the control of epidemics.

Joklik, Wolfgang K., et al. *Zinsser Microbiology*. 20th ed. Norwalk, Conn.: Appleton and Lange, 1997. The information presented in this textbook is thorough, logical, and supplemented by interesting diagrams, photographs, and charts. Contains a thorough description of Bancroft's filariasis.

Ransford, Oliver. *"Bid the Sickness Cease."* London: John Murray, 1983. Discusses the effect of disease on the development of Africa. Chapter 6, "The Father of Tropical Medicine," describes how Patrick Manson made the original discoveries of the cause of elephantiasis.

Roberts, Larry S., and John Janovy, Jr., eds. *Gerald D. Schmidt and Larry S. Roberts' Foundations of Parasitology.* 7th ed. Boston: McGraw-Hill Higher Education, 2005. Gives a good general description of all parasitic diseases and their causes, effects, and treatments. Deals specifically with diseases caused by filariae, including *Wuchereria bancrofti*.

Salyers, Abigail A., and Dixie D. Whitt. *Bacterial Pathogenesis: A Molecular Approach.* 2d ed. Washington, D.C.: ASM Press, 2002. Examines the molecular mechanism involved in bacterial-host interactions that can produce infectious disease. Introductory chapters discuss host-parasite relationships.

EMBOLISM

DISEASE/DISORDER

ANATOMY OR SYSTEM AFFECTED: Blood vessels, brain, circulatory system, lungs, lymphatic system

SPECIALTIES AND RELATED FIELDS: Cardiology, internal medicine, neurology, vascular medicine

DEFINITION: A mass of undissolved matter traveling in the blood or lymphatic current.

CAUSES AND SYMPTOMS

An embolism is a mass of undissolved matter traveling in the vascular or lymphatic system. Although an embolism can be solid, liquid, or gaseous, the majority of emboli are solid. Likewise, emboli may consist of air bubbles, bits of tissue, globules of fat, tumor cells, or many other materials. The majority of emboli, however, are blood clots (thrombi) that originate in one portion of the body, then break loose and travel, eventually lodging in another part of the body. Where the traveling blood clot lodges will determine what kind of damage is done.

If the thrombus starts in the veins of the legs, it may break loose, travel up the veins of the leg and abdomen, pass through the right side of the heart, and lodge in the arteries in the lungs. This condition, called a pulmonary embolism, is often fatal. If the embolism is small, it may cause only shortness of breath and chest pain. If it is even smaller, the embolism may produce no symptoms at all.

INFORMATION ON EMBOLISM

CAUSES: Blood clot, air bubble, tissue, fat globules, tumor cells, or other material lodging in part of the body

SYMPTOMS: If in the lung, shortness of breath and chest pain; if in the heart, symptoms of heart attack; if in the brain, symptoms of stroke; if in the leg, pain, cold, numbness

DURATION: Acute

TREATMENTS: Depends on system affected; may include blood-thinners (heparin), thrombolytic drugs, bypass surgery

---

If a blood clot forms in the chambers of the heart, breaks loose, and eventually lodges in an artery in the brain, then the patient will experience a stroke. If a clot breaks loose and lodges in an artery in the leg, then the patient will experience pain, coldness, or numbness in that leg. A blood clot that lodges in the coronary arteries, the arteries that feed the heart muscle, may cause a heart attack.

TREATMENT AND THERAPY

Treatment will vary depending on what system has been affected by the embolus. If the clot lodges in the lungs, then the patient will likely be placed on a blood-thinning drug such as heparin. In severe cases, thrombolytic drugs, which dissolve clots, may be used. If the clot lodges in a coronary artery, then open-heart surgery may be performed to bypass the occluded artery. If the clot lodges in the leg, a surgeon may remove the clot from the artery. This procedure is possible only when the clot is discovered early, when it has not yet formed a strong attachment to the vessel wall. Another approach to this problem may be to bypass the occluded artery using an artificial artery or a graft.

PERSPECTIVE AND PROSPECTS

The prevention and treatment of emboli are constantly improving. Venous thrombosis, the most common cause of pulmonary emboli, is becoming easier to diagnose thanks to major advances in ultrasound imaging. Also, magnetic resonance imaging (MRI) is being used to make the identification of emboli in the lungs more accurate and safer. Imaging procedures of the chambers of the heart, a common spot where emboli form, are improving as well, making prevention easier.

—*Steven R. Talbot, R.V.T.*

See also Arteriosclerosis; Blood and blood disorders; Blood vessels; Cholesterol; Circulation; Embolization; Heart; Heart attack; Lungs; Phlebitis; Pulmonary diseases; Pulmonary medicine; Pulmonary medicine, pediatric; Respiration; Strokes; Thrombolytic therapy and TPA; Thrombosis and thrombus; Varicose vein removal; Varicose veins; Vascular medicine; Vascular system.

FOR FURTHER INFORMATION:

Bick, Roger L. *Disorders of Thrombosis and Hemostasis: Clinical and Laboratory Practice.* 3d ed. Philadelphia: Lippincott Williams & Wilkins, 2002.

Kroll, Michael H. *Manual of Coagulation Disorders.* Malden, Mass.: Blackwell Science, 2001.

Reader's Digest, editors of. *ABC's of the Human Body: A Family Answer Book.* Pleasantville, N.Y.: Author, 1987.

Verstrate, Marc, Valentin Fuster, and Eric Topol, eds. *Cardiovascular Thrombosis: Thrombocardiology and Thromboneurology.* 2d ed. Philadelphia: Lippincott-Raven, 1998.

Virchow, Rudolf L. K. *Thrombosis and Emboli.* Translated by Axel C. Matzdorff and William R. Bell. Canton, Mass.: Science History, 1998.

EMBOLIZATION

PROCEDURE

ALSO KNOWN AS: Catheter or coil embolization, endovascular embolization, embolotherapy

ANATOMY OR SYSTEM AFFECTED: Blood vessels, brain, gastrointestinal system, genitals, liver, uterus

SPECIALTIES AND RELATED FIELDS: Critical care, emergency medicine, gynecology, oncology, pathology, radiology, vascular medicine

DEFINITION: A procedure used to block specific blood vessels in order to stop blood flow to a certain region—for example, to a tumor—by way of introducing special substances called emboli.

KEY TERMS:

arteriovenous malformation (AVM): a genetic disorder in which the capillary beds that connect the arteries and the veins are abnormal or defective, resulting in malnourishment of tissues, especially in the brain and spinal cord

catheter: a thin tube that is inserted into the groin area and pushed through arteries during embolization procedure

emboli: substances that are released into the blood vessel for the purpose of their occlusion

interventional radiology: the specialty of radiology in which techniques such as X-ray imaging, computed tomography (CT) scans, ultrasounds, or magnetic resonance imaging (MRI) are used for guidance to navigate and introduce catheters or electrodes for various purposes

uterine fibroid embolization (UFE): embolization procedure to stop blood supply for uterine fibroids (benign tumors in the uterus)

varicocele: the condition in which the varicose vein of the scrotum enlarges and causes extreme pain; this condition is also associated with infertility

INDICATIONS AND PROCEDURES

Embolization is used in a variety of circumstances. In cases such as the uterine fibroids where the tumor is rarely malignant, UFE is a preferred option compared to an invasive surgery. The procedure stops blood supply to the fibroids, which eventually shrink and disintegrate. In cerebral or brain aneurysms, the cerebral artery inflates or ruptures due to dilations of its wall, resulting in bleeding into the brain or in the space between the brain and the membrane. Embolization of an aneurysm using a platinum coil is performed to block the blood flow to it and to prevent its rupture.

In conditions like varicocele, embolization is used to occlude the abnormal blood vessel and divert the blood flow from that region. Other cases where this procedure can be used are AVM, arteriovenous fistula, or hemangiomas, all of which concern abnormalities in blood vessels. In some cases such as liver cancers where there are a number of small tumors, arterial embolization is the most effective treatment option. In such cases, either the artery is occluded by embolization procedure or is used to deliver drugs into the tumors. The latter process is called chemoembolization.

Embolization involves the insertion of a small catheter from the groin area, navigation through the vascular system to the appropriate region, and delivery of emboli, which block the desired blood vessel. In general, a fluoroscope or an X-ray camera is used to guide the physician to visualize the movement of emboli along with a tracking dye or a contrasting agent and also to ensure the exact location of their delivery. A variety of particles are used as emboli. Chief among them are polyvinyl alcohol, gelatin-coated microspheres, absolute alcohol, N-butyl-2-cyanoacrylate (NBCA), gelfoam, or some platinum coils. These particles are pushed through the catheter and delivered to the affected region under anesthesia. The emboli are delivered by the application of a very small voltage current once the catheter reaches its destination. The procedure is usually performed at the doctor's office by an interventional radiologist and the patient may be required to stay overnight after the procedure.

USES AND COMPLICATIONS

Like in any procedure, there are both advantages and risks associated with embolization. Embolization of uterine fibroids is less invasive and complicated compared to a surgical procedure to remove them. Damage to blood vessels because of the insertion of the catheter is a possible complication, as is infection of the punctured site. Allergic reactions to the tracking dye are also a risk. Discharge of submucosal fibroids has been observed in a small percentage of women. However, the benefits associated with this procedure outweigh the risks and therefore UFE is widely adapted around the world.

Embolization is also used in emergency situations, such as in traumatic hemorrhage, where there is severe blood loss. Embolization provides a viable solution to regions that possibly cannot be operated upon, like some deep AVM or tumors that cannot be surgically removed. Coil embolization for brain aneurysms is another commonly used procedure. After the procedure, some patients might experience pain, numbness, or strokelike symptoms. With larger aneurysms, the chances of recurrence increase and a complete cure is not achieved through this procedure. Sometimes this procedure might have to be followed by surgery.

PERSPECTIVE AND PROSPECTS

Embolization has been practiced since the 1960's, and the medical field has witnessed many advances in this procedure over the years. Interventional radiology was established by Charles Dotter in the 1960's and was applied in cardiac procedures, but it subsequently has been adapted in several other fields. UFE was developed in the 1990's and has emerged as a procedure that is now adapted worldwide with great success. Many emboli such as microspheres and platinum coils have been developed since and have been approved by the Food and Drug Administration (FDA) for use in patients. In a breakthrough development in the treatment of brain aneurysms, detachable coils called Guglielmi coils were developed in the early 1990's and are widely used today. Portal vein embolization, a procedure to shrink a liver affected by cancer before its surgical removal, has gained enormous acceptance in the medical field in recent years.

The embolization procedure is a viable and safe alternative to surgery and is less invasive. Side effects and recurrence rates have been reported to be quite low. This procedure indeed has revolutionized medicine in recent years because of its simplicity compared to surgery and its reliability. Embolization is growing in its applicability in the medical field and its usefulness is increasing with the advent of new technologies.

—*Geetha Yadav, Ph.D.*

See also Aneurysms; Blood vessels; Embolism; Liver cancer; Testicular surgery; Tumors; Uterus; Vascular medicine; Vascular systems.

FOR FURTHER INFORMATION:

Bradley, L. D. "Uterine Fibroid Embolization: A Viable Alternative to Hysterectomy." *American Journal of Obstetrics and Gynecology* 201, no. 2 (August, 2009): 127-135.

Golzarian, Jafar, Sun Shiliang, and Sharfuddin Melhelm, eds. *Vascular Embolotherapy: A Comprehensive Approach.* Vol. 1. New York: Springer, 2006.

Ravina, Jacques. "History of Embolization of Uterine Myoma." In *Uterine Fibroids: Embolization and Other Treatments*, edited by Tulandi Togas. New York: Cambridge University Press, 2003.

EMBRYOLOGY

SPECIALTY

ANATOMY OR SYSTEM AFFECTED: All

SPECIALTIES AND RELATED FIELDS: Genetics, neonatology, obstetrics, perinatology

DEFINITION: The study of prenatal development from conception until the moment of birth.

KEY TERMS:

blastocyst: a small, hollow ball of cells which typifies one of the early embryonic stages in humans

cleavage: the process by which the fertilized egg undergoes a series of rapid cell divisions, which results in the formation of a blastocyst

congenital malformation: any anatomical defect present at birth

embryo: the developing human from conception until the end of the eighth week

fetus: the developing human from the end of the eighth week until the moment of birth

neural tube: the embryonic structure that gives rise to the central nervous system *teratogens:* substances that induce congenital malformations when embryonic tissues and organs are exposed to them

zygote: the fertilized egg; the first cell of a new organism

SCIENCE AND PROFESSION

The study of human embryology is the study of human prenatal development. The three stages of development are cleavage (the first week), embryonic development (the second through eighth weeks), and fetal development (the ninth through thirty-eighth weeks).

After an egg is fertilized by sperm in the uterine, or Fallopian, tube, the resulting zygote begins to divide rapidly. This period of rapid cell division is known as cleavage. By the third day, the zygote has divided into a solid ball containing twelve to sixteen cells. The small ball of cells resembles a mulberry and is called the morula, which is Latin for "mulberry." The morula moves from the uterine tube into the uterus.

The morula develops a central cavity as spaces begin to form between the inner cells. At this stage, the developing human is called a blastocyst. The ring of cells on the outer edge of the hollow ball is called the trophoblast and will form a placenta, while the cluster of cells within becomes the inner cell mass and will form the embryo. By the end of the first week, the surface of the inner cell mass has flattened to form an embryonic disc, and the blastocyst has attached to the lining of the uterus and begun to embed itself.

During the second week of development, the trophoblast makes connections with the uterus into which it has burrowed to form the placenta. Blood vessels from the embryo link it to the placenta through the umbilical cord, through which the embryo receives food and oxygen and releases wastes. Two sacs develop around the embryo: the fluid-filled amniotic sac that surrounds and cushions the embryo and the yolk sac that hangs beneath to provide nourishment. Finally, a large chorionic sac develops around the embryo and the two smaller sacs.

During the third week, the cells of the embryo are arranged in three layers. The outer layer of cells is called the ectoderm, the middle layer is the mesoderm, and the inner layer is the endoderm. The ectoderm gives rise to the epidermis (outer layer) of the skin and to the nervous system; the mesoderm gives rise to blood, bone, cartilage, and muscle; and the endoderm gives rise to body organ linings and glands.

Other significant events of the third week are the development of the primitive streak and notochord. The primitive streak is a thickened line of cells on the embryonic disk indicating the future embryonic axis. Development of the primitive streak stimulates the formation of a supporting rod of tissue beneath it called the notochord. The presence of the notochord triggers the ectoderm in the primitive streak above it to thicken, and the thickened area will give rise to the brain and spinal cord. Later, when vertebrae and muscles develop around the neural tissue, the notochord will disappear, leaving the center of the vertebral disk as its remnant.

The important event of the fourth week is the formation of the neural tube. After the thickened neural plate tissue has formed, an upward folding forms a groove, finally closing to form a neural tube. Closure begins at the head end and proceeds backward. The neural tube then sinks beneath surrounding ectodermal surface cells, which will become the skin covering the embryo.

Blocks of mesoderm cells line up along either side of the notochord and neural tube. These blocks are called

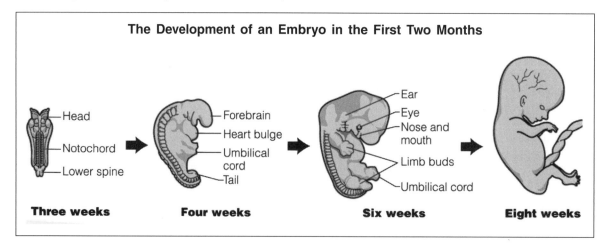

The Development of an Embryo in the First Two Months

Head
Notochord
Lower spine

Three weeks

Forebrain
Heart bulge
Umbilical cord
Tail

Four weeks

Ear
Eye
Nose and mouth
Limb buds
Umbilical cord

Six weeks

Eight weeks

somites, and eventually forty-two to forty-four pairs will form. They give rise to muscle, the cartilage of the head and trunk, and the inner layer of skin. At the same time, embryonic blood vessels develop on the yolk sac. Because the human embryo is provided little yolk, there is need for early development of a circulatory system to provide nutrition and gas exchange through the placenta.

The heart is formed and begins to beat in the fourth week, though it is not yet connected to many blood vessels. During the fourth through eighth weeks, all the organ systems develop, and the embryo is especially vulnerable to teratogens (environmental agents that interfere with normal development). A noticeable change in shape is seen during the fourth week because the rapidly increasing number of cells causes a folding under at the edges of the embryonic disk. The flattened disk takes on a cylindrical shape, and the folding process causes curvature of the embryo and it comes to lie on its side in a C-shaped position.

The beginnings of arms and legs are first seen in the fourth week and are called limb buds, appearing first as small bumps. The lower end of the embryo resembles a tail, and the swollen cranial part of the neural tube constricts to form three early sections of the brain. The eyes and ears begin to develop from the early brain tissue.

During the fifth through eighth weeks, the head enlarges as a result of rapid brain development. The head makes up almost half the embryo, and facial features begin to appear. Sexual differences exist but are difficult to detect. Nerves and muscles have developed enough to allow movement. By the end of the eighth week the limb buds have grown and differentiated into appendages with paddle-shaped hands and feet and short, webbed digits. The tail disappears, and the embryo begins to demonstrate human characteristics. By convention, the embryo is now called a fetus.

The fetal stage of development is the period between the ninth and thirty-eighth weeks, until birth. Organs formed during the embryonic stage grow and differentiate during the fetal stage. The body has the largest growth spurt between the ninth and twentieth weeks, but the greatest weight gain occurs during the last weeks of pregnancy.

In the third month, the difference between the sexes becomes apparent, urine begins to form and is excreted into the amniotic fluid, and the fetus can blink its eyelids. The fetus nearly doubles in length during the fourth month, and the head no longer appears to be so disproportionately large. Ossification of the skeleton begins, and by the end of the fourth month, ovaries are differentiated in the female fetus and already contain many cells destined to become eggs.

During the fifth month, fetal movements are felt by the mother, and the heartbeat can be heard with a stethoscope. Movements until this time usually go unnoticed. The average length of time that elapses between the first movement felt by the mother and delivery is twenty-one weeks.

During the sixth month, weight is gained by the fetus, but it is not until the seventh month that a baby usually can survive premature birth, when the body systems, particularly the lungs, are mature enough to function. During the eighth month, the eyes develop the ability to control the amount of light that enters them. Fat accumulates under the skin and fills in wrinkles. The skin becomes pink and smooth, and the arms and legs may become chubby. In the male fetus, the testes descend into the scrotal sac. Growth slows as birth approaches. The usual gestation length is 266 days, or thirty-eight weeks, after fertilization.

DIAGNOSTIC AND TREATMENT TECHNIQUES

Knowledge of normal embryonic development is very important both in helping women provide optimal prenatal care for their children and in promoting scientific research for improved prenatal treatment, better understanding of malignant growths, and insight into the aging process.

Environmental stress to the embryo during the fourth through eighth weeks can cause abnormal development and result in congenital malformation, which may be defined as any anatomical defect present at birth. Environmental agents that cause malformations are known as teratogens. Malformations may develop from genetic or environmental factors, but most often they are caused by a combination of the two. Some of the common teratogens are viral infections, drug use, a poor diet, smoking, alcohol consumption, and irradiation.

The genetic makeup of some individuals makes them particularly sensitive to certain agents, while others are resistant. The abnormalities may be immediately apparent at birth or hidden within the body and discovered later. Embryos with severe structural abnormalities often do not survive, and such abnormalities represent an important cause of miscarriages. In fact, up to half of all conceptions spontaneously abort, with little or no notice by the prospective mother.

Genetic birth defects are passed on from one generation to another and result from a gene mutation at some time in the past. Mutations are caused by accidental rearrangement of deoxyribonucleic acid (DNA), the material of which genes are made, and range in severity from mild to life-threatening. They may cause such conditions as extra fingers and toes, cataracts, dwarfism, albinism, and cystic fibrosis. Gene mutations on a sex chromosome are described as sex-linked and are usually passed from mother to son; these include hemophilia, hydrocephalus (an excessive amount of cerebrospinal fluid), color blindness, and a form of baldness.

Abnormalities in the embryo may result because of unequal distribution of chromosomes in the formation of eggs or sperm. This imbalance can cause a variety of problems in development, such as Down syndrome and abnormal sexual development. The normal human cell contains twenty-three chromosomes, twenty-two pairs of which are nonsex chromosomes, or autosomes. The last pair consists of the two sex chromosomes. Females normally have two X chromosomes, and males have an X and a Y chromosome.

When females have only one X, a set of conditions known as Turner syndrome results. The embryo will develop as a normal female, though ovaries will not fully form and there may be congenital heart defects. Because the single X chromosome does not cause enough estrogen to be produced, sexual maturity will not occur. If a male embryo should receive only the Y chromosome, it cannot survive. Sometimes a male will receive two (or more) X chromosomes along with a Y chromosome (XXY), producing Klinefelter syndrome. The appearance of the child is normal, but at puberty the breasts may enlarge and the testes will not mature, causing sterility. Males receiving two Y chromosomes (XYY) develop normally, but they may be quite tall and find controlling their impulses to be difficult.

Viral infections in the mother during the embryonic stages can cause problems in organ formation by disturbing normal cell division, fetal vascularization, and the development of the immune system. The organs most vulnerable to infection will be those undergoing rapid cell division and growth at the time of infection. For example, the lens of the eye is forming during the sixth week of development, and infection at this time could cause the formation of cataracts.

While most microorganisms cannot pass through the placenta to reach the embryo or fetus, those that can are capable of causing major problems in embryonic development. Rubella, the virus that causes German measles, often causes birth defects in children should infection occur shortly before or during the first three months of pregnancy. The developing ears, eyes, and heart are especially susceptible to damage during this time. When a rubella infection occurs during the first five weeks of pregnancy, interference with organ development is most pronounced. After the fifth week, the risks of infection are not as great, but central nervous system impairment may occur as late as the seventh month.

The most common source of fetal infection may be the cytomegalovirus (CMV), a form of herpes which causes abortion during the first three months of pregnancy. If infection occurs later, the liver and brain are especially vulnerable and impairment in vision, hearing, and mental ability may result. Evidence has also suggested that the immune system of the fetus is adversely affected.

Other viruses may affect fetal development as well. When herpes simplex infects the fetus several weeks before birth, blindness or mental retardation may result. *Toxoplasma gondii*, a parasite of animals often kept as pets, may adversely affect eye and brain development without the mother having known that she had the infection. Syphilis infection in the mother leads to death or serious fetal abnormalities unless it is treated before the sixteenth week of pregnancy; if it is untreated, the fetus may possess hearing impairment, hydrocephalus, facial abnormalities, and mental retardation. Women infected with acquired immunodeficiency syndrome (AIDS) may transmit the virus to their infants before or during birth.

Certain chemicals can cross the placenta and produce malformation of developing tissues and organs. During an embryo's first twenty-five days, damage to the primitive streak can cause malformation in bone, blood, and muscle. While bones and teeth are being formed, they may be adversely affected by antibiotics such as tetracycline.

At one time, thalidomide was widely used as an antinauseant in Great Britain and Germany and to some extent in the United States. Large numbers of congenital abnormalities began to appear in newborns, and the drug was withdrawn from the market after two years. Thalidomide caused failure of normal limb development and was especially damaging during the third to seventh weeks.

Exposure to other chemicals causes central nervous system disorders when the neural tube fails to close.

When the anterior end of the tube does not close, development of the brain and spinal cord will be absent or incomplete and anencephaly results. Babies can live no more than a few days with this condition because the higher control centers of the brain are undeveloped. If the posterior end of the tube fails to close, one or more vertebrae will not develop completely, exposing the spinal cord; this condition is called spina bifida. This condition varies in severity with the level of the defect and the amount of neural tissue that remains exposed, because exposed tissue degenerates.

It has been long believed that neural tube disorders accompanied maternal depletion of folic acid, one of the B vitamins, and research has substantiated that relationship. Anencephaly and spina bifida rarely occur in the infants of women taking folic acid supplements. One of the harmful effects of alcohol and anticonvulsants is their depletion of the body's natural folic acid. A decrease in the mother's folic acid levels in the first through third months of pregnancy can cause abortion or growth deformities.

Maternal smoking is strongly implicated in low infant birth weights and higher fetal and infant mortality rates. Cigarette smoke may cause cardiac abnormalities, cleft lip and palate, and a missing brain. Nicotine decreases blood flow to the uterus and interferes with normal development, allowing less oxygen to reach the embryo.

Alcohol use may be the number one cause of birth defects. Exposure of the fetus to alcohol in the blood results in fetal alcohol syndrome. Symptoms may include growth deficiencies, an abnormally small head, facial malformation, and damage to the heart and the nervous and reproductive systems. Behavioral disorders such as hyperactivity, attention deficit, and inability to relate to others may accompany fetal alcohol syndrome.

Radiation treatments given to pregnant women may cause cell death, chromosomal injury, and growth retardation in the developing embryo. The effect is proportional to the dosage of radiation. Malformations may be visible at birth, or a condition such as leukemia may develop later. Abnormalities caused by radiation include cleft palate, an abnormally small head, mental retardation, and spina bifida. Diagnostic X rays are not believed to emit enough radiation to cause abnormalities in embryonic development, but precautions should be taken.

Oxygen deficiency to the embryo or fetus occurs when mothers use cocaine. Maternal blood pressure fluctuates with the use of this drug, and the embryonic brain is deprived of oxygen, resulting in vision problems, lack of coordination, and mental retardation. Too little oxygen to the fetus may also cause death from lung collapse soon after birth.

Obvious physical malformations resulting from embryonic exposure to drugs have been recognized for a number of years, but recent investigators have found there are more subtle levels of effect that may show up later as behavioral problems. Physical abnormalities have been easily documented, but more attention is needed regarding the behavioral effects caused by teratogens.

PERSPECTIVE AND PROSPECTS

The first recorded observations of a developing embryo were performed on a chick by Hippocrates in the fifth century B.C.E. In the fourth century B.C.E., Aristotle wondered whether a preformed human unfolded in the embryo and enlarged with time, or whether a very simple embryonic structure gradually became more and more complex. This question was debated for nearly two thousand years until the early nineteenth century, when microscopic studies of chick embryos were carefully conducted and described.

Understanding human embryology is foundational for recognizing the relationships that exist between the body systems and congenital malformations in newborns. This field of study takes on new importance in the light of advances of modern technology, which have made prenatal diagnosis and treatment a reality.

The study of embryology is also making contributions toward finding the causes of malignant growth. Malignancy is a breakdown in the mechanisms for normal growth and differentiation first seen in the early embryo. Questions about uninhibited malignant growth may be answered by studying embryonic tissues and organs.

The study of old age is another area in which embryological research is valuable. Understanding the clock mechanisms of embryonic cells has led to greater understanding of the "winding down" of cells in old age. It is also important that researchers discover how environmental conditions modify rates of growth and affect the cell's clock. The degree to which the human life span can be expanded remains one of the most challenging questions in the area of aging.

In addition to the health benefits that may be derived from embryological research, this field is an important source of insight into some of the moral and ethical dilemmas facing humankind. Artificial insemination, contraception, and abortion regulations are some of the problems that will require close collaboration between ethicists and scientists, especially embryologists.

—*Katherine H. Houp, Ph.D.;*
updated by Alexander Sandra, M.D.

See also Abortion; Amniocentesis; Assisted reproductive technologies; Birth defects; Brain disorders; Cerebral palsy; Cesarean section; Chorionic villus sampling; Cloning; Conception; Down syndrome; Fetal alcohol syndrome; Fetal surgery; Gamete intrafallopian transfer (GIFT); Genetic counseling; Genetic diseases; Genetics and inheritance; Growth; Gynecology; In vitro fertilization; Miscarriage; Multiple births; Neonatology; Obstetrics; Perinatology; Placenta; Pregnancy and gestation; Premature birth; Reproductive system; Rh factor; Rubella; Sexual differentiation; Spina bifida; Stillbirth; Teratogens; Toxoplasmosis; Ultrasonography; Uterus.

FOR FURTHER INFORMATION:

Mader, Sylvia S. *Inquiry into Life.* Dubuque, Iowa: William C. Brown, 2010. An introductory-level college text designed to cover the entire range of biological topics. Gives a clear description of typical early developmental stages of all vertebrates and offers a section on human embryology and fetal development, adulthood, and aging.

Marieb, Elaine N. *Essentials of Human Anatomy and Physiology.* 9th ed. San Francisco: Pearson/Benjamin Cummings, 2009. This introductory anatomy and physiology textbook, easily accessible to those with little science background, is richly illustrated with diagrams and photographs, which help to illuminate body systems and processes.

Moore, Keith L., and T. V. N. Persaud. *The Developing Human.* 8th ed. Philadelphia: Saunders/Elsevier, 2008. An outstanding textbook on human embryonic development, with specific information about the causes of congenital malformations and common defects occurring in each of the body's systems. This widely used textbook gives a clear and careful description of normal human development during the entire prenatal period.

Riley, Edward P., and Charles V. Vorhees, eds. *Handbook of Behavioral Teratology.* New York: Plenum Press, 1986. An informative compilation of learning in the field of behavioral teratology. Covers historical context, general principles, and specific drugs and environmental agents that act as behavioral teratogens. Effects are listed for each agent that has been studied.

Tortora, Gerard J., and Bryan Derrickson. *Principles of Anatomy and Physiology.* 12th ed. Hoboken, N.J.: John Wiley & Sons, 2009. An intermediate-level college text widely used in fields of allied health. Chapters include overview of human prenatal development from fertilization through birth. Written in a very readable fashion; has excellent color diagrams and photographs on every page.

Tsiaras, Alexander, and Barry Werth. *From Conception to Birth: A Life Unfolds.* New York: Doubleday, 2002. Using state-of-the-art medical imaging technology, traces the development of a human life from conception through birth in spectacular, highly detailed photographs.

EMERGENCY MEDICINE
SPECIALTY

ANATOMY OR SYSTEM AFFECTED: All

SPECIALTIES AND RELATED FIELDS: Cardiology, critical care, gastroenterology, geriatrics and gerontology, neurology, nursing, obstetrics, pediatrics, pharmacology, psychiatry, public health, pulmonary medicine, radiology, sports medicine, toxicology

DEFINITION: The care of patients who are experiencing immediate health crises, a field defined by twenty-four-hour availability, the management of multiple patients simultaneously, and the need for broad-based skills and interventions.

KEY TERMS:

diagnostic: relating to the determination of the nature of a disease

emergency medical services: the complete chain of human and physical resources that provides patient care in cases of sudden illness or injury

heuristics: methods used to aid and guide in the discovery of a disease process when incomplete knowledge exists

paramedic: a person trained and certified to provide prehospital emergency medical care

pathologic: pertaining to the study of disease and the development of abnormal conditions

pathophysiology: an alteration in function as seen in disease

patient assessment: the systematic gathering of information in order to determine the nature of a patient's illness

triage: the medical screening of patients to determine their relative priority for treatment

SCIENCE AND PROFESSION

The field of emergency medicine is defined as care to acutely ill and injured patients, both in the prehospital setting and in the emergency room. It is practiced as patient-demanded and continuously accessible care and is defined by the location of its practice rather than by an anatomical concern. Emergency medicine encompasses all medical specialties and physical systems. The commitment to rapid, prudent intervention under stressful and often chaotic conditions is of paramount importance to the critically ill patient. This branch of medicine is characterized by its complexity of problems, its twenty-four-hour availability to a variety of patients, and its effective and broad-based understanding of disease and injury. These features are used to orchestrate the response of multiple hands with the ultimate goal of referring the patient to ongoing care.

The hourglass is an appropriate symbol of the nature of this medical division. It not only portrays the importance of time and the need for quick intervention, but its shape—wide at either end and narrowing in the middle—also is an appropriate visualization of the pattern of emergency medical treatment. A large number of patients converge on a single area, the emergency room, where they are diagnosed, treated, and eventually released to other appropriate care, diverging on a wide range of follow-up options.

Unique to the field of emergency medicine is the importance of rapid definition and comprehension of the pathophysiology of the critically ill patient. Emergency care physicians must have a unique understanding of the practice of medicine, the nature of disease and injury, availing themselves of a host of clinical skills needed for the treatment of the variety of physical and psychological problems that require treatment. Emergency rooms are a melting pot of problems; most are medical, many are not. All of them reflect some person's perception of an emergency. Success in the emergency medical field often depends on the ability of personnel to use not only their medical knowledge but their knowledge of people as well.

Most often those seeking the assistance of emergency medical providers are people suffering from pain of illness or trauma; however, any patient may seek treatment at the emergency room. Often loneliness, disability, or homelessness serves as the motivation to seek treatment. Regardless of what brought the patient, the emergency physician strives to recognize and deal with the patient's "emergency," remembering that not all patients are as ill as they might think and that not all are as well as they might appear. Physicians of this specialty sift through a multitude of information. It is necessary to know the patient's pertinent medical history and the history of the present illness or complaint before appropriate and effective treatment can be prescribed. Patients rarely follow a preconceived plan. Emergency medicine works best, therefore, when its practitioners follow heuristics—that is, incomplete guides that lead to greater knowledge, a holistic approach.

Emergency medicine is primarily a hospital-based specialty; however, it also involves extensive prehospital responsibilities. Many times, patients seeking emergency care are first the responsibility of police, fire, or ambulance personnel. In these situations, the role of emergency medicine must be viewed under the wider context of the emergency medical system. This system—beginning with the first aid administered by bystanders leading to initial treatment and transportation by trained certified emergency medical technicians, paramedics, or flight nurses and culminating with care at an emergency room or a highly equipped trauma center—forms a uniquely structured unit. The emergency medical system is designed to provide rapid quality intervention regardless of prehospital conditions. The emergency medical physician is best viewed as a central part of a team whose knowledge and understanding of the whole allow the best possible care to patients undergoing health crises.

Emergency physicians are charged with the responsibility of providing the highest standard of care in the hospital setting. They ensure that both staff members and equipment are maintained at their utmost level of quality. Trends, breakthroughs, and advances are monitored via journals and other medical publications. Training of personnel must keep pace with medical advancement. Developing an overall program depends as much on its planning as its dissemination. The emergency physician often plays the role of teacher, actively influencing the overall quality of the program through education and skills development. Thus, the exercise of emergency medicine is truly a team effort, with all members acting in accordance with their training and level of competence in order to minimize further injury or discomfort.

In practice, emergency medicine encompasses any person or structure involved in the immediate decision making and/or actions necessary to prevent death or further disability of a patient in the midst of a health crisis. It represents a chain of human and physical resources brought together for the purpose of providing

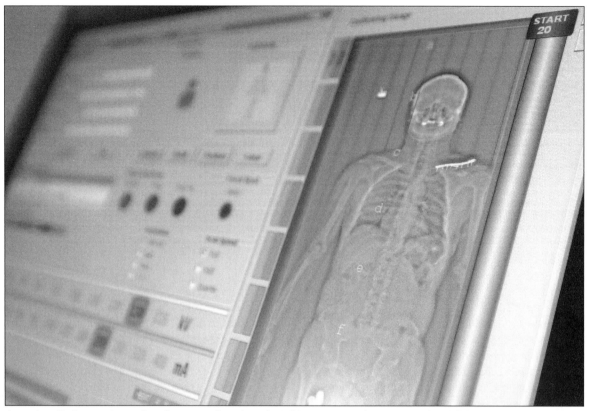

A monitor displays an image from Statscan, a low-dose, digital X-ray system that can provide a full-body scan in thirteen seconds without movement required from the patient. Such technology could prove lifesaving in emergency rooms. (AP/Wide World Photos)

total patient care. In this respect, everyone has a part to play in the delivery of emergency care. The bottom line of emergency medicine is the welfare of the patient. Thus, it is most appropriate to view the practice of emergency medicine in the context of the entire emergency medical system.

The components of the emergency medical system include recognition of the emergency, initiation of emergency medical response, treatment at the scene, transport by members of an emergency medical team to the appropriate facility, treatment in the emergency room or trauma center, and release of the patient. These components are only as strong as the weakest link.

DIAGNOSTIC AND TREATMENT TECHNIQUES

Recognition of an emergency is the first step in emergency care. Often this step is complicated by the patient's own denial and ignorance of basic symptoms. "Emergency" is in part defined by the patient's ability to identify, accept, and respond to a given situation. Regardless of the nature of the illness or injury, the sooner

an emergency is defined, the sooner care can be provided. The typical heart attack victim, for example, waits an average of three hours after experiencing symptoms before seeking help. In such cases, treatment by bystanders who have been trained in first aid and cardiopulmonary resuscitation (CPR) has proven effective.

In the United States, the response of emergency medical personnel has been aided by the implementation of the 911 emergency system. While not all communities have this capability, its use is increasing. It has been documented that patients who receive treatment at an appropriate facility within sixty minutes of the onset of a life-threatening emergency are more likely to survive. This "golden hour" is precious time.

Operating under protocols developed and approved by the emergency medical director and emergency medical councils of a given locale, emergency medical technicians (EMTs) and paramedics are trained and authorized to deliver care to the patient in need at the scene. EMTs and paramedics are charged with the initial assessment of the patient's condition, immediate stabilization prior to transport, delivery of care as far as their training allows, and the transport of the patient.

Unique to the field of emergency medicine is the special relationship of the paramedic with the doctor. Many people in need of emergency care are first treated outside the hospital. In these cases, emergency caregivers on the scene act as the eyes, ears, and hands of the physician. Through the EMT or paramedic, using telecommunications, an emergency doctor can speed the process of diagnosis. Signs and symptoms relayed through these trained professionals enable a doctor to make an accurate assessment of the patient's condition and to request a variety of treatments for a patient whom they cannot see or touch. Linked by telephone or radio, the medic and doctor can capitalize on the golden hour with the initiation of quality care.

Paramedics operate under the medical license of a medical command physician who has met all criteria set forth by the Department of Health and has been approved to provide medical directives to prehospital and interhospital providers. Protocols are the recognized practices that are within the training of the EMT and paramedic. They serve as standard procedures for prehospital treatment. While it is recognized that situations will arise which call for deviation from particular aspects of a given protocol, they are the standards under which the doctor and emergency personnel on the scene operate.

Treatment at the scene is followed by transport with advanced life support by members of the emergency medical system in 85 percent of all emergency cases. This requires much-needed equipment for the further treatment of patients. Deficiencies in the vehicle, equipment, or training of medical personnel can seriously endanger a patient. Thus, government agencies have been designated to grant permission for ambulance services and hospitals to engage in the practice of emergency medicine. This licensure process is designed to demand a level of competency for health care providers and ensure the public's protection.

Since only about 5 percent of all emergency department admissions constitute life-threatening situations, not all facilities stand at the same level of readiness for a given emergency. Transportation to the appropriate facility, therefore, requires a matching of the patient's need to the hospital's capabilities. Hospitals are categorized according to their ability to render emergency intensive care, as well as to provide needed support services on a patient-demand basis. In general, they are viewed as emergency facilities and trauma centers designed to provide twenty-four-hour, comprehensive emergency intensive care, including operating rooms and intensive care nurses.

When the patient reaches the emergency facility, during the first five to fifteen minutes of care, many important decisions are made by the physician on duty. The process continues to overlap with needed diagnostic tests and consultations in an effort to provide quality care directed at the source of the illness or injury. The patient's immediate needs are cared for by emergency department staff until the patient is moved to a site of continued care or released to his or her own care.

Questions correctly phrased and sharply directed are effective tools for the rapid diagnosis needed in emergency medicine. The key to this field is the ability to triage, stabilize, prioritize, treat, and refer.

Triage is the system used for categorizing and sorting patients according to the severity of their problems. Emergency practitioners seek to ascertain the nature of the patient's problem and consider any life-threatening consequences of the present condition. This stage of triage allows for immediate care to the more seriously endangered person, relegating the more stable, less seriously ill or wounded patients to a waiting period. The emergency room, in other words, does not operate on a first come, first served basis.

Secondary to triage is stabilization. This term refers to any immediate treatment or intervening steps taken to alleviate conditions that would result in greater pain or defect and/or lead to irreversible or fatal consequences. Primary stabilization steps include ensuring an unobstructed airway and providing adequate ventilation and cardiovascular function.

Once patients have been stabilized, all illnesses must be looked at on the scale of their hierarchical importance. Life-threatening diseases or injuries are treated before more moderate or minor conditions. This system of prioritization can be illustrated from patient to patient: A heart attack victim, for example, is treated prior to the patient with an ankle sprain. It can also be applied for multiple conditions within the same patient. The heart attack victim with a sprained ankle receives treatment first for the life-threatening cardiovascular incident.

Treatment of the critically ill patient often poses a series of further questions. What is the primary disorder? Is there more than one active pathologic process present? How does the patient appear? Is the patient's presentation consistent with the initial diagnosis? Is a hospital stay warranted? What consultations are needed to diagnose and treat this patient?

The emergency physician's approach is to consider the most serious disease consistent with the patient's presentation and chief complaint. By rule of thumb, thinking the worst and hoping for the best is often the psychological stance of the emergency care provider. Only when more severe conditions have been ruled out are more minor processes considered. Often too, this broad view of patient assessment allows for multiple diagnosis. Through continued probing, alternate and additional conditions are often uncovered. It is not unlikely that the patient who seeks treatment for a head injury after a fall is diagnosed with a more serious condition which caused the fall. Focusing only on the immediate condition would endanger the patient. Success in this medical field therefore demands broad-based medical knowledge and diagnostic tools.

Emergency medicine is not practiced in a vacuum. Its very nature necessitates its interfacing with a variety of medical specialties. The emergency room is often only the first step in patient recovery. Initial diagnosis and stabilization must be coupled with plans for ongoing treatment and evaluation. Consultations and referrals play important roles in the overall care of a patient.

Perspective and Prospects

Historians are unable to document specific systems for emergency patients before the 1790's. The need to provide care to the battlefield wounded is seen as the first implementation of emergency response. Early wartime treatment did not, however, include prehospital treatment. Clara Barton is credited with providing the first professional-level prehospital emergency care for the wounded as part of the American Red Cross. Ambulance services began in major cities of the United States at the beginning of the twentieth century, but it was not until 1960 that the National Academy of Sciences' Na-

In the News: Exemption from Informed Consent Requirements for Emergency Research

Informed consent is a patient's competent, voluntary permission to undergo a proposed treatment plan or procedure. To obtain a patient's informed consent, the physician or clinician must provide the patient with sufficient information to assist the patient in making an informed decision. The information provided should include indications for the procedure, any risks, and any available alternatives. The patient should be given an opportunity to ask questions and to deny consent if, after a thorough explanation, the patient feels that denying consent is the best option.

Federally mandated Institutional Review Boards (IRBs) must approve any research involving human subjects, including research in emergency departments. The IRBs aim to protect patients by ensuring that people who participate in research give adequate informed consent. In a medical emergency, however, it is unclear whether consent is sufficiently informed. So that critically ill and injured patients are not denied an opportunity to participate in beneficial research trials, the Food and Drug Administration (FDA) and the U.S. Department of Health and Human Services issued regulations that allow "emergency research" without informed consent. These regulations create an exception to the informed consent requirement when subjects are in a life-threatening situation, when obtaining informed consent is not feasible, when the research offers possible direct therapeutic benefit to the subjects, when the investigation could not be carried out without the waiver, and when additional protections of the rights and welfare of the subjects are provided. Because a waiver of informed consent undermines one of the most significant protections of human subjects, the guidelines attempt to compensate by providing additional precautions, including community consultation, public disclosure, and intensive oversight by an independent data and monitoring committee. The basis for these regulations is the premise that if the proposed research is not harmful, and particularly if it is potentially helpful, most "reasonable" patients would give their consent. Another instance in which consent may be waived involves minimal risk research, provided that the waiver will not adversely affect the rights and welfare of the subjects.

—*Marcia J. Weiss, M.A., J.D.*

tional Research Council actually studied the problem of emergency care.

Emergency medicine as a specialty is relatively new. Not until 1975, when the House of Delegates of the American Medical Association defined the emergency physician, did the medical community even recognize this branch of medicine. In 1981, the American College of Emergency Physicians added further recognition through the development of the definition of emergency medicine. Since then, growth and changes have enabled this field to develop as a major specialty, evolving to accept greater responsibility in both education and practice.

The development of emergency medicine and the increasing number of health care providers in this field have been dramatic. In 1990, there were a total of 23,000 emergency physicians, 85,000 emergency nurses, and 521,734 emergency technicians. These health care providers delivered care to the nearly 87 million emergency department patients seen that year.

Emergency medicine developed at a time when both the general public and the medical community recognized the need for quality accessible care in the emergency situation. It has grown to include a gamut of services provided by a community. In addition to responding to the acutely ill or injured, emergency medicine has grown to accept responsibilities of education, administration, and advocacy.

Included in the role of today's emergency medical providers is the administration of the entire emergency medical system within a community. This system includes the development of public education programs such as CPR instruction, poison control education, and the introduction of the 911 system. Emergency management systems and coordinators are now part of every state and local government. Disaster planning for both natural and human-made accidents also comes under the heading of emergency medicine.

Research, too, plays an important role in emergency medicine. The desire to identify, understand, and disseminate scientific rationale for basic resuscitative interventions, as well as the need to improve preventive medical techniques, are often driving forces in scientific research.

Finally, emergency medicine plays a key role in many of society's problems. Homelessness, drug use and abuse, acquired immunodeficiency syndrome (AIDS), and rising health costs have all contributed to the increase in the number of patients seen in the emergency room. In response, those administering emergency medical care have tried to communicate such problems to the general public and legislative bodies, as well as educate them regarding preventive measures. Being on the front line of medicine brings a special obligation to improve laws and services to ensure public safety and well-being.

—*Mary Beth McGranaghan*

See also Abdominal disorders; Altitude sickness; Amputation; Aneurysms; Antibiotics; Appendectomy; Appendicitis; Asphyxiation; Avian influenza; Biological and chemical weapons; Bites and stings; Bleeding; Botulism; Burns and scalds; Cardiac arrest; Cardiology; Cardiology, pediatric; Cardiopulmonary resuscitation (CPR); Catheterization; Cesarean section; Choking; Coma; Concussion; Critical care; Critical care, pediatric; Drowning; Electrical shock; Electrocardiography (ECG or EKG); Electroencephalography (EEG); Emergency medicine, pediatric; Emergency rooms; First aid; Fracture and dislocation; Fracture repair; Frostbite; Grafts and grafting; Head and neck disorders; Heart attack; Heat exhaustion and heatstroke; Hospitals; Hyperbaric oxygen therapy; Hyperthermia and hypothermia; Intensive care unit (ICU); Intoxication; Intravenous (IV) therapy; Laceration repair; Meningitis; Nursing; Obstetrics; Paramedics; Peritonitis; Pneumonia; Poisoning; Radiation sickness; Resuscitation; Reye's syndrome; Salmonella infection; Shock; Snakebites; Spinal cord disorders; Splenectomy; Sports medicine; Staphylococcal infections; Streptococcal infections; Strokes; Thrombolytic therapy and TPA; Tracheostomy; Transfusion; Unconsciousness; Veterinary medicine; Wounds.

FOR FURTHER INFORMATION:

Bledsoe, Bryan E., Robert S. Porter, and Bruce R. Shade. *Brady Paramedic Emergency Care*. 3d ed. Upper Saddle River, N.J.: Brady/Prentice Hall, 1997. A comprehensive guide to the practice of emergency medicine as it applies to and is practiced by the paramedic. A solid overview of the basics of prehospital care. This text focuses on advanced life support practices.

Caroline, Nancy L. *Nancy Caroline's Emergency Care in the Streets*. 6th ed. Sudbury, Mass.: Jones and Bartlett, 2010. This text provides a sophisticated understanding of the fundamental concepts of advanced life support and the underlying physiology. A focused approach written by a physician who has spent many hours in the field as a prehospital care provider.

Hamilton, Glenn C., et al. *Emergency Medicine: An Approach to Clinical Problem-Solving*. 2d ed. New York: W. B. Saunders, 2003. Addressed to students of medicine, this text provides a detailed, well-written script for the clinical setting. Facilitates the reader's understanding of the emergency scene. Actual medical cases are integrated into the chapters in order to reinforce concepts.

Limmer, Daniel, et al. *Emergency Care*. 11th ed. Upper Saddle River, N.J.: Pearson/Prentice Hall Health, 2009. This simple text has been acclaimed for its comprehensive, accurate, and up-to-the-minute treatment of emergency care. Easy to read, this book provides the contemporary standards on CPR from the American Heart Association and a full treatment on many emergency medical protocols for prehospital treatment.

Markovchick, Vincent J., and Peter T. Pons, eds. *Emergency Medicine Secrets*. 4th ed. Philadelphia: Mosby/Elsevier, 2006. Details all aspects of emergency medicine in a question-and-answer format. Topics include nontraumatic illness, hematology/oncology, infectious disease, environmental emergencies, neonatal and childhood disorders, toxicologic emergencies, emergency medicine administration and risk management, and disaster management.

Marx, John A., et al., eds. *Rosen's Emergency Medicine: Concepts and Clinical Practice*. 7th ed. Philadelphia: Mosby/Elsevier, 2010. A logical and straightforward presentation of current standards of emergency medicine. Intended to be a reference in busy emergency rooms. The writing is clear and to the point.

Tintinalli, Judith E., ed. *Emergency Medicine: A Comprehensive Study Guide*. 6th ed. New York: McGraw-Hill, 2004. This bible of emergency medicine provides a basic understanding of the field. Describes in detail key diagnostic techniques and treatments.

EMERGENCY MEDICINE, PEDIATRIC
SPECIALTY

ANATOMY OR SYSTEM AFFECTED: All

SPECIALTIES AND RELATED FIELDS: Critical care

DEFINITION: The decision making and actions necessary to prevent death or any further disability in children with life-threatening injuries, illnesses, and other health crises.

KEY TERMS:

abc's: the basics of survival—*a* is for airway obstruction/choking, *b* is for breathing/respiratory distress, and *c* is for circulatory collapse/shock

pediatric emergency specialists: emergency physicians who focus their practices on emergency care for children, including research and teaching pediatric emergency medicine

triage: the process of choosing who will receive medical treatment first because of dire illness or injury

SCIENCE AND PROFESSION

Physicians who specialize in pediatric emergency medicine have been trained to diagnose and treat patients in order to prevent death or any further disability for children in health crises. They are also skilled at health promotion and injury prevention efforts. For some young patients, emergency departments are increasingly the only source of routine medical care. Pediatric emergency physicians represent the front line of medicine.

Emergency medicine emphasizes the anticipation and recognition of a life-threatening process, rather than seeking a definitive diagnosis. The emergencies that these physicians treat are often the type parents hope never to see. The perceptions and complaints of the patients or the people who bring them to the emergency department or pediatric trauma center define the emergencies themselves. Most children treated in an emergency department will be seen in a general hospital whose staff is unlikely to include pediatric specialists. Each year, about one-third of the children who visit the emergency department are there because of an injury. Two-thirds of the visits are the result of illnesses such as debilitating asthma or life-threatening meningitis. Services are available twenty-four hours a day, seven days a week, 365 days a year in the hospital and in the field. They are provided by a network of health specialists, nurses, paramedics, emergency medical technicians, police officers, firefighters, and others dedicated to offering emergency medical services to children and adults.

Pediatric emergency specialists are needed because children are not little adults. The differences between children and adults are so great that they exist in virtually every organ system, body part, physiological process, and disease syndrome. For example, children's lungs are smaller and more fragile than those of adults, so that they require gentler thrusts during cardiopulmonary resuscitation (CPR). Children have faster heart and respiration rates than do adults, so that what may look like normal adult rates may be a sign of serious trouble in a child. Children require different and special equipment, different-sized instruments, different doses of different medicines, and different approaches to the psychological support and remedial care given to the ill or injured patient.

Physicians and other health care providers who lack pediatric emergency medical training and experience may find it difficult to recognize children who are critically ill and require the most urgent care. For example, infants may not develop a fever to signal infection. In children, respiratory arrest or shock signals the risk of cardiopulmonary arrest, rather than the arrhythmias that typically precede cardiac arrest in adults.

DIAGNOSTIC AND TREATMENT TECHNIQUES

A good medical outcome depends on the prompt identification and treatment of serious illness or injury in children. Emergency services personnel use a system called triage to decide whether patients are at risk for severe illness or imminent death, whether they have less urgent but still serious medical problems, or whether they have routine problems. Health care professionals use a system called the *abc*'s. Children who are choking (*a* for airway obstruction), in respiratory distress (*b* for breathing), or in shock (*c* for circulatory collapse) are treated immediately. The sickest patients always come first.

Doctors often make the most important decisions about a patient within the first five to fifteen minutes of care. The physician first determines whether the patient is in need of treatment and confirms or rules out the presence of catastrophic disease as quickly as possible. The doctor then stabilizes the patient's vital signs to reduce the risk of worsening symptoms or death. Next, the physician acts to relieve the most acute symptoms. The patient may then be hospitalized or discharged with directions about what to do next.

PERSPECTIVE AND PROSPECTS

Physicians have been treating pediatric emergencies for centuries. Only recently, however, has there been much recognition among the medical community or the public that pediatric emergency care requires unique training, equipment, and procedures.

Emergency medicine as a discipline in the United States dates to 1968, when the American College of Emergency Physicians was formed. During the 1970's, pediatricians and pediatric surgeons recognized that children's emergency care needs were not receiving adequate attention. The American Medical Association (AMA) and the American Board of Medical Specialties recognized emergency medicine as the twenty-third medical specialty in 1979. In the early 1980's, growing numbers of pediatric specialists and professional societies began to participate in the development of emergency medical systems. In 1993, a committee of the Institute of Medicine published a major study on the state of emergency care for children. The committee focused on standardizing the emergency care system so that the quality of emergency care would be consistent from state to state and community to community. It encouraged the creation of a nationwide 911 emergency response system and the establishment of minimum standards of care.

The tools, technologies, treatments, and problem-solving methods used by pediatric emergency physicians have been advancing rapidly. These specialists have gotten better at coping with the gamut of children's emergencies, including the medical and behavioral crises of newborns, infants, toddlers, young children, and adolescents. Emergency physicians have been and continue to be responsible for the development of new treatment techniques and the widespread availability of specialized pediatric equipment.

—*Fred Buchstein*

See also Allergies; Asthma; Biological and chemical weapons; Bites and stings; Bleeding; Burns and scalds; Cardiac arrest; Cardiology, pediatric; Cardiopulmonary resuscitation (CPR); Cardiovascular system; Choking; Critical care, pediatric; Dizziness and fainting; Drowning; Electrical shock; Emergency rooms; Fever; Food poisoning; Fracture and dislocation; Frostbite; Heat exhaustion and heatstroke; Hospitals; Intensive care unit (ICU); Meningitis; Physical examination; Pneumonia; Poisoning; Poisonous plants; Pulmonary medicine, pediatric; Rabies; Respiration; Respiratory distress syndrome; Seizures; Snakebites; Suicide.

FOR FURTHER INFORMATION:

Durch, Jane S., and Kathleen N. Lohr, eds. *Emergency Medical Services for Children*. Washington, D.C.: National Academy Press, 1993. This report of an Institute of Medicine study examines the nature and extent of acute illness and injury among children, reviews the origins and organization of emergency medical services (EMS) systems, describes the current state of effective care, and addresses data and standards needed for surveillance and evaluation of services and outcomes.

Hamilton, Glenn C., et al. *Emergency Medicine: An Approach to Clinical Problem-Solving*. 2d ed. New York: W. B. Saunders, 2003. A comprehensive textbook, in concise format, for residents and medical students.

Lynn, Stephan G., with Pamela Weintraub. *Medical Emergency! The St. Luke's-Roosevelt Hospital Center Book of Emergency Medicine*. New York: Hearst Books, 1996. This most helpful, informative, and well-arranged book tells how to be personally prepared for emergencies by having basic records and documents in a wallet or purse and others in known places for easy location. It clarifies emergency tests and treatments and explains how family members and friends can act as emergency patient advocates.

Soud, Treesa E., and Janice Steiner Rogers. *Manual of Pediatric Emergency Nursing*. St. Louis, Mo.: Mosby, 1998. A portable handbook summarizing most of the conditions seen in a pediatric emergency department. Includes the essential points and priorities for diagnosis, management, and follow-up care, as well as indications for hospitalization.

Strange, Gary R., et al., eds. *Pediatric Emergency Medicine: A Comprehensive Study Guide*. 2d ed. New York: McGraw-Hill, 2002. A handbook for a range of emergency situations encountered in pediatric care.

EMERGENCY ROOMS

HEALTH CARE SYSTEM

ALSO KNOWN AS: ERs, trauma centers

ANATOMY OR SYSTEM AFFECTED: All

SPECIALTIES AND RELATED FIELDS: All

DEFINITION: Sites that provides twenty-four-hour emergency medical care. Metropolitan trauma centers often have more than fifty patient care areas and treat hundreds of patients daily. Rural or community hospital ERs may be as small as several rooms but usually have many treatment areas available.

KEY TERMS:

American Board of Emergency Medicine (ABEM): the agency certifying medical doctors as emergency medicine specialists; sets criteria for training and knowledge to become board certified in emergency medicine

American College of Emergency Physicians (ACEP): supports quality emergency care and promotes the interests of emergency physicians

emergency medicine: one of twenty-four medical specialties recognized by the American Board of Medical Specialties

trauma center: an ER that meets certain criteria for the delivery of emergent care to those suffering severe injuries

triage: from French word meaning "to pick or cull"; in ER triage, health care personnel, usually nurses, make an initial determination regarding the severity of a person's illness

BACKGROUND

Emergency medicine is one of twenty-four medical specialties recognized by the American Board of Medi-

cal Specialties (ABMS). A board-certified specialist in emergency medicine meets training and certification requirements established by the American Board of Emergency Medicine (ABEM). Emergency medicine became a medical specialty in 1979 and is well established as a recognized body of medical specialists and knowledge.

After World War II, emergency rooms became primary health care access points for an increasing number of people. Many factors contributed to this change, including increasing specialization among physicians along with decreasing numbers of primary care and general practitioners. The resultant decrease in hospital on-call physicians available to treat ER patients fostered the concept of full-time ER specialists, whose primary duties involved treating patients coming to ERs.

The first plans for full-time emergency room physician coverage originated in the 1960's. A model featuring dedicated ER doctors proved to be the most attractive among hospitals and patients. Emergency physicians limit their practice to the emergency department while providing 24/7 coverage. Emergency physicians treat all patients, regardless of ability to pay, while establishing contractual relationships with hospitals. This model for emergency care fostered the development of emergency medicine, setting standards of care for the new specialty. (Michael T. Rapp and George Podgorny provide a detailed consideration of the many factors in the developmental history of emergency medicine in their 2005 article "Reflections on Becoming a Specialist and Its Impact on Global Emergency Medical Care: Our Challenge for the Future" in *Emergency Medicine Clinics of North America*.)

The National Academy of Sciences and the National Research Council raised concern with a 1966 report titled *Accidental Death and Disability: The Neglected Disease of Modern Society*. More rapid prehospital response along with better emergency care standards were needed to improve emergency care in the United States. Emergency physicians from Michigan, including John Wiegenstein, founded an organization fostering the national development of Emergency Medicine, the American College of Emergency Physicians (ACEP), in 1968.

Emergency physicians integrate medical care in a variety of settings, including military, disaster, community, and academic settings. Emergency physicians are experts in emergent cardiovascular care, including resuscitative medicine and the various highly specialized procedures that accompany that care. Accident and trauma stabilization is another area of ER expertise. Emergency medicine residency training is three to four years in length. This training occurs after a doctor has completed medical school and undergraduate education. During that time, a well-trained ER doctor becomes proficient in many complex, lifesaving procedures, such as thoracotomies (opening the chest to correct emergent heart and lung problems), pacemaker placement (correcting heart rate and rhythm problems), intubation (allowing airway access), chest tube insertion (draining blood and fluid from the lungs), and lumbar puncture (assessing neurological problems). Rapid recognition, prompt emergent care, and effective triage are emergency medicine physician characteristics.

Emergency physicians treat life-threatening and severe emergent medical problems, such as myocardial infarctions (heart attacks), strokes, drug overdoses, and diabetic ketoacidosis. Traumatic injuries, such as stabbings, shootings, industrial accidents, and automobile accidents, are also treated and stabilized in the Emergency Department, which is the major care location for disaster care. Emergency physicians treat all age groups and all conditions, at all hours of the day, simultaneously. This ability to treat the variety and breadth of emergent problems stands ER doctors out as the group of specialists best suited to assess and properly treat the greatest number of acutely ill patients.

FEATURES AND PROCEDURES

Emergency rooms vary in size, but most share uniform characteristics. The first ER assessment is triage, a term with French roots meaning "to pick or cull." In triage, health care personnel, usually nurses, determine the severity of a patient's injury or illness and record the patient's chief complaint or medical problem. They measure and record vital signs, including pulse, temperature, respiratory rate, and blood pressure. If the patient's condition is stable, then triage personnel obtain other important information, such as medications taken, a brief medical history, and any patient allergies.

The most important triage duty determines the severity of an illness. Usually, there are three main categories: critical and immediately life threatening, such as a myocardial infarction; urgent but not immediately life threatening, such as most abdominal pain; and less urgent, such as a minor leg laceration, known as the "walking wounded" in military triage. ER personnel often refer to these categories as Cat I, Cat II, or Cat III. After assessing the patient's condition, triage person-

nel advance patients to appropriate care areas. A new category I patient may be wheeled on a gurney directly to the critical area, with the nurse announcing to any doctors on the way, "new Cat I patient in 101." These patients need immediate emergency care.

A stable patient is registered by front-desk personnel. Registration clerks obtain insurance and contact information. New medical charts are generated for new patients, or old records are requested if they already exist at that hospital. Patients arriving by ambulance or critically ill category I patients bypass this step until after treatment or stabilization in the critical care area of the emergency room.

Most emergency departments have many patient care areas, reflecting the wide variety of patients seen in the ER. These areas include resuscitation rooms for patients needing cardiopulmonary resuscitation; trauma care areas for patients with severe injuries like gunshot wounds or accident victims; critical care areas for patients needing cardiac monitoring along with ongoing critical care; pediatric ERs for the care of children; chest-pain evaluation areas; and suture rooms for the repairs of lacerations (cuts). Rooms for the examination of women with gynecological problems are available. ERs usually have a fast track or urgent care area for minor illness (such as sore throats) and an observation unit for patients waiting for hospital admission or diagnostic tests.

Many personnel contribute to the wide variety of care provided in emergency departments. Emergency physicians, nurses, physician assistants, medical technologists, and medical assistants have specified health care roles. Unit clerks help with the paperwork, and laboratory personnel assist with radiological and laboratory procedures. Administrative people help with staffing issues, equipment purchasing, facility maintenance, and scheduling of workers. These are some of the important roles necessary to deliver emergency care. To a varying degree, ERs will also have social workers, psychological care providers, and patient advocates available as full-time ER personnel.

PERSPECTIVE AND PROSPECTS

Many agencies promote effective, more standardized emergency and trauma care. In addition to the American Board of Emergency Medicine and the American College of Emergency Physicians, many other agencies promote effective emergency care, such as the American Academy of Emergency Medicine. The American Heart Association takes a lead in cardiopulmonary resuscitation (CPR) guidelines. The American College of Surgeons (ACS) develops standards for trauma care. Nursing organizations, emergency medical technician (EMT) agencies, and other professional organizations develop standards for improving emergency care.

The American College of Surgeons provides trauma center designation guidelines. Trauma center designation requires various important resources and characteristics. Although the ACS provides consultants and guidelines for this process, other agencies designate trauma centers, such as local or state governments. Three main trauma center levels exist in ACS guidelines.

In level I, comprehensive 24/7 trauma care specialists are available in the hospital, including emergency medicine, general surgery, and anesthesiology. Various surgical specialists are available, including neurosurgery, orthopedic surgery, and plastic surgery. Level I designation requires intensive care units (ICUs) along with operating rooms staffed and ready to go twenty-four hours daily all year round. These are major referral centers, often known as tertiary care facilities.

Level II offers comprehensive trauma and critical care, but the full array of specialists may not be as readily available as those found in a level I trauma center. Trauma volume levels are usually lower than the level I trauma centers.

In level III, resources are available for critical care and stabilization of trauma victims. Patient volume, array of specialists, and 24/7 availability vary. Transfer protocols with level II and I trauma centers allow comprehensive care after stabilization. Community or rural hospitals may have this designation.

The efforts of all these groups enhance emergency care, in all of its various forms. Emergency medicine is at the front lines of medical care. Like any forward-moving group, backup and support improve the ultimate goal—available and effective emergency care delivered when needed the most.

—*Richard P. Capriccioso, M.D.*

See also Accidents; Critical care; Emergency medicine; Hospitals; Intensive care unit (ICU).

FOR FURTHER INFORMATION:

American Board of Emergency Medicine. www.abem.org/public. The agency that certifies medical doctors as emergency medicine specialists. Sets criteria for training and knowledge to become board certified in emergency medicine.

American College of Emergency Physicians. www

.acep.org. ACEP supports quality emergency care and promotes the interests of emergency physicians. Many resources related to emergency medicine are available at this site.

American College of Surgeons Committee on Trauma. *Consultation/Verification Programs for Hospitals.* http://www.facs.org/trauma/verificationhosp.html. Includes lists of verified trauma centers and multiple resources for the treatment of trauma patients.

_____. *Resources for Optimal Care of the Injured Patient: 2006.* http://web4.facs.org/ebusiness/product catalog/product.aspx?ID=194. Requirements outlined for ACS trauma center designations.

Arnold J. L. "International Emergency Medicine and the Recent Development of Emergency Medicine Worldwide." *Annals of Emergency Medicine* 33 (1999): 97-103. Many countries use the U.S. model for establishing emergency medicine in their own countries.

National Academy of Sciences and the National Research Council. *Accidental Death and Disability: The Neglected Disease of Modern Society.* Washington, D.C.: Government Printing Office, 1966. A report raising concern and demonstrating need for development of better emergent and accident care.

Rapp, Michael T., and George Podgorny. "Reflections on Becoming a Specialist and Its Impact on Global Emergency Medical Care: Our Challenge for the Future." *Emergency Medicine Clinics of North America* 23, no. 1 (February, 2005): 259-269. A well-considered exploration of the development of emergency medicine. Also available at http://www.acep.org.

EMERGING INFECTIOUS DISEASES

DISEASE/DISORDER

ANATOMY OR SYSTEM AFFECTED: All

SPECIALTIES AND RELATED FIELDS: All

DEFINITION: First introduced by Nobel laureate Joshua Lederberg, the phrase "emerging infectious diseases" applies to those diseases that newly appear in a populace or have been in existence for some time but are rapidly increasing in incidence, geographic range, or surface as new drug-resistant strains of viruses, bacteria, or parasitic species.

KEY TERMS:

endemic: a disease that is constantly present in a particular region or country and is usually under control

epidemic: a contagious disease that is prevalent and rapidly spreading in a community *pandemic:* rapidly spreading disease over a whole area, country, continent or the globe

vector: an animal, especially an insect, that transmits a pathogenic organism from a host to a noninfected animal

zoonosis: a disease or infection transmitted to humans by vertebrate animals

INTRODUCTION

Most emerging infectious diseases are of zoonotic (animal) origin, and a variety of insect vectors such as mosquitoes help to spread the infections. While "new" infectious diseases continue to emerge, many of the old plagues remain, often appearing in more virulent and drug-resistant forms. While some outbreaks inexplicably appear, often specific identifiable ecologic factors such as climate change, agricultural development, and demographic changes such as urbanization place individuals at increased risk through exposure to unfamiliar microbes or their natural zoonotic hosts; the rise of megacities with their high population densities, dearth of potable water, and foodstuffs makes urbanites particularly vulnerable to emerging infectious diseases. Moreover, modern humans have the capability to rapidly spread contagious disease halfway around the world through air travel. Mostly these are global problems and are viewed as "global infectious disease threats."

BACKGROUND

Throughout history, populations have been afflicted by major outbreaks of emerging infectious diseases such as the bubonic plague or Black Death, a zoonosis caused by the bacterium *Yersinia pestis* that is spread by fleas which feed off rodents. The Black Plague emerged in the fourteenth century and decimated Europe and Asia, obliterating a third of the European population within a few years. More deadly than *Y. pestis*, however, was the variola virus, the etiologic agent of smallpox which evolved from poxviruses in cattle and emerged into human populations thousands of years ago. From the fourteenth to sixteenth centuries, the Spanish conquered Central America by causing a smallpox epidemic through introduction of the virus into indigenous populations, thereby disabling their armies. In 1980, the World Health Organization (WHO) declared that smallpox had been eradicated. However, in 2003, as the United States entered into war with Iraq, U.S. president George W. Bush decreed that the armed forces be vaccinated against smallpox in anticipation of

a bioterrorism attack. This pronouncement came on the heels of similar attacks in the United States wherein anthrax infection caused by *Bacillus anthracis* was intentionally spread in Florida and New York. In 2009, another bacterial infection continued to emerge, methicillin-resistant *Staphylococcus aureus* (MRSA) due to the apparent overuse of the antibiotic methicillin.

Influenza, known as a human disease for hundreds of years, emerged in the pandemic of 1918 that killed 20 million to 40 million persons, more than died in World War I. Other influenza pandemics included the Asian flu in 1957, the Hong Kong flu in 1968, and swine flu in 1977. Avian influenza, or bird flu, which rarely infects people, emerged in 2004. The H1N1 influenza (formerly called swine flu) emerged in Mexico in 2009 and rapidly spread throughout the Northern hemisphere, infecting millions in the United States alone and countless others across the globe, sickening and killing a disproportionate number of young children and pregnant women in its wake and rarely affecting those over age sixty-five. Human immunodeficiency virus (HIV), a retrovirus, is the causative agent of acquired immunodeficiency syndrome (AIDS), one the world's deadliest infectious diseases; according to the WHO, about 2 million people die from AIDS-related diseases each year, more than from tuberculosis or malaria. In 2008, sub-Saharan Africa accounted for 71 percent of all new HIV infections. In 2009, multi-drug resistant tuberculosis (MDR-TB) and extensively multi-drug resistant tuberculosis (XMDR-TB) continued to emerge, especially in those living with HIV infection. Malaria, a parasitic scourge, causes approximately 881,000 deaths every year, with 90 percent of deaths occurring in sub-Saharan Africa. Malaria continues to emerge with strains of its most lethal species, *Plasmodium falciparum*, resistant to antimalarial drugs.

EXAMPLES

Three diseases serve as important recent examples of epidemics and pandemics: H1N1 influenza, HIV/AIDS, and resistant tuberculosis.

A zoonotic disease resulting from a mix of swine, avian, and human flu viruses, H1N1 influenza emerged in the United States following the regular 2008-2009 flu season wherein influenza A (H1), A (H3), and B viruses all circulated. In mid-April, 2009, the Centers for Disease Control and Prevention (CDC) documented the first two cases of influenza A pandemic (H1N1) in the United States; after September 1, 2009, the CDC characterized the antigens of collected flu viruses: 412 2009 influenza A (H1N1); 4 influenza B; 3 influenza A (H3N2); and 1 seasonal influenza A (H1N1). In December 2009, 99 percent of flu strains were comprised of pandemic H1N1 2009. According to WHO, as of November 22, 2009, there were more than 40,617 commulative "confirmed and probable" cases of pandemic H1N1 2009, and 7,826 deaths worldwide. However, these statistics are significantly lower than the actual morbidity and mortality because they are based on just 20 percent of the countries, territories, and communities that provided laboratory confirmed evidence. Moreover, pandemic H1N1 2009 infections in which the virus mutated to a strain more virulent and/or less sensitive to drug treatment are being studied across the globe; five patients in the United Kingdom had strains of H1N1 resistant to the antiviral oseltamivir (Tamiflu), and four other cases were under scrutiny. Another type of mutation that may trigger more severe illness was found in Norway in two patients who died from the disease; between April and December, 2009, there were fifty-seven U.S. cases of Tamiflu resistance and reported mutations akin to those that occurred in Norway.

HIV and AIDS. Since HIV, the virus that causes AIDS, was first isolated in the early 1980's, the virus has continued to emerge into new populations and new geographic locations while morphing into new strains and variants, becoming resistant to available antiretroviral therapies (ART). Therefore, new drugs and combinations of old and new therapies must continually be produced to help keep alive the more than 33.4 million persons living with HIV and AIDS in 2008, up from 29 million in 2001. Moreover, while HIV infection is now treated like a chronic disease in many developed countries, the developing nations continue to struggle to obtain adequate drugs and preventive programs to treat all those infected with the virus while the world awaits the first vaccine that can prevent the disease. Moreover, despite the advent of highly active antiretroviral therapy (HAART) in 1996, a range of comorbidities continues to plague those living with HIV and AIDS (1.3 million in North America of the 33.4 million across the globe) including liver disease (hepatitis B and C), non-Hodgkin's lymphoma, neurological illnesses, malignancy, malnutrition, alcoholism, and increased susceptibility to TB and MDR-TB, in addition to socioeconomic factors such as poverty, unemployment, stigmatization, and undocumented status. In addition, there has been a resurgence of HIV infection in men who have sex with men (MSM) and other vulnerable populations such as sex-workers, the incarcerated, mobile workers, and injection drug users (IDUs). Nevertheless, according to the WHO and Joint United Nations Programme on HIV/AIDS (UNAIDS), new HIV infections declined by 18 percent worldwide from 2001 to 2008 due to preventive measures.

MDR-TB/XMDR-TB. The emergence and spread of Mycobacterium tuberculosis strains resistant to multiple drugs represent an emerging threat for the global control of both tuberculosis and HIV, which often coinfect patients. WHO estimates that almost 500,000 cases of MDR-TB emerged in 2006. MDR-TB is defined as resistance to a minimum of the anti-TB drugs isoniazid and rifampin; in certain regions of the world, prevalence of MDR-TB may be greater than 20 percent. While HIV may or may not be directly associated with the risk of developing MDR-TB, nosocomial outbreaks in individuals living with HIV and AIDS have been noted. HIV/AIDS has also been linked to an increased risk for rifampin-monoresistant TB. In addition, new cases of XMDR-TB, defined as MDR-TB resistant to a fluoroquinolone and a minimum of one second-line injectable agent, have been widely reported across the globe. Treatment of MDR-TB is complex, sometimes requiring the use of less effective and more toxic drugs that mandate treatment over longer periods of time, thereby lessening the chance of successful outcomes and posing serious problems for developing countries, especially those with a high prevalence of HIV-1 infection. MDR-TB and XMDR-TB is also a concern in wealthier countries where massive immigration and global travel is commonplace.

—*Cynthia F. Racer, M.A., M.P.H.*

See also Acquired immunodeficiency syndrome (AIDS); Antibiotics; Avian influenza; Bacterial infections; Centers for Disease Control and Prevention (CDC); Drug resistance; Ebola virus; Epidemics and pandemics; Epidemiology; H1N1 influenza; Human immunodeficiency virus (HIV); Immunization and vaccination; Influenza; Insect-borne diseases; Malaria; National Institutes of Health (NIH); Parasitic diseases; Plague; Severe acute respiratory syndrome (SARS); Tuberculosis; Viral infections; West Nile virus; World Health Organization; Zoonoses.

FOR FURTHER INFORMATION:

Garrett, Laurie. *Betrayal of Trust: The Collapse of Global Public Health.* New York: Hyperion Books, 2001.

Hill, Stuart. *Emerging Infectious Diseases*. San Francisco: Benjamin Cummings, 2005.

Leslie, T., et al. "Epidemic of *Plasmodium falciparum* Malaria Involving Substandard Anti-malarial Drugs, Pakistan, 2003." *Emerging Infectious Diseases* 15 (2009): 1753-1759.

MacPherson, D. W., et al. "Population Mobility, Globalization, and Antimicrobial Drug Resistance." *Emerging Infectious Diseases* 15 (2009): 1727-1732.

EMOTIONS: BIOMEDICAL CAUSES AND EFFECTS

BIOLOGY

ANATOMY OR SYSTEM AFFECTED: Brain, endocrine system, gastrointestinal system, immune system, muscles, musculoskeletal system, nerves, nervous system, psychic-emotional system

SPECIALTIES AND RELATED FIELDS: Neurology, psychiatry, psychology

DEFINITION: Experiential events not characterized by any one sense and accompanied by complex physiological and mental changes.

KEY TERMS:

autonomic nervous system: the division of the nervous system that regulates involuntary action; comprises the sympathetic and parasympathetic systems

bipolar disorders: syndromes characterized by alternating periods of elevated and depressed mood; also discussed as manic-depressive disorder

Kluver-Bucy syndrome: a series of symptoms first observed in monkeys following temporal lobe removal, such as psychic blindness, abnormal oral tendencies, and changes in sexuality

loss-of-control syndrome: a pattern of behavior characterized by violent and emotional outbursts, occasionally associated with temporal lobe seizures

major depressive syndrome: a syndrome characterized by profound sadness and loss of pleasure in normal activities

sympathetic nervous system: the division of the autonomic nervous system concerned primarily with preparing the individual to expend energy

STRUCTURE AND FUNCTIONS

A central characteristic of being human is the ability to experience and express a wide range of emotions. Just what happens in the human brain and body to generate these feelings, however, is not completely clear. Over the years, it has been demonstrated that activity in the sympathetic nervous system is important in the expression and experience of emotional states, although the role of various regions of the brain in emotion has proved to be more elusive.

No consensus exists on how many different emotions humans are capable of experiencing, as so much depends on definitions and the type of evidence admitted. Most experts agree, however, that emotions have a significant impact on human behavior. The term "emotion" usually means some subjectively experienced effect. In addition, at least three other factors can be considered part of emotion: physiological arousal (increased heart rate, sweating palms), expressive changes of the muscles of the face and body (smiles, frowns), and behavior (striking with a fist, cringing). Debates persist about the degree to which there is a distinction between feelings and emotions; others argue about the degree to which cognition, or thinking, also affects emotion.

The best-studied physical responses characteristic of emotional states are those produced by the sympathetic nervous system, which controls many different internal organs of the body, as well as the salivary and sweat glands. Several of the responses produced by this system occur in emotional states. These responses are recorded in an attempt to study, measure, and evaluate emotion. The most commonly used responses include changes in heart rate, blood pressure, dilation of the pupils, and sweat gland activity. Physiological arousal in emotion also includes changes in the secretion of some hormones such as adrenaline, testosterone, and cortisol, measured from their presence in such body fluids as urine, saliva, and blood plasma.

The nervous system provides for rapid communication in the body, as it is concerned with events that occur on the order of milliseconds. Its structural and functional unit is the neuron, or nerve cell. Neurons have certain distinctive regions. The dendrites, or bushy protrusions, are the part specialized in receiving excitation, whether from an external stimulus or from another cell. The axon, or elongated part of the cell, takes care of distributing excitation away from the dendrite zone. Axons can be very long and form bundles that make up nerves.

The entire nervous system is a functional unit, and an impulse arising in any receptor can be transmitted to every effector in the body. Synapses are the functional junctions where connections between neurons form. In this region, one cell comes into contact, or near contact, with another cell, thus influencing it. Nerve impulses are propagated by electrochemical reactions. The neural message must jump from the axon of one neuron to the dendrite of another for transmission to occur. The most common way of achieving this is through a chemical transmitter substance, also called a neurotransmitter. Chemical transmission at a synapse involves two steps. The first is the release of the specific chemical or neurotransmitter on the arrival of a nerve impulse. The chemical is released from its storage place in the tip of the axon into the narrow space between adjacent neurons. Once this has taken place, the specific transmitter substance is attached to a specific molecular site in the dendrite of the other neuron. This attachment produces a change in the properties of its cell membrane so that a new nerve impulse is set up, and the transmission continues.

The rapidly acting neurotransmitters include norepinephrine, epinephrine, dopamine, serotonin, acetylcholine, gamma aminobutyric acid (GABA), glycine, glutamate, and probably aspartate and adenosine triphosphate (ATP). The action of these neurotransmitters depends on the chemistry of the receptor to which they bind, and there are several types of receptor for each neurotransmitter. Receptors for neurotransmitters are important targets for toxins and drugs. For example, psychoactive drugs exert their effects at synapses, mostly by binding to specific receptors, but also by interfering with the degradation or removal of the transmitter from the synaptic cleft so that it lingers longer in the system.

From research on people with spinal cord injuries, it was found that while emotions may not be caused by feedback from sympathetic activity, this activity does play an important role in reinforcing emotional feelings, making them more intense and longer lasting.

Many different regions of the brain participate in emotions. The neocortex is responsible for dealing with symbolic manipulation, and bodily responses to emotion involve circuits located in lower brain regions such as the hypothalamus. Hormonal changes bring the endocrine system into play.

Dramatic changes in personality and emotional expression often occur following damage to various areas of the brain, such as weakening of emotional control with an injury to the frontal lobes. There is controversy, however, regarding where in the brain emotion is actually experienced. Research has pointed to certain parts of the brain below the cerebral cortex, such as the hypothalamus and the amygdala, as possible key participants. Two syndromes corroborate this finding. In loss-of-control syndrome, emotional outbursts are caused by abnormal electrical discharges in the region of the temporal lobe and amygdala. These spontaneous discharges are characteristic of epilepsy and are thought to result from congenital defects, high fever, brain infection, or trauma. Epilepsy can be controlled with drugs that inhibit the electrical discharges, since uncontrolled discharges result in epileptic seizures. Violent behavior and periods of intense emotion are common prior to an epileptic attack, although in some cases the sensations that take place before the seizure are interpreted by the individual as ecstasy of the highest order. Kluver-Bucy syndrome refers to a series of symptoms first observed in monkeys following temporal lobe removal: psychic blindness, abnormal oral tendencies, changes in sexuality, tameness (a significant lack of emotion), and hypermetamorphosis (a tendency to examine and react to virtually everything in the environment). Some or all of the symptoms described have been seen in human patients following strokes, brain injury, brain infections such as herpes, dementias, and other traumas, although the presence of all five in a single individual is very rare. Subsequent research has suggested that changes in emotionality and sexuality are probably caused by damage to the amygdala, while psychic blindness is more likely attributable to the removal of the neocortex of the temporal lobe.

Besides the temporal lobe and the amygdala, portions of the limbic system such as the septal area and the hypothalamus are involved in emotional responses. The pleasure centers of the brain are found in the limbic system (which includes the septal area, amygdala, cingulate cortex, and hippocampus), the hypothalamus, and the brain stem. Brain regions can be classified as positive, negative, or neutral with respect to whether animals will work to turn on or turn off electrical stimulation of these particular areas. Virtually all the cerebral neurocortex and cerebellum is neutral, much of the limbic system and hypothalamus is positive, and some regions of the brain stem and hippocampus are negative. In some cases, electrical stimulation of positive sites mimics the effects of a naturally rewarding event so well that animals prefer the electrical stimulation to the actual experience.

Some research has indicated possible differences between the brain hemispheres in the understanding and expression of emotion. Such data come from the examination of neurological patients having brain damage confined to either side of the brain. Those patients with damage to the left hemisphere are more likely to suffer catastrophic reaction, characterized by intense fear, depressions, and a generally negative outlook on life. The ones with damage on the right side show an attitude of indifference or even unusual cheerfulness. One possible interpretation is that the observed emotions are a result of dominance by the healthy hemisphere, suggesting that the right side is responsible for negative emotional states such as fear, anger, and depression and that the left side produces more positive emotional states. Another possible explanation can reverse this conclusion, simply by stating that the damaged hemisphere becomes dominant in these cases. Identifying emotions with one side of the brain or the other, however, ignores some important data. For example, some patients with frontal lobe damage in either hemisphere will display changes in personality and emotional reactions.

The relationship between behavioral and physiological response processes has long provided an important focus for both laboratory and clinical studies of emotion. For example, research concerned with shyness in children is aimed at investigating the role of sympathetic arousal in emotion. It has been shown that children who are inhibited and quiet when placed in an unfamiliar social situation show larger sympathetic responses than more relaxed, spontaneous children.

Emotions are also the focus of research in the detection of deception, especially as it relates to criminal investigations. A polygraph is a device used to measure involuntary body responses such as changes in respiration, heart rate, and blood pressure in relation to various kinds of questions. It can determine whether the individual is trying to be deceptive. The use of a polygraph is based on two main assumptions: first, that physiological responses during emotional arousal are involuntary, and second, that only individuals with guilty knowledge will display emotional arousal to certain questions asked by the tester. There are three types of questions: irrelevant questions, such as "What is your name?"; control questions, which deal with issues similar to those under consideration but not directly relevant; and relevant questions. The questions are asked in an unpredictable order, sometimes more than once. It is assumed that the person is being deceptive if the polygraph shows more arousal to relevant questions than to control ones. In a controlled laboratory setting, the polygraph is 80 to 90 percent effective in identifying guilty individuals and 90 to 95 percent effective in identifying innocent individuals. It is a process filled with interpretive problems that have to be solved.

Almost every drug found to be effective in altering affective states in humans has also been found to exert effects upon catecholamines (such as norepinephrine and epinephrine) in the brain. These effects would suggest that catecholamines are involved in the mediation of affective states and in the action of the drugs that affect them. Drugs that are associated with depressive phenomena in humans normally cause the loss of catecholamines, while drugs that elevate the mood (antidepressants) have the opposite effect by blocking the mechanisms that destroy the compounds.

DISORDERS AND DISEASES

Disorders of emotion may involve any of a variety of psychological disorders. The formal diagnostic class of mood disorders is one example. Mood disorders generally fall into one of two categories: those involving primarily depressed mood (such as major depression) and those involving both depressed and elevated mood (such as bipolar disorders).

Major depressive syndrome can often be treated without drugs. In many cases, however, drugs accelerate the recovery process. Three main families of antidepressant drugs are the tricyclics, the monoamine oxidase inhibitors (MAOIs), and the selective serotonin reuptake inhibitors (SSRIs). All these drugs help lift depression by increasing the availability of monoamine neurotransmitters at synapses in critical circuits in the brain. Monoamine neurotransmitters include norepinephrine, epinephrine, dopamine, and serotonin. Tricyclic compounds increase the time that the neurotransmitter is available in the synapse, and thus the duration of neurotransmitter action. MAOIs inhibit the action of the enzyme that normally degrades monoamines. SSRIs inhibit serotonin, thus making more of it available to brain cells.

Antidepressants, like any other drugs, can have bothersome side effects that may include constipation, urinary retention, blurred vision, and weight gain. More severe side effects include abnormalities in heart function and blood pressure. SSRIs have fewer and more easily tolerated side effects. As is evident from the list of symptoms, these drugs affect many systems in the body, raising again the question of where emotions reside and underscoring how profound their influence is on the body.

Bipolar mood disorder is much less common than major depressive syndrome. The main method of treatment is to administer lithium salts, although their mechanism of action is not known.

Anxiety disorders are another common emotional

disorder. Included in this group is panic disorder. A panic attack includes shortness of breath, dizziness, acceleration of heart rate, and sweating. It can take place by anticipation of something or for no reason at all. Although attacks last only a few minutes, they are very disturbing. These symptoms involve activation of the sympathetic division of the nervous system.

Other anxiety disorders include conditions like phobias (chronic fears of certain situations), post-traumatic stress disorder, and obsessive-compulsive disorder. The benzodiazepines are drugs that are effective in the treatment of panic disorder. They include alprazolam (Xanax), chlordiazepoxide (Librium), and diazepam (Valium). These drugs enhance the inhibitory effect of GABA, a major inhibitory neurotransmitter, at synapses throughout the brain. Obsessive-compulsive disorder is characterized by stereotyped rituals or compulsions that develop in an attempt to deal with the anxiety produced by obsessions (such as the fear of germs). It has been successfully treated with some of the tricyclic drugs and also with SSRIs.

Perspective and Prospects

The word "passion" was frequently used by early philosophers to connote roughly what is now referred to as emotion: the phenomena of anger, fear, love, jealousy, and so on. In the fourth century B.C.E., Aristotle made a distinction between experiences that involve concurrent activity of both soul and body (such as appetites and passions) and those that involve activity of the soul alone (thinking). In the thirteenth century, Saint Thomas Aquinas was more explicit in affirming this belief in such a distinction, placing his argument within the context of Christian theology. In the seventeenth century, René Descartes directed his attention specifically to the passions. He reiterated that every passion experienced by the soul has its physical counterpart, and he emphasized the role of environmental stimulation in the generation of a passion and proposed a mechanism by which the environment created the passions. Descartes also established conceptual distinctions among passion (of the soul), bodily commotion (activity of the visceral organs), and action (motion of the somatic musculature) and indicated close correspondence among the three.

About two centuries passed without significant development in theoretical ideas about emotion. Interest was renewed, however, as a result of the publication of Charles Darwin's *The Expression of Emotions in Man and Animals* (1872), in which he drew attention to emotional behavior as the biologically significant aspect of emotion and pointed out the causal role of stimulus events or situations in producing behavior.

The American philosopher and psychologist William James proposed the first explicit psychological theory of emotion in 1884. He claimed that emotions are the result, not the cause, of bodily arousal. According to James, bodily arousal is produced by the actions of the sympathetic system. These reactions he believed to be reflexive responses to emotion-provoking situations. The emotion would then be produced by feedback from nerves bringing input from various internal organs (the heart and stomach) and blood vessels affected by the sympathetic system. This theory triggered the serious experimental study of emotion. Danish physiologist Carl Lange independently published a similar theory in 1885, and as a result, the theory is known as the James-Lange theory of emotion. Although it was frequently criticized, this theory dominated the field of emotion research for more than fifty years.

In 1915, Walter Cannon provided convincing experimental evidence of endocrine and autonomic participation in emotional response patterns. In 1927, he conducted a dramatic experiment by removing the sympathetic nervous system of a few cats. All the nerve connections between sympathetic neurons and internal organs and blood vessels were eliminated. According to the James-Lange theory, the cats should feel no emotions. They still displayed clear-cut emotional behaviors, however, and Cannon proposed that external stimuli caused emotion by simultaneously activating neural circuits in the neocortex and triggering responses in the sympathetic nervous system. Most modern theories are more closely aligned with Cannon's work than with the James-Lange hypothesis.

In 1962, Stanley Schachter and Jerome Singer followed up on Gregorio Maranon's 1924 experiment on the role of bodily responses in emotion. They proposed that people need to attribute their feelings to some emotional state and that the complete emotional experience is a joint product of cognition and feedback from sympathetic arousal. The role of sympathetic activity in emotion is still an active topic of research.

Various experiments have sought to discover the functions of certain regions of the brain, as they relate to emotional responses. In 1939, psychologist Heinrich Kluver and neurosurgeon Paul Bucy were interested in identifying the regions of the brain where drugs produce hallucinations. They speculated that the temporal lobe might be involved since brief hallucinations precede temporal lobe epileptic attacks. Both temporal lobes of monkeys were removed, and a constellation of dramatic behavioral changes was observed, proving their theory. In 1954, James Olds and Peter Milner published a report that rats would press a lever for the sole reward of passing electrical current into certain regions of their brains. This phenomenon is known as self-stimulation, and it led to the discovery of the pleasure centers of the brain. Fearlike responses have been elicited from electrical stimulation of three regions of a cat's brain: the tectum, the thalamus, and portions of the hippocampus. Such sites are called negatively reinforcing regions.

As additional information is accumulated, the complexity of the human brain becomes increasingly evident. Emotion is no exception. The biochemical aspects of emotional states have been studied extensively, and considerable information has been acquired, largely in terms of the biochemical changes that accompany and feed back into the central emotional state. Yet there are still many areas to be explored, including complete elucidation of the mechanism of action of some drugs and thus better treatment options for certain disorders.

—Maria Pacheco, Ph.D.;
updated by Nancy A. Piotrowski, Ph.D.

See also Addiction; Aging; Alcoholism; Antianxiety drugs; Antidepressants; Anxiety; Asperger's syndrome; Autism; Bipolar disorders; Bonding; Brain; Brain disorders; Death and dying; Depression; Developmental stages; Endocrinology; Endocrinology, pediatric; Epilepsy; Grief and guilt; Hormones; Hyperhidrosis; Hypochondriasis; Light therapy; Midlife crisis; Nervous system; Nightmares; Obsessive-compulsive disorder; Panic attacks; Paranoia; Phobias; Postpartum depression; Post-traumatic stress disorder; Psychiatric disorders; Psychiatry; Psychiatry, child and adolescent; Psychiatry, geriatric; Psychoanalysis; Psychosis; Psychosomatic disorders; Puberty and adolescence; Schizophrenia; Seasonal affective disorder; Separation anxiety; Sexual dysfunction; Shock therapy; Sibling rivalry; Stress; Thumb sucking; Toilet training.

FOR FURTHER INFORMATION:

Anders, S., et al., eds. *Understanding Emotions.* Boston: Elsevier Science, 2006. Provides overviews of different aspects of emotional perception and the underlying brain mechanisms. For researchers and advanced students.

Borod, Joan C. *The Neuropsychology of Emotion.* New York: Oxford University Press, 2000. Provides a discussion of the neural basis of emotional process, covering techniques, theory, emotional disorders, and treatments.

Breedlove, S. Marc, Mark R. Rosenzweig, and Neil V. Watson. *Biological Psychology: An Introduction to Behavioral, Cognitive, and Clinical Neuroscience.* 5th rev. ed. Sunderland, Mass.: Sinauer, 2007. This new edition examines each major topic in psychobiology from the perspectives of the description, evolution, and development of behavior as well as biological mechanisms underlying it.

Cooper, J. R., F. E. Bloom, and R. H. Roth. *The Biochemical Basis of Neuropharmacology.* 8th ed. New York: Oxford University Press, 2003. A fine treatise on the drugs that affect the nervous system, such as psychotropic drugs that affect mood and behavior, sedatives, and other drugs that affect the autonomic nervous system.

Heilman, K. M., and Paul Satz, eds. *Neuropsychology of Human Emotion.* New York: Guilford Press, 1983. This book contains chapters by different authors on right-hemisphere involvement in emotion, the emotional changes associated with epilepsy, and other neurological and psychiatric diseases.

Henry, Helen L., and Anthony W. Norman, eds. *Encyclopedia of Hormones.* 3 vols. San Diego, Calif.: Academic Press, 2003. A comprehensive overview of the role of hormones, the major physiological systems in which they operate, and the biological consequences of an excess or deficiency of a particular hormone.

EMPHYSEMA

DISEASE/DISORDER

ANATOMY OR SYSTEM AFFECTED: Chest, lungs, respiratory system

SPECIALTIES AND RELATED FIELDS: Internal medicine, pulmonary medicine

DEFINITION: A disease of the lung characterized by enlargement of the small bronchioles or lung alveoli, the destruction of alveoli, decreased elastic recoil of these structures, and the trapping of air in the lungs, resulting in shortness of breath, reduced oxygen to the body, and a variety of serious and eventually fatal complications.

KEY TERMS:

alveoli: tiny, delicate, balloonlike air sacs composed of blood vessels that are supported by connecting tissue and enclosed in a very thin membrane; these sacs are found at the ends of the bronchioles

bronchioles: small branches of the bronchi, which are extensions of the trachea (the central duct that conducts air from the environment to the pulmonary system)

bullous emphysema: localized areas of emphysema within the lung substance

centrilobular (centriacinar) emphysema: a type of emphysema that destroys single alveoli, entering directly into the walls of terminal and respiratory bronchioles

diffusion: the passage of oxygen into the bloodstream from the alveoli and the return or exchange of carbon dioxide across the membrane between the blood vessels and the alveoli

panlobular (panacinar) emphysema: a type of emphysema that involves weakening and enlargement of the air sacs, which are clustered at the end of respiratory bronchioles

perfusion: the flow of blood through the lungs or other vessels in the body

ventilation: the transport of air from the mouth through the bronchial tree to the air sacs and back through the nose or mouth to the outside; ventilation includes both inspiration (breathing in) and expiration (breathing out)

INFORMATION ON EMPHYSEMA
CAUSES: Long-term exposure to dry air, smoke, or other environmental toxins; infection; allergies
SYMPTOMS: Shortness of breath, labored breathing, discolored skin, wheezing, difficulty coughing and talking
DURATION: Chronic
TREATMENTS: Eliminating causes of irritation, cleaning out airways via nebulizers and intermittent positive pressure breathing machine, medications (theophylline, antibiotics, steroids)

CAUSES AND SYMPTOMS

Emphysema is a lung disease in which damage to these organs causes shortness of breath and can lead to heart or respiratory failure. A discussion of the structure and function of the normal lung can illuminate the nature and effects of this damage.

Gases, smoke, germs, allergens, and environmental pollutants pass from the nose and mouth into a large duct called the trachea. The trachea branches into smaller ducts, the bronchi and bronchioles (small branches of the bronchi), which lead to tiny air sacs called alveoli. The respiratory system is like a tree: The trachea is the trunk, the bronchi and bronchioles are similar to the branches, and the alveoli are similar to the leaves. The blood vessels of the alveoli carry red blood cells, which pick up oxygen and transport it to the rest of the body. The cellular waste product, carbon dioxide, is released to the alveoli from the bloodstream and then exhaled. The alveoli are supported by a framework of delicate elastic fibers and give the lung a very distensible quality and the ability to "snap back," or recoil.

The lungs and bronchial tubes are surrounded by the chest wall, composed of bone and muscle and functioning like a bellows. The lung is elastic and passively increases in size to fill the chest space during inspiration and decreases in size during expiration. As the lung (including the alveoli) enlarges, air from the environment flows in to fill this space. During exhalation, the muscles relax, the elasticity of the lung returns it to a normal size, and the air is pushed out. Air must pass through the bronchial tree to the alveoli before oxygen can get into the bloodstream and carbon dioxide can get out, because it is the alveoli that are in contact with blood vessels. The bronchial tree has two kinds of special lining cells. The first type can secrete mucus as a sticky protection against injury and irritation. The second type of cell is covered with fine, hairlike structures called cilia. These cells are supported by smooth muscle cells and elastic and collagen fibers. The cilia wave in the direction of the mouth and act as a defense system by physically removing germs and irritating substances. The cilia are covered with mucus, which helps to trap irritants and germs.

When alveoli are exposed to irritants such as cigarette smoke, they produce a defensive cell called an alveolar macrophage. These cells engulf irritants and bacteria and call for white blood cells, which aid in the defense against foreign bodies, to come into the lungs. The lung tissue also becomes a target for the enzymes or chemical substances produced by the alveolar macrophages and leukocytes (white blood cells). In a healthy body, natural defense systems inhibit the enzymes released by the alveolar macrophages and leukocytes, but it seems that this inhibiting function is impaired in smokers. In some cases, an individual may inherit a deficiency in an enzyme inhibitor. The enzymes vigorously attack the elastin and collagen of the lungs, the lung loses its elastic recoil, and air is trapped.

Emphysema, and a related disease, bronchitis, often work in concert. They are often lumped under the term "chronic obstructive pulmonary disease." Chronic bronchitis weakens and narrows the bronchi. Often, bronchial walls collapse, choking off the vital flow of air. Air is also trapped within the bronchial walls. Weakened by enzymes, the walls of the alveoli rupture and blood vessels die. Lung tissue is replaced with scar tissue, leaving areas of destroyed alveoli that appear as "holes" on an X ray. Small areas of destroyed alveoli are called blebs, and larger ones are called bullae.

As emphysema progresses, a patient has a set of large, overexpanded lungs with a weakened and partially plugged bronchial tree subject to airway collapse and air trapping with blebs and bullae. Breathing, especially exhalation, becomes a slow and difficult process. The patient often develops a "barrel chest" and is known, in medical circles, as a "blue bloater." The scientific world calls the mismatching of breathing to blood distribution a ventilation-to-perfusion imbalance; that is, when air arrives in the alveolus, there are no blood vessels there to transport the vital gaseous cargo to the cells (as a result of enzymatic damage). A person with chronic obstructive pulmonary disease has a bronchial tree with a narrow, defective trunk and sparse leaves.

The loss of elasticity of the lung and alveoli is a critical problem in the emphysemic patient. About one-half of the lungs' elastic recoil force comes from surface tension. The other half comes from the elastic nature of certain fibers throughout the lungs' structure. Emphysema weakens both of these forces because it destroys the elastic fibers and interferes with the surface tension. Fluid, a saline solution, bathes all the body's cells and surfaces. In the lung, this fluid contains surfactant, a substance that interferes with water's tendency to form a spherical drop with a pull into its center (and ultimate collapse). The tissue that gives shape to the lungs is composed of specialized fibers which contain a protein called elastin. These elastic fibers are also found in the alveolar walls and in the elastic connective tissue of the airways and air sacs. The amount of elastin in lung tissue determines its behavior. Healthy lungs maintain a proper balance between destruction of elastin and renewal. (Other parts of the body, such as bones, do this as well.) If too little elastin is destroyed, the lungs have difficulty expanding. If too much is destroyed, the lungs overexpand and cannot recoil properly.

The process of elastin destruction and renewal involves complex regulation. Specialized lung cells pro-

duce new elastin protein. Others produce elastase, an enzyme that destroys elastin. The liver plays a role in the production of a special enzyme known as alpha-1-antitrypsin, which controls the amount of elastase so that too much elastin is not digested. In emphysema, these regulatory systems fail: Too much elastin is destroyed because elastase is no longer controlled, apparently because alpha-1-antitrypsin production has been reduced to a trickle.

The loss of elastin (and thus elastic recoil) means

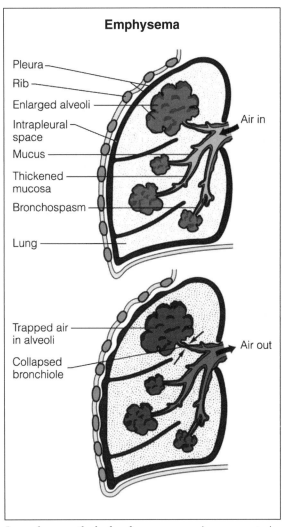

In emphysema, the body releases enzymes in response to inhaling irritants in the air, such as cigarette smoke; these enzymes reduce the lungs' elasticity, compromising the bronchioles' ability to expand and contract normally. Air becomes trapped in the alveoli upon inhalation (top) and cannot escape upon exhalation (bottom). Over time, breathing becomes extremely difficult.

that the lungs expand beyond the normal range during inspiration and cannot resume their resting size during expiration. Thus, alveoli overinflate and rupture. This further reduces elasticity because the loss of each alveolus further impairs the surface tension contribution to the lungs' ability to recoil. Thus, a state of hyperinflation is assumed in the emphysemic patient. This leads to stretched and narrowed alveolar capillaries, loss of elastic tissue, and dissolution of alveolar walls. The lungs increase in size, the thoracic (chest) cage assumes the inspiratory position, and the diaphragm becomes low and flat instead of convex. The patient becomes short of breath with any type of exertion. As the disease worsens, the patient's skin takes on a cyanotic color, as a result of poor oxygenation and perfusion. Wheezing is often present, and coughing is difficult and tiring. In the worst cases, even talking is enough exertion to produce a spasmodic cough. The hyperinflated chest causes inspiration to become a major effort, and the entire chest cage lifts up, resulting in considerable strain. The head moves with each inspiration while the chest remains relatively fixed.

Emphysema may be diagnosed by the early symptom of dyspnea (shortness of breath) on exertion. In advanced cases, the distended chest, depressed diaphragm, increased blood carbon dioxide content, and severe dyspnea clearly point to the disease.

TREATMENT AND THERAPY

The initial step in treating emphysema is to open the airways by eliminating the causes of irritation: smoke, dry air, infection, and allergies. The second treatment is to clean out the airways. There are several techniques and medicines for loosening airway mucus and expelling it. In most chronic obstructive lung diseases, including emphysema, the mucus becomes thick and purulent; coughing up mucus of this type is difficult. In addition, in emphysema the natural cleansing action of the cilia and lung elasticity are impaired. Thus, treatment is aimed at the patient consciously taking over the function of cleaning out the lungs. Coughing is nature's way of bringing up mucus (phlegm), and the emphysemic patient is urged to cough. Since the mucus is thick, one needs to do whatever is necessary to thin it out and to lubricate the airways so that the mucus slips up easily with coughing. The cough must come from deep within the chest in order to be "productive" (to raise mucus).

Moisture is helpful in loosening up thick mucus; hence, drinking large amounts of fluid is encouraged.

Adding a humidifier or a vaporizer to a home is often helpful to the emphysemic patient. There are also machines known as nebulizers and intermittent positive pressure breathing (IPPB) machines that can help to add moisture to the airway of the patient with emphysema. Nebulizers are more effective in getting moisture beyond the throat and major airways than cold vaporizers. Nebulizers, which get their name from the Latin word for cloud or mist, create a mist that is a profusion of tiny droplets that keep themselves apart, even as they bump into one another. Nebulizers release only the smallest droplets—those which can penetrate far down into air passages, where thick mucus is likely to be. (Atomizers produce small droplets as well, but they also spray large droplets.) IPPBs have a special kind of valve that opens when one begins to breathe and allows the air to move into the lungs under mild pressure. As soon as the patient has come to the end of the inhalation, the valve closes and allows the patient to exhale freely.

When phlegm cannot be brought up by breathing mist, a technique called postural drainage is often combined with chest wall percussion or vibration. The idea is to move one's body to a position such that airways are perpendicular to the floor, or at least tilted down, so that gravity can help pull the mucus toward the larger airways, from which the phlegm can be coughed up. Percussion, or clapping the chest, is another way to loosen the mucus in the airways so that it can be coughed up.

A number of medications are useful in the treatment of emphysema. The bronchodilator drugs are xanthines, such as theophylline (Theo-Dur), that relieve bronchospasms, reduce wheezing and dyspnea, and improve respiratory muscle function. Theophylline is a drug that is similar chemically to caffeine. Whereas caffeine stimulates the skeletal muscles and the central nervous system, however, theophylline is potent as a cardiac stimulant and a smooth muscle relaxer. It has also been learned that theophylline stimulates mucociliary clearance of the airways, strengthens the diaphragm, and suppresses edema. Theophylline holds two benefits for the chronic obstructive pulmonary diseased patient: It helps get rid of mucus, and it strengthens the diaphragm, the main respiratory muscle. Common side effects are nausea, stomach pain, vomiting, insomnia, rapid heartbeat, loss of appetite, and restlessness. Another category of bronchodilator are the beta adrenergic stimulants such as metaproterenol (Alupent). Their side effects include nervousness, headache, nausea, and muscle cramps.

The antibiotics sometimes prescribed for emphysemic patients are used to combat bacterial infection. Common antibiotics include tetracycline, penicillin, cephalosporin, erythromycin, and sulfa drugs. Their side effects include a burning sensation in the stomach, vomiting, diarrhea, increased sensitivity to sunlight, rashes, itching, hives, fever, and weakness.

The steroid hormones, such as prednisone, decrease swelling, inflammation, and bronchospasms; they also relieve wheezing. Side effects include blurred vision, frequent urination, thirst, black stools, bone pain, mood changes, weight gain, swelling of the feet, muscle weakness, hoarseness, and a sore mouth.

Other drugs given for emphysema include digitalis, cardiac glycosides, diuretics, mast cell inhibitors, expectorants, and parasympatholytics. Digitalis and cardiac glycosides, such as digoxin, improve the strength of heart contractions and treat disturbances in heart rhythm. Side effects are loss of appetite, abdominal pain, nausea, slow uneven pulse, blurred vision, diarrhea, mood changes, and weakness. Diuretics, such as furosemide (Lasix), are often given to prevent excessive fluid retention. Such drugs cause loss of hearing, skin rashes, hives, bleeding, bruising, jaundice, an irregular or fast heartbeat, muscle cramps, light-headedness, dizziness, and weakness. Mast cell inhibitors are a unique category of drugs that inhibit the release of body chemicals that cause wheezing and bronchospasm; however, they also cause weakness, nosebleeds, and nasal congestion. Expectorants, such as Robitussin, are used to thin secretions and have no known side effects. The parasympatholytics are a type of bronchodilator drug that inhibits the nerves that cause bronchospasm. They are apparently free from the many side effects associated with other bronchodilator drugs.

The emphysemic patient should avoid both excessive heat and excessive cold. If body temperature rises above normal, the heart works faster, as do the lungs. Excessive cold stresses the body to maintain its normal temperature. Smog, air pollution, dusts, powders, and hairspray should be avoided. Finally, a healthy diet consisting of foods high in calcium, vitamins, complex carbohydrates, proteins, and fiber is advised for the patient with lung disease.

A healthy core diet is high in complex carbohydrates; is low in sugars, fats, and cholesterol; and has adequate protein for moderate stress. It should be high in fiber and contain approximately 1,000 milligrams of calcium, 15,000 milligrams of vitamin A, and 250 milligrams of vitamin C. Snack foods can include skim milk, fruit, popcorn, and fresh salads. The respiratory distress of the emphysemic patient uses vast amounts of energy, and the patient should eat several small meals a day so as not to distend the stomach and limit movement of the diaphragm. Liquids are important in keeping airways clear. Good nutrition is helpful in maintaining strength and improving the quality of life for the patient with lung disease.

PERSPECTIVE AND PROSPECTS

Chronic bronchitis and emphysema are responsible for at least fifty thousand deaths a year in the United States alone. An increase in air pollution and cigarette consumption are apparent causes for this rise. In males over forty, chronic obstructive pulmonary disease (COPD) is second to heart disease as a cause of disability. With more females and young people smoking, the incidence of lung disease is likely to increase. Aside from death, a disease such as emphysema can cause long years of disability, joblessness, loss of income, depression, hospitalization, and an inability to perform normal activities.

Smoking is, by far, the single most important risk factor for emphysema. In the United States especially, social acceptance of women smokers began after World War II and has increased the number of women being diagnosed with COPD. Socioeconomic status also influences smoking habits. In many countries in Europe, the mortality rate from lung disease for the lowest socioeconomic class has been six times higher than for the highest. In the United States, the COPD mortality rate among unskilled and semiskilled laborers is twice as high as among professionals. Families with lower incomes usually live in small, often overcrowded apartments; such overcrowding makes respiratory infections more frequent. Often, family members of the COPD patient also smoke, increasing the surrounding air pollution.

In the United States, COPD causes 3 percent of all deaths. In some cases, it causes another 100,000 Americans to be too weak to survive other, unrelated medical conditions. Therefore, an annual figure of 150,000 deaths from COPD-related diseases is more realistic. The expanding COPD population is a growing market for pharmaceutical firms. For example, greater amounts of bronchodilator medications will be needed; hence, pharmaceutical firms are eager to find longer-acting and more effective drugs for these patients to buy.

A number of economic pressures are likely to move COPD treatment from the hospital to the home. When effectively carried out by a well-trained health team, home care can lower medical costs. The COPD patient who finds a knowledgeable doctor and who begins a comprehensive rehabilitation program is the one who can look forward to a life that is more productive and more comfortable.

—*Jane A. Slezak, Ph.D.*

See also Asbestos exposure; Aspergillosis; Bronchi; Chronic obstructive pulmonary disease (COPD); Coughing; Cyanosis; Environmental diseases; Lungs; Oxygen therapy; Pulmonary diseases; Pulmonary medicine; Respiration; Smoking; Wheezing.

FOR FURTHER INFORMATION:

American Lung Association. http://www.lungusa.org. Includes in-depth information and recent research findings, a guide to local events and programs, and a section to share personal stories, among other features.

Bates, David V. *Respiratory Function in Disease.* 3d ed. Philadelphia: W. B. Saunders, 1989. Summarizes the effects of disease on pulmonary function. Also discussed are some of the more sophisticated pulmonary function tests. Exercise testing, obesity, and the effects of drugs are other topics reviewed in this work.

Decker, Caroline D. "Room to Breathe." *Saturday Evening Post* 266, no. 6 (November/December, 1994): 48-49. This article on emphysema discusses lung surgery. Illustrated with photographs.

Haas, François, and Sheila Sperber Haas. *The Chronic Bronchitis and Emphysema Handbook.* Rev. ed. New York: John Wiley & Sons, 2000. Helps patients with COPD learn to lead full and productive lives. Provides information pertinent to their disease and describes the treatments and medications available to them in order to improve their quality of life.

Hedrick, Hannah L., and Austin K. Kutscher, eds. *The Quiet Killer: Emphysema, Chronic Obstructive Pulmonary Disease.* Lanham, Md.: Scarecrow Press, 2002. Clinicians, researchers, and health educators combine their expertise in twenty-five chapters that discuss such topics as managing dyspnea, traveling with mechanical ventilation, encouraging patients to quit smoking, self-help groups, and hospice care.

Matthews, Dawn D. *Lung Disorders Sourcebook.* Detroit, Mich.: Omnigraphics, 2002. A comprehensive overview of lung anatomy, physiology, and dysfunc-

tions taken from government agencies, the American Academy of Family Physicians, the American Lung Association, and the Mayo Foundation. Discusses thirty-five lung disorders in depth.

National Emphysema Foundation. http://www.emphysemafoundation.org. Site offers tips on exercises, inhaler uses, and other helpful items for those with emphysema.

West, John B. *Pulmonary Pathophysiology: The Essentials.* 7th ed. Philadelphia: Wolters Kluwer/Lippincott Williams & Wilkins, 2008. Examines lungs afflicted with obstructive, restrictive, vascular, and environmental diseases.

Wolff, Ronald K. "Effects of Airborne Pollutants on Mucociliary Clearance." *Environmental Health Perspectives* 66 (April, 1986): 223-237. The role of mucociliary clearance as a lung defense mechanism is described in this article. The abnormal elimination of bronchial mucus is considered a possible factor in the pathogenesis of COPD. The role of certain pollutants, which pose a challenge to the mucociliary system, is detailed.

ENCEPHALITIS

DISEASE/DISORDER

ANATOMY OR SYSTEM AFFECTED: Brain, circulatory system, neck, nerves, nervous system, psychic-emotional system

SPECIALTIES AND RELATED FIELDS: Bacteriology, epidemiology, internal medicine, neurology, public health, virology

DEFINITION: A disease that involves inflammation of the brain.

KEY TERMS:

arbovirus: a virus transmitted by the bite of an arthropod, particularly a mosquito or a tick

central nervous system (CNS): in vertebrates, consisting of the brain and spinal cord

enterovirus: a virus that tends to multiply in the intestinal tract

CAUSES AND SYMPTOMS

In the United States, about twenty thousand cases of encephalitis are reported each year. The disease is sometimes classified according to the causative agent or the anatomic structures affected. Limbic encephalitis, for example, affects structures in the brain known as the limbic system. Exposure to lead often produces cerebral inflammation and edema (swelling) and is referred to as lead encephalitis. If the agent is bacterial, then the disease is referred to as bacterial encephalitis. In amebic encephalitis, patients with weakened immune systems become infected through certain protozoa (*Acanthamoeba*) found in water and moist soil.

The principal cause of encephalitis, however, is viral. In primary encephalitis, the virus directly invades the brain and spinal cord. Secondary encephalitis occurs as an aftereffect of such airborne diseases as measles and influenza (postinfectious) or of certain vaccinations (postvaccinal).

Though many viruses can produce encephalitis, only a limited number tend to recur. They fall into three major groups: enteroviruses; arboviruses, which include the four main agents common in the United States; and nonarthropod viruses. Nonarthropod viruses, transmitted without an insect vector, include the very common herpes simplex virus 1 (HSV-1).

Enteroviruses infect the gastrointestinal tract and are spread by a fecal-oral route. Hands come into contact with feces or bodily fluids in which the virus is present. If unwashed, the hands can transfer the virus to the mouth. Once ingested, the virus replicates in the intestines and then moves to the nervous system.

Arboviruses, which are responsible for epidemics, are spread by mosquitoes (such as in eastern equine encephalitis) and ticks (as in Powassan encephalitis, which occurs in the northeastern United States). For natural reasons related to their vectors (carriers), these infections, at least in northerly climes, peak in late summer. In 2002, West Nile virus caused the largest epidemic ever recorded, with nearly 4,200 cases and 300 deaths.

If a mosquito ingests a blood meal from an infected vertebrate, over a period of one to three weeks, the virus replicates in the mosquito's gut and then moves to its salivary glands. When the mosquito bites a human, the virus lurks in the person's visceral organs and then passes by means of the blood to the nervous system. A possible route to the central nervous system (CNS) is through the brain capillaries. Infection of neurons, and glial cells, which constitute the non-nervous tissue of the brain and spinal cord, follows, leading to cell dysfunction and death. The body's own immune response, which includes infusing white blood cells into the cerebrospinal fluid, contributes to the brain edema and inflammation.

In diagnosis, physicians use blood and deoxyribonucleic acid (DNA) tests and analyze the cerebrospinal fluid for a too-high count of white blood cells and elevated protein levels and fluid pressure. Neuroimaging

---

INFORMATION ON ENCEPHALITIS

CAUSES: Viral infection, complications from another disease
SYMPTOMS: Headache, fever, stiff neck, loss of consciousness, seizures, sleep disturbances, blurred or double vision, vomiting, body aches
DURATION: Acute or chronic
TREATMENTS: Alleviation of symptoms

---

and electroencephalograms (EEGs), which record electrical activity in the brain, are used to eliminate other possibilities, such as clotting because of the rupture of a blood vessel (hematoma). Isolation of the virus itself, with some exceptions, is difficult. Biopsy of brain tissue for evidence of the virus has largely been replaced by less invasive procedures.

Symptoms may occur within a few hours or over the course of several days and initially are nonspecific, which complicates the diagnosis. Although they vary depending on the virus and the extent and length of infection, symptoms generally include fever, headache, muscle ache, stiff neck, respiratory symptoms, sensitivity to light, abdominal pain, vomiting, dizziness, an altered level of consciousness that may range from lethargy to coma, personality changes which may progress to behavior that appears psychotic, intellectual deficit, and a host of neurological deficiencies, such as tremors, loss of muscular coordination, partial paralysis, and ocular (eye) fixation.

TREATMENT AND THERAPY

For some types of encephalitis, such as Japanese encephalitis, effective vaccines exist. In bacterial cases, antibiotics are prescribed. In patients in whom the herpes simplex virus is implicated, the antiviral acyclovirin is useful. In general, however, treatment, often initially in an intensive care unit (ICU), is supportive and designed to control complications. For example, steroids are sometimes administered to reduce brain swelling and anticonvulsants, if seizures occur.

The disease runs its course in one to two weeks. Mortality rates depend on the type of virus and the age of the patient, the very young and elderly being more vulnerable. In eastern equine encephalitis, the mortality rate is about 33 percent; in western equine encephalitis, it is about 3 percent in older patients and as high as 30 percent in younger patients. Residual symptoms after recovery vary, again according to the agent and extent of infection. In eastern equine encephalitis, 80 percent of patients suffer neurologic aftereffects.

PERSPECTIVE AND PROSPECTS

Some historians of medicine believe that viral encephalitis appeared early in the Mediterranean area. The evidence is indirect, with the mention in the *Hippocratic corpus* (fifth century B.C.E. and later) of genital and labial lesions consistent with herpesvirus, a leading cause of the disease. It was not until the nineteenth and twentieth centuries that the numerous agents and vectors for encephalitis were successfully identified, such as the rabies virus (isolated by Louis Pasteur's dog experiments), the spirochete of syphilis, and more recently human immunodeficiency virus (HIV).

A firm connection between the great influenza pandemic of 1918 and the repeated global outbreaks of encephalitis lethargica in the 1920's was not established until 1982. In the 1990's, aspirin therapy in children's influenza was implicated in the sometimes fatal brain edema known as Reye's syndrome.

Research has focused on oral antiviral drug therapy. Interferon alpha-2b therapy and ribovarin, related to the vitamin B complex, have been tested on patients with West Nile virus, but their value has not been conclusively established. Emphasis therefore has remained on prevention: proper vaccinations and, for arboviruses, mosquito spraying campaigns, application of effective insect repellents, and limited outside exposure during the early evening hours.

—*David J. Ladouceur, Ph.D.*

See also Bites and stings; Brain; Brain damage; Brain disorders; Dementias; Hemiplegia; Inflammation; Insect-borne diseases; Lice, mites, and ticks; Nervous system; Neuroimaging; Neurology; Neurology, pediatric; Parasitic diseases; Sleeping sickness; Viral infections; West Nile virus.

FOR FURTHER INFORMATION:

American Medical Association. *American Medical Association Family Medical Guide.* 4th rev. ed. Hoboken, N.J.: John Wiley & Sons, 2004.

Goldman, Lee, and Dennis Ausiello, eds. *Cecil Textbook of Medicine.* 23d ed. Philadelphia: Saunders/ Elsevier, 2007.

Kasper, Dennis L., et al., eds. *Harrison's Principles of Internal Medicine.* 16th ed. New York: McGraw-Hill, 2005.

Professional Guide to Diseases. 9th ed. Philadelphia: Lippincott Williams & Wilkins, 2008.

END-STAGE RENAL DISEASE
DISEASE/DISORDER

ANATOMY OR SYSTEM AFFECTED: Blood, blood vessels, circulatory system, endocrine system, heart, kidneys, urinary system

SPECIALTIES AND RELATED FIELDS: Cardiology, endocrinology, geriatrics and gerontology, internal medicine, nephrology, vascular medicine

DEFINITION: Stage 5 of chronic kidney disease, which causes irreversible damage to and near-complete failure of the kidneys.

KEY TERMS:

creatinine clearance: a test that measures levels of the waste product creatinine in blood and in a twenty-four-hour urine sample

diabetic nephropathy: a kidney disease associated with long-standing diabetes

dialysis: a mechanical means of cleansing the blood; an exchange of water and solute filters waste products out through diffusion

fistula: a surgically created opening that joins an artery and vein

glomerular filtration rate: the amount of glomerular filtrate formed each minute in nephrons of both kidneys; calculated from the rate of creatinine clearance and adjusted for body-surface area

renal osteodystrophy: a bone disease of chronic renal failure

uremia: a syndrome occurring with deteriorating renal function and characterized by combination of metabolic, fluid, electrolyte, and hormone imbalances

CAUSES AND SYMPTOMS

End-stage renal disease (ESRD) is stage 5 of chronic kidney disease, defined as kidney function at less than 10 percent of normal and a glomerular filtration rate of less than 15 milliliters per minute. Both diseases are characterized by the inability to remove wastes and concentrate urine, have poor outcomes, and are usually the result of long-standing diabetes and/or uncontrolled hypertension.

ESRD is a serious, life-threatening systematic disease characterized by renal failure, decreased production of red blood cells and active vitamin D_3, and excess excretion of acid, potassium, salt, and water. Many metabolic abnormalities and imbalances occur, causing complications, such as anemia, acidemia or acidosis, hyperkalemia, hyperphosphatemia, hyperparathyroidism, and hypocalcemia. Symptoms include swollen feet and ankles, fatigue, lethargy or weakness, itching, skin color changes, loss of mental alertness, shortness of breath, and recurrent or chronic heart failure.

Tests that measure the level of creatinine and urea in blood and urine are conducted to determine the extent of kidney damage and the filtration capacity of the kidneys. High levels of these waste products found in the blood but not in the urine, are signs of kidney damage. ESRD may be suspected when very high levels of protein are detected in the urine (proteinuria). The results of a creatinine clearance are used to determine the glomerular filtration rate, the standard measurement used to assess kidney function.

Diabetes mellitus is the most common cause of ESRD in the United States, due to its underlying kidney disease—diabetic nephropathy. Approximately 40 percent of patients with diabetes develop the disease, and nearly half of them progress to ESRD within five to ten years. Diabetic nephropathy develops with changes in the microvasculature (tiny blood vessels) of the glomerulus and is characterized by a progressive and aggressive disease course: Wastes increase, building up in the blood; kidneys leak larger amounts of albumin, causing proteinuria; and nodular glomerulosclerosis lesions proliferate and destroy the glomeruli.

Hypertension (high blood pressure) is a major cause of ESRD, estimated at 30 percent of all cases. Although arteries are elastic, they can become overstretched from hypertension and narrow, weaken, or harden. This is especially deadly in the kidneys, which are highly vascular and carry large volumes of blood. Damaged blood vessels and filters prevent the kidneys from functioning adequately, including reducing the hormone that they normally produce to help the body regulate its own blood pressure. Thus, hypertension is both a cause and a symptom of ESRD.

Uremia is a syndrome that develops with ESRD when metabolic, fluid, electrolyte, and hormone imbalances emerge concurrently. Clinical symptoms include nausea or vomiting, fatigue, weight loss, muscle cramps, pruritus (itching), mental status changes, visual disturbances, and increased thirst.

Renal osteodystrophy is a degenerative bone disease that develops with metabolic imbalances in the minerals phosphorus and calcium. High levels of phosphorus in the blood draw calcium out of the bones, causing them to become brittle and break. The excess of phosphorus and calcium salts in the blood deposit and harden, forming metastatic calcifications in the skin, blood vessels, and other soft tissues.

TREATMENT AND THERAPY

Dialysis and kidney transplantation are the only treatments for ESRD and provide a means of prolonging a patient's life span and maintaining quality of life.

Dialysis is a means of cleansing the blood when the kidneys do not function and is done by the process of diffusion, in which blood is passed through a filter in contact with a dialysate (salt solution), separating the smaller molecules (solute particles) from the larger molecules (colloid particles). There are two types of dialysis—hemodialysis and peritoneal dialysis—each of which has several variants.

In hemodialysis, blood is filtered by diverting it outside the body through a fistula and flows across a semipermeable membrane in the dialysis unit in a direction countercurrent to the dialysate. Hemodialysis takes three to four hours to complete and must be done three to five times a week, usually in a dialysis clinic. In peritoneal dialysis, blood is filtered internally through the peritoneum, a thin membrane inside the abdomen and peritoneal dialysis fluid is infused into the cavity via a catheter. Exchanges are repeated four to six times a day by the patient, and the process must be done every day.

Kidney transplants are another option for most ESRD patients. The United Network for Organ Sharing recommends that patients be put on the cadaveric renal transplant list when their glomerular filtration rate is less than 18 milliliters per minute. Improvements in their policies provide for a more equitable allocation system, broaden the classification of expanded donor criteria, and are expected to increase the donor pool. Unfortunately, thousands of patients die each year waiting for an available kidney.

PERSPECTIVE AND PROSPECTS

Chronic kidney disease and ESRD represent a growing public health problem in the United States and reflect the disturbing health profile of present-day society—

INFORMATION ON END-STAGE RENAL DISEASE

CAUSES: Diabetes and hypertension
SYMPTOMS: Swollen feet and ankles, fatigue/lethargy/weakness, itching, pale skin, loss of mental alertness, shortness of breath, recurrent or chronic heart failure
DURATION: Variable, fatal if not treated
TREATMENTS: Dialysis or kidney transplant

rising numbers of people with obesity, diabetes, hypertension, cardiovascular disease, and metabolic syndrome. The prevalence of chronic kidney disease has risen steadily since the 1980's and affects approximately 11 percent of the adult population, 2 percent of which are patients with ESRD. The National Kidney Foundation Disease Outcomes Quality Initiative expects the prevalence of ESRD in 2010 to be nearly 600,000, a projection double that of ten years earlier. Changes in lifestyle and increased awareness of disease risk are key to preventing chronic kidney disease and reducing the number of patients who progress to ESRD.

—*Barbara Woldin*

See also Diabetes mellitus; Dialysis; Hypertension; Kidney disorders; Kidney transplantation; Kidneys; Nephrology; Polycystic kidney disease; Proteinuria; Pyelonephritis; Renal failure; Transplantation; Uremia.

FOR FURTHER INFORMATION:

Offer, Daniel, Marjorie Kaiz Offer, and Susan Offer Szafir. *Dialysis Without Fear: A Guide to Living Well on Dialysis for Patients and Their Families.* New York: Oxford University Press, 2007.

Townsend, Raymond R., and Debbie Cohen. *One Hundred Q&A About Kidney Disease and Hypertension.* Sudbury, Mass.: Jones & Bartlett, 2008.

Walser, Mackenzie, and Betsy Thorpe. *Coping with Kidney Disease: A Twelve-Step Treatment Program to Help You Avoid Dialysis.* Hoboken, N.J.: John Wiley & Sons, 2004.

Wein, Alan, et al., eds. *Campbell-Walsh Urology.* 9th ed. Philadelphia: Saunders/Elsevier, 2007.

ENDARTERECTOMY

PROCEDURE

ANATOMY OR SYSTEM AFFECTED: Blood vessels, circulatory system, neck

SPECIALTIES AND RELATED FIELDS: General surgery, vascular medicine

DEFINITION: A surgical procedure used to remove plaque from the lining of the carotid arteries in the neck.

INDICATIONS AND PROCEDURES

The internal carotid artery lies in the side of the neck, slightly in front of and beneath the sternocleidomastoid muscle. A skin incision is made anterior to this muscle. The branches of the carotid artery, adjacent blood vessels, and nerves are freed and inspected. A clamp is applied to the common carotid artery. Two additional

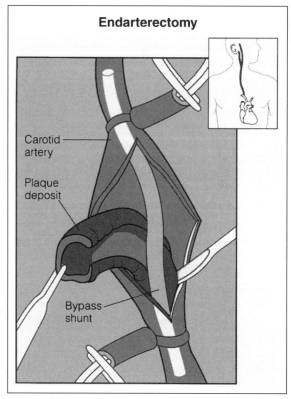

The excision of plaque deposits from the carotid artery in the neck is called endarterectomy; the inset shows the location of the carotid artery.

clamps are applied to the external and internal carotid arteries to prevent bleeding and to prevent emboli from migrating to the brain during the procedure.

A lengthwise incision is made in the internal carotid artery from a point about 3.8 centimeters (1.5 inches) above the beginning of the vessel into the common carotid artery, about 2.5 centimeters (1 inch) below the beginning of the vessel. The edges of the artery are retracted, and the interior is exposed. The plaque can usually be scraped off the walls of the artery. The internal lining of the artery is carefully closed, and any tears are sutured. The carotid artery is then sewed together with fine suture material. If the underlying disease has been extensive or if the lining of the artery is damaged, a portion of the saphenous vein in the patient's leg is used to repair the arterial wall.

Restoring blood flow is crucial; it is important to avoid both leaks in the artery and the formation of emboli. The clamp on the external carotid artery is briefly released, and a small amount of blood is allowed to flow back into the repaired area to check for leaks under low pressure. This clamp is reapplied. The clamp on the common carotid artery is removed to check for leaks under high pressure. The clamp to the external carotid artery is removed next. Blood is allowed to flow, flushing any emboli from the operative site and away from the brain. If all is well, the clamp on the internal carotid artery is removed.

The structures that were pulled away from the carotid artery are released and briefly inspected to ensure that no damage has been done. The edges of the skin are then brought together and closed with sutures. The patient returns in about a week for a checkup and removal of the sutures.

USES AND COMPLICATIONS

Endarterectomy is used to restore adequate blood flow to the brain, thus preventing periods of ischemia that can result in loss of consciousness or strokes. However, complications can include emboli, which can also cause strokes by blocking important blood vessels. Endarterectomy is successful in most patients and restores more normal circulation. It has decreased the incidence of strokes in younger patients.

—*L. Fleming Fallon, Jr., M.D., Ph.D., M.P.H.*

See also Angioplasty; Arteriosclerosis; Blood vessels; Bypass surgery; Carotid arteries; Circulation; Embolism; Strokes; Vascular medicine; Vascular system.

FOR FURTHER INFORMATION:

Ancowitz, Arthur. *Strokes and Their Prevention: How to Avoid High Blood Pressure and Hardening of the Arteries.* New York: Jove, 1980.

Browse, Norman L., A. O. Mansfield, and C. C. R. Bishop. *Carotid Endarterectomy: A Practical Guide.* Boston: Butterworth-Heinemann, 1997.

Loftus, Christopher M. *Carotid Endarterectomy: Principles and Technique.* 2d ed. New York: Informa Healthcare, 2007.

Loftus, Christopher M., and Timothy F. Kresowik. *Carotid Artery Surgery.* New York: Thieme, 2000.

Rutherford, Robert B., ed. *Vascular Surgery.* 6th ed. Philadelphia: Saunders/Elsevier, 2005.

ENDOCARDITIS

DISEASE/DISORDER

ANATOMY OR SYSTEM AFFECTED: Circulatory system, heart

SPECIALTIES AND RELATED FIELDS: Bacteriology, cardiology, internal medicine, vascular medicine

DEFINITION: Inflammatory lesions of the endocardium, the lining of the heart.

INFORMATION ON ENDOCARDITIS

CAUSES: Bacterial infection
SYMPTOMS: Fever, malaise, fatigue, dyspnea, chest pain, heart murmurs
DURATION: Temporary
TREATMENTS: Antibiotics

CAUSES AND SYMPTOMS

The lesions of endocarditis may be noninfective, as in some autoimmune conditions, or infective. The latter are characterized by direct invasion of the endocardium by microorganisms, most often bacteria. Bacterial endocarditis may occur on normal or previously damaged heart valves and also on artificial (prosthetic) heart valves. Rarely, endocarditis may occur on the wall (mural surface) of the heart or at the site of an abnormal hole between the pumping chambers of the heart, called a ventricular septal defect.

In areas of turbulent blood flow, platelet-fibrin deposition can occur, providing a nidus for subsequent bacterial colonization. Transient bacteremia may accompany infection elsewhere in the body or some medical and dental procedures, and these circulating bacteria can adhere to the endocardium, especially at platelet-fibrin deposition sites, and produce endocarditis. Intravenous drug abusers using unsterile equipment and drugs often inject bacteria along with the drugs, which can result in endocarditis. The lesions produced by these depositions plus bacteria are called vegetations. Clinical symptoms and signs usually begin about two weeks later.

Bacterial endocarditis usually involves either the mitral or the aortic heart valve. In intravenous drug abusers, the tricuspid heart valve is more commonly affected because it is the first valve to be reached by the endocardium-damaging drugs and contaminating bacteria. The pulmonic valve is only rarely the site of endocarditis. Occasionally, more than one heart valve is infected; this occurs most often in intravenous drug abusers or patients with multiple prosthetic heart valves.

Gram-positive cocci are the most common cause of bacterial endocarditis. Different species predominate in various conditions or situations: *Streptococcus viridans* in native valves, *Staphylococcus aureus* in the valves of intravenous drug abusers, and *Staphylococcus epidermidis* in prosthetic heart valves. Gram-negative bacilli are found in association with prosthetic heart valves or intravenous drug addiction.

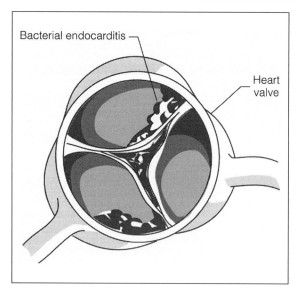

Bacterial endocarditis of a heart valve occurs when bacteria invade and cause inflammatory lesions; untreated, the condition is usually fatal.

The clinical manifestations of endocarditis are varied and often nonspecific. Early symptoms are similar to those encountered in most infections: fever, malaise, and fatigue. As the disease progresses, more cardiovascular and renal-related symptoms may appear: dyspnea, chest pain, and stroke. Fever and heart murmurs are found in most patients. Enlargement of the spleen, skin lesions, and evidence of emboli are commonly present.

The key to the diagnosis of bacterial endocarditis is to suspect the presence of the illness and obtain blood cultures. Febrile patients who have a heart murmur, cardiac failure, a prosthetic heart valve, history of intravenous drug abuse, preexisting valvular disease, stroke (especially in young adults), multiple pulmonary emboli, sudden arterial occlusion, unexplained prolonged fever, or multiple positive blood cultures are likely to have endocarditis. The hallmark of bacterial endocarditis is continuous bacteremia; thus, nearly all blood cultures will be positive. Other nonspecific blood tests, such as an erythrocyte sedimentation rate, or specific blood tests, such as tests for teichoic acid antibodies, may be helpful in establishing a diagnosis.

TREATMENT AND THERAPY

Endocarditis may be prevented by administering prophylactic antibiotics to patients with preexisting heart abnormalities that predispose them to endocarditis when they are likely to have transient bacteremia. An example would be a patient with an artificial heart valve scheduled to have a dental cleaning.

Endocarditis is one of the few infections that is nearly always fatal if mistreated. Antibacterial therapy with agents capable of killing the offending bacteria, along with supportive medical care and cardiac surgery when indicated, cures most patients.

PERSPECTIVE AND PROSPECTS

The first demonstration of bacteria in vegetations associated with endocarditis was by Emmanuel Winge of Oslo, Norway, in 1869. Fifty years later, a fresh section was cut from the preserved heart valve described by Winge, and staining by modern methods revealed a chain of streptococci verifying his discovery. It was not until 1943, when Leo Loewe successfully treated seven cases of bacterial endocarditis with penicillin, that the era of modern therapy of this serious illness began.

Endocarditis accounts for approximately one case in every one thousand hospital admissions in the United States. The incidence remained fairly constant between the 1960's and the 1990's, but the type of patient has changed: Heroin addicts, the elderly, and patients with prosthetic heart valves constitute an increasing percentage of endocarditis cases.

—*H. Bradford Hawley, M.D.*

See also Bacterial infections; Cardiac arrest; Cardiology; Cardiology, pediatric; Circulation; Echocardiography; Heart; Heart disease; Heart valve replacement; Mitral valve prolapse; Rheumatic fever; Vascular medicine; Vascular system.

FOR FURTHER INFORMATION:

American Heart Association. http://www.american heart.org. A group dedicated to reducing disability and death from cardiovascular diseases and stroke. Offers thorough information on a wide range of cardiovascular diseases, referrals to emergency cardiovascular care classes, and research statistics and articles.

Crawford, Michael, ed. *Current Diagnosis and Treatment—Cardiology.* 3d ed. New York: McGraw-Hill Medical, 2009. Discusses advances in cardiac diagnostics, treatments, and prognostic indicators and includes extensive information on prevention techniques.

Durack, David T., and Michael H. Crawford, eds. *Infective Endocarditis.* Philadelphia: W. B. Saunders, 2003. Covers all the features of endocarditis in the modern era.

Eagle, Kim A., and Ragavendra R. Baliga, eds. *Practical Cardiology: Evaluation and Treatment of Common Cardiovascular Disorders*. 2d ed. Philadelphia: Lippincott Williams & Wilkins, 2008. Details advances in cardiac medicine.

Giessel, Barton E., Clint J. Koenig, and Robert L. Blake, Jr. "Information from Your Family Doctor: Bacterial Endocarditis, a Heart at Risk." *American Family Physician* 61, no. 6 (March 15, 2000): 1705. This patient handout sheet contains information about bacterial endocarditis, an infection of the valves and inner lining of the heart. It includes information on prevention, complications, and treatment.

Magilligan, Donald J., Jr., and Edward L. Quinn, eds. *Endocarditis: Medical and Surgical Management*. New York: Marcel Dekker, 1986. Discusses the treatment of endocarditis and its complications.

Muirhead, Greg. "Targeting Therapy for Infective Endocarditis." *Patient Care* 33, no. 16 (October 15, 1999): 127-149. The diagnosis of infective endocarditis remains difficult, as does the treatment of this uncommon but potentially deadly disease. Discussed here are the better diagnostic criteria, developed in recent years, which allow for more effective therapy.

ENDOCRINE DISORDERS

DISEASE/DISORDER

ANATOMY OR SYSTEM AFFECTED: Endocrine system, glands

SPECIALTIES AND RELATED FIELDS: Endocrinology

DEFINITION: The endocrine system controls the metabolic processes of the body. Endocrine disorders occur when the normal function of the endocrine system is disrupted.

KEY TERMS:

cyclic AMP: a chemical that acts as a second messenger to bring about a response by the cell to the presence of some hormones at their receptors

endocrine: the secretion of hormones directly into the bloodstream, rather than by way of a duct

feedback: the mechanism whereby a hormone inhibits its own production; often involves the inhibition of the hypothalamus and tropic hormones

hypothalamohypophysial: relating to the hypothalamus and the hypophysis (pituitary gland)

target cell or organ: a cell or organ possessing the specific hormone receptors needed to respond to a given hormone

tropic: hormones that feed a particular physiological state

tropin: hormones that cause a "turning toward" a particular physiological state

PROCESS AND EFFECTS

Endocrine disorders include disturbances in the production of hormones that result from either insufficient or excessive activity and tissues unable to respond to hormones. To understand endocrine disorders, it is necessary to review briefly the location of the principal endocrine glands, the hormones secreted, and the normal functions of the hormones. The hormones are released into the bloodstream and are carried throughout the body, where they affect target cells or organs that have receptors for the given hormone.

The pituitary gland, or hypophysis, is sometimes called the master gland because of its widespread influences on many other endocrine glands and the body as a whole. It is located in the midline on the lower part of the brain just above the posterior part of the roof of the mouth. The pituitary has three lobes: the posterior lobe, the intermediate lobe, and the anterior lobe.

The posterior lobe does not synthesize hormones, but it does have nerve fibers coming into it from the hypothalamus of the brain. The ends of these axons release two hormones that are synthesized in the hypothalamus, oxytocin and antidiuretic hormone (ADH). Oxytocin causes the contraction of the smooth muscles of the uterus during childbirth and the contraction of tissues in the mammary glands to release milk during nursing. ADH causes the kidneys to reabsorb water and thereby reduce the volume of urine to normal levels when necessary.

The intermediate lobe of the pituitary secretes melanocyte-stimulating hormone (MSH), a hormone with an uncertain role in humans but known to cause the darkening of melanocytes in animals. Sometimes, the intermediate lobe is considered to be a part of the anterior lobe.

The anterior lobe of the pituitary is under the control of releasing hormones produced by the hypothalamus and carried to the anterior lobe by special blood vessels. In response to these releasing hormones, some stimulatory and some inhibitory, the anterior lobe produces thyroid-stimulating hormone (TSH), adrenocorticotropic hormone (ACTH), follicle-stimulating hormone (FSH), luteinizing hormone (LH), prolactin, and somatotropin or growth hormone (GH). TSH stimulates the thyroid to produce thyroxine, ACTH stimu-

---

INFORMATION ON ENDOCRINE DISORDERS

CAUSES: Malfunction of endocrine system
SYMPTOMS: Wide ranging and dependent on region; may include precocious puberty, dwarfism, thyroid problems, diseases such as diabetes
DURATION: Chronic
TREATMENTS: Hormonal therapy, medications

---

lates the adrenal cortex to produce some of its hormones, FSH stimulates the growth of the cells surrounding eggs in the ovary and causes the ovary to produce estrogen, LH induces ovulation (the release of an egg from the ovary) and stimulates the secretion of progesterone by the ovary, prolactin is essential for milk production and various metabolic functions, and GH is needed for normal growth.

The pineal gland, or epiphysis, is a neuroendocrine gland attached to the roof of the diencephalon in the brain. It produces melatonin, which is released into the bloodstream during the night and has important functions related to an individual's biological clock.

The thyroid gland is located below the larynx in the front of the throat. It produces the hormones triiodothyronine (T_3) and thyroxine (T_4), which are essential for maintaining a normal level of metabolism and heat production, as well as enabling normal development of the brain in young children. Specialized cells called C cells are scattered throughout the thyroid, parathyroid, and thymus glands. These cells secrete the hormone calcitonin, which is involved in maintaining the correct blood levels of calcium. The thymus, located under the breast bone or sternum, produces the hormone thymosin that stimulates the immune system. Even the heart is an endocrine gland: It produces atrial natriuretic factor, which stimulates sodium excretion by the kidneys. The pancreas, located near the stomach and small intestine, produces digestive enzymes that pass to the duodenum, but also it produces insulin and glucagon in special cells called pancreatic islets. Insulin causes blood sugar (glucose) to be taken up from the blood into the tissues of the body, and glucagon causes stored glycogen to be broken down in the liver and thereby increases blood glucose levels.

The pair of adrenal glands, located on the kidneys, are made up of two components: first, a cortex that produces glucocorticoids, mineralocorticoids, and sex steroids or androgens; and second, a medulla, or inner part, that secretes adrenaline and noradrenaline. The gonads, testes or ovaries, are located in the pelvic region and produce several hormones, including the estrogen and progesterone that are essential for reproduction in females and the testosterone that is essential for reproduction in males. The kidneys and digestive tract also produce hormones that regulate red blood cell formation and the functioning of the digestive tract, respectively.

COMPLICATIONS AND DISORDERS

A wide variety of endocrine disorders can be treated successfully. In fact, the ability to restore normal endocrine function with replacement therapy has long been one of the techniques for showing the existence of hypothesized hormones.

The posterior pituitary releases both oxytocin and ADH. Chemicals similar to oxytocin are sometimes given to induce contractions in pregnant women so that birth will occur at a predetermined time. The other hormone released from the posterior pituitary, ADH, normally causes the reabsorption of water within the tubules of the kidney. A deficiency of ADH leads to diabetes insipidus, a condition in which many liters of water a day are excreted by the urinary system; the patient must drink huge quantities of water simply to stay alive. A synthetic form of ADH, desmopressin acetate, can be given in the form of a nasal spray that diffuses into the bloodstream and thus restores the reabsorption of water by the kidneys.

The anterior lobe of the pituitary produces six known hormones. The production of these hormones is stimulated and/or inhibited by special releasing hormones secreted by the hypothalamus and carried to the anterior lobe by the hypothalamohypophysial portal system of blood vessels. Thus, the source of some anterior pituitary disorders can reside in the hypothalamus. Tumors of anterior pituitary cells can result in the overproduction of a hormone, or if the tumor is destructive, the underproduction of a hormone. Radiation or surgery can be used to destroy tumors and thereby restore normal pituitary functioning.

Anterior pituitary hormones can be the basis of a variety of disorders. As with other hormones, there may be below-normal production of the hormone (hyposecretion) or overproduction of the hormone (hypersecretion). Because the pituitary hormones are often supportive of hormone secretion by the target organ or tissue, hyposecretion or hypersecretion of the tropic or supportive hormone leads to a similar change in the production of hormones by the target organ or tissue.

For example, hyperthyroidism, or Graves' disease, can be caused by excessive secretion of TSH by the pituitary, leading to hypersecretion of thyroxine, or by nodules within the thyroid that produce excessive thyroxine. In the diagnosis process, blood levels of both TSH and thyroxine are usually measured to determine the specific cause of the disorder. Similarly, hypothyroidism can be induced by deficits at several levels. The lack of iodine in the diet can prevent the production of thyroxine, which requires iodide as part of its molecular composition. The production of thyroxine usually has a negative feedback effect on the hypothalamus and pituitary, reducing TSH production. The failure to produce thyroxine causes high blood levels of TSH and an abnormal growth of the thyroid that results in a greatly enlarged thyroid, called a goiter. The addition of iodine to salt has eliminated the incidence of goiter in developed countries. Even with an adequate supply of iodine in the diet, however, hypothyroidism can still develop from other sources. The usual treatment is to ingest a dose of thyroxine daily.

Other examples of anterior pituitary disorders include those involving changes in GH secretion. Undersecretion of GH can lead to short stature or even a type of dwarfism called pituitary dwarfism, in which an individual has normal body proportions but is smaller than normal. Now it is possible to obtain human GH from bacteria genetically engineered to produce it. Replacement GH can be given during the normal growth years to enhance growth. A tumor sometimes develops in the pituitary cells that produce GH, and this can cause abnormally increased growth or gigantism. If the tumor develops during the adult years, only a few areas of abnormal growth can occur, such as in the facial bones and the bones of the hands and feet. This condition is called acromegaly. Abraham Lincoln is thought to have had abnormal levels of GH that caused gigantism in his youth and then acromegaly in his later years. Acromegaly can be treated by radiation or surgery of the anterior pituitary.

Pineal gland tumors have been associated with precocious puberty, in which children become sexually developed in early childhood. It is thought that melatonin normally inhibits sexual development during this period. The pineal gland is influenced by changes in the daily photo-period, so that the highest levels of melatonin appear in the blood during the night, especially during the long nights of winter. Seasonal affective disorder (SAD), a mental depression that occurs during the late fall and winter, has been linked to seasonally high melatonin levels. Daily exposure to bright lights to mimic summer has been used to treat SAD. The pineal gland and melatonin are also being studied with regard to jet lag and disorders associated with shift work. The pineal gland thus seems to be involved in the functioning of the body's biological clock.

The pancreatic islets, also called the islets of Langerhans, produce insulin and glucagon. Diabetes mellitus is caused by insufficient insulin production (type 1 or juvenile-onset diabetes) or by the lack of functional insulin receptors on body cells (type 2 diabetes). Type 1 diabetes can be treated with insulin injections, an implanted insulin pump, or even a transplant of fetal pancreatic tissue. Type 2 diabetes is treated with diet and weight loss. Weight loss induces an increase in insulin receptors. Long-term complications resulting from high blood-sugar levels include damage to the kidneys, to the blood vessels in the retina (diabetic retinopathy), to the legs and feet, and to the nerves (diabetic neuropathy).

Changes in the levels of steroid hormones (glucocorticoids, mineralocorticoids, or androgens) secreted by the adrenal cortex can lead to disease. For example, hypersecretion of the glucocorticoid cortisol results in Cushing's syndrome and hyposecretion of cortisol results in Addison's disease. Similar to the thyroid, the hormones produced by the adrenal cortex participate in a feedback loop mechanism with the pituitary and hypothalamus. Thus, when levels of hormones released by the adrenal glands are low, the pituitary and hypothalamus try to compensate by secreting higher levels of their own hormones. In Addison's disease, low levels of adrenal glucocorticoids causes increased ACTH release from the pituitary. Addison's disease is characterized by low blood pressure and a poor physiological response to stress: It can be treated by the administration of exogenous glucocorticoids. Extreme cases of adrenal insufficiency can bring about an "adrenal crisis." In this situation, an immediate injection of glucocorticoid hormone is given to prevent death.

In addition to treating Addison's disease, glucocorticoids, particularly cortisone, are used to treat inflammation; however, overuse can lead to adrenal cortex suppression by the negative feedback mechanism. When athletes abuse the androgen sex hormones for the purpose of increasing muscle mass, adrenal suppression can develop along with sterility and damage to the heart. Masculinization is observed in women who have tumors of the androgen-producing cells of the adrenal glands. These women display several changes associated with increased male sex hormones, changes that include beard growth and increased muscle development.

Perspective and Prospects

The early history of endocrinology noted that boys who were castrated failed to undergo the changes associated with puberty. A. A. Berthold in 1849 described the effects of castration in cockerels. The birds failed to develop large combs and wattles and failed to show male behavior. He noted that these effects could be reversed if testes were transplanted back into the cockerels. W. M. Bayliss and E. H. Starling in 1902 first introduced the term "hormone" to refer to secretin. They found that secretin is produced by the small intestine in response to acid in the chyme and that secretin causes the pancreas to release digestive enzymes into the small intestine. Most important, F. G. Banting and G. H. Best in 1922 reported their extraction of insulin from the pancreas of dogs and their success in alleviating diabetes in dogs by means of injections of the insulin. Frederick Sanger in 1953 established the amino acid sequence for insulin and later won a Nobel Prize for this achievement.

Another Nobel Prize was awarded to Earl W. Sutherland, Jr., in 1971 for his demonstration in 1962 of the role of cyclic AMP as a second messenger in the sequence involved in the stimulation of cells by many hormones. Andrew V. Schally and Roger C. L. Guillemin in 1977 received a Nobel Prize for their work in isolating and determining the structures of hypothalamic regulatory peptides.

More recent achievements in endocrinological research have centered on the identification of receptors that bind with the hormone when the hormone stimulates a cell and on the genetic engineering of bacteria to produce hormones such as human growth hormone. The use of fetal tissues in endocrinological research and therapy—the host usually does not reject fetal implants—continues to be an area for future research.

—John T. Burns, Ph.D.;
updated by Sharon W. Stark, R.N., A.P.R.N., D.N.Sc.

See also Addison's disease; Adrenalectomy; Amenorrhea; Corticosteroids; Cushing's syndrome; Diabetes mellitus; Dwarfism; Dysmenorrhea; Endocrine glands; Endocrinology; Endocrinology, pediatric; Endometriosis; Fructosemia; Gigantism; Glands; Goiter; Growth; Hashimoto's thyroiditis; Hormone therapy; Hormones; Hyperhidrosis; Hyperparathyroidism and hypoparathyroidism; Hypoglycemia; Infertility, female; Infertility, male; Insulin resistance syndrome; Liver; Menopause; Menorrhagia; Metabolic disorders; Ovarian cysts; Pancreas; Pancreatitis; Parathyroidectomy; Pregnancy and gestation; Prostate gland; Prostate gland removal; Puberty and adolescence; Steroids; Testicular surgery; Thyroid disorders; Thyroid gland; Thyroidectomy.

For Further Information:

Griffin, James E., and Sergio R. Ojeda, eds. *Textbook of Endocrine Physiology.* 5th ed. New York: Oxford University Press, 2004. A detailed account of normal and abnormal functioning of the endocrine system written by specialists. Intended for first year medical students.

Hadley, Mac E., and Jon E. Levine. *Endocrinology.* 6th ed. Upper Saddle River, N.J.: Pearson/Prentice Hall, 2007. A college-level text covering the endocrine system, primarily in humans and mammals. Recommended for a technical but understandable coverage of the field.

Henry, Helen L., and Anthony W. Norman, eds. *Encyclopedia of Hormones.* 3 vols. San Diego, Calif.: Academic Press, 2003. A comprehensive overview of the role of hormones, the major physiological systems in which they operate, and the biological consequences of an excess or deficiency of a particular hormone.

Kronenberg, Henry M., et al., eds. *Williams Textbook of Endocrinology.* 11th ed. Philadelphia: Saunders/Elsevier, 2008. Comprehensive information regarding endocrine diseases—their pathophysiology, diagnoses, treatment, and prognoses.

Martini, Frederic. *Fundamentals of Anatomy and Physiology.* 7th ed. Upper Saddle River, N.J.: Prentice Hall, 2006. A good place to start for a solid overview of the anatomy and physiology of the endocrine system before considering the details of disease states.

Scanlon, Valerie, and Tina Sanders. *Essentials of Anatomy and Physiology.* 5th ed. Philadelphia: F. A. Davis, 2007. A text designed around three themes: the relationship between physiology and anatomy, the interrelations among the organ systems, and the relationship of each organ system to homeostasis.

Shaw, Michael, ed. *Everything You Need to Know About Diseases.* Springhouse, Pa.: Springhouse Press, 1996. This well-illustrated consumer reference, compiled by more than one hundred doctors and medical experts, describes five hundred illnesses and conditions, listing their causes, symptoms, diagnosis, treatment, and prevention. Of particular interest is chapter 12, "Hormone and Gland Disorders."

Wells, Ken R. "Endocrine System." In *Gale Encyclopedia of Nursing and Allied Health*, edited by Kristine Krapp. Detroit, Mich.: Gale Group, 2002. A thorough examination of the endocrine system—its organs, role in health, and diseases and disorders.

ENDOCRINE GLANDS

ANATOMY

ANATOMY OR SYSTEM AFFECTED: Brain, endocrine system, glands, pancreas, reproductive system

SPECIALTIES AND RELATED FIELDS: Biochemistry, endocrinology, internal medicine

DEFINITION: Organs that send chemical messages through the blood to target cells. They are responsible for maintaining homeostasis by tightly regulating physiological processes.

KEY TERMS:

exocrine gland: a gland that releases its secretions via ducts to external surfaces

homeostasis: the process by which a constant internal environment is maintained

hormones: signaling molecules secreted into the blood by endocrine glands

negative feedback: the mechanism whereby the output of a process acts on the original input, resulting in a dampening of the process

STRUCTURE AND FUNCTION

Endocrine glands produce chemical messenger molecules called hormones. Hormones bind to receptors on the cells of the target organ, which causes the cells to respond internally by modifying their biochemical pathways. Unlike exocrine glands, which secrete their products via ducts, endocrine glands secrete hormones directly into the bloodstream: They are ductless. Together, the endocrine glands form the endocrine system.

The glands of the endocrine system and their target organs work in concert; many target organs of endocrine glands are, themselves, endocrine glands. In this way, relatively small signals can be amplified until the desired response takes place in the target organs. This response often leads to a signal being sent to the initiating endocrine gland, which reduces secretion of the original hormone, dampening the entire pathway. This process is called negative feedback.

The hypothalamus and the pituitary gland are located next to each other at the base of the brain. They are the master regulators of the endocrine system. The hypothalamus receives input from nerves in the brain. This triggers the hypothalamus to secrete hormones that act directly on the pituitary, causing it to secrete its own hormones. Depending on the original stimulus, the output of the hypothalamus and pituitary regulates the thyroid gland, adrenal glands, or the gonads.

The thyroid gland is in the neck wrapped around the trachea. The thyroid maintains control of metabolism, the rate at which the body uses energy. Associated with the thyroid gland are four parathyroid glands. These secrete parathyroid hormone, which is important for maintaining correct calcium levels in the blood.

There are two adrenal glands one on top of each kidney. They are responsible for the secretion of glucocorticoids, mineralocorticoids, and androgens. Adrenal glands are important in fluid and electrolyte homeostasis and in the stress response.

The gonads (ovaries and testes) are located in the pelvic region. In addition to producing the gametes (eggs and sperm), these glands secrete androgens and estrogens, hormones that are essential for the development and maintenance of sexual characteristics.

The pancreas is in the abdominal cavity, underneath the stomach, closely associated with the digestive tract. A majority of the pancreas acts as an exocrine gland secreting digestive enzymes. However, scattered throughout the pancreas are groups of endocrine cells called islets of Langerhans. The two major hormones secreted by these islets are insulin and glucagon; they are crucial for the maintenance of constant glucose levels in the body.

The pineal gland is located in the center of the brain. It secretes melatonin, a hormone that regulates sleep pattern.

DISORDERS AND DISEASES

Endocrinology is the medical field in which endocrine glands are studied. Diagnosis of endocrine gland disorders involves testing the levels of hormones in the blood of the patient. This can be difficult, because most hormones are secreted in pulses. Testing must be performed over hours, days, or weeks, depending on the hormone.

Most diseases that involve the endocrine glands are a result of either oversecretion or undersecretion of hormones. This upsets the optimal physiological homeostasis and forces negative feedback loops to work inappropriately. Three examples of endocrine disorders are diabetes mellitus, hyperthyroidism, and hypothyroidism.

Diabetes mellitus is the most common endocrine disorder in the United States. The pancreas of an individual suffering from diabetes mellitus produces either too little insulin or insulin that cannot be used by the target cells. The result is abnormally high levels of glucose in the blood. Symptoms of diabetes mellitus include increased thirst and urination, fatigue, and blurred vision. Long-term complications of high blood-glucose levels include blindness, numbness in the feet, kidney failure, and heart disease. Treatment for diabetes mellitus includes insulin injection, drugs that improve the ability of target cells to react to glucose, and drugs that lower glucose levels in the blood.

Thyroid disorders are the second most common endocrine gland problem. Hyperthyroidism is the oversecretion of thyroid hormones caused, for example, by an enlarged thyroid gland (Graves' disease), or by nodules on the thyroid. Symptoms include a fast heart rate, weight loss, and intolerance of heat. Treatment includes drugs that reduce thyroid hormone production, surgery, or radiation therapy.

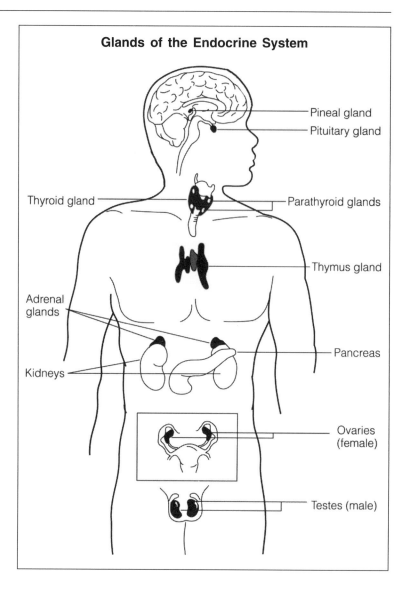

Glands of the Endocrine System

Hypothyroidism, insufficient thyroid hormone production, is more common. It is usually caused by inflammation of the thyroid (for example, Hashimoto's thyroiditis), or by over-compensatory medical treatment (for example, too much thyroid being removed during surgery to treat thyroid nodules). Symptoms include weight gain, cold intolerance, and hair loss. Hypothyroidism is usually treated with levothyroxine, a synthetic form of thyroxine which is one of the major thyroid hormones.

PERSPECTIVE AND PROSPECTS

Carvings from ancient Egyptian times have been identified that show people with enlarged thyroid glands (goiter) and acromegaly (a disorder in which the pituitary gland produces too much growth hormone). However, it was in the eighteenth century that scientists and clinicians really began to understand the concept of endocrine glands and identified them as ductless glands that secrete hormones.

The revolution in the treatment of endocrine gland dysfunction came with the ability to synthesize human hormones in the laboratory. A few examples of synthetic hormones now available are insulin, growth hormone, and thyroxine. Previously, these hormones were purified from animal, or even cadaver, organs. Synthetic hormones are cheaper and safer and the doses are more easily regulated than the hormones available previously.

Currently, new testing methods and treatments for

endocrine disorders are being researched. One example is the possibility of an insulin drug that can be administered orally instead of by injection. An exciting prospect for the future is the use of stem cell therapy to provide replacement hormones within the affected individual's own body.

—*Claire L. Standen, Ph.D.*

See also Addison's disease; Adrenalectomy; Corticosteroids; Cushing's syndrome; Diabetes mellitus; Endocrine disorders; Endocrinology; Endocrinology, pediatric; Gestational diabetes; Glands; Goiter; Growth; Hair loss and baldness; Hashimoto's thyroiditis; Hormone therapy; Hormones; Hyperparathyroidism and hypoparathyroidism; Obesity; Obesity, childhood; Pancreas; Pancreatitis; Parathyroidectomy; Thyroid disorders; Thyroid gland; Thyroidectomy; Weight loss and gain.

FOR FURTHER INFORMATION:

Gardner, Dave, and Delores Shoback. *Greenspan's Basic and Clinical Endocrinology.* 8th ed. New York: McGraw-Hill Medical, 2007.

Koeppen, Bruce, and Bruce Stanton. *Berne and Levy Physiology.* 6th ed. Philadelphia: Elsevier, 2008.

Neal, Matthew. *How the Endocrine System Works.* Malden, Mass.: Blackwell Science, 2001.

ENDOCRINOLOGY

SPECIALTY

ANATOMY OR SYSTEM AFFECTED: Brain, endocrine system, glands, immune system, nervous system, pancreas, psychic-emotional system, reproductive system, uterus

SPECIALTIES AND RELATED FIELDS: Biochemistry, genetics, gynecology, immunology

DEFINITION: The science dealing with how the internal secretions from ductless glands in the body act both in normal physiology and in disease states.

KEY TERMS:

adrenal gland: an endocrine gland situated immediately above the upper pole of each kidney; it consists of an inner part or medulla, which produces epinephrine and norepinephrine, and an outer part or cortex, which produces steroid hormones

endocrine pancreas: specialized secretory tissue dispersed within the pancreas called islets of Langerhans, which are responsible for the secretion of glucagon and insulin

hypothalamus: the region of the brain called the diencephalon, forming the floor of the third ventricle, including neighboring associated nuclei

metabolism: the process of tissue change, which may be synthetic (anabolic) or degradative (catabolic)

parathyroid gland: one of four small endocrine glands situated underneath the thyroid gland, whose main product is parathyroid hormone, which regulate serum calcium levels

pituitary gland: a small (0.5-gram), two-lobed endocrine gland that is attached by a stalk to the brain at the level of the hypothalamus

thyroid gland: a 20-gram endocrine gland that sits in front of the trachea and consists of two lateral lobes connected in the middle by an isthmus

SCIENCE AND PROFESSION

The rates of metabolic pathways in the body are controlled mainly by the endocrine system, in conjunction with the nervous system. These two systems are integrated in the neuroendocrine system, which controls the secretion of hormones by the endocrine glands. The study of endocrinology deals with the normal physiology and pathophysiology of endocrine glands. The endocrine glands that are typically the main focus of clinical endocrinologists are the hypothalamus, pituitary gland, thyroid, parathyroid, adrenal glands, endocrine pancreas, ovaries, and testes. The endocrine system regulates virtually all activities of the body, including growth and development, homeostasis, energy production, and reproduction.

The hypothalamus is a highly specialized endocrine organ that sits at the base of the brain and that functions as the master gland of the endocrine system. It is the main integrator for the endocrine and nervous systems. The hypothalamus produces a number of chemical mediators which have direct control over the pituitary gland. These chemicals are made in the cells of the hypothalamus and reach the pituitary gland, which sits just below it, by a special hypophyseoportal blood system. In adult humans, the pituitary is divided into two lobes: the anterior lobe (adenohypophysis) and the posterior lobe (neural lobe).

Vasopressin and oxytocin are the two main hormones that are made in the hypothalamus but stored in the posterior lobe of the pituitary for release when needed. Vasopressin (also known as antidiuretic hormone, or ADH) is a hormone that maintains a normal water concentration in the blood and is a regulator of circulating blood volume. Oxytocin is a hormone that is involved in lactation and obstetrical labor.

The hypothalamic-pituitary-thyroid axis is important in the control of basal metabolic rate. There are a number of releasing hormones secreted from the hypothalamus that control the release of anterior pituitary hormones, which then cause the release of hormones at the end organ. Most of these hormones have the chemical structures of peptides. Thyrotropin-releasing hormone (TRH) was the first hypothalamic releasing hormone that was synthesized and used clinically. TRH, secreted in nanogram quantities, is a cyclic tripeptide that causes release of thyrotropin-stimulating hormone (TSH) from the thyrotropic cells of the anterior pituitary gland. The release of TSH is in microgram quantities and leads to an increase in thyroid hormone release by the thyroid gland. The amount of thyroid hormone synthesized is on the order of milligrams. Therefore, the secretion of minute amounts of TRH allows for the production of thyroid hormone that is a millionfold greater than the amount of TRH itself. This is an example of an amplifying cascade, a system by which the central nervous system can control all metabolic processes with the secretion of very small amounts of hypothalamic releasing hormones. This intricate system possesses controls to stop the production of too much hormone as well. Such negative feedback is an important concept in endocrinology.

In the case of the thyroid, an increased amount of thyroid hormone produced by the thyroid gland will cause the pituitary and hypothalamus to decrease the amounts that they produce of TSH and TRH, respectively. Many hormones are subject to the laws of negative feedback control. TRH also causes potent release of the anterior pituitary hormone called prolactin. Thyroid hormone is important in determining basal metabolism and is needed for proper development in the newborn child. The thyroid gland produces both thyroxine (T_4, also called tetraiodothyronine) and triiodothyronine (T_3), both of which it synthesizes from iodine and the amino acid tyrosine.

The hypothalamic-pituitary-adrenal axis is critical in the reaction to stress, both physical and emotional. Corticotropin-releasing hormone (CRH) is a polypeptide, consisting of forty-one amino acids, that causes the production of the proopiomelanocortin molecule by the corticotropic cells of the anterior pituitary. The proopiomelanocortin molecule is cleaved by proteolytic enzymes to yield adrenocorticotropic hormone (ACTH, also called corticotropin), melanocyte-stimulating hormone, and lipotropin. It is ACTH made by the anterior pituitary which then stimulates the adrenal cortex to produce steroid hormones. The main stress hormone produced by the adrenal cortex in response to ACTH is the glucocorticoid cortisol. ACTH also has some control over the production of the mineralocorticoid aldosterone and the androgens dehydroepiandrosterone and testosterone. These steroids are synthesized from cholesterol. The production of cortisol (also known as hydrocortisone) is subject to negative feedback by CRH and ACTH.

The hypothalamic-pituitary-gonadal axis is involved in the control of reproduction. Gonadotropin-releasing hormone (GnRH), also known as luteinizing hormone-releasing hormone (LHRH), is produced by the hypothalamus and stimulates the release of luteinizing hormone (LH) and follicle-stimulating hormone (FSH) from the gonadotrophic cells of the anterior pituitary. LH and FSH have different effects in men and women. In men, LH controls the production and secretion of testosterone by the Leydig's cells of the testes. The release of LH is regulated by negative feedback from testosterone. FSH along with testosterone acts on the Sertoli cells of the seminiferous tubule of the testis at the time of puberty to start sperm production. In women, LH controls ovulation by the ovary and also the development of the corpus luteum, which produces progesterone. Progesterone is a steroid hormone that is critically important for the maintenance of pregnancy. FSH in women stimulates the development and maturation of a primary follicle and oocyte. The ovarian follicle in the nonpregnant woman is the main site of production of estradiol. Estradiol is the principal estrogen made in the reproductive years by the ovary and is responsible for the development of female secondary sexual characteristics.

Growth hormone-releasing hormone (GHRH) is a polypeptide with forty-four amino acids that stimulates the release of growth hormone (GH) from the somatotrophic cells of the anterior pituitary. The regulation of GH secretion is under dual control. While GHRH positively releases GH, somatostatin (a polypeptide with fourteen amino acids, also released from the hypothalamus) inhibits the release of GH. Somatostatin has a wide variety of functions, including the suppression of insulin, glucagon, and gastrointestinal hormones. GH released from the pituitary circulates in the bloodstream and stimulates the production of somatomedins by the liver. Several somatomedins are produced, all of which have a profound effect on growth, with the most important one in humans being somatomedin C, also called insulin-like growth factor I (IGF I). Molecular biological techniques have shown that many cells outside the liver also produce IGF I; in these cells, IGF I acts in autocrine or paracrine ways to cause the growth of the cells or to affect neighboring cells.

Prolactin is a peptide hormone that is secreted by the lactotrophs of the anterior pituitary. It is involved in the differentiation of the mammary gland cells and initiates the production of milk proteins and other constituents. Prolactin may also have other functions, as a stress hormone or growth hormone. Prolactin is under tonic negative control. The inhibition of prolactin release is caused by dopamine, which is produced by the hypothalamus. Thus, while dopamine is normally considered to be a neurotransmitter, in the case of prolactin release it acts as an inhibitory hormone. Serotonin, also classically thought of as a neurotransmitter, may cause the stimulation of prolactin release from the anterior pituitary.

DIAGNOSTIC AND TREATMENT TECHNIQUES

One of the most common medical problems seen by specialists in the field of endocrinology is a patient with type 1 diabetes mellitus, sometimes also called juvenile-onset or insulin-dependent diabetes mellitus. "Insulin-dependent" is probably more appropriate, as not all patients with type 1 diabetes mellitus develop the disease in childhood. Type 1 diabetes is an autoimmune disease in which antibodies to different parts of the pancreatic beta cell, the cell that normally produces insulin, are produced. Some of these antibodies are cytotoxic; that is, they actually destroy the pancreatic beta cell. The most striking characteristic of patients with type 1 diabetes is that they produce very little insulin. The symptoms of type 1 diabetes include increased thirst, increased urination, blurring of vision, and weight loss. A doctor would confirm the diagnosis by running blood tests for glucose and insulin. The glucose level would be high, and the insulin level would be low. The treatment includes controlled diet, exercise, insulin therapy, and self-monitoring of blood glucose. With proper control of blood glucose, patients with type 1 diabetes can lead normal, productive lives.

Graves' disease is another autoimmune disease that is commonly seen by endocrinologists. Graves' disease is caused by the production of thyroid-stimulating immunoglobulin antibodies that bind to and activate TSH receptors. As a result, the thyroid gland produces too much thyroid hormone and the thyroid gland enlarges in size. The antibodies also commonly affect the eyes, causing a characteristic bulging. The clinical symptoms of hyperthyroidism include increased heart rate, anxiety, heat sensitivity, sleeplessness, diarrhea, and abdominal pain. Patients often lose considerable weight, despite having a great appetite and eating large amounts of food. Sometimes, the diagnosis is missed, leading to an extensive evaluation for a variety of other diseases. Often, a family history of thyroid disease or other endocrine disease can be found.

The usual method of screening for Graves' disease is with a simple blood test for thyroid function, which includes testing for T_4, T_3, and TSH. In patients with Graves' disease, both T_4 and T_3 will be elevated, and TSH will be very low. If the blood test reveals this pattern, the next usual step is to proceed to a radioactive iodine uptake and scan test, which involves giving a very small amount of radioactive iodine by mouth and having the patient return twenty-four hours later for a scan. The thyroid gland normally accumulates iodine and thus will accumulate the radioactive iodine as well. The radioactive iodine emits a gamma-ray energy that can be picked up by a solid-crystal scintillation counter placed over the thyroid gland. With this device, one can determine the percentage of iodine uptake and also obtain a picture of the thyroid gland. The normal radioactive iodine uptake is about 10 to 30 percent of the dose, depending somewhat on the amount of total body iodine, which is derived from the diet. Patients with Graves' disease will have high radioactive iodine uptakes.

Those who suffer from Graves' disease can be treated by three different means, depending on the circumstances. The first treatment that is often tried is antithyroid drugs, either propylthiouracil or methimazole. These drugs belong to the class of sulfonamides and inhibit the production of new thyroid hormone by blocking the attachment of iodine to the amino acid tyrosine. Another mode of therapy is the use of radioactive iodine. A dose of radioactive iodine (on the order of 5 to 10 millicuries) is used to destroy part of the thyroid gland. The gamma-ray energy emitted from the iodine molecule that has traveled to the thyroid gland is enough to kill some thyroid cells. An alternative way to destroy the thyroid gland is to remove it surgically (thyroidectomy). Endocrinologists rarely send patients for surgery, as the other therapies are often effective. The goal of all treatments is to bring the level of thyroid hormone into the normal range, as well as to shrink the thyroid gland. After treatment, the patient's level of thyroid hormone sometimes falls to levels that are below normal. The symptoms of hypothyroidism are the opposite of hyperthyroidism and include fatigue, weight gain, cold sensitivity, constipation, and dry skin. If this happens, the patient is treated with thyroid hormone replacement. The dose is adjusted for each individual to produce normal levels of T_4, T_3, and TSH.

A less common but important endocrine disorder is the existence of a pituitary tumor that secretes prolactin, called a prolactinoma. Prolactinomas are diagnosed earlier in women than in men, as women with the disorder often complain of a lack of menstrual periods and spontaneous milk production from the breasts, known as galactorrhea. These tumors, which can be quite small, are called microadenomas because they are less than 10 millimeters in size. They can affect men as well, causing decreased sex drive and impotence. Macroadenomas are tumors greater than 10 millimeters in size. When the tumors increase in size, they can cause symptoms such as headache and decreased vision. It is important to note that most microadenomas never progress to macroadenomas. Vision loss and/or decreased eye movement can be seen with a macroadenoma and are reason for immediate treatment.

Doctors screen patients for a prolactinoma by running a blood test for prolactin. There are other reasons for mild elevations in prolactin levels, including the use of certain psychiatric drugs such as phenothiazines or the antihypertensive drugs reserpine and methyldopa, primary hypothyroidism, cirrhosis, and chronic renal failure. If a pituitary tumor is suspected, then other biochemical tests of pituitary function are conducted to determine if the rest of the gland is functioning normally. At that time, imaging tests are often done to get a picture of the hypothalamic-pituitary area; this can be done with either computed tomography (CT) scanning or magnetic resonance imaging (MRI). Patients with macroadenomas will require treatment. In patients with little neurological involvement, medical therapy may be initiated. Bromocriptine, a semisynthetic ergot alkaloid which is an inhibitor of prolactin secretion, may be used. It has been shown that patients treated with this drug have reduction in tumor size. Patients can be maintained on the drug indefinitely because prolactin levels return to pretreatment levels when the drug is stopped. If there is severe neurologic involvement, with loss of vision and other eye problems, immediate surgery may be indicated. There is a very high incidence of tumor recurrence after surgery, requiring medical and/ or radiation therapy.

PERSPECTIVE AND PROSPECTS

The field of endocrinology is a continuously evolving one. Advances in biomedical technology, including molecular biology and cell biology, have made it a de-

manding job for the clinician to keep up with all the breakthroughs in the field. The challenge for endocrinology will be to apply many of these new technologies to novel treatments for patients with endocrine diseases.

An example of the progression of the field of endocrinology can be seen in the history of pituitary diseases. The start of pituitary endocrinology is ascribed to Pierre Marie, the French neurologist who in 1886 first described pituitary enlargement in a patient with acromegaly (enlargement of the skull, jaw, hands, and feet) and linked the disease to a pituitary abnormality. During the first half of the twentieth century, many of the hypothalamic and pituitary hormones were isolated and characterized. The field of endocrinology was revolutionized by the development of the radioimmunoassay, which allows sensitive and specific measurements of hormones. The radioimmunoassay replaced bioassay techniques, which were laborious, time-consuming, and not always precise. This technique has allowed for rapid measurement of hormones and improved screening for endocrine diseases involving hormone deficiency or hormone excess.

The development of new hormone assays has been complemented by the development of noninvasive imaging techniques. Before the advent of CT scanning in the late 1970's, it was an ordeal to diagnose a pituitary tumor. Pneumoencephalography was often performed, which involved injecting air into the fluid-containing structures of the brain, with associated risk and discomfort to the patient. In the 1980's, with new generations of high-resolution CT scanners that were more sensitive than early scanners, smaller pituitary lesions could be detected and diagnosed. That decade also ushered in the use of MRI to diagnose disorders of the hypothalamic-pituitary unit. MRI has allowed doctors to evaluate the hypothalamus, pituitary, and nearby structures very precisely; it has become the method of choice for evaluating patients with pituitary disease. MRI can easily visualize the optic chiasm in the forebrain and the vascular structures surrounding the pituitary.

In patients who require surgery, advances have helped decrease mortality rates. Harvey Cushing pioneered the transsphenoidal technique in 1927 but abandoned it in favor of the transfrontal approach. This involves reaching the pituitary tumor by retracting the frontal lobes to visualize the pituitary gland sitting underneath. The modern era of transsphenoidal pituitary surgery was developed by Gérard Guiot and Jules Hardy in the late 1960's. Transsphenoidal surgery done with an operating microscope to visualize the pituitary contents allows for selective removal of the tumor, leaving the normal pituitary gland intact. The advantage of this approach from below, instead of from above, includes minimal movement of the brain and less blood loss. This technique requires a neurosurgeon with much skill and experience. There are also new drug treatments for patients with pituitary diseases, such as bromocriptine for use in patients with prolactinomas and octreotide (a somatostatin analogue) to lower growth hormone levels in patients with acromegaly.

—RoseMarie Pasmantier, M.D.

See also Addison's disease; Adrenalectomy; Chronobiology; Corticosteroids; Cushing's syndrome; Diabetes mellitus; Dwarfism; Endocrine disorders; Endocrine glands; Endocrinology, pediatric; Enzymes; Fructosemia; Gender reassignment surgery; Gestational diabetes; Gigantism; Glands; Goiter; Growth; Gynecology; Hair loss and baldness; Hashimoto's thyroiditis; Hormone therapy; Hormones; Hot flashes; Hyperhidrosis; Hyperparathyroidism and hypoparathyroidism; Hypoglycemia; Hysterectomy; Melatonin; Menopause; Menstruation; Metabolic disorders; Obesity; Obesity, childhood; Paget's disease; Pancreas; Pancreatitis; Parathyroidectomy; Pharmacology; Pharmacy; Prostate gland; Prostate gland removal; Puberty and adolescence; Sexual differentiation; Steroids; Thyroid disorders; Thyroid gland; Thyroidectomy; Weight loss and gain.

FOR FURTHER INFORMATION:

Bar, Robert S., ed. *Early Diagnosis and Treatment of Endocrine Disorders.* Totowa, N.J.: Humana Press, 2003. Reviews the early signs and symptoms of common endocrine diseases, surveys the clinical testing needed for a diagnosis, and presents recommendations for therapy.

Braverman, Lewis E., and Robert D. Utiger, eds. *Werner and Ingbar's The Thyroid: A Fundamental and Clinical Text.* 9th ed. Philadelphia: Lippincott Williams & Wilkins, 2005. An exhaustive textbook on all aspects of the thyroid, including history, anatomy, biology, pathology, basic and clinical research, and the thyroid in development and pregnancy.

Harmel, Anne Peters, and Ruchi Mathur. *Davidson's Diabetes Mellitus: Diagnosis and Treatment.* 5th ed. Philadelphia: W. B. Saunders, 2004. A very good, practical approach to the overall management of the endocrine patient with diabetes mellitus.

Imura, Hiroo, ed. *The Pituitary Gland.* 2d ed. New York: Raven Press, 1994. Good discussion of the master gland, the hypothalamic-pituitary unit.

Kronenberg, Henry M., et al., eds. *Williams Textbook of Endocrinology.* 11th ed. Philadelphia: Saunders/Elsevier, 2008. Text that covers the spectrum of information related to the endocrine system, including thyroid disorders, diabetes, endocrinology and aging, female reproduction and fertility control, sexual function and dysfunction, kidney stones, and endocrine hypertension.

Lebovitz, Harold E., ed. *Therapy for Diabetes Mellitus and Related Disorders.* 5th ed. Alexandria, Va.: American Diabetes Association, 2009. A comprehensive treatise on the treatment of various aspects of diabetes mellitus. The different chapters are written by experts in the field.

Speroff, Leon, and Marc A. Fritz. *Clinical Gynecologic Endocrinology and Infertility.* 7th ed. Philadelphia: Lippincott Williams & Wilkins, 2005. An excellent textbook which brings together all aspects of endocrinology in women from embryology to old age. Good discussion of the problems seen in infertile couples.

ENDOCRINOLOGY, PEDIATRIC
SPECIALTY

ANATOMY OR SYSTEM AFFECTED: Brain, endocrine system, glands, immune system, nervous system, pancreas, psychic-emotional system

SPECIALTIES AND RELATED FIELDS: Biochemistry, genetics, immunology, neonatology, pediatrics

DEFINITION: The study of the normal and abnormal function of the endocrine (ductless) glands in children and adolescents.

KEY TERMS:

hormone: a chemical molecule produced in either the hypothalamus or one of the endocrine glands that is secreted and travels (usually via the bloodstream) to a target organ or to specific receptor cells, causing a specific response

insulin: a hormone that is essential in regulating blood glucose, as well as in assimilating carbohydrates for growth and energy

pancreas: a large gland near the stomach which has both exocrine and endocrine functions and which produces insulin

pituitary gland: a very small gland at the base of the brain that is referred to as the master gland; with the hypothalamus, it regulates most of the endocrine systems

thyroid: a gland in the anterior neck which regulates the level of the body's metabolism and which is instrumental in normal physical and mental growth

SCIENCE AND PROFESSION

Pediatric endocrinology is a major subspecialty, limited to children and adolescents, which involves the study of normal as well as abnormal functions of the endocrine system, which comprises the glands of internal or ductless secretions. These practitioners, referred to as endocrinologists or pediatric endocrinologists, are doctors of medicine or osteopathy who have completed three years of pediatric residency training and an additional two to three years of fellowship training in endocrinology.

Endocrinology is one of the most interesting and challenging fields in pediatrics because it requires a blend of basic science and technology in the clinical setting. Some of the diagnoses are very difficult, yet they are almost always completely logical. Endocrinology is tightly related to other areas of pediatrics, such as adolescent medicine, genetics, growth, development, nutrition, and metabolism. These relationships make this field even more complex and intellectually stimulating.

Pediatric endocrinology and adult endocrinology are relatively young fields, probably beginning with the discovery in 1888 that "myxedema" (hypothyroidism) could be improved by feeding the patient thyroid extract. Both fields deal with the major endocrine glands and their disorders, such as diabetes mellitus or hypothyroidism, but there are several key differences, most related to growth (both physical and mental), potential, and genetics. Some major areas of specific emphasis in pediatric endocrinology include diabetes mellitus (which presents very differently in children), disorders of growth, disorders of sexual maturation and differentiation, genetic disorders, and adolescent medicine.

DIAGNOSTIC AND TREATMENT TECHNIQUES

In pediatric endocrinology, as in all medical fields, history taking and physical examination are the starting points and usually the most useful tools for diagnosis. Endocrinology is a specialty that is particularly aided by science. Blood and urine chemistries, hormone assays, chromosomal analyses, X rays, computed tomography (CT) scans, magnetic resonance imaging (MRI), and a host of other sophisticated tests have advanced diagnosis and treatment and have made this specialty one of the favorites for physicians who like science. Virtu-

ally all the known hormones can be assayed accurately and quickly.

Since insulin was first available for injection in 1922, there have been amazing advances in treatment. Many of the treatments in endocrinology involve hormone therapy. In 1985, recombinant growth hormone was synthesized for the first time. This development has allowed endocrinologists to treat not only pituitary dwarfism but also other kinds of growth deficiencies, such as Turner syndrome.

Turner syndrome is a relatively common chromosomal abnormality affecting females and resulting in short stature and lack of sexual development. While these girls will never become fertile, the combination of growth hormone for stature and other hormonal therapy for the development of secondary sexual characteristics enables them to have a normal female body. Studies have shown that normal body image and the presence of menstruation is essential for the self-esteem of these patients.

Diabetes mellitus is the most common significant endocrine disorder in both adults and children. What was commonly referred to as juvenile diabetes years ago is now called diabetes mellitus, type 1. Unlike type 2, which usually presents insidiously in middle-aged and older adults, type 1 presents rapidly, and the patient will need daily injectable insulin treatments. Diabetes in children is complex to manage not only because of the insulin treatment but also because of the patients' growth, metabolism, fluctuating activity levels, and physiologic and psychological changes that occur, especially in adolescence.

Now small portable and quite accurate glucometers allow patients to measure blood glucose (sugar) at home, making diabetes management much simpler. Tighter control of blood glucose will decrease or delay the onset of long-term complications of the disease, such as blindness, heart disease, and kidney disease. In the United States, newborn screening, which is now performed in all fifty states, has virtually eliminated cretinism, which tragically resulted when congenital hypothyroidism was not diagnosed until later in childhood. These children were irreversibly mentally retarded.

Enhanced techniques in pediatric surgery and neurosurgery, greatly aided by scans, play a role in the treatment of some endocrine disorders. Very small tumors and masses can be identified and often removed successfully. Often, endocrinologists and oncologists work together in concert with the surgeon.

Although this subspecialty is one of the most scientific and laboratory-based in pediatrics, it is also a field where emotional support, counseling, and often mental health care are given. Children do not like being "different," and body image is very important in children and particularly in teenagers. Even when a child appears absolutely normal, the frustration of ongoing monitoring and treatment is resented and can result in rebellion, especially in children with diabetes. Often, a team approach is needed, which involves professionals, teachers, family, and peers.

PERSPECTIVE AND PROSPECTS
The future promises ever-advancing and dramatic tools for the diagnosis and treatment of endocrine disorders, as well as for their prevention. On the immediate horizon, an implantible glucose pump, which can serve as a substitute pancreas, can change the lives of diabetic patients dramatically. A method for rapidly analyzing blood glucose using the surface of the skin has been developed. In addition, genetic engineering may revolutionize the approaches to treating many of these diseases.

—*C. Mervyn Rasmussen, M.D.*

See also Addison's disease; Adrenalectomy; Chronobiology; Corticosteroids; Diabetes mellitus; Dwarfism; Endocrine disorders; Endocrine glands; Endocrinology; Enzymes; Fructosemia; Gigantism; Glands; Growth; Gynecology; Hormone therapy; Hormones; Hyperparathyroidism and hypoparathyroidism; Hypoglycemia; Melatonin; Menstruation; Metabolic disorders; Obesity; Obesity, childhood; Pancreas; Pancreatitis; Parathyroidectomy; Pediatrics; Pharmacology; Pharmacy; Puberty and adolescence; Steroids; Thyroid disorders; Thyroid gland; Thyroidectomy; Weight loss and gain.

FOR FURTHER INFORMATION:
Bar, Robert S., ed. *Early Diagnosis and Treatment of Endocrine Disorders*. Totowa, N.J.: Humana Press, 2003. Reviews the early signs and symptoms of common endocrine diseases, surveys the clinical testing needed for a diagnosis, and presents recommendations for therapy.
Handwerger, Stuart, ed. *Molecular and Cellular Pediatric Endocrinology*. Totowa, N.J.: Humana Press, 1999. The chapters in this book reflect the genetic and molecular bases of many of the fundamental problems of differentiation and growth in a manner appropriate for a pediatrics textbook.
Kronenberg, Henry M., et al., eds. *Williams Textbook of Endocrinology*. 11th ed. Philadelphia: Saunders/Elsevier, 2008. Text that covers the spectrum of information related to the endocrine system, including thyroid disorders, diabetes, endocrinology and aging, female reproduction and fertility control, sexual function and dysfunction, kidney stones, and endocrine hypertension.
Little, Marjorie. *Diabetes*. New York: Chelsea House, 1991. A clearly written overview directed toward a nonspecialized audience. Includes a fourteen-page chapter on type 1 (juvenile) diabetes.
Sperling, Mark A., ed. *Pediatric Endocrinology*. 3d ed. Philadelphia: Saunders/Elsevier, 2008. Discusses endocrine diseases in infancy and childhood. Includes a bibliography and an index.
Wales, Jeremy K. H., and Jan Maarten Wit. *Pediatric Endocrinology and Growth*. 2d ed. Philadelphia: W. B. Saunders, 2004. An illustrated text that outlines specific endocrine problems, from growth disorders to glucose homeostasis, early or late sexual development, abnormal genitalia, goiter, failure to thrive, and obesity.

ENDODONTIC DISEASE
DISEASE/DISORDER
ANATOMY OR SYSTEM AFFECTED: Mouth, teeth
SPECIALTIES AND RELATED FIELDS: Dentistry
DEFINITION: Disease of the dental pulp and sometimes also the soft tissues and bone around the tip of the root.

CAUSES AND SYMPTOMS
The most common cause of endodontic disease is infection of the dental pulp by the bacteria that cause tooth decay. The pulp is composed of connective tissue, nerves, blood vessels, and tooth regenerative cells. It fills the root canal, a narrow channel in the center of the tooth root, which is embedded in the jawbone. Teeth usually contain one to four root canals. Decay-causing bacteria reach the pulp after dissolving their way through the two, hard outer layers of the tooth—the enamel and dentin. Bacteria may also reach the pulp through a crack or fracture in a tooth and through tooth wear or abrasion. Many kinds of bacteria can infect the pulp.

Pulp infected by bacteria becomes inflamed and has no place to swell because it is surrounded by dentin, which is rigid. Pain may result. Eventually, the entire pulp may become infected and die. If not treated, the in-

INFORMATION ON ENDODONTIC DISEASE

CAUSES: Bacterial infection of dental pulp
SYMPTOMS: Gum inflammation and pain, which is severe if abscess forms
DURATION: Chronic if untreated
TREATMENTS: Root canal treatment

fection can spread to the soft tissue and bone surrounding the tip of the root and form an abscess, which often produces severe pain.

TREATMENT AND THERAPY

To treat damaged or dead pulp tissue and preserve the tooth, endodontic therapy, or root canal treatment, is required. Endodontists specialize in this procedure. One or two visits are usually required. A small hole is made in the top (crown) of the infected tooth, and all the pulp tissue is removed. Then an inert material, usually a piece of rubberlike gum called gutta percha, is inserted in place of the pulp and secured in place with a sealer or cement. A tooth that has had root canal treatment is commonly considered to be dead, but the fibers of the periodontal ligament that hold the tooth in the jawbone are still alive. Following this procedure, additional dental treatments are necessary to preserve the weakened tooth.

PERSPECTIVE AND PROSPECTS

Historically, the only remedy for endodontic disease was tooth extraction. Since the mid-twentieth century, endodontic research has yielded treatments that preserve infected teeth. Furthermore, there has been an increased appreciation of the role of dental hygiene in preventing tooth decay and the endodontic infections that can result from it. Research on the causes and prevention of endodontic disease, and treatments for it, is being conducted at dental schools and at the National Institute of Dental and Cranio-Facial Research.

—*Jane F. Hill, Ph.D.*

See also Bacterial infections; Cavities; Dental diseases; Dentistry; Gingivitis; Gum disease; Periodontal surgery; Periodontitis; Root canal treatment; Teeth; Tooth extraction; Toothache.

FOR FURTHER INFORMATION:

Christensen, Gordon J. *A Consumer's Guide to Dentistry.* 2d ed. St. Louis, Mo.: Mosby, 2002.
Connecticut Consumer Health Information Network. "Your Dental Health: A Guide for Patients and Families." http://library.uchc.edu/departm/hnet/dental health.html.
Kim, Syngcuk, ed. *Modern Endodontic Practice.* Philadelphia: W. B. Saunders, 2004.
Porter, Robert S., et al., eds. *The Merck Manual Home Health Handbook.* Whitehouse Station, N.J.: Merck Research Laboratories, 2009.
Smith, Rebecca W. *The Columbia University School of Dental and Oral Surgery's Guide to Family Dental Care.* New York: W. W. Norton, 1997.

ENDOMETRIAL BIOPSY
PROCEDURE

ANATOMY OR SYSTEM AFFECTED: Genitals, reproductive system, uterus

SPECIALTIES AND RELATED FIELDS: Gynecology, histology, obstetrics, preventive medicine

DEFINITION: A procedure in which a tissue sample is taken from the lining of the uterus and then examined.

KEY TERMS:

cervix: the entrance to the uterus

dilation and curettage (D&C): a procedure in which the cervix is stretched and the lining of the uterus is scraped

endometrium: tissue lining the inside of the uterus

hysteroscopy: a procedure using a thin, lighted tube with a camera and tool to examine visually and remove part of the endometrium

uterus: the part of the reproductive tract that supports the development and nourishment of a developing fetus; also called the womb

vagina: the tube leading from the uterus to the outside of the body

INDICATIONS AND PROCEDURES

An endometrial biopsy is usually performed to identify the cause of abnormal uterine bleeding. Abnormal bleeding is that which is excessive in duration, frequency, or amount for the particular woman, and it includes bleeding at the wrong times (between menstrual periods) or after menopause. The biopsy may also be performed when there is no bleeding (or menstruation), or if a woman is having difficulty becoming pregnant.

Approximately 90 percent of women who have endometrial cancer have abnormal bleeding, so the biopsy is performed to rule out both cancer and hyperplasia, an excessive growth of tissue that could become cancerous. Women who are perimenopausal (prior to the actual end of menstrual cycles) may experience changes in their cycle that make it difficult to determine if there is abnormal bleeding or simply normal changes. Perimenopause usually lasts six to eight years, and then women become menopausal when menstrual cycles end. Women on hormone therapy are at greater risk of endometrial cancer, because they usually take the hormones estrogen and progesterone that their body is no longer producing at sufficient levels. Women who take estrogen but cannot take progesterone are at an even greater risk of endometrial cancer.

The biopsy may also be used as part of an infertility examination to determine if there are problems with the development of the endometrium. If the endometrium does not thicken in time to accept and support a fertilized egg, then the egg cannot implant properly, a condition called luteal phase defect (LPD). The biopsy can show whether the uterine lining is thickening and maturing by developing more blood vessels before menstruation, a definite sign that ovulation (the maturation and release of an egg by the ovary) has occurred and that the lining can support a pregnancy. Additionally, the biopsy may be performed to help evaluate the problem of repeated early miscarriages. Another use of the procedure is to obtain a sample for patients with suspected endometritis or polycystic ovary disease.

An obstetrician or gynecologist, or in some cases a nurse practitioner or nurse midwife, will perform the procedure, which is usually done in an office setting. The procedure takes about two minutes, and no anesthesia is needed, although a mild over-the-counter painkiller such as ibuprofen is often recommended about one hour before the procedure to ease discomfort. In cases of cervical stenosis, cervical softening may be accomplished by administration of the medication misoprostel. Additionally, a local anesthetic may occasionally be injected into the cervix to decrease pain and discomfort.

After a pelvic examination, the clinician will insert a speculum into the vagina to hold the walls open. After the cervix is cleaned with antiseptic, a tiny hollow plastic tube is inserted into the vagina, through the cervix, and into the uterus. A plunger attached to the tube will suction out a sample of the inner layer of tissue in the uterine wall. The tube is turned clockwise or counterclockwise while being moved in and out of the uterine cavity in order to obtain specimens. The cells are then sent to a laboratory for testing and microscopic examination.

Uses and Complications

Mild cramping may occur during and after the procedure. Cramping, pressure, and discomfort may also occur when the instruments are inserted and the samples collected. A small amount of bleeding, or spotting, may occur afterward, although normal activities can be resumed immediately.

After the procedure, there are slight risks of infection or heavy bleeding. Heavy bleeding, severe pain or cramping, or a fever over 100 degrees Fahrenheit (about 38 degrees Celsius) requires immediate medical attention. Extremely rarely, the uterus may be injured or punctured by the tool, or the cervix torn, during the procedure. The procedure should not be performed if the patient is pregnant or suffers from acute pelvic inflammatory disease or acute cervical or vaginal infections.

Abnormal cells may indicate endometrial cancer, LPD, the presence of fibroids (benign, or noncancerous, excessive growths of the smooth muscle wall of the uterus), or polyps (a usually benign growth of normal tissue attached to the lining of the uterus). Surgery and/or medication may be necessary to treat these conditions.

Ultrasound is often utilized along with endometrial sampling for initial evaluation. Patients with persistent symptoms may need additional tests and procedures. Because an endometrial biopsy often misses polyps and fibroids, alternative procedures such as dilation and curettage (D&C) or hysteroscopy may be used for further diagnostic purposes.

Perspective and Prospects

The use of endometrial sampling to diagnose and treat problems has been practiced since at least 1843. The earliest tools were wide and required scraping the uterine lining. Later devices, such as the stainless-steel Novak, or Kevorkian, curet or Vabra aspirator, cause significant discomfort. The Novak curet requires a syringe to apply suction. The Vabra aspirator is a disposable device that uses an electric suction pump to obtain the sample.

By 2006, the most used tool for endometrial biopsies was the Pipelle curet, developed in France. The curet is narrower, more flexible, and easier to insert through the cervix, and it removes the sample by suction. This device is relatively inexpensive, causes little to no discomfort to the patient, and has been shown to obtain adequate specimens in 87 to 100 percent of patients.

—*Virginia L. Salmon*

See also Biopsy; Cancer; Cervical, ovarian, and uterine cancers; Cervical procedures; Diagnosis; Genital disorders, female; Gynecology; Infertility, female; Oncology; Polyps; Reproductive system; Uterus; Women's health.

FOR FURTHER INFORMATION:

Berek, Jonathan S., ed. *Berek and Novak's Gynecology.* 14th ed. Philadelphia: Lippincott Williams & Wilkins, 2007.

Cherath, Lata. "Endometrial Biopsy." In *The Gale Encyclopedia of Medicine*, edited by Jacqueline L. Longe. 3d ed. Farmington Hill, Mich.: Thomson Gale, 2006.

Cunningham, F. Gary, et al., eds. *Williams Obstetrics.* 23d ed. New York: McGraw-Hill, 2010.

"Endometrial Biopsy: Finding the Cause of Uterine Bleeding." *Mayo Clinic Health Letter* 19, no. 8 (August, 2001): 6.

Minkin, Mary Jane, and Carol V. Wright. *The Yale Guide to Women's Reproductive Health: From Menarche to Menopause.* New Haven, Conn.: Yale University Press, 2003.

ENDOMETRIOSIS
DISEASE/DISORDER

ANATOMY OR SYSTEM AFFECTED: Reproductive system, uterus

SPECIALTIES AND RELATED FIELDS: Gynecology

DEFINITION: Growth of cells of the uterine lining at sites outside the uterus, causing severe pain and infertility.

KEY TERMS:

cervix: an oval-shaped organ that separates the uterus and the vagina

dysmenorrhea: painful menstruation

dyspareunia: painful sexual intercourse

endometrium: the tissue that lines the uterus, builds up, and sheds at the end of each menstrual cycle; when it grows outside the uterus, endometriosis occurs

Fallopian tubes: two tubes extending from the ovaries to the uterus; during ovulation, an egg travels down one of these tubes to the uterus

hysterectomy: surgery that removes part or all of the uterus

implant: an abnormal endometrial growth outside the uterus

laparoscopy: a surgical procedure in which a small incision made near the navel is used to view the uterus and other abdominal organs with a lighted tube called a laparoscope

laparotomy: a surgical procedure, often exploratory in nature, carried out through the abdominal wall; it may be used to correct endometriosis

laser: a concentrated, high-energy light beam often used to destroy abnormal tissue

oophorectomy (or ovariectomy): removal of the ovaries, which is often necessary in cases of severe endometriosis

prostaglandins: fatlike hormones that control the contraction and relaxation of the uterus and other smooth muscle tissue

CAUSES AND SYMPTOMS

Endometriosis is the presence of endometrial tissue outside its normal location as the lining of the uterus. It can be asymptomatic, mild, or a disabling disease causing severe pain. The classic symptoms of endometriosis are very painful menstruation (dysmenorrhea), painful intercourse (dyspareunia), and infertility. Some other common endometriosis symptoms include nausea, vomiting, diarrhea, and fatigue.

It has been estimated that endometriosis affects between five million and twenty-five million American women. Often, it is incorrectly stereotyped as being a disease of upwardly mobile, professional women. According to many experts, the incidence of endometriosis worldwide and across most racial groups is probably very similar. They propose that the reported occurrence rate difference for some racial groups, such as a lower incidence in African Americans, has been a socioeconomic phenomenon attributable to the social class of women who seek medical treatment for the symptoms of endometriosis and to the highly stratified responses of many health care professionals who have dealt with the disease.

The symptoms of endometriosis arise from abnormalities in the effects of the menstrual cycle on the endometrial tissue lining the uterus. The endometrium normally thickens and becomes swollen with blood (engorged) during the cycle, a process controlled by fe-

---

INFORMATION ON ENDOMETRIOSIS

CAUSES: Unknown

SYMPTOMS: Painful menstrual periods, discomfort during sexual intercourse, localized pain, infertility

DURATION: Chronic

TREATMENTS: Chemotherapy, surgery

male hormones called estrogens and progestins. This engorgement is designed to prepare the uterus for conception by optimizing conditions for implantation in the endometrium of a fertilized egg, which enters the uterus via one of the Fallopian tubes leading from the ovaries.

By the middle of the menstrual cycle, the endometrial lining is normally about ten times thicker than at its beginning. If the egg that is released into the uterus is not fertilized, pregnancy does not occur and decreases in production of the female sex hormones result in the breakdown of the endometrium. Endometrial tissue mixed with blood leaves the uterus as the menstrual flow and a new menstrual cycle begins. This series of uterine changes occurs repeatedly, as a monthly cycle, from puberty (which usually occurs between the ages of twelve and fourteen) to the menopause (which usually occurs between the ages of forty-five and fifty-five).

In women who develop endometriosis, some endometrial tissue begins to grow ectopically (in an abnormal position) at sites outside the uterus. The ectopic endometrial growths may be found attached to the ovaries, the Fallopian tubes, the urinary bladder, the rectum, other abdominal organs, and even the lungs. Regardless of body location, these implants behave as if they were still in the uterus, thickening and bleeding each month as the menstrual cycle proceeds. Like the endometrium at its normal uterine site, the ectopic tissue responds to the hormones that circulate through the body in the blood. Its inappropriate position in the body prevents this ectopic endometrial tissue from leaving the body as menstrual flow; as a result, some implants grow to be quite large.

In many cases, the endometrial growths that form between two organs become fibrous bands called adhesions. The fibrous nature of adhesions is attributable to the alternating swelling and breakdown of the ectopic tissue, which yields fibrous scar tissue. The alterations in size of living portions of the adhesions and other endometrial implants during the monthly menstrual cycle cause many afflicted women considerable pain. Because the body location of implants varies, the site of the pain may be almost anywhere, such as the back, chest, thighs, pelvis, rectum, or abdomen. For example, dyspareunia occurs when adhesions hold a uterus tightly to the abdominal wall, making its movement during intercourse painful. Many women report significant pain on a monthly basis with ovulation as well.

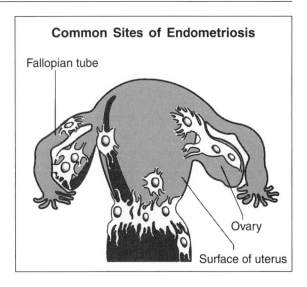

Common Sites of Endometriosis

Fallopian tube

Ovary

Surface of uterus

The presence of endometriosis is usually confirmed by laparoscopy, viewed as being the most reliable method for its diagnosis. Laparoscopy is carried out after a physician makes an initial diagnosis of probable endometriosis from a combined study including an examination of the patient's medical history and careful exploration of the patient's physical problems over a period of at least six months. During prelaparoscopy treatment, the patient is very often maintained on pain medication and other therapeutic drugs that will produce symptomatic relief.

For laparoscopy, the patient is anesthetized with a general anesthetic, a small incision is made near the navel, and a flexible lighted tube—a laparoscope—is inserted into this incision. The laparoscope, equipped with fiber optics, enables the examining physician to search the patient's abdominal organs for endometrial implants. Visibility of the abdominal organs in laparoscopic examination can be enhanced by pumping harmless carbon dioxide gas into the abdomen, causing it to distend. Women who undergo laparoscopy usually require a day of postoperative bed rest, followed by seven to ten days of curtailed physical activity. After a laparoscopic diagnosis of endometriosis is made, a variety of surgical and therapeutic drug treatments can be employed to manage the disease.

About 40 percent of all women who have endometriosis are infertile; contemporary wisdom evaluates this relationship as one of cause and effect, which should make this disease the second most common cause of fertility problems. The actual basis for this infertility is not always clear, but it is often the result of damage to the ovaries and Fallopian tubes, scar tissue produced by implants on these and other abdominal organs, and hormone imbalances.

Because the incidence of infertility accompanying endometriosis increases with the severity of the disease, all potentially afflicted women are encouraged to seek early diagnosis. Many experts advise all women with abnormal menstrual cycles, dysmenorrhea, severe menstrual bleeding, abnormal vaginal bleeding, and repeated dyspareunia to seek the advice of a physician trained in identifying and dealing with endometriosis. Because the disease can begin to present symptoms at any age, teenagers are also encouraged to seek medical attention if they experience any of these symptoms.

John Sampson coined the term "endometriosis" in the 1920's. Sampson's theory for its causation, still widely accepted, is termed retrograde menstruation. Also called menstrual backup, this theory proposes that the backing up of some menstrual flow into the Fallopian tubes, and then into the abdominal cavity, forms the endometrial implants. Evidence supporting this theory, according to many physicians, is the fact that such backup is common. Others point out, however, that the backup is often found in women who do not have the disease. A surgical experiment was performed on female monkeys to test this theory. Their uteri were turned upside down so that the menstrual flow would spill into the abdominal cavity. Sixty percent of the animals developed endometriosis postoperatively—an inconclusive result.

Complicating the issue is the fact that implants are also found in tissues (such as in the lung) that cannot be reached by menstrual backup. It has been theorized that the presence of these implants results from the entry of endometrial cells into the lymphatic system, which returns body fluid to the blood and protects the body from many other diseases. This transplantation theory is supported by the occurrence of endometriosis in various portions of the lymphatic system and in tissues that could not otherwise become sites of endometriosis.

A third theory explaining the growth of implants is the iatrogenic, or nosocomial, transmission of endometrial tissue. These terms both indicate an accidental creation of the disease through the actions of physicians. Such implant formation is viewed as occurring most often after cesarean delivery of a baby when passage through the birth canal would otherwise be fatal to mother and/or child. Another proposed cause is episiotomy—widening of the birth canal by an incision between the anus and vagina—to ease births.

Any surgical procedure that allows the spread of endometrial tissue can be implicated, including surgical procedures carried out to correct existing endometriosis, because of the ease with which endometrial tissue implants itself anywhere in the body. Abnormal endometrial tissue growth, called adenomyosis, can also occur in the uterus and is viewed as a separate disease entity.

Other theories regarding the genesis of endometriosis include an immunologic theory, which proposes that women who develop endometriosis are lacking in antibodies that normally cause the destruction of endometrial tissue at sites where it does not belong, and a hormonal theory, which suggests the existence of large imbalances in hormones such as the prostaglandins that serve as the body's messengers in controlling biological processes. Several of these theories—retrograde menstruation, the transplantation theory, and iatrogenic transmission—all have support, but none has been proved unequivocally. Future evidence will identify whether one cause is dominant, whether they all interact to produce the disease, or whether endometriosis is actually a group of diseases that simply resemble one another in the eyes of contemporary medical science.

TREATMENT AND THERAPY

Laparoscopic examination most often identifies endometriosis as chocolate-colored lumps (chocolate cysts) ranging from the size of a pinhead to several inches across or as filmy coverings over parts of abdominal organs and ligaments. Once a diagnosis of the disease is confirmed by laparoscopy, endometriosis is treated by chemotherapy, surgery, or a combination of both methods. The only permanent contemporary cure for endometriosis, however, is the onset of the biological menopause at the end of a woman's childbearing years. As long as menstruation continues, implant development is likely to recur, regardless of its cause. Nevertheless, a temporary cure of endometriosis is better than no cure at all.

The chemotherapy that many physicians use to treat mild cases of endometriosis (and for prelaparoscopy periods) is analgesic painkillers, including aspirin, acetaminophen, and ibuprofen. The analgesics inhibit the body's production of prostaglandins, and the symptoms of the disease are merely covered up. Therefore, analgesics are of quite limited value except during a prelaparoscopy diagnostic period or with mild cases of endometriosis. In addition, the long-term administration of aspirin will often produce gastrointestinal bleeding, and excess use of acetaminophen can lead to severe liver damage. In some cases of very severe endometriosis pain, narcotic painkillers are given, such as codeine, Percodan (oxycodone and aspirin), or morphine. Narcotics are addicting and should be avoided unless absolutely necessary.

More effective for long-term management of the disease is hormone therapy. Such therapy is designed to prevent the monthly occurrence of menstruation—that is, to freeze the body in a sort of chemical menopause. The hormone types used, made by pharmaceutical companies, are chemical cousins of female hormones (estrogens and progestins), male hormones (androgens), and a brain hormone that controls ovulation (gonadotropin-releasing hormone, or GnRH). Appropriate hormone therapy is often useful for years, although each hormone class produces disadvantageous side effects in many patients.

The use of estrogens stops ovulation and menstruation, freeing many women with endometriosis from painful symptoms. Numerous estrogen preparations have been prescribed, including the birth control pills that contain them. Drawbacks of estrogen use can include weight gain, nausea, breast soreness, depression, blood-clotting abnormalities, and elevated risk of vaginal cancer. In addition, estrogen administration may cause endometrial implants to enlarge.

The use of progestins arose from the discovery that pregnancy—which is maintained by high levels of a natural progestin called progesterone—reversed the symptoms of many suffering from endometriosis. This realization led to the utilization of synthetic progestins to cause prolonged false pregnancy. The rationale is that all endometrial implants will die off and be reabsorbed during the prolonged absence of menstruation. The method works in most patients, and pain-free periods of up to five years are often observed. In some cases, however, side effects include nausea, depression, insomnia, and a very slow resumption of normal menstruation (such as lags of up to a year) when the therapy is stopped. In addition, progestins are ineffective in treating large implants; in fact, their use in such cases can lead to severe complications.

In the 1970's, studies showing the poten-

tial for heart attacks, high blood pressure, and strokes in patients receiving long-term female hormone therapy led to a search for more advantageous hormone medications. An alternative developed was the synthetic male hormone danazol (Danocrine), which is very effective. Danazol works by decreasing the amount of estrogen which is produced by the ovaries on a monthly basis to close to that which is present at menopause. The lack of estrogen prevents endometrial cells from growing, thereby eliminating most of the symptoms associated with endometriosis. One of its advantages over female hormones is the ability to shrink large im-

---

IN THE NEWS: LINK BETWEEN ENDOMETRIOSIS AND OTHER DISEASES

In the October, 2002, issue of *Human Reproduction*, the Endometriosis Association and the National Institutes of Health (NIH) announced the results of a study involving 3,680 women who were members of the Endometriosis Association and who had been diagnosed with endometriosis. The study suggested that women with endometriosis are significantly more likely than other women to contract a number of serious autoimmune diseases including lupus, Sjögren's syndrome, rheumatoid arthritis, and multiple sclerosis.

Although a study conducted in 1980 established a link between endometriosis and immune dysfunctions, the new study sought to identify specific diseases for which women with endometriosis are at higher risk. In addition to the connection between endometriosis and autoimmune diseases, researchers found that the women in the study were more than one hundred times more likely than women in the general population to suffer from chronic fatigue syndrome; twice as likely to suffer from fibromyalgia (recurrent debilitating pain in the muscles, tendons, and ligaments), and seven times as likely to suffer from hypothyroidism (which can also be an autoimmune disorder). Researchers also found that the women studied reported higher rates of allergies and asthma than women in the general population.

Researchers warn that the study may not be representative of all patients with endometriosis, both because members of the Endometriosis Association are most probably those patients suffering pain from their condition and because the survey was completed predominantly by white, educated women. Even so, this new information provides more light on an enigmatic disease and should help health care professionals treat patients.

—*Cassandra Kircher, Ph.D.*

plants and restore fertility to those patients whose problems arise from nonfunctional ovaries or Fallopian tubes. Danazol has become the drug of choice for treating millions of endometriosis sufferers. Problems associated with danazol use, however, can include weight gain, masculinization (decreased bust size, increased muscle mass, muscle cramping, facial hair growth, and deepened voice), fatigue, depression, and baldness. Those women contemplating danazol use should be aware that it can also complicate pregnancy.

Because of the side effects of these hormones, other chemotherapy was sought. Another valuable drug that has become available is GnRH, which suppresses the function of the ovaries in a fashion equivalent to surgical oophorectomy (removal of the ovaries). This hormone produces none of the side effects of the sex hormones, such as weight gain, depression, or masculinization, but some evidence indicates that it may lead to osteoporosis.

Thus, despite the fact that hormone therapy may relieve or reduce pain for years, contemporary chemotherapy is flawed by many undesirable side effects. Perhaps more serious, however, is the high recurrence rate of endometriosis that is observed after the therapy is stopped. Consequently, it appears that the best treatment of endometriosis combines chemotherapy with surgery.

The extent of the surgery carried out to combat endometriosis is variable and depends on the observations made during laparoscopy. In cases of relatively mild endometriosis, conservative laparotomy surgery removes endometriosis implants, adhesions, and lesions. This type of procedure attempts to relieve endometriosis pain, to minimize the chances of postoperative recurrence of the disease, and to allow the patient to have children. Even in the most severe cases of this type, the uterus, an ovary, and its associated Fallopian tube are retained. Such surgery will often include removal of the appendix, whether diseased or not, because it is very likely to develop implants. The surgical techniques performed are the conventional excision of diseased tissue or the use of lasers to vaporize it. Many physicians prefer lasers because it is believed that they decrease the chances of recurrent endometriosis resulting from retained implant tissue or iatrogenic causes. In a new procedure, following the removal of endometrial tissue by surgical means, an intrauterine device containing Levonogestrel (a hormone which will decrease estrogen levels) is placed in order to prevent recurrence of endometriosis.

In more serious cases, hysterectomy is carried out. All visible implants, adhesions, and lesions are removed from the abdominal organs, as in conservative surgery. In addition, the uterus and cervix are taken out, but one or both ovaries are retained. This allows female hormone production to continue normally until the menopause. Uterine removal makes it impossible to have children, however, and may lead to profound psychological problems that require psychiatric help. Women planning to elect for hysterectomy to treat endometriosis should be aware of such potential difficulties. In many cases of conservative surgery or hysterectomy, danazol is used, both preoperatively and postoperatively, to minimize implant size.

The most extensive surgery carried out on the women afflicted with endometriosis is radical hysterectomy, also called definitive surgery, in which the ovaries and/or the vagina are also removed. The resultant symptoms are menopausal and may include vaginal bleeding atrophy (when the vagina is retained), increased risk of heart disease, and the development of osteoporosis. To counter the occurrence of these symptoms, replacement therapy with female hormones is suggested. Paradoxically, this hormone therapy can lead to the return of endometriosis by stimulating the growth of residual implant tissue.

Recently, more women have turned to complementary and alternative medicine in an attempt to relieve the symptoms of endometriosis. Acupuncture, homeopathy, and herbal therapy are currently being explored as means of treatment for endometriosis.

Perspective and Prospects

Modern treatment of endometriosis is viewed by many physicians as beginning in the 1950's. A landmark development in this field was the accurate diagnosis of endometriosis via the laparoscope, which was invented in Europe and introduced into the United States in the 1960's. Medical science has progressed greatly since that time. Physicians and researchers have recognized the wide occurrence of the disease and accepted its symptoms as valid; realized that hysterectomy will not necessarily put an end to the disease; utilized chemotherapeutic tools, including hormones and painkillers, as treatments and as adjuncts to surgery; developed laser surgery and other techniques that decrease the occurrence of formerly ignored iatrogenic endometriosis; and understood that the disease can ravage teenagers as well and that these young women should be examined as early as possible.

Research into endometriosis is ongoing, and the efforts and information base of the proactive American Endometriosis Association, founded in 1980, have been very valuable. As a result, a potentially or presently afflicted woman is much more aware of the problems associated with the disease. In addition, she has a source for obtaining objective information on topics including state-of-the-art treatment, physician and hospital choice, and both physical and psychological outcomes of treatment.

Many potentially viable avenues for better endometriosis diagnosis and treatment have become the objects of intense investigation. These include the use of ultrasonography and radiology techniques for the predictive, nonsurgical examination of the course of growth or the chemotherapeutic destruction of implants; the design of new drugs to be utilized in the battle against endometriosis; endeavors aimed at the development of diagnostic tests for the disease that will stop it before symptoms develop; and the design of dietary treatments to soften its effects.

Regrettably, because of the insidious nature of endometriosis—which has the ability to strike almost anywhere in the body—some confusion about the disease still exists. New drugs, surgical techniques, and other aids are expected to be helpful in clarifying many of these issues. Particular value is being placed on the study of the immunologic aspects of endometriosis. Scientists hope to explain why the disease strikes some women and not others, to uncover its etiologic basis, and to solve the widespread problems of iatrogenic implant formation and other types of endometriosis recurrence.

—*Sanford S. Singer, Ph.D.;*
updated by Robin Kamienny Montvilo, R.N., Ph.D.

See also Amenorrhea; Cervical, ovarian, and uterine cancers; Childbirth complications; Dysmenorrhea; Endometrial biopsy; Genital disorders, female; Gynecology; Hormone therapy; Hysterectomy; Infertility, female; Menorrhagia; Menstruation; Pregnancy and gestation; Reproductive system; Uterus; Women's health.

FOR FURTHER INFORMATION:

Berek, Jonathan S., ed. *Berek and Novak's Gynecology.* 14th ed. Philadelphia: Lippincott Williams & Wilkins, 2007. A standard text covering all aspects of gynecology with an emphasis on diagnosis and treatment. Topics include biology and physiology, family planning, sexuality, evaluation of pelvic infections, early pregnancy loss, benign breast disease, benign gynecologic conditions, malignant diseases of the reproductive tract, and breast cancer.

Endometriosis.org. http://www.endometriosis.org. A Web site that offers FAQs about the disease, research articles, case histories, information about local support groups, diagnosis and treatment information, and a glossary.

Fernandez, I., C. Reid, and S. Dziurawiec. "Living with Endometriosis: The Perspective of Male Partners." *Journal of Psychosomatic Research* 61, no. 4 (October, 2006): 433-438. This study explores the experience of the male partners of women with endometriosis.

Henderson, Lorraine, and Ros Wood. *Explaining Endometriosis*. 2d ed. St. Leonards, N.S.W.: Allen and Unwin, 2000. Details possible causes, diagnosis, surgeries, and current treatment options for endometriosis.

Phillips, Robert H., and Glenda Motta. *Coping with Endometriosis*. New York: Avery, 2000. Educates the reader on current research and addresses the psychological and emotional concerns brought on by a diagnosis.

Physicians' Desk Reference. 64th ed. Montvale, N.J.: PDR Network, 2009. This classic reference source on prescription drugs includes the drugs used against endometriosis, the companies that produce them, their useful dose ranges, their effects on metabolism and toxicology, and their contraindications.

Shaw, Michael, ed. *Everything You Need to Know About Diseases*. Springhouse, Pa.: Springhouse Press, 1996. This well-illustrated consumer reference, compiled by more than one hundred doctors and medical experts, describes five hundred illnesses and conditions, including their causes, symptoms, diagnosis, treatment, and prevention. Of particular interest is chapter 9, "Gynecologic Disorders."

Sherwood, Lauralee. *Human Physiology: From Cells to Systems*. 7th ed. Pacific Grove, Calif.: Brooks/Cole/Cengage Learning, 2010. This college text contains much useful biological information. Included are details about the menstrual cycle, hormones, the endometrium, and many helpful definitions. Clearly written, the book is a mine of information for interested readers.

Weinstein, Kate. *Living with Endometriosis*. Reading, Mass.: Addison-Wesley, 1991. The main divisions of this handy book are medical aspects, treatments and outcomes, emotional problems, and pain and psychiatric problems. Highlights include the complete description of the female reproductive system and menstruation, the glossary, and appendixes on organizations, literature, and pain management centers.

Weschler, Toni. *Taking Charge of Your Fertility.* Rev. ed. New York: Collins, 2001. Explores common health issues of women and their role in preventing pregnancy.

Endoscopic retrograde cholangiopancreatography (ERCP)

Procedure

Anatomy or system affected: Abdomen, gallbladder, gastrointestinal system, liver, pancreas, stomach

Specialties and related fields: Gastroenterology, internal medicine, radiology

Definition: A procedure combining elements of an X ray with an endoscope to look into the digestive system.

Key terms:

duodenum: the first part of the small intestine

endoscope: a hollow, flexible, telescope-like tube about the size of a pen in diameter and about 2.5 feet long with a lens, light, and holes on the end

gastroenterologist: a doctor specializing in the digestive system

sphincterotomy: a small cut made in a muscle surrounding the opening of a duct, usually made by cauterization

stent: a small, hollow device left in a duct or tube to keep it open

INDICATIONS AND PROCEDURES

Endoscopic retrograde cholangiopancreatography (ERCP) is usually performed if a patient is experiencing jaundice, unexplained pain in the upper abdomen, or unexplained weight loss. It is used to determine the sources of these conditions. ERCP can be used to find tumors, blockages, cysts, tissue irregularities, or gallstones. It may also be used to discover the source of inflammation in the liver, bile ducts (which drain the liver, gallbladder, and pancreas), gallbladder, or pancreas. If imaging or blood tests are confusing or inconclusive, this procedure may be used to clarify those inconsistencies. ERCP may also help to plan surgery for a patient who is already known to be suffering from gallbladder or pancreatic disease or who has a mass or tumor shown in imaging processes.

ERCP is usually performed by a gastroenterologist who has had further training specifically in ERCP procedures. It may be performed in a hospital or a clinic. The patient lies down on a radiology bed and is sedated, usually through an IV, to relax the involuntary muscles. An anesthetic is sprayed in the patient's throat to counteract any gag reflex, and a guard may be placed over the teeth and gums to protect them during the procedure. The endoscope is inserted into the throat, and the patient is asked to swallow to help the endoscope into the correct position. The endoscope is then guided through the digestive system to the duodenum. Then a small catheter is inserted into the hollow endoscope until it reaches the duct system. Iodine or another type of contrast solution (dye) is put into the catheter so that the duct system can be shown on X rays. X rays are then taken and examined while the endoscope remains in place. The patient may be asked to change positions so the doctor can view different structures.

Usually, this procedure is performed in an outpatient setting, and the patient is released to go home (with a designated driver) after the sedative wears off. Occasionally, a patient may stay in the hospital for a longer period, particularly when further procedures, as described below, are performed at the time of the ERCP or when complications develop.

USES AND COMPLICATIONS

Some problems can be identified and solved during the ERCP procedure. Depending what is shown on the X rays taken during this procedure, the doctor may be able to perform further procedures, such as removing gallstones (which may involve crushing the stones and removing them or simply leaving them in the intestines to pass through the digestive system naturally), taking tissue biopsies, dilating a duct with a balloon, performing a sphincterotomy, or inserting a stent. Other problems, such as possible cancers, will need to be identified through tissue samples and treated later.

Serious complications from ERCP are rare. One possible serious complication is aspiration (inhaling) of saliva, which may lead to pneumonia. Other serious complications may include perforation, inflammation, bleeding, injury, or infection of any of the organs examined or the stomach, esophagus, or intestines. Complications from sedation and contrast dyes, such as allergies, are also possible. More common complications are nausea and stomach pain. One may feel discomfort (such as a sore throat), tenderness, or bloating, depending on whether air is blown into the endoscope during the process to open up the structures that the doctor wishes to view.

Factors that complicate this procedure include obesity, allergies, diabetes, hypertension, or certain drugs, especially anticlotting drugs. Another complicating factor may be that the patient has not fasted for at least six hours prior to this procedure as instructed.

PERSPECTIVE AND PROSPECTS

Endoscopic procedures were first reported in 1968. Improvements to the procedure, then called endoscopic cholangiopancreatography (ECPG), occurred throughout the early 1970's, when Japanese doctors worked with engineers to develop better instruments to use during the procedure. The procedure spread through Europe during the 1970's and soon became known as a valuable diagnostic tool despite its potential for serious complications in its early stages. From the mid-1970's, it was recognized as a cost-saving alternative to surgical procedures with a much quicker recovery time for the patient. With the addition of X ray technology, it became an often used diagnostic and therapeutic tool.

With improvements in imaging technology, such as high-quality ultrasound, computed tomography (CT) scans, endoscopic ultrasonography, and magnetic resonance imaging (MRI), the use of this procedure for solely diagnostic purposes has diminished somewhat. Its use as a therapeutic tool is still acknowledged, however, and it is still an alternative diagnostic procedure when noninvasive procedures result in inconclusive diagnosis.

—*Marianne M. Madsen, M.S.*

See also Abdomen; Abdominal disorders; Arthritis; Arthroscopy; Biopsy; Cholecystectomy; Colon and rectal polyp removal; Colon cancer; Colonoscopy and sigmoidoscopy; Cystoscopy; Endoscopy; Gallbladder diseases; Gastrointestinal disorders; Gastrointestinal system; Invasive tests; Laparoscopy; Pulmonary diseases; Stone removal; Stones.

FOR FURTHER INFORMATION:

Aronson, Naomi. *Endoscopic Retrograde Cholangiopancreatography.* Washington, D.C.: Department of Health and Human Services, Public Health Service, Agency for Healthcare Research and Quality, 2002.

Cotton, P. B., and J. W. Leung, eds. *Advanced Digestive Endoscopy: ERCP.* Hoboken, N.J.: Wiley-Blackwell, 2006.

Seigel, J. H., J. Delmont, and A. G. Harris. *Endoscopic Retrograde Cholangiopancreatography: Technique,* *Diagnosis, and Therapy.* New York: Raven Press, 1991.

Talley, N. J., and C. J. Martin. *Clinical Gastroenterology: A Practical Problem-Based Approach.* Philadelphia: Churchill-Livingstone/Elsevier, 2006.

ENDOSCOPY
PROCEDURE

ANATOMY OR SYSTEM AFFECTED: Abdomen, anus, bladder, gastrointestinal system, intestines, joints, knees, lungs, stomach, urinary system

SPECIALTIES AND RELATED FIELDS: Gastroenterology, gynecology, obstetrics, orthopedics, proctology, pulmonary medicine, urology

DEFINITION: The use of a flexible tube to look into body structures in order to inspect and sometimes correct pathologies.

KEY TERMS:

biopsy: the collection and study of body tissue, often to determine whether it is cancerous

fiber optics: the transmission of light through thin, flexible tubes

pathology: a disease condition; also the study of diseases

INDICATIONS AND PROCEDURES

Early endoscopes were simply rigid hollow tubes with a light source. They were inserted into body orifices, such as the anus or the mouth, to allow the physician to look directly at structures and processes within. Modern instruments are more sophisticated. They use fiber optics in flexible cables to penetrate deep into body structures. For example, one form of colonoscope can be threaded though the entire lower intestine, allowing the physician to search for pathologies all the way from the anus to the cecum of the colon (large intestine).

There are eight basic types of endoscope: gastroscope, colonoscope, bronchoscope, cystoscope, laparoscope, colposcope, arthroscope, and amnioscope. Their primary uses are diagnostic; however, they can be fitted with special instruments to perform many different tasks, including taking bits of tissue for biopsy and carrying out surgical procedures.

USES AND COMPLICATIONS

The gastroscope and its variants are used to inspect structures of the gastrointestinal system. The name of one class of procedure gives an idea of how sophisticated the gastroscope has become: esophagogastro-

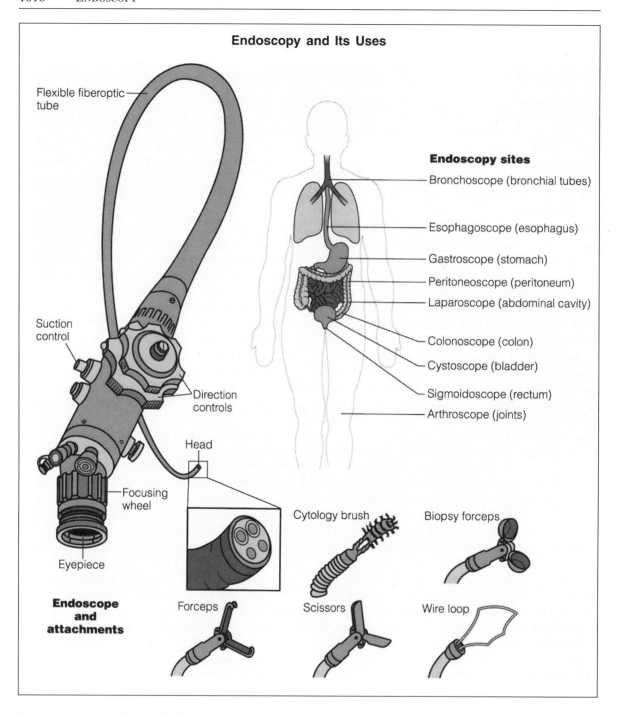

Endoscopy and Its Uses

Flexible fiberoptic tube

Suction control

Direction controls

Head

Focusing wheel

Eyepiece

Endoscope and attachments

Forceps

Cytology brush

Scissors

Biopsy forceps

Wire loop

Endoscopy sites

Bronchoscope (bronchial tubes)

Esophagoscope (esophagus)

Gastroscope (stomach)

Peritoneoscope (peritoneum)

Laparoscope (abdominal cavity)

Colonoscope (colon)

Cystoscope (bladder)

Sigmoidoscope (rectum)

Arthroscope (joints)

duodenoscopy. As the term implies, this technique can be used to investigate the esophagus (the tube leading to the stomach), the stomach itself, and the intestines all the way into the duodenum (the first link of the small intestine). Furthermore, in a procedure called endoscopic retrograde cholangiopancreatography, the endoscope can be used to investigate processes in the gall-bladder, the cystic duct, the common hepatic duct, and the common bile duct. By far the most common use of the gastroscope is in the diagnosis and management of esophageal and stomach problems. The gastroscope is used to confirm the suspicion of stomach ulcers and other gastroesophageal conditions and to monitor therapy.

The colonoscope and its variants are critical in the diagnosis of diseases in the lower intestine and in some aspects of therapy. The long, flexible fiber-optic tube can be threaded through the anus and rectum into the S-shaped sigmoid colon (flexible fiber-optic sigmoidoscopy). The tube can be made to rise up the descending colon, across the transverse colon, and down the ascending colon to the cecum. With the colonoscope, the physician can discover abnormalities such as polyps, diverticula, and blockages and the presence of cancer, Crohn's disease, ulcerative colitis, and many other diseases. The physician can also use the colonoscope to remove polyps; this is the major therapeutic use of colonoscopy.

Like most other forms of endoscopy, bronchoscopy is used for both diagnosis and treatment. The bronchoscope allows direct visualization of the trachea (the tube leading from the throat to the lungs) and the bronchi (the two main air ducts leading into the lungs). It will show certain forms of lung cancer, various infectious states, and other pathologies. The bronchoscope can also be used to remove foreign objects, excise local tumors, remove mucus plugs, and improve bronchial drainage.

The cystoscope is used for visual inspection of the urethra and bladder. The bladder stores urine; the urethra is the tube through which it is eliminated. Cystoscopy discovers many of the conditions that can afflict these organs: obstruction, infection, cancer, and other disorders.

The laparoscope is used to look into the abdominal cavity for evidence of a wide variety of conditions. It can inspect the liver, help evaluate liver disease, and take tissue samples for biopsy. Laparoscopy can confirm the diagnosis of ectopic pregnancy (a condition in which a fetus develops outside the womb, usually in one of the Fallopian tubes). It can confirm the presence or absence of abdominal cancers and diagnose disease conditions in the gallbladder, spleen, peritoneum (the membrane that surrounds the abdomen), and the diaphragm, as well as give some views of the small and large intestine. In an important, relatively new development, the laparoscope is being used to remove gallbladders (cholecystectomy). This procedure is far less traumatic than the old surgery, often permitting release of the patient a day or two after the operation rather than requiring weeks of recuperation.

The colposcope is used to inspect vaginal tissue and adjacent organs. Common reasons for colposcopy include abnormal bleeding and suspicion of tumors.

Arthroscopy, the investigation of joint structures by endoscopy, is now the most common invasive technique used on patients with arthritis or joint damage. In addition to viewing the area, the arthroscope can be fitted with various instruments to perform surgical procedures.

The term "amnioscope" comes from the amnion, the membrane that surrounds a fetus. This type of endoscope is used to enter the uterus and inspect the growing fetus in the search for any visible abnormalities.

Endoscopy is one of the most useful and most-used techniques for diagnosis because it permits the investigation of many internal body organs without surgery. It is extraordinarily safe in the hands of experienced practitioners and is relatively free of pain and discomfort. In addition, specialized endoscopes are assuming greater roles in therapy. Many procedures that once involved major surgery can now be conducted through the endoscope, saving the patient pain, trauma, and expense.

PERSPECTIVE AND PROSPECTS

Endoscopes have become highly sophisticated instruments with enormous range throughout the body and enormous potential. Colonoscopy, for example, promises to revolutionize the treatment of cancerous and precancerous polyps by helping physicians attain a clearer understanding of the polyp-to-cancer progression. The laparoscope has revolutionized gallbladder removal, as the arthroscope has revolutionized joint surgery. The gastroscope gives the physician new security and control in the management of gastrointestinal conditions, and the bronchoscope facilitates many lung procedures.

Similarly throughout the entire range of endoscopy, new opportunities are opening and leading to significant improvements in therapy, and these improvements will continue. Electronic and video techniques are being introduced into endoscopy, and this new technology promises to widen the applications and therapeutic range of endoscopy still further.

—*C. Richard Falcon*

See also Abdomen; Abdominal disorders; Arthritis; Arthroscopy; Biopsy; Cholecystectomy; Colonoscopy and sigmoidoscopy; Colorectal cancer; Colorectal polyp removal; Cystoscopy; Endoscopic retrograde cholangiopancreatography (ERCP); Gallbladder diseases; Gastrointestinal disorders; Gastrointestinal system; Invasive tests; Laparoscopy; Pulmonary diseases; Stone removal; Stones.

FOR FURTHER INFORMATION:

Classen, Meinhard, G. N. J. Tytgat, and C. J. Lightdale, eds. *Gastroenterological Endoscopy.* 2d ed. New York: Thieme Medical, 2010. Text that examines such topics as the impact of endoscopy, its history of use, diagnostic procedures and techniques, therapeutic procedures, descriptions of diseases involving the upper and lower intestine, endoscopic features of infectious diseases of the GI tract, and pediatric endoscopy.

Emory, Theresa S., et al. *Atlas of Gastrointestinal Endoscopy and Endoscopic Biopsies.* Washington, D.C.: Armed Forces Institute of Pathology, 2000. This resource is divided into four major sections that correspond to the major endoscopic divisions of the gastrointestinal tract. Each section begins with an overview of the endoscopic examination and the histology.

Litin, Scott C., ed. *Mayo Clinic Family Health Book.* 4th ed. New York: HarperResource, 2009. Perhaps the best general medical text for the layperson, this book covers the entire medical field. While the information is derived from a wide variety of highly technical sources, the articles are written to be easily understood by a general audience.

Scott-Conner, Carol E. H., ed. *The SAGES Manual: Fundamentals of Laparoscopy, Thoracoscopy, and GI Endoscopy.* 2d ed. New York: Springer, 2006. Explains the major laparoscopic and flexible endoscopic procedures.

ENEMAS

PROCEDURE

ANATOMY OR SYSTEM AFFECTED: Abdomen, anus, gastrointestinal system, intestines

SPECIALTIES AND RELATED FIELDS: Gastroenterology

DEFINITION: A procedure to assist the body in evacuating fecal material from the bowel.

INDICATIONS AND PROCEDURES

Enemas are used primarily for two purposes: cleansing and retention. Many solutions have been used to promote cleansing. The most commonly used is made up of mild soapsuds and tap water. Commercially prepared solutions containing premeasured mild soap and water are also available.

To receive an enema, the patient should lie on the left side of the body with the upper thigh drawn up to the abdomen. The solution should be slightly above body temperature. The source of the enema fluid should be 30 to 45 centimeters (12 to 18 inches) above the anus. All air should be removed from the tubing that connects the enema reservoir and the tip. The tip is warmed in the hands, lubricated with a commercial preparation or a bit of soapy water, and gently inserted into the anus with a combination of soft pressure and a twisting motion. The tip should not be inserted more than 10 centimeters (4 inches) into the rectum. The solution is allowed to flow slowly into the rectum to prevent cramping.

A towel may be held gently against the rectum to prevent leakage. If cramping does occur, the flow should be interrupted by pinching the tubing. For an adult, approximately 1 liter (1 quart) of solution is probably sufficient; the patient should hold the solution for two to three minutes. The enema tube is tightly clamped and slowly withdrawn; a towel is again held against the anus to catch any leakage. A readily available bedpan or toilet stool is used while the patient evacuates the bowel. Depending on the need for the enema, the procedure may be repeated.

The procedure for administering a retention enema is similar except that the solution is instilled very slowly to promote retention. Lubricants or medicines are administered in this fashion. The patient holds the instilled solution as long as possible before evacuating the bowel.

USES AND COMPLICATIONS

Cleansing enemas are used to promote bowel evacuation by softening fecal material and stimulating the movement by bowel walls (peristalsis). Retention enemas are used to lubricate or soothe the mucosal lining of the rectum, to apply medication to the bowel wall or for absorption by the colon, and to soften feces.

There is no physiological need to have a bowel movement every day; normality is defined as from three to ten per week. Enemas should not be used routinely for cleansing because the bowel quickly becomes dependent on them. This problem is especially common among older individuals.

—*L. Fleming Fallon, Jr., M.D., Ph.D., M.P.H.*

See also Anus; Colon; Colonoscopy and sigmoidoscopy; Colorectal cancer; Colorectal polyp removal; Colorectal surgery; Gastroenterology; Gastrointestinal disorders; Gastrointestinal system; Hemorrhoid banding and removal; Hemorrhoids; Internal medicine; Intestines; Peristalsis; Proctology; Rectum; Surgery, general.

FOR FURTHER INFORMATION:

Heuman, Douglas M., A. Scott Mills, and Hunter H. McGuire, Jr. *Gastroenterology*. Philadelphia: W. B. Saunders, 1997.

Icon Health. *Enemas: A Medical Dictionary, Bibliography, and Annotated Research Guide to Internet References*. San Diego, Calif.: Author, 2003.

Mitsuoka, Tomotari. *Intestinal Bacteria and Health*. Translated by Syoko Watanabe and W. C. T. Leung. Tokyo: Harcourt Brace Jovanovich, 1978.

Peikin, Steven R. *Gastrointestinal Health*. Rev. ed. New York: Quill, 2001.

ENTEROCOLITIS
DISEASE/DISORDER

ALSO KNOWN AS: Acute infectious diarrhea

ANATOMY OR SYSTEM AFFECTED: Gastrointestinal system, intestines

SPECIALTIES AND RELATED FIELDS: Family medicine, gastroenterology, pediatrics

DEFINITION: Inflammation of the small and large intestines, which may be caused by a severe bacterial infection.

CAUSES AND SYMPTOMS

Enterocolitis is characterized by copious and sometimes bloody diarrhea, abdominal pain, vomiting, and dehydration. A high fever usually exists in young children. Cultures of the stool and blood can establish the exact organism involved.

Campylobacter enterocolitis, resulting from infection with *Campylobacter* bacteria, is the most common bacterial cause of diarrhea. It is endemic in developing countries, and epidemics are seen in Western countries in daycare centers. Salmonella enterocolitis is an infection in the lining of the small intestine caused by *Salmonella* bacteria acquired through the ingestion of contaminated food or water or exposure to reptiles. This type of enterocolitis can range from mild to severe and lasts from one to two weeks.

A different type of enterocolitis is necrotizing enterocolitis (NEC), the most common gastrointestinal medical emergency occurring in newborns. It is more prevalent in premature infants. NEC may begin with poor feeding, abdominal distention or tenderness, and decreased bowel sounds. If it becomes systemic, then symptoms can include apnea, lethargy, shock, and cardiovascular collapse. Outbreaks of NEC seem to follow an epidemic pattern, suggesting an infectious disease, but a specific causative organism has not been identified. Research suggests that several factors may be involved.

TREATMENT AND THERAPY

The treatment of bacterial enterocolitis involves rehydration and, in some cases, antibiotics. In underdeveloped countries, where medical care is poor, enterocolitis causes more than 60 percent of all deaths in children under age five.

Infants with NEC cannot take food by mouth and often must be fed through a central venous catheter. Those with severe disease may require surgical intervention such as intestinal resection. The mortality rate for NEC approaches 50 percent in infants weighing less than 1,500 grams.

—Connie Rizzo, M.D., Ph.D.;
updated by Tracy Irons-Georges

See also Antibiotics; Bacterial infections; *Campylobacter* infections; Dehydration; Diarrhea and dysentery; Fever; Gastroenterology, pediatric; Gastrointestinal disorders; Gastrointestinal system; Intestinal disorders; Intestines; Nausea and vomiting; Salmonella infection.

INFORMATION ON ENTEROCOLITIS

CAUSES: Bacterial infection; unknown for necrotizing enterocolitis

SYMPTOMS: For bacterial infection, copious and sometimes bloody diarrhea, abdominal pain, vomiting, dehydration, high fever in young children; for necrotizing enterocolitis, poor feeding, abdominal distention or tenderness, decreased bowel sounds, apnea, lethargy, shock, cardiovascular collapse

DURATION: Acute

TREATMENTS: For bacterial infection, intravenous fluids and antibiotics; for necrotizing enterocolitis, surgery (intestinal resection)

FOR FURTHER INFORMATION:

Gilchrist, Brian F., ed. *Necrotizing Enterocolitis*. Georgetown, Tex.: Landes Bioscience, 2000.

Janowitz, Henry D. *Your Gut Feelings: A Complete Guide to Living Better with Intestinal Problems*. Rev. and updated ed. New York: Oxford University Press, 1995.

Stoll, Barbara J., and Robert M. Kliegman, eds. *Necrotizing Enterocolitis*. Philadelphia: W. B. Saunders, 1994.

Thompson, W. Grant. *Gut Reactions: Understanding Symptoms of the Digestive Tract.* New York: Plenum Press, 1989.

ENTEROVIRUSES
DISEASE/DISORDER

ANATOMY OR SYSTEM AFFECTED: Brain, eyes, heart, nervous system, skin

SPECIALTIES AND RELATED FIELDS: Cardiology, dermatology, environmental health, internal medicine, microbiology, neurology, virology

DEFINITION: A class of viruses capable of infecting multiple organ systems, such as the central nervous system, the skin, the eyes, and the heart.

KEY TERMS:

lesion: an abnormal area of tissue

meningitis: the inflammation of the protective tissues surrounding the brain and spinal cord

syndrome: a constellation of different symptoms or signs that are associated with a certain illness

vesicle: a fluid-filled blister

wild type: the form of species that occurs in nature

CAUSES AND SYMPTOMS

The enteroviruses is a class of viruses that includes the well known poliovirus but also includes the coxsackieviruses, echoviruses, and enteroviruses. Genetically, they are small, nonenveloped, single-stranded deoxyribonucleic acid (DNA) viruses that belong to the family Picornaviridae. These viruses are ubiquitous and infections occur year-round.

Enteroviruses cause a variety of clinical syndromes with different clinical manifestations depending on the specific viruses involved. Typically, transmission is through direct contact with fecal matter and contaminated food or water. The virus usually replicates initially in the throat and the small intestine, from where it then spreads to other organs.

Rash is a symptom common in all enterovirus infections. A maculopapular rash (mixture of flat and raised spots) can be seen in echovirus and poliovirus infections. Coxsackieviruses can cause the hand-foot-mouth syndrome in children, which presents as fever and vesicles in the oral cavity, hands, feet, buttocks, and sometimes genitalia. Transmission is through direct contact, and the illness usually resolves in two to three days. Herpangina is another syndrome caused by coxsackieviruses; it presents with painful vesicular lesions on the tonsils and soft palates in children. Echovirus

and coxsackievirus can both cause a petechial rash (small, red or purple spots), which sometimes may be confused with a meningococcal infection.

The central nervous system (CNS) is a well-known site of enteroviral infections. Enteroviruses as a group is the most common cause of viral meningitis in adults, which is usually due to echoviruses and coxsackieviruses. Because infants are not able to verbalize, they usually exhibit signs of irritability and fever, whereas in adults the common complaints are fever, headache, stiff neck, nausea, and vomiting. Encephalitis, the swelling and inflammation of the brain, is usually also the result of coxsackieviruses and echoviruses. It can develop either as a complication of meningitis or as an isolated event. Encephalitis typically presents as fever, lethargy, headache, seizures, or confusion. Paralytic poliomyelitis is the well-known syndrome due to polioviruses, but this presentation is the least common, since most people who have been infected with poliovirus do not have symptoms and only a minority of patients develop meningitis. Those who do develop paralysis usually present with a progressive, asymmetric weakness. The legs are commonly involved, followed by arms, abdominal, chest, or throat muscles. It is the involvement of respiratory and throat muscles that may be life threatening since these patients are prone to respiratory failure. While muscle paralysis is the hallmark of poliovirus infection, a similar picture may also be seen with echovirus infections, although the symptoms are not as severe or persistent.

Enterovirus and coxsackievirus are also capable of causing eye infections, commonly known as acute hemorrhagic conjunctivitis (AHC), with red eyes, pain, and swelling of the eyelids.

Coxsackieviruses can affect the chest and abdominal muscles, causing what is known as pleurodynia, which presents as fever and spasms of the chest and abdominal muscles. Coxsackievirus infection of the heart muscles and its surrounding tissues, known as myopericarditis, can present with mild symptoms such as chest pain or severe and rapid progression to heart failure and death.

TREATMENT AND THERAPY

Because most enteroviral infections are self-limited and resolve spontaneously, specific treatments are not warranted. In cases of severe infections—such as paralytic disease, meningitis, or myocarditis—supportive therapies are needed as life preservation measures. Even in such severe cases, no specific antiviral agents are available. Serum intravenous immunoglobulin has been tested in patients with certain immunodeficiencies and in neonates, although results have been mixed.

As in most infections, prevention is just as important as treatment. Because enteroviral infections are transmitted through contaminated sources, it is imperative to exercise good judgment regarding handwashing and hygienic practices.

PERSPECTIVE AND PROSPECTS

As one of the most recognized members of the enteroviral class, poliovirus has come a long way since its isolation in 1909 by Karl Landsteiner and Erwin Popper. The development of polio vaccines along with implementation of polio eradication programs have largely eliminated the disease due to wild-type poliovirus. The virus has been largely eradicated in the United States and other developed countries, and it is targeted for imminent global eradication.

The first polio vaccine was developed in 1952 by Jonas Salk. It was developed as an injectable vaccine using dead virus and is known as the inactivated polio vaccine (IPV). Doses are given at two, four, and six to eighteen months and at four to six years of age. Albert Sabin subsequently developed an oral polio vaccine (OPV) in 1962 which utilizes an attenuated but live poliovirus. Dosing is the same as that for the inactivated polio vaccine. A major concern of the oral polio vaccine is its ability to cause vaccine-induced polio, although the likelihood is very low, with rates of approximately 1 in 2.5 million vaccine recipients. Since most wild-type poliovirus have been eradicated, most cases of poliomyelitis in the twenty-first century are attributed to vaccine-induced poliomyelitis.

—*Andrew Ren, M.D.*

See also Childhood infectious diseases; Encephalitis; Epidemiology; Hand-foot-and-mouth disease; Immunization and vaccination; Meningitis; Paralysis; Poliomyelitis; Viral infections.

FOR FURTHER INFORMATION:

Fauci, Anthony, eds. "Enteroviruses and Reoviruses." In *Harrison's Principles of Internal Medicine*, edited by Jeffrey Cohen. 17th ed. New York: McGraw-Hill, 2008.

Mandell, Gerald, eds. *Mandell, Douglas, and Bennett's Principles and Practice of Infectious Diseases*. 5th ed. Philadelphia: Churchill Livingstone, 2000.

Richman, Douglas, eds. *Clinical Virology*. 3d ed. Washington, D.C.: ASM Press, 2009.

ENURESIS. *See* BED-WETTING.

ENVIRONMENTAL DISEASES
DISEASE/DISORDER

ANATOMY OR SYSTEM AFFECTED: All
SPECIALTIES AND RELATED FIELDS: All
DEFINITION: Sicknesses caused or exacerbated by human exposure to physical, chemical, biological, or social environmental conditions, the duration and intensity of the exposure typically affecting the manifestation of symptoms and fatality-case ratios. Acute environmental diseases may result in rapid decline of health status and warrant emergency response, while chronic conditions often result from long-term exposures to low levels of environmental risk factors.

KEY TERMS:

acute: referring to exposure to hazardous environmental agents or conditions that occur once or over a short period of time (typically fourteen days or less); environmental disease symptoms that appear rapidly

chronic: referring to exposure to environmental risk factor or agent occurring over a long period of time, typically more than one year; symptoms of environmental diseases that take a long time to appear after first contact with the causative agent

dose-response: the relationship between the dose (a quantitative measurement of exposure usually expressed in terms of concentration and duration) and the quantitative expression of change to the status of human health and well-being resulting in disease

environmental epidemiology: the systematic study of the distribution and determinants of environmental diseases in a population

environmental infection: human exposure to infectious agents of diseases (including bacteria, fungi, parasites, and viruses) through contact with environmental media such as contaminated water, air, food, and soil

environmental radiation: human exposure to electromagnetic radiation at doses and durations that can produce adverse impacts on human health

environmental toxicity: human exposure to chemical or biochemical substances at doses that produce harmful modification to the body's physiological mechanisms, leading to diseases

exposure assessment: a systematic process of discovering the pathway through which humans are exposed to specific environmental agents and risk factors, and of ascertaining the quantity and duration of that exposure

CAUSES AND SYMPTOMS

The modern word "miasma" comes from the Greek *miasma* or *miainein,* meaning "pollution" or "to pollute." Before scientific theories of disease became entrenched in medical practice, miasma was used to connote bad environments to which human exposure led to various diseases. Even today, one of the most devastating human diseases, malaria, draws its name from references to "bad air." There is clearly a rich historical record of human recognition of the intimate connection between environmental quality and diseases. It is now known that serious human diseases are caused by numerous chemical, physical, and biological agents (risk factors) that occur naturally or as a result of human actions that modify the environment. In fact, the more that is learned about disease etiology, the more the complex interplay between environmental conditions and root causes of diseases within the body are recognized. Furthermore, some people are more sensitive to environmental risk factors because of their age, gender, occupation, culture, or genetic characteristics.

Environmental diseases are those illnesses for which cause and effect can be reasonably associated through epidemiological studies, preferably verified through laboratory experiments. Therefore, the recognition of environmental diseases draws upon two traditional postulates regarding causation in the study of human diseases, one ascribed to Robert Koch (1843-1910) and the other ascribed to Austin Bradford Hill (1897-1991). The more important set of guidelines for environmental diseases is generally known in epidemiology as Hill's criteria of causation, based on his landmark 1965 publication entitled "The Environment and Disease: Association or Causation?" Hill warned in the article that cause-effect decisions should not be based on a set of rules. Instead, he supported the view that cost-benefit analysis is essential for policy decisions on controlling environmental quality in order to avoid diseases. It is arguable that Hill's treatise initiated current trends characterized by the precautionary principle in environmental health science. Nevertheless, Hill's nine viewpoints for exploring the relationship between environment and disease are worth emphasizing. They are precedence, correlation, dose-response, consistency, plausibility, alternatives, empiricism, specificity, and coherence.

According to the precedence viewpoint, exposure must always precede the outcome in every case of the environmental disease. One of the most famous examples here is the classic epidemiological study of John Snow (1813-1858) on the spread of cholera and its association with exposure to contaminated water in the densely populated city of London.

According to the correlation viewpoint, a strong association or correlation should exist between the exposure and the incidence of the environmental disease. The clustering of diseases within neighborhoods or among workers at a specific occupation is frequently the beginning of investigations into environmental diseases. Clusters can provide strong evidence of correlations. Bernardino Ramazinni (1633-1714), considered by many to be one of the founders of the discipline of occupational and environmental health sciences, published his treatise *De Morbis Artificum* in 1700 following critical observations regarding the correlation between environmental exposures of and diseases in workers.

According to the dose-response viewpoint, the relationship between exposure and the severity of environmental disease should be characterized by a dose-response relationship, in which an increase in the intensity and/or duration of exposure produces a more severe disease outcome. "The dose makes the poison" is one of the central tenets of environmental toxicology. This phrase is attributed to Paracelsus (1493-1541). This tenet has proven difficult to interpret for formulating health policy in the case of environmental diseases because the variation in human genetics and physiology means that, in many situations, a single threshold of toxicity cannot be established as safe for every person. Exposure to ionizing radiation is an example of a situation in which it is difficult to establish dose-response relationships that are useful for setting uniformly applicable preventive health policy.

According to the consistency viewpoint, there should be consistent findings in different populations, across different studies, and at different times regarding the association between exposure and environmental disease. This means that the relationship should be reproducible. For example, exposure of people to mercury across civilizations, occupations, and age groups has been consistently associated with certain health effects that allowed the recognition of the special hazards posed by this toxic metal. Mercury was used in various manufacturing processes for several centuries, and where precautions are not taken to prevent human exposure, disease invariably results.

Consistency should cut across not only generations but also occupations and different doses of exposure. For example, "mad hatter's" disease was associated with the use of mercury in the production of fur felt, in which mercurous nitrate was used to add texture to smooth fibers such as rabbit fur to facilitate matting (the process is called carroting because of the resulting orange color). More recently, the exposure of pregnant women to fish contaminated with methyl mercury from industrial sources in Japan produced developmental diseases in fetuses. The societal repercussions of the so-called Minamata disease are still not completely settled after more than forty years. Mercury is now widely recognized as a cumulative toxicant with systemic effects and organ damage, with symptoms including trembling, dental problems, ataxia, depression, and anxiety.

According to the plausibility viewpoint, compelling evidence of "biological plausibility" should exist that a physiological pathway leads from exposure to a specific environmental risk factor to the development of a specific environmental disease. This does not exclude the possibility of multiple causes, some acquired through environmental exposures and others through genetic processes. For example, lead poisoning has been recognized since the 1950's as a pervasive and devastating environmental disease. The symptoms of lead poisoning vary, from specific organ effects such as kidney disease to systemic effects such as anemia and to cognitive effects such as intelligence quotient (IQ) deficiency. How a single environmental toxicant can produce such wide-ranging diseases was a puzzle until the molecular mechanisms underpinning lead poisoning and the pharmacokinetic distribution of lead in the human body was understood. Lead is temporarily stored in the blood, where it binds to a key enzyme, aminolevulinate dehydratase, which participates in the synthesis of heme. The by-products of that reaction produce anemia and organ effects, including kidney and brain diseases. Long-term storage of lead in the body occurs in bony tissue, where other effects are possible. These biological understandings have helped activists and scientists agitate for environmental policy to reduce lead exposure worldwide.

According to the alternatives viewpoint, alternative explanations for the development of diseases should be considered alongside the plausible environmental causes. These alternative explanations should be ruled out before conclusions are reached about causal relationships between environmental exposures and disease. For example, the typically low doses to which populations are exposed to pesticides and the long time period between exposure and the typical chronic disease outcomes such as cancers and neurodegenerative disorders make it difficult to reconstruct the disease pathways and pinpoint causative agents. This is where it is important to consider all alternatives and to eliminate them before compelling arguments can be made about the effects of pesticide toxicity. Sometimes observing wildlife response to environmental risk factors help narrow down alternative explanations, as Rachel Carson taught in her timeless book *Silent Spring* (1965).

According to the empiricism viewpoint, the course of environmental disease should be alterable by appropriate intervention strategies verifiable through experimentation. In other words, the disease can be preventable or curable following manipulation of the environment and/or human physiology. For acute exposures, the emergency response is to eliminate the source of exposure. However, this is not always possible in cases where patients are unconscious or otherwise unable to articulate clearly the source of exposure, as is the case for many children. Nevertheless, standardized procedures exist for responding to environmental exposure beyond eliminating the source. For example, therapy based on chelation (from the Greek *chele*, meaning "claw") works for toxic metal exposure because the mode of action of the therapeutic agent, ethylene diamine tetra-acetic acid (EDTA), is well understood. It is possible to establish empirically the relative effectiveness of EDTA in dealing with various forms of toxic metal exposures. For example, under normal physiological conditions, EDTA binds metals in the following order: iron (ferric ion), mercury, copper, aluminum, nickel, lead, cobalt, zinc, iron (ferrous ion), cadmium, manganese, magnesium, and calcium. Based on this information, it is possible to design therapeutic processes that minimize adverse side effects.

In the News:
Iraq War Increases Disease Risks

Throughout the history of warfare, diseases have often caused more casualties among both soldiers and civilians than weaponry itself. The conflict in Iraq is no exception. A rare type of lung infection, acute eosinophilic pneumonia (AEP), is occurring at a higher rate among U.S. soldiers in Iraq than in any other segment of the population. The illness, characterized by fever, serious lung impairment, and eventually respiratory failure, has killed a number of soldiers since the war began in 2003. Of the individuals who contracted this pneumonia, all reported exposure to fine sand and dust particles, a common hazard in the desert environments of the Middle East. Administration of corticosteroids proved life-saving for most patients, but many who have recovered complain of residual lung problems.

Veterans of Operation Iraqi Freedom are not alone in fighting disabling illnesses. Brain cancer, amyotrophic lateral sclerosis (ALS), fibromyalgia, and multiple sclerosis are among the serious ailments plaguing the earlier Gulf War veterans from 1991. The demolition of weapons dumps in Iraq in March, 1991, released the deadly nerve agents sarin and cyclosarin. Many Gulf War veterans claim that this incident is to blame for the diseases from which they now suffer. A U.S. Department of Defense-sponsored study conducted by the Institute of Medicine of the National Academy of Sciences and published in the *American Journal of Public Health* (August, 2005), focused on the nerve gas release event at Al Khamisiyah and subsequent increase in neurological illnesses in those exposed to the chemical contamination that followed.

Inflamed joints, heat and chemical sensitivities, severe headaches, hair loss, and recurrent skin rashes are just a few of the symptoms endured by affected troops who have returned from both Iraq conflicts. Thousands of Gulf War veterans are currently receiving disability payments from the Veterans Administration, and many of those payments are for battle-related illness rather than for injury.

—Lenela Glass-Godwin, M.WS.

ally, new ideas about causation challenge orthodox theories. According to the coherence viewpoint, it is important to conduct a rigorous assessment of coherence with existing information and scientific ideas before such causes are accepted in the case of environmental diseases. For example, the origin of neurodegenerative diseases currently associated with exposure to prion protein remains mysterious, and some environmental causes have been proposed, including exposure to toxic metal ions. Another example is the current concern with the introduction of nanoparticles into commercial products, with concomitant environmental dissemination. Although much has been learned from an understanding of the human health effects of respirable particulate matter, researchers should be sufficiently open-minded to the possibility that nanoparticles will behave differently in the environment and in the human body.

Hill's nine viewpoints were presented in the context of pitfalls associated with overreliance on statistical tests of "significance" as a justification to base health policy on epidemiological observations. Hill's viewpoints have been debated extensively, and it is worth noting the following caveats presented in the 2004 article "The Missed Lessons of Sir Austin Bradford Hill," by Carl V. Phillips and Karen J. Goodman: Statistical significance should not be mistaken for evidence of substantial association, association does not prove causation, precision should not be mistaken for validity, evidence that a causal relationship exists is not sufficient to suggest that action should be taken, and uncertainty about causation or association is not sufficient to suggest that action should not be taken.

The second set of guidelines regarding causality derives from what is generally known as Koch's postulates, but it is perhaps only useful for precautionary ap-

According to the specificity viewpoint, when an environmental disease is associated with only one environmental agent, the relationship between exposure and environmental disease is said to be specific. This strengthens the argument for causality, but this situation is extremely rare. For example, the rarity of mesothelioma, a lung disease that afflicts people who have been exposed to asbestos fibers, made it possible to use epidemiological evidence quickly to support policy in restricting the use of asbestos in commercial products and to protect employees from occupational exposures.

The recognition of new diseases often leads to speculation about causative agents or conditions. Occasion-

proaches to proactive assessment of potential health impacts of new agents about to be introduced into the environment. This approach complements the epidemiology-based inferences described by Hill, but further refinement is warranted to deal with complicated issues such as interactions between multiple environmental agents, which could have additive, neutral, or canceling effects. The question of dose is also difficult to subject to simple conclusions because of phenomena such as hormesis, in which small doses may show beneficial effects.

For environmental diseases, a modified version of Koch's postulates can be expressed as follows. First, exposure to an environmental agent must be demonstrable in all organisms suffering from the disease, but not in healthy organisms (assuming predisposition factors). Second, the identity, concentrations in different environmental and physiological compartments, and transformation pathways of the agent must be known as much as possible. Third, the agent should cause disease when introduced into healthy organisms. Fourth, biomarkers showing modification of the physiological target affected by the environmental agent must be observable in experimentally exposed organisms.

TREATMENT AND THERAPY

The symptoms of environmental diseases vary widely, and physiological, anatomical, and behavioral characteristics can succumb to the effects of environmental agents. In evaluating treatment and therapy, it is useful to consider two categories of symptoms. Acute symptoms are exhibited in response to human exposure to high doses of toxic agents within a short period of time. Essentially, the body is overwhelmed, and emergency therapy is necessary to avoid death or permanent disability. For toxic air contaminants, respiratory distress is a common symptom, and mortality can occur rapidly. Conversely, chronic symptoms of human exposures to low levels of environmental (particularly air) pollutants are difficult to diagnose, as in the case of cancers attributable to secondhand tobacco smoke or ambient exposure to respirable particulate matter. Similarly, exposure of the skin to rapidly absorbed toxins can produce rapid mortality, but the development of skin cancer due to ultraviolet (UV) light exposure may take decades to manifest. Ingestion of contaminated liquids or food may take minutes to provoke distress and vomiting, whereas it may take years for chronic symptoms to manifest in cases of carcinogenic water pollutants.

Treatment and therapy of environmental diseases requires accurate diagnosis of the causative agent. The first line of response is to limit exposure through flushing the body with clean air or liquids. Chelation therapy can be used to reduce the body burden of certain toxic metals. Curative measures follow the established procedures developed for specific organs. For example, chemotherapy, radiotherapy, and surgery are used to treat cancers regardless of the involvement of known environmental factors in their etiology. Skin diseases such as chloracne associated with exposure to chlorinated aromatic hydrocarbon pollutants, including polychlorinated biphenyls (PCBs), are managed to reduce the severity of lesions and enhance natural healing processes. Cognitive deficits associated with exposure to metals and other environmental pollutants are believed to be reversible as long further exposures are avoided. Finally, environmental diseases associated with infectious agents such as bacteria can be controlled through a combination of source disinfection and antibiotic therapy.

PERSPECTIVE AND PROSPECTS

There has been a resurgence of interest in environmental diseases because of societal changes at regional and international levels. Industrialization demands the use of thousands of potentially hazardous chemicals that ultimately end up polluting human environments and remain an important source of causative agents for environmental diseases. Recent threats associated with global environmental change, bioterrorism, and chemical warfare have all contributed to the need for rapid detection of hazardous environmental agents and tougher laws to protect air, water, soil, and food resources. Prevention is still the crucial solution to reducing the human burden of environmental diseases worldwide.

On June 16, 2006, the World Health Organization (WHO) issued a landmark report estimating that environmental risk factors play a role in more than 80 percent of diseases regularly reported by WHO across fourteen regions globally. The environment has an impact on human health through exposures to physical, chemical, and biological risk factors and through changes in human behavior in response to environmental change at local and global levels. Globally, nearly 25 percent of all deaths and of the total disease burden (measured in disability-adjusted life years, or DALYs) can be attributed to environmental quality. The situation is more dire for children, with environmental risk factors accounting for more than 33 percent of the disease burden. These discoveries have important implications for national and international health policy, because many of the implicated environmental risk factors can be modified by established interventions. The lack of understanding on how to deploy these interventions globally has inspired the involvement of well-funded organizations and institutions in environmental health issues.

In the United States, the National Institute of Environmental Health Sciences (NIEHS), a subsidiary of the National Institutes of Health (NIH), studies environmental diseases and guides policy on how to protect vulnerable populations. A comprehensive five-year strategic plan developed by the NIEHS in 2006 outlined seven specific goals aimed at curtailing environmental exposures and reducing societal burden of environmental diseases.

The first goal is to expand the role of clinical research in environmental health sciences by emphasizing the use of environmental exposures to understand and better characterize complex diseases. This includes the development of research models for human diseases based on the coordinated knowledge of environmental sciences and human biology.

The second goal is to use environmental toxins to gain more insight into the basic mechanisms in human biology. This goal involves tapping into the rapidly expanding knowledge of the biochemical mechanisms of disease progression and the influence of genetic factors in the path from environmental exposures to disease symptoms.

The third goal is to build an integrative multidisciplinary understanding of complex environmental systems and the various ways in which human diseases are manifested. The fourth goal is to improve the quality of community-based environmental health research. Much can be learned from studying populations that are exposed to high concentrations of environmental agents believed to cause human disease. The hope is to better understand disease clusters in communities and to link the understanding of regional prevalence of environmental diseases to global environmental health concerns.

The fifth goal is to improve the understanding and use of sensitive markers of exposure, susceptibility, and effects of environmental agents. There is also an urgent need to develop technologies for measuring exposures more accurately in order to link exposures more tightly to assessments of toxicity and other physiological impacts.

The sixth goal is to engage the broader biomedical community in research on environmental diseases and to support a pipeline for encouraging new researchers to enter the discipline of environmental health.

The seventh goal is to encourage pathways by which the results of research can inform policy quickly in order to protect vulnerable populations. This requires fostering cooperation with other agencies and organizations such as the U.S. Environmental Protection Agency (EPA), the Food and Drug Administration (FDA), the U.S. Department of Agriculture, and the Occupational Safety and Health Administration (OSHA). In addition, there must be straightforward communication paths between manufacturing industries where environmental agents of disease originate and the community of environmental health physicians, researchers, and regulatory agencies to ensure successful implementation of these laudable goals.

—*Oladele A. Ogunseitan, Ph.D., M.P.H.*

See also Allergies; Asbestos exposure; Aspergillosis; Asthma; Bronchitis; Cancer; Carcinogens; Carpal tunnel syndrome; Chronic obstructive pulmonary disease (COPD); Coccidioidomycosis; Dengue fever; *E. coli* infection; Emerging infectious diseases; Emphysema; Environmental health; Epidemics and pandemics; Epidemiology; Food poisoning; Gulf War syndrome; Lead poisoning; Lung cancer; Melanoma; Mercury poisoning; Mesothelioma; Multiple chemical sensitivity syndrome; Occupational health; Poisoning; Pulmonary diseases; Radiation sickness; Respiration; Rocky Mountain spotted fever; Skin cancer; Skin lesion removal; Teratogens; Toxicology; Tularemia.

FOR FURTHER INFORMATION:

Carson, Rachel. *Silent Spring.* 40th anniversary ed. New York: Houghton Mifflin, 2002. A classic book that began the tradition of connecting ecosystems, environmental quality, and human health.

Hill, Austin Bradford. "The Environment and Disease: Association or Causation?" *Proceedings of the Royal Society of Medicine* 58 (1965): 295-300. A classic publication on causality in environmental epidemiology.

McMichael, Tony. *Human Frontiers, Environments, and Disease.* New York: Cambridge University Press, 2003. A general textbook on environmental quality and human diseases.

National Institute of Environmental Health Sciences (NIEHS). *New Frontier in Environmental Sciences and Human Health: The 2006-2011 NIEHS Strate-*

gic Plan. http://www.niehs.nih.gov/external/plan 2006. The comprehensive five-year strategic plan developed by the NIEHS.

Phillips, Carl V., and Karen J. Goodman. "The Missed Lessons of Sir Austin Bradford Hill." *Epidemiologic Perspectives and Innovations* 1, no. 3 (October 4, 2004). Presents the caveats on inferring causation based on epidemiological data. Also available at http://www.epi-perspectives.com/content/1/1/3.

Solomon, Gina, Oladele A. Ogunseitan, and Jan Kirsch. *Pesticides and Human Health: A Resource for Health Care Professionals.* San Francisco: Physicians for Social Responsibility, 2000. A compendium on environmental diseases associated with pesticides in the human environment.

World Health Organization. *Preventing Disease Through Healthy Environments: Towards an Estimate of the Environmental Burden of Disease.* Edited by A. Pruss-Ustun and C. Corvalan. Geneva: Author, 2006. Provides a global outlook on environmental diseases.

ENVIRONMENTAL HEALTH

SPECIALTY

ANATOMY OR SYSTEM AFFECTED: All

SPECIALTIES AND RELATED FIELDS: Epidemiology, occupational health, preventive medicine, psychology, public health, toxicology

DEFINITION: The control of all factors in the physical environment that exercise, or may exercise, a deleterious effect on human physical development, health, and survival and correcting and preventing those effects from adversely affecting future generations. The study of the influence of environment on health and disease.

KEY TERMS:

community: a group of people living in the same locality

hygiene: the science of health and the prevention of disease

pollutant: a noxious substance that contaminates the environment

remediation: correcting an evil, fault, or error

sanitation: the application of measures designed to protect public health

SCIENCE AND PROFESSION

The environment is the sum of all external influences and conditions affecting the life and development of an organism. For humans, a healthy environment means that the surroundings in which humans live, work, and play meet some predetermined quality standard. The field of environmental health encompasses biological, chemical, physical, and psychosocial factors in the environment. This is the air that humans breathe, the water that they drink, the food that they consume, and the shelter that they inhabit. The definition also includes the identification of pollutants, waste materials, and other environmental factors that adversely affect life and health. The study of environmental health investigates how human health and disease are influenced by the environment. It encompasses the fields of environmental engineering and sanitation, public health engineering, and sanitary engineering. The majority of professionals working in the field of environmental health are trained as civil engineers, environmental engineers, geologists, toxicologists, or preventive medicine specialists. Many are also qualified in subspecialties such as hydrogeology, epidemiology, public sanitation, and occupational health.

Environmental health deals with the control of factors in the physical environment that cause (or may cause) a negative effect on the health and survival of communities. Consideration is given to the physical, economic, and social impact of the controlling measures. These measures include controlling, modifying, or adapting the physical, chemical, and biological factors of the environment in the interest of human health, comfort, and social well-being. Environmental health is concerned not only with simple survival and the prevention of disease and poisoning but also with the maintenance of an environment that is suited to efficient human performance and that preserves human comfort and enjoyment.

DIAGNOSTIC AND TREATMENT TECHNIQUES

The field of environmental health covers an extremely broad area of human living space. For practical purposes, those involved in the profession of environmental health concern themselves with the impact of humans on the environment and the impact of the environment on humans, balancing their appraisals and allocations of available resources. The scope of environmental health research and community environmental health planning usually involves the following topics: water supplies, water pollution and wastewater treatment, solid waste disposal, pest control, soil pollution, food hygiene, air pollution, radiation control, noise control, transportation control, safe housing, land use planning, public recreation, abuse of controlled substances, resource conservation, postdisaster sanitation, accident prevention, medical facilities, and occupational health, particularly the control of physical, chemical, and biological hazards.

The implementation of effective environmental health strategies must take place within the context of comprehensive regional or area-wide community planning. Planning considerations for a community's environmental health are based on individual community aspirations and goals, priorities, local resources, and the availability of outside resources required to meet projected health standards. The planning and implementation of environmental health activities directly involve engineers, sanitarians, medical specialists, planners, architects, geologists, biologists, chemists, geophysicists, technicians, naturalists, and related personnel. The natural and physical scientists provide research necessary for communities to locate and use available resources responsibly, and they also identify potential and existing health hazards. The engineering specialties provide know-how to communities concerning the design, installation, and operation of equipment. When a problem is identified or an emergency occurs, it is often the engineering professionals who direct remediation efforts. Medical specialists, with scientific backup, determine dangers to a community's physical health; if health problems arise, they concern themselves with treating and preventing disease and restoring health. The implementation of any environmental health strategy is clearly a team effort.

Perspective and Prospects

The concept of environmental health in modern society is considerably expanded from that of the past. Activities in the field of environmental health were once controlled only because they were known to be disease-related. The present concept of environmental health aims to provide a high quality of living.

The field of environmental health concerns itself with the control of physical factors affecting the health of humans and is different from the prevention and control of individual illness and the preservation of human health. Most environmental health problems are the direct result of human activities and interactions with natural and manufactured resources. Human manipulation of natural resources causes changes to the environment. These changes can be local or global, anticipated or unanticipated. At the present time, humans are living in a polluted environment, the result of centuries of lack of concern for and appreciation of the ecologic consequences of human activities. The cumulative effects of human actions on the environment have risen steeply and continuously, while human response to mounting problems of environmental quality has been sporadic and targeted toward high-profile or emergency problems. As a result, environmental programs have been developed to preserve wildlife, maintain clean groundwater supplies, manage resources, combat communicable disease, increase agricultural production, and ensure healthy and sanitary living conditions for human populations.

As a direct reflection of the public's concern about environmental degradation, environmental health has become a rapidly growing specialty in the fields of engineering, medicine, environmental science, geology, and resource management. As public awareness of the devastating effects of pollution and resource depletion grows, the demand for qualified environmental health professionals and administrators increases. Whether these sought-after professionals are asked to offer stopgap measures for environmental problems that have already progressed to dangerous, possibly unresolvable levels or whether they are employed to foster a new, more holistic approach to the natural world will depend on the environmental conscience of modern civilization.

—*Randall L. Milstein, Ph.D.;* *updated by Sharon W. Stark, R.N., A.P.R.N., D.N.Sc.*

See also Allergies; Asbestos exposure; Aspergillosis; Asthma; Bacteriology; Biological and chemical weapons; Carcinogens; Cholera; Chronic obstructive pulmonary disease (COPD); Dengue fever; Emerging infectious diseases; Environmental diseases; Epidemics and pandemics; Epidemiology; Food poisoning; Frostbite; Gulf War syndrome; Heat exhaustion and heatstroke; Hyperthermia and hypothermia; Immune system; Immunization and vaccination; Immunology; Insect-borne diseases; Interstitial pulmonary fibrosis (IPF); Lead poisoning; Legionnaires' disease; Lice, mites, and ticks; Lung cancer; Lungs; Lyme disease; Malaria; Mercury poisoning; Mesothelioma; Microbiology; Nasopharyngeal disorders; Occupational health; Parasitic diseases; Plague; Poisoning; Poisonous plants; Preventive medicine; Pulmonary diseases; Pulmonary medicine; Pulmonary medicine, pediatric; Rocky Mountain spotted fever; Salmonella infection; Skin cancer; Snakebites; Stress; Stress reduction; Teratogens; Toxicology; Tropical medicine; Tularemia.

FOR FURTHER INFORMATION:

Environmental Defense Fund. http://www.environmental defense.org.

Friis, Robert H. *Essentials of Environmental Health.* Sudbury, Mass.: Jones and Bartlett, 2007.

Moeller, Dade W. *Environmental Health.* 3d ed. Cambridge, Mass.: Harvard University Press, 2005.

Morgan, Monroe T. *Environmental Health.* 3d ed. Belmont, Calif.: Thomson/Wadsworth, 2003.

National Institute of Environmental Health Sciences. "What Is Environmental Health?" http://www.niehs .nih.gov/health/topics.

Philp, Richard B. *Ecosystems and Human Health: Toxicology and Environmental Hazards.* 2d ed. Boca Raton, Fla.: Lewis, 2001.

Raven, Peter H., and Linda R. Berg. *Environment.* 6th ed. Hoboken, N.J.: John Wiley & Sons, 2009.

World Health Organization. "Public Health and Environment." http://www.who.int/phe/en.

Yassi, Annalee, et al. *Basic Environmental Health.* New York: Oxford University Press, 2001.

ENZYME THERAPY

TREATMENT

ALSO KNOWN AS: Enzyme replacement therapy

ANATOMY OR SYSTEM AFFECTED: All

SPECIALTIES AND RELATED FIELDS: Alternative medicine, biochemistry, genetics

DEFINITION: The use of enzymes as drugs to treat specific medical problems.

INDICATIONS AND PROCEDURES

Enzymes are large, complex protein molecules that catalyze chemical reactions in living organisms. The phrase "enzyme therapy" is sometimes used to refer to enzyme preparations given as dietary supplements, often as digestive aids. Such treatment is of questionable value because enzymes, like all proteins, are degraded in the stomach. Legitimate enzyme therapy is an innovative procedure based on emerging technology. Enzymes used to treat various medical conditions are delivered intravenously.

Enzyme therapy is used to dissolve clots in stroke and cardiac patients. Enzymes such as streptokinase, plasmin, and human tissue plasminogen activator (TPA) are able to dissolve clots when injected into the bloodstream.

Some types of adult leukemia can be treated by injection of the enzyme asparaginase, which destroys asparagine. Tumors in these patients require aspara-gine, and the asparaginase removes it from the blood, thus inhibiting the ability of these tumors to grow.

Enzyme therapy can also be used to treat certain inherited diseases. One of these is Fabry's disease. Patients with this disease are deficient in an enzyme called alpha-galactosidase A. Without this enzyme, harmful levels of a substance called ceremide trehexoside accumulate in the heart, brain, and kidneys. If left untreated, patients usually die in their forties or fifties after a lifetime of pain. On the other hand, patients injected with alpha-galactosidase A once every two weeks lead nearly normal lives.

Gaucher's disease is another severe inherited disease characterized by a deficiency in an enzyme that normally prevents the buildup of a chemical to injurious levels. It can be treated by injections of the enzyme glucocerebrosidase.

USES AND COMPLICATIONS

The use of enzymes to treat clotting problems and genetic diseases started in the early 1990's; thus, the long-term effects are unknown. Enzyme therapy does not cure genetic disease, so the therapy must be lifelong.

Some people are encouraged to swallow enzyme preparations to aid digestion. For example, the enzyme papain is promoted as a digestive aid. Although papain is very effective at breaking down proteins in the laboratory or as a meat tenderizer in the kitchen, it does not function well in the stomach. Papain is most effective at a nearly neutral pH of 6.2, whereas the stomach is highly acidic with a pH of about 2.0. On the other hand, papain is active in the more neutral esophagus. Although normally little or no food is found in the esophagus, papain has the potential to damage the esophageal lining, especially in people with esophageal disorders.

—*Lorraine Lica, Ph.D.*

See also Blood and blood disorders; Digestion; Enzymes; Fatty acid oxidation disorder; Fructosemia; Galactosemia; Gaucher's disease; Genetic diseases; Glycogen storage diseases; Heart attack; Leukemia; Metabolism; Mucopolysaccharidosis (MPS); Niemann-Pick disease; Oncology; Pharmacology; Strokes; Tay-Sachs disease; Thrombolytic therapy and TPA; Thrombosis and thrombus; Tumors.

FOR FURTHER INFORMATION:

Cichoke, Anthony J. *The Complete Book of Enzyme Therapy.* Garden City Park, N.Y.: Avery, 1999.

Devlin, Thomas M., ed. *Textbook of Biochemistry:*

With Clinical Correlations. 6th ed. Hoboken, N.J.: Wiley-Liss, 2006.

Rimoin, David L., et al., eds. *Emery and Rimoin's Principles and Practice of Medical Genetics*. 5th ed. Philadelphia: Churchill Livingstone/Elsevier, 2007.

Scriver, Charles R., et al., eds. *The Metabolic and Molecular Bases of Inherited Disease*. 8th ed. New York: McGraw-Hill, 2001.

Enzymes

Biology

Anatomy or system involved: Cells, immune system

Specialties and related fields: Biochemistry, cytology, endocrinology, genetics, pharmacology

Definition: Large molecules, produced by cells, that catalyze chemical reactions inside living organisms.

Key terms:

active site: the part of an enzyme where the substrate is bound; this is the site where the reaction occurs

activity: a measure of the ability of an enzyme to catalyze its reaction

amino acid: the fundamental building blocks of proteins; there are twenty amino acids, each with a different chemistry

catalysis: increasing the speed of a chemical reaction

molecule: a collection of atoms bonded together; normally neutral because it has an equal number of protons and electrons

mutation: a substitution of one amino acid for another in the amino acid sequence of a protein

protein: large molecules made up of amino acids connected by peptide bonds; the sequence of amino acids in a protein determines its three-dimensional structure

substrates: reactants that enzymes convert into products; every enzyme is specific for one specific substrate

Structure and Functions

Enzymes are remarkable molecules because they increase rates of biochemical reactions. Each enzyme within a cell selectively speeds up, or catalyzes, one particular reaction or type of reaction. The vast majority of enzymes belong to the class of large molecules known as proteins. Proteins are built by combining amino acids. There are twenty amino acids, which can be divided into three classes: hydrophobic, charged, and polar. Hydrophobic amino acids behave chemically like oils, avoiding contact with water. Charged amino acids are ionic, containing one extra or one less electron than do neutral molecules. Polar amino acids are attracted to water and other polar amino acids. Each of these three classes of amino acids has a distinct chemistry. The specific order of the amino acid sequence defines the structure and function of every protein. Inside cells, enzymes catalyze reactions so that they occur millions of times faster than they would without the presence of these proteins. Each cell in the body produces many different enzymes. Different sets of enzymes are found in different tissues, reflecting the specialized function of each particular enzyme. Thousands of different enzymes are at work in the body; many have yet to be discovered.

Protein enzymes work by bringing the reactants in a chemical reaction together in the most favorable geometrical arrangement, so that bonds can be easily broken and reformed. This is possible because different enzymes have different three-dimensional shapes. It is the shape of the enzyme that determines its chemistry. Each enzyme combines with a specific substrate, or reactant, and catalyzes its characteristic reaction. When the reaction is over, the substrate has been converted into products. The enzyme remains unchanged, ready to catalyze another reaction with the next substrate molecule it encounters.

Enzymes play a significant role in treating diseases. Because enzymes have specific functions, a particular enzyme that has the required function to treat the disorder can be administered. Modern methods of genetic engineering allow the production of desired enzymes. Scientists can use bacteria as factories to produce large amounts of enzyme from an organism by copying the gene from the organism of interest into bacterial cells. The bacteria are then grown in culture, producing the enzyme of interest as they grow. This procedure is a much safer method than the old procedure of isolating enzymes from animal tissues, because the enzymes produced are free of viruses and other contaminants present in animal tissues. Proteins produced by genetic engineering techniques are called recombinant proteins.

Sometimes enzymes can be used as drugs for the treatment of specific diseases. Streptokinase is an enzyme mixture that is useful in clearing blood clots that occur in the heart and the lower extremities. Another useful enzyme for dissolving blood clots that occur as a result of heart attacks is human tissue plasminogen activator (TPA). Recombinant TPA is produced by genetic engineering techniques, using bacteria cultures to produce large quantities of human TPA. The administration of TPA within an hour of the formation of a blood clot in a coronary artery dramatically increases survival rates of heart attack victims. Some types of adult leukemia are treated by intravenous administration of the asparaginase enzyme. Tumor cells require the molecule asparagine to grow, and they scavenge it from the bloodstream. Asparaginase drastically reduces the amount of asparagine in the blood, thus slowing the growth of the tumor. Because most enzymes do not last long in blood, huge amounts of enzymes are required for therapeutic effects. In classic hemophilia, the factor VIII enzyme is missing or is genetically mutated so that it has a very low activity. This enzyme is essential for inducing the formation of blood clots. In the past, it was a laborious task to collect a concentrated blood plasma sample containing factor VIII, which was administered to hemophiliacs to stop hemorrhages. This treatment carried the risk of infecting the patient with viruses that cause acquired immunodeficiency syndrome (AIDS), hepatitis, and other diseases. Purified recombinant factor VIII is now available. Because the recombinant human factor VIII is produced by bacteria, it cannot be infected with the viruses that cause hepatitis and AIDS.

A classic enzyme inhibitor used as a drug is penicillin. Penicillin was discovered in 1928 by Alexander Fleming, after he noticed that bacterial growth was prevented by a contaminating mold known as *Penicillium*. Ten years later, Howard Florey and Ernst Chain performed the key experiments that led to the isolation, characterization, and clinical use of this wonder drug antibiotic. In 1957, Joshua Lederberg showed that penicillin interferes with the synthesis of the cell walls of bacteria. In 1965, James Park and Jack Strominger independently discovered that penicillin blocks the last step in cell wall synthesis. The last step is the crosslinking of different strands of the wall and is catalyzed by the enzyme glycopeptide transpeptidase. The shape of penicillin resembles that of the normal substrate of glycopeptide transpeptidase, so that penicillin binds to the active site of the transpeptidase enzyme. Once bound to the active site, penicillin forms a permanent bond with one of the amino acid residues. This chemical reaction permanently inhibits the glycopeptide transpeptidase enzyme, thus preventing the transpeptidase from cross-linking the bacterial wall.

Several anticancer drugs work by blocking the synthesis of deoxythymidylate (dTMP), as an abundant supply of dTMP is required for rapid cell division to be sustained. Drugs that inhibit the enzymes thymidylate synthase and dihydrofolate reductase are very effective agents in cancer chemotherapy. Thymidylate synthase, which makes dTMP from deoxyuridylate, is irreversibly inhibited by the drug fluorouracil. This drug is converted into fluorodeoxyuridylate (F-dUMP), which chemically reacts with thymidylate synthase so that the enzyme can no longer function in its normal role of making dTMP from deoxyuridylate. The synthesis of dTMP can also be blocked by drugs that inhibit the enzyme dihydrofolate reductase. The normal substrate for dihydrofolate reductase is the molecule dihydrofolate. Drugs such as aminopterin and methotrexate bind to the active site of the reductase enzyme, inhibiting rapid cell growth. Methotrexate is very effective at inhibiting rapidly growing tumors such as acute leuke-

The Function of Some Enzymes

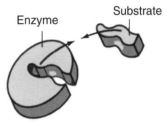

Enzyme · Substrate

An enzyme combines with a substrate that has molecules of a complementary shape.

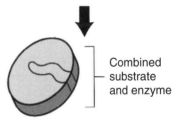

Combined substrate and enzyme

The interaction between the enzyme and substrate causes a chemical change in the substrate, splitting it in two.

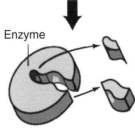

Enzyme

The enzyme is unchanged and can repeat the process with another substrate molecule.

mia and choriocarcinoma. Unfortunately methotrexate kills all rapidly dividing cells, including stem cells in bone marrow, epithelial cells of the intestinal tract, and hair follicles, which explains the many toxic side effects of this drug. Computer-aided drug design has been applied to the dihydrofolate reductase enzyme, with encouraging results.

The activity of an enzyme is a measure of how efficiently a particular enzyme catalyzes its reaction. A loss in activity corresponds to a decrease in catalytic efficiency, and an increase in activity corresponds to an increase in catalytic efficiency. Many drugs increase enzyme activity (enzyme induction), and many decrease enzyme activity (enzyme inhibition). Both enzyme induction and enzyme inhibition result from the interaction of the drug with the enzyme, altering the surface of the enzyme where the substrate normally is bound during catalysis. In enzyme induction, the surface is altered such that the substrate is bound tighter than usual, while in enzyme inhibition, the surface is altered so that the substrate cannot bind to the enzyme. The structures of many enzyme inhibitors are similar to the structures of substrates. Inhibitors bind at active sites of enzymes. Drugs that are enzyme inhibitors are very powerful medical tools, as they bind to the enzyme and are not easily removed.

Universities, government agencies, and pharmaceutical companies are continually seeking to develop drugs that specifically bind and inhibit enzymes responsible for disease. Much effort is spent trying to design drugs in a rational manner, using the most powerful tools of chemistry. Techniques such as X-ray crystallography, nuclear magnetic resonance (NMR) spectroscopy, and computational chemistry allow researchers to determine the shapes of enzymes, their substrates, and their inhibitors. These efforts allow the research team to design drugs that bind more specifically to the target enzyme, thus increasing the effectiveness and lowering the toxicity of the drug.

DISORDERS AND DISEASES

Defects in enzymes, known as mutations, can cause disease. A protein molecule is mutated when one or more of the original amino acids in the protein is replaced by a different amino acid. For example, if an enzyme consists of one hundred amino acids, and amino acid number 35 is changed from one kind of amino acid to a different kind, the protein is now a mutant. A mutated enzyme has a slightly altered shape compared to the original enzyme. If the change in shape causes the

enzyme to perform its chemistry more slowly than the original enzyme, then the cell and tissue have an impaired function. In particular, if an amino acid is changed from one of the three classes (hydrophobic, charged, or polar) to a different class, then the mutation is more likely to cause a change in the structure and function of the enzyme. Not all mutations are harmful, but a single mutation in a key region of an enzyme can be fatal to a living organism.

Many diseases are diagnosed by measuring enzyme concentrations and activities in the body. Enzyme concentration refers to the amount of enzyme present, while enzyme activity refers to the ability of the enzyme to perform its chemistry. Enzyme concentrations and activities can be measured in blood or in tissue. Disease of tissues and organs can cause cellular damage, so that enzymes that are normally not present in significant quantities in blood are raised to very high levels as they flow from the damaged tissue into the blood plasma. Detection of particular enzymes in blood plasma indicates a diseased organ. The higher the concentration of enzyme in the blood, the more extensive the damage to that tissue or organ. The detection of these enzymes in the blood is a diagnostic tool, indicating a particular disorder. Genetic diseases caused by a mutation in an enzyme can be detected by laboratory tests that measure enzyme activity or enzyme shape.

Disease diagnosis is often made by measuring the concentration or activity of enzymes. Isozymes are enzymes that catalyze the same reaction but have slightly different structures. Most isozymes are enzymes consisting of two or more subunits, with different combinations of the subunits differentiating the isozymes. Isozymes of the enzymes lactate dehydrogenase, creatine kinase, and alkaline phosphatase are used for clinical applications. Monitoring of the isozyme concentrations and activities of lactate dehydrogenase and creatine kinase in the blood shows whether a patient has suffered a heart attack.

Creatine kinase consists of two subunits. The two possible subunits are M, which stands for muscle type, and B, which stands for brain type. There are three possible isozymes: MM, BB, and MB. The MM isozyme consists of two M subunits and is the only isozyme found in skeletal muscle, the BB isozyme consists of two B subunits and is the only isozyme found in the brain, and the MB isozyme consists of one M and one B subunit and is found only in the heart. Lactate dehydrogenase consists of four subunits, made from five combinations of two subunits. The two subunits are the heart subunit, designated by H, and the muscle subunit, designated by M. The HHHH and HHHM isozymes are found in the heart and in red blood cells, the HHMM isozyme is found in the brain and kidney, and the MMMM isozyme is found in the liver and skeletal muscle.

After a heart attack, the cellular breakup of heart tissue releases the MB isozyme of creatine kinase into the bloodstream within six to eighteen hours. Release of lactate dehydrogenase into the blood is slower than that of creatine kinase, occurring one to two days after the appearance of creatine kinase. In a healthy person, the activity of the HHHM isozyme of lactate dehydrogenase is higher than that of the HHHH isozyme. In heart attack victims, however, the activity of the HHHH isozyme becomes greater than that of the HHHM isozyme between twelve and twenty-four hours after the attack. Measurement of increased concentration of the MB isozyme a short while after a suspected heart attack, followed by the switch in lactate dehydrogenase activity between the HHHH and HHHM isozymes, indicates that a heart attack occurred. Secondary complications of a heart attack can also be followed with isozyme measurements. For example, increased activity of the MMMM isozyme of lactate dehydrogenase is an indication of liver congestion.

Certain medical conditions can be screened by using immobilized enzymes as reagents in desktop clinical analyzers. For example, screening tests for cholesterol and triglycerides can be completed in a few minutes using 0.01 milliliter of blood plasma. The enzymes cholesterol oxidase and lipase are immobilized, or fixed in place, in a detection kit. If cholesterol is present, cholesterol oxidase breaks off hydrogen peroxide from the cholesterol. The enzyme peroxidase and a colorless dye are included in the detection kit, and peroxidase catalyzes the reaction of the colorless dye and hydrogen peroxide to form a colored dye that can be easily measured from the amount of light reflected from the solution. The enzyme lipase allows the accurate determination of triglycerides in blood.

A mutation in a protein that acts as a natural inhibitor of an enzyme can cause disease. For example, emphysema is a destructive lung disease in which the alveolar walls of the lungs are destroyed by an enzyme known as elastase. A person with emphysema breathes much harder to exchange the same volume of air because the alveoli, or air pockets, have become much less efficient. Normally, the elastase enzyme is prevented from destroying lung tissue by the protein antitrypsin. Anti-trypsin is made in the liver and flows to the lungs, where it binds to the active site of elastase and prevents it from digesting lung tissue. Emphysema can occur when the negatively charged amino acid at position 53 of the amino acid sequence of antitrypsin is replaced with a positively charged amino acid. This mutation changes the chemical nature of antitrypsin such that the mutant antitrypsin is released from the liver at a much slower rate. The level of this mutant antitrypsin in the lungs is 15 percent of the normal level. The net result of this one amino acid mutation in the antitrypsin protein is that most of the elastase enzyme is free to destroy lung tissue. Cigarette smoking dramatically increases the incidence of emphysema in people who have the mutant antitrypsin. Cigarette smoke reacts with the hydrophobic amino acid at position 358 of antitrypsin, adding one oxygen atom at this position in the amino acid sequence. The addition of this one extra oxygen atom at this critical place in antitrypsin changes the chemical nature of the hydrophobic amino acid so that the antitrypsin no longer can bind to elastase. Because only 15 percent of the mutant antitrypsin gets from the liver to the lungs in the first place, cigarette smoking puts people with this particular mutation at grave risk for developing emphysema.

Perspective and Prospects

Enzymatic reactions have been used by humankind since prehistoric times. It has been known for more than six thousand years that fermentation processes transform grapes into wine, but it was not until the nineteenth century that it was understood that the conversion of grape sugar to alcohol is a process catalyzed by enzymes found in yeast. In the eighteenth century, Antoine Lavoisier showed that a solution of sugar could be fermented if provided with the sediment of a previous fermentation and that the sugar was converted to alcohol and carbon dioxide in this process. At this time, it was thought that there was a vital force responsible for the workings of a living cell. This notion of a vital force slowed the development of the discipline of biochemistry considerably, as many good scientists struggled to understand the fermentation process. In 1828, Friedrich Wöhler synthesized urea in a test tube, providing strong evidence against the concept of a vital force. In 1833, Anselme Payen and Jean Persoz discovered the first enzyme, diastase (now known as amylase), which converted starch into sugar. The next year, Johann Eberle showed that the presence of a stomach is not required for gastric digestion to take place. In 1836,

Theodor Schwann made the very important discovery that the active ingredient in digestion, which he called pepsin, could be extracted from the stomach wall.

The next year, Jöns Jakob Berzelius developed the idea of catalysis, making the point that both living and inorganic systems had catalysts. In the late 1850's, Louis Pasteur confirmed and extended the earlier experiments of Schwann. Despite his brilliant experimental abilities, however, Pasteur was handicapped in his research by his belief that fermentation could happen only within a living organism. In 1860, Marcelin Berthelot showed that a living being was not the ferment, but produced the ferment, in sharp contrast to Pasteur's vitalist ideas. Pasteur's response to this work was that Berthelot and he meant different things by the use of the word "ferment." Moritz Traube, a German wine merchant, realized that chemical processes and living bodies were mostly based on ferment actions, and he published these ideas in 1858 and again in 1878. In 1878, Friedrich Kühne proposed that to remove the discrepancy over the meaning of the word "ferment," the word "enzyme" should be used, as it means "in yeast." It was not until 1897 that Eduard Buchner showed that living cells are not essential for fermentation to occur, as he extracted from yeast a cell-free juice containing the entire fermentation system.

From 1894 to 1898, Emil Fischer used synthetic organic chemistry for the preparation of substrates of known structure and configuration. He showed that enzymes have a very high degree of specificity for their own particular substrate and developed the famous "lock-and-key" hypothesis. This theory, which has been only slightly modified, states that the shape of a substrate and the enzyme's active site must be complementary for catalysis to occur. Purification of enzymes remained a difficult problem, and it was not until 1926 that James Summer crystallized the first enzyme, jack bean urease. The sequence of protein enzymes could be determined experimentally after 1952, when Frederick Sanger developed his methods for amino acid sequencing. In 1965, David Phillips produced the first three-dimensional picture of an enzyme, determining the shape of lysozyme. The advent of genetic engineering techniques in the 1970's revolutionized the field of enzyme research and the use of enzymes in medical applications by enabling the production of copious amounts of recombinant proteins.

—*George C. Shields, Ph.D.*

See also Antibiotics; Bacteriology; Blood and blood disorders; Blood testing; Cholesterol; Digestion; Emphysema; Enzyme therapy; Fatty acid oxidation disorders; Food biochemistry; Fructosemia; Gaucher's disease; Genetic diseases; Genetic engineering; Genetics and inheritance; Glycogen storage diseases; Glycolysis; Hemophilia; Laboratory tests; Leukemia; Maple syrup urine disease (MSUD); Metabolic disorders; Metabolism; Mucopolysaccharidosis (MPS); Mutation; Niemann-Pick disease; Oncology; Pharmacology; Pulmonary medicine; Screening; Tay-Sachs disease; Thrombolytic therapy and TPA.

FOR FURTHER INFORMATION:

Campbell, Neil A., et al. *Biology: Concepts and Connections.* 6th ed. San Francisco: Pearson/Benjamin Cummings, 2008. This classic introductory textbook provides an excellent discussion of essential biological structures and mechanisms. Its extensive and detailed illustrations help to make even difficult concepts accessible to the nonspecialist. Of particular interest is the chapter on enzymes, titled "An Introduction to Metabolism."

Copeland, Robert A. *Enzymes: A Practical Introduction to Structure, Mechanism, and Data Analysis.* 2d ed. New York: Wiley, 2000. An introductory text that examines the structural complexities of proteins and enzymes and the mechanisms by which enzymes perform their catalytic functions.

Fruton, Joseph S. *Molecules and Life.* New York: Wiley-Interscience, 1972. Fruton, a Yale biochemist, has filled his book with historical essays on the interplay of chemistry and biology. The first part of the book, "From Ferments to Enzymes," is an interesting account of how science progressed from the known results of fermentation to the chemical knowledge that enzymes were the molecules responsible for this and all other biochemical processes.

Kornberg, Arthur. *For the Love of Enzymes: The Odyssey of a Biochemist.* Cambridge, Mass.: Harvard University Press, 1989. Both an autobiography of a great biochemist and a history of the study of enzymes. Arthur Kornberg won a Nobel Prize for the laboratory synthesis of deoxyribonucleic acid (DNA). An excellent scientific biography.

Liska, Ken. *Drugs and the Human Body, with Implications for Society.* 8th ed. Upper Saddle River, N.J.: Pearson/Prentice Hall, 2009. An easy-to-read book about the effects of drugs on the human body. A good overview of how drugs interact with various molecules in the body, including many cases in which enzymes are drug targets.

Palmer, Trevor. *Understanding Enzymes*. 4th ed. New York: Prentice Hall, 1995. A standard text on enzymes and how they function. Includes a bibliography and an index.

Silverman, Richard B. *Organic Chemistry of Enzyme-Catalyzed Reactions*. Rev. ed. San Diego, Calif.: Academic Press, 2002. A text that examines the general mechanisms used by enzymes and stresses that enzymology is simply a biological application of physical organic chemistry.

Voet, Donald, and Judith G. Voet. *Biochemistry*. 3d ed. Hoboken, N.J.: John Wiley & Sons, 2004. A text that approaches biochemistry via organic chemistry reactions.

EPIDEMICS AND PANDEMICS

DISEASE/DISORDER

ANATOMY OR SYSTEMS AFFECTED: All

SPECIALTIES AND RELATED FIELDS: Bacteriology, critical care, epidemiology, gastroenterology, hematology, immunology, internal medicine, microbiology, nursing, otorhinolaryngology, pathology, pharmacology, public health, pulmonary medicine, serology, virology

DEFINITION: An epidemic is a widespread, rapid occurrence of an infectious disease in a community or region at a particular time. A pandemic is an epidemic prevalent throughout a country, a continent, or the world.

KEY TERMS:

coronavirus: a member of the family Coronaviridae, characterized by a viral envelope that looks like a crown and has a positive-sense single-stranded ribonucleic acid (RNA) genome

filovirus: a member of the family Filoviridae, characterized by a filamentous form of the virus and causing severe hemorrhagic fever in humans; it has a negative-sense single-stranded RNA genome; these viruses are so pathological that they require biosafety level four (BSL-4) containment

hemorrhagic fever: a disease in humans or other animals characterized by a high fever and a bleeding disorder, affecting multiple organ systems and, if severe, leading to death

negative-sense RNA virus: a virus in which the virion-enclosed genome is a single strand of RNA that requires transcription to a positive messenger RNA strand before protein synthesis can occur; these viruses enclose a RNA-dependent RNA polymerase to carry this out

orthomyxovirus: a member of the family Orthomyxoviridae, characterized by a spherical (or occasionally filamentous) form and having two major surface glycoproteins, N (neuraminidase) and H (hemagglutinin), that vary from strain to strain; it has a negative-sense single-stranded RNA genome of seven to eight segments

pathogen: an agent that is capable of causing a disease, including viruses, bacteria, protozoa, rickettsia, or parasitic worms

positive-sense RNA virus: a virus in which the virion-enclosed genome is a single strand of RNA that acts directly as a messenger RNA and can be translated directly into protein

CAUSES AND SYMPTOMS

Epidemics, those caused by old diseases that have been around for centuries or newly identified diseases, break out regularly in the human population. Whether they become full-scale pandemics depends on several factors, including how contagious the pathogen; the number of pathogens needed to initiate a disease; how the pathogen is transmitted; the period during which a person is infectious before and after symptoms appear; how long the pathogen can survive in the environment; if an intermediate or alternate host for the pathogen exists; whether vaccines are available, effective, and have been widely used; whether there are any drugs or medications to treat the disease; and whether the contagion can be isolated and contained. Some examples can illustrate these points.

Ebola, one of the most deadly diseases known, is a hemorrhagic fever first identified in 1976 along the Ebola River in the Democratic Republic of the Congo (formerly Zaire). It is caused by a filovirus, a negative-sense single-stranded RNA virus that, in the electron microscope, looks like string, or thread, or filament. Infection leads to a disruption of connective tissues, in-

---

INFORMATION ON EPIDEMICS AND PANDEMICS

CAUSES: Often viruses or bacteria
SYMPTOMS: Depend upon particular disease
DURATION: Some pandemics run their course in three to four months; others last for years
TREATMENTS: Depend upon individual disease; antibiotics for bacterial infections, antiviral medications for viral diseases

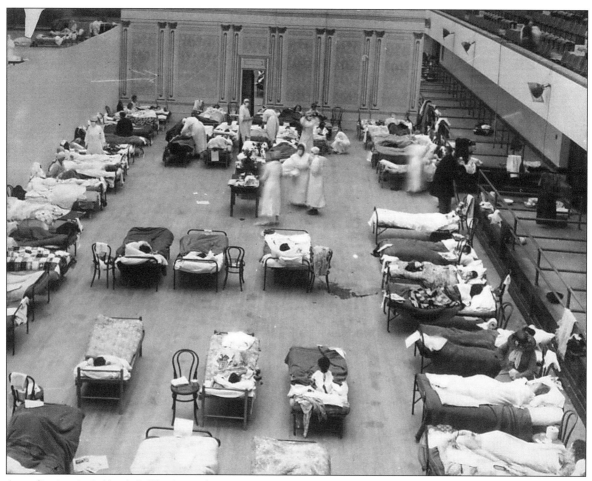

An auditorium in Oakland, California, used as a temporary hospital during the 1918 influenza pandemic. (Courtesy, Oakland Public Library)

cluding that of the blood vessel wall. This results in hemorrhaging from all orifices of the body and rapid death. The death rate for Ebola hemorrhagic fever is greater than 80 percent. There is no treatment or cure. Fortunately, the virus is not airborne; it is transmitted only by direct contact with contaminated bodily fluids. There is an alternate host, believed to be another mammal, possible bats. Thus periodic, local outbreaks occur. However, despite it being extremely deadly, Ebola can be contained by isolation. It has never led to a widespread epidemic or pandemic.

Severe acute respiratory syndrome (SARS) is another example of a recent disease that did lead to an epidemic. SARS was first identified in Guangdong Province, China, in 2003. It is caused by a coronavirus, a positive-sense RNA virus that, in the electron microscope has a ring of viral spikes somewhat like a crown from which this type of virus gets its name. The virus

infects the epithelia of the upper respiratory tract. The symptoms are similar to influenza (fever, headache, muscle ache, fatigue, coughing, sneezing). However, in a significant number of cases, the lungs become involved. This causes severe respiratory distress. There is no cure for SARS, and the disease needs to run its course. The body will produce antibodies against the virus. Antivirals can reduce the severity, and when appropriate, antibiotics are used to treat secondary bacterial infections. Nevertheless, the death rate is estimated at about 10 percent, but more than 50 percent in those over sixty-five.

The disease is spread by virus-containing droplets from coughing or sneezing. Unlike influenza, however, fairly close contact is needed, and the virus does not remain viable in the environment for more than a few hours. SARS quickly spread to twenty-nine countries in 2003 because of air travel, but a rapid and effective global public health response with isolation of SARS cases prevented the disease from becoming a severe pandemic. Although SARS was widespread, a total of only 8,096 cases worldwide were reported to the World Health Organization (WHO); the organization declared SARS to be eradicated in 2005. Because the virus can infect mammals and birds, however, some scientists believed that new outbreaks of the disease could occur in the future.

In contrast, a disease becomes a pandemic when it is both widespread and affects a significant percentage of the population. The best example is the seasonal influenza (flu). The well-known symptoms are fever (often elevated), head and general body aches, sore throat, cough, nasal congestion, and fatigue. It may or may not be accompanied by diarrhea and/or vomiting, symptoms more often seen in young children. It usually runs its course in a week to ten days. Influenza is caused by orthomyxoviruses, which in the electron microscope appear as a spherical or ovoid particles, or occasionally as a filament. These viruses have a negative-sense, single-stranded RNA genome, but it is segmented into several RNA molecules. Infection reaches a peak during the winter months (December through March in the Northern Hemisphere, June through September in the Southern Hemisphere). Estimates indicate that 5 to 30 percent of the world population may become infected in any given year. The reasons that flu pandemics are so common is because flu viruses are highly contagious, survive in the environment for long periods, and frequently mutate so that immunity to one strain of influenza virus does not protect against the same but mutated virus in the future. Moreover, influenza viruses can infect other organisms, which act as a reservoir and in which the virus can mutate or recombine with other coinfected influenza viruses, producing a new strain. The mortality rate for seasonal influenza is about 0.1 percent, usually in the very young, the elderly, and those with other underlying medical conditions such as asthma, diabetes, or cardiovascular disease. Flu vaccines are effective in preventing or reducing the severity of the disease, if they have been made against the type of influenza virus circulating in the world that year. Antiviral medications such as Tamiflu reduce severity of the disease.

TREATMENT AND THERAPY

Treatment and therapies for various contagions will depend on the specific disease, but usually includes antibiotics for bacterial infections and antiviral medications for viral diseases.

PERSPECTIVE AND PROSPECTS

Epidemics and pandemics have plagued humans throughout history. Approximately forty thousand years ago, humans began to domesticate plants and animals for food. Clearing land for crops exposed them to new pathogens, and the close proximity to domesticated animals allowed for transmission of animal pathogens to people. Ancient diseases including smallpox, tuberculosis, measles, and influenza probably arose from animal pathogens adapting to humans. In more recent times, human immunodeficiency virus (HIV) probably adapted to humans in the past fifty years and can be traced to similar simian viruses (SIV) of the chimpanzee and the sooty mangebey monkey. Monkeys are common pets in Africa. Chimpanzees have been used as bush meat, and the transmission of SIV probably occurred during butchering of the animal. The gathering of ancient peoples into larger groups and forming villages with close proximity of inhabitants allowed for pathogens to spread easily. Later, diseases spread along trade routes from Asia and Africa to Europe. Wars have always contributed to the spread of disease as a result of unsanitary conditions, malnutrition, rape, susceptibility of the new population to the pathogen, and lack of sufficient medical care.

History records many epidemics and pandemics. Homer wrote of pestilence devastating the Greeks in the siege of Troy. Thucydides described the Athenian plague of 430-427 B.C.E. The so-called father of medicine Hippocrates has one of the earliest descriptions of an influenza epidemic in 412 B.C.E. The Bible records pestilences in the books of Numbers and in Exodus, the latter most likely being an epidemic of Black Plague in Egypt. In Rome, the physician Pliny the Elder described epidemics of smallpox (165-185 C.E.) and measles (251-266). Probably the best-known pandemic is the Black Plague that devastated Europe in the fourteenth century. In December, 1347, three spice ships from China disembarked at Messina, Italy, carrying plague-infected rats. The plague spread quickly throughout Europe. Ultimately an estimated 25 million died of plague by 1352, amounting to as much as 42 percent of the European population. This pandemic led to great social changes, including the end of the feudal system and the rise of the middle class. Lesser epidemics of plague reappeared in the seventeenth century in Europe and each century since, including one of pneumonic plague in India in the 1990's.

The greatest pandemic in recorded history is that of the influenza pandemic of 1918. Indeed, 80 percent of all Americans who died in Europe during World War I died of influenza, not in direct combat. The 50 to 100 million people worldwide died of what has been called the Spanish flu not because it originated in Spain but because Spain was particularly hard hit by the pandemic. This virus, a mixture of avian and human influenza components, was one hundred times more lethal than the typical seasonal flu. This has caused concern over a reemergence of a highly contagious form of avian flu.

In the past thirty-five years, many new or reemerging diseases, or old pathogens that have developed drug resistance, have been identified. They include Lyme disease; Ebola hemorrhagic fever; Marburg hemorrhagic fever; Lassa fever; Legionnaire's disease; toxic shock syndrome; acquired immunodeficiency syndrome (AIDS), caused by HIV; hantavirus pulmonary syndrome; E. coli O157:H7, a Shigella toxin-producing strain of E. coli; variant Creutzfeldt-Jakob disease (vCJD), the human equivalent of mad cow disease; hepatitis C; cryptosporidiosis; cyclospiridosis; Whitewater arroyo virus; enterovirus 71; hendra virus; West Nile virus; Malaysian Nipah virus; human monkeypox; pneumonic plague; SARS; avian flu; methicillin-resistant *Staphlococcus aureus* (MRSA); vancomycin-resistant *Staphlococcus aureus*; drug-resistant malaria; and multi-drug resistant tuberculosis.

Finally, there is great concern that many of these highly contagious and deadly agents could be "weaponized" and used as biological agents for bioterrorism. Moreover, using biotechnology, new viruses with the contagion of smallpox or influenza along with the lethality of something like Ebola could be developed.

—*Ralph R. Meyer, Ph.D.*

See also Acquired immunodeficiency syndrome (AIDS); Antibiotics; Avian influenza; Bacterial infections; Centers for Disease Control and Prevention (CDC); Drug resistance; Ebola virus; Emerging infectious diseases; Epidemiology; H1N1 influenza; Human immunodeficiency virus (HIV); Immunization and vaccination; Influenza; Insect-borne diseases; Malaria; National Institutes of Health (NIH); Parasitic diseases; Plague; Severe acute respiratory syndrome (SARS); Tuberculosis; Viral infections; West Nile virus; World Health Organization; Zoonoses.

FOR FURTHER INFORMATION:

Barry, John M. *The Great Influenza: The Story of the Deadliest Pandemic in History.* New York: Penguin Books, 2005. Although there are several books describing the great 1918 influenza pandemic, this is clearly one of the best. Written more like a novel and easily understandable by the nontechnical reader.

Krause, Richard M. "The Origin of Plagues: Old and New." *Science* 257 (August 21, 1992): 1073-1078. Although dated, this is an excellent and concise overview of the origin of diseases in an easy-to-read format.

Morens, David M., Gregory K. Folkers, and Anthony S. Fauci. "The Challenge of Emerging and Re-emerging Infectious Diseases." *Nature* 430 (July 8, 2004): 242-249. Although more technical, this short review article looks at emerging diseases from a public health point of view.

Oldstone, Michael B. A. *Viruses, Plagues, and History: Past, Present, and Future.* New York: Oxford University Press, 2010. This excellent book is easily comprehensible to the general public, providing a detailed and fascinating account of historical epidemics and pandemics, including the most recent ones HIV/AIDS, SARS, and West Nile virus encephalitis. Each chapter deals with the history of an individual disease, epidemiology, treatments, and the effect of the disease on course of human history. Well documented with an extensive bibliography.

Sherman, Irwin W. *Twelve Diseases That Changed Our World.* Washington D.C.: ASM Press, 2007. A small, easy-to-read book chronicling a dozen diseases, not all of which infect humans but all of which greatly influenced human history, such as the Irish potato blight. The author does provide useful sources in the chapter notes.

Tucker, Jonathan B. *Scourge: The Once and Future Threat of Smallpox.* New York: Atlantic Monthly Press, 2001. A detailed account of the history of smallpox, the eradication of the disease from the earth, and the controversy surrounding whether the remaining smallpox stocks should be destroyed. The potential of smallpox as a bioweapon is also addressed.

EPIDEMIOLOGY

SPECIALTY

ANATOMY OR SYSTEM AFFECTED: All

SPECIALTIES AND RELATED FIELDS: Public health

DEFINITION: The study of the distribution and determinants of diseases or health-related events in the human population. The main purpose of epidemiology is to prevent and control health problems.

KEY TERMS:

case-control study: an epidemiological study that starts with identification of a group of cases with the disease of interest and a control group of persons without the disease; the association between risk factors and the disease is examined by comparing the two groups with regard to how frequently the risk factors are present in each group

cohort study: an epidemiological study in which groups are identified by the status of exposure to risk factors of the disease of interest; the occurrences of the disease are observed during a follow-up and compared between different groups

cross-sectional study: an epidemiological study that describes disease distribution or frequency by person, place, and time in order to identify a population at risk

epidemiological triangle model: a model used to explain the interrelationship between agent, host, and environment, the three essential factors in the development of disease

population at risk: a group of people who have an increased risk for a particular disease

public health: the effort organized by society to protect, promote, and restore people's health through programs that emphasize the prevention of diseases

risk factor: an aspect of behaviors, lifestyle, environmental exposure, or heredity that is known to be associated with a particular disease

SCIENCE AND PROFESSION

Although epidemiology is closely related to medicine, there are significant differences between the two fields. The main focus of medicine is to diagnose and to treat diseases in individuals, while the core purpose of epidemiology is to identify factors that cause health problems and to control diseases in populations. The health of a population is the responsibility of the field of public health, and epidemiology is a tool for public health. Epidemiology studies disease distribution in populations (for example, how often a disease occurs in different groups of people), examines determinants of diseases or risk factors that increase the risk for disease development, and evaluates strategies to prevent and control diseases in communities.

Diseases have certain patterns in populations. Some groups of people are at a higher risk for a particular disease. For example, smokers are at a higher risk for lung cancer. A key feature of epidemiology is the measurement of disease outcomes in relation to a population

at risk. The concept of a population at risk can be explained by the traditional epidemiological triangle model. In this model, the three angles are agent, host, and environment. The interrelationship of these three factors is the basis of development of disease in the population.

In the triangle model, the agent is the cause of the disease and includes four main categories: biological, physical, chemical, and nutritive. Biological agents are often infectious. The common infectious agents that cause disease are bacteria, viruses, and parasites. Physical agents are related to mechanics, temperature, radiation, noise, and so forth. Chemical agents are often linked to poisons and air or water pollution. Nutritive agents are the macronutrients and micronutrients that the human body needs. Excess or deficiencies in these nutrients can cause health problems.

The second aspect in the triangle model is the host—the intrinsic factors that influence exposure, susceptibility, or response of an individual to an agent. Such intrinsic factors include age, gender, ethnic group, immunity, heredity, and personal behavior. For example, older age increases the risk for many diseases, such as heart disease and stroke. Certain ethnic groups also have increased risks for certain diseases, such as a high incidence of breast cancer in Jewish women.

The third component of the triangle model is the environment, which consists of the surroundings and conditions external to the individual that allow disease transmission or occurrence. The environment consists of physical, biologic, and socioeconomic components. Geology and climate are some examples of physical environment. Biologic environment may include population density, age distribution, and food sources. Socioeconomic environment may include degrees of industrialization and urbanization, use of technology, job security, cultural practices, and availability of health care.

The primary mission of epidemiology is to investigate the interrelationship among agent, host, and environment of a disease in a population and to disrupt the connection at some point in the triangle, so that the disease can be prevented. Some typical epidemiological activities include identification and surveillance of individuals and populations at risk for diseases, monitoring of diseases over time, identification of risk factors associated with diseases, recognition of disease transmission mode, and evaluation of the effectiveness of public health programs.

A specialist of epidemiology is an epidemiologist,

who usually possesses a graduate degree in epidemiology with additional training in disease, public health, and biostatistics. The main responsibility of an epidemiologist is to investigate all elements contributing to the occurrence or absence of a disease in populations. Epidemiologists may work at all levels of communities, including academic or research institutions, federal governmental agencies, state health departments, or local health organizations or medical centers.

Diagnostic and Treatment Techniques
The techniques or methods that epidemiologists use to investigate diseases in populations are epidemiological studies, which mainly consists of cross-sectional studies, case-control studies, and cohort studies.

Cross-sectional studies are also called descriptive epidemiology, because this method describes the distribution of diseases or health-related events and the exposure status of risk factors in terms of person, place, and time. Describing disease distribution by person allows discovery of disease frequency and the populations at greatest risk for the disease. Populations at a high risk can be identified by investigating such characteristics as age, gender, race, education, occupation, income, living arrangement, health status, smoking status, physical activity level, medication use, and access to health care. Disease frequencies can be observed specifically for any of these characteristics by different classifications. For example, hypertension occurrence can be observed by physical activity levels, such as low, medium, and high. Through comparisons of hypertension frequency among the three levels of physical activity, the group with the highest hypertension rate can be identified. Describing disease distribution by place can provide information associated with the geographic extent of the disease. This information includes county, state, country, birthplace, and workplace. Identifying place allows epidemiologists to examine where the causal agent of disease resides and how the disease is transmitted and spread. Describing distribution by time can reveal any seasonality of the disease and trends over time. Some diseases may be more common during a certain season; for example, influenza is more likely to be seen in winter and early spring. By tracking disease trends over time, changes in disease distribution, either emerging or declining, can be documented and corresponding measures can be taken to accompany these changes.

From a cross-sectional study, a group of people with an increased risk for a disease may be identified. Then, one would ask why this group of people has a higher risk for the disease. To answer this question, epidemiologists use case-control studies and cohort studies. Both of these methods are considered analytical studies, as they examine the relationship between a disease and its possible risk factors.

Case-control studies are one of the commonly used epidemiologic designs. A case-control study begins with the selection of a group of cases—the case group, individuals who have the disease or health-related outcome of interest. Then, through interviews or medical records, epidemiologists collect information about the previous exposure of cases (case group members) to possible risk factors. Because case-control studies obtain the information about risk factors in the past, they are also called retrospective studies. Certain demographic variables, such as age, gender, race, occupation, education, and residence, are collected as well and are used as the criteria to select the control group by matching the control subjects to the cases as closely as possible with respect to the demographic variables. No individuals of the control group exhibit the disease or health-related outcome under investigation. The information on previous exposure to risk factors is also collected from the controls.

Matching controls to cases allows the investigators to ignore the demographic variables and focus on risk factors in the analysis. Control subjects can match the cases individually or as a group. The ratio of cases to controls can be one to one or one to two or more. Increasing the number of controls can increase the power of the study to detect the differences between cases and controls; however, a large number of controls can increase the cost of the study as well.

The case and control groups are then compared for previous exposure to the risk factors of the disease using statistical analyses. The association and the strength of association between risk factors and the disease under investigation are evaluated. The results of a case control study may be a positive association, in which the risk factors increase the chance of seeing the disease; a negative association, in which the risk factors decrease the frequency of the disease; or no association, in which no relationship is found between the risk factors and the disease. For example, to study whether obesity is associated with type 2 diabetes, the researcher would select a group of diabetic cases and a group of controls who do not have diabetes but have similar demographic variables, such as age, gender, and occupation. Then, the history of weight would be assessed though interviews of both cases and controls. The information on weight history would then be compared between diabetic cases and nondiabetic controls. For this example, it is likely to see a positive association between obesity and diabetes, which means that obesity is more frequently seen in the diabetic cases.

Cohort studies are another type of analytical design of epidemiology. They are used to examine the causal relationship between a disease or health-related outcome and its risk factors. The cohorts or study groups in a cohort study are identified by characteristics of risk factors exhibited by subjects prior to the appearance of the disease under investigation. Thus, one cohort may consist of subjects with risk factors for a disease, and another cohort may include subjects without such risk factors. In both cohorts, no subjects have the disease under investigation at the beginning of the study. Then, the research would follow both cohorts for a set period of time; therefore, cohort studies are also called prospective studies or longitudinal studies.

During the follow-up time, the difference in the occurrence of the disease under investigation will be recorded and compared between the two cohorts. The results of a cohort study may also be positive, negative, or no association, recognized through statistical analyses. A positive association means the incidence of the disease is increased in the cohort with the risk factors. A negative association indicates that the incidence of the disease is decreased in the cohort with the risk factors, which protect individuals from getting the disease— "good" risk factors. If no statistical differences are identified between the two cohorts, then the risk factors are not associated with the disease. A cohort study might study the relationaship between cholesterol level and coronary artery disease. Individuals with a high cholesterol level would be included in one cohort, and individuals with a normal cholesterol level would be included in another cohort. Then, both cohorts would be followed up for a period of ten years. At the end of ten years, the incidence of coronary artery disease that is diagnosed during those ten years, would be evaluated and compared between the two cohorts. For this study, it is very likely that the cohort with a high cholesterol level would have a higher incidence of coronary artery disease during the ten years of follow-up. A cohort study with only two cohorts is the simplest design. A study may use more than two cohorts, as long as each cohort has the unique risk factor characteristics.

There are advantages and disadvantages for both case-control studies and cohort studies. Cohort studies

observe a disease from cause to effect and thus generate more accurate results; however, they are time-consuming and expensive. On the other hand, case-control studies are quick and inexpensive, but their results are less accurate since they are based on self-reported past experiences, which often encounter recall biases. In practice, epidemiologists often carry out a case-control study first. If a significant association is found from a case-control study, then a cohort study is used to confirm the association.

PERSPECTIVE AND PROSPECTS

Literally translated from Greek, "epidemiology" means "the study of people"—the population-level study of disease. The origins of epidemiology began with John Snow, a physician of London in the eighteenth century who investigated an epidemic of cholera. By observing and plotting the location of deaths related to the disease, Snow was able to legitimize his finding that cholera was spread through contaminated water and food.

In its early years, epidemiology was mainly used to study epidemics of infectious diseases, because infectious diseases were the major cause of death in populations at that time. Through improvements in nutrition and living standards, as well as advances in medicine, the major cause of death has been shifted from infectious diseases to noninfectious or chronic diseases, accompanied by a longer life expectancy in developed countries such as the United States. Epidemiology has now been applied to chronic diseases and other conditions as well, such as cancer, heart disease, diabetes, and injuries. The Framingham Heart Study is a famous epidemiological study of cardiovascular disease in the U.S. population. Epidemiologic methods have been approved as a powerful tool to study diseases or other conditions in populations and have been also applied to other fields, such as sociology.

In the future, the use of epidemiologic methods will continue to expand and allow an understanding of more human diseases and their causes. Because of improved medical technologies, epidemiology has been able to combine traditional observational methods with laboratory tests. New branches of epidemiology have been created, such as molecular epidemiology and genetic epidemiology. Research in these areas will yield knowledge about human diseases at a new level.

—*Kimberly Y. Z. Forrest, Ph.D.*

See also Acquired immunodeficiency syndrome (AIDS); Anthrax; Avian influenza; Bacterial infections; Bacteriology; Biological and chemical weapons; Biostatistics; Centers for Disease Control and Prevention (CDC); Childhood infectious diseases; Cholera; Creutzfeldt-Jakob disease (CJD); Department of Health and Human Services; Disease; *E. coli* infection; Ebola virus; Elephantiasis; Environmental diseases; Environmental health; Epidemics and pandemics; Epstein-Barr virus; Food poisoning; Forensic pathology; Hanta virus; Hepatitis; H1N1 influenza; Human papillomavirus (HPV); Influenza; Insect-borne diseases; Kawasaki disease; Laboratory tests; Legionnaires' disease; Leprosy; Lice, mites, and ticks; Malaria; Marburg virus; Measles; Mercury poisoning; Microbiology; National Institutes of Health; Necrotizing fasciitis; Noroviruses; Occupational health; Parasitic diseases; Pathology; Plague; Poisoning; Poliomyelitis; Prion diseases; Pulmonary diseases; Rabies; Salmonella infection; Severe acute respiratory syndrome (SARS); Sexually transmitted diseases (STDs); Stress; Teratogens; Tropical medicine; Tularemia; Veterinary medicine; Viral infections; World Health Organization; Yellow fever; Zoonoses.

FOR FURTHER INFORMATION:

Day, Ian N. M., ed. *Molecular Genetic Epidemiology: A Laboratory Perspective.* New York: Springer, 2002. This book describes approaches to a series of methodologies in laboratories engaged in molecular and genetic epidemiological studies of population samples. It contains overviews of core topics and techniques that are widely available to researchers.

Fletcher, Robert H., and Suzanne W. Fletcher. *Clinical Epidemiology: The Essentials.* 4th ed. Baltimore: Lippincott Williams & Wilkins, 2005. Provides students and clinicians with the basic principles and concepts of clinical epidemiology, which helps develop a system observing and assessing outcomes in patients for the improvement of care for future patients.

Last, John M., et al., eds. *A Dictionary of Epidemiology.* 4th ed. New York: Oxford University Press, 2001. A standard English-language dictionary of epidemiology and many other related fields, including biostatistics, infectious disease control, health promotion, genetics, and medical ethics.

Lilienfeld, David E., and Paul D. Stolley. *Foundations of Epidemiology.* 3d ed. New York: Oxford University Press, 1994. A textbook commonly used by graduate students of epidemiology, with comprehensive information about concepts and methods of epidemiology. It provides numerous classical epidemiological study examples.

Newman, Stephen C. *Biostatistical Methods in Epidemiology.* New York: John Wiley & Sons, 2003. This book introduces the statistical methods used to analyze epidemiologic data. A reference book for students, health professionals, and epidemiologists.

EPIGLOTTITIS
DISEASE/DISORDER

ALSO KNOWN AS: Supraglottitis

ANATOMY OR SYSTEM AFFECTED: Respiratory system, throat

SPECIALTIES AND RELATED FIELDS: Bacteriology, emergency medicine, family medicine, internal medicine, pediatrics

DEFINITION: An acute, life-threatening inflammation of the epiglottis.

CAUSES AND SYMPTOMS

Epiglottitis is an acute, severe infection that commonly affects children between ages two and six. It is most commonly caused by the bacterium *Haemophilus influenzae*, but it can also be caused by other bacteria such as *Staphylococcus aureus* or *Streptococcus pneumoniae*, fungi such as *Candida albicans*, and viruses.

Epiglottitis presents classically with a fever and sore throat in a young child, who progresses rapidly within a few hours to an inability to eat and drooling, with signs of respiratory obstruction such as stridor. The epiglottis is a thin flap of cartilage at the back of the tongue that closes the respiratory tract while swallowing. When it is inflamed, considerable swelling and consequent respiratory obstruction result. Drooling occurs as the child is unable to swallow his or her own saliva. This is an emergency situation, as the respiratory distress can progress rapidly and become life-threatening within minutes.

INFORMATION ON EPIGLOTTITIS

CAUSES: Usually bacterial infection; sometimes fungal or viral infection

SYMPTOMS: Sore throat, fever, inability to eat, drooling, stridor

DURATION: Acute

TREATMENTS: Hospitalization, humidified oxygen, antibiotics, intravenous fluids, corticosteroids, emergency tracheostomy if needed

It is strongly advised that the mouth and larynx not be examined using a tongue depressor, as this could precipitate a spasm of the epiglottis and exacerbate respiratory distress. Epiglottitis is diagnosed by a clinician through laryngoscopy, with efforts made to secure the airway first. Neck X rays reveal a characteristic "thumbprint" sign caused by an enlarged epiglottis. A blood culture may reveal the causative organism, and an elevated white blood cell count may be observed.

TREATMENT AND THERAPY

In most cases of epiglottitis, hospitalization is required, and the patient is usually admitted to the intensive care unit (ICU). The foremost concern is to secure and maintain an airway as soon as possible. Humidified oxygen, which has been moistened to help the patient breathe better, is administered. An emergency tracheostomy or needle cricothyrotomy may be needed to secure the airway. Antibiotics, intravenous fluids, and corticosteroids may also be administered to decrease the swelling. With proper and prompt treatment, the prognosis is very good.

PERSPECTIVE AND PROSPECTS

Epiglottitis, which was first described in 1848, is an acute inflammation of the epiglottis that should be distinguished from laryngotracheobronchitis or croup. Also, children ingesting hot liquids may present with similar symptoms. The disease must be managed efficiently and in a clinical setting only. Since the causative agent of the disease is infectious, family members must also be screened and treated for the disease. The aggressive immunization of children against *Haemophilus influenzae B* by the Hib vaccine has resulted in a significant decrease in the incidence of epiglottitis.

—*Venkat Raghavan Tirumala, M.D., M.H.A.*

See also Antibiotics; Bacterial infections; Cartilage; Childhood infectious diseases; Choking; Croup; Otorhinolaryngology; Pulmonary medicine, pediatric; Respiration; Sore throat; Tracheostomy.

FOR FURTHER INFORMATION:

Kasper, Dennis L., et al., eds. *Harrison's Principles of Internal Medicine.* 16th ed. New York: McGraw-Hill, 2005.

Rakel, Robert E., ed. *Textbook of Family Practice.* 6th ed. Philadelphia: W. B. Saunders, 2002.

Tapley, Donald F., et al., eds. *The Columbia University College of Physicians and Surgeons Complete Home Medical Guide.* Rev. 3d ed. New York: Crown, 1995.

EPILEPSY

DISEASE/DISORDER

ANATOMY OR SYSTEM AFFECTED: Brain, head, nerves, nervous system

SPECIALTIES AND RELATED FIELDS: Neurology

DEFINITION: A serious neurologic disease characterized by seizures, which may involve convulsions and loss of consciousness.

KEY TERMS:

anticonvulsant: a therapeutic drug that prevents or diminishes convulsions

aura: a sensory symptom or group of such symptoms that precedes a grand mal seizure

clonic phase: the portion of an epileptic seizure that is characterized by convulsions

electroencephalogram (EEG): a graphic recording of the electrical activity of the brain, as recorded by an electroencephalograph

grand mal: a type of epileptic seizure characterized by severe convulsions, body stiffening, and loss of consciousness during which victims fall down; also called tonic-clonic seizure

idiopathic disease: a disease of unknown origin

petit mal: a mild type of epileptic seizure characterized by a very short lapse of consciousness, usually without convulsions; the epileptic does not fall down

psychomotor epilepsy: condition of impairment of consciousness with amnesia of the episode which may include movements of the arms and legs and hallucinations

seizure: a sudden convulsive attack of epilepsy that can involve loss of consciousness and falling down

seizure discharges: characteristic brain waves seen in the EEGs of epileptics; their strength and frequency depend upon whether a seizure is occurring and its type

status epilepticus: a rare, life-threatening condition in which many sequential seizures occur without recovery between them

tonic-clonic seizure: another term for a grand mal seizure

tonic phase: the portion of an epileptic seizure characterized by loss of consciousness and body stiffness

CAUSES AND SYMPTOMS

Epilepsy is characterized by seizures, commonly called fits, which may involve convulsions and the loss of consciousness. It was called the "falling disease" or "sacred disease" in antiquity and was mentioned in 2080 B.C.E. in the laws of the famous Babylonian king

Hamurabi. Epilepsy is a serious neurologic disease that usually appears between the ages of two and fourteen. It does not affect intelligence, as shown by the fact that the range of intelligence quotients (IQs) for epileptics is quite similar to that of the general population. In addition, many suspected epileptics have achieved fame, such as Alexander the Great, Julius Caesar, Russian novelist Fyodor Dostoevski, and Dutch artist Vincent van Gogh.

In 400 B.C.E., Hippocrates of Cos proposed that epilepsy arose from physical problems in the brain. This origin of the disease is now known to be unequivocally true. Despite many centuries of exhaustive study and effort, however, only a small percentage (20 percent) of cases of epilepsy caused by brain injuries, brain tumors, and other diseases are curable. This type of epilepsy is called symptomatic epilepsy. In contrast, 80 percent of epileptics can be treated to control the occurrence of seizures but cannot be cured of the disease, which is therefore a lifelong affliction. In these cases, the basis of the epilepsy is not known, although the suspected cause is genetically programmed brain damage that still evades discovery. Most epilepsy is, therefore, an idiopathic disease (one of unknown origin), and such epileptics are thus said to suffer from idiopathic epilepsy.

A common denominator in idiopathic epilepsy, and also in symptomatic epilepsy, is that it is evidenced by unusual electrical discharges, brain waves, seen in the electroencephalograms (EEGs) of epileptics. These brain waves are called seizure discharges. They vary in both their strength and their frequency, depending on whether an epileptic is having a seizure and what type of seizure is occurring. Seizure discharges are almost always present and recognizable in the EEGs of epileptics, even during sleep.

There are four types of common epileptic seizures. Two of these are partial (local) seizures called focal motor and temporal lobe seizures, respectively. The others, grand mal and petit mal, are generalized and may involve the entire body. A focal motor seizure is characterized by rhythmic jerking of the facial muscles, an arm, or a leg. As with other epileptic seizures, it is caused by abnormal electrical discharges in the portion of the brain that controls normal movement in the body part that is affected. This abnormal electrical activity is always seen as seizure discharges in the EEG of the affected part of the brain.

In contrast, temporal lobe seizures (also known as psychomotor epilepsy), again characterized by seizure

---

INFORMATION ON EPILEPSY

CAUSES: Brain injury, brain tumors, disease, possible genetic factors
SYMPTOMS: Seizures, loss of consciousness
DURATION: Typically chronic
TREATMENTS: Surgery to remove tumor or causative brain tissue abnormality, anticonvulsant drugs

---

discharges in a distinct portion of the cerebrum of the brain, are characterized by sensory hallucinations and other types of consciousness alteration, a meaningless physical action, or even a babble of some incomprehensible language. Thus, for example, temporal lobe seizures may explain some cases of people "speaking in tongues" in religious experiences or in the days of the Delphic oracles of ancient Greece.

The term "grand mal" refers to the most severe type of epileptic seizure. Also called tonic-clonic seizures, grand mal attacks are characterized by very severe EEG seizure discharges throughout the entire brain. A grand mal seizure is usually preceded by sensory symptoms called an aura (probably related to temporal lobe seizures), which warn an epileptic of an impending attack. The aura is quickly followed by the grand mal seizure itself, which involves the loss of consciousness, localized or widespread jerking and convulsions, and severe body stiffness.

Epileptics suffering a grand mal seizure usually fall to the ground, may foam at the mouth, and often bite their tongues or the inside of their cheeks unless something is placed in the mouth before they lose consciousness. In a few cases, the victim will lose bladder or bowel control. In untreated epileptics, grand mal seizures can occur weekly. Most of these attacks last for only a minute or two, followed quickly by full recovery after a brief sense of disorientation and feelings of severe exhaustion. In some cases, however, grand mal seizures may last for up to five minutes and lead to temporary amnesia or to other mental deficits of a longer duration. In rare cases, the life-threatening condition of status epilepticus occurs, in which many sequential tonic-clonic seizures occur over several hours without recovery between them.

The fourth type of epileptic seizure is petit mal, which is often called generalized nonconvulsive seizure or, more simply, absence. A petit mal seizure consists of a brief period of loss of consciousness (ten to forty seconds) without the epileptic falling down. The epileptic usually appears to be daydreaming (absent) and shows no other symptoms. Often a victim of a petit mal seizure is not even aware that the event has occurred. In some cases, a petit mal seizure is accompanied by mild jerking of hands, head, or facial features and/or rapid blinking of the eyes. Petit mal attacks can be quite dangerous if they occur while an epileptic is driving a motor vehicle.

Diagnosing epilepsy usually requires a patient history, a careful physical examination, blood tests, and a neurologic examination. The patient history is most valuable when it includes eyewitness accounts of the symptoms, the frequency of occurrence, and the usual duration range of the seizures observed. In addition, documentation of any preceding severe trauma, infection, or episodes of addictive drug exposure provides useful information that will often differentiate between idiopathic and symptomatic epilepsy.

Evidence of trauma is quite important, as head injuries that caused unconsciousness are often the basis for later symptomatic epilepsy. Similarly, infectious diseases of the brain, including meningitis and encephalitis, can cause this type of epilepsy. Finally, excessive use of alcohol or other psychoactive drugs can also be a causative agent for symptomatic epilepsy.

Blood tests for serum glucose and calcium, electroencephalography, and computed tomography (CT) scanning are also useful diagnostic tools. The EEG will nearly always show seizure discharges in epileptics, and the location of the discharges in the brain may localize problem areas associated with the disease. CT scanning is most useful for identifying tumors and other serious brain damage that may cause symptomatic epilepsy. When all tests are negative except for abnormal EEGs, the epilepsy is considered idiopathic.

It is thought that the generation of epileptic symptoms occurs because of a malfunction in nerve impulse transport in some of the billions of nerve cells (neurons) that make up the brain and link it to the body organs that it innervates. This nerve impulse transport is an electrochemical process caused by the ability of the neurons to retain substances (including potassium) and to excrete substances (including sodium). This ability generates the weak electrical current that makes up a nerve impulse and that is registered by electroencephalography.

A nerve impulse leaves a given neuron via an outgoing extension (or axon), passes across a tiny synaptic gap that separates the axon from the next neuron in line,

and enters an incoming extension (or dendrite) of that cell. The process is repeated until the impulse is transmitted to its site of action. The cell bodies of neurons make up the gray matter of the brain, and axons and dendrites (white matter) may be viewed as connecting wires.

Passage across synaptic gaps between neurons is mediated by chemicals called neurotransmitters, and it is now believed that epilepsy results when unknown materials cause abnormal electrical impulses by altering neurotransmitter production rates and/or the ability of sodium, potassium, and related substances to enter or leave neurons. The various nervous impulse abnormalities that cause epilepsy can be shown to occur in the portions of the gray matter of the cerebrum that control high-brain functions. For example, the frontal lobe—which controls speech, body movement, and eye movements—is associated with temporal lobe seizures.

TREATMENT AND THERAPY

Idiopathic epilepsy is viewed as the expression of a large group of different diseases, all of which present themselves clinically as seizures. This is extrapolated from the various types of symptomatic epilepsy observed, which have causes that include faulty biochemical processes (such as inappropriate calcium levels), brain tumors or severe brain injury, infectious diseases (such as encephalitis), and the chronic overuse of addictive drugs. As to why idiopathic epilepsy causes are not identifiable, the general biomedical wisdom states that present technology is too imprecise to detect its causes.

Symptomatic epilepsy is treated with medication and either by the extirpation of the tumor or other causative brain tissue abnormality that was engendered by trauma or disease or by the correction of the metabolic disorder involved. The more common, incurable idiopathic disease is usually treated entirely with medication that relieves symptoms. This treatment is essential because without it most epileptics cannot attend school successfully, maintain continued employment, or drive a motor vehicle safely.

A large number of anticonvulsant drugs are presently available for epilepsy management. It must, however, be made clear that no one therapeutic drug will control all types of seizures. In addition, some patients require several such drugs for effective therapy, and the natural history of a given case of epilepsy may often require periodic changes from drug to drug as the disease evolves. Furthermore, every therapeutic antiepilepsy drug has dangerous side effects that may occur when it is present in the body above certain levels or after it is used beyond some given time period. Therefore, each epileptic patient must be monitored at frequent intervals to ascertain that no dangerous physical symptoms are developing and that the drug levels in the body (monitored by the measurement of drug content in blood samples) are within a tolerable range.

More than twenty antiepilepsy drugs are widely used. Phenytoin (Dilantin) is very effective for grand mal seizures. Because of its slow metabolism, phenytoin can be administered relatively infrequently, but this slow metabolism also requires seven to ten days before its anticonvulsant effects occur. Side effects include cosmetically unpleasant hair overgrowth, swelling of the gums, and skin rash. These symptoms are particularly common in epileptic children. More serious are central nervous effects including ataxia (unsteadiness in walking), drowsiness, anemia, and marked thyroid deficiency. Most such symptoms are reversed by decreasing the drug doses or by discontinuing it. Phenytoin is often given together with other antiepi-

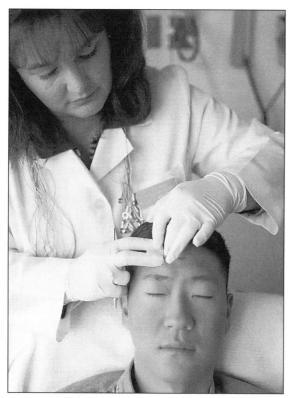

A doctor attaches electrodes to a patient's head in order to monitor his epilepsy. (PhotoDisc)

lepsy drugs to produce optimum seizure prevention. In those cases, great care must be taken to prevent dangerous synergistic drug effects from occurring. High phenytoin doses also produce blood levels of the drug that are very close to toxic 25 micrograms per milliliter values.

Carbamazepine (Tegretol) is another frequently used antiepileptic drug. Chemically related to the drugs used as antidepressants, it is useful against both psychomotor epilepsy and grand mal seizures. Common carbamazepine side effects are ataxia, drowsiness, and double vision. A more dangerous, and fortunately less common, side effect is the inability of bone marrow to produce blood cells. Again, very serious and unexpected complications occur in mixed-drug therapy that includes carbamazepine, and at high doses toxic blood levels of the drug may be exceeded.

Phenobarbital, a sedative hypnotic also used as a tranquilizer by nonepileptics, is a standby for treating epilepsy. It too can have serious side effects, including a lowered attention span, hyperactivity, and learning difficulties. In addition, when given with phenytoin, phenobarbital will speed up the excretion of that drug, lowering its effective levels.

Four major lessons can be learned from these three drugs. First, individual antiepilepsy drugs have many different side effects. Second, there are concrete reasons that epileptics taking therapeutic drugs must be monitored carefully for physical symptoms. Third, at high antiepileptic drug doses, the blood levels attained may closely approximate and even exceed toxic values. Fourth, drug interactions in mixed-drug therapy can be counterproductive.

A new generation of antiepileptic medications that act by various mechanisms is now available. These drugs, which include gabapentin, lamotrigine, topiramate, tiagabine, levetiracetam, zonisamide, oxcarbazepine, and pregabalin, are often better tolerated, safer, and faster acting than the older generation of antiepileptics. However, the efficacy of both the newer and older drugs to prevent seizures remains highly dependent on the individual patient.

About 20 percent of idiopathic epileptics do not achieve adequate seizure control after prolonged and varied drug therapy. Another option for some—but not all—such people is brain surgery. This type of brain surgery is usually elected after two conditions are met. First, often-repeated EEGs must show that most or all of the portion of the brain in which the seizures develop is very localized. Second, these affected areas must be in a brain region that the patient can lose without significant mental loss (often in the prefrontal or temporal cerebral lobes). When such surgery is carried out, it is reported that 50 to 75 percent of the patients who are treated and given chronic, postoperative antiepilepsy drugs become able to achieve seizure control.

The most frequent antiepilepsy surgery is temporal lobectomy. The brain has two temporal lobes, one of which is dominant in the control of language, memory, and thought expression. A temporal lobectomy is carried out by removing the nondominant temporal lobe, when it is the site of epilepsy. About 6 percent of temporal lobectomies lead to a partial loss of temporal lobe functions, which may include impaired vision, movement, memory, and speech.

Another common type of antiepilepsy surgery is called corpus callosotomy. This procedure involves partially disconnecting the two cerebral hemispheres by severing some of the nerves in the corpus callosum that links them. This surgery is performed when an epileptic has frequent, uncontrollable grand mal attacks that cause many dangerous falls. The procedure usually results in reduced numbers of seizures and decreases in their severity.

Physicians now believe that many cases of epilepsy may be prevented by methods aimed at avoiding head injury (especially in children) and the use of techniques such as amniocentesis to identify potential epileptics and treat them before birth. Furthermore, the prophylactic administration of antiepilepsy drugs to nonepileptic people who are afflicted with encephalitis and other diseases known to produce epilepsy is viewed as wise.

Perspective and Prospects

A great number of advances have occurred in the treatment of epilepsy via therapeutic drugs and surgical techniques. With the exception of symptomatic epilepsy, drug therapy has been the method of choice because it is less drastic than surgery, is easier to manage, and rarely has the potential for irreversible damage to patients that can be caused by the removal of a portion of the brain. The main antiepileptic drugs are phenytoin, carbamazepine, and phenobarbital, but a tremendous variety of other chemical therapies has been investigated and utilized successfully.

Such treatments include the new generation of antiepileptic drugs, high doses of vitamins, injections of muscle relaxants, and changes in diet. The variety is unsurprising, considering the vast number of disease states that can cause seizures. For example, the rare genetic disease phenylketonuria (PKU) can cause epilepsy. Phenylketonuric epilepsy is often treated by use of a ketogenic diet rich in fats; the clear value of this treatment is unexplained. Readers are encouraged to investigate the many epilepsy treatments that have not been noted. Such an examination may be quite valuable because there are about a million epileptics in the United States alone, and some estimates indicate that four of every thousand humans are likely to develop some epileptic symptoms during their lifetime.

Modern surgical treatment of epilepsy reportedly began in 1828, with the efforts of Benjamin Dudley, who removed epilepsy-causing blood clots and skull fragments from five patients, who all survived despite primitive and nonsterile operating rooms. The next landmark in such surgery was the removal of a brain tumor by the German physician R. J. Godlee, in 1884, without the benefit of X rays or EEG techniques, which did not then exist.

By the 1950's EEGs were used to locate epileptic brain foci, and physicians such as the Canadians Wilder Penfield and Herbert Jasper pioneered their use to locate brain regions to remove for epilepsy remission without damaging vital functions. After considerable evolution over the course of forty years, antiepilepsy surgery by the 1990's had become widespread, commonplace, and relatively safe.

Nevertheless, because of the imperfections of all available methodologies, 5 to 8 percent of epileptics cannot achieve seizure control by any method or method combination, and even the "well-managed" epilepsy treatment regimen has its flaws. There is still much to be learned about curing epilepsy. Clinical and experimental perioperative studies are now possible during epilepsy surgery to examine the bioelectrical activity and molecular events of the affected neurons. It is hoped that the efforts of ongoing biomedical research, both in basic science and in clinical settings, will eliminate epilepsy through the development of new therapeutic drugs and sophisticated advances in surgery and other nondrug methods.

—Sanford S. Singer, Ph.D.;
updated by W. Michael Zawada, Ph.D.

See also Auras; Brain; Brain damage; Brain disorders; Brain tumors; Computed tomography (CT) scanning; Electroencephalography (EEG); Nervous system; Neuroimaging; Neurology; Neurology, pediatric; Neurosurgery; Phenylketonuria (PKU); Seizures; Unconsciousness.

FOR FURTHER INFORMATION:

Appleton, Richard, and Anthony G. Marson. *Epilepsy: The Facts*. 3d ed. New York: Oxford University Press, 2009. The author wishes to eliminate misunderstanding about epilepsy and educate people about it. This is done nicely by clear coverage of topics including explanation of epilepsy, seizure types and causes, epilepsy treatment methods, and information on living with the disease.

Beers, Mark H., et al., eds. *The Merck Manual of Diagnosis and Therapy*. 18th ed. Whitehouse Station, N.J.: Merck Research Laboratories, 2006. Contains a compendium of data on the characteristics, etiology, diagnosis, and treatment of adult epilepsy. Also discusses seizure disorders of children and newborns. Designed for physicians, the material is also useful to less specialized readers.

Bloom, Floyd E., M. Flint Beal, and David J. Kupfer, eds. *The Dana Guide to Brain Health*. New York: Dana Press, 2006. An easy-to-understand health guide to the brain from neuroscience, neurology, and psychiatry perspectives. More than seventy psychiatric and neurological disorders, their diagnoses, and their treatments are covered.

Devinsky, Orrin. *Epilepsy: Patient and Family Guide*. 3d ed. New York: Demos Medical, 2008. An excellent lay guide to the medical and social topics relevant to epilepsy. Topics include diagnosis and treatment, epilepsy in children and adults, legal and financial issues, and research resources.

Epilepsy Foundation. http://www.epilepsyfoundation .org. A national organization dedicated to education, research, and advocacy. Web site offers information on careers and employment, parent support groups and children's programs, and online "Interest Groups," among many other features.

Freeman, John M., Eileen P. G. Vining, and Diana J. Pillas. *Seizures and Epilepsy in Childhood: A Guide*. 3d ed. Baltimore: Johns Hopkins University Press, 2002. Designed for parents, an overall guide to the symptoms, diagnosis, and treatment of children with epilepsy. Third edition includes new chapters on alternative therapies and medicines, routine health care, insurance issues, and research resources.

Gumnit, Robert J. *Living Well with Epilepsy*. 2d ed. New York: Demos Vermande, 1997. Designed to give people with epilepsy the outlook necessary to live successfully with the disease. Among the topics covered are causes and treatment, high-quality care, medical and surgical options, the problems of epi-

leptic children, sexuality and pregnancy, the workplace, rights, and resources.

Nolte, John. *Human Brain: An Introduction to Its Functional Anatomy*. 6th ed. Philadelphia: Mosby/ Elsevier, 2009. Text covering major concepts and structure-function relationships in the human neurological system.

Weaver, Donald F. *Epilepsy and Seizures: Everything You Need to Know*. Toronto, Ont.: Firefly Books, 2001. A lay guide covering research advances, history of the disease, different types, the mechanisms, diagnosis and treatment, and special situations, such as epilepsy in pregnant women, children, and the elderly.

EPISIOTOMY
PROCEDURE

ANATOMY OR SYSTEM AFFECTED: Anus, genitals, reproductive system

SPECIALTIES AND RELATED FIELDS: Gynecology, obstetrics

DEFINITION: A surgical cut made in the pelvic floor to enlarge the vagina for the facilitation of childbirth.

INDICATIONS AND PROCEDURES

An episiotomy is performed to enlarge the vaginal opening and ease the delivery of a baby during childbirth. While not a routine procedure, some circumstances that indicate the need for an episiotomy include macrosomia (large fetal size), rapid delivery, breech delivery, and presentation of the baby with face to the front of the birth canal, all of which prevent the perineum (the area between the vagina and the anus) from stretching rapidly enough to prevent tearing. Scarring from vaginal surgeries also limits the ability of the vagina to expand.

During the procedure, a local anesthetic is injected into the perineum. The provider uses straight-bladed blunt scissors to snip the tissue between the vagina and anus diagonally, avoiding the anal sphincter muscle and preventing tearing into the anal sphincter. After delivery, the incision is carefully stitched together, along with any minor tears in the birth canal. Delivery by a nurse midwife as opposed to a private obstetrician is far less likely to result in an episiotomy, as episiotomies are not done routinely by nurse midwives. Furthermore, with a nurse midwife, techniques such as vaginal-perineal massage with warm oil are employed to help stretch the perineum and avoid the need for episiotomy.

USES AND COMPLICATIONS

The birth canal has very limited space to accommodate an infant, and situations such as feetfirst or faceforward presentation can lead to compression of the umbilical cord and interruption of the oxygen supply to the baby, or even to potential crushing of the infant. An episiotomy can facilitate a rapid delivery in these circumstances, thereby preventing serious injury to the infant. Failure of the perineum to stretch sufficiently to accommodate the child can result in severe, irregular tears of the vagina and even of the anal sphincter muscles. Ragged tears are very difficult to repair surgically and are much more prone to infection. Tearing of the anal sphincter could lead to permanent incontinence. The easily repaired incisions of episiotomy eliminate these potential difficulties.

Healing of the incisions is rapid and straightforward, but the area may itch and be somewhat painful for a few weeks. Painkilling drugs may be prescribed, and ice packs can be used to alleviate pain. Women who do not desire episiotomies and have controlled, problem-free deliveries may try to stretch the perineum gradually by massaging it with warm oil during the delivery. While in the past, episiotomies were considered a routine part of delivery, they are now done less commonly, only as necessitated for conditions like those indicated above. Additionally, maternal satisfaction is increasing as episiotomies are being done more when they are necessary and to a lesser extent when they are avoidable.

—*Karen E. Kalumuck, Ph.D.;*
updated by Robin Kamienny Montvilo, R.N., Ph.D.

See also Anus; Childbirth; Childbirth complications; Incontinence; Obstetrics; Women's health.

FOR FURTHER INFORMATION:

Carlson, Karen J., Stephanie A. Eisenstat, and Terra Ziporyn. *The New Harvard Guide to Women's Health.* Cambridge, Mass.: Harvard University Press, 2004.

Cunningham, F. Gary, et al., eds. *Williams Obstetrics.* 23d ed. New York: McGraw-Hill, 2010.

Goldberg, Roger P. *Ever Since I Had My Baby: Understanding, Treating, and Preventing the Most Common Physical After-Effects of Pregnancy and Childbirth.* New York: Crown, 2003.

Gonik, Bernard, and Renee A. Bobrowski. *Medical Complications in Labor and Delivery.* Cambridge, Mass.: Blackwell Scientific, 1996.

Machisio, Sara, et al. "Care Pathways in Obstetrics: The Effectiveness in Reducing the Incidence of Episiotomy in Childbirth." *Journal of Nursing Management* 14, no. 7 (October, 2006): 538-543.

Reynolds, Karina, Christoph Lees, and Grainne McCarten. *Pregnancy and Birth: Your Questions Answered.* Rev. ed. New York: DK, 2007.

Sears, William, and Martha Sears. *The Birth Book: Everything You Need to Know to Have a Safe and Satisfying Birth.* Boston: Little, Brown, 1994.

Simkin, Penny, Janet Whalley, and Ann Keppler. *Pregnancy, Childbirth, and the Newborn: The Complete Guide.* 3d ed. Minnetonka, Minn.: Meadowbrook Press, 2008.

Stoppard, Miriam. *Conception, Pregnancy, and Birth.* Rev. ed. New York: DK, 2005.

Warhus, Susan. *Countdown to Baby: Answers to the One Hundred Most Asked Questions About Pregnancy and Childbirth.* Omaha, Nebr.: Addicus Books, 2003.

EPSTEIN-BARR VIRUS

DISEASE/DISORDER

ALSO KNOWN AS: Human herpesvirus 4 (HHV-4)

ANATOMY OR SYSTEM AFFECTED: Blood, cells, glands, immune system, lymphatic system, mouth, muscles, nose, throat

SPECIALTIES AND RELATED FIELDS: Cytology, hematology, immunology, microbiology, oncology, pathology, pediatrics, virology

DEFINITION: An extensively occurring virus which infects almost all humans during their lifetime, often remaining latent in their systems but sometimes causing malignant tumors and various types of cancer.

KEY TERMS:

antibodies: protein molecules that detect antigens and destroy infected host cells

antigens: viral proteins that attract antibodies, which the immune system designs to attack them

B cells: also known as B lymphocytes; white blood cells that create antibodies

oncoviruses: viruses causing the growth of cancerous cells

replication: the viral insertion of genetic information into host cell nuclei to create additional similar viruses

T cells: also known as cytotoxic T lymphocytes; white blood cells that destroy cells hosting antigens or infected by pathogens which eluded antibodies

virion: a viral particle that contains genetic information inside a protective structure

CAUSES AND SYMPTOMS

Present only in humans, Epstein-Barr virus was the first documented oncovirus. The virus, resembling other human herpesviruses, consists of sphere-shaped, barbed virions approximately 120 to 220 nanometers in diameter. Each Epstein-Barr virus genome contains two strands of deoxyribonucleic acid (DNA). A protein shell protects the genome, and an envelope surrounds the protein shell. Various Epstein-Barr virus strains have evolved that can infect an individual at the same time.

The Epstein-Barr virus typically infects salivary gland cells or B cells. Usually, Epstein-Barr viral infections are transmitted through saliva. Seeking host cells in order to replicate, the Epstein-Barr virus proliferates, creating approximately one hundred types of antigens, including nuclear antigen EBNA 1, which the Epstein-Barr virus uses to put its DNA into new cells created during cell division.

T cells fight Epstein-Barr virus antigens by destroying infected host cells. T cells and antibodies stay in the immune system to continue protecting against infection, regulating latency, and developing immunity. EBNA1 is necessary for the Epstein-Barr virus genomes to endure being latent. T cells cannot detect the antigen EBNA1 and attack those host cells, which results in the Epstein-Barr virus often being invisible to immune protection. Latent infections are not apparent, usually remaining passive, but they can become active, potentially resulting in tumors and diseases.

The Epstein-Barr virus usually infects throat, blood, or immune system cells. Infectious mononucleosis, also known as glandular fever, is the most widely known Epstein-Barr viral infection. Physicians determine if people have been infected by Epstein-Barr virus by performing laboratory tests analyzing blood samples to detect if any of the antibodies to combat Epstein-Barr virus antigens are present and, if so, how many are present. Such antibodies might have existed for years and are not proof of an active infection.

People can contract the virus as children, adolescents, or adults, depending on their geographic location and socioeconomic factors. Some infants are born with the virus transmitted by their mothers. The Epstein-Barr virus usually infects people when they are children, without obvious signs. Often, these individuals never know that they are infected. Approximately half of the people who contract the Epstein-Barr virus as an adolescent or at an older age, however, develop infectious mononucleosis.

INFORMATION ON EPSTEIN-BARR VIRUS

CAUSES: Viral infection spread primarily through saliva

SYMPTOMS: In children, usually none; in adolescents and adults, often mononucleosis; associated with a number of cancers and other diseases

DURATION: Acute and then chronic

TREATMENTS: None for viral infection; chemotherapy and radiation for resulting cancers

---

Activated Epstein-Barr virus can result in several serious diseases, and people with suppressed immune systems are vulnerable to developing such malignancies as cancerous tumors in smooth muscle tissue, stomach carcinomas, lymphomas, and sarcomas. Epstein-Barr virus often causes nasal and throat cancers known as nasopharyngeal carcinoma. In some individuals with acquired immunodeficiency syndrome (AIDS), Epstein-Barr virus replicates in tongue cells, resulting in oral hairy leukoplakia. Epstein-Barr virus has also been associated with leukemia.

Weak immune systems cause people to be vulnerable to Epstein-Barr virus infections, particularly after organ transplantation and the use of immunosuppressive drugs to lower the immune reaction and encourage acceptance of the new organ. In those cases, Epstein-Barr virus sometimes causes post-transplant lymphoproliferative disease to occur.

When it infects the nodes, Epstein-Barr virus might be a factor in people affected by Hodgkin's disease. Researchers have considered a possible role of Epstein-Barr virus in the development of multiple sclerosis and breast cancer. They have eliminated it as a factor in chronic fatigue syndrome.

TREATMENT AND THERAPY

Approximately 90 to 95 percent of humans globally at any time have been infected with Epstein-Barr virus, which remains latent and endures in their bodies until death. There is currently no way to eliminate the virus once infection has occurred. Treatment focuses instead on the diseases that Epstein-Barr virus causes.

Researchers have attempted to develop antiviral vaccines to stop the replication of Epstein-Barr virus. In the early twenty-first century, scientists at Queensland Institute of Medical Research developed a vaccine prototype to strengthen T cells combatting Epstein-Barr virus antigens.

PERSPECTIVE AND PROSPECTS

The Epstein-Barr virus was located as a result of researchers seeking viruses possibly associated with cancer in humans, In 1961, London researcher M. Anthony Epstein attended a lecture at which Denis P. Burkitt discussed his work with tumors, later called Burkitt's lymphoma, in African children's facial bones. Epstein, experienced with investigating viruses causing animal tumors, wanted to examine Burkitt's lymphoma tumor tissues to detect any viruses. The British Empire Cancer Campaign funded Epstein's travel to Uganda to acquire a consistent supply of tumor samples for his Middlesex Hospital Medical School laboratory. Epstein tried unsuccessfully to locate a virus for a couple of years.

The U.S. National Cancer Institute presented Epstein $45,000 for his investigations, and he hired doctoral student Yvonne M. Barr and colleague Bert G. Achong to expand his laboratory work attempting to culture viruses. The trio successfully grew a Burkitt's lymphoma cell line in culture. When cells from that sample were examined with an electron microscope, the London scientists saw viral particles with structural elements of herpesvirus. Scrutinizing the virions, the trio declared that they had isolated a previously unknown human herpesvirus. They published their results in a 1964 *Lancet* article. After Epstein-Barr virus was identified, additional investigators studied the virus to expand knowledge of its structure, replication, and the diseases associated with it, determining that it was an oncovirus.

Research into ways to fight Epstein-Barr virus is ongoing. Scientists at the European Molecular Biology Laboratory and Institut de Virologie Moléculaire et Structurale have focused on controlling a protein molecule known as ZEBRA that accompanies Epstein-Barr virus, helping activate it from the latent phase.

—*Elizabeth D. Schafer, Ph.D.*

See also Acquired immunodeficiency syndrome (AIDS); Burkitt's lymphoma; Cancer; Carcinoma; Carcinogens; Ewing's sarcoma; Herpes; Leukemia; Lymphadenopathy and lymphoma; Lymphatic system; Mononucleosis; Oncology; Sarcoma; Transplantation; Tumors; Viral infections.

FOR FURTHER INFORMATION:

Epstein, M. Anthony, and Bert G. Achong, eds. *The Epstein-Barr Virus.* New York: Springer, 1979.

Robertson, Erle S., ed. *Epstein-Barr Virus.* Wymondham, England: Caister Academic Press, 2005.

Tselis, Alex C., and Hal B. Jenson, eds. *Epstein-Barr Virus.* New York: Taylor & Francis, 2006.

Umar, Constantine S., ed. *New Developments in Epstein-Barr Virus Research.* New York: Nova Science, 2006.

Wilson, Joanna B., and Gerhard H. W. May, eds. *Epstein-Barr Virus Protocols.* Totowa, N.J.: Humana Press, 2001.

ERECTILE DYSFUNCTION

DISEASE/DISORDER

ALSO KNOWN AS: Impotence

ANATOMY OR SYSTEM AFFECTED: Blood vessels, cells, genitals, reproductive system

SPECIALTIES AND RELATED FIELDS: Urology

DEFINITION: A disorder whereby a male cannot achieve an erection suitable for sexual intercourse.

KEY TERMS:

atherosclerosis: a condition in which the artery wall becomes thickened due to a buildup of fatty materials such as cholesterol; the arteries become less elastic because of the formation of plaques within the arteries

corpora cavernosa: two spongelike regions of erectile tissue that run the length of the penis and fill with blood during a penile erection

phosphodiesterase type 5 inhibitors: phosphodiesterases are enzymes within cells that degrade phosphodiesterase; in the penis, phosphodiesterase type 5 degrades the substance cGMP made by another enzyme, guanylate cyclase; when levels of cGMP are allowed to increase, it causes the smooth muscle cells in the penile vasculature to relax

CAUSES AND SYMPTOMS

When a human male is sexually aroused, the brain sends a signal through the nervous system to the penis. The signal tells the blood vessels in the penis to relax so that the vessels get larger and fill with blood. Two spongy, cylinder-shaped chambers called the corpora cavernosa run the length of the penis. It is these chambers filled with blood vessels and blood sinuses that become engorged with blood. The same nerve signals that tell the vessels entering the penis to fill with blood also slow down the rate of blood leaving the penis, such that the penis fills with blood and becomes erect. In most males with erectile dysfunction (ED), the blood flow or nerve signals to the penis are reduced or damaged such that one cannot achieve an erection suitable for sexual intercourse.

Erectile dysfunction is more common with advancing age. The prevalence of any degree (mild to complete) of erectile dysfunction in men forty years of age and older is about 40 percent. Age is strongly associated with erectile dysfunction, but men with heart disease, hypertension, diabetes, and depression are more likely to experience erectile dysfunction than are men of the same age without these health problems. Men who have surgery of the prostate gland, located near the base of the penis, might have damage to the nerves that go to the penis and might experience erectile dysfunction that is either temporary or permanent.

Erectile dysfunction seems to be associated with cardiovascular diseases, leading to speculation that vascular causes for erectile dysfunction might be due to a process similar to atherosclerosis that occurs in the penile blood vessels and keeps them from being able to relax and enlarge. Sometimes drugs taken for other disorders can cause erectile dysfunction. They include drugs taken for depression (amitriptyline, doxepin), psychosis (phenothiazines, haloperidol, benzisoxazole), and high blood pressure (beta blockers, thiazide diuretics, methyldopa, clonidine).

Although complete erectile dysfunction, defined as no hardening of the penis with sexual stimulation, may be easily recognized as erectile dysfunction, the subtler symptoms of milder erectile dysfunction are not always identified as such by men. Additionally, despite the publicity and advertisements for ED medications, some men are still reluctant to discuss erection problems with their health care provider or are concerned that treatments for ED are unsafe.

TREATMENT AND THERAPY

Lifestyle changes such as weight loss, which can improve high blood pressure and type 2 diabetes, can also improve erectile dysfunction. Oral therapy with phosphodiesterase type 5 inhibitors (Viagra, Cialis, or Levitra) are the treatment options usually tried first in men with erectile dysfunction. These drugs act by stimulating the blood vessels in the penis to relax. Phosphodiesterase inhibitors have a good safety record, but some men experience visual or other side effects after taking these drugs. Men who take nitrates for chest pain should not take phosphodiesterase inhibitors, because the combination of nitrates and phosphodiesterase inhibitors can cause the blood pressure to drop below normal and cause blackouts.

> ## INFORMATION ON ERECTILE DYSFUNCTION
>
> **CAUSES:** Physical (nerve damage or vascular disease), psychological
> **SYMPTOMS:** Inability to achieve a penile erection suitable for sexual intercourse
> **DURATION:** Chronic
> **TREATMENTS:** Pharmaceuticals (phosphodiesterase inhibitors), mechanical vacuum devices, intracavernous injection therapy, intraurethral suppositories, penile implants, and surgery

Other treatments include mechanical vacuum devices, intracavernous injection therapy, intraurethral suppositories, penile implants, and surgery. Mechanical vacuum devices create a vacuum around the penis, which draws blood into the penis to cause an erection. The penis is placed in a plastic cylinder and then a pump pulls the air out of the cylinder. Once an erection is achieved, an elastic band is placed at the base of the penis to maintain the erection after the cylinder is removed. With intracavernous injection therapy, drugs are injected directly into the penis to cause an erection. Intraurethral suppositories are prostaglandin-containing pellets that are inserted into the urethra. Occasional side effects include pain in the penis and sometimes in the testicles, mild urethral bleeding, and dizziness. After inserting the pellet, the man must remain standing to increase blood flow to the penis. It can take about fifteen minutes to achieve an erection. This method can also have consequences for a man's female sex partner by causing vaginal itching and possibly uterine contractions. The latter reason is why men should not use this method when having intercourse with a pregnant woman unless a condom or other type of barrier device is also used.

Penile implants are inflatable inserts surgically implanted on either side of the penis. The implants are attached to a pump placed in the scrotum and a reservoir fitted just below the groin muscles. The implants are inflated with saline solution from the reservoir to make the penis erect. There is some risk of mechanical failure with these kinds of devices.

Vascular reconstructive surgery for erectile dysfunction is rarely performed and considered experimental. The surgery involves taking a vein from the leg and attaching it so that it allows blood to bypass areas of vascular blockage in the penis. Venous ligation is performed to keep the veins going out of the penis from leaking so that enough blood stays in the penis to keep it erect.

Perspective and Prospects

Before the approval of Viagra, the subject of erectile dysfunction or impotence was rarely discussed. To market the drug, Pfizer, the company that produces and markets Viagra, launched an advertising campaign that included several celebrities who acknowledged that they had ED. This advertising campaign brought the subject of erectile dysfunction into the public domain, and soon erectile dysfunction was no longer a forbidden topic of conversation. Viagra was originally developed as a medicine intended to treat the heart disease angina pectoris. Viagra was not effective as a treatment for that condition, but one of the side effects reported during clinical trials in angina was that of erections.

Phosphodiesterase inhibitors have also become drugs of abuse, because these drugs can also enhance erections in persons who do not have erectile dysfunction. Some men take a phosphodiesterase inhibitor after taking illicit recreational drugs that can cause erection problems to counteract the effect on their sexual performance.

—Nancy E. Price, Ph.D.

See also Alcoholism; Anxiety; Aphrodisiacs; Genital disorders, female; Genital disorders, male; Hormones; Hypertension; Men's health; Psychiatry; Psychiatry, geriatric; Psychosomatic disorders; Sexual dysfunction; Sexuality; Stress; Urinary disorders.

For Further Information:

Kirby, Michael. *Erectile Dysfunction and Vascular Disease.* Malden, Mass.: Blackwell, 2003. Includes a discussion of vascular causes of erectile dysfunction and the safety of sex for men with cardiovascular diseases.

Kirby, Roger S. *An Atlas of Erectile Dysfunction.* 2d ed. New York: Parthenon, 2003. Covers the epidemiology, anatomy and physiology, risk factors, clinical evaluation, and treatment of erectile dysfunction.

Kirby, Roger S., Culley C. Carson, and Irwin Goldstein. *Erectile Dysfunction: A Clinical Guide.* Oxford, England: Isis Medical Media, 1999. Covers the epidemiology, anatomy and physiology, clinical evaluation, and treatment of erectile dysfunction.

Ergogenic aids
Biology

Also known as: Blood doping, steroids, caffeine, growth hormone, creatine

Anatomy or system affected: Blood, brain, cells, circulatory system, endocrine system, genitals, glands, heart, joints, kidneys, liver, musculoskeletal system

Specialties and related fields: Biochemistry, endocrinology, ethics, exercise physiology, family medicine, hematology, internal medicine, nephrology, orthopedics, pharmacology, psychology, sports medicine, toxicology

Definition: Substances used by athletes in an effort to gain an advantage. Most of these substances are illegal and unethical within competitive sports.

Introduction

In the history of sport, athletes have attempted to find a competitive advantage through advanced techniques in training, nutrition, and even in ergogenic aids, such as nutritional supplements and pharmacological aids. The use of these substances—such as anabolic-androgenic steroids (AAS), testosterone precursors (such as androstenedione), and nonsteroidal aids such as human growth hormone (GH) and creatine—have become increasingly popular in recent years, even without thorough scientific data supporting their efficacy and safety.

The population using such performance-enhancing drugs ranges from collegiate to professional athletes to adolescents and high school students. Recent meta-analyses estimate that 3 to 12 percent of adolescent boys have used an anabolic steroid at least once, and 28 percent of collegiate athletes admit to taking creatine. Other studies have suggested that the number may be closer to 41 percent.

Though such ergogenic aids are thought to improve strength, endurance, agility, and overall performance, most athletic improvement is anecdotal at best. Scientific evidence supporting these ideas is scarce and incomplete. Even with aids that may improve strength and/or performance, the safety of these substances has been seriously questioned, such as with the use of AAS, GH, and ephedra.

Types of Ergogenic Aids

Anabolic-androgenic steroids (AAS) as ergogenic aids in sports are chemical compounds that resemble the structure of testosterone, the naturally occurring male sex hormone that affects muscle growth and strength.

"Anabolic" refers to the growth of cells, and "androgenic" refers to the stimulation of the growth of male sex organs and masculine sex characteristics. AAS bind to cells that are used for muscle repair and that can transform into muscle fibers.

AAS has been one of the most studied ergogenic aids, yet many of its mechanisms and adverse effects are still not well understood. Studies have shown that increased doses of testosterone can decrease total body adipose tissue in the body and can increase strength and fat-free mass. Adverse effects of AAS use include hypothalamic-pituitary dysfunction, gynecomastia, severe acne, infection as a result of sharing needles, aggressive and depressive behavior, and a possible association with premature death.

Androstenedione (andro) is a testosterone precursor produced by the adrenal glands and gonads. Its ergogenic effect occurs after it is converted to testosterone in the testes as well as in other tissues. It can also be converted to estrone and estradiol, which are steroid compounds that are primary female sex hormones (found in both men and women). The creation of testosterone is regulated by the amount of testosterone precursors in the body. Theoretically, an increase in androstenedione would increase the production of testosterone and thus can increase protein synthesis, lean body mass, and strength.

Older studies showed that andro supplementation results in increased serum testosterone levels. However, more recent studies have shown that andro supplementation fails to directly improve lean body mass, muscular strength, or serum testosterone levels. Possible side effects to andro use are suppressed testosterone production, liver dysfunction, cardiovascular disease, testicular atrophy, baldness, acne, and aggressive behavior.

Similar to androstenedione, dihydroepiandrosterone (DHEA) is a precursor of testosterone and is also formed in the adrenal glands and gonads. DHEA is the most abundant steroid hormone in circulation and is a precursor to androstenedione and other testosterone precursors (such as androstenediol). Studies of DHEA supplementation have not been shown to increase lean body mass, strength, or testosterone levels. Possible side effects are similar to andro and AAS use.

Human growth hormone (GH) is a metabolic hormone that is secreted into the blood by cells found in the anterior pituitary gland. After its secretion, GH stimulates the production of insulin-like growth factor (IGF)-1 in the liver. These hormones stimulate bone growth, protein synthesis, and the conversion of fat to energy. Athletes have been attracted to GH not only because of such theoretical benefits but also because of the limited techniques in detecting GH in the urine. GH levels vary in individuals of different, ages, sex, and activity and can vary throughout the day, so no reliable benchmark can be made to determine if illicit use has taken place.

Scientific studies have been unable to show that GH leads to increased muscle strength and exercise performance or changes in protein synthesis. Because of ethical limitations, it is difficult to study the effect of larger doses of GH on healthy individuals. Adverse effects of GH use include cosmetic damage, joint pain, muscle weakness, fluid retention, impaired glucose regulation (which may lead to diabetes mellitus), cardiomyopathy, hyperlipidemia, and possibly death.

Erythropoieten (EPO) is a hormone secreted by the kidneys that is a precursor to bone marrow. EPO increases the oxygen-carrying capacity of blood and, as a result, aids in endurance and aerobic respiration. The appeal of EPO among athletes is this endurance-enhancing effect. As a result, many abusers have been found to be skiers, cyclists, and other athletes who require high levels of endurance. Early use of EPO as an ergogenic aid, termed "blood doping," came in the form of autologous blood transfusions, in which athletes would harvest their own red blood cells and reintroduce them into their systems before events. Recently, the use of recombinant human erythropoietin (r-HuEPO) via injection has become more widespread.

Scientific studies have shown that EPO and r-HuEPO treatments do increase certain blood concentrations and can aid in endurance. EPO may also have serious and dangerous side effects, however, such as hypertension, seizures, thromboembolic events, and possibly death.

Creatine monohydrate is an amine synthesized in the kidneys, pancreas, and liver, and it can also be obtained through the diet from meat and fish. Approximately 90 to 95 percent of creatine in the body is found in skeletal muscle. Creatine, which is converted to creatine phosphate (PCr), is an important limiting factor in the resynthesis of adenosine triphosphate (ATP), which plays a significant role in energy reserves within the body. Theoretically, an increase of PCr in the body would increase the regeneration of ATP, resulting in an increase in sustained maximal energy production for short-term exercise. This could lead to increased intensity and repetition frequency, and thus possible increases in skeletal muscle mass.

In 2002, A. M. Bohn and colleagues argued in an article in *Current Sports Medicine Reports* that there are "no studies demonstrating benefit with the relatively indiscriminant use of variable amounts of creatine by large numbers of athletes on a specific team." Nevertheless, creatine has been shown to enhance performance in small populations of athletes of various sports. Possible adverse effects of creatine include muscle cramping, dehydration, gastrointestinal distress, weight gain, increased risk of muscle tears, inhibited insulin and creatine production, renal damage, and possibly nephropathy.

Stimulants are drugs that increase nervous system activity. Examples of stimulants commonly used as ergogenic aids include the class of drugs called amphetamines, as well as specific chemical compounds such as caffeine and ephedrine. The use of caffeine has been shown to improve exercise time to exhaustion and may even significantly increase intestinal glucose absorption. It has been suggested that caffeine increases fat utilization for energy and delays the depletion of glycogen (the stored form of glucose). As a result, caffeine and other stimulants are popular ergogenic aids for extended aerobic activity.

Caffeine in small doses has been shown to increase performance. Possible adverse effects of caffeine may include anxiety, dependency, withdrawal, and possibly a diuretic effect (dehydration). Ephedrine may have similar adverse affects. Other stimulants, such as amphetamines or cocaine, have more serious and detrimental effects.

PERSPECTIVE AND PROSPECTS

The use of ergogenic aids in the history of sport has progressively moved from primitive aids to more sophisticated performance enhancers. Crude natural concoctions and stimulants have paved the way for complex pharmacological agents (such as erythropoietin) and designer anabolic steroids (such as tetrahydrogestrinone). Athletes and trainers have utilized any and all means to gain a competitive edge, even if that results in damage to health and even a risk of death.

The biggest problem stemming from the use of such aids is the difficulty in detecting them. This is evident in recent media attention given to ergogenic aids and their popularity, as seen through the 1995 congressional hearings regarding steroid use in Major League Baseball as well as the recent discoveries of abuse by high-profile cyclists and track-and-field athletes. This media attention has also shown the difficulties among investigators, such as the International Olympic Committee (IOC) and United States Anti-Doping Agency, in detecting the use of new designer steroids and new ergogenic aids among elite athletes.

—*Julien M. Cobert and Jeffrey R. Bytomski, D.O.*

See also Blood and blood disorders; Blood testing; Caffeine; Ethics; Exercise physiology; Hormones; Hypertrophy; Metabolism; Muscles; Pharmacology; Sports medicine; Steroid use; Steroids.

FOR FURTHER INFORMATION:

Bhazin, S., et al. "The Effects of Supraphysiologic Doses of Testosterone on Muscle Size and Strength in Normal Men." *New England Journal of Medicine* 335 (1996): 1-7.

Bohn, Amy Miller, Stephanie Betts, and Thomas L. Schwenk. "Creatine and Other Nonsteroidal Strength-Enhancing Aids." *Current Sports Medicine Reports* 1, no. 4 (August, 2002): 239-245.

Foster, Zoë J., and Jeffrey A. Housner. "Anabolic-Andogenic Steroids and Testosterone Precursors: Ergogenic Aids and Sport." *Current Sports Medicine Reports* 3, no. 4 (August, 2004): 234-241.

Graham, T. E. "Caffeine and Exercise: Metabolism, Endurance, and Performance." *Sports Medicine* 31, no. 11 (November 1, 2001): 785-807.

Juhn, Mark S. "Ergogenic Aids in Aerobic Activity." *Current Sports Medicine Reports* 1, no. 4 (August, 2002): 233-238.

Powers, Michael E. "The Safety and Efficacy of Anabolic Steroid Precursors: What Is the Scientific Evidence?" *Journal of Athletic Training* 37, no. 3 (2002): 300-305.

Shekelle, Paul G., et al. "Efficacy and Safety of Ephedra and Ephedrine for Weight Loss and Athletic Performance: A Meta-analysis." *Journal of the American Medical Association* 289, no. 12 (March 26, 2003): 1537-1545.

Singbart, G. "Adverse Events of Erythropoietin in Long-Term and in Acute/Short-Term Treatment." *Clinical Investigation* 72 (1994): S36-S43.

Stacy, Jason J., Thomas R. Terrell, and Thomas D. Armsey. "Ergogenic Aids: Human Growth Hormone." *Current Sports Medicine Reports* 3, no. 4 (August, 2004): 229-233.

Yesalis, C. E., and M. S. Bahrke. "Doping Among Adolescent Athletes." *Baillieres Best Practice and Research in Clinical Endocrinology and Metabolism* 14, no. 1 (March, 2000): 25-35.

ESOPHAGEAL CANCER. *See* **MOUTH AND THROAT CANCER.**

ESOPHAGUS

ANATOMY

ANATOMY OR SYSTEM AFFECTED: Gastrointestinal system, mouth, stomach, throat

SPECIALTIES AND RELATED FIELDS: Gastroenterology, otorhinolaryngology

DEFINITION: A muscular tube, approximately 10 inches in length, that carries food from the mouth or pharynx to the stomach.

STRUCTURE AND FUNCTION

The esophagus lies between the spine and the trachea and is part of the digestive system. The esophagus, however, does not produce or secrete any digestive enzymes, and absorption of nutrients in this part of the digestive system is almost nil. The esophagus pierces the diaphragm as it moves through the thoracic cavity and into the abdominopelvic cavity, where it joins with the stomach.

All parts of the digestive system have four tunics (tissues): from superficial to deep, tunica serosa, tunica muscularis, tunica submucosa, and tunica mucosa. Tunica serosa anchors the esophagus in the mesentery. Tunica muscularis is composed of smooth muscle fibers arranged in circular and longitudinal fibers. These two layers of muscles are important as they are able to squeeze the food bolus (chewed mass of food) and move it down toward the stomach. The muscles are involuntary and perform peristaltic contractions behind the bolus, pushing it downward, as if a tennis ball were being pushed through a leg of panty hose. Tunica submucosa is a layer of loose connective tissue; blood vessels and nerves, including the important submucosa plexus, are found in this layer. The innermost layer, tunica mucosa, is comprised of epithelial cells and is the layer in contact with the bolus. Of all the tunics, tunica mucosa is the most variable along the length of the digestive system. The epithelium here is stratified squamous epithelial tissue to protect the esophagus from sharp or dangerous food items, such as bones, hot pizza, or insufficiently chewed carrots.

The esophagus has an upper and a lower sphincter. When one swallows, the upper sphincter relaxes. In a coordinated effort, the larynx pulls forward and the epiglottis clamps down to cover this opening into the respiratory system (lungs). Glands produce mucus to lubricate food as it passes along the lumen. The lower sphincter closes once the bolus has passed into the stomach. Failure to do so would allow stomach acids to leak up into the esophagus, causing what is commonly called heartburn or acid indigestion, more properly known as gastroesophageal reflux disease.

DISORDERS AND DISEASES

The most common medical problem with the esophagus is gastroesophageal reflux disease (GERD), which is caused when the lower sphincter fails to close properly. Stomach contents, which are acidic, then leak into the esophagus and irritate it. Left untreated, GERD can damage the esophagus.

Barrett's esophagus is a disease often is found in patients with GERD. In Barrett's esophagus, the tissue that lines the esophagus, tunica mucosa, is replaced by tissue that is more similar to tissue lining the intestines. The process is called intestinal metaplasia. Barrett's esophagus may lead to the development of esophageal cancer, but this is a rare event. It should be emphasized that not all patients with GERD develop Barrett's esophagus and that very few people with Barrett's esophagus develop cancer. The cause of Barrett's esophagus is unknown, as is the cause of esophageal cancer.

—*M. A. Foote, Ph.D.*

See also Acid reflux disease; Bile; Digestion; Enzymes; Gastroenterology; Gastroenterology, pediatric; Gastrointestinal disorders; Gastrointestinal system; Heartburn; Indigestion; Peristalsis.

FOR FURTHER INFORMATION:

Johnson, Leonard R., ed. *Gastrointestinal Physiology.* 7th ed. Philadelphia: Mosby/Elsevier, 2007.

Mayo Clinic. *Mayo Clinic on Digestive Health: Enjoy Better Digestion with Answers to More than Twelve Common Conditions.* 2d ed. Rochester, Minn.: Author, 2004.

Scanlon, Valerie, and Tina Sanders. *Essentials of Anatomy and Physiology.* 5th ed. Philadelphia: F. A. Davis, 2007.

ESTROGEN REPLACEMENT THERAPY. *See* **HORMONE THERAPY.**

ETHICS

ALSO KNOWN AS: Bioethics, medical ethics

DEFINITION: Ethics is a code of conduct based on established moral principles. Medical ethics is the study of the conduct of professionals in the field of medicine.

KEY TERMS:

autonomy: independence and self-reliance, especially referring to decision making

beneficence: doing good

informed consent: the dialogue between physician and patient prior to an invasive procedure

justice: the rationing of scarce resources according to a prearranged plan

nonmaleficence: avoiding evil

paternalism: acting in the manner of a father to his children

PRINCIPLES

Ethics deals with a code of conduct based on established moral principles. When applied to a particular professional field, abstract theories as well as concrete principles are considered. Often the consequences of a particular course of action dictate its rightness or wrongness. Bioethics is the study of ethics by professionals in the fields of medicine, law, philosophy, or theology. Some also refer to this area as applied ethics. The term "bioethics" is often used interchangeably with "medical ethics," but purists would define medical ethics as the study of conduct by professionals in the field of medicine. Codes of ethics promulgated by professional groups or associations define obligations governing members of a given profession.

Initial questions concerning medical ethics entail purpose, to whom a duty is owed (legal or moral) and how far that duty extends. Does it extend solely to patients, or does it extend to their families or to society as a whole? For example, public health obligations to society involve a duty to prevent disease, maintain the health of the populace, and oversee the delivery of health care.

In the 1972 article "Models for Ethical Practice in a Revolutionary Age," Robert M. Veatch proposed four models for ethical medicine. The first is the engineering model, in which the physician becomes an applied scientist interested in treating disease rather than caring for a patient. The Nazi physicians during World War II acting as so-called scientists and technicians are examples of the engineering model taken to its extreme. The second is the priestly model, in which the physician assumes a paternalistic role of moral dominance, treating the patient as a child. The main principle of this model is the traditional one of *primum non nocere*, or "first do no harm." It neglects principles of patient autonomy, dignity, and freedom. The third is the collegial model, in which physician and patient are colleagues cooperat-

ing in pursuing a common goal, such as preserving health, curing illness, or easing pain. This model requires mutual trust and confidence, demanding a continued dialogue between the parties. The fourth is the contractual model, in which the relationship between health care provider and patient is analogous to a legal contract, with rights and obligations on both sides. The contractual model can be modified to provide for shared decision making and cooperation between physician and patient and tailored to the particular physician-patient relationship involved, resulting in a collegial association.

Autonomy and informed consent. Since the Nuremberg trials, which presented horrible accounts of medical experimentation in Nazi concentration camps, the issue of consent has been one of primary importance. These basic concepts recognize an individual's uniqueness and inherent decision-making ability without coercion or undue influence from others. Respect for privacy and freedom are fundamental to human dignity. Even when people present difficult problems, such as being unconscious or in a coma, they must continue to be respected. Rational decision making by patients or their surrogates must be followed, and those with specialized knowledge or expertise are not authorized to impose their will on another person or limit that person's freedom.

Informed consent seeks to encourage open communication between patient and health care provider, to protect patients and research subjects from harm, and to encourage health care providers to act responsibly vis-à-vis patients and subjects, ultimately preserving autonomy and rational decision making. Especially applicable in invasive procedures, such as those involving surgery or treatments with serious risks, informed consent requires the presence of certain conditions, including a patient's competency or decision-making capacity, in order to understand the relative consequences of a proposed course of treatment and its effect on a patient's life and health. (Absent informed consent, an invasive procedure would constitute a legal cause of action in battery, or a harmful or offensive touching.) The health care provider must inform patients of alternative courses of action, if any, and the fact that patients have the option to refuse treatment, even if that alternative is contrary to the recommendation of the physician. The information conveyed to the patient must include the diagnosis, nature of the proposed treatment, known risks and consequences (excluding those that are too remote or improbable to bear significantly on the ultimate decision whether to proceed on a course of treatment, as well as those that are so well known that they are obvious to everyone), benefits from the proposed treatment, alternatives, prognosis without treatment, economic cost, and how the treatment plan will impact the patient's lifestyle. The patient should also be made aware that once given, an informed consent can be withdrawn. Hospital consent forms do not provide this type of information.

The information conveyed must be material and important to this patient, not a fictional reasonable and prudent person. A factor is material if it could change the decision of that patient. Inherent problems include speculation into the factors that would have a dramatic impact on the patient's life, requiring a dialogue between patient and health care provider. It is also important to recognize the role of the physician's time constraints as well as the patient's overall stress level while the information is being conveyed, including possible information overload. Not only must the information be conveyed adequately, but it must also be assimilated and understood. The ability of an individual to process information raises substantial issues about understanding. Comprehension is not always easily ascertainable. Sometimes a person's ability to make decisions is affected by problems of nonacceptance of information, even if it was comprehended. A patient may voluntarily waive informed consent, so that the patient asks not to be informed, thereby relieving the physician of the obligation to obtain informed consent and ultimately delegating decision-making authority to the physician.

Medical emergencies constitute exceptions to the informed consent requirement, provided that four conditions are met: The patient, whose wishes are unknown because no advance directive or living will exists, is incapable of giving consent because of the emergency; no surrogate is available; the medical condition poses a danger to the patient's life or seriously impairs the patient's health; and immediate treatment is required to avert the danger to life or health. This exception is justified on the grounds that consent can be assumed in cases in which a reasonable person would consent if informed. If the patient is not in imminent danger, or if consent can be obtained at a later time, the emergency exception does not apply. The second exception is the therapeutic privilege in which health care providers are justified in legitimately withholding information from a patient when they reasonably believe that disclosure will have an adverse effect on the patient's condition or health, as in the case of a depressed, emotionally

drained, or unstable patient. Again, the decision is subjective, referring to this patient, decided on a case-by-case basis. The privilege does not apply if the health care provider withholds information based on the belief that the patient will refuse consent if told all the facts. In that instance, withholding information amounts to misrepresentation or deception.

Another ethical dilemma involving intentional deception or incomplete disclosure concerns the therapeutic use of placebos. One defense is that deception is moral when it is used for the patient's welfare.

Paternalism. From the Latin word *pater*, meaning "father," paternalism refers to controlling others as a father acts in his relationship with his children. In medical ethics, paternalism involves overriding one's own wishes in order to act to benefit or avert harm to the patient. Intervention by a health care provider to prevent competent patients from harming themselves is called strong paternalism. Strong paternalism is generally rejected by ethicists because of the view that health care providers do not know all the factors influencing the life of another person and therefore lack the competence to decide what is best for another person. Weak paternalism exists when the health care provider overrules the wishes of an incompetent or questionably competent patient. It is sometimes justified in nonemergencies without informed consent to relieve serious pain and suffering. Another example of weak paternalism is the temporary use of restraints, justified on the grounds that confused and disoriented patients are otherwise likely to injure themselves. When restraints are necessary, the surrogate is generally asked to give consent, recognizing that restraints, albeit temporary, constitute a limitation of one's liberty.

Beneficence and nonmaleficence. The principles of beneficence (doing good) and nonmaleficence (avoiding evil) are both expressed in the Hippocratic oath: "I will use treatment to help the sick according to my ability and judgment, but I will never use it to injure or wrong them." Each principle has a bearing on the other, and each is limited by the other. The obligations in beneficence are also limited by obligations to avoid evil. One may perform an act that risks evil if the following conditions are present (the principle of double effects): The action is good or morally indifferent; the agent intends a good effect; the evil effect is not the means to achieving good; and proportionality exists between good and evil. The principle of proportionality states that provided that an action does not go directly against the dignity of the individual, there must be a proportionate good to justify risking evil consequences. Items to be considered are the possible existence of an alternative means with less evil or no evil, the level of good intended and the level of evil risked, and the certitude or probability of good or evil. The latter is called the wedge principle, referring to the fact that putting the tip of a wedge into a crack in a log and striking the wedge will split the log and destroy it; by analogy, in defending a given position, even a small concession can destroy that position. The last element is the causal influence of the agent, recognizing that most effects result from many causes and that a particular agent is seldom the sole cause. For example, as noted by Thomas M. Garrett and colleagues in *Health Care Ethics: Principles and Problems* (2001), lung cancer can be triggered not only by smoking but also by conditions in the workplace, the environment, and heredity.

Obligations are imposed on the patient that demand the use of ordinary but not extraordinary means of preserving and restoring health. In other words, the patient should use means that produce more good than harm and evaluate the effects on the self, family, and society, including pain, cost, and health benefits to life, its meaning and quality. The health care provider's obligation demands that the benefits outweigh the burdens on the patient. An overarching obligation to society exists to provide health care information and leadership to ensure the equitable distribution of scarce medical resources accomplished in ways that allow the goals of health care to be achieved. Finally, the surrogate's obligation depends on whether the wishes of the once-competent patient are known or can be ascertained. If so, the surrogate should decide accordingly (the substituted judgment principle). Overruling the person's wishes would constitute a denial of the patient's autonomy. If the person has never been competent or has never expressed his or her wishes, the surrogate should act in the best interests of the patient alone, disregarding the interests of family, society, and the surrogate. Another approach requires the surrogate to choose what the patient would have chosen if and when competent after having considered all relevant information and the interests of others.

Certain conditions justify the decision to omit treatment, such as pointless or futile treatment, especially with regard to the dead or those who are dying, and situations in which the burdens of treatment outweigh the benefits. It should be noted that no bright line exists here because these cases are not decided easily. Ethicists as well as those in the medical professions debat-

ing these issues have not reached a clear-cut solution that applies in every case.

Justice. Also called distributive justice, justice establishes principles for the distribution of scarce resources in circumstances where demand outstrips supply and rationing must occur. Needs are to be considered in terms of overall needs and the dignity of members of society. Aside from the biological and physiological elements, the social context of health and disease may influence a given problem and its severity. Individual prejudices and presuppositions may enlarge the nature and scope of the disease, creating a demand for health care that makes it even more difficult to distribute scarce resources for all members of society. Principles of fair distribution in society often supersede and become paramount to the concerns of the individual. Questions about who shall receive what share of society's scarce resources generate controversies about a national health policy, unequal distributions of advantages to the disadvantaged, and the rationing of health care.

Similar problems recur with regard to access to and distribution of health insurance, medical equipment, and artificial organs. The lack of insurance as well as the problem of underinsurance constitutes a huge economic barrier to health care access in the United States. In *Principles of Biomedical Ethics* (6th ed., 2009), Tom L. Beauchamp and James F. Childress point out that the acquired immunodeficiency syndrome (AIDS) crisis has presented dramatic instances of the problems of insurability and underwriting practices, in which insurers often appeal to actuarial fairness in defending their decisions while neglecting social justice. Proposals to alleviate the unfairness to those below the poverty line have been based on charity, compassion, and benevolence toward the sick rather than on claims of justice. The ongoing debate over the entitlement to a minimum of health care in the United States involves not only government entitlement programs but also complex social, political, economic, and cultural beliefs.

Decisions concerning the allocation of funds will dictate the type of health care that can be provided and for which problems. Numerous resources, supplies, and space in intensive care units (ICUs) have been allocated for specific patients or classes of patients. A life-threatening illness complicates this decision. In the United States, health care has often been allocated by one's ability to pay rather than by other criteria; rationing has at times been based on ranking a list of services or a patient's age.

Confidentiality and privacy. In the United States, the medical profession has always strived to maintain the confidentiality of physician-patient communications, as well as the privacy of a patient's medical records. While admirable, these values have not been absolute, and no uniformity exists among the fifty states regarding access to one's medical records. As technology improved, with computers and fax machines transmitting health care data to distant locations and medical records themselves existing in electronic form, no laws had been created to protect medical records adequately. In the late twentieth and early twenty-first centuries, the administrations of Bill Clinton and George W. Bush sought to enact legislation that would bridge the privacy gaps and create uniform standards, at the same time eliminating discrimination in employment and insurance coverage based on one's genetic predisposition. The Health Insurance Portability and Accountability Act (HIPAA) became law in 1997.

APPLICATION OF ETHICAL PRINCIPLES

Advances in medical technology have expanded the scope of what medicine can accomplish. As capabilities grow and become more sophisticated, medical ethics also seeks to resolve age-old dilemmas and to evaluate the use of new technologies. Certain ethical dilemmas have garnered sharp disagreement. Chief among these is the issue of death and dying, which brings into controversy two theories about the nature of health care. The "curing" approach is based on traditional medical ethical principles that date back to Hippocrates and include the principles of beneficence, nonmaleficence, and justice. The "caring" approach focuses on patient autonomy, proper bedside manners by health care providers, the preparation of advance directives, and the hospice movement.

The "curing" approach to medical ethics equates medicine with healing. The sanctity of life is important because it is a gift from God and must be sustained to the extent reasonably possible. All ordinary measures must be taken to preserve life. This tradition holds that only God can decide the time of death, and even in the face of suffering, the health care provider must not take measures to shorten life. Physicians are the primary decision makers and in the best position to recommend and advise the patient and to direct the treatment plan. The model is paternalistic.

In the "caring" approach, the health care provider's role is to minimize pain, to present alternatives and the relative consequences of various options, and ulti-

mately to proceed according to the patient's determination. The "caring" approach is subjective, as each case is decided individually. The quality of life rather than the sanctity of life becomes the guiding principle.

Issues regarding futility of treatment arise, as well as the recognition that prolonging life does not always benefit patients. Physicians are not obligated to provide futile treatment, which may violate the physician's duty not to harm patients because such treatments are often burdensome and invasive, exacerbating the patient's pain and discomfort. Patients cannot ethically compel health care workers to provide treatment that violates the worker's own personal beliefs or the standards of the profession. Other issues in this area deal with physician-assisted suicide and whether to provide or withhold lifesaving treatments.

The transplantation of vital organs—notably the heart, liver, and kidney—raises difficult ethical questions. As organ transplantation has become routine at many medical centers, its success has opened a Pandora's box of ethical questions involving the allocation of scarce donor organs. One example is whether the sickest person on the waiting list for an organ should be the recipient, or whether it should go to someone more robust who may live longer. Another is whether live donors should be compensated for donating an organ, just as blood donors are compensated. Many countries outside the United States and the United Kingdom condone the sale of organs; the 1984 National Organ Transplant Act makes selling organs illegal in the United States. Ethicists are debating animal-to-human organ transplants to alleviate the scarcity of human donor organs for transplantation.

Assisted reproduction in the form of in vitro fertilization (IVF), egg freezing, and sperm banking is largely an unregulated industry. Couples seeking help must make complex ethical decisions dealing with the preselection of embryos based on genetic traits through screening of a single cell. Other decisions deal with how many eggs should be fertilized and whether the remainder should be disposed of or frozen. The rights of the participants and the children created through assisted reproduction remain undefined. State laws vary widely regarding whether a child conceived by IVF or donor eggs or sperm has the right to know the identity of the biological parents.

The identification of human embryonic stem cells has been widely acknowledged as extremely valuable because it will assist scientists in understanding basic mechanisms of embryo development and gene regulation. It also holds the promise of allowing the development of techniques for manipulating, growing, and cloning stem cells to create designer cells and tissues. Stem cells are created in the first days of pregnancy. Scientists hope to direct stem cells to grow into replacement organs and tissues to treat a wide variety of diseases. Embryos are valued in research for their ability to produce stem cells, which can be harvested to grow a variety of tissues for use in transplantation to treat serious illnesses such as cancer, heart disease, and diabetes. In so doing, however, researchers must destroy days-old embryos, a procedure condemned by the Catholic Church, some antiabortion activists, and some women's rights organizations. Other research points to similar promise using stem cells harvested from adults, so that no embryos are destroyed.

PERSPECTIVE AND PROSPECTS

Medical ethics in Western culture has its roots in ancient Greek and Roman medicine, the Greek physician Hippocrates and the Roman physician Galen. In ancient Greece, as in most early societies, healing wounds and treating disease first appeared as folk practice and religious ritual. The earliest statement about ethics appears in a clinical and epidemiological book entitled *Epidemics I*, attributed to Hippocrates. It is in this work that the admonition "to help and not to harm" first appeared. The book itself deals with prognosis rather than treatment, which is the approach taken by Hippocrates. Galen asserted that any worthwhile doctor must know philosophy, including the logical, the physical, and the ethical, and be skilled at reasoning about the problems presented to him, understanding the nature and function of the body within the physical world.

From the fourth to the fourteenth centuries, medicine became firmly established in the universities and in the public life of the emerging nations of Europe. During this time, the Roman Catholic Church had a strong influence on Western civilization. Medicine was deeply touched by the doctrine and discipline of the Church, and its theological influence shaped the ethics of medicine. The early Church endorsed the use of human medicine and encouraged care of the sick as a work of charity. One of the greatest physicians during this period was the Jewish Talmudic scholar Maimonides, whose writings sometimes dealt with ethical questions in medicine.

The duty to comfort the sick and dying was a moral imperative in Christianity and Judaism. As the bubonic plague swept across Europe over the following several centuries, Protestant leader Martin Luther urged doctors and ministers to fulfill the obligation of Christian charity by faithful service, but John Calvin argued that physicians and ministers could depart if the preservation of their lives was in the common interest.

The ethical debates surrounding the plague moved medical ethics ahead. As noted by Albert R. Jonsen in *A Short History of Medical Ethics* (2000), the question became, "Under what circumstances does a person who has medical skills have a special obligation to serve the community?" When syphilis emerged in epidemic proportions at the end of the fifteenth century, a similar question regarding service to the sick at the cost of danger to oneself resurfaced, and members of the medical profession struggled with the link between medical necessity and moral correctness. Not until the nineteenth century did a consensus appear, mandating that the physician should take personal risks to serve the needy without appraising the morality of a patient's behavior.

—*Marcia J. Weiss, M.A., J.D.*

See also Abortion; Aging: Extended care; Animal rights vs. research; Assisted reproductive technologies; Cloning; Contraception; Ergogenic aids; Euthanasia; Fetal tissue transplantation; Genetic engineering; Hippocratic oath; Hospice; In vitro fertilization; Law and medicine; Living will; Malpractice; Medicare; Palliative medicine; Resuscitation; Screening; Stem cells; Suicide; Terminally ill: Extended care; Transplantation; Xenotransplantation.

FOR FURTHER INFORMATION:

Beauchamp, Tom L., and James F. Childress. *Principles of Biomedical Ethics*. 6th ed. New York: Oxford University Press, 2009. Regarded as one of the basic texts of bioethics. An excellent source for a detailed discussion of fundamental principles.

Beauchamp, Tom L., and LeRoy Walters, eds. *Contemporary Issues in Bioethics*. 7th ed. Belmont, Calif.: Thomson/Wadsworth, 2008. A compilation of scholarly articles and major legal cases in bioethics.

Garrett, Thomas M., Harold W. Baillie, and Rosellen M. Garrett. *Health Care Ethics: Principles and Problems*. 5th ed. Upper Saddle River, N.J.: Prentice Hall, 2010. A basic and succinct text outlining the principles and problems of health care ethics.

Jonsen, Albert R. *A Short History of Medical Ethics*. New York: Oxford University Press, 2000. A concise and comprehensive chronicle of the history of ethics and medicine.

Pence, Gregory E. *Re-creating Medicine: Ethical Issues at the Frontiers of Medicine.* Lanham, Md.: Rowman & Littlefield, 2007. A subjective and skeptical (not balanced) discussion of the major bioethical issues at the beginning of the twenty-first century, such as organ donation, reproduction and its progeny, genetics, and other controversial subjects.

Torr, James D., ed. *Medical Ethics.* San Diego, Calif.: Greenhaven Press, 2000. Part of the Current Controversies series, this book presents reprints of articles illustrating both sides of controversial and contested issues in medical ethics.

Veatch, Robert M. "Models for Ethical Practice in a Revolutionary Age." *Hastings Center Report* 2, no. 3 (June, 1972): 5-7. A major figure in the bioethics movement, Veatch outlines four ethical medical models.

EUTHANASIA

ETHICS

DEFINITION: The intentional termination of a life, which may be active (resulting from specific actions causing death) or passive (resulting from the refusal or withdrawal of life-sustaining treatment), and voluntary (with the patient's consent) or involuntary (on behalf of infants or others who are incapable of making this decision, such as comatose patients).

KEY TERMS:

active euthanasia: administration of a drug or some other means that directly causes death; the motivation is to relieve patient suffering

durable power of attorney: designation of a person who will have legal authority to make health care decisions if the patient becomes incapable of making decisions for himself or herself

living will: a legal document in which the patient states a preference regarding life-prolonging treatment in the event that he or she cannot choose

nonvoluntary euthanasia: a decision to terminate life made by another when the patient is incapable of making a decision for himself or herself

passive euthanasia: ending life by refusing or withdrawing life-sustaining medical treatment

voluntary euthanasia: a patient's consent to a decision which results in the shortening of his or her life

THE CONTROVERSY SURROUNDING EUTHANASIA

In the past, the role of the doctor was clear: The physician should minimize suffering and save lives whenever possible. In the present, it is possible for these two goals to be at odds. Saving lives in some situations seems to prolong the misery of the patient. In other cases, procedures or treatments may only marginally postpone the time of death. Advances in medical technology enable many to live who would have died just a few years ago, and massive amounts of money are spent each year on medical research with the goal of prolonging life. Experts in U.S. population trends indicate that by the year 2030, those over the age of sixty-five will comprise about 20 percent of the country's total population. These people will probably be healthy and alert well into their eighties; however, in the last years of their lives they will probably require significant medical care, putting financial stress on the health care system.

The complex issues surrounding death, suffering, and economics create demands for answers to difficult ethical questions. Does all life have value? Should one fight against death even when suffering is intense? Should suffering be lessened if the time of death is brought nearer? Should a patient be given the right to refuse medical treatment if the result is death? Should others be allowed to make this decision for the patient? Should other factors such as the financial or emotional burden on the family be part of the decision-making process? Once a decision has been made to terminate suffering by death, is there any ethical difference between discontinuing medical treatment and giving a lethal dosage of painkilling medication? Should laws be put into place that offer guidelines in these situations, or should each case be decided on an individual basis? And who should decide? There is a wide range of opinion and much uncertainty involving euthanasia and what constitutes a "good" death.

Euthanasia comes from a Greek word that can be translated as "good death" and is defined in several ways, depending on the philosophical stance of the one giving the definition. Tom Beauchamp, in his book *Health and Human Values* (1983), defines euthanasia as

> putting to death or failing to prevent death in cases of terminal illness or injury; the motive is to relieve comatoseness, physical suffering, anxiety or a serious sense of burdensomeness to self and others. In euthanasia at least one other person causes or helps to cause the death of one who desires death or, in the case of an incompetent person, makes a substituted decision, either to cause death directly or to withdraw something that sustains life.

Most patients who express a wish to die more quickly are terminally ill; however, euthanasia is sometimes considered as a solution for nonterminal patients as well. An example of the latter would be seriously deformed or retarded infants whose futures are judged to have a poor "quality of life" and who would be a serious burden on their families and society.

When discussing the ethical implications of euthanasia, the types of cases have been divided into various classes. A distinction is made between voluntary and nonvoluntary euthanasia. In voluntary euthanasia, the patient consents to a specific course of medical action in which death is hastened. Nonvoluntary euthanasia would occur in cases in which the patient is not able to make decisions about his or her death because of an inability to communicate or a lack of mental facility. Each of these classes has advocates and antagonists. Some believe that voluntary euthanasia should always be allowed, but others would limit voluntary euthanasia to only those patients who have a terminal illness. Some, although agreeing in principle that voluntary euthanasia in terminal situations is ethically permissible, nevertheless oppose euthanasia of any type because of the possibility of abuses. With nonvoluntary euthanasia, the main ethical issues deal with when such an action should be performed and who should make the decision. If a person is in an irreversible coma, most agree that that person's physical life could be ended; however, arguments based on "quality of life" can easily become widened to include persons with physical or mental disabilities. Infants with severe deformities can sometimes be saved but not fully cured with medical technology, and some individuals would advocate nonvoluntary euthanasia in these cases because of the suffering of the infants' caregivers. Some believe that family members or those who stand to gain from the decision should not be allowed to make the decision. Others point out that the family is the most likely to know what the wishes of the patient would have been. Most believe that the medical care personnel, although knowledgeable, should not have the power to decide, and many are reluctant to institute rigid laws. The possibility of misappropriated self-interest from each of these parties magnifies the difficulty of arriving at well-defined criteria.

The second type of classification is between passive and active euthanasia. Passive euthanasia occurs when sustaining medical treatment is refused or withdrawn and death is allowed to take its course. Active euthanasia involves the administration of a drug or some other means that directly causes death. Once again, there are many opinions surrounding these two types. One position is that there is no difference between active and passive euthanasia because in each the end is premeditated death with the motive of prevention of suffering. In fact, some argue that active euthanasia is more compassionate than letting death occur naturally, which may involve suffering. In opposition, others believe that there is a fundamental difference between active and passive euthanasia. A person may have the right to die, but not the right to be killed. Passive euthanasia, they argue, is merely allowing a death that is inevitable to occur. Active euthanasia, if voluntary, is equated with suicide because a human being seizes control of death; if nonvoluntary, it is considered murder.

Passive euthanasia, although generally more publicly acceptable than active euthanasia, has become a topic of controversy as the types of medical treatment that can be withdrawn are debated. A distinction is sometimes made between ordinary and extraordinary means. Defining these terms is difficult, since what may be extraordinary for one patient is not for another, depending on other medical conditions that the patient may have. In addition, what is considered an extraordinary technique today may be judged ordinary in the future. Another way to assess whether passive euthanasia should be allowed in a particular situation is to weigh the benefits against the burdens for the patient. Although most agree that there are cases in which high-tech equipment such as respirators can be withdrawn, there is a question about whether administration of food and water should ever be discontinued. Here the line between passive and active euthanasia is blurred.

RELIGIOUS AND LEGAL IMPLICATIONS

Decisions about death concern everyone because everyone will die. Eventually, each individual will be the patient who is making the decisions or for whom the decisions are being made. In the meantime, one may be called upon to make decisions for others. Even those not directly involved in the hard cases are affected, as taxpayers and subscribers to medical insurance, by the decisions made on the behalf of others. In a difficult moral issue such as this, individuals look to different institutions for guidelines. Two sources of guidance are the church and the law.

In 1971, the Roman Catholic Church issued *Ethical and Religious Directives for Catholic Health Facilities*. Included in this directive is the statement that

[I]t is not euthanasia to give a dying person sedatives and analgesics for alleviation of pain, when such a measure is judged necessary, even though they may deprive the patient of the use of reason or shorten his life.

This thinking was reaffirmed by a 1980 statement from the Vatican that considers suffering and expense for the family legitimate reasons to withdraw medical treatment when death is imminent. Bishops from The Netherlands, in a letter to a government commission, state that

[B]odily deterioration alone does not have to be unworthy of a man. History shows how many people, beaten, tortured and broken in body, sometimes even grew in personality in spite of it. Dying becomes unworthy of a man, if family and friends begin to look upon the dying person as a burden, withdraw themselves from him....

When speaking of passive euthanasia, the bishops state, "We see no reason to call this euthanasia. Such a person after all dies of his own illness. His death is neither intended nor caused, only nothing is done anymore to postpone it." Christians from Protestant churches may reflect a wider spectrum of positions. Joseph Fletcher, an Episcopal priest, defines a person as one having the ability to think and reason. If a patient does not meet these criteria, according to Fletcher, his or her life may be ended out of compassion for the person he or she once was. The United Church of Christ illustrates this view in its policy statement:

When illness takes away those abilities we associate with full personhood . . . we may well feel that the mere continuance of the body by machine or drugs is a violation of their person. . . . We do not believe simply the continuance of mere physical existence is either morally defensible or socially desirable or is God's will.

These varied positions generally are derived from differing emphases on two truths concerning the nature of God and the role of suffering in the life of the believer. First is the belief that God is the giver of life and that human beings should not usurp God's authority in matters of life and death. Second, alleviation of suffering is of critical importance to God, since it is not loving one's neighbor to allow him or her to suffer. Those who give more weight to the first statement believe as well that God's will allows for suffering and that the suffering can be used for a good purpose in the life of the believer. Those who emphasize the second princi-

ple insist that a loving God would not prolong the suffering of people needlessly and that one should not desperately fight to prolong a life which God has willed to die.

C. Everett Koop, former surgeon general of the United States, differentiates between the positive role of a physician in providing a patient "all the life to which he or she is entitled" and the negative role of "prolonging the act of dying." Koop has opposed euthanasia in any form, cautioning against the possibility of sliding down a slippery slope toward making choices about death that reflect the caregivers' "quality of life" more than the patient's.

Jack Kevorkian, a Michigan physician, became the best-known advocate of assisted suicide in the United States. From 1990 to 1997, Kevorkian assisted at least sixty-six people in terminating their lives. According to Kevorkian's lawyer, many other assisted suicides have not been publicized. Kevorkian believes that physician-assisted suicide is a matter of individual choice and should be seen as a rational way to end tremendous pain and suffering. Most of the patients assisted by him spent many years suffering from extremely painful and debilitating diseases, such as multiple sclerosis, bone cancer, and brain cancer.

The American Medical Association (AMA) has criticized this view, calling it a violation of professional ethics. When faced with pain and suffering, the AMA asserts that it is a doctor's responsibility to provide adequate "comfort" care, not death. In the AMA's view, Kevorkian served as "a reckless instrument of death." Three trials in Michigan for assisting in suicide resulted in acquittals for Kevorkian before another trial delivered a guilty verdict on the charge of second-degree murder in March, 1999.

During the course of reevaluating the issues involved in terminating a life, the law has been in a state of flux. The decisions that are made by the courts act on the legal precedents of an individual's right to determine what is done to his or her own body and society's position against suicide. The balancing of these two premises has been handled legally by allowing refusal of treatment (passive euthanasia) but disallowing the use of poison or some other method that would cause death (active euthanasia). The latter is labeled "suicide," and anyone who assists in such an act can be found guilty of assisting a suicide, or of murder. Following the Karen Ann Quinlan case in 1976, in which the family of a comatose woman secured permission to withdraw life-sustaining treatment, the courts routinely allowed family members to make decisions regarding life-sustaining treatment if the patient could not do so. The area of greatest legal controversy involves the withdrawal of food and water. Some courts have charged doctors with murder for the withdrawal of basic life support measures such as food and water. Others have ruled that invasive procedures to provide food and water (intravenously, for example) are similar to other medical procedures and may be discontinued if the benefit to the patient's quality of life is negligible.

In 1994, 51 percent of the voters in Oregon passed the world's first "death with dignity" law. It allowed physician-assisted suicide. Doctors could begin prescribing fatal overdoses of drugs to terminally ill patients. The vote was reaffirmed in 1997 by 60 percent of the state's voters, despite opposition from the Catholic Church, the AMA, and various anti-abortion and right-to-life groups. The Ninth United States Circuit Court of Appeals in San Francisco then lifted a lower court order blocking implementation of the law. Since 1999, several states, including Hawaii, Vermont, New Hampshire, Maine, and North Carolina, have witnessed attempts to legalize physician-assisted suicide, but the cases have either been withdrawn or defeated by voters or in state legislature.

Doctors in Oregon became free to prescribe fatal doses of barbiturates to patients with less than six months to live. Physicians were required to file forms with the Oregon Health Division before prescribing the overdose. Then, there would be a fifteen-day waiting period between the request for suicide assistance and the approval of the prescription. Opponents of the Oregon law charged that it perverted the practice of medicine and forced many suffering people to "choose" an early death to save themselves from expensive medical care or pain that could be manageable if physicians were aware of new methods of pain control. The National Right to Life Committee indicated that it would continue to fight implementation of the law in federal courts.

Although the laws vary from state to state, most states allow residents to make their wishes known regarding terminal health care either by writing a living will or by choosing a durable power of attorney. A living will is a document in which one can state that some medical treatments should not be used in the event that one becomes incapacitated to the point where one cannot choose. Living wills allow the patient to decide in advance and protect health care providers from lawsuits. Which treatment options can be terminated and when this action can be put into effect may be limited in some states. Most states have a specific format that should be followed when drawing up a living will and require that the document be signed in the presence of two witnesses. Often, qualifying additions can be made by the individual that specify whether food and water may be withdrawn and whether the living will should go into effect only when death is imminent or also when a person has an incurable illness but death is not imminent. A copy of the living will should be given to the patient's physician and become a part of the patient's medical records. The preparation or execution of a living will cannot affect a person's life insurance coverage or the payment of benefits. Since the medical circumstances of one's life may change and a person's ethical stance may also change, a patient may change the living will at any time by signing a written statement.

A second way in which a person can control what kind of decisions will be made regarding his or her death is to choose a decision maker in advance. This person assumes a durable power of attorney and is legally allowed to act on the patient's behalf, making medical treatment decisions. One advantage of a durable power of attorney over a living will is that the patient can choose someone who shares similar ethical and religious values. Since it is difficult to foresee every medical situation that could arise, there is more security with a durable power of attorney in knowing that the person will have similar values and will therefore probably make the same judgments as the patient. Usually a primary agent and a secondary agent are designated in the event that the primary agent is unavailable. This is especially important if the primary agent is a spouse or a close relative who could, for example, be involved in an accident at the same time as the patient.

PERSPECTIVE AND PROSPECTS

Although large numbers of court decision, articles, and books suggest that the issues involved in euthanasia are recent products of medical technology, these questions are not new. Euthanasia was widely practiced in Western classical culture. The Greeks did not believe that all humans had the right to live, and in Athens, infants with disabilities were often killed. Although in general they did not condone suicide, Pythagoras, Plato, and Aristotle believed that a person could choose to die earlier in the face of an incurable disease and that others could help that person to die. Seneca, the Roman Stoic philosopher, was an avid proponent of euthanasia, stating that

Against all the injuries of life, I have the refuge of death. If I can choose between a death of torture and one that is simple and easy, why should I not select the latter? As I choose the ship in which I sail and the house which I shall inhabit, so I will choose the death by which I leave life.

The famous Hippocratic oath for physicians acted in opposition to the prevailing cultural bias in favor of euthanasia. Contained in this oath is the statement, "I will never give a deadly drug to anybody if asked for it . . . or make a suggestion to this effect." The AMA has reaffirmed this position in a policy statement:

the intentional termination of the life of one human being by another—"mercy killing"—is contrary to that for which the medical profession stands and is contrary to the policy of the American Medical Association.

The great English poet John Donne, in his *Devotions Upon Emergent Occasions*, wrote extensively on the concept of suffering in the severely ill. He wrote, "Affliction is a treasure, and scarce any man hath enough of it." In addition, Jewish and Christian theology have traditionally opposed any form of euthanasia or suicide, avowing that since God is the author of life and death, life is sacred. Therefore, a man would rebel against God if he prematurely shortens his life, because he violates the Sixth Commandment: "Thou shalt not kill." Suffering was viewed not as an evil to be avoided but as a condition to be accepted. The apostle Paul served as an example for early Christians. In 2 Corinthians, he prayed for physical healing, yet when it did not come, he accepted his weakness as a way to increase his dependence on God. This position was affirmed by Saint Augustine in his work *De Civitate Dei* (413-426; *The City of God*) when he condemned suicide as a "detestable and damnable wickedness" that was worse than murder because it left no room for repentance. These strong indictments from the Church against suicide and euthanasia were largely responsible for changing the Greco-Roman attitudes toward the value of human life. They were accepted as society's position until the advent of technologies in the late twentieth century that made it possible to extend life beyond what would have been the point of death.

Although these issues have been debated by physicians and philosophers for centuries, there remains a heightened need for thoughtful discussion and resolution. The majority of nations, as well as major medical organizations such as the AMA, oppose euthanasia as contrary to the proper role of the physician and society. However, closely related and complex issues such as the treatment of pain in the terminally ill leave much room for development in human understanding.

—*Katherine B. Frederich, Ph.D.;*
updated by Leslie V. Tischauser, Ph.D.

See also Aging: Extended care; Critical care; Critical care, pediatric; Death and dying; Ethics; Hippocratic oath; Hospice; Law and medicine; Living will; Pain management; Palliative medicine; Psychiatry; Psychiatry, geriatric; Suicide; Terminally ill: Extended care.

FOR FURTHER INFORMATION:

Corr, Charles A., Clyde M. Nabe, and Donna M. Corr. *Death and Dying, Life and Living.* 6th ed. Belmont, Calif.: Wadsworth/Cengage Learning, 2009. This book provides perspective on common issues associated with death and dying for family members and others affected by life-threatening circumstances.

Dowbiggin, Ian Robert. *A Merciful End: The Euthanasia Movement in Modern America.* New York: Oxford University Press, 2003. Blends social history, medical knowledge, and political analysis to trace the evolution of euthanasia and its perception in the United States throughout the twentieth century.

Gorovitz, Samuel. *Drawing the Line: Life, Death, and Ethical Choices in an American Hospital.* Philadelphia: Temple University Press, 1993. This book reflects on the author's sabbatical-in-residence at Beth Israel Hospital. Gorovitz presents numerous insights drawn from conversations with patients and medical personnel.

Harron, Frank, John Burnside, and Tom Beauchamp. *Health and Human Values.* New Haven, Conn.: Yale University Press, 1983. Using a case-study approach, the authors consider the different types of euthanasia and report on policy statements from interested social groups.

Leone, Daniel A. *The Ethics of Euthanasia.* San Diego, Calif.: Greenhaven Press, 1998. This volume includes ten essays on the ethics and morality of euthanasia, potential abuse, distinctions between active and passive euthanasia, and whether euthanasia is consistent with Christian belief.

Magnusson, Roger, and Peter H. Ballis. *Angels of Death: Exploring the Euthanasia Underground.* New Haven, Conn.: Yale University Press, 2002. Explores the existence of a euthanasia underground in Australia and the United States using firsthand accounts of health professionals who have been involved in assisted death.

Rebman, Renée C. *Euthanasia and the Right to Die: Pro/Con Issues*. Berkeley Heights, N.J.: Enslow, 2002. Part of the Hot Pro/Con Issues series for young adults, offers a balanced perspective on a range of issues surrounding euthanasia.

Spring, Beth, and Ed Larson. *Euthanasia*. Portland, Oreg.: Multnomah Press, 1988. This book considers the spiritual, medical, and legal issues in terminal health care, citing numerous perspectives from the religious community. Contains two chapters detailing practical guidelines for writing living wills and durable powers of attorney.

Torr, James D. *Euthanasia: Opposing Viewpoints*. San Diego, Calif.: Greenhaven Press, 2000. Designed for students in grades nine through twelve, this volume brings together essays by authorities in diverse vocations. The four chapters explore whether euthanasia is ethical, if it should be legalized, if legalization would lead to involuntary killing, and under what circumstances, if any, doctors should assist in suicide.

Wennberg, Robert N. *Terminal Choices: Euthanasia, Suicide, and the Right to Die*. Grand Rapids, Mich.: Wm. B. Eerdmans, 1989. The author presents a helpful history of the euthanasia debate and also discusses possible moral distinctions between treatment refusal and treatment withdrawal.

EWING'S SARCOMA
DISEASE/DISORDER

ALSO KNOWN AS: Bone cancer

ANATOMY OR SYSTEM AFFECTED: Bones, musculoskeletal system

SPECIALTIES AND RELATED FIELDS: Oncology, orthopedics, pediatrics, radiology

DEFINITION: A rare bone cancer involving any part of the skeleton but found commonly in the long bones (60 percent), the pelvis (18 percent), and the ribs (15 percent) of children and young adults.

CAUSES AND SYMPTOMS

The specific cause of Ewing's sarcoma is unknown, but it may be associated with recurrent trauma, metal implants, congenital anomalies, unrelated tumors, or exposure to ionizing radiation. Approximately 90 percent of patients are between five and twenty-five years of age; rarely are patients younger than five or older than forty.

The initial symptom is pain, discontinuous at first

> ### INFORMATION ON EWING'S SARCOMA
>
> **CAUSES:** Unknown; possibly related to recurrent trauma, metal implants, congenital anomalies, unrelated tumors, exposure to ionizing radiation
>
> **SYMPTOMS:** Pain in long bones, vertebra, or pelvis; swelling; neurological disorders; weight loss; fever; mild anemia
>
> **DURATION:** Long-term
>
> **TREATMENTS:** Surgery, chemotherapy, radiation

and then intense, in the long bones, vertebra, or pelvis. Swelling may follow. Neurological signs involving the nerve roots or spinal cord depression are characteristic of nearly one-half of patients with involvement of the axial skeleton. Weight loss may occur, with remittent fever and mild anemia.

The phases of Ewing's sarcoma are based on degree of metastasis: the local phase (a nonmetastatic tumor), the regional phase (lymph node involvement), and the distant phase (involvement of the lungs, bones, and sometimes the central nervous system).

TREATMENT AND THERAPY

Patients are of two types, those with localized tumors and those with metastasized tumors. Depending on where the tumor is located, the treatment of Ewing's sarcoma is complex in all stages of disease and requires a multidisciplinary perspective. It is best treated when diagnosed early. Obtaining a bone biopsy is recommended in nearly all cases.

Surgery may be used to remove a tumor, followed by chemotherapy administered to kill any remaining cancer cells. Radiation may be prescribed to kill cancer cells and shrink tumors.

PERSPECTIVE AND PROSPECTS

Ewing's sarcoma is one of the most malignant of all tumors. It may be localized or metastasize to the lungs and other bones. The primary tumor can be controlled by irradiation, but the prognosis is poor. Often, amputation is not justifiable. Recent developments in multiagent chemotherapy, however, are encouraging. Long-term survival of patients with Ewing's sarcoma is 50 to 70 percent or more with localized disease; the rate drops to less than 30 percent for metastatic disease.

—John Alan Ross, Ph.D.

See also Bone cancer; Bone disorders; Bones and the skeleton; Cancer; Orthopedics, pediatric.

FOR FURTHER INFORMATION:

Cady, Blake, ed. *Cancer Manual.* 7th ed. Boston: American Cancer Society, 1986.

Dollinger, Malin, et al. *Everyone's Guide to Cancer Therapy.* 5th ed. Kansas City, Mo.: Andrews McMeel, 2008.

Dorfman, Howard D., and Bogdan Czerniak. *Bone Tumors.* St. Louis, Mo.: Mosby, 1998.

Eyre, Harmon J., Dianne Partie Lange, and Lois B. Morris. *Informed Decisions: The Complete Book of Cancer Diagnosis, Treatment, and Recovery.* 2d ed. Atlanta: American Cancer Society, 2002.

Grealy, Lucy. *Autobiography of a Face.* New York: Perennial, 2003.

Holleb, Arthur I., ed. *The American Cancer Society Cancer Book: Prevention, Detection, Diagnosis, Treatment, Rehabilitation, Cure.* Garden City, N.Y.: Doubleday, 1986.

Janes-Hodder, Honna, and Nancy Keene. *Childhood Cancer: A Parent's Guide to Solid Tumor Cancers.* 2d ed. Cambridge, Mass.: O'Reilly, 2002.

Morra, Marion, and Eve Potts. *Choices: Realistic Alternatives in Cancer Treatment.* Rev. ed. New York: Viking, 1997.

EXERCISE PHYSIOLOGY

SPECIALTY

ANATOMY OR SYSTEM AFFECTED: Circulatory system, heart, joints, knees, lungs, muscles, musculoskeletal system, respiratory system, tendons

SPECIALTIES AND RELATED FIELDS: Cardiology, family medicine, nutrition, physical therapy, preventive medicine, sports medicine

DEFINITION: The science that studies the effects on the body of various intensities and types of physical activity, including cellular metabolism, cardiovascular responses, respiratory responses, neural and hormonal adaptations, and muscular adaptations to exercise.

KEY TERMS:

adenosine triphosphate (ATP): a high-energy compound found in the cell which provides energy for all bodily functions

aerobic: metabolism involving the breakdown of energy substrates using oxygen

anaerobic: metabolism involving the breakdown of energy substrates without using oxygen

electrocardiogram (ECG): a graphic record of electrical currents of the heart

glycogen: the form that glucose takes when it is stored in the muscles and liver

heart rate: the number of times the heart contracts, or beats, per minute

maximal oxygen uptake: the maximum rate of oxygen consumption during exercise

metabolic equivalent (MET): a unit used to estimate the metabolic cost of physical activity; 1 MET is equal to 3.5 milliliters of oxygen consumed per kilogram of body weight per minute

SCIENCE AND PROFESSION

The primary focus of research in the field of exercise physiology is to gain a better understanding of the quantity and type of exercise needed for health maintenance and rehabilitation. A major goal of professionals in exercise physiology is to find ways to incorporate appropriate levels of physical activity into the lifestyles of all individuals.

Physiology is the science of physical and chemical factors and processes involved in the function of living organisms. The study of exercise physiology examines these factors and processes as they relate to physical exertion. The physical responses that occur are specific to the intensity, duration, and type of exercise performed.

Low or moderate exercise intensity relies on oxygen to release energy for work. This process is often referred to as aerobic exercise. In the muscles, carbohydrates and fats are broken down to produce adenosine triphosphate (ATP), the basic molecule used for energy. Aerobic exercise can be sustained for several minutes to several hours.

Higher-intensity exercise is predominantly fueled anaerobically (in the absence of oxygen) and can be sustained for up to two minutes only. Muscle glycogen is broken down without oxygen to produce ATP. Anaerobic metabolism is much less efficient at producing ATP than is aerobic metabolism.

During anaerobic metabolism, a by-product called lactic acid begins to accumulate in the blood as blood lactate. The point at which this accumulation begins is called the anaerobic threshold (AT), or the onset of blood lactate accumulation (OBLA). Blood lactate can cause muscle soreness and stiffness, but it also can be used as fuel during aerobic metabolism.

A third and less often used energy system is the creatine phosphate (ATP-CP) system. Utilizing the very

The Effects of Exercise on the Body

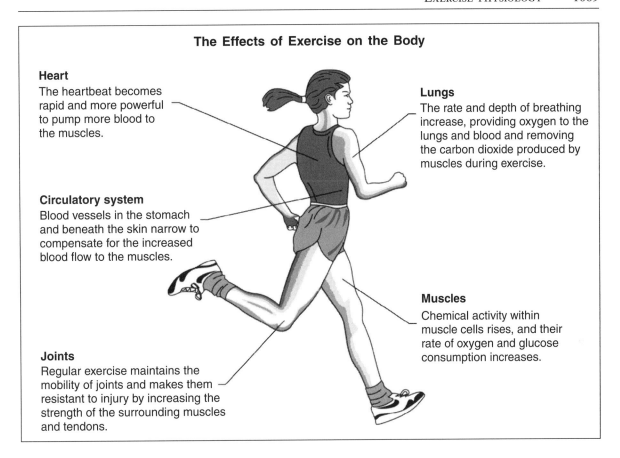

Heart
The heartbeat becomes rapid and more powerful to pump more blood to the muscles.

Circulatory system
Blood vessels in the stomach and beneath the skin narrow to compensate for the increased blood flow to the muscles.

Joints
Regular exercise maintains the mobility of joints and makes them resistant to injury by increasing the strength of the surrounding muscles and tendons.

Lungs
The rate and depth of breathing increase, providing oxygen to the lungs and blood and removing the carbon dioxide produced by muscles during exercise.

Muscles
Chemical activity within muscle cells rises, and their rate of oxygen and glucose consumption increases.

limited supply of ATP that is stored in the muscles, phosphate molecules are exchanged between ATP and CP to provide energy. This system provides only enough fuel for a few seconds of maximum effort.

The type of muscle fiber recruited to perform a specific type of exercise is also dependent on exercise intensity. Skeletal muscle is composed of "slow-twitch" and two types of "fast-twitch" muscle fibers. Slow-twitch fibers are more suited to using oxygen than are fast-twitch fibers, and they are recruited primarily for aerobic exercise. One type of fast-twitch fiber also functions during aerobic activity. The second type of fast-twitch fiber serves to facilitate anaerobic, or high-intensity, exercise.

Exercise mode is also a factor in the physiological responses to exercise. Dynamic exercise (alternating muscular contraction and relaxation through a range of motion) using many large muscles requires more oxygen than does activity utilizing smaller and fewer muscles. The greater the oxygen requirement of the physical activity, the greater the cardiorespiratory benefits.

Many bodily adaptations occur over a training period of six to eight weeks, and other benefits are gradu-ally manifested over several months. The positive adaptations include reduced resting and working heart rates. As the heart becomes stronger, there is a subsequent increase in stroke volume (the volume of blood the heart pumps with each beat), which allows the heart to beat less frequently while maintaining the same cardiac output (the volume of the blood pumped from the heart each minute). Another beneficial adaptation is increased metabolic efficiency. This is partially facilitated by an increase in the number of mitochondria (the organelles responsible for ATP production) in the muscle cells.

One of the most recognized representations of aerobic fitness is the maximum volume of oxygen (VO_{2max}) an individual can use during exercise. VO_{2max} is improved through habitual, relatively high-intensity aerobic activity. After three to six months of regular training, levels of high-density lipoproteins (HDLs) in the blood increase. HDL molecules remove cholesterol (a fatty substance) from the tissues to aid in protecting the heart from atherosclerosis.

Various internal and external factors influence the metabolic processes that take place during and after exercise. Internally, nutrition, degree of hydration, body composition, flexibility, sex, and age are some of the variables that play a role in the physiological responses. Other internal variables include medical conditions such as heart disease, diabetes, and hypertension (high blood pressure). Externally, environmental conditions such as temperature, humidity, and altitude alter how the exercising body functions.

Various modes of exercise testing and data collection are used to study the physiological responses of the body to exercise. Treadmills and cycle ergometers (instruments used to measure work and power output) are among the most common methods of evaluating maximum oxygen consumption. During these tests, special equipment and computers analyze expired air, heart rate is monitored with an electrocardiograph (ECG), and blood pressure is taken using a sphygmomanometer. Blood samples and muscle fiber samples can also be extracted to aid in identifying the fuel system and type of muscle fibers being used. Other data sometimes collected, such as skin temperatures and body core temperatures, can provide pertinent information.

Metabolic equivalent units, or METs, are often used to translate a person's capability into workloads on various pieces of exercise equipment or into everyday tasks. For every 3.5 milliliters of oxygen consumed per kilogram of body weight per minute, the subject is said to be performing at a workload of one MET. One MET is approximately equivalent to 1.5 kilocalories per minute, or the amount of energy expended per kilogram of body weight in one minute when a person is at rest.

Another factor greatly affecting the physical response to exercise is body composition. The three major structural components of the body are muscle, bone, and fat. Body composition can be evaluated using a combination of anthropometric measurements. These measurements include body weight, standard height, measurements of circumferences at various locations using a tape measure, measurements of skeletal diameters using a sliding metric stick, and measurements of skinfold thicknesses using calipers.

Body fat can be estimated using several methods, the most accurate of which is based on a calculation of body density. This method is called hydrostatic weighing, which involves weighing the subject under water while taking into account the residual volume of air in the lungs. The principle underlying this measurement of body density is based on the fact that fat is less dense than water and will float, whereas bone and muscle, which are denser than water, will sink. One biochemi-

cal technique often used to determine levels of body fat is based on the relatively constant level of potassium 40 naturally existing in lean body mass. Another method utilizes ultrasound waves to measure the thickness of fat layers. X rays and computed tomography (CT) scanning can be used to provide images from which fat and bone can be measured. Bioelectrical impedance (BIA) is a method of estimating body composition based on the resistance imposed on a low voltage electrical current sent through the body. The most widely used and easily assessable method, however, involves measurement of skinfolds at various sites on the body using calipers. In all cases, mathematical formulas have been devised to interpret the collected data and provide the best estimate of an individual's body composition.

Other tests have been developed to determine muscular strength, muscular endurance, and flexibility. Muscular strength is often measured by performance of one maximal effort produced by a selected muscle group. Muscular endurance of a muscle or muscle group is often demonstrated by the length of time or number of repetitions a particular, submaximal workload or skill can be performed.

Two major types of flexibility have been identified. One type consists of the flexibility through the range of motion of a muscle group or joint. This is called static flexibility. It can be measured using a metric stick or a protractor-type instrument called a goniometer. Dynamic flexibility is the other major identified type of flexibility. It is the torque of or resistance to movement. Methods to measure dynamic flexibility have not been developed.

Overlapping the science of exercise physiology are the studies of biomechanics or kinesiology (sciences dealing with human movement) and nutrition. Only through an understanding of efficient body mechanics and proper nutrition can the physiological responses of the body to exercise be identified correctly.

Diagnostic and Treatment Techniques

Exercise prescription is the primary focus in the application of exercise physiology. General health maintenance, cardiac rehabilitation, and competitive athletics are three major areas of exercise prescription.

Before making recommendations for an exercise program, an exercise physiologist must evaluate the physical limitations of the exerciser. In a normal, health maintenance setting—often called a "wellness" program—a health-related questionnaire can reveal relevant information. Such a questionnaire should include questions about family medical history and the subject's history of heart trouble or chest pain, bone or joint problems, and high blood pressure. The presence of any of these problems suggests the need for a physician's consent prior to exercising. After the individual has been deemed eligible to participate, an assessment of the level of physical fitness should be performed. Determining or estimating VO_{2max}, muscular strength, muscular endurance, flexibility, and body composition is usually included in this assessment. It is then possible to design a program best suited to the needs of the individual.

For the healthy adult participant, the American College of Sports Medicine (ACSM), a widely recognized authoritative body on exercise prescription, recommends three to five sessions of aerobic exercise weekly. Each session should include a five- to ten-minute warm-up period, twenty to sixty minutes of aerobic exercise at a predetermined exercise intensity, and a five- to ten-minute cool-down period.

To recommend an appropriate aerobic exercise intensity, the exercise physiologist must determine an individual's maximum heart rate. The best way to obtain this maximum heart rate is to administer a maximal ex-

ercise test. Such a test can be supervised by an exercise physiologist or an exercise test technician; it is advisable, especially for the older participant, that a cardiologist also be in attendance. An ECG is monitored for irregularities as the subject walks, runs, cycles, or performs some dynamic exercise to exhaustion or until the onset of irregular symptoms or discomfort.

Exercise prescription using heart rate as a measure can be achieved by various methods. A direct correlation exists between exercise intensity, in terms of oxygen consumption, and heart rate. From data collected during a maximal exercise test, a target heart rate range of 40 percent to 85 percent of functional capacity can be calculated. Another method used to determine an appropriate heart rate range is based on the difference between an individual's resting heart rate and maximum heart rate, called the heart rate reserve (HRR). Values representing 60 percent and 80 percent of the heart rate reserve are calculated and added to the resting heart rate, yielding the individual's target heart rate range. A third method involves calculating 70 percent and 85 percent of the maximum heart rate. Although this method is less accurate than the other two methods, it is the simplest way to estimate a target heart rate range.

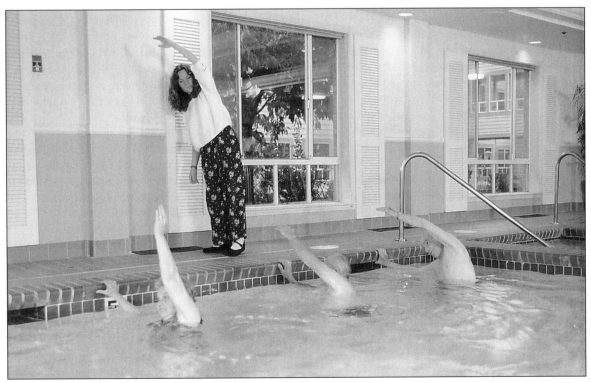

Elderly individuals may find low-impact exercise, such as swimming, to be a safer and easier way to stay fit. (PhotoDisc)

Intensity of exercise can also be prescribed using METs. This method relies on the predetermined metabolic equivalents required to perform activities at various intensities. Activity levels reflecting 40 percent to 85 percent of functional capacity can be calculated.

The rating of perceived exertion (RPE) is another method of prescribing exercise intensity. Verbal responses by the participant describing how an exercise feels at various intensities are assigned to a numerical scale, which is then correlated to heart rate. Through practice, the participant can correlate heart rate with the RPE, reducing the necessity of frequent pulse monitoring in the healthy individual.

Adequate physical fitness can be defined as the ability to perform daily tasks with enough reserve for emergency situations. All aspects of health-related fitness direct attention toward this goal. Aerobic exercise often provides some conditioning for muscular endurance, but muscular strength and flexibility need to be addressed separately.

The ACSM recommends resistance training using the "overload principle," which involves placing habitual stress on a system, causing it to adapt and respond. For this training, it is suggested that eight to twelve repetitions of eight to ten strengthening exercises of the major muscle groups be performed a minimum of two days per week.

Flexibility of connective tissue and muscle tissue is essential to maximize physical performance and to limit musculoskeletal injuries. At least one stretching exercise for each major muscle group should be executed three to four times per week while the muscles are warm. Three methods of stretching that have been designed to improve flexibility are ballistic stretching, static stretching, and proprioceptive neuromuscular facilitation (PNF). Ballistic stretching incorporates a bouncing motion and is generally prescribed only in sports that replicate this type of movement. During a static stretch, the muscles and connective tissue are passively stretched to their maximum lengths. PNF involves a contract-relax sequence of the muscle.

In addition to exercise prescription for cardiorespiratory fitness, muscular fitness, and flexibility, it is appropriate for the exercise physiologist to make recommendations concerning body composition. Exercise is an effective tool in fat loss. Dietary caloric restriction without exercise results in a greater loss of muscle mass along with fat loss than if exercise is part of a weight loss program.

For persons with special health concerns, such as di-abetes mellitus or high blood pressure, the exercise physiologist works with the participant's physician. The physician prescribes necessary medications and often decides which modes of exercise are contraindicated (those that should be avoided).

A second application, cardiac rehabilitation, takes exercise prescription a step further. Participation of the heart patient is more individualized than in wellness programs. The condition of the circulatory system, pulmonary system, and joints are only a few of the special concerns. Secondary conditions such as obesity, diabetes, and hypertension must also be considered. The responsibilities of cardiac rehabilitation specialists include monitoring blood sugar in diabetic patients and blood pressure in all patients, especially those with hypertension. Many drugs affect heart rate or blood pressure, and most of these participants are taking more than one type of medication. Patients with heart damage caused by a heart attack may display atypical heart rhythms, which can be seen on an ECG monitor. Furthermore, the stage of recovery of the postsurgical patient is a major factor in recommending the type, frequency, intensity, and duration of exercise.

Patient education is also important. Lifestyle is usually the main factor in the development of heart disease. Cardiac patients often have never participated in a regular exercise program. Frequently, they are smokers, are overweight, and have poor eating habits. Helping them to identify and correct destructive health-related behaviors is the focus of education for the heart patient.

A third application of the study of exercise physiology involves dealing with the competitive athlete. In this case, findings from the most recent research are constantly applied to yield the best athletic performance possible. A delicate balance of aerobic training, anaerobic training, strength training, endurance training, and flexibility exercises are combined with the optimum percentage of body fat, proper nutrition, and adequate sleep. The program that is designed must enhance the athletic qualities that are most beneficial to the sport in which the athlete participates.

The competitive athlete usually pushes beyond the boundaries of general exercise prescription in terms of intensity, duration, and frequency of exercise performance. As a result, the athlete risks suffering more injuries than the individual who exercises for health benefits. If the athlete sustains an injury, the exercise physiologist may work in conjunction with an athletic trainer or sports physician to return the athlete to competition as soon as possible.

PERSPECTIVE AND PROSPECTS

The modern study of exercise physiology developed out of an interest in physical fitness. In the United States, and possibly much of the world, that interest was primarily driven by a desire to prepare soldiers for war adequately.

In the United States, the concern for development and maintenance of physical fitness was well established by the end of the twentieth century. As early as 1819, Stanford and Harvard universities offered professional physical education programs. At least one textbook on the physiology of exercise was published by that time.

Much of the pioneer work in this field, however, was done in Europe. Nobel Prize-winning European research on muscular exercise, oxygen utilization as it relates to the upper limits of physical performance, and production of lactic acid during glucose metabolism dates back to the 1920's.

In the early 1950's, poor performance by children in the United States on a minimal muscular fitness test helped lead to the formation of what is now known as the President's Council on Physical Fitness and Sport. Concurrently, a significant number of deaths of middle-aged American males were found to be caused by poor health habits associated with coronary artery disease. A need for more research in the areas of health and physical activity was recognized by the mid-1960's. The subsequent research was facilitated by the existence of fifty-eight exercise physiology research laboratories in colleges and universities throughout the country. Organizations such as the American Physiological Society (APS), the American Alliance of Health, Physical Education, Recreation and Dance (AAHPERD), and the American College of Sports Medicine (ACSM) were established by the mid-1950's. In an effort to ensure that well-trained professionals were involved in cardiac rehabilitation programs, the ACSM developed a certification program in 1975. Certifications for fitness personnel were added later.

A better understanding of fundamental physiological mechanisms should stem from increasingly sophisticated testing equipment, allowing practitioners to be more effective in measuring physical fitness and in prescribing exercise programs. Health maintenance has become a priority as the number of adults over the age of fifty continues to increase. Advances in medical techniques also increase the survival rate of victims of heart attacks, creating a need for more cardiac rehabili-tation programs and practitioners. Health care professionals and the general population need to be made more aware of the benefits of exercise in the maintenance of good health and in the rehabilitation of individuals with medical problems.

—Kathleen O'Boyle;
updated by Bradley R. A. Wilson, Ph.D.

See also Biofeedback; Bones and the skeleton; Braces, orthopedic; Cardiac rehabilitation; Cardiology; Electrocardiography (ECG or EKG); Ergogenic aids; Glycolysis; Heart; Hyperbaric oxygen therapy; Kinesiology; Lungs; Metabolism; Muscle sprains, spasms, and disorders; Muscles; Nutrition; Orthopedics; Orthopedics, pediatric; Overtraining syndrome; Oxygen therapy; Physical rehabilitation; Physiology; Preventive medicine; Pulmonary medicine; Respiration; Sports medicine; Steroid abuse; Sweating; Tendinitis; Vascular system.

FOR FURTHER INFORMATION:

American College of Sports Medicine. *ACSM's Guidelines for Exercise Testing and Prescription.* 8th ed. Philadelphia: Lippincott Williams & Wilkins, 2010. This manual provides guidelines for professionals working in preventive exercise programs or in cardiac rehabilitation. The recommendations are based on updated research.

_____. *ACSM's Resource Manual for Guidelines for Exercise Testing and Prescription.* 6th ed. Baltimore: Lippincott Williams & Wilkins, 2010. Based on the objective of providing safe and effective exercise programs for all individuals, this publication provides an excellent overview of many of the topics of concern to the exercise physiologist. Specific recommendations regarding stress testing and exercise prescription are included in the text.

Brooks, George A., and Thomas D. Fahey. *Fundamentals of Human Performance.* Mountain View, Calif.: Mayfield, 2000. This textbook was written for students of physical education, nursing, nutrition, and physical therapy who need a practical introduction to exercise physiology. The theoretical basis and practical application of physical activity are explained through a discussion of metabolic phenomena.

McArdle, William, Frank I. Katch, and Victor L. Katch. *Exercise Physiology: Energy, Nutrition, and Human Performance.* 7th ed. Boston: Lippincott Williams & Wilkins, 2010. A wide-ranging text on exercise and the human body, covering topics such as nutrition, energy transfer, exercise training, systems of energy delivery and utilization, enhancement of energy capacity, the effect of environmental stress, and the effect of exercise on successful aging and disease prevention.

Powers, Scott K., and Edward T. Howley. *Exercise Physiology: Theory and Application to Fitness and Performance.* 7th ed. New York: McGraw-Hill, 2009. The upper-level undergraduate or beginning graduate student will find detailed information concerning exercise physiology in this useful textbook. Designed for students who are serious about the study of exercise science.

EXTENDED CARE FOR THE AGING. *See* AGING: EXTENDED CARE.

EXTENDED CARE FOR THE TERMINALLY ILL. *See* TERMINALLY ILL: EXTENDED CARE.

EXTREMITIES. *See* FEET; FOOT DISORDERS; LOWER EXTREMITIES; UPPER EXTREMITIES.

EYE INFECTIONS AND DISORDERS
DISEASE/DISORDER

ANATOMY OR SYSTEM AFFECTED: Blood vessels, brain, cells, eyes, glands, head, ligaments, muscles, nerves

SPECIALTIES AND RELATED FIELDS: Bacteriology, cytology, general surgery, geriatrics and gerontology, histology, neurology, nursing, nutrition, ophthalmology, optometry, pathology, pediatrics, radiology, virology

DEFINITION: Eye infections involve the invasion, multiplication, and colonization of microorganisms in the tissues of the eye. Eye disorders are derangement or abnormality of the functions of parts of the eye and the general impairment of function of the eye for precise and clear vision.

KEY TERMS:

allergy: abnormal reaction or increased sensitivity to a foreign substance

infection: invasion and multiplication of microorganisms in body tissues

inflammation: localized protective response provoked by injury or destruction of tissues

laser: an extremely intense small beam producing immense heat

ocular: pertaining to the eye

ophthalmologist: a physician who specializes in diagnosing and treating eye diseases and disorders

sign: a doctor's objective evidence of disease or dysfunction

symptom: any indication of disease perceived by the patient

CAUSES AND SYMPTOMS

Several varieties of eye problems exist worldwide. Among the most important are corneal infections, ocular herpes, trachoma, conjunctivitis, iritis, cataracts, glaucoma, macular degeneration, diabetic retinopathy, styes, ptosis, ectropion, entropion, either watery or dry eyes, astigmatism, myopia, hyperopia, presbyopia, amblyopia, and keratoconus.

Many organisms can infect the eye. In corneal infections, bacteria, fungi, or viruses invade the cornea and cause painful inflammation and corneal infections called keratitis. Visual clarity is reduced, and the cornea produces a discharge or becomes destroyed, resulting in corneal scarring and vision impairment.

Ocular herpes is a recurrent viral infection by the herpes simplex virus. Symptoms are a painful sore on the eyelid or eye surface and inflammation of the cornea. More severe infection destroys stromal cells and causes stromal keratitis, cornea scarring, and vision loss or blindness. It is the most common infectious cause of corneal blindness in the United States.

Trachoma is a chronic and contagious bacterial disease of the conjunctiva and cornea. The eye becomes inflamed, painful, and teary. Small gritty particles develop on the cornea. Conjunctivitis is the inflammation of the conjunctiva caused by virus or bacteria infection, chemical irritations, physical factors, and allergic reactions. Inflammation of the cornea accompanies viral forms. The eyes become very sensitive to light. The infectious form is highly contagious, especially acute contagious conjunctivitis (pinkeye). Signs are red, extremely itching, and irritating eyes with a gritty feeling; tearing; nasal discharge; sinus congestion; swollen eyelids (in severe cases); and eyelids that may stick together from dry mucus formed during the night.

Iritis is inflammation of the iris. The cause is still under investigation, but it is associated with rheumatoid arthritis, diabetes mellitus, syphilis, diseased teeth, tonsillitis, trauma, and infections. Symptoms are red eyes, contracted and irregularly shaped pupil, extreme sensitivity to light, tender eyeball, and blurred vision.

A cataract is a clouding of the lens that causes a progressive, slow, and painless loss of vision. Symptoms are reduced night vision, blurriness, poor depth perception, color distortion, problems with glare, and frequent eyeglass prescription changes. Cataracts are the world's leading cause of blindness. Causes are under investigation, but it could result from eye injury, prolonged exposure to drugs such as corticosteroids or to X rays, inflammatory and infectious eye diseases, complications of diseases such as diabetes, prolonged exposure to direct sunlight, poor nutrition, and smoking. Babies can be born with congenital cataracts.

Glaucoma is an optic nerve disease caused by fluid pressure that builds up abnormally within the eye because of very slow fluid production and draining. This can damage the optic nerve, retina, or other parts of the eye and result in vision loss. Early stages have no symptoms. Side (peripheral) vision is lost at an advanced point when irreversible damage makes vision restoration impossible. Blindness results if the condition is left untreated.

In macular degeneration, often called age-related macular degeneration (AMD or ARMD), the light-sensing cells of the macula, which is responsible for sharp and clear central vision, degenerates. The result is a slow, painless loss of central vision necessary for important activities such as driving and reading. Early signs are shadowy areas in the central vision, or fuzzy, blurry, or distorted vision. About 90 percent of cases are "dry" AMD, without bleeding, and 10 percent cases a more severe "wet" type, in which new blood vessels grow and leak blood and fluid under the macula, causing the most vision loss.

Diabetic retinopathy is damage to the blood vessels of the retina caused by uncontrolled diabetes. Early signs may not be exhibited, but blurred vision, pain in the eye, floaters, and gradual vision loss are the symptoms in advanced cases.

A number of disorders can affect the eyelids. A stye, or hordeolum, is a painful localized swelling produced by infection or inflammation in a sweat gland of the eyelids or the sebaceous glands that secrete oil to stop the eyelids from sticking together. Ptosis is drooping of the upper eyelid that obstructs the upper field of vision for one or both eyes. It produces blurred vision, refractive errors, astigmatism, strabismus (in which the eyes are not properly aligned), or amblyopia (lazy eye). Symptoms include aching eyebrows, difficulty in keeping the eyelids open, eyestrain, and eye fatigue, especially during reading.

With an ectropion, the lower eyelid and eyelashes turn outward and sag, usually because of aging. Scar-

> ## INFORMATION ON EYE INFECTIONS AND DISORDERS
>
> **CAUSES:** Bacteria, viruses, or fungi in the eye; abnormal function of parts of the eye impairing vision
> **SYMPTOMS:** Various; may include redness, itching, irritation, pain, swelling, sensitivity to light, blurred vision, vision loss, blindness
> **DURATION:** Acute or chronic
> **TREATMENTS:** Depends on cause; may include eyedrops or ointments, warm compresses, corrective lenses, surgery

ring of the eyelid caused by thermal and chemical burns, skin cancers, trauma, or previous eyelid surgery can also cause the problem. Symptoms are eye irritation, excessive tearing, mucus discharge, and crusting of the eyelid. With an entropion, the lower eyelid and eyelashes roll inward toward the eye and rub against the cornea and conjunctiva. This condition is also primarily the result of aging. Symptoms are irritation of the cornea, excessive tearing, mucus discharge, crusting of the eyelid, a feeling of something in the eye, and impaired vision. It can also be caused by allergic reactions, inflammatory diseases, and scarring of the inner surface of the eyelid caused by chemical and thermal burns.

Watery eyes are caused by the blockage of the lacrimal puncta (two small pores that drain tear secretions from lacrymal glands that bathe the conjunctival surfaces of the eye) or oversecretion of the lacrimal glands. Dry eyes result from inadequate tear production due to malfunction of the lacrymal (tear) glands, more common in women, especially after menopause. Symptoms are a scratchy or sandy feeling in the eye, pain and redness, excessive tearing following dry sensations, a stinging or burning feeling, discharge, heaviness of the eyelids, and blurred, changing, or decreased vision. Causes include dry air; the use of drugs such as tranquilizers, nasal decongestants, antidepressants, and antihistamines; connective tissue diseases such as rheumatoid arthritis; or the aging process.

Several refractive vision disorders are common. Astigmatism is blurred vision caused by a misshapen lens or cornea that makes light rays converge unevenly without focusing at any one point on the retina. In hyperopia (farsightedness), the eye can see distant objects normally but cannot focus at short distances because the eyeball is shorter than normal, causing the lens to focus images behind the retina. Presbyopia is farsightedness that develops with age. The lens gradually loses its ability to change shape and focus on nearby objects, creating difficulty in reading. In myopia (nearsightedness), the eye cannot focus properly on distant objects, although it can see well at short distances, because the eyeball is longer than normal. The lens cannot flatten enough to compensate and focuses distant objects in front of, instead of on, the retina.

Amblyopia, commonly called lazy eye, is a neurologic disorder in which the brain favors vision in one eye. Misalignment of the eyes (strabismus) creates two different images for the brain. If the condition goes untreated, then the weaker eye ceases to function.

Keratoconus is the progressive thinning of the cornea, producing conical protrusion of the central part of the cornea. It results in astigmatism or myopia and swelling or scarring of cornea tissue that ultimately impairs sight. Its causes are heredity, eye injury, and systemic diseases.

TREATMENT AND THERAPY

The treatment of eye infections and disorders depends on their cause and severity. Minor corneal infections are treated with antibacterial eyedrops. Intensive antibiotic, antifungal, and steroid eyedrop treatments eliminate the infection and reduce inflammation in severe cases. With ocular herpes, prompt treatment with antiviral drugs stops the herpesvirus from multiplying and destroying epithelial cells. The resulting stromal keratitis, however, is more severe and therefore difficult to treat. The primary treatment for trachoma consists of three to four weeks of antibiotic therapy. Severe cases require surgical correction.

A conjunctivitis infection can clear without medical care, but sometimes treatment is necessary to avoid long-term effects of corneal inflammation and loss of

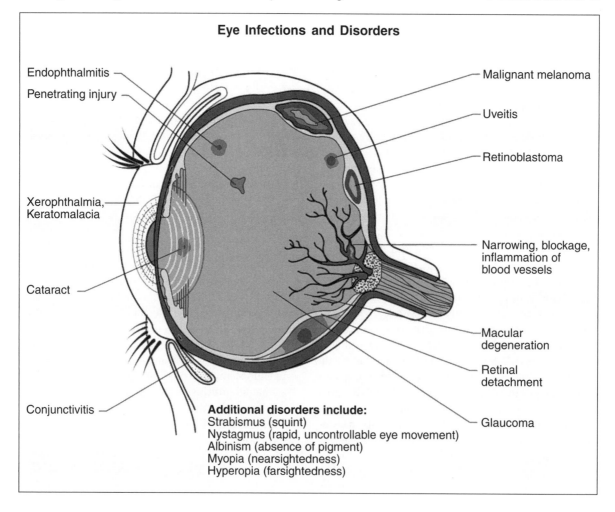

Eye Infections and Disorders

Endophthalmitis
Penetrating injury
Xerophthalmia, Keratomalacia
Cataract
Conjunctivitis

Malignant melanoma
Uveitis
Retinoblastoma
Narrowing, blockage, inflammation of blood vessels
Macular degeneration
Retinal detachment
Glaucoma

Additional disorders include:
Strabismus (squint)
Nystagmus (rapid, uncontrollable eye movement)
Albinism (absence of pigment)
Myopia (nearsightedness)
Hyperopia (farsightedness)

vision. Treatment includes antibiotic eyedrops or ointments, antihistamine eyedrops or pills, decongestants, nonsteroidal anti-inflammatory drugs (NSAIDs), or mast-cell stabilizers. Artificial tears and warm compresses offer some relief. Tinted glasses reduce the discomfort of bright light.

With iritis, warm compresses can lessen the inflammation and pain. Certain steroid drugs produce quick reduction of the inflammation. A protective covering enables the eye to rest, and atropine drops could be used to dilate the pupils and prevent scarring or adhesions.

For cataracts, a stronger eyeglass prescription is recommended, but surgery that replaces the clouded lens with an artificial one is the only real cure. Drugs that keep the pupil dilated may help with vision.

Glaucoma detection is challenging because the disease is asymptomatic until it is advanced. Medical therapy is the first step for treatment. Glaucoma is difficult to cure, but some medications successfully lower pressure in the eye. If medication is ineffective, then laser surgery is applied to create openings and facilitate fluid draining in the eye.

One way to diagnose macular degeneration is by viewing a chart of black lines arranged in a graph pattern (Amsler grid). Early signs can be detected through retinal examination. No outright cure has been discovered, but some drug treatments may delay its progression or even improve vision.

Some cases of diabetic retinopathy can be treated with laser surgery that shrinks or seals leaking and abnormal vessels on the retina. Vision already lost cannot be restored. A vitrectomy is recommended for some advanced cases, in which the vitreous component of the eye is surgically removed and replaced with a clear solution.

In treating a stye, applying hot compresses for fifteen minutes every two hours may help localize the infection and promote drainage. Mild antiseptics may be applied to prevent spread of the infection. A small surgical incision may be necessary in some cases.

Surgery is the treatment for congenital ptosis. The procedure tightens the levator muscle to lift the upper eyelid to the required position, allowing a full field of vision. For ectropion and entropion, surgery, under local anesthesia, is used to repair the abnormal eyelid before the cornea becomes infected and scarred. This is followed by an overnight patch and application of antibiotics for a week.

For dry eyes, lubricating artificial tears in the form of eyedrops are the usual answer. Serious cases of watery eyes may be treated by surgically closing the lacrimal puncta (tear drain) temporarily or permanently. Sterile ointments prevent the eye from drying at night.

Astigmatism is corrected with asymmetrical lenses that compensate for the asymmetry in the eye. Surgery and laser treatments are used to reshape the cornea and change its focusing power. Myopia is corrected by concave-shaped glasses or contact lenses that diverge light rays from distant objects to focus on the retina. Hyperopia and presbyopia are corrected with convex-shaped eyeglasses or contact lenses that converge light rays from nearby objects slightly before entering the eye, in order to focus on the retina. For those with amblyopia, a patch over the preferred eye forces the brain to use the other eye, but the drug atropine, which temporarily blurs vision in the preferred eye, offers a better medical alternative to eye patches.

For keratoconus, vision is corrected with eyeglasses initially, followed by special contact lenses that reduce distortion if astigmatism worsens. Corneal transplantation becomes necessary when scarring becomes too severe. Preventive measures in strong sunlight are protective eyeglasses, sunglasses, and hats with brims.

Perspective and Prospects

Ancient papyri indicate that physicians of Egypt were the first to establish clinical practices for the treatment of eye infections and disorders. Herbs and eye paints with bacteriocidal properties, such as malachite, were used to prevent infections. Medicated ointments were used by Arab and Greek physicians to treat trachoma. Leukoma (a white spot on the cornea) was treated with animal galls, especially the gall of tortoise. Antimony sulfite and copper solutions were used to treat eyelid disorders. Herbs have been used in Africa, Asia, and Latin America to treat eye problems since ancient times.

In the twenty-first century, improved antibiotics and other chemicals are widely used to treat eye diseases. Technological advances in surgical procedures and laser techniques have provided additional options for treating vision disorders. Cataract surgery that once required several days of hospitalization is performed in less than thirty minutes on an outpatient basis. Multifocal lenses are designed to provide both near and distant vision that eliminates the use of reading glasses, advanced lens technology provide more foldable and flexible lens materials, and doctors use lasers to reduce secondary opacification in lenses. Immunotherapy is used to treat allergies that cause conjunctivitis.

Innovative research provides new knowledge and treatments for eye disorders. The Collaborative Longitudinal Evaluation of Keratoconus Study by the National Eye Institute (NEI) is investigating factors that influence the progression and severity of keratoconus. The NEI supported the clinical trials of the Herpetic Eye Disease Study that investigated treatments for severe ocular herpes, the most common infectious cause of corneal blindness in the United States.

Research that explored ayurvedic herbs of India has produced the isotine eyedrop, which effectively treats different eye disorders without surgery, including early stages of cataracts.

Functional MRI (fMRI) techniques allow researchers to create images of neurological activity in real time and to obtain insight into neurological eye diseases such as amblyopia. Scientists are conducting research to obtain implanted lens material that is able to form a new lens within the eye and that works efficiently with the original eye muscles. Investigations are in progress for glaucoma medications that reduce eye pressure and also protect the optic nerve. Research shows that antioxidants and nutrients such as zeaxanthin and lutein (found in green, leafy vegetables), zinc, and vitamins A, C, and E help to control AMD, and omega-3 fatty acids (abundant in coldwater fish) have a protective and healing effect against AMD.

The Food and Drug Administration (FDA) approved Lucentis in 2006 for treating the more severe "wet" AMD by monthly injections into the eye. Macugen (pegaptanib sodium), another AMD treatment medication that improves vision with six-week interval injections, was FDA-approved in 2004. In 2006, it was reported that a team of international research scientists discovered a protein called sVEGFR-1 that prevents blood vessels from forming in the cornea; it could become the basis of new treatments for cancer and macular degeneration.

Also in 2006, the *HealthDay News* reported that a visual aid invented by U.S. scientists comprising a tiny camera, a pocket-sized computer, and a transparent computer display mounted on a pair of glasses provides better vision and mobility for people with tunnel vision, who have lost their peripheral vision. Such innovations are welcome, since one in 200 Americans over age fifty-five has tunnel vision, which is caused by diseases such as retinitis pigmentosa and glaucoma.

Early detection of signs and symptoms is a primary key to the treatment of all eye infections and disorders. As preventive measures, people must avoid eyestrain, exercise their bodies, eat healthy foods, control their sugar levels and blood pressure, avoid smoking, protect the eyes from sunlight, and have regular medical checkups.

—*Samuel V. A. Kisseadoo, Ph.D.*

See also Albinos; Astigmatism; Blindness; Cataract surgery; Cataracts; Chlamydia; Color blindness; Conjunctivitis; Corneal transplantation; Diabetes mellitus; Dyslexia; Eye surgery; Eyes; Face lift and blepharoplasty; Glaucoma; Gonorrhea; Herpes; Jaundice; Keratitis; Laser use in surgery; Macular degeneration; Microscopy, slitlamp; Myopia; Ophthalmology; Optometry; Optometry, pediatric; Pigmentation; Ptosis; Refractive eye surgery; Sense organs; Sjögren's syndrome; Strabismus; Styes; Systems and organs; Trachoma; Transplantation; Vision; Vision disorders.

FOR FURTHER INFORMATION:

Boron, Walter F., and Emile L. Boulpaep. *Medical Physiology: A Cellular and Molecular Approach.* 2d ed. Philadelphia: Saunders/Elsevier, 2009. Updated information on human functional and medical information, including that pertaining to the eye, for better understanding of structural and functional disorders.

Jenkins, Gail W., Christopher P. Kemnitz, and Gerard J. Tortora. *Anatomy and Physiology: From Science to Life.* Hoboken, N.J.: John Wiley & Sons, 2009. Treats human body function, including the eye. With color photographs, illustrations, a DVD, an index, and a glossary.

McKinley, Michael P., and Valerie D. O'Loughlin. *Human Anatomy.* 2d ed. Dubuque, Iowa: McGraw-Hill, 2009. Provides updated anatomical information and describes the adaptive functions of the eye and other human organs. With an appendix, a glossary, and an index.

Marieb, Elaine N., Jon Mallatt, and Patricia Brady Wilhelm. *Human Anatomy.* 4th ed. San Francisco: Pearson/Benjamin Cummings, 2005. Comprehensive treatment of parts and uses of the eye, with practice questions, color photographs, an appendix, a glossary, and an index.

Saladin, Kenneth S. *Human Anatomy.* 3d ed. Dubuque, Iowa: McGraw-Hill, 2010. Updated treatment of eye anatomy and function. With color photographs, illustrations, an appendix, a glossary, and an index.

Tortora, Gerard J., and Bryan Derrickson. *Principles of Anatomy and Physiology.* 12th ed. Hoboken, N.J.: John Wiley & Sons, 2009. Excellent information on the structure and function of the eye and other organs. Includes color photographs, good illustrations, critical thinking exercises, an appendix, a glossary, and an index.

Van De Graaff, Kent M. *Human Anatomy*. 6th ed. New York: McGraw-Hill, 2002. Excellent information on the eye and internal human structures. Includes an appendix listing useful Web sites, a glossary, and an index.

Eye surgery

Procedure

Anatomy or system affected: Eyes

Specialties and related fields: General surgery, geriatrics, ophthalmology, optometry

Definition: Surgical removals from or repairs to the eye.

Key terms:

choroid: the vascular, intermediate coat furnishing nourishment to parts of the eyeball

cornea: the clear, transparent portion of the eye's outer coat, forming the covering of the aqueous chamber

iris: a colored circular membrance suspended behind the cornea and in front of the lens, regulating the amount of light entering the eye by changing the size of the pupil

lens: the transparent biconvex body of the eye

retina: the innermost coat of the eye, formed from sensitive nerve elements and connected with the optic nerve

sclera: the white part of the eye; with the cornea, it forms the eye's external protective coat

trabeculae: the portion of the eye in front of the canal of Schlemm and within the angle created by the iris and cornea

Indications and Procedures

Compared to surgery performed on internal organs and any number of outpatient procedures, eye surgery can fill patients with added fears, often concerned with great suffering and the possibility of permanent sight loss. Surgery to an internal organ is usually perceived as happening in a remote location in an unseen portion of the body, and most patients have little idea of the organ's function. Often, if an internal growth or organ is removed, the body continues to function quite well. Most patients have some knowledge of the eye, unlike most internal organs, and thus are more likely to develop anxiety about even common surgical procedures involving it. Patients know what eyes are and what they

are used for and that they are extremely sensitive and painful to touch. A grain of sand or a hair touching the eye is painful, so the thought of contacting the eye with a needle or making an incision in it with a scalpel or laser can be almost unimaginable. Patients with ocular problems requiring surgery fear damage to the eye and know all too well the consequences of removal. In most instances, the general public has little to no knowledge or understanding of the function and mechanics of eye surgery. Common eye surgeries include, but are not limited to, cataract surgery, corneal transplantation, vision correction, pterygium removal, retinal detachment repair, and tear duct surgery.

A cataract is an opacity on the eye's lens. A cataract may be minimal in size and low in density, so that light transmission is not appreciably affected, or it may be large and opaque so that light cannot gain entry into the interior eye. When the cataract is pronounced, the interior of the patient's eye cannot be seen with clarity, and the patient cannot see out clearly. Over time, the lens takes on a yellowish hue and begins to lose transparency. As the lens thus becomes "cloudy," the patient needs brighter and brighter lights for visual clarity. If the lens becomes completely opaque, then the patient is functionally blind. A cataract is removed when it endangers the health of the eye or interferes with a patient's ability to function. Conditions such as contrast sensitivity, glare, pupillary constriction, and ambient light may significantly affect a patient's functionality.

The objective of cataract surgery is to remove the crystalline lens of the eye that has become cloudy. Modern surgical procedures involve removing the lens, either intact or in pieces after shattering it with high-frequency sound. The surgery is usually performed under an operating microscope because magnification is necessary. Many methods are used for cataract surgery, including an extracapsular procedure, an intracapsular procedure, and phacoemulsification. Most surgeons perform cataract surgery in freestanding surgical centers on an outpatient basis.

In extracapsular surgery, an incision is made at the superior limbus and a small opening is made into the anterior chamber. A viscoelastic substance is introduced and then a small, bent needle, or cystotome, is introduced. An incision is made into the anterior capsule in a circular, triangular, or D-shaped fashion. The wound is enlarged to a diameter of 10 to 11 millimeters, allowing removal of the cataractous nucleus.

The most common cataract surgical procedure is phacoemulsification, or small-incision cataract surgery.

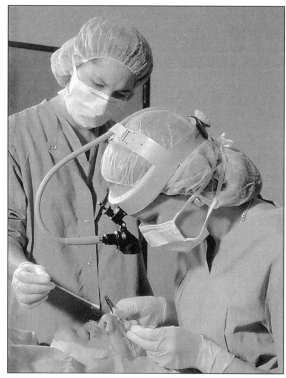

An eye surgeon performs an operation. (Digital Stock)

A stair-stepped incision of between 1.5 and 4.0 millimeters is made in the front of the eye. A cystotome is inserted to cut the anterior capsule of the lens. An emulsifier and aspirator is inserted to remove the collapsed lens. The missing lens is then replaced by an artificial substitute that is folded and inserted through the incision and rotated into place. The wound is sealed with a single suture or no suture at all. This procedure has become favored because it causes less tissue destruction, less wound reaction, and less astigmatism, and patients can resume normal activities immediately after surgery. Vision is then fine-tuned with glasses or contact lenses, if needed.

Another common eye surgery is corneal transplantation. The cornea is the clear portion in the front part of that eye. When injured, degenerated, or infected, the cornea can become cloudy and vision disrupted. Corneal surgery restores lost vision by replacing a portion of the cornea with a clear window taken from a donor eye. Usually, the donor cornea is taken from a recently deceased person. However, not everyone with corneal disease can be helped by corneal transplantation.

The cornea was one of the first structures of the body to be transplanted. Because the cornea is devoid of blood vessels, it is one of the few tissues in the human body that may be transplanted from one human to another with a high degree of success. The absence of blood vessels in the donor cornea reduces immune system reactions.

Two types of corneal transplants are performed: partial penetration, in which a half thickness of the cornea is transplanted, and penetrating transplantation, which involves the full thickness of the cornea. In partial penetration, the anterior of the eye is not entered; only the outer half or two-thirds of the cornea is transplanted. Union is made by several sutures around the periphery of the donor tissue. Depending on the extent of the disease, the donor tissue may be 6 to 10 millimeters in diameter. In a penetrating transplantation, surgery involves entering the anterior chamber of the eye, inserting the donor cornea, and establishing a tight fit with a continuous suture.

Glaucoma is an ocular disease affecting roughly 2 percent of the population over forty. The major characteristic of the condition is a sustained increase in intraocular pressure so great that the fibrous scleral coat cannot expand significantly and the eye cannot withstand the increasing pressures against surrounding soft tissue without damage to its structure and vision impairment. The results of this pressure increase include excavation of the optic disc, hardness of the eyeball, reduced vision, the appearance of colored halos around lights, visual field defects, and headaches. Surgical procedures are performed to relieve this pressure. Although many types of surgical procedures are performed to treat glaucoma, they are all basically fistulizing surgeries, attempting to create an opening between the anterior chamber and the subconjunctival space or between the surgically prepared layers of the sclera.

Glaucoma surgery involves a small incision made either directly through the cornea at the upper limbus or under a flap of conjunctival tissue. The iris is grasped with small forceps and pulled out of the eye, and a small portion of the trabecular meshwork is partially removed, allowing the aqueous fluid to filter out of the anterior chamber. The cornea is then sutured and the eye bandaged. The most popular procedure of this type is trabeculectomy. As a whole, glaucoma surgeries are performed less often today because of the success of nonsurgical treatments and management with drug therapies. A major consequence of some glaucoma surgery is the development of cataracts.

A common early stage nonincisive procedure in treating glaucoma is laser trabeculoplasty. This procedure involves lasing the middle to anterior portion of the trabecular meshwork with eighty to one hundred equally spaced burns. The argon laser reopens blocked drainage channels and reduces fluid pressure in the eye. More than 90 percent of patients experience successful outcomes from this treatment. Surgery is performed only if patients continue to lose the visual field.

A pterygium is a fibrovascular membrane that extends from the medial aspect of the bulbar conjunctiva and invades the cornea. It is a progressive growth related to overexposure to ultraviolet (UV) light. In time, it can make its way to the central portion of the cornea and interfere with vision. Pterygia are most common in southern climates, where people have greater exposure to UV light. In northern regions, people who work outdoors, especially in open fields or on open water, are most prone to developing a pterygium growth.

The purpose of removing a pterygium is to excise the membrane before it can interfere with vision. The operation requires incision into the cornea as well as the conjunctiva, then removal of the pterygium tissue or its transplantation to another position to redirect its growth.

In a normal eye, the retina lies against the choroidal layer, from which it receives part of its blood supply and nourishment. The retina is loosely attached to the choroid, but when it becomes separated from the choroid, it flaps and hangs within the eye's vitreous fluid. Retinal detachment does not allow adequate nutrients to reach the retina and thus causes poor function, and it eventually leads to vision loss. Retinal detachment may be caused by injury, myopia, or previous eye surgeries. Often, a tear or hole permits fluid to collect under the retina, causing the detachment.

Retinal detachment surgery corrects the loose retina by bringing it back to the choroid or by pushing the choroid up to the retina. To bring the retina back into place, scleral punctures are made to drain fluids that lay between the retina and the choroid. When the retina returns to lie against the choroid, either electrocoagulation or cryotherapy with a cold probe against the sclera unites the retina to the choroid. Then the retina and choroid are brought together with a silicone buckling band to exert inward pressure. If the retina is not attached at this point, then air, special gas, or oil is injected into the vitreous fluid to push the retina back against the choroid.

Surgery involving corrective procedures to tear ducts is common, especially in older patients. A blockage in the nasolacrimal passage may result in a condition called epiphora, in which the tear ducts water constantly. Such a blockage of the tear canal may result from some form of obstruction. These obstructions are cleared by a surgical procedure called dacryocystorhinostomy. In this procedure, a large incision of 8 to 10 millimeters is made in the wall of the nose, and a union is created between the mucosal lining of the nose and the lacrimal sac. In this way, the lacrimal sac opens directly into the nose. The operation is usually successful in curing the tearing and infection problems arising from stagnation in the blocked tear duct.

Elective refractive eye surgery for the purpose of vision correction began in the Soviet Union in the 1970's and gained popularity in the United States in the 1990's with the use of lasers. It is performed for the relief of myopia, hypermyopia, and astigmatism, with the goal of eliminating the need for either eyeglasses or contact lenses. It is also used to correct refractive errors caused by cataract surgery and corneal transplantation.

Two of the most common refractive surgeries are radial keratotomy (RK) and photorefractive keratectomy (PRK), also known as excimer laser surgery. Myopic patients suffer from a cornea that is either too convex or has an axial length that is too long, causing light to converge at a focal point anterior to the retina. In refractive surgery, corneal reshaping is the important concept. The surgical goal is to flatten the center of the cornea so that light will focus more posteriorly.

RK reshapes the cornea by radial incisions made with a diamond knife. This process weakens the cornea, so normal intraocular pressure pushes the center of the cornea outward, flattening the central cornea. PRK uses a laser to remove the superficial layers of the central cornea, about 50 to 100 microns of tissue, to achieve a similar reshaping of the cornea.

Uses and Complications

The introduction of lasers to eye surgery has proved both beneficial and controversial, depending on its use. An excimer laser can remove any opacifications of the superficial layers of the cornea while retaining the health and clarity of deeper corneal layers. The laser can be used to remove injury-related and surgical corneal scars and to treat astigmatism that may follow implant cataract surgery. The excimer laser also enables surgeons to treat diseases such as fungal ulcers and to smoothe out pterygium irregularities.

Patients interested in pursuing elective refractive surgeries, however, should be aware of the inherent risks of the procedures and that some ophthalmologists are hesitant to use these procedures to correct nearsightedness. The leading cause of skepticism is a reluctance to operate on an essentially healthy eye, thus putting it at risk. These operative procedures have been developed to correct only refractive vision errors. Refractive surgery does not treat glaucoma, cataracts, or other disorders that affect or damage vision.

PERSPECTIVE AND PROSPECTS

As experience and long-term results from the use of laser energy as a surgical tool increase, other forms of therapy will be investigated. Noninvasive glaucoma procedures and laser disruptions of vitreous opacitites and retinal traction bands are already being performed. Ablation procedures to control late-stage glaucoma and techniques to emulsify and remove cataract lenses with lasers in a noninvasive procedure have undergone positive trials.

Today, lasers share space in many clinics and operating rooms along with traditional surgical techniques. Laser technology is providing new types of therapy and is treating more challenging forms of eye disease.

—*Randall L. Milstein, Ph.D.*

See also Blindness; Blurred vision; Cataract surgery; Cataracts; Corneal transplantation; Eye infections and disorders; Eyes; Glaucoma; Keratitis; Laser use in surgery; Myopia; Ophthalmology; Optometry; Refractive eye surgery; Sense organs; Surgery, general; Vision; Vision disorders.

FOR FURTHER INFORMATION:

Bartlett, Jimmy D., and Siret D. Jaanus, eds. *Clinical Ocular Pharmacology*. 5th ed. Boston: Butterworth-Heinemann/Elsevier, 2008. A well-illustrated and descriptive account of diseases of the eye, as well as surgical and pharmacological treatments. Though aimed at medical professionals, the book is a valuable reference for any interested reader.

Eden, John. *The Physician's Guide to Cataracts, Glaucoma, and Other Eye Problems*. Yonkers, N.Y.: Consumer Reports Books, 1992. A book about eye problems and surgeries aimed at the general reader. The explanations and descriptions are easy to read and follow. The book contains no illustrations.

Johnson, Gordon J., et al., eds. *The Epidemiology of Eye Disease*. 2d ed. New York: Oxford University Press, 2003. A university-level text concerning eye disease. Very descriptive and richly illustrated with color images. The book is well referenced and provides researchers and interested readers with timely data sources.

Newell, F. W. *Ophthalmology: Principles and Concepts*. 8th ed. St. Louis, Mo.: Mosby, 1996. A medical textbook of general ophthalmology. Written for the medical professional, it describes diagnostic and operational techniques for disorders of the eye.

Riordan-Eva, Paul, and John P. Whitcher. *Vaughan and Asbury's General Ophthalmology*. 17th ed. New York: Lange Medical Books/McGraw-Hill, 2007. An in-depth medical text on the general practice and science of ophthalmology. It is very technical and not for the general reader, though rich in information and illustrations.

Stein, Harold A., Raymond M. Stein, and Melvin I. Freeman. *The Ophthalmic Assistant: A Text for Allied and Associated Ophthalmic Personnel*. 8th ed. Philadelphia: Mosby/Elsevier, 2006. A teaching text for ophthalmic surgical assistants. Very descriptive and well illustrated, with overviews of diseases, disorders, and infections, as well as most surgical procedures. Though written for students training in the field, the text is well referenced to the appendix and glossary.

EYES

ANATOMY

ANATOMY OR SYSTEM AFFECTED: Nervous system

SPECIALTIES AND RELATED FIELDS: Ophthalmology, optometry

DEFINITION: The body structures that receive and transform information about objects into neural impulses that can be translated by the brain into visual images.

KEY TERMS:

accommodation: adjustments of the crystalline lens that are necessary for clear vision at various distances

cornea: the transparent structure forming the anterior part of the fibrous tunic of the eye; light must pass through this structure to reach the retina

crystalline lens: the transparent focusing mechanism of the eye; it is a biconvex structure situated between the posterior chamber and the vitreous body of the eye

diopter: a unit of power of a lens equal to the reciprocal of the focal length of the lens in meters

iris: the circular pigmented membrane behind the cornea, perforated by the pupil; the most anterior portion of the vascular tunic of the eye

photoreceptor: a light-responsive nerve cell or receptor located in the retina of the eye *pupil:* the opening at the center of the iris through which light passes

retina: the innermost of the three tunics of the eyeball, which is situated around the vitreous body and is continuous posteriorly with the optic nerve; it contains the photoreceptors

sclera: the tough outer coat or fibrous tunic of the eyeball, which covers the posterior five-sixths of its surface and is continuous anteriorly with the cornea

visual acuity: clarity or clearness in vision

STRUCTURE AND FUNCTIONS

The eye captures pictures from the environment and transforms them into neural impulses that are processed by the brain into visual images. The retina, with its light-sensitive cells, acts as a camera to "put the picture on film," while neural processing in the brain "develops the film" and forms a visual image that is meaningful and informative for the individual.

The human eye originates during development, that is, while the individual is being formed as an embryo in the uterus. Eye formation begins during the end of the third week of development when outgrowths of brain neural tissue, called the optic vesicles, form at the sides of the forebrain region. The optic vesicle induces overlying embryonic tissue to thicken in one region, forming a primitive lens structure called the lens placode. The lens placode, in turn, induces the optic vesicles to form a cuplike structure, the optic cup, while the brain's connection of the vesicles narrows into a slender stalk that forms the optic nerve. The inner part of the optic cup forms the neural or sensory retina, with its photoreceptors, while the outer part of the optic cup develops into the layers of tissues, or tunics, that make up the wall of the eyeball. The lens placode further condenses and solidifies by forming lens fibers that become transparent. The function of the lens will eventually be to focus light onto the retina. The major structures of the eye—the retina, lens, and eyeball coats—are initially formed by the fifth month of fetal development. During the remainder of the prenatal period, eye structures continue to enlarge, mature, and form increasingly complex neural networks with the visual processing regions of the brain.

At birth, an infant's eyes are about two-thirds the size of adult eyes. Until after their first month of life, most newborns lack complete retinal development, especially in the area that is responsible for visual acuity. As a result, infants cannot focus their eyes properly and typically have a vacant stare during their first weeks of life. Most of the subsequent eye growth occurs rapidly during the remainder of the first year of life. From the second year of life until puberty, the rate of eye growth progressively slows. After puberty, eye growth is negligible.

The adult human eye weighs approximately 7.5 grams and measures approximately 24.5 millimeters in its anterior-to-posterior diameter. All movement of the eyeball, or globe, is accomplished by six voluntary muscles attached anteriorly by ligaments to the outer coat of the globe and posteriorly to a tendinous ring located behind the globe. One voluntary muscle elevates the upper lid.

Three concentric tunics form the globe itself. The outermost fibrous tunic consists of two portions. In the small, anterior portion, the tunic fibrils are arranged in a regular pattern, forming the transparent cornea. Posteriorly, the tunic fibrils are irregularly spaced, forming the opaque, white sclera. The innermost tunic, or nervous tunic, consists of two parts: the pars optica, or retina, containing photoreceptor cells, and the pars ceca lining the iris and ciliary body. Tucked between the outer and inner tunics lies the vascular tunic, consisting of the pigmented iris, which gives the eye its distinctive color; the ciliary body, which forms the aqueous humor to provide nourishment for the anterior structures of the globe; and the highly vascular choroid, which provides nourishment for the retina and also acts as a cooling system by regulating blood flow to the chemically active retina. In the center of the circular, pigmented iris lies the pupil, which is a small opening into the posterior parts of the eyeball.

The cavity that contains the globe, circumscribed by the concentric tunics, is filled with a clear, jellylike substance called the vitreous body. This substance is anteriorly bounded in the vitreous cavity by the transparent crystalline lens that lies just posterior to the pupil. The crystalline lens is elastic in structure, allowing for variations in thickness that change the focusing power of the eye.

The eye can refract, or bend, light rays because of the curved surfaces of two transparent structures, the cornea and the crystalline lens, through which light rays must pass to reach the retina. Any curved surface, or lens, will refract light rays to a greater or lesser degree depending on the steepness or flatness of the surface curve. The steeper the curve, the greater the refracting power. If a curved surface refracts light rays to an intersection point one meter away from the refracting lens, this lens is defined as having 1 diopter of power. The

The Anatomy of the Human Eye

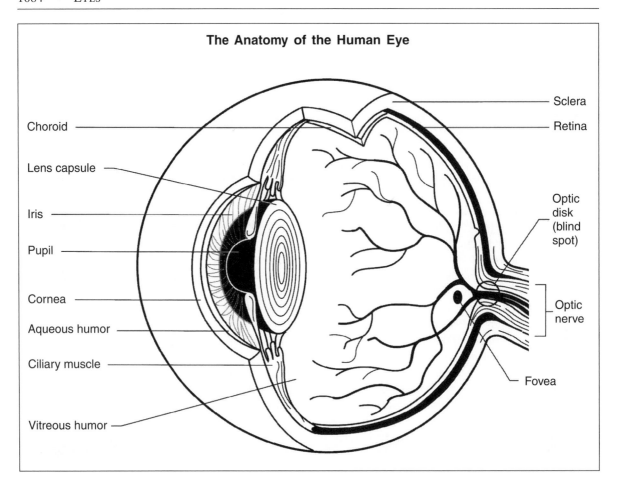

human eye has approximately 59 diopters of power in its constituent parts, including the cornea and crystalline lens.

Light rays emitted from a distant point of light enter the eye in a basically parallel pattern and are bent to intersect perfectly at the retina, forming an image of the distant point of light. If the point of light is near the eye, the rays that are emitted are divergent in pattern. These divergent rays must also be refracted to meet at a point on the retina, but these rays require more bending—hence, a steeper curved surface is needed. By a process called accommodation, the human eye automatically adjusts the thickness of the crystalline lens, forming a steeper curve on its surface and thereby creating a perfect image on the retina. Variations from the normal in either the length of an eyeball or the curves of the cornea and crystalline lens will result in a refractive error or blurred image on the retina.

The major task of the eye is to focus environmental light rays on the photoreceptor cells, the rods and cones of the retina. These photoreceptors absorb the light energy, transforming it into electrical signals that are carried to the visual center of the brain. Cones are specialized for color or daylight vision and have greater visual discrimination or acuity than the rods, which are specialized for black-and-white or nighttime vision.

The fovea is a pin-sized depression in the center of the retina that contains only cone cells in high concentrations. This makes the fovea the point of the most distinct vision, or greatest visual acuity. When the eye focuses on an object, the object's image falls on the retina in the area of the fovea. Immediately surrounding the fovea is a larger area called the macula lutea that contains a relatively high concentration of cones. Macula lutea acuity, while not as great as in the fovea, is much greater than in the retina's periphery, which contains fewer cones. The concentration of cones is greatest in the fovea and declines toward the periphery of the retina. Conversely, the concentration of the rods is greater at the more peripheral areas of the retina than in the macula luteal area. The retina of each eye contains about 100 million rod cells and about 300 million cone cells.

The optic nerve carries impulses from the photoreceptors to the brain. This nerve exits the retina in a central location called the blind spot. No image can be detected in this area because it contains neither rods nor cones. Normally, an individual is not aware of the retinal blind spot because the brain's neural processing compensates for the missing information when some portion of a peripheral image falls across this part of the retina.

On a cellular level, rod and cone photoreceptors consist of three parts: an outer segment that detects the light stimulus, an inner segment that provides the metabolic energy for the cell, and a synaptic terminal that transmits the visual signal to the next nerve cell in the visual pathway leading to the brain. The outer segment is rodshaped in the rods and cone-shaped in the cones (hence their names). This segment is made of a stack of flattened membranes containing photopigment molecules that undergo chemical changes when activated by light.

The rod photopigment, called rhodopsin, cannot discriminate between various colors of light. Thus rods provide vision only in shades of gray by detecting different intensities of light. Rhodopsin is a purple pigment (a combination of blue and red colors), and it transmits light in the blue and red regions of the visual spectrum while absorbing energy from the green region of the spectrum. The light that is absorbed best by a photopigment is called its absorption maximum. Thus at night, when rods are used for vision, a green car is seen far more easily than a red car, because red light is poorly absorbed by rhodopsin. Only absorbed light produces the photochemical reaction that results in vision.

When rhodopsin absorbs light, the photopigment dissociates or separates into two parts: retinene, which is derived from vitamin A, and opsin, a protein. This separation of retinene from opsin, called the bleaching reaction, causes the production of nerve impulses in the photoreceptors. In the presence of bright light, practically all the rhodopsin undergoes the bleaching reaction and the person is in a light-adapted state. When a light-adapted person initially enters a darkened room, vision is poor since the light sensitivity of the rod photoreceptors is very low. After some time in the dark, however, a gradual increase in light sensitivity, called dark adaptation, occurs as increased amounts of retinene and opsin are recombined by the rods to form rhodopsin. The increased level of rhodopsin occurs after a few minutes in the dark and reaches a maximum sensitivity in about twenty minutes.

Each kind of cone—red, green, and blue—is distinguished by its unique photopigment, which responds to a particular wavelength or color of light. Combinations of cone colors provide the basis for color vision. While each type of cone is most sensitive to the particular wavelength of light indicated by its color—red, green, or blue—cones can respond to other colors with varying degrees. One's perception of color rests on the differential response of each cone type to a particular wavelength of light. The extent that each cone type is activated is coded and sent in separate parallel pathways to the brain. A color vision center in the brain combines and processes these parallel inputs to create the perception of color. Color is thus a concept in the mind of the viewer.

The intricacies of the human visual system require various methods to assess eye structure and function. Visual acuity is a measure of central cone function. Clinically, the most common method for testing visual acuity is by the use of a Snellen chart, consisting of a white background with black letters. All symbols on the chart create, or subtend, a visual angle at the approximate center of the eye. The smaller the symbol, the smaller the angle and the more difficult cone recognition becomes. At the standard distance of twenty feet, the smallest letters on the Snellen chart subtend an angle of five minutes of arc at the eye's center. The larger letters on the chart are calibrated such that each consecutively larger letter subtends a multiple unit of five minutes of arc. If the eye can detect the smallest letters on the chart, the patient is said to have normal (20/20) vision. The numerator of the clinical fraction designates the test distance of twenty feet. The denominator varies with the patient's visual function, identifying the distance at which the smallest letter recognized by the patient subtends an angle of five minutes of arc. For example, if the smallest letter recognized is fifty minutes of arc in size, the fraction used to record this visual acuity is 20/200 because the letter with fifty minutes of arc is ten times as large as the smallest letters on the chart. Therefore, the distance needed for this letter to create five minutes of arc at the eye is ten times as far as the normal twenty feet. In this example, the patient is said to have a refractive error.

DISORDERS AND DISEASES

Commonly existing refractive errors are astigmatism, myopia, hyperopia, and presbyopia. Presbyopia is an anomaly that occurs with aging when the crystalline lens loses its ability to accommodate. Causes include thickening of the lens and changes in the attachment fibers that anchor the lens. Because of these alterations, the lens is not able to change its shape and the eye remains focused at a specific distance. To compensate for this problem, bifocal spectacles are normally prescribed, with the upper region of the lens focused for distant vision and the lower lens focused for near vision. Hyperopia, also called farsightedness, results when an eyeball is too short. Because light rays are not bent sufficiently by the lens system, the image is focused not on the retina but behind the retina. To compensate for this problem, spectacles with convex lenses are prescribed, which bring the focus point back on the retina. Conversely, myopia, or nearsightedness, results from an abnormally long eyeball. In this case, the lens system focuses in front of the retina. This abnormal vision can be corrected by spectacles with a concave lens. Astigmatism results from a refractive error of the lens system, usually caused by an irregular shape in the cornea or less frequently by an irregular shape in the lens. The consequence of this anomaly is that some light rays are focused in front of the retina and some behind the retina, creating a blurred image. To correct the focusing error, a special irregular spectacle must be made to correct the abnormal irregularity of the eye's lens system.

An examiner can assess the amount of refractive error based on a patient's verbal choice as to which of a given series of lenses sharpens the retinal image of the letters on the Snellen chart. Refractive error can also be determined when a patient is not capable of response. A retinoscope is often used to shine a light through the pupil onto the retina. An image of the light is reflected back out to the examiner who, in turn, can assess refractive error by the movement and shape of the image.

Visual field testing is a measure of the integrity of the neural pathways to the vision center in the brain. To test visual fields clinically, the patient focuses on a central target. While continuing to focus centrally, test targets are serially brought into the patient's peripheral vision, or visual field. The smaller and dimmer the test target, the more sensitive the test. The simplest visual field test technique is by confrontation. The patient and examiner sit facing each other one meter apart. If both patient and examiner cover their right eyes, the patient's left visual field is being tested. Since the patient's left visual field is congruent to the examiner's left visual field, the examiner can detect visual field defects when the pa-

tient is not responsive to a test target brought into view from the side. Lesions to some portion of the visual pathway to the brain will result in a scotoma, or blind area, in the corresponding visual field.

A biomicroscope, or slitlamp microscope, is commonly used to assess external eye structures, including the eyelids, lashes, conjunctiva, cornea, sclera, and one internal structure, the crystalline lens. The white part of the eye, or sclera, is covered with a thin, transparent covering called the conjunctiva. Infections and tumors often invade this external structure. Though the normally transparent crystalline lens is essentially free of infections and tumors, it can become cloudy or opaque and develop a cataract. Causes for cataract formation are multiple, the most common being the aging process; less frequently, trauma to the lens or a secondary symptom of systemic disease can result in cataracts. When the cataract is so dense that it obstructs vision, the crystalline lens is surgically removed and replaced with an artificial, plastic lens.

To view internal eye structures, the pupil is dilated to allow more light to be introduced into the interior and posterior regions of the eyeball. Two commonly used instruments are the handheld ophthalmoscope and the head-mounted indirect ophthalmoscope. Diseases of the retina include retinal tears, detachments, artery or vein occlusions, degenerations, and retinopathies secondary to systemic disease.

Glaucoma is an eye disease characterized by raised pressure inside the eye. Normal eye pressure is stabilized by the balance between the production and removal of the aqueous humor, the solution that bathes the internal, anterior structures of the eye. Abnormal pressures are often associated with defects in the visual, or optic, nerve and in the visual field. Approximately 300 people per 100,000 are affected by glaucoma. Clinically, intraocular pressure is assessed by numerous methods in a process called tonometry.

Abnormalities of the eye muscles constitute a significant portion of visual problems. Binocular vision and good depth perception are present when both eyes are aligned properly toward an object. A weakness in any of the six rotatory eye muscles will result in a tendency for that eye to deviate away from the object, resulting in an obvious or latent eye turn called strabismus. Associated signs are eye fatigue, abnormal head postures, and double vision. To alleviate objectionable double vision, a patient often suppresses the retinal image at the brain level, resulting in functional amblyopia (often called lazy eye), in which visual acuity is deficient.

Color blindness, a trait that occurs more frequently in men than in women, is caused by a hereditary lack of one or more types of cones. For example, if the green-sensitive cones are not functioning, the colors in the visual spectral range from green to red can stimulate only red-sensitive cones. This person can perceive only one color in this range, since the ratio of stimulation of the green-red cones is constant for the colors in this range. Thus this individual is considered to be green-red color-blind and will have difficulty distinguishing green from red.

PERSPECTIVE AND PROSPECTS

Early physicians recognized the importance of good eyesight, but because of limited understanding they had minimal means to treat major eye disorders. During the Middle Ages, surgeons performed eye operations, including ones for cataracts in which the lens was pushed down and out of the way with a needle inserted into the eyeball. In the eighteenth century, this operation was improved when cataract lenses were extracted from the eye. In the early seventeenth century, Johannes Kepler described how light was focused by the lens of the eye on the retina, thus providing insight into why spectacles are valuable in cases of poor eyesight. In 1801, Thomas Young published a foundational text entitled *On the Mechanics of the Eye*. Hermann von Helmholtz in the nineteenth century invented the first ophthalmoscope, which allowed inspection of the interior structures of the eye. Young and Helmholtz also developed theories to explain the phenomenon of color vision. From the invention of the ophthalmoscope, the range of clinical observation was extended to the inside of the eyeball, allowing the diagnosis of eye disorders. The modern understanding of eyesight and vision is increasing with contributions from ongoing research.

Ophthalmology is the study of the structure, function, and diseases of the eye. An ophthalmologist is a physician who specializes in the diagnosis and treatment of eye disorders and diseases with surgery, drugs, and corrective lenses. An optometrist is a specialist with a doctorate in optometry who is trained to examine and test the eyes and treats defects in vision by prescribing corrective lenses. An optician is a technician who fits, adjusts, and dispenses corrective lenses that are based on the prescription of an ophthalmologist or optometrist.

Vision care personnel are vital to industry, public health, recreation, highway safety, education, and the community. Since 85 percent of learning is visual-based, good vision is extremely important in education, work, and play. Good vision enhances the production and morale of workers, and athletic performance is improved when vision problems are corrected. Vision care specialists work to promote the prevention of eye injuries and diseases while supporting practices that enhance good health and vision. Vision therapy may be used to correct many disorders of the eye such as amblyopia, reduced visual perception, reading disorders, poor eye coordination, and reduced visual acuity.
—*Elva B. Miller, O.D., and Roman J. Miller, Ph.D.*

See also Albinos; Astigmatism; Blindness; Cataract surgery; Cataracts; Chlamydia; Color blindness; Conjunctivitis; Corneal transplantation; Diabetes mellitus; Dyslexia; Eye infections and disorders; Eye surgery; Face lift and blepharoplasty; Glaucoma; Gonorrhea; Jaundice; Keratitis; Laser use in surgery; Macular degeneration; Microscopy, slitlamp; Myopia; Ophthalmology; Optometry; Optometry, pediatric; Pigmentation; Ptosis; Refractive eye surgery; Sense organs; Sjögren's syndrome; Strabismus; Styes; Systems and organs; Trachoma; Transplantation; Vision; Vision disorders.

FOR FURTHER INFORMATION:

Buettner, Helmut, ed. *Mayo Clinic on Vision and Eye Health: Practical Answers on Glaucoma, Cataracts, Macular Degeneration, and Other Conditions.* Rochester, Minn.: Mayo Foundation for Medical Education and Research, 2002. A helpful handbook on all the medical, social, and emotional facets of vision impairment.

Guyton, Arthur C., and John E. Hall. *Human Physiology and Mechanisms of Disease.* 6th ed. Philadelphia: W. B. Saunders, 1997. Guyton is a nationally recognized authority on medical physiology, having written and edited numerous college-level and medical school textbooks on the subject. His writing style is understandable to the nonmedical specialist and student. This college-level text contains two chapters on the eye: The first deals with the optics of vision and the function of the retina; the second emphasizes the neurophysiology of vision.

Litin, Scott C., ed. *Mayo Clinic Family Health Book.* 4th ed. New York: HarperResource, 2009. Perhaps the best general medical text for the layperson, this book covers the entire medical field. While the information is derived from a wide variety of highly technical sources, the articles are written to be easily understood by a general audience.

National Foundation for Eye Research. http://www .nfer.org. Site provides consumers and professionals with access to developing technology for treating impaired vision.

Prevent Blindness America. http://www.preventblind ness.org. Founded in 1908, this group is dedicated to fighting blindness and saving sight. Its efforts are focused on promoting a continuum of vision care, public and professional education, certified vision screening training, and community and patient service programs and research.

Riordan-Eva, Paul, and John P. Whitcher. *Vaughan and Asbury's General Ophthalmology.* 17th ed. New York: Lange Medical Books/McGraw-Hill, 2007. This well-illustrated textbook is an excellent reference for the serious student who desires more in-depth information on any aspect of the eye or its diseases.

Tortora, Gerard J., and Bryan Derrickson. *Principles of Anatomy and Physiology.* 12th ed. Hoboken, N.J.: John Wiley & Sons, 2009. An outstanding textbook of human anatomy and physiology, containing a well-written chapter on the special senses, emphasizing eyesight and vision.

FACE LIFT AND BLEPHAROPLASTY

PROCEDURES

ANATOMY OR SYSTEM AFFECTED: Eyes, skin

SPECIALTIES AND RELATED FIELDS: General surgery, plastic surgery

DEFINITION: Techniques used to remove unwanted wrinkles and other indicators of aging from the face.

INDICATIONS AND PROCEDURES

Aging may create serious problems among individuals for whom success in their occupations depends on appearance. Premature wrinkling of skin on the face and eyelids or premature looseness of these tissues can create an insurmountable psychological barrier. In these situations, cosmetic surgery such as face lift (rhytidectomy) and/or blepharoplasty (the removal of excess tissue around the eyelids) is indicated.

Surgical face lifting involves making an incision at the hairline and extending it downward in front of the ear toward the angle of the jaw; the length of the incision is dependent on the amount of skin sagging that is present. The skin is gently separated from the underlying fascia and is pulled back and tightened until the desired degree of wrinkle elimination is achieved. Excess skin at the posterior (back) margins is removed. The edges are carefully brought together and secured with fine sutures or adhesive closures. The patient returns to the plastic surgeon in seven to ten days for follow-up evaluation.

Blepharoplasty refers to the surgical alteration of the eyelids. The surgery is similar to that described for a total face lift. An incision is made along the lower margin

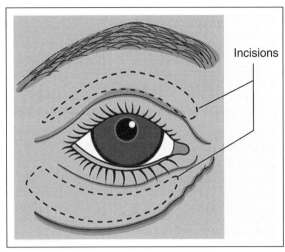

Blepharoplasty is the removal of excess, baggy skin around the eyes.

of the eyebrow. Skin is separated from the fascia. Sometimes, small amounts of fat are also removed. The skin of the upper eyelid is tightened. After excess tissue is removed, the free edges are attached with fine sutures. Cosmetic alteration of the lower eyelid can also be accomplished surgically. The incision is made along a natural crease in the skin just below the lower eyelid. The skin above the incision is separated from its underlying fascia. Some fat may be removed. Typically, excess skin is removed before the edges are reattached, again using very fine sutures. The patient returns to the plastic surgeon in approximately one week for removal of the sutures. Chemical peeling or dermabrasion are additional techniques that can be used to remove fine wrinkles and lines in skin.

USES AND COMPLICATIONS

A face lift is a form of cosmetic surgery and is usually undertaken for aesthetic reasons. Short-term problems include bruising and swelling. Possible long-term complications include infection, scarring, and insufficient removal of unwanted wrinkles. Proper techniques can reduce the first two problems. Realistic expectations can minimize disappointment.

Because of the eyelid's good blood circulation blepharoplasty performed under sterile conditions seldom results in serious infection. However, the procedure can result in a number of other complications: continued bleeding that requires reopening the eyelid wound and either the cauterization of the bleeding vessel or evacuation of a clot; the edges of the eyelid skin closure may separate, requiring either support tape or

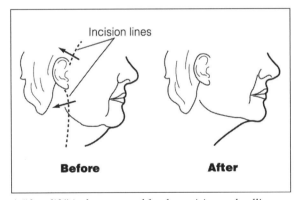

A "face lift" is the term used for the excision and pulling upward of sagging skin on the face. This cosmetic procedure can smooth wrinkles and provide a more attractive profile, but there are drawbacks: The patient's appearance may be changed too dramatically, and the procedure must be repeated periodically to maintain the desired results.

sutures; eyelid asymmetry, whereby the eyelids look fine individually but do not match as a pair; and finally, either insufficient or excessive skin removal.

PERSPECTIVE AND PROSPECTS

At birth, human skin contains relatively large amounts of a molecule called collagen. Collagen provides strength to the skin; this is technically called turgor. The function of collagen is similar to the fibers in fiberglass or steel reinforcement in concrete: strength. Living on Earth, people are constantly subjected to the effects of gravity and ultraviolet radiation, which over time cause slight damage to the collagen in skin. The turgor is slowly lost. Without sufficient collagen, the skin starts to sag under the influence of gravity. Excessive exposure to the sun accelerates this process. The use of tanning beds in salons can increase the amount of harmful ultraviolet radiation, which also accelerates the aging process. With sufficient time and exposure, the typical appearance of skin in old age is seen.

There is no way to stop the human body from aging; accepting this inevitable reality can reduce both stress and anxiety. Cosmetic surgical procedures such as blepharoplasty and face lifts are temporary and enable an individual to maintain only an approximation of youthfulness. Over time, the skin will continue to change, necessitating repeat procedures. Each time the procedure is repeated, the result is diminished in comparison to an earlier procedure. Cosmetic surgery can thus only retard the appearance of aging rather than recreate youth.

—*L. Fleming Fallon, Jr., M.D., Ph.D., M.P.H.*

See also Aging; Botox; Collagen; Facial transplantation; Plastic surgery; Skin; Skin disorders.

FOR FURTHER INFORMATION:

Aston, Sherrell J., Robert W. Beasley, and Charles H. M. Thorne, eds. *Grabb and Smith's Plastic Surgery.* 6th ed. Philadelphia: Lippincott-Raven, 2007.

Bosniak, Stephen L., and Marian Cantisano Zilkha. *Cosmetic Blepharoplasty and Facial Rejuvenation.* 2d ed. Philadelphia: Lippincott-Raven, 1999.

Henry, Kimberly A. *The Face-Lift Sourcebook.* Los Angeles: Lowell House, 2000.

Lewis, Wendy. *The Beauty Battle: The Insider's Guide to Wrinkle Rescue and Cosmetic Perfection from Head to Toe.* Berkeley, Calif.: Laurel Glen Books, 2003.

Loftus, Jean. *The Smart Woman's Guide to Plastic Surgery.* 2d ed. Dubuque, Iowa: McGraw-Hill, 2010.

Marfuggi, Richard A. *Plastic Surgery: What You Need to Know Before, During, and After.* New York: Berkeley, 1998.

Narins, Rhoda, and Paul Jarrod Frank. *Turn Back the Clock Without Losing Time: Everything You Need to Know About Simple Cosmetic Procedures.* New York: Three Rivers Press, 2002.

Turkington, Carol, and Jeffrey S. Dover. *The Encyclopedia of Skin and Skin Disorders.* 3d ed. New York: Facts On File, 2007.

Wyer, E. Bingo. *The Unofficial Guide to Cosmetic Surgery.* New York: Wiley, 1999.

FACIAL PALSY. *See* BELL'S PALSY.

FACIAL TRANSPLANTATION
PROCEDURE

ANATOMY OR SYSTEM AFFECTED: Blood vessels, bones, circulatory system, ears, eyes, head, immune system, mouth, muscles, neck, nerves, nervous system, nose, skin

SPECIALTIES AND RELATED FIELDS: Dermatology, ethics, physical therapy, plastic surgery, psychology

DEFINITION: A surgical procedure to transplant all or part of the face from a donor's corpse onto the severely disfigured face of a living person in order to provide a dramatic improvement in the appearance of the recipient.

KEY TERMS:

composite tissue allotransplantation (CTA): the grafting of several structures (such as skin, bones, muscles, and nerves) between two or more individuals

immunosuppressants: medications used to prevent the body from rejecting transplanted tissue and organs

transplant: to transfer organs or tissue from one part or individual to another

INDICATIONS AND PROCEDURES

Facial transplantation is a procedure that is reserved for people with extensive facial disfigurements who have exhausted all other options, including reconstructive surgery. Accidents such as burns, trauma, maulings, and gunshot wounds; diseases such as cancer and infection; and birth defects affect thousands of people each year, causing disfigurement to the face. For most people, surgery can correct all or most of the disfigurement. For the few people who experience a great loss of tissue, however, reconstructive surgery is very limited in returning normal function and appearance.

Facial transplantation is technically easier than other

facial reconstruction surgeries, should involve fewer surgeries, and can improve appearance and mobility. In traditional facial reconstruction, tissue is surgically reattached or taken from another part of the person's own body. These reconstructions, however, do not transfer the subtle muscles needed for expression, which creates an expressionless, masklike appearance.

People with severe facial disfigurement may have limited facial movement, which can cause difficulty talking, eating, and even closing the eyes. People with facial disfigurement often have low self-esteem and experience social isolation, depression, anxiety, and poor quality of life. They may have difficulty making friends and finding employment.

The transplantation involves three separate surgeries. The first surgery, which takes ten to twelve hours, degloves the corpse of the donor. Degloving involves the removal of the face, whereby an incision is made across the hairline, down the temples, behind or around the ears, and around the jaw line. The face, including the eyebrows, eyelids, nose, mouth, and lips, is then detached, as is underlying fat and connective tissue. Surgeons must be careful not to damage the nerves controlling facial expression, eye movement, and facial sensation. If the donor's face is healthy enough for the transplant, then the surgeons begin the second surgery, in which they deglove the patient's face. This surgery takes longer, since the surgeons must clamp off the veins and arteries and take special care not to damage the nerves. Bone grafts would be performed if the patient needs bone replacement. The third surgery involves reattaching the face, including veins, arteries, and nerves, and could take twenty-four hours to complete.

Temporary tubing and drains are installed to remove fluid buildup. The patient would take immunosuppressants for life. After about two months, the patient's face would return to normal size. Depending on the nerve damage before the transplant and the success in nerve reattachment, the patient's facial movements may not be normal for several months to over a year.

USES AND COMPLICATIONS

Few facial transplantations have been performed worldwide, and no one yet knows of all the risks involved. In general, skin grafts are more susceptible to rejection than are most organ or other tissue transplants. In addition, skin transplants carry a life-threatening risk, and a rejected facial transplant would leave the patient in worse condition physically, emotionally, and psychologically.

Other risks include tissue damage that occurs because of cell death from the time of removal to reattachment, and a 10 percent loss of facial cells could result in lifelong sores. If the sensory nerves are not properly reconnected, then permanent numbness would occur. Long-term risks, including tissue mutation or psychological impact, are unknown. Short-term risks include infection, additional scarring, potential tissue rejection, and long-term healing. The side effects of immunosuppressants include infections, metabolic disorders

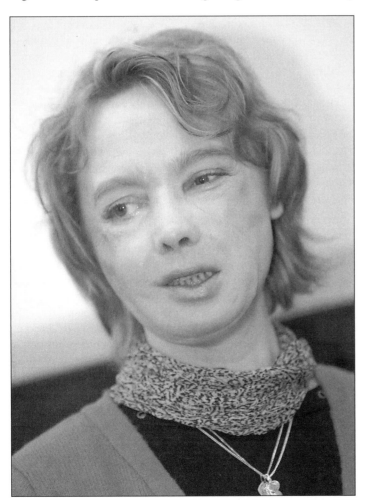

Isabelle Dinoire, the first person to undergo a partial face transplant. (AP/Wide World Photos)

such as diabetes, malignancies, and decreased kidney and lung function.

The new face would be a hybrid, a cross between the donor and recipient's faces. Most surgeons believe that, instead of completely removing any sign of disfigurement, a facial transplant would dramatically improve the appearance of the patient.

PERSPECTIVE AND PROSPECTS

With the introduction of immunosuppressive drugs in the 1980's, composite tissue allotransplantation (CTA) became possible. Prior to the introduction of these drugs, hand and face transplants had been considered almost impossible because of the tissue involved and the high risk of rejection.

In 1994, a surgeon successfully reattached the face of a nine-year-old in India whose face and scalp were ripped off by a threshing machine. Two other surgeries, one in Australia and one in the United States in 2002, also reattached entire faces. Facial transplantation was discussed as a serious therapeutic option in a 2002 meeting of the Plastic Surgical Research Council in Boston, Massachusetts, and, by early 2006, teams in the United States, France, and Great Britain had been working for years to develop surgical techniques, protocols for immunosuppression, psychological assessment, and informed consent for potential patients.

In France, on November 27, 2005, doctors transplanted a chin, lips, and nose onto Isabelle Dinoire, a woman who had been mauled by her dog while she was unconscious. In April, 2006, doctors in China grafted a nose, cheeks, and upper lip onto a man mauled by a bear years before. In December 2008, doctors in the United States performed the first near-total face transplant on a woman who had been shot in the face four years earlier.

Despite these successes, the procedure is still very experimental, involves great risks, and raises numerous ethical questions. Patients are participating in research, not receiving traditional medical care. The results are promising, however, and will likely inspire further procedures.

—*Virginia L. Salmon*

See also Bone grafting; Dermatology; Ethics; Grafts and grafting; Immune system; Oral and maxillofacial surgery; Plastic surgery; Skin; Transplantation.

FOR FURTHER INFORMATION:

Baylis, Françoise. "Changing Faces: Ethics, Identity, and Facial Transplantation." In *Cutting to the Core*, edited by David Benatar. New York: Rowman & Littlefield, 2006.

Concar, David. "The Boldest Cut." *New Scientist* 182 (May 29, 2004): 32-37.

"Crossing New Frontier: Paving the Way to Make Face Transplantation Reality." *Medical Ethics Advisor*, July 1, 2006.

McLaughlin, Sabrina. "Face to Face." *Current Science* 89, no. 2 (September 12, 2003): 8-9.

Wilson, Jim. "Trading Faces." *Popular Mechanics* 180, no. 11 (November, 2003): 76-79.

FACTITIOUS DISORDERS

DISEASE/DISORDER

ANATOMY OR SYSTEM AFFECTED: Psychic-emotional system, most bodily systems

SPECIALTIES AND RELATED FIELDS: Family medicine, internal medicine, psychiatry, psychology

DEFINITION: Psychophysiological disorders in which individuals intentionally produce their symptoms in order to play the role of patient.

CAUSES AND SYMPTOMS

Although factitious disorders cover a wide array of physical symptoms and are believed to be closely related to a subset of psychophysiological disorders (somatoform disorders), they are unique in all of medicine for two reasons. The first distinguishing factor is that whatever the physical disease for which treatment is sought and regardless of how serious, the patients who seek its treatment have deliberately and intentionally produced the condition. They may have done so in one of three ways, or in any combination of these three ways. First, patients fabricate, invent, lie about, and make up symptoms that they do not have; for example, they claim to have fever and night sweats or severe back pain that they actually do not have. Second, patients have the actual symptoms that they describe, but they intentionally caused them; for example, they might inject human saliva into their own skin to produce an abscess or ingest a known allergic food to cause the predictable reaction. Third, someone with a known condition such as pancreatitis has a pain episode but exaggerates its severity, or someone else with a history of migraines claims his or her headache to be yet another migraine when it is not. Factitious disorders may manifest as complaints about psychological problems, physical problems, or both.

The second element that makes these disorders unique (and at the same time both fascinating to study and frustrating to treat) is that the sole motivation for causing or claiming the symptoms is for these patients to become and remain patients, to assume the sick role wherein little can be expected from them. These patients are not malingerers, individuals who consciously use actual or feigned symptoms for some other gain (such as claiming a fever so one does not have to go to work or school, or insisting that one's post-traumatic stress is worse than it is to enhance the judgment in a lawsuit). In fact, it is the absence of any discernible external benefit that makes these disorders so intriguing.

Technically, psychiatrists and psychologists understand factitious disorders as having three subtypes. In the first, patients claim to have predominantly psychological symptoms such as memory loss, depression, contemplation of suicide, the hearing of voices, or false memory of childhood molestation. Characteristically, the symptoms worsen whenever the patients know themselves to be under observation. In the second, patients have predominantly physical symptoms that at least superficially suggest some general medical condition. In a more extreme form called Münchausen syndrome, individuals will have spent much of their lives getting admitted to medical facilities and, once there, remaining as long as possible. While common complaints include vomiting, dizziness, blacking out, generalized rashes, and bleeding, the symptoms can involve any organ and seem limited only to the individuals' medical knowledge and experience with the medical system. The third subtype combines both psychological and physical complaints in such a way that neither predominates.

Regardless of subtype, factitious disorders are difficult to diagnose. Usually, the diagnosis is considered when the course of treating either a medical or a mental illness becomes atypical and protracted. Often, the person with a factitious disorder will present in a way which seems odd to the experienced clinician. The person may have an unusually extensive history of traveling, much familiarity with medical procedures and terminology, a complex medical and surgical history, few visitors during the hospitalization, behavioral disruptions and disturbances while hospitalized, exacerbation of symptoms while under observation, and/or fluctuating illness with new symptoms and complications arising as the workup proceeds. When present, these traits along with others make suspicion of factitious disorders reasonable.

No one knows how many people suffer with factitious disorders, but the condition is generally regarded as uncommon. It is certainly rarely reported, but this in part may be attributable to the difficulties in determining the diagnosis. While brief episodes of the condition occur, most people who claim a factitious disorder have it chronically, and they usually move on to another physician or facility when they are confronted with the true nature of their illness. It is therefore likely that some individuals are reported more than once by different hospitals and providers.

There is little certainty about what causes factitious disorders. This is true in large measure because those who know the most about the subject—patients with the disorder—are notoriously unreliable in providing information about their psychological state and often seem only dimly aware of what they are doing to themselves. It may be that they are generally incapable of putting their feelings into words. They are unaware of having inner feelings and may not know, for example, that they are sad or angry. It is possible that they experience emotions more physically, behaviorally, and concretely than do most others.

Another view suggests that people learn to distinguish their primitive emotional states through the responsivity of their primary caretaker. A normal, healthy, average mother responds appropriately to her infant's differing affective states, thereby helping the infant, as he or she develops, to distinguish, define, and eventually name what he or she is feeling. When a primary caretaker is, for any of several reasons, incapable of responding in consistently appropriate ways, the infant's emotional awareness remains undifferentiated and the child experiences confusion and emotional chaos.

It is possible, too, that factitious disorder patients are motivated to assume what sociology defines as a sick role wherein people are required to acknowledge that they are ill and are required to relinquish adult responsibilities as they place themselves in the hands of designated caretakers.

TREATMENT AND THERAPY

In the United States, estimates suggest that factitious disorders may result in costs totaling well over $40 million per year. Understanding how to identify individuals with factitious disorders early in their treatment process is crucial to public health for three important reasons. First, early identification will help the individual obtain a more appropriate referral. Second, it will conserve valuable health care resources, so that clients who have pressing medical needs get the treatment that they deserve. Third, the earlier in the process these individuals can be identified, the sooner valuable health care dollars can be saved, lowering the cost of health care as a whole.

Internists, family practitioners, and surgeons are the specialists most likely to encounter patients with factitious disorder, although psychiatrists and psychologists are often consulted in the management of these patients. These patients pose a special challenge because, in a real sense, they do not wish to become well even as they present themselves for treatment. They are not ill in the usual sense, and their indirect communication and manipulation often make them frustrating to treat using standard goals and expectations.

Sometimes mental and medical specialists' joint, supportive confrontation of these patients results in a disappearance of the troubling and troublesome behavior. During these confrontations, the health professionals are acknowledging that such extreme behavior evidences extreme distress in these patients, and as such is its own reason for psychotherapeutic intervention. These patients are not psychologically minded, however; they also have trouble forming relationships that foster genuine self-disclosure, and they rarely accept the recommendation for psychotherapeutic treatment. Because they believe that their problems are physical, not psychological, they often become irate at the suggestion that their problems are not what they believe them to be. Taken from the patient's perspective, this anger makes some sense. For them, they have endured significant time in evaluation and often also a good bit of money, and if they are lacking insight into their condition, such a confrontation may leave them feeling helpless and misunderstood. As such, even in these circumstances, empathy remains an important element in successful intervention.

—*Paul Moglia, Ph.D.;*
updated by Nancy A. Piotrowski, Ph.D.

See also Hypochondriasis; Münchausen syndrome by proxy; Psychiatric disorders; Psychiatry; Psychiatry, child and adolescent; Psychiatry, geriatric; Psychoanalysis; Psychosomatic disorders.

FOR FURTHER INFORMATION:

American Psychiatric Association. *Diagnostic and Statistical Manual of Mental Disorders: DSM-IV-TR.* 4th ed. Arlington, Va.: Author, 2000. This reference book lists the clinical criteria for psychiatric disorders, including mood disorders.

Feldman, Marc D. *Playing Sick? Untangling the Web of Munchausen Syndrome, Munchausen by Proxy,* *Malingering, and Factitious Disorder.* New York: Brunner-Routledge, 2004. Fascinating case histories of people whose conditions lead them to fake illnesses, in themselves and others, sometimes to the point of death.

Phillips, Katherine A., ed. *Somatoform and Factitious Disorders.* Washington, D.C.: American Psychiatric Association, 2001. A comprehensive examination of such topics as epidemiology, etiology/pathology, and treatment modalities for somatoform and factitious disorders.

FAILURE TO THRIVE
DISEASE/DISORDER

ALSO KNOWN AS: Growth impairment, stunting, wasting

ANATOMY OR SYSTEM AFFECTED: Bones, brain, endocrine system, psychic-emotional system

SPECIALTIES AND RELATED FIELDS: Endocrinology, family medicine, gastroenterology, genetics, neonatology, pediatrics, psychiatry, psychology

DEFINITION: A disorder of early childhood growth that includes disturbances in psychosocial skills and development.

CAUSES AND SYMPTOMS

Failure to thrive may be organic or inorganic; in many children, the etiology is multifactorial. The onset of growth problems may be prenatal as a result of maternal substance abuse, most notably alcohol use, or of maternal infection, particularly with rubella, cytomegalovirus (CMV), or toxoplasmosis. Small size in infants secondary to prematurity resolves by two to three years of age unless there are complications.

Many children with failure to thrive are both stunted (linear growth-affected) and wasted (weight-affected). Assessing which of the two conditions predominates can be done using the body mass index (BMI), which is

---

**INFORMATION ON
FAILURE TO THRIVE**

CAUSES: Maternal substance abuse or infection during prenatal phase, familial short stature, constitutional delay

SYMPTOMS: Stunted growth, weight impairment

DURATION: Two to three years

TREATMENTS: Nurturing environment, nutritional intervention, family counseling

calculated by dividing weight in kilograms by height in meters squared. A low BMI is a sign of malnutrition. Children with environmental failure to thrive fall into this category.

A child who is small but has an appropriate BMI has short stature rather than failure to thrive. The two leading causes of short stature are familial short stature and constitutional delay.

TREATMENT AND THERAPY

The main focus of the medical intervention with failure to thrive is to ensure a nurturing environment and adequate nutrition. Nutritional intervention can be achieved in many ways, such as by securing adequate access to food for the family and offering concentrated formulas, nutritional supplementation, and calorie-dense food, depending on the age of the child. Developmental intervention should also be provided if delay is detected. Likewise, family counseling, especially focusing on parenting skills, may be indicated.

PERSPECTIVE AND PROSPECTS

The term "failure to thrive" originated in 1933; it replaced the term "cease to thrive," which appeared in 1899. Initially, the condition was reported in institutionalized children, including those in orphanages. In the 1940's, it was recognized as a condition that could also affect children living at home with their biological or adoptive parents.

Although the list of conditions that can cause growth impairment in children is quite extensive, a systematic approach using history and both physical and psychosocial assessment will provide clues to the diagnosis. Intervention ensures an adequate outcome, with improved prospects for physical growth and brain development.

—*Carol D. Berkowitz, M.D.*

See also Bonding; Cognitive development; Cytomegalovirus (CMV); Developmental disorders; Developmental stages; Fetal alcohol syndrome; Growth; Malnutrition; Neonatology; Nutrition; Pediatrics; Rubella; Toxoplasmosis; Weight loss and gain.

FOR FURTHER INFORMATION:

Berk, Laura E. *Child Development*. 8th ed. Boston: Pearson/Allyn & Bacon, 2009.

Geissler, Catherine A., and Hilary J. Powers, eds. *Human Nutrition*. 12th ed. New York: Churchill Livingstone/Elsevier, 2010.

Kreutler, Patricia A., and Dorice M. Czajka-Narins. *Nutrition in Perspective*. 2d ed. Englewood Cliffs, N.J.: Prentice Hall, 1987.

Nathanson, Laura Walther. *The Portable Pediatrician: A Practicing Pediatrician's Guide to Your Child's Growth, Development, Health, and Behavior from Birth to Age Five*. 2d ed. New York: HarperCollins, 2002.

Shore, Rima. *Rethinking the Brain: New Insights into Early Development*. Rev. ed. New York: Families and Work Institute, 2003.

Whitney, Ellie, and Sharon Rady Rolfes. *Understanding Nutrition*. 12th ed. Belmont, Calif.: Wadsworth, 2009.

Winick, Myron, et al. *The Columbia Encyclopedia of Nutrition*. New York: G. P. Putnam's Sons, 1988.

FAINTING. *See* DIZZINESS AND FAINTING.

FAMILY MEDICINE
SPECIALTY
ALSO KNOWN AS: Family practice

ANATOMY OR SYSTEM AFFECTED: All

SPECIALTIES AND RELATED FIELDS: Geriatrics and gerontology, internal medicine, obstetrics, osteopathic medicine, pediatrics, preventive medicine, psychiatry, psychology

DEFINITION: The specialty concerned with the primary health maintenance and medical care of an undifferentiated patient population, in the context of family and community.

KEY TERMS:

ambulatory care: health care provided outside the hospital, usually in a clinic or office and sometimes in the patient's home

biopsychosocial model: a model that examines the effects of illness on all spheres in which the patient functions—the biological sphere, the psychological sphere, and the social sphere

general practice: a primary care field with care provided by physicians who usually have completed less than three years of residency training; the organization from which family medicine evolved

generalism: a medical and political movement concerned with primary care, often associated with the medical specialties of family medicine, general internal medicine, general pediatrics, and sometimes obstetrics and gynecology

health maintenance: the practice of anticipating, finding, preventing, and/or dealing with potential or established medical problems at the earliest possible stage to minimize adverse effects on the patient

internship: a synonym for the first year of residency training

patient advocacy: the representation of the patient's interest in medical diagnosis and treatment decisions, in which the physician acts as an information source and counselor for the patient

primary care: first-line or entry-level care; the health care that most people receive for most illnesses

residency training: medical training provided in a specialty after graduation from medical school; similar to an apprenticeship and designed to mimic real-life practice as closely as possible

specialist: any physician who practices in a specialty other than the generalist areas of family medicine, general internal medicine, general pediatrics, and obstetrics and gynecology

undifferentiated patient population: patients seen by family physicians regardless of age, sex, or type of problem

SCIENCE AND PROFESSION

From cradle to grave, family physicians have the ability to take care of patients from all age groups and manage a great variety of medical problems on a daily basis. As the primary care provider, they are central to a patient's care, either by providing it directly (85 percent of all medical problems) or by consulting specialists and following their management recommendations. They act as the patient's advocate even when healthy by providing preventive care services to find disease earlier in an attempt to eliminate it or slow its progression.

In the United States, there are 70,000 practicing family physicians, accounting for more than 200 million annual office visits. More than a third of all U.S. counties have access to only family physicians to provide medical care to their communities.

Family medicine is the direct descendant of general practice. For many years, most physicians were general practitioners. In the mid- to late twentieth century, however, the explosion of medical knowledge led to the specialization of medicine. For example, increased knowledge of the function and diseases of the heart seemed to demand creation of the specialty of cardiology. The model of the country doctor or jack-of-all-trades physician taking care of a wide range of medical problems seemed doomed to sink in the sea of subspecialization in medicine. The general practitioner, the venerable physician who hung out his or her shingle after medical school and one or more years of internship or residency training, appeared to be headed for

extinction. Indeed, in their then-existent forms, the general practitioner and general practice would not have survived. Several forces came into play which did result in the passing of general practice but which also changed general practice into family medicine.

The primary force pushing for general practice to survive and improve was the desire of the general public to retain the family doctor. The services that these physicians rendered and the relationships developed between physician and patients were held in high esteem. Through such voices as the Citizen Commission on Graduate Medical Education appointed by the American Medical Association (AMA), the public requested the rescue of the family doctor.

Other major players in the movement to revive and reshape general practice included the AMA itself and the American Academy of General Practice. On February 8, 1969, approval was granted for the creation of family medicine as medicine's twentieth official specialty. The American Academy of General Practice became the American Academy of Family Physicians (AAFP), and a certifying board, the American Board of Family Practice (ABFP), was established. The name has since been changed to the American Board of Family Medicine (ABFM). After these steps were completed, three-year training programs (residencies) in family medicine were established in medical universities and larger community hospitals to provide the necessary training for family physicians.

Family physicians are trained to provide comprehensive ongoing medical care and health maintenance for their patients. Those people who choose to become family physicians tend to value relationships over technology and service over high financial rewards. Many family physicians find themselves providing service to underserved populations and in mission work both inside and outside the United States. Family physicians often become advocates, providing counseling and advice to patients who are trying to sort out medical treatment options. They generally enjoy close relationships with their patients, who often hold them in high esteem.

Following graduation from medical school, students interested in a career in family medicine begin a three-year residency in the specialty. During the residency, these physicians train in actual practice settings under the supervision of faculty physicians. Family medicine residency training consists of three years of rotations with other medical specialties, such as internal medicine, pediatrics, surgery, and psychiatry. The unifying thread in family medicine residency training is the continuity clinic. Throughout their training, the residents see their own patients several days a week under the supervision of family medicine faculty physicians. Every effort is made to make this training as close as possible to experiences in the real world. Family medicine residents will deliver their patients' babies, hospitalize their patients, and deal with the emotional issues of death and dying, chronic illness, and disability.

Family medicine residents receive intensive training in behavioral and psychosocial issues, as well as "bedside manner" training. Scientific research has shown that many patients who seek care from family physicians have problems that require the physician to be a good listener and a skilled counselor. Family medicine residency training emphasizes these skills. It also emphasizes the functioning (or malfunctioning) of the family as a system and the effect of major changes (such as the birth of a child or retirement) on the health and functioning of the family members.

The length of training (three years versus one year) and the emphasis on psychosocial and family systems training are two of the major differences in the training of a family physician and the training of a general practitioner. Moreover, family physicians spend up to 30 percent of their training time outside the hospital in a clinic. Family medicine was the first medical specialty to emphasize this type of training, and family physicians spend more time in ambulatory (clinic) training than virtually any other specialist.

Following the successful completion of a residency program, a family physician may take a competency examination devised and administered by the ABFM. Passing this examination allows the physician to assume the title of Diplomate of the American Board of Family Medicine and makes him or her eligible to join the American Academy of Family Physicians, the advocacy and educational organization of family medicine.

There are about 250 fellowships now available to graduating family medicine residents: faculty development (16 percent), geriatrics (14 percent), obstetrics (9 percent), preventive medicine (1 percent), research (19 percent), rural medicine (3 percent), sports medicine (28 percent), and others (24 percent) such as occupational medicine.

If family physicians wish to retain their diplomate status, they must take at least fifty hours per year of medical education. After a family physician fulfills all educational and other requirements of the ABFM, that physician must then retake the certifying examination every seven years or the certification will lapse. This periodic retesting is required by the ABFM to make sure that family physicians keep up their medical education and maintain their knowledge level and clinical skills. Family medicine was the first specialty to require periodic reexamination of its physicians. In fact, since family medicine has mandated reexaminations, many other medical specialty organizations now require periodic reexamination of their members or are considering such a move. Many former general practitioners who did not have a chance to do a three-year family medicine residency took the ABFM certifying examination and became diplomates based on their years of practice experience and successful completion of the certifying examination. This option was closed to general practitioners in 1988.

A new recertification program, called the Maintenance of Certification Program for Family Physicians (MC-FP), is being required by the ABFM starting with diplomates who recertified in 2003 and all diplomates phased in by 2010. To maintain certification, candidates must perform the following every seven years: submit an online application, maintain a valid medical license, verify completion of three hundred credits of accepted CME credits, and pass the cognitive exam.

Currently, the American Academy of Family Physicians requires new active physician members to be residency-trained in family medicine. Diplomate status reflects only an educational effort by the physician and does not directly affect medical licensure. Medical licensure is based on a different testing mechanism, and license requirements vary from state to state. There are more than fifty thousand family physicians providing health care in the United States, the District of Columbia, the Virgin Islands, Guam, and Puerto Rico. Family medicine residency programs are approximately four hundred in number and usually have about seven thousand residents in training.

DIAGNOSTIC AND TREATMENT TECHNIQUES

Service to patients is the primary concern of family medicine and all those who practice, teach, administer, or foster the specialty. Of all the family physicians in practice, more than 93 percent are involved in direct patient care. While family physicians by no means constitute a majority of physicians, they are among the busiest when measured in terms of ambulatory patient visits. Family physicians see 30 percent of all ambulatory patients in the United States, which is more than the number of ambulatory visits to the next two specialty groups combined. Because of their training, family physicians can successfully care for more than 85 percent of all patient problems they encounter. Consultation with other specialty physicians is sought for the problems that are outside the scope of the family physician's knowledge or abilities. This level of consultation is not unique to family physicians, as other specialty physicians find it necessary to seek consultation for 10 to 15 percent of their patients as well.

Family physicians can be found in all areas of the United States and in virtually all types of practice situations, providing a wide range of medical services. Family physicians can successfully practice in metropolitan areas or rural communities of one thousand people (or less), and they can be found teaching or doing research in medical colleges. Because of their training and the fact that they see a truly undifferentiated patient population, family physicians deliver a wide range of medical services. Besides seeing many patients in their offices, family physicians care for patients in nursing homes, make house calls, and admit patients to the hospital. Within the hospital, many family physicians care for patients in intensive care and other special care units and assist in surgery when their patients have operations. A small number perform extensive surgical procedures in the hospital setting. A sizable minority of family physicians take care of pregnant women and deliver their children; some of these physicians also perform cesarean sections. Because family physicians see anyone that walks through the door, it is not unheard of for a family physician to deliver a child in the morning, see the siblings in the office in the afternoon, and make a house call to the grandparents in the evening. Over 80 percent of family physicians perform dermatologic procedures, musculoskeletal injections, and electrocardiograms (EKGs) in their own offices.

The thing that makes family physicians different from other physicians is their attention to the physician-patient relationship. The family physician has first contact with the patient and is in a position to bond with the patient. The family physician evaluates the patient's complete health needs and provides personal care in one or more areas of medicine. Such care is not limited to any particular type of problem, be it biological, behavioral, or social, and the patients seen are not screened according to age, sex, or illness. The family physician utilizes knowledge of the patient's functioning in the family and community and maintains continuity of care for the patient in a hospital, clinic, or nurs-

ing home or in the patient's own home. Thus, in family medicine, the patient-physician relationship is initiated, established, and nurtured for both sexes, for all ages, and across time for many types of problems.

Because of their training, family physicians are highly sought-after care providers. Small rural communities, insurance companies, and government agencies at all levels actively seek family physicians to care for patients in a wide variety of settings. In this respect, family medicine is the most versatile medical specialty. Family physicians are able to practice and live in communities that are too small to support any other types of physician.

In two reports released by Merritt Hawkins, a national recruiting company, requests for family physicians surged by 55 percent, more than all other specialties. According to data from the Massachussetts Medical Society, community hospitals reported family physicians constituted their "most critical shortage."

While the vast majority of family physicians find themselves providing care for patients, there is a minority of family physicians who serve in other, equally important roles. Roughly 3.5 percent of family physicians serve as administrators and educators. They can be found working in state, federal, and local governments; in the insurance industry; and in residency programs and medical schools. Family physicians in residency programs provide instruction and role modeling for family medicine residents in community-based and university-based residency programs. Family physicians in medical colleges design, implement, administer, and evaluate educational programs for medical students during the four years of medical school. The Society of Teachers of Family Medicine (STFM) is the organization that supports family physicians in their teaching role.

One problem facing the specialty of family medicine is the very small percentage who are dedicated to research: only 0.3 percent of all family physicians. There is a large need for research in family medicine to determine the natural course of illnesses, how best to treat them, and the effects of illness on the functioning of the family unit. The need for research in the ambulatory setting is especially acute because, while most medical research is done in the hospital setting, most medical care in the United States is provided in clinics and offices. This problem will not be easily solved because of the service focus of family medicine training and the small number of family physicians dedicated to research.

PERSPECTIVE AND PROSPECTS

Family medicine developed as a medical specialty because of the demands of the citizens of the United States; it is the only medical specialty with that claim. The ancestor of family medicine was general practice, and there is a direct link from the family physician to the general practitioner. Family medicine has grown and evolved into the specialty best suited to provide for the primary health care needs of most patients. Because of their broad scope of practice, cost-effective methods, and versatility, family physicians are found in virtually every type of medical and administrative setting. Family physicians provide a large portion of all ambulatory health care in the United States, and in some settings they are the sole providers of health care. General practice has been around as long as there have been physicians—Hippocrates was a general practitioner—but family medicine has a definite point of origin. It was created from general practice on February 8, 1969.

In January, 2000, a leadership team consisting of seven national family medicine organizations began the Future of Family Medicine (FMM) Project with its goal being "to develop a strategy to transform and renew the specialty of family medicine to meet the needs of patients in a changing health care environment." Six task forces were created as a result, with each one formed to address specific issues that aid in meeting the core needs of the people receiving care, the family physicians delivering that care, and shaping a quality health care delivery system. The FFM Leadership Committee has focused on improving the American health care system by implementing the following strategies:

> taking steps to ensure that every American has a personal medical home, has health care coverage for basic services and protection against extraordinary health care costs, promoting the use and reporting of quality measures to improve performance and service, advancing research that supports the clinical decision making of family physicians, developing reimbursement models to sustain family medicine and primary care offices, and asserting family medicine's leadership to help transform the U.S. health care system.

The present role of the family physician is and will continue to be to seek to improve the health of the people of the United States at all levels. Major problems exist for family medicine, including attrition as older family physicians retire or die, lack of medical student interest in family medicine as a career choice, and the lack of a solid cadre of researchers to advance medical knowledge in family medicine. The major strengths supporting family medicine are its service ethic, attention to the physician-patient relationship, and cost-effectiveness.

After their near demise as a recognizable group in the mid-twentieth century, family physicians have a number of reasons to expect that they will have expanded opportunities to provide for the health care needs of their patients in the future. As the United States, for example, examines its system of health care, which is the most costly and the least effective of any health care system in the developed world, many medical and political leaders look to generalism, and particularly family medicine, to provide answers. Research has shown that, for many medical problems, family physicians can provide outcomes very similar to those provided by specialists. When one couples that fact with the versatility and cost-effectiveness of generalist physicians, it can be argued that to save health care dollars the nation must reverse the 30 percent to 70 percent ratio of generalist to specialist physicians. A ratio of 50 percent to 50 percent generalist to specialist physicians has been proposed at many levels in medicine and government.

As the population ages due to improved mortality statistics and the addition of baby boomers to the geriatric age group, a further shortage of general practitioners such as family physicians is inevitable. This situation will force the United States to deal with its health care issues in order to provide its citizens with cost-effective and adequate coverage. The shortage of family physicians specifically in rural areas has led to 22 million Americans living in federally designated rural health professions shortage areas (HPSAs), defined as less than 1 primary care physician per 3,500 people. A growing challenge exists for those physicians living in rural areas as a lack of training and preparation for practice in their medical education and residency training has led to a steady decline in their choosing to practice there.

—Paul M. Paulman, M.D.;
updated by Kenneth Dill, M.D.

See also African American health; Allergies; American Indian health; Anemia; Asian American health; Athlete's foot; Bacterial infections; Bronchitis; Bruises; Chickenpox; Childhood infectious diseases; Cholesterol; Common cold; Constipation; Coughing; Cytomegalovirus (CMV); Death and dying; Diarrhea and dysentery; Diagnosis; Digestion; Dizziness and fainting; Domestic violence; Ear infections and disorders; Exercise physiology; Eye infections and disorders; Fatigue; Fever; Fungal infections; Geriatrics and gerontology; Grief and guilt; Halitosis; Headaches; Healing; Heartburn; Hypercholesterolemia; Hyperlipidemia; Hypertension; Hypoglycemia; Indigestion; Infection; Inflammation; Influenza; Laryngitis; Measles; Men's health; Mercury poisoning; Mononucleosis; Mumps; Muscle sprains, spasms, and disorders; Nutrition; Obesity; Obesity, childhood; Osteopathic medicine; Over-the-counter medications; Pain; Pediatrics; Pharmacology; Pharmacy; Physical examination; Pneumonia; Poisonous plants; Preventive medicine; Psychology; Puberty and adolescence; Rashes; Rheumatic fever; Rubella; Scabies; Scarlet fever; Sciatica; Shingles; Shock; Signs and symptoms; Sinusitis; Sleep disorders; Sore throat; Strep throat; Stress; Telemedicine; Tetanus; Tonsillitis; Toxicology; Ulcers; Viral infections; Vitamins and minerals; Wheezing; Whooping cough; Women's health; Wounds.

FOR FURTHER INFORMATION:

American Academy of Family Physicians. http://www.aafp.org. A Web site with a wealth of information regarding the field of family medicine and the organization as well as links to the journals *Family Practice Management* and *Journal of Family Practice.*

American Board of Family Medicine. http://www.theabfm.org. A Web site detailing the ABFM membership requirements for family physicians.

Behrman, Richard E., Robert M. Kliegman, and Hal B. Jenson, eds. *Nelson Textbook of Pediatrics.* 18th ed. Philadelphia: Saunders/Elsevier, 2007. Text covering all medical and surgical disorders in children with authoritative information on genetics, endocrinology, etiology, epidemiology, pathology, pathophysiology, clinical manifestations, diagnosis, prevention, treatment, and prognosis.

Rakel, Robert E., ed. *Essential Family Medicine: Fundamentals and Case Studies.* 3d ed. Philadelphia: Saunders/Elsevier, 2006. This book outlines the core content essentials for family medicine training.

Scherger, Joseph E., et al. "Responses to Questions by Medical Students About Family Practice." *Journal of Family Practice* 26, no. 2 (1988): 169-176. Although aimed at medical students, this popular medical article provides good background information about the scope and socioeconomic aspects of family medicine.

Sloane, Philip D., et al., eds. *Essentials of Family Medicine.* 5th ed. Philadelphia: Lippincott Williams & Wilkins, 2008. A basic introductory reference text to family medicine with three sections: "Principles of Family Medicine," "Preventive Care," and "Common Problems."

FASCIA

ANATOMY

ALSO KNOWN AS: Connective tissue

ANATOMY OR SYSTEM AFFECTED: All

SPECIALTIES AND RELATED FIELDS: Exercise physiology, neurology, orthopedics, osteopathic medicine, physical therapy

DEFINITION: A network of connective tissue that extends throughout the body. It functions as a shock absorber, a structural component of the body, and a medium that permits intracellular communication.

KEY TERMS:

connective tissue: the tissue in the body that binds and supports body parts

parasympathetic nervous system: part of the autonomic nervous system that restores and conserves the body's resources

synovial: related to or producing synovial fluid; many of the body's joints have a sack of synovial fluid that surrounds the joint and provides lubrication

STRUCTURE AND FUNCTIONS

There are three layers of fascia: the superficial fascia, the deep fascia, and the visceral fascia. The superficial fascia, also known as the subcutaneous tissue, is a layer of adipose or fatty tissue that lies under the skin. The deep fascia is a layer of dense, fibrous tissue that lies under the superficial fascia, surrounding and penetrating the muscles, bones, nerves, body organs, and blood vessels. The deep fascia has extensions that stretch from the tendons that attach muscles to bone and lie in broad, flat sheets, called an aponeurosis. The deep fascia is so strong that it is rarely damaged, even in traumatic injuries. The visceral fascia surrounds the body organs, suspends them, and wraps them in a protective layer of connective tissue.

The superficial fascia has the capability of stretching to accommodate pregnancy and weight gain. Usually, it slowly reverts to its normal tension level after pregnancy or weight loss. The visceral fascia lacks the elastic properties of the superficial fascia, since its role is to protect the body organs. It provides for limited movement of the organs within their cavities, while not constricting the organs. Deep fascia contains many sensory receptors that are able to report pain and changes in body movement, in pressure and vibration within the body, in the chemicals produced by the body, and in body temperature.

The deep fascia contracts during the response to a threat, known as the "fight or flight" reflex. This increased tension increases the strength of it. The deep fascia relaxes at times when the body is stressed beyond what it can tolerate and when the body is put in a relaxing position. If the tension on the deep fascia persists, then it responds by adding collagen and other proteins, which bind to the existing proteins. While this increases the strength of the body, it can restrict the structures that it is supposed to protect. Hormones produced by the body can relax the deep fascia. For example, parasympathetic nervous system hormones can trigger its relaxation.

DISORDERS AND DISEASES
Due to the presence of fascia throughout the body, many conditions can be caused by its disorders. Some examples are adhesions, carpal tunnel syndrome, compartment syndrome, fibromyalgia, hernia, Marfan syndrome, meningitis, mixed connective tissue disease, myofascial pain syndrome, necrotizing fasciitis, pericardial effusion, plantar fasciitis, pleural effusion, polyarteritis nodosa, rheumatoid arthritis, scleroderma, and tendinitis.

Common conditions that affect the fascia are carpal tunnel syndrome, inguinal hernia, plantar fasciitis (heel spur), rheumatoid arthritis, and tendonitis. Carpal tunnel syndrome affects a small opening through the wrist into the hand. The median nerve and the carpal ligament pass through this opening. Narrowing of the opening pinches these structures and causes pain and numbness in the hand. The treatment includes physical therapy, wrist splints, and, possibly, surgery. An inguinal hernia is the protrusion of part of the bowel through an opening in the fascia. An inguinal hernia protrudes through the openings in the abdominal aponeurosis for the two saphenous veins. Inguinal hernias are treated by surgery to support the aponeurosis in the area of these openings.

Plantar fasciitis is caused by chronic inflammation of the fascia that supports the arch of the foot, leading to calcification on the bottom of the heel. This condition is treated with orthotics or surgery. Rheumatoid arthritis is an autoimmune condition that affects symmetric joints in the body and causes chronic inflammation of the synovial membranes in the joints, leading to joint damage. Many medications are available to treat rheumatoid arthritis, but they suppress the immune response of the body and so have risks. Tendinitis is inflammation of a tendon, often as a result of injury or repetitive use, such as tennis elbow. This condition is treated with corticosteroid injections into the joint, application of ice or heat, and rest.

PERSPECTIVE AND PROSPECTS
The importance of the fascia has been embraced by practitioners other than traditional medicine. The fascia forms the basis for therapies such as Rolfing, massage, chiropractic, physical therapy, osteopathy, yoga, and Tai Chi Chuan. In the late 1800's, Sweden's Pehr Henrik Ling, with his associates, wrote of the relationship of mind and body. His therapy was aimed at improving the mental status of a person by improving their ability to move their body. In 1984, Raymond Nimmo wrote of the importance of treating the fascia, as well as trigger points in the body.

Ida P. Rolf (1896-1979) was a notable pioneer in the understanding of the importance of the body fascia. Rolf felt that the fascia had been largely ignored by medicine. She developed her technique of structural integrity and the importance of gravity. Structural integrity deals with the property of the fascia that causes it to adapt to changes in the body, even when the change puts the body off balance, out of alignment, or causes pain. She devoted much of her life to treating the disabled who had not responded to medical treatment. Her therapy is called Rolfing.

Medical doctors specializing in exercise physiology, neurology, and orthopedics are becoming more cognizant of the role of the fascia in the body. However, chiropractors continue to have the primary role in dealing with problems of the fascia that do not respond to medical treatment. In 2007, the first Fascia Research Congress was held in Boston.

—*Christine M. Carroll, R.N., B.S.N., M.B.A.*

See also Carpal tunnel syndrome; Chiropractic; Connective tissue; Hernia; Rheumatoid arthritis; Stress; Tendinitis; Tendons.

FOR FURTHER INFORMATION:
Lindsay, Mark. *Fascia: Clinical Applications for Health and Human Performance.* Clifton Park, N.Y.: Delmar Cengage Learning, 2008.

Paoletti, Serge. *The Fasciae: Anatomy, Dysfunction, and Treatment.* Lisbon, Maine: Eastland Press, 2006.

Schultz, R. Louis, and Rosemary Feltis. *The Endless Web: Fascial Anatomy and Physical Reality.* Berkeley, Calif.: North Atlantic Books, 1996.

FATIGUE

DISEASE/DISORDER

ANATOMY OR SYSTEM AFFECTED: All

SPECIALTIES AND RELATED FIELDS: Family medicine, geriatrics and gerontology, internal medicine, psychiatry

DEFINITION: A general symptom of tiredness, malaise, depression, and sometimes anxiety associated with many diseases and disorders; in some cases, no specific cause can be found.

KEY TERMS:

physical deconditioning: a condition that results when a person who has previously been exercising (has become conditioned) stops exercising

psychogenic fatigue: fatigue caused by mental factors, such as anxiety, and not attributable to any physical cause

sleep apnea: cessation of breathing during sleep, which may result from either an inhibition of the respiratory center (central apnea) or an obstruction to the flow of air (obstructive apnea)

sleep disorders: conditions resulting in sleep interruption, interfering with the restorative functions of sleep

syndrome: a collection of complaints (symptoms) and signs (abnormal findings on clinical examination) that do not match any specific disease

CAUSES AND SYMPTOMS

Almost all people suffer from fatigue at some point in their lives. It is a nonspecific complaint including tiredness, lack of energy, listlessness, or malaise. Patients often confuse fatigue with weakness, breath-

---

INFORMATION ON FATIGUE

CAUSES: Disease, depression, sleep disorders, physical and/or mental overactivity, excessive intake of stimulants, medications

SYMPTOMS: Tiredness, malaise, depression, anxiety, withdrawal

DURATION: Typically short-term but can be chronic

TREATMENTS: Rest and relaxation, medications, counseling

---

lessness, or dizziness, which indicate the existence of other physical disorders. Rest or a change in the daily routine ordinarily alleviates fatigue in healthy individuals. Though normally short in duration, fatigue occasionally lasts for weeks, months, or even years in some individuals. In such cases, it limits the amount of physical and mental activity in which the person can participate.

Long-term fatigue can have serious consequences. Often, patients begin to withdraw from their normal activities. They may withdraw from society in general and may gradually become more apathetic and depressed. As a result of this progression, a patient's physical and mental capabilities may begin to deteriorate. Fatigue may be aggravated further by a reduced appetite and inadequate nutritional intake. Ultimately, these symptoms lead to malnutrition and multiple vitamin deficiencies, which intensify the fatigue state and trigger a vicious circle.

This fatigue cycle ends with a person who lacks interest and energy. Such patients may lose interest in daily events and social contacts. In later stages of fatigue, they may neglect themselves and lose track of their goals in life. The will to live and fight decreases, making them prime targets for accidents and repeated infections. They may also become potential candidates for suicide.

Physical and/or mental overactivity commonly cause recent-onset fatigue. Management of such fatigue is simple: Adequate physical and/or mental relaxation typically relieve it. Fortunately, many persistent fatigue states can be easily diagnosed and successfully treated. In some cases, however, fatigue does not respond to simple measures.

Fatigue can stem from depression. Depressed individuals often reflect boredom and a lack of interest, and frequently express uncertainty and/or anxiety about the future. These people usually appear "down." They may walk slowly with their head down, slump their shoulders, and sigh frequently. They often take unusually long to respond to questions or requests. They also show little motivation. Depressed individuals typically relate feelings of dejection, sadness, worthlessness, or helplessness. Often, they complain of feeling tired when they wake up in the morning, and no amount of sleep or rest improves their condition. In fact, they feel weary all day and frequently complain of feeling weak. They often have poor appetites and sometimes lose weight. Once these patients are questioned by a physician, however, it may become apparent that their state of fatigue actually fluctuates. At times they feel exhausted, while at other times (sometimes only minutes later) they feel refreshed and full of energy.

Other manifestations of depression include sleep disorders (particularly early morning waking), reduced appetite, altered bowel habits, and difficulty concentrating. Depressed individuals sometimes fail to recognize their condition. They may channel their depression into physical complaints such as abdominal pain, headaches, joint pain, or vaguely defined aches and pains. In older people, depression sometimes manifests itself as impaired memory.

Anxiety, another major cause of fatigue, interferes with the patient's ability to achieve adequate mental and physical rest. Anxious individuals often appear scared, worried, or fearful. They frequently report multiple physical complaints, including neck muscle tension, headaches, palpitations, difficulty in breathing, chest tightness, intestinal cramping, and trouble falling asleep. In some cases, both depression and anxiety may be present simultaneously.

Medications also constitute a major cause of fatigue. All drugs—prescription, over-the-counter, or recreational—can cause fatigue. Sleeping medications, antidepressants, antianxiety medications, muscle relaxants, allergy medications, cold medications, and certain blood pressure medications can lead to problems with fatigue.

An excessive intake of stimulants, paradoxically, sometimes leads to easy fatigability. Stimulants can interfere with proper sleeping habits and relaxation. Common culprits include caffeine and medications (such as some diet pills and nasal decongestants) that can be purchased without a prescription. Recreational drugs can also contribute to chronic fatigue. Depending on their tendencies, they function to cause fatigue in much the same way as the prescription and over-the-counter drugs already discussed. Cocaine and amphetamines, for example, act as stimulants. Narcotics such as heroin and barbiturates (downers) possess strong sedative qualities. Alcohol consumption in an attempt to escape loneliness, depression, or boredom may further exacerbate a sense of fatigue. Alcohol produces fatigue in two ways. It has sedative qualities, and it also intensifies the sedative effects of other medications, if taken with them.

Other drugs that may induce fatigue include diuretics and those that lower blood pressure. These medications increase the excretions of many substances through the kidneys. If inappropriately given or regulated, these drugs may alter the blood concentration of other medications taken concurrently.

Painkillers can lead to fatigue in a different way. In some individuals, they irritate the lining of the stomach and cause it to bleed. Such bleeding usually occurs in small amounts and goes unnoticed by the patient. This slight blood loss can gradually lead to anemia and fatigue.

Medications are particularly likely to cause fatigue in elderly individuals. With many drugs, their elimination from the body through metabolism or excretion may decrease with age. This often leads to higher drug concentrations in the blood than intended, resulting in a state of constant sedation and lethargy. Also, elderly individuals' brains may be more sensitive to sedation than those of younger individuals. Finally, the elderly tend to take more medication for more illnesses than younger adults. The additive side effects of multiple medicines can add to fatigue problems.

Sleep deprivation or frequent sleep interruptions lead to fatigue. A change in environment can induce sleep disorders, especially if accompanied by unfamiliar noises, excessive lighting, uncomfortable temperatures, or an excessive degree of humidity or dryness. Total sleep time may be adequate under such conditions, but quality of sleep is usually poor. Nightmares can also interrupt sleep, and if numerous and recurring, they also cause fatigue.

Some sleep interruptions are not so readily apparent. In sleep apnea, a specific and increasingly diagnosed sleep disorder, the patient temporarily stops breathing while sleeping. This results in reduced oxygen levels and increased carbon dioxide levels in the blood. When a critical level is reached, the patient awakens briefly, takes a few deep breaths, and then falls asleep again. Many episodes of sleep apnea may occur during the night, making the sleep interrupted and less refreshing than it should be. The next day, the patient often feels tired and fatigued but may not recognize the source of the problem. Obstructive sleep apnea normally develops in grossly overweight patients or in those with large tonsils or adenoids. Patients with obstructive sleep apnea usually snore while sleeping, and typically they are unaware of their snoring and/or sleep disturbance.

A number of diseases can lead to easy fatigability. In most illnesses, rest relieves fatigue and individuals awake refreshed after a nap or a good night's sleep. Unfortunately, they also tire quickly. Unlike psychogenic fatigue or fatigue induced by drugs, disease-related fatigue is not usually the patient's main symptom. Other symptoms and signs frequently reveal the underlying diagnosis. Individuals who suffer from severe malnutrition, anemia, endocrine system malfunction, chronic infections, tuberculosis, Lyme disease, bacterial endocarditis (a bacterial infection of the valves of the heart), chronic sinusitis, mononucleosis, hepatitis, parasitic infections, and fungal infections may all experience chronic fatigue.

In early stages of acquired immunodeficiency syndrome (AIDS), fatigue may be the only symptom. Persons at high risk for contracting the human immunodeficiency virus (HIV)—those with multiple sexual partners, homosexual men, those with a history of blood transfusion, or intravenous drug users—who complain of persistent fatigue should be tested for HIV infection.

Abnormalities of mineral or electrolyte concentrations—potassium, sodium, chloride, and calcium are the most important of these—may also cause fatigue. Such abnormalities may result from medications (diuretics are frequently responsible), diarrhea, vomiting, dietary fads, and endocrine or bone disorders.

Some less common medical causes of chronic fatigue include dysfunction of specific organs such as kidney failure or liver failure. Allergies can also produce chronic fatigue. Cancer can cause fatigue, but other symptoms usually surface and lead to a diagnosis before the patient begins to notice chronic weariness.

Treatment and Therapy

When an individual's fatigue persists in spite of adequate rest, medical help becomes necessary in order to determine the cause. Common diseases known to be associated with fatigue should be considered. Initially, the physician makes detailed inquiries about the severity of the fatigue and how long ago it started. Other important questions include whether it is progressive, whether there are any factors that make it worse or relieve it, or whether it is worse during specific times of the day. An examination of the patient's psychological state may also be necessary.

The physician should ask about the presence of any symptoms that occur along with the general sense of fatigue. For example, breathlessness may indicate a cardiovascular or respiratory disease. Abdominal pain might arouse the suspicion of a gastrointestinal disease. Weakness may point to a neuromuscular collagen disease. Excessive thirst and increased urine output may suggest diabetes mellitus, and weight loss may accompany metabolic or endocrinal abnormalities, chronic infections, or cancer.

Whether they have been prescribed by a physician or purchased over the counter, the medications taken regularly by a patient should be reviewed. The doctor should also inquire about alcohol and tobacco use and dietary fads. A thorough physical examination may be required. During an examination, the doctor sometimes uncovers physical signs of fatigue-inducing diseases. Blood tests and other laboratory investigations may also be needed, especially because a physical examination does not always reveal the cause.

Often, however, despite an extensive workup, no specific cause for the persistent fatigue appears. At this stage, the diagnosis of chronic fatigue syndrome should be considered. To fit this diagnosis, patients must have several of the symptoms associated with this syndrome. They must have complained of fatigue for at least six months, and the fatigue should be of such an extent that it interferes with normal daily activities. Since many of the symptoms associated with chronic fatigue syndrome overlap with other disorders, these other fatigue-inducing conditions must be considered and ruled out.

To fit the diagnosis of chronic fatigue syndrome, patients must have at least six of the classic symptoms. These include a mild fever and/or sore throat, painful lymph nodes in the neck or axilla, unexplained generalized weakness, and muscle pain or discomfort. Patients may describe marked fatigue lasting for more than twenty-four hours that is induced by levels of exercise that would have been easily tolerated before the onset of fatigue. They may suffer from generalized headaches of a type, severity, or pattern that is different from headaches experienced before the onset of chronic fatigue. Patients may also have joint pain without swelling or redness and/or neuropsychologic complaints such as a bad memory and excessive irritability. Confusion, difficulty in thinking, inability to concentrate, depression, and sleep disturbances are also on the list of associated symptoms.

No one knows the exact cause of chronic fatigue syndrome. Researchers continue to study the disease and come up with hypotheses, though none have proven entirely satisfactory. One theory argues that since patients with chronic fatigue syndrome appear to have a reduced aerobic work capacity, defects in the muscles may cause the condition. This, however, constitutes only one of many theories concerning the syndrome and its origin.

Many patients with chronic fatigue syndrome relate that they suffered from an infectious illness immediately preceding the onset of fatigue. This pattern causes some scientists to suspect a viral origin. Typically, the illness that precedes the patient's problems with fatigue is not severe, and resembles other upper respiratory tract infections experienced previously. The implicated viruses include the Epstein-Barr virus, Coxsackie B virus, herpes simplex virus, cytomegalovirus, human herpesvirus 6, and the measles virus. It should be mentioned, however, that some patients with long-term fatigue do not have a history of a triggering infectious disease before the onset of fatigue.

Patients with chronic fatigue syndrome sometimes have a number of immune system abnormalities. Laboratory evidence exists of immune dysfunction in many patients with this syndrome, and there have been reports of improvement when immunoglobulin (antibody) therapy was given. The significance of immunological abnormalities in chronic fatigue syndrome, however, remains uncertain. Most of these abnormalities do not occur in all patients with this syndrome. Furthermore, the degree of immunologic abnormality does not always correspond with the severity of the symptoms.

Some researchers believe that the acute infectious disease that often precedes the onset of chronic fatigue syndrome forces the patient to become physically inactive. This inactivity leads to physical deconditioning, and the progression ends in chronic fatigue syndrome. Experiments in which patients with chronic fatigue syndrome were given exercise testing, however, do not support this theory completely. In the case of physical deconditioning, the heart rates of patients with chronic fatigue syndrome should have risen more rapidly with exercise than those without the syndrome. The exact opposite was found. The data were not determined consistent with the suggestion that physical deconditioning causes chronic fatigue syndrome.

A high prevalence of unrecognized psychiatric disorders exists in patients with chronic fatigue, especially depression. Depression affects about half of chronic fatigue syndrome patients and precedes other symptoms in about half of them as well. Yet a critical question remains unanswered concerning chronic fatigue syndrome: Are patients with this syndrome fatigued because they have a primary mood disorder, or has the mood disorder developed as a secondary component of the chronic fatigue syndrome?

No completely satisfactory treatment exists for chronic fatigue syndrome, since the cause remains a mystery. A group of researchers using intravenous immunoglobulin therapy met with varying degrees of success, but other investigators could not reproduce these results. Other therapeutic trials used high doses of medications such as acyclovir, liver extract, folic acid, and cyanocobalamine. A mixture of evening primrose oil and fish oil was also administered with some degree of success. Claims have also been made that patients administered magnesium sulfate improved to a larger extent than those receiving a placebo. Other therapeutic options include cognitive behavioral therapy, programs of gradually increasing physical activity, analgesics, nonsteroidal anti-inflammatory drugs (NSAIDs), and antidepressants. Finally, a number of self-help groups exist for chronic fatigue sufferers.

The prognosis and natural history of chronic fatigue syndrome are still poorly defined. Chronic fatigue syndrome does not kill patients, but it does significantly decrease the quality of life for sufferers. For the physician, management of this syndrome remains challenging. In addition to correcting any physical abnormalities present, the physician should attempt to find an activity that interests the patient and encourage him or her to become involved in it.

Perspective and Prospects

Fatigue is generally considered a normal bodily response, protecting the individual from excessive physical and/or mental activity. After all, the normal levels of performance for individuals who do not rest usually decline. In the case of overactivity, fatigue should be viewed as a positive warning sign. Using relaxation and rest (mental and/or physical), the individual can often alleviate weariness and optimize performance.

In some cases, however, fatigue does not derive from physical or mental overactivity, nor does it respond adequately to relaxation and rest. In these instances, it interferes with an individual's ability to cope with everyday life and enjoy usual activities. The patient begins referring to fatigue as the reason for not participating in normal physical, mental, and social activities.

Unfortunately, physicians, health care professionals, society, and even the patients themselves dismiss fatigue as a trivial complaint. As a result, sufferers seek medical help only after the condition becomes advanced. This dangerous, negative attitude can delay the correct diagnosis of the underlying pathology and threaten the patient's chances for a quick recovery.

The diagnosis and management of chronic fatigue

syndrome prove challenging for both physician and patient. It is important to note that chronic fatigue syndrome often stems from nonmedical causes. While the possibility of a serious medical illness should be addressed, illness-related fatigue usually occurs along with other, more prominent symptoms. The causes of chronic fatigue syndrome are numerous and can take time to define. Patients need to answer all questions related to their complaints as thoroughly and accurately as possible, so that their physicians can reach accurate diagnoses using the minimum number of tests. Extensive testing for rare medical causes of fatigue can become extraordinarily expensive and uncomfortable, so doctors select the tests that they are ordering cautiously. They must balance the benefit, the cost, and the risk of each test to the patient. Such decisions should be based on their own experience and on the available data.

Open communication between the patient and doctor is of paramount importance. It ensures a correct diagnosis, followed by the most effective treatment. Follow-up visits and reassurance may be the best therapy in many cases. Professional counselors can offer assistance with fatigue-inducing psychological disorders. Examination of sleep and relaxation habits can reveal potential problems, and steps can be taken to ensure adequate rest.

Persistent fatigue should not be regarded lightly, and serious attempts should be made to determine its underlying causes. In this respect, it may be appropriate to recall one of Hippocrates' aphorisms, "Unprovoked fatigue means disease."

—*Ronald C. Hamdy, M.D., Mark R. Doman, M.D., and Katherine Hoffman Doman*

See also Aging; Anemia; Anxiety; Apnea; Chronic fatigue syndrome; Depression; Dizziness and fainting; Epstein-Barr virus; Fibromyalgia; Malnutrition; Multiple chemical sensitivity syndrome; Narcolepsy; Overtraining syndrome; Sleep; Sleep disorders; Sleeping sickness; Stress; Stress reduction.

FOR FURTHER INFORMATION:

Archer, James, Jr. *Managing Anxiety and Stress.* 2d ed. New York: Routledge, 1991. Anxiety is a common cause of persistent fatigue. This text examines the nature of anxiety. Contains several methods to combat anxiety and stress, ranging from management skills, personal relations, nutrition, and exercise to meditation and relaxation techniques.

DePaulo, J. Raymond, Jr., and Leslie Ann Horvitz. *Understanding Depression: What We Know and What You Can Do About It.* New York: Wiley, 2003. A leading expert on depression examines the disease's nature, causes, effects, and treatments.

Feiden, Karyn. *Hope and Help for Chronic Fatigue Syndrome: The Official Guide of the CFS-CFIDS Network.* New York: Prentice Hall, 1990. A complete review of chronic fatigue syndrome, presenting the many aspects of this disease. The history of this syndrome, symptomatology, theories of causation, and experimental therapies are addressed.

Goroll, Allan H., and Albert G. Mulley, eds. *Primary Care Medicine.* 5th ed. Philadelphia: Lippincott Williams & Wilkins, 2006. The essential text for the medical office practice of adult medicine. It is problem-oriented and easily read even by individuals without medical training. The section on the causes of fatigue is one of the best available.

Patarca-Montero, Roberto. *Chronic Fatigue Syndrome and the Body's Immune Defense System.* New York: Haworth Medical Press, 2002. Patarca-Montero, a leading immunologist, examines the connections between the disease and immunology, reviews how therapeutic tools such as herbal medicine, vaccines, and cell therapy are being used in CFS research, and discusses the connection between CFS and fibromyalgia, Gulf War syndrome, sick building syndrome, and multiple chemical sensitivity.

Talley, Joseph. *Family Practitioner's Guide to Treating Depressive Illness.* Chicago: Precept Press, 1987. Depression is probably the most common cause of persistent fatigue. This well-written text examines the multiple facets of depression. It also reviews the various therapies available, different philosophies of depressive treatments, and the use of psychotherapy.

Wilson, James L. *Adrenal Fatigue: The Twenty-first Century Stress Syndrome.* Petaluma, Calif.: Smart, 2004. The author, a clinician for more than two decades, helps readers assess their condition and symptoms and determine causes, and suggests treatment of the condition through lifestyle and dietary modification.

Zgourides, George D., and Christie Zgourides. *Stop Feeling Tired! Ten Mind-Body Steps to Fight Fatigue and Feel Your Best.* Oakland, Calif.: New Harbinger, 2003. A self-help book that stresses holistic tools for eliminating tension and improving quality of life. Explores relaxation methods adapted from both Western and Eastern disciplines, such as cognitive-behavioral strategies, simple meditation, visualization, and energy-balancing techniques.

Fatty acid oxidation disorders

Disease/disorder

Anatomy or system affected: Heart, liver, muscles

Specialties and related fields: Biochemistry, biotechnology, nutrition, pediatrics, perinatology

Definition: Inherited metabolic defects that prevent the breakdown of fatty acids in the liver, muscles, and heart.

Causes and Symptoms

Fatty acid oxidation disorders are inherited defects in the enzymes that break down fatty acids to generate metabolic energy. Defects in at least eleven of the twenty enzymes involved with this process have been identified and can be diagnosed by enzymatic analysis of a tissue biopsy. Some generate unique profiles of metabolites in the blood or urine that can be used for diagnosis. These disorders are inherited as autosomal recessive traits, and, in many cases, the causative deoxyribonucleic acid (DNA) mutations have been determined. Fatty acid oxidation disorders can affect the liver, which breaks down fatty acids for its own needs and, by converting them to ketone bodies, for energy generation in other body tissues; they can also affect muscles and the heart, which use fatty acids as a source of energy.

Symptoms appear only under fasting conditions, either overnight or when exacerbated by infection or fever. Under these conditions, as glycogen stores are depleted, the body depends increasingly on fatty acids for energy. If fatty acids cannot be broken down completely, an energy deficit and the accumulation of deleterious intermediates lead to vomiting, coma, and, in severe cases, death. The levels of blood glucose are low because the energy needed for its synthesis is lacking. The first episode may occur in the first two years of life; such an episode can be fatal and may be mistakenly attributed to sudden infant death syndrome (SIDS). Some fatty acid oxidation disorders, however, are largely asymptomatic.

Treatment and Therapy

The general treatment for fatty acid oxidation disorders is to minimize fasting, as by snacking before sleep, and, in acute episodes, to administer intravenous glucose. This treatment restores depleted blood glucose and reduces the demand for fatty acid oxidation. Some defects also benefit from a low intake of dietary fat. Fasting or low carbohydrate diets, for weight loss or other

---

Information on Fatty Acid Oxidation Disorders

Causes: Genetic enzyme deficiency

Symptoms: Only under fasting conditions (overnight or when exacerbated by infection or fever), vomiting, coma, and sometimes death; some disorders largely asymptomatic

Duration: Chronic with acute episodes

Treatments: Minimizing of fasting (snacking before sleep), intravenous glucose for acute episodes

---

reasons, are contraindicated for individuals with these disorders.

One of these diseases is attributable to the defective cellular uptake of carnitine, which is needed to transport fatty acids into mitochondria, where they are oxidized; this type can be treated with supplemental carnitine. In acute episodes with some other disorders, treatment with carnitine has proven beneficial in increasing the urinary excretion of deleterious intermediates.

Perspective and Prospects

The first observation of a defect in fatty acid oxidation was made in 1972. Although not reported until 1982, one such disorder, medium-chain acyl-coenzyme A dehydrogenase (MCAD) deficiency, is among the most common inborn errors of metabolism, with a frequency of 1 in 9,000 live births. Each disorder of fatty acid oxidation is a candidate for enzyme replacement therapy or gene replacement therapy, although these remain experimental treatments.

—James L. Robinson, Ph.D.

See also Enzyme therapy; Enzymes; Food biochemistry; Glycogen storage diseases; Metabolic disorders; Metabolism.

For Further Information:

Devlin, Thomas M., ed. *Textbook of Biochemistry: With Clinical Correlations.* 6th ed. Hoboken, N.J.: Wiley-Liss, 2006.

Hay, William W., Jr., et al., eds. *Current Diagnosis and Treatment in Pediatrics.* 18th ed. New York: Lange Medical Books/McGraw-Hill, 2009.

Roe, C. R., and J. Ding. "Mitochondrial Fatty Acid Oxidation Disorders." In *The Metabolic and Molecular Bases of Inherited Disease,* edited by Charles R. Scriver et al. 8th ed. New York: McGraw-Hill, 2001.

FEET

ANATOMY

ANATOMY OR SYSTEM INVOLVED: Bones, musculo-skeletal system

SPECIALTIES AND RELATED FIELDS: Orthopedics, podiatry

DEFINITION: The lowest extremities, composed of a complex system of muscles and bones, that act as levers to propel the body and that must support the weight of the body in standing, walking, or running.

KEY TERMS:

distal: referring to a particular body part that is farther from the point of attachment or farther from the trunk than another part

extension: movement that increases the angle between the bones, causing them to move farther apart; straightening or extension of the ankle occurs when the toes point away from the shin

flexion: a bending movement that decreases the angle of the joint and brings two bones closer together; flexion of the ankle pulls the foot closer to the shin

hallucis: a term referring to the big toe; the flexor hallucis longus is a muscle that flexes the big toe

inferior: situated below another part; the ankle bones are inferior to the bones of the lower leg

lateral: toward the side with respect to the body's imaginary midline; away from the midline of the body, a limb, or any understood point of reference

medial: closer to an imaginary midline dividing the body into equal right and left halves than another part

plantar: having to do with the sole of the foot (for example, a plantar wart)

podiatry: the branch of medicine that deals with the study, examination, diagnosis, treatment, and prevention of diseases and malfunctions of the foot

proximal: referring to a particular body part that is closer to a point of attachment than another part

superior: above another part or closer to the head; the ankle bones are superior to the bones of the feet

STRUCTURE AND FUNCTIONS

The anatomy of the foot is very similar to that of the hand; however, the foot is adapted to perform very different functions. The human hand has the ability to perform fine movements such as grasping and writing, while the foot is involved mainly in support and movement. Therefore, the bones and muscles of the foot tend to be heavier and function without the same dexterity as the hand.

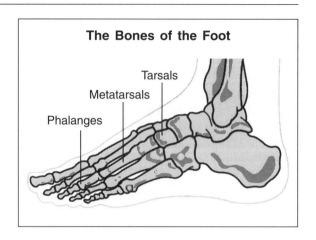

The Bones of the Foot

The twenty-six bones of the foot include the tarsals, metatarsals, and phalanges. The proximal portion of the foot next to the ankle is composed of seven tarsal bones: the calcaneus, talus, navicular, cuboid, medial cuneiform, intermediate cuneiform, and lateral cuneiform. The bones are rather irregular in shape and form gliding joints; these joints allow only a limited movement when compared to other joints in the body. The calcaneus forms the large heel bone, which serves as a major attachment for the muscles that are located in the back of the lower leg. Just above the calcaneus is another large foot bone called the talus. The talus rests between the tibia and the fibula, the two lower leg bones. Interestingly, the talus is the single bone that receives the entire weight of the body when an individual is standing; it must then transmit this weight to the rest of the foot below. The cuboid and the three cuneiform bones meet the proximal end of the long foot bones, the metatarsals.

The five separate metatarsal bones are relatively long and thin when compared to the tarsal bones. Anatomists distinguish between the five metatarsals by number. If one begins numbering from the medial (or inside) part of the foot, that metatarsal is number one and the lateral (or outside) metatarsal is number five. The distal portion of each metatarsal articulates (meets) with the toe bones, or phalanges.

Humans have toes that are very similar to their fingers. In fact, the numbers and names of the toe and finger bones, phalanges, are identical. The major differences lie in the fact that the finger phalanges are longer than the phalanges that make up toes. Hinge joints are located between each phalanx and allow for flexion and extension movements only. Human toes (or fingers) are made up of fourteen different phalanges. Each toe (or finger) has three phalanges except for the big toe (or thumb), which has only two. The toes are named in a similar way as the metatarsals; that is, the big toe is number one and the little toe is number five. The three phalanges that make up each toe (except for the big toe) are named according to location. The phalanx meeting the metatarsal is referred to as the proximal phalanx. The bone at the tip of the toe is the distal phalanx, and the one in between is the middle phalanx. Since the big toe only has two phalanges, they are called proximal and distal phalanges.

Although it seems that there is only a single arch in each foot, podiatrists and anatomists identify three arches: the medial and lateral longitudinal arches and the transverse, or metatarsal, arch. The medial longitudinal arch, as the name implies, is located on the medial surface of the foot and follows the long axis from the calcaneus to the big toe. Likewise, the lateral longitudinal arch is on the lateral surface and runs from the heel to the little toe. The transverse, or metatarsal, arch crosses the width of the foot near the proximal end of the metatarsals. The bones are only one factor that maintains arches in the feet and prevents them from flattening under the weight of the body. Ligaments (which connect bones), muscles, and tendons (which attach muscles to bones) are primarily responsible for the support of the arches. The arches function to distribute body weight between the calcaneus and the distal end of the metatarsals (the balls of the feet). They also are flexible enough to absorb some of the shock to the feet from walking, running, and jumping.

While the feet seem to be composed of only bones, tendons, and ligaments, the movements of the toes and feet require an extensive system of muscles. Most of the larger muscles that act on the foot and toes are actually located in the lower leg. Anatomists divide these muscles into separate compartments: anterior, posterior, and lateral.

The muscles of the anterior compartment move the foot upward (dorsiflex) and extend the toes. These muscles include the tibialis anterior, extensor digitorum longus, extensor hallucis longus, and peroneus tertius. The tibialis anterior is attached to the top of the first metatarsal and pulls the medial part of the foot upward and slightly lateral. All the toes except the big toe are pulled up (extended) by the extensor digitorum longus. The extensor hallucis longus moves only the big toe upward, while the peroneus tertius is attached to the fifth metatarsal and moves the foot upward.

The muscles of the lateral compartment act to move the foot in a lateral or outward direction. The peroneus

longus and peroneus brevis are attached to the first and fifth metatarsal, respectively. Using these attachments, the muscles can pull the foot laterally.

The muscles of the posterior compartment are the largest group and act to flex the foot and toes. All these muscles share a common tendon, the calcaneus (or Achilles) tendon. As the name suggests, this large tendon attaches to the calcaneus bone. The larger, more superficial muscles include the gastrocnemius, soleus, and plantaris; these powerful muscles are commonly called the calf muscles. Also in the posterior compartment are four smaller muscles located beneath the calf muscles: the popliteus (located directly behind the knee joint), flexor hallucis longus, flexor digitorum longus, and tibialis posterior. The popliteus rotates the lower leg medially. The flexor hallucis longus flexes the big toe. The remaining toes are flexed by the flexor digitorum longus, while the tibialis posterior acts opposite the tibialis anterior to flex the foot.

Within the foot itself are some muscles known as the intrinsic foot muscles. All but one of these muscles are located on the bottom surface of the foot. This one muscle extends all the toes except the little toe. The remaining intrinsic muscles are on the plantar (bottom) surface and serve to flex the toes.

The major vessels that provide blood to the foot include branches from the anterior tibial artery. This relatively large artery is located along the anterior surface of the lower leg and branches into the dorsalis pedis artery, which serves the ankle and upper part of the foot. Physicians often check for a pulse in this foot artery to provide information about circulation to the foot and circulation in general, as this is the point farthest from the heart. The bottom parts of the feet are supplied with blood by branches of the peroneal artery. At the ankle, this artery branches into plantar arteries, which supply the structures on the sole of the foot. The human toes receive most of their blood from branches of the plantar arteries called the digital arteries.

DISORDERS AND DISEASES

Even though the anatomy of the foot is resistant to the tremendous amount of force that the body places on it, it can be injured. Force injuries to the foot commonly result in fractures or breaks of the metatarsals and phalanges. Occasionally, the calcaneus may fracture from a fall on a hard surface. More commonly, patients complain of painful heel syndrome.

Because the shock-absorbing pads of tissue on the heel become thinner with age, repeated pressure on the heel can cause pain. Prolonged standing, walking, or running can add to the pressure, as can being overweight. One cause of pain is plantar fasciitis, an inflammation of the tough band of connective tissue on the sole. The inflammation occurs when the muscles located on the back of the lower leg that are attached to the connective tissue at the calcaneus pull under stress. This may even be associated with small fractures. X rays may show small spurs of bone near the site of stress; however, these spurs are not believed to be the cause of pain.

Deformities of the foot at birth are fairly common and include clubfoot, flat foot, and clawfoot. The cause of these anomalies is abnormal development. The foot of the fetus normally goes through stages where it is turned outward and inward but gradually assumes a normal position by about the seventh month of gestation. In the case of clubfoot, arrested development in the stage when the foot is turned inward causes the muscles, bones, and joints to develop in this abnormal anatomical position. At the time of birth, the deformity is readily observable and the foot immobile. Treatment includes splints, casting, and surgery. If treatment is begun at birth, the foot may look relatively normal after approximately one year.

Almost everyone is born with feet that are flat because the arches do not begin to develop until the ligaments and muscles function normally. In most people, the arches are fully formed by the age of six. In some individuals, however, the ligaments and muscles remain weak and the feet do not develop a normal arch. Flat feet can also develop in adult life, at which time they are called "fallen arches." Body weight moves along a precise path during walking or running, beginning with the heel touching the ground. Then, as the foot steps, the arch receives the forces pushing down on the foot. Because the bones, muscles, and ligaments form an arch in the foot, the arch can deform slightly and absorb some of the downward force. With further movement, the weight passes to the ball of the foot (the distal metatarsals). A fallen arch has lost this flexibility and shock-absorbing capability. The arch "falls" because of improper weight distribution along the foot, causing the arch to stretch excessively and to weaken with time. Without proper arch support, the foot begins to twist inward, or medially, causing the body weight to be transmitted to the inside of the foot rather than in a straight line toward the toes. This problem often occurs in runners who have improperly fitted shoes or a poor running style (although anyone can suffer from fallen longitudinal arches, regardless of the individual's level of physical activity). As a runner increases distance and speed without correcting his or her shoes or running form, the force applied to the feet increases. Fallen arches appear to occur particularly in runners or joggers who exercise on hard surfaces without proper technique or arch support.

A number of disorders can affect the skin of the foot. Corns are small areas of thickened skin on a toe that are usually caused by tight-fitting shoes. People with high arches are affected most because the arch increases the pressure applied to the toes during walking. If the corn becomes painful, the easiest treatment is for the person to wear better-fitting shoes. If the pain persists, a clinician can pare down the growth with a scalpel.

Plantar warts appear on the skin of the sole and are caused by a papillomavirus. Because of pressure from the weight of the body, the plantar wart is often flattened and forced into the skin of the sole. The wart may disappear without treatment. If it persists, surgery or chemical therapy can be used to relieve the discomfort.

Athlete's foot is a common fungal infection which causes the foot to become itchy, sore, and cracked. It is usually treated with antifungal agents such as miconazole. Preventive measures including keeping the feet dry and disinfecting areas where the fungus may live, such as shower stalls.

Another common deformity is a bunion, which is a bursa (fluid-filled pad) overlying the joint at the base of the big toe. Normal structure of the first metatarsal, first phalange, and their joint is necessary to withstand the force applied to them in everyday activities. A bunion is caused by an abnormal outward projection of the joint and an inward projection of the big toe. Treatment involves correcting the position of the big toe and keeping it in a normal position. Sometimes surgery is necessary if the tissues become too swollen. In fact, some severe cases of bunions have required complete reconstruction of the toe. Unless treated, a bunion will get progressively worse.

Gout is a metabolic disorder, mainly found in men, which causes uric acid crystals to form in joints. Even though any joint can be affected, the big toe joint is likely the major site for gout because it is under chronic stress from walking. The joint is usually red, swollen, and very tender and painful. The first attack usually involves only one joint and lasts a few days. Some patients never experience another attack, but most have a second episode between six months and two years after the first. After the second attack, more joints may become involved. Treatment includes anti-inflammatory drugs and colchicine. These drugs help reduce the pain by decreasing the amount of inflammation around the joint. Physicians may also prescribe allopurinol to reduce the amount of uric acid that the body produces. Drugs are also available that increase the kidneys' ability to excrete uric acid; examples of these agents are probenecid and sulfinpyrazone.

Perspective and Prospects

Even though the feet constitute a relatively small area of the body, ailments of the feet afflict more than half the world's population. For a long time, disorders of the foot were not taken as seriously as those found in other parts of the body. It is now known, however, that poor foot health can have serious effects. For example, in children a painful foot condition not properly diagnosed and treated can result in lost school days and decreased participation in other activities. More important, an uncorrected congenital abnormality, if neglected, could have irreversible consequences. For the elderly, foot problems hinder or prevent normal activities such as taking care of personal needs, exercising, and socializing. Anything that affects the feet affects that individual's overall health and well-being.

Because of the potentially devastating problems of improper foot care, a branch of medicine developed that specifically addresses problems of the feet. Physicians known as podiatrists practice a specialized branch of medicine called podiatry. It is the job of the podiatrist to assess the cause of the foot problem and the patient's general medical condition in determining the need for and the course of treatment. This assessment often calls for contact with the patient's primary care physician for access to the patient's medical records, as many diseases affect the whole body but present signs and symptoms in the feet. The podiatrist or other physician, such as an orthopedist, will evaluate a disorder through physical exams, laboratory tests, and anatomical tests to examine the internal structures; the latter may include X rays, computed tomography (CT) scans, or magnetic resonance imaging (MRI). The physician will then diagnose and begin treating the disorder using surgery, medical therapy, or physical therapy.

As more individuals become physically active throughout their lives, clinicians who practice sports medicine are paying closer attention to problems of the foot. Many people seek to improve their health by walking, jogging, and bicycling. All these activities have proven to be excellent for maintaining cardiovascular health, but all place additional stress on the foot.

Physicians who counsel patients on physical fitness programs attempt to identify individuals who may be injury-prone. Failure to recognize an anatomical anomaly of the feet could lead to an injury or series of injuries that restrict certain activities or even cause permanent damage. Occasionally, individuals are too enthusiastic about their exercise program and experience overuse injuries involving the feet. Such injuries may cause a sudden cessation of the physical activity and may have a significant demoralizing effect on individuals who finally decide to take steps to improve their health and well-being.

People commonly neglect their feet and underemphasize the importance of the normal functional anatomy of the foot. Individuals who experience a foot injury, however, begin to appreciate the absolute importance of this rather complex but often overlooked structure.

—*Matthew Berria, Ph.D.*

See also Anatomy; Athlete's foot; Bones and the skeleton; Bunions; Cysts; Flat feet; Foot disorders; Frostbite; Ganglion removal; Gout; Hammertoe correction; Hammertoes; Heel spur removal; Lower extremities; Nail removal; Nails; Orthopedic surgery; Orthopedics; Orthopedics, pediatric; Podiatry; Sports medicine; Tendon repair; Warts.

For Further Information:

Currey, John D. *Bones: Structures and Mechanics*. Princeton, N.J.: Princeton University Press, 2002. Very accessible overview of a range of information related to whole bones, bone tissue, and dentin and enamel. Topics include stiffness, strength, viscoelasticity, fatigue, fracture mechanics properties, buckling, impact fracture, and properties of cancellous bone.

Hales, Dianne. *An Invitation to Health Brief.* Updated ed. Belmont, Calif.: Wadsworth/Cengage Learning, 2010. This updated text should be read by anyone who wishes an overview of health topics. Chapter 4 deals with exercise and fitness and contains a section on the importance of wearing the correct shoes for a given activity.

Lippert, Frederick G., and Sigvard T. Hansen. *Foot and Ankle Disorders: Tricks of the Trade.* New York: Thieme, 2003. Details common foot disorders and their causes and treatment.

Mader, Sylvia S. *Human Biology.* Dubuque, Iowa: McGraw-Hill, 2009. Provides an excellent overview of lower limb anatomy and physiology. It also addresses common medical terminology relating to foot movement.

Marieb, Elaine N., and Katja Hoehn. *Human Anatomy and Physiology*. 9th ed. San Francisco: Pearson/ Benjamin Cummings, 2010. This text discusses the functional significance of various anatomical structures, including the foot. Readers will enjoy the excellent pictures and diagrams of the foot and associated body parts.

Shier, David N., Jackie L. Butler, and Ricki Lewis. *Hole's Essentials of Human Anatomy and Physiology*. 10th ed. Boston: McGraw-Hill, 2009. The authors do an excellent job of describing the rather complex anatomy of the foot and lower leg. Several views of the internal and external anatomy of the foot are given.

Van De Graaff, Kent M., and Stuart I. Fox. *Concepts of Human Anatomy and Physiology*. 5th ed. Dubuque, Iowa: Wm. C. Brown, 2000. Van De Graaff has taught human anatomy for years, and anyone would appreciate the approach that he has taken in presenting human structures. Chapters 7, 9, and 10 cover the anatomy of the foot and some problems that can occur if the anatomy is abnormal. Chapter 10 includes the surface anatomy of the lower leg and foot.

FETAL ALCOHOL SYNDROME
DISEASE/DISORDER

ALSO KNOWN AS: Fetal alcohol spectrum disorder (FASD), alcohol-related neurodevelopmental disorder (ARND), alcohol-related birth defects (ARBD), fetal alcohol effects (FAE)

ANATOMY OR SYSTEM AFFECTED: Brain, ears, eyes, hands, head, heart, mouth

SPECIALTIES AND RELATED FIELDS: All

DEFINITION: Prenatal alcohol exposure of the fetus, resulting in specific facial and central nervous system abnormalities, impairment of physical growth (especially linear growth), and other associated anomalies.

CAUSES AND SYMPTOMS

Fetal alcohol syndrome was first described in 1973 after recognition of a specific pattern of craniofacial, limb, and cardiac defects in unrelated infants born to alcoholic mothers.

Alcohol is a potent teratogen. Ethanol toxicity was initially suspected and has since been proven as the etiology of this syndrome. Fetal alcohol syndrome is not genetically inherited but rather is an acquired syndrome.

> ### INFORMATION ON FETAL ALCOHOL SYNDROME
>
> **CAUSES:** Alcohol consumption by mother during pregnancy
>
> **SYMPTOMS:** Growth retardation, certain facial anomalies, central nervous system impairment, clumsiness, behavioral problems, brief attention span, poor judgment, impaired memory, diminished capacity to learn from experience
>
> **DURATION:** Chronic
>
> **TREATMENTS:** None; preventive measures during pregnancy

Alcohol induces abnormalities in neurogenesis and synaptogenesis and is the leading cause of preventable mental retardation in the United States. These processes result in central nervous system structural anomalies and microcephaly (small head size). Attention deficit, hyperactivity, and behavioral and learning difficulties; planning difficulties; memory problems; receptive language skill deficits; and math and verbal processing difficulties are common with fetal alcohol syndrome. Alcohol also has lifelong negative effects on fine motor coordination and balance. Prenatal and postnatal growth is below the 10th percentile for age and ethnicity.

Additionally, prenatal alcohol exposure results in numerous cardiovascular problems and facial and limb anomalies. Distinguishing features include short palpebral (eyelid) fissures, a thin vermilion (upper edge of the lip), and a long, smooth philtrum (vertical groove in the upper lip). Underdeveloped ears, clinodactyly (curvature of the little fingers), camptodactyly (bent fingers that cannot straighten), "hockey stick" palmar creases, and cardiac defects are common.

TREATMENT AND THERAPY

Primary prevention is the optimal treatment. Programs to educate health care providers and the general public regarding the adverse effects of alcohol usage during pregnancy may be effective in reducing the incidence of fetal alcohol syndrome. For individuals with this disorder, lifelong therapy directed toward educational planning, including improving cognitive, motor, behavioral, and psychosocial skills, is warranted. In addition, medical care is required for various associated anomalies such as cardiac defects.

PERSPECTIVE AND PROSPECTS

Alcohol exposure—as a fetus, adolescent, or adult—leads to an increased probability of further alcohol ingestion at other developmental stages. An interruption of this cycle is imperative in order to reduce the incidence of fetal alcohol syndrome. Prevention of alcohol-affected pregnancies depends on developing and implementing evidence-based tools for fetal alcohol syndrome prevention, diagnosis, and treatment. There is no safe dose of alcohol during pregnancy, and current recommendations note that no alcohol should be ingested at conception and throughout gestation.

—*Wanda Todd Bradshaw,*
M.S.N., N.N.P., P.N.P., C.C.R.N.

See also Addiction; Alcoholism; Birth defects; Brain disorders; Childbirth; Childbirth complications; Embryology; Learning disabilities; Mental retardation; Neonatology; Obstetrics; Perinatology; Pregnancy and gestation.

FOR FURTHER INFORMATION:

Calhoun, Faye, et al. "National Institute on Alcohol Abuse and Alcoholism and the Study of Fetal Alcohol Spectrum Disorders: The International Consortium." *Annali dell'Istituto superiore di sanità* 42, no. 1 (2006): 4-7.

Chudley, Albert, et al. "Fetal Alcohol Spectrum Disorder: Canadian Guidelines for Diagnosis." *Canadian Medical Association Journal* 172, suppl. 5 (2005): S1-21.

Gerberding, Julie Louise, Jose Cordero, and R. Louise Floyd. *Fetal Alcohol Syndrome: Guidelines for Referral and Diagnosis.* Atlanta: CDC National Task Force on Fetal Alcohol Syndrome and Fetal Alcohol Effect, 2004.

Hoyme, H. Eugene, et al. "A Practical Clinical Approach to Diagnosis of Fetal Alcohol Spectrum Disorders: Clarification of the 1996 Institute of Medicine Criteria." *Pediatrics* 115, no. 1 (2005): 39-47.

National Organization on Fetal Alcohol Syndrome. http://www.nofas.org.

Wattendorf, Daniel, and Maximilian Muenke. "Fetal Alcohol Spectrum Disorders." *American Family Physician* 72 (2005): 279-282, 285.

FETAL SURGERY

PROCEDURE

ANATOMY OR SYSTEM AFFECTED: Bladder, blood, brain, liver, lungs, respiratory system, urinary system

SPECIALTIES AND RELATED FIELDS: Cardiology, ethics, genetics, neonatology, obstetrics, pediatrics, urology

DEFINITION: Surgical intervention in utero, before birth, if the fetus has a life-threatening condition or congenital abnormality that can be alleviated.

KEY TERMS:

amniocentesis: the drawing of amniotic fluid through the abdominal wall of a pregnant woman in the fifteenth or sixteenth week of pregnancy to test for fetal abnormalities, particularly Down syndrome

diaphragmatic hernia: a protrusion of the stomach into the diaphragm

hiatal hernia: a protrusion of the stomach into the opening normally occupied in the diaphragm by the esophagus

hydronephrosis: swelling (distension) of the kidney

hypotonic: the presence of a low osmotic pressure

in utero: the Latin term for "inside or within the womb"

neonatologist: a physician who specializes in treating newborn infants

osmotic pressure: the pressure between two solutions separated by a membrane

teratoma: a tumor composed of tissue not normally found at that site

thorax: the bone and cartilage cage attached to the sternum; generally referred to as the rib cage

uropathy: any disease of the urinary tract

INDICATIONS AND PROCEDURES

As early as the 1960's, some unborn infants suffering from progressive anemia caused by antibodies that drew away their strength were saved by receiving blood transfusions in utero. These early procedures marked the beginnings of invasive medical intervention in dealing with fetal problems.

Not until the technical advances of the 1970's and beyond, however, was it possible to observe human fetuses in the uterus. With the development of ultrasound imaging, it became possible to examine in considerable detail the size, growth, and contour of fetuses. The use of ultrasound enabled physicians to assess with considerable accuracy the age of fetuses, their probable date of birth, and a number of congenital abnormalities, such as spina bifida.

Laparoscopes with diameters of less than 0.1 inch make it possible to examine the fetal stomach. The use of lasers and tiny instruments guided by computers has allowed methods of fetal surgery that were inconceivable at mid-twentieth century. These instruments greatly reduce blood loss in all types of surgery, including fetal surgery, and greatly improve the prognosis in such procedures. They are used to repair ruptured membranes in fetuses, to install shunts to relieve blockages, and, with the laser excision of placental vessels, to equalize osmotic pressure in twin-twin transfusion syndrome.

It has become possible for obstetricians to observe all significant fetal organs. Whereas physicians earlier could barely hear the beat of the fetal heart, they now can monitor all four of its chambers in the unborn to detect defects early, and, in some cases, to repair them surgically. Ultrasound enables physicians to observe fetal movement within the uterus and to monitor fetal breathing and swallowing.

Because physicians can now gather specific information about the fetus and its health, abnormalities and life-threatening physical problems can be detected several months prior to delivery. Whereas neonatologists have regularly encountered such problems as intestinal and urinary tract obstructions, heart defects, protrusions of the wall of the stomach into the thorax (diaphragmatic hernia) or into the esophageal region (hiatal hernia), swelling of the kidney (hydronephrosis), tumors (sacrococcygeal teratomas), hydrocephalus

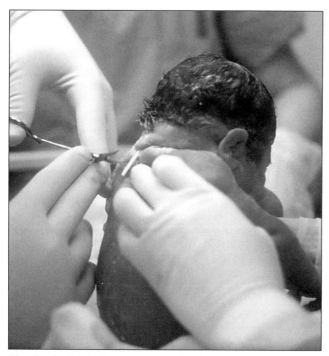

Shortly after birth, doctors examine the shunt that was inserted into a baby two months earlier in an effort to correct his hydrocephalus. (AP/Wide World Photos)

(water on the brain), and defects of the chromosomes shortly after the birth of a child, it is now possible to detect and, in some cases, to treat these defects surgically in utero.

In cases where fetal surgery appears to offer the most reasonable solution to a difficult problem, the mother may be sent to one of the few centers in the United States where this highly specialized and controversial form of surgery is performed regularly. With the development of sophisticated computer-operated instrumentation, surgeons geographically distant from their patients can perform highly specialized surgery on them. Eventually, such surgery will likely be performed without uprooting mothers.

The current success rate of fetal surgery is not encouraging, although some remarkable outcomes have occurred through its use. Fetal surgical procedures often result in miscarriages and sometimes in the death of both the mother and the fetus.

Two conditions that frequently require fetal surgery are obstructions in the urinary tract that, if untreated until birth, may lead to kidney failure, and hydrocephalus, in which cerebral swelling makes it difficult or impossible for brain cerebrospinal fluid to circulate. Both conditions, which occur in 1 of every 5,000 to 10,000 births, require immediate attention to prevent long-term problems or death. Stents can overcome blockages. Instruments have been developed to drain fluid from the brain in instances of hydrocephalus.

When surgery is performed to allow fetal lungs to develop normally, the fetus, attached to the mother through the umbilical cord, exists in the most protective environment it is ever likely to know. If corrections are made in the uterus, then the fetal lungs are in the safest possible environment for becoming stronger before they are forced to function on their own.

In cases of obstructive uronopathy (obstruction of the urinary tract), surgery may help injured kidneys to recover and develop. Hypotonic urine found in fetal samples indicates that normal kidney function might be restored and suggests that surgery may permit the affected kidneys to gain strength within the uterus. On the other hand, the presence of isotonic urine in fetal samples indicates kidneys that are too badly compromised to regain normal function. Treatments currently available offer no solution to this problem.

One of the more routine procedures connected with pregnancy is amniocentesis, testing for chromosomal abnormalities through the analysis of amniotic fluid drawn through the abdominal wall of the mother and of blood drawn from the umbilical cord. This procedure is not without risks to mothers and fetuses. It is commonly used, however, because the benefits derived from it are generally thought to outweigh the risks.

Nevertheless, amniocentesis remains a controversial procedure, and major ethical questions surround its use. If the test reveals a chromosomal abnormality, the parents are left with the decision of whether to seek a therapeutic abortion to terminate the pregnancy, which in many jurisdictions would be considered a realistic option. With many such abnormalities, however, the fetus might be delivered alive and, although significantly handicapped, have a life expectancy of many years.

Fetal surgery is indicated when physicians are convinced that a fetus will not survive long enough to be delivered or when it appears certain that the newborn will be unable to survive long after its birth. For example, if it appears through ultrasound that a fetus suffers from a severe kind of congenital diaphragmatic hernia in which the liver is in the chest, then it is obvious that the development of the lungs will be seriously compromised without surgical intervention. Fetal surgery becomes a stopgap measure in such cases to lessen the severity of the problem so that the fetus can grow to term and be delivered, after which corrective surgery outside the uterus can be undertaken. This procedure involves substantial risk, however, because the liver can be destroyed in the process of trying to restore it to its normal position below the diaphragm.

Sometimes ultrasound reveals noncancerous sacrococcygeal tumors. Such tumors, if untreated, can become large enough in a fetus to put a strain on the heart sufficient to cause heart failure. This severely compromises the survival of the fetus. Guided by ultrasound imagery, surgeons can cut off the blood supply to such tumors and starve them before they do irreparable damage to the fetus. When this procedure is used, the destroyed tumor can be removed surgically after birth.

Another growing use of fetal surgery is in cases where spina bifida, usually identified through ultrasound around the sixteenth week of pregnancy, is present. This congenital defect involves a malformation in the vertebral arch, in which the neural tube connected to the brain and the spine is exposed. When this condition is diagnosed and treated early in the development of the fetus, considerable spinal cord function can be preserved. This makes postnatal treatment more effective than it would be were the condition not discovered until after delivery.

There are essentially two major forms of fetal surgery. The more drastic of these involves performing a cesarean section, after which the fetus is carefully removed from the uterus and treated. It is then returned to the uterus, which is closed with sutures. The umbilical cord is not cut, so that the fetus is still receiving oxygen and need not breathe on its own before its lungs have developed sufficiently. This procedure is indicated when some congenital defect, possibly a teratoma (tumor), blocks the airway. Clearing the fetal airway enables the baby to breathe independently upon delivery. The other form of fetal surgery is done without removing the fetus from the uterus and is made possible by the use of laparoscopes and other specialized instruments. This is the preferred method if a choice is offered.

USES AND COMPLICATIONS

As fetal surgery becomes more significant and more common in the treatment and elimination of many threatening prenatal conditions, numerous complications, both ethical and physical, necessarily arise. Any surgery involves risk, and in fetal surgery a dual risk exists: risk to the fetus and risk to the mother. Therefore, physicians who perform fetal surgery have simultaneously as patients both prospective mothers and fetuses. Because fetuses cannot speak for themselves or make their own decisions, fetal surgeons often find themselves in an ethical quagmire. Most physicians hesitate to recommend fetal surgery except in such extreme cases that fetal death or severe disability without such surgery seems inevitable.

Sometimes wrenching decisions must be made about whether to save the life of the mother or the life of the fetus. Questions also arise about whether to allow a fetus to come to term if it is obvious that it will suffer from birth defects that will either severely limit the length of its life or adversely compromise its quality of life, which in some cases may involve a normal life span. Many notable people who suffered from severe birth defects have made significant contributions to society and have led productive and rewarding lives.

One of the more significant uses of fetal surgery is in the treatment of twin-twin transfusion syndrome. In the United States, this syndrome occurs in about one thousand pregnancies each year. Twin-twin transfusion syndrome results in a pair of twins being of unequal size in the fetal state because of abnormal circulation of amniotic fluid between them within the placenta that they share. The larger of the two is surrounded by considerably more amniotic fluid than the smaller one. This disproportion can result in the death of one or both of the fetuses. Attempts can be made to equalize the amniotic fluid by inserting a hollow needle through the mother's abdomen and drawing out excess fluid, a procedure that can threaten the viability of one or both of the fetuses.

Another more sophisticated treatment of twin-twin transfusion syndrome involves inserting a fetoscope into the uterus and using heat from a laser to seal off the blood vessels between the fetuses. This treatment is directed toward separating the circulation between the twins, which accounts for the condition. Regardless of which treatment is employed, the mortality rate is currently quite high in such cases, and premature delivery is a virtual certainty in them. Without intervention, however, these fetuses inevitably die in the uterus.

One of the greatest complications of fetal surgery is premature delivery. Fetuses were once thought to be viable only in the seventh month and beyond. Now the means are available to make survival outside the uterus possible earlier than that, although extraordinary care, attention, and equipment are required for extended periods following the delivery of a baby short of seven months and hospitalization in the neonatal intensive care unit (NICU) may continue for many months following such a birth.

When fetal surgery is performed, the mother is routinely medicated with drugs that will both reduce her pain and substantially decrease the possibility of miscarriage or premature delivery. As the field grows and becomes increasingly sophisticated, many of the current problems that it poses will surely be overcome.

PERSPECTIVE AND PROSPECTS

The development of highly specialized instruments, including fiber-optic telescopes and instruments specially designed to enter the uterus through minute incisions, has made possible the field of fetal surgery. Obstetrical surgeons can now correct life-threatening defects and malformations through the smallest, least invasive of openings while the fetus remains within the protection of the mother's body. This procedure, referred to as fetoscopic surgery, is the method preferred whenever it is possible because it reduces substantially the danger of bringing about premature labor at a time when the fetus cannot breathe on its own.

Because fetal surgery is in its infancy, relatively few surgeons specialize in it and the full range of its uses

and promises has yet to be explored. The two major centers in the United States that have pioneered development in this field are the Children's Hospital in Philadelphia and the University of California Hospital in San Francisco.

Considerable research in fetal surgery is being conducted at both of these institutions and in laboratories and hospitals throughout the country. It is a matter of time before improved technology will exist to eradicate some of the major barriers to more extensive fetal surgery. Surgery of all kinds is becoming less invasive, which reduces considerably the shock that it delivers to patients' bodies, including blood loss and recovery time. Noninvasive fetal surgery is particularly important to ensure the physical welfare of both the fetus and the mother.

—R. Baird Shuman, Ph.D.;
updated by Alexander Sandra, M.D.

See also Abortion; Amniocentesis; Birth defects; Brain disorders; Cesarean section; Chorionic villus sampling; Down syndrome; Embryology; Ethics; Genetic diseases; Genetics and inheritance; Hernia; Hernia repair; Hydrocephalus; Laparoscopy; Miscarriage; Multiple births; Neonatology; Obstetrics; Perinatology; Pregnancy and gestation; Premature birth; Spina bifida; Stillbirth; Teratogens; Ultrasonography; Umbilical cord.

FOR FURTHER INFORMATION:

Barron, S. L., and D. F. Roberts, eds. *Issues in Fetal Medicine: Proceedings of the Twenty-ninth Annual Symposium of the Galton Institute, London, 1992.* New York: St. Martin's Press, 1995. Chapter 7, "Fetal Surgery," by Don K. Nakauyama, and chapter 8, "Fetal Therapy," by Martin J. Whittle, deal directly with matters relating to fetal surgery, clearly outlining the medical problems that it is generally directed toward treating. In chapter 1, "The Galton Lecture for 1992: The Changing Status of the Fetus," Barron also touches briefly on intravenous transfusion and limited exchange transfusion in utero.

Harrison, Michael, et al. *The Unborn Patient: The Art and Science of Fetal Therapy.* 3d ed. Philadelphia: W. B. Saunders, 2001. Deals with correcting hydrocephalus through fetal surgery that results in the reduction of fluid in the brain.

O'Neill, J. A., Jr. "The Fetus as a Patient." *Annals of Surgery* 213 (1991): 277-278. This brief editorial raises cogent ethical concerns surrounding fetal surgery.

Wise, Barbara, et al., eds. *Nursing Care of the General Pediatric Surgical Patient.* Gaithersburg, Md.: Aspen, 2000. Of particular relevance is chapter 9, "Fetal Surgery," by Lori J. Howell, Susan K. Von Nessen, and Kelli M. Burns, which explores the varieties of surgeries generally performed on fetuses.

FETAL TISSUE TRANSPLANTATION

PROCEDURE

ANATOMY OR SYSTEM AFFECTED: Blood, brain, eyes, immune system, nervous system, pancreas, spine

SPECIALTIES AND RELATED FIELDS: Embryology, ethics, immunology, neurology

DEFINITION: The experimental and controversial use of tissue from aborted human fetuses to replace damaged tissue in patients with diseases in which the patient's own tissue has been destroyed (such as Parkinson's disease or diabetes mellitus).

KEY TERMS:

allograft: a transplanted tissue or organ from a genetically different member of the same species as the recipient

autograft: tissue transplanted from one site to another in the same patient

cannula: a narrow tube used in surgery to drain fluid or to deliver cell suspensions for a transplant

fetal: in humans, a term normally referring to the developmental period following eight weeks of gestation; in fetal tissue transplantation, refers to tissue from earlier developmental stages as well

in utero: a Latin term meaning "in the womb"

isograft: a transplanted tissue or organ from a genetically identical individual (identical twin)

Parkinson's disease: a disease in which the dopamine-secreting cells of the midbrain degenerate, resulting in reduced levels of the neurotransmitter dopamine, tremors, uncontrolled and slow movement, and rigidity

stereotaxic computed tomography (CT): a method of imaging using a series of X rays that are compiled by a computer to give a three-dimensional image of internal structures

xenograft: a transplanted tissue or organ obtained from a member of a species different from that of the recipient

INDICATIONS AND PROCEDURES

Advances in technology sometimes catapult a society into ethical arenas that are not yet circumscribed by laws and clear moral boundaries. Fetal tissue transplan-tation is one of these advances. It is a technology that carries the hope of curing a diverse array of severe, often tragic, ailments but one that raises many difficult questions. Tissues from aborted fetuses have been shown in experimental trials to be an excellent source of replacement tissue for patients whose diseases have destroyed their own vital tissues. Parkinson's, Huntington's, and Alzheimer's diseases (in which regions of the brain deteriorate) or juvenile-onset diabetes mellitus (in which insulin-secreting cells of the pancreas degenerate) theoretically could be cured with suitable tissue replacement.

The two sources of tissue used in transplantations, donations from adult cadavers and from aborted fetuses, differ significantly in their suitability. Tissues from cadavers have the severe disadvantage of being immunologically rejected when grafted into anyone who is not an identical twin. The body's surveillance system that protects against infection is designed to attack and destroy any cells that carry molecular markers identifying them as foreign. Patients receiving tissue transplants from other individuals, therefore, will tolerate the tissue graft only if their immune systems are first suppressed with a battery of potent drugs, leaving the patient dangerously unarmed against infection.

Other disadvantages of cadaveric tissues are cell death due to extended postmortem interval (time between individual's death and collection of the tissue) and poor integration into the recipient organ. Porcine xenografts into patients with Parkinson's disease have also been attempted, but they were unsuccessful because of the rejection of the majority of transplanted cells despite aggressive immunosuppression. Taken together, allografts, a transplanted tissue or organ from a genetically different member of the same species, are generally much better tolerated than are xenografts, a transplanted tissue or organ obtained from a member of a species different from that of the recipient. In contrast, isografts, which utilize tissue from a genetically identical twin, are not rejected. Of note is that transplant rejection decreases with the recipient's age, possibly due to immunosenescence and the increased effectiveness of immunosuppressive drugs.

Fetal tissues, however, do not induce a full-scale immune response when transplanted. This is particularly true when cells are transplanted into an organ such as the brain, which is considered an immunologically privileged site along with other locations in the body, such as the anterior chamber of the eye, testis, renal tubule, and uterus. At these sites, the immune response to antigens is reduced and/or not destructive to the transplanted tissue. Nevertheless, transplanted fetal tissues do attract lymphocytes (a type of white blood cell of the immune system) and other immune cells, but the role of this process in graft survival and function is not well understood.

Other properties add to the suitability of fetal tissue for transplantation. Because it is not yet fully differentiated, fetal tissue is said to be very plastic in its abilities to adapt to new locations. Moreover, once placed in a patient, it secretes factors that promote its own growth and those of the new blood vessels at the site. Tissue from an adult source does not have these properties and consequently is slow-growing and poorly vascularized. Though growth factors can be added along with the graft, adult tissue is less responsive to these hormones than is fetal tissue.

It is the source of fetal tissue that has fired such debate over its use for transplantation. Though there has been general acceptance of using tissue from spontaneous abortions or from ectopic pregnancies which, because of their location outside the womb, endanger the life of the mother and must be terminated, these sources are not well suited to transplantation. Spontaneous abortions rarely produce viable tissue, since in most cases the fetus has died two to three weeks before it is expelled. In addition, there are usually major genetic defects in the aborted fetus. In ectopic pregnancies as well, more than 50 percent of the fetuses are genetically abnormal, and most resolve themselves in spontaneous abortion outside a clinic setting. These types of abortions are almost always accompanied by a sense of tragic loss felt by the parents. Many researchers find it unacceptable to request permission from these parents to transplant tissue from the lost fetus.

The alternative source of fetal tissue is elected abortions. One-and-a-half million of these abortions occur in the United States every year. The debate over the ethical correctness of elected abortions has left a cloud of confusion over the issue of using this tissue for transplantation.

When an elective abortion is performed in a clinic, the tissue is removed by suction through a narrow tube. Normally, the tissue would be thrown away. If it is to be used for transplantation, written permission must be obtained from the woman after the abortion is completed. No discussion of transplantation is to take place prior to the abortion, and no alteration in the abortion procedure, except to keep the tissue sterile during collection, is to be made. The donor may not be paid for the tissue, and both the donor and the recipient of the tissue must remain anonymous to each other.

Once collected, the tissue is searched through to locate suitable tissue for transplantation. Although the size of the transplanted tissue varies depending on the type of cell replacement, often only a small block of tissue is used, about eight cubic millimeters (the size of a thin slice of pencil eraser). The tissue is screened for infectious diseases such as hepatitis B and human immunodeficiency virus (HIV). Tissue that is collected is washed a number of times in a sterile solution to ensure that there is no bacterial contamination, and then it is maintained in a sterile, buffered salt solution until it is used. To increase the amount of usable tissue, the tissue may be grown in culture on a nutritive medium under carefully controlled conditions of humidity (95 percent), temperature (37 degrees Celsius), and gas (5 percent carbon dioxide in air) to stimulate normal growing conditions. Preservation of the tissue for long-term storage has been made possible by the highly refined technique of freezing the tissue in liquid nitrogen (cryostorage). Fetal tissue has been kept for as long as ten months in this manner before being used successfully in transplantation. Although the technique should provide methods of maintaining tissue indefinitely, not all types of cells contained in such tissues survive cryopreservation well. For example, despite many attempts to optimize storage conditions, fetal neurons are severely harmed by freezing.

The actual transplantation of the tissue is usually relatively quick and in some cases relatively noninvasive. Often the tissue is injected into the patient as a suspension of individual cells. This permits the use of a small-bore tube called a cannula to deliver the cells to the target organ, thereby avoiding large surgical incisions. Because of modern stereotaxic imaging equipment such as computed tomography (CT) scanning and ultrasound, the physician is able to determine with extreme precision exactly where the cells are to be delivered and can visualize the position of the transplant cannula as the cells are injected. In this way, an entire region of an organ can be seeded with fetal cells. Often the patient is under only a local anesthetic. This aspect of the surgery is especially important when fetal cells are being inserted into the brain, since the physicians can then monitor the patient's ability to speak and move, to ensure that no major damage to the brain is occurring. Usually, antibiotics are given on the day of the transplantation procedure and for two additional days to avoid infection. Although the procedure is relatively safe and recovery is quick—patients often go home in less than three days—transplantation into the central nervous system (CNS) carries risk of hemorrhage (bleeding) and blood clot formation that can damage neurons in the affected area.

Fetal tissue transplantation is still considered an experimental procedure, and further trials are needed to fine-tune the techniques. For example, the precise age of fetal tissue that would be most effective in various cases is uncertain, though it is generally agreed that tissue from a first-trimester fetus is optimal, and six to eight weeks of gestation is most suitable for grafts into brains of Parkinson's sufferers. Often it is not known which patients would respond best to the therapy, but in case of neurotransplantation in Parkinson's disease patients, those with good response to levodopa (L-dopa), a precursor of dopamine, benefit the most. Researchers are also uncertain about whether immunosuppressive drugs should be administered. In animal trials using mice, rats, and monkeys, fetal tissue allografts, but not xenografts, have been well tolerated in the absence of immunosuppression. In humans as well, fetal tissue appears to be readily accepted, with no signs of rejection, and in one study, patients did better without immunosuppression. Some surgeons, however, unwilling to risk tissue rejection, routinely give the transplant patient immunosuppressive drugs, such as cyclosporine and prednisone.

USES AND COMPLICATIONS

The major focus for fetal tissue transplantation has been the treatment of patients with Parkinson's disease, and results have been encouraging. The disease is caused by a deterioration of dopamine-producing regions of the midbrain, the substantia nigra, so named because of the presence of pigmented neurons, which secrete dopamine, in the putamen and caudate nucleus of the basal ganglia. There these neurons send their processes (projecting parts). There is an accompanying loss of motor control causing slowness of movement (bradykinesia), tremors, rigidity, and finally paralysis. Death is most typically a result of accompanying illnesses, such as infections, or caused by the loss of balance and falls. The key drug used to treat the disorder, L-dopa, produces side effects that cause unrelenting and uncontrolled movement of the limbs (dyskinesias) and hallucinations, and the drug loses its effectiveness over time. Advanced patients, who are no longer taking the medication, often remain in a "frozen" state.

A number of patients who have received fetal tissue transplants have shown remarkable improvement and diminished requirements for drug treatment. The first case in the United States to be treated was a man with a twenty-year history of parkinsonian symptoms. He had frequent freezing spells, could not walk without a cane, and suffered from chronic constipation. He also was unable to whistle, a beloved hobby of his. He was operated on by Curt R. Freed and his associates in 1988. Following the operation, initial improvement was slow, but within a year, he was walking without a cane, his speed of movement had considerably improved, and his constipation had resolved itself. He also had regained his ability to whistle. Even after four years, improvements continued. Such results have occurred with many parkinsonian patients receiving fetal tissue transplants.

Beneficial effects of transplants have also been obtained in patients with induced Parkinson-like symptoms. In 1982, some intravenous drug users developed Parkinson-like symptoms after using a homemade preparation of "synthetic heroin" that was contaminated with 1-methyl-4-phenyl-1,2,5,6-tetrahydropyridine (MPTP). MPTP destroys dopamine-secreting cells of the substantia nigra. Two of these patients received fetal tissue transplants in Sweden. Within a year after their operation, they were able to walk with a normal gait, resume chores, and be virtually free of their previously uncontrollable movements.

Because no patient with Parkinson's disease or with Parkinson-like symptoms has yet been cured by a fetal tissue transplant, some have considered the results of such experiments to be disappointing. The expectation of complete cures from a technique that is still in its early experimental phase, however, is overly optimistic. Many patients themselves are encouraged, and many have resumed driving and the other tasks of normal daily life. Altogether, more than two hundred patients with Parkinson's disease have received fetal tissue transplants worldwide. It is important to note that fetal tissue transplants are not stem cell transplants, or grafts of tissue produced from stem cells. Coincidentally, fetal tissue usually contains some stem cells, but the transplant effects are thought to be mostly mediated by the mature or maturing cells in the donor tissue (dopamine neurons or pancreatic beta cells, for example).

That transplanted fetal brain tissue can replace damaged brain tissue to any extent has opened the doors of hope for many diseases. For example, Huntington's disease, a genetic disorder that destroys a different set of neurons but in the same region as that affected by parkinsonism, brings a slow death to those carrying the dominant trait. Its severe dementia and uncontrollable jerking and writhing that steadily progress have had no treatment and no cure. In animal studies in which fetal brain tissue was transplanted into rats with symptoms mimicking Huntington's disease, results have been encouraging enough to warrant human trials, and one human trial, reported by a surgeon in Mexico, has shown limited success. Another such study is ongoing in France. Researchers are hopeful, though less optimistic, that Alzheimer's disease, a form of dementia that is characterized by neuronal death within the brain, also may be treatable with fetal tissue transplants. Because the destruction is so widespread, however, it is difficult to determine where the transplants should be placed.

Type 1 insulin-dependent diabetes, often called juvenile-onset diabetes, also has been treated with fetal tissue transplants. More than a million people in the United States suffer from this disease caused by the destruction of pancreatic beta cells, the insulin-secreting cells that regulate sugar metabolism. Though the disease can be controlled with regular insulin shots, the long-term effects of diabetes can lead to blindness, premature aging, and renal and circulatory problems. After animal tests showed a complete reversal of the disease when fetal pancreatic tissue was transplanted into diabetic rats, human trials were initiated with great expectations. Though complete success has not been achieved, the sixteen diabetic patients who were given fetal pancreatic tissue transplants by Kevin Lafferty between 1987 and 1992 all showed significant drops in the amount of insulin needed to manage their disease. The transplanted tissue continued to pump out insulin.

An unusual variation of such procedures has been to transplant fetal tissue into fetuses diagnosed with severe metabolic diseases. It is more effective to treat the condition while the fetus is still in the womb than to wait until after birth, when damage from the disease may already be extensive. Fetuses with Hurler's syndrome and similar "storage" diseases have been treated in this way. Hurler's syndrome is a lethal condition in which tissues become clogged with stored mucopolysaccharides, long-chain sugars that the body is unable to break down because it lacks the appropriate enzyme. One of the fetuses to receive this treatment was the child of a couple who had lost two children to the disease. With the transplanted tissue, the child lived and by one year of age was producing therapeutic levels of the enzyme. It has been estimated that there are at least 155 other genetic disorders that could be similarly treated by fetal tissue transplants in utero.

The list of ailments that fetal tissue transplants may alleviate includes some of the major concerns of modern medicine. In addition to those already mentioned are macular degeneration, sickle cell disease, thalassemias, metabolic disorders, immune deficiencies, myelin disorders, and spinal cord injuries. In interpreting the value of these applications, however, it is important to separate the politics of abortion from the medical issue of fetal tissue transplantation.

PERSPECTIVE AND PROSPECTS

Though controversy surrounds the use of fetal tissue for transplantation, such controversy has not included all facets of fetal tissue research. Indeed, fetal cells were used in the 1950's to develop the Salk polio vaccine and later the vaccine against rubella (German measles). With the scourge of acquired immunodeficiency syndrome (AIDS), in the 1990's fetal cells were first used to help design treatments against the AIDS virus. Even the early attempts at fetal tissue transplantation occurred quietly. Reports date as far back as 1928, when Italian surgeons attempted unsuccessfully to cure a patient with diabetes using fetal pancreatic tissue, a procedure repeated, again unsuccessfully, in the United States in 1939. In 1959, American physicians tried to cure leukemia with fetal tissue transplants, but again without success.

The first real indicator that such techniques might work came in 1968, when fetal liver cells were used to treat a patient with DiGeorge syndrome. The success of this procedure resulted in its becoming the accepted treatment for this usually fatal genetic disorder, which results from a deletion of a part of chromosome 22. Because many of the DiGeorge patients are athymic (fail to develop a thymus), they lack T cells, making them immunodeficient. Because the fetal liver supports hematopoiesis (the production of blood cells, including immune cells) during development, fetal liver cells have some value in the treatment of immunodeficiency. However, fetal thymus transplantation can promote more complete immune system reconstitution and is now used as a treatment in athymic patients.

Because suitable fetal tissues are often very difficult to obtain, recently the focus on donor cells for transplantation has shifted toward stem cell-derived cells. Stem cells can be relatively easily expanded in numbers in culture and have the potential to generate a large supply of different cell types for transplantation, thereby averting some of the issues that have decelerated the field of fetal transplantation. Donor cells differentiated from one's own stem cells could be used in an autograft and thereby circumvent both immunological and ethical issues. Studies to explore the potential of such technologies are ongoing. Thus the next chapter in the fetal tissue transplantation story may involve the fast-evolving fields of stem cell research and regenerative medicine.

It was not until 1987 that ethical issues over fetal tissue transplants truly surfaced in the United States. Debate was precipitated when the director of the National Institutes of Health (NIH) submitted a request to the Department of Health and Human Services to transplant fetal tissue into patients with Parkinson's disease. Rather than receiving approval, the request was tabled, pending a thorough study of the issue by an NIH panel on fetal tissue transplantation. The panel made a detailed report on the ethical, legal, and scientific implications of fetal tissue transplantation, concluding that it was acceptable public policy. Despite the report, however, the Secretary of Health and Human Services instituted a ban against the use of government funds for transplanting fetal tissue derived from elective abortions. While in effect, the ban influenced private funding as well. Physicians who performed fetal tissue transplants, unable to obtain grant money, were forced to charge their patients—a bill that could reach as high as forty thousand dollars per transplant. President Bill Clinton's lifting of the ban in 1993, on his third day in office, paved the way for research advances, including isolating and propagating human stem cells. The opposition of Clinton's successor, George W. Bush, to the use of fetal tissue and stem cells for scientific purposes led to several legislative battles and cast some doubts on the future of this field. President Barack Obama restored the use of government funds for stem cell research upon taking office in 2009.

The debates over fetal tissue transplantation are far from over. Though a strict set of guidelines are in place concerning the procurement of fetal tissue, ensuring that the needs never influence decisions concerning abortion, other issues have not been addressed. Some ask whether a fetal tissue bank should be established and, if so, whether it should be government-funded to avoid commercialization. As technology continues to create increasingly complicated ethical issues, society's responsibility increases, as does its need to be scientifically informed.

—Mary S. Tyler, Ph.D.;
updated by W. Michael Zawada, Ph.D.

See also Abortion; Alzheimer's disease; Brain; Brain disorders; Diabetes mellitus; Ethics; Genetic diseases; Genetic engineering; Neurology; Pancreas; Parkinson's disease; Stem cells; Transplantation.

FOR FURTHER INFORMATION:

Beardsley, Tim. "Aborting Research." *Scientific American* 267, no. 2 (August, 1992): 17-18. An excellent encapsulation of the debate over fetal tissue transplantation and the instances in which it has been used.

Beauchamp, Tom, and James F. Childress. *Principles of Biomedical Ethics.* 6th ed. New York: Oxford University Press, 2009. A classic text that introduces the field of ethics, its theories, and their application to biomedical issues and presents ten cases covering a wide range of issues in biomedical ethics, some of which have led to landmark decisions.

Begley, Sharon. "From Human Embryos, Hope for 'Spare Parts.'" *Newsweek*, November 16, 1998, 73. Researchers have teased out clumps of cells from human embryos and induced them to burst into a veritable cellular symphony, forming most of the 210 kinds of cells that constitute the human body. These colonies could revolutionize transplantation medicine.

Brundin, Patrik, and C. Warren Olanow, eds. *Restorative Therapies in Parkinson's Disease.* New York: Springer, 2006. Covers in depth the ethical, clinical, and scientific issues surrounding neural grafting in Parkinson's disease and prospects for the future use of stem cell-derived grafts. The book is appropriate for clinicians, scientists, and anyone interested in restorative therapies for the brain.

Clinical Trials. http://www.clinicaltrials.gov. A Web site of the National Institutes of Health (NIH) and the National Library of Medicine that provides information on current and completed federally and privately supported clinical trials in human volunteers. The purposes of the research, as well as details on how to participate, are included.

"Fetal Cell Study Shows Promise for Parkinson's." *Los Angeles Times*, April 22, 1999, p. 29. The first federally funded trial to study the effectiveness of fetal cell transplants for Parkinson's disease has proved that it works for some patients, mainly those under the age of sixty.

Freed, Curt R., Robert Breeze, and Neil Rosenberg. "Transplantation of Human Fetal Dopamine Cells for Parkinson's Disease." *Archives of Neurology* 47, no. 5 (May 1, 1990): 505-512. A historically important paper describing the techniques used by Freed, an American doctor who has been a pioneer in the technique of fetal tissue transplantation. Though written for a medical audience, most of the paper is readily understandable to a lay audience.

Freed, Curt R., and Simon LeVay. *Healing the Brain: A Doctor's Controversial Quest for a Cell Therapy to Cure Parkinson's Disease.* New York: Times Books/ Henry Holt, 2002. A thrilling story about the development of a new cell transplantation therapy for Parkinson's disease and the controversies surrounding it. A must read for anyone interested in cell replacement therapies.

Holland, Suzanne, Karen Lebacqz, and Laurie Zoloth, eds. *The Human Embryonic Stem Cell Debate: Science, Ethics, and Public Policy.* Cambridge, Mass.: MIT Press, 2001. Tackles difficult questions such as the nature of human life, the limits of intervention into human cells and tissues, who should approve controversial research, and what constitutes human dignity, respect, and justice.

Lindvall, Olle, Patrik Brundin, and Håkan Widner. "Grafts of Fetal Dopamine Neurons Survive and Improve Motor Function in Parkinson's Disease." *Science* 247 (February 2, 1990): 574-577. A landmark reference describing the technique of a group of physicians led by Lindvall of Sweden. This and the paper by Freed's group encompass the extent of variation in the technique, and the degrees of success.

Marshak, Daniel R., Richard L. Gardner, and David Gottlieb, eds. *Stem Cell Biology.* Cold Springs Harbor, N.Y.: Cold Springs Harbor Press, 2002. An excellent, multidisciplinary examination of advances in the field and their impact on medicine and science.

Singer, Peter, et al., eds. *Embryo Experimentation.* New York: Cambridge University Press, 1993. This text provides an excellent discussion of the moral questions raised by the use of fetal tissue for transplantation.

U.S. Congress. Senate. Committee on Labor and Human Resources. *Finding Medical Cures: The Promise of Fetal Tissue Transplantation Research.* 102d Congress, 1st session, 1992. Senate Report 1902. A surprisingly readable and gripping set of testimonies from physicians, interest groups, and citizens concerning the debate over the use of fetal tissue for transplantations.

Wade, Nicholas. "Primordial Cells Fuel Debate on Ethics." *The New York Times*, November 10, 1998, p. 1.

Two groups of scientists, one led by James A. Thomson of the University of Wisconsin at Madison and the other led by John D. Gearhart of Johns Hopkins University in Baltimore, have reported success in the attempt to grow primordial human cells outside the body.

FEVER
DISEASE/DISORDER
ANATOMY OR SYSTEM AFFECTED: All

SPECIALTIES AND RELATED FIELDS: Family medicine, internal medicine, pediatrics, virology

DEFINITION: A symptom associated with a variety of diseases and disorders, characterized by body temperature above normal (98.6 degrees Fahrenheit, or 37 degrees centigrade or Celsius); considered very serious at 104 degrees Fahrenheit (40 degrees Celsius) and higher.

KEY TERMS:

antipyretic drugs: drugs that are employed to reduce fevers, such as sodium salicylate, indomethacin, and acetaminophen

ectotherms: organisms that rely on external temperature conditions in order to maintain their internal temperature

endotherms: organisms that control the internal temperature of their bodies by the conversion of calories to heat

febrile response: an upward adjustment of the thermoregulatory set point

metabolic rate: a measurement of the Calories (kilocalories) that are converted into heat energy in order to maintain body temperature and/or for physical exertion

pyrogens: protein substances that appear at the outset of the process that leads to a fever reaction

thermoregulatory set point: the ultimate neural control that maintains the human internal body temperature at 37 degrees Celsius and can either raise or lower it

CAUSES AND SYMPTOMS

Although the symptoms that often accompany a fever are familiar to everyone—shivering, sweating, thirst, hot skin, and a flushed face—what causes fever and its function during illness are not fully clear even among medical specialists. Considerable literature exists on the differences between warm-blooded organisms (endotherms) and cold-blooded organisms (ectotherms) in what is called the normal state, when no symptoms of disease are present. Cold-blooded organisms depend

INFORMATION ON FEVER

CAUSES: Infection, various diseases
SYMPTOMS: Shivering, sweating, thirst, hot skin, flushed face
DURATION: Acute
TREATMENTS: Medication, comfort measures (e.g., cool compress), rest

on temperature conditions in their external environment to maintain various levels of temperature within their bodies. These fluctuations correspond to the various levels of activity that they need to sustain at given moments. Thus, reptiles, for example, may "recharge" themselves internally by moving into the warmth of the sun. Warm-blooded organisms, on the other hand, including all mammals, utilize energy released from the digestion of food to maintain a constant level of heat within their bodies. This level—a "normal" temperature—is approximately 37 degrees Celsius (98.6 degrees Fahrenheit) in humans. An internal body temperature that rises above this level is called a febrile temperature, or a fever.

If the temperature in the surrounding environment is low, warm-blooded organisms must raise their metabolic rate (a measurement, in Calories, of converted energy) accordingly to maintain a normal internal body temperature. In humans, this rate of energy expenditure is about 1,800 Calories per day. If insufficient food is taken in to supply the necessary potential energy for this metabolic conversion into heat, the body will draw on its storage resource—fat—to fulfill this vital need. The potentially fatal condition called hypothermia, in which the body is too fatigued to maintain metabolic functions or has exhausted all of its stores of Calories, occurs when the internal temperature falls below normal. Although cold-blooded animals must also protect themselves against the danger that their body heat may fall too low to sustain life functions, they can support adjustments in their own internal temperature down to about 20 degrees Celsius. At the same time, metabolic expenditures, as measured in Calories, are very low in cold-blooded animals; for example, alligators must expend only 60 Calories per day to create the same amount of heat as 1,800 Calories per day in warm-blooded humans.

The question of internal temperature in warm-blooded animals is closely tied to management efficiency in the body. This function becomes critical

when one considers abnormally high internal temperature, or fever. Generally speaking, all essential biochemical functions in the human body can be carried out at optimal levels of efficiency at the set point of 37 degrees Celsius. In the simplest of terms, any increase or decrease in temperature creates either more or less kinetic energy and has the potential to affect the chemistry of all body functions.

Endotherms are able to tolerate a certain range of involuntary change in their internal body temperature (brought about by disease or illness), but there is an upper limit of 45 degrees Celsius, which constitutes a high fever. If the self-regulating higher set point associated with fever goes beyond this point, destructive biochemical phenomena will occur in the body—in particular, a breaking down of protein molecules. If these phenomena are not checked, they can bring about death.

Modern scientific approaches to the internal body processes that lead to fever, like a medical discussion of the effects that occur once fever is operating in the body, are much more complicated. They revolve around the concept of a change in the set point monitored in the brain. When this change in the brain's normal (37 degree) thermostatic signal is called for, a process called phagocytosis begins, leading to a higher internal body heat level throughout the organism.

Phagocytosis, the ingestion of a solid substance (especially foreign material such as invading bacteria), involves the appearance in the host's system of large numbers of leukocyte cells. When these cells ingest the bacteria, small quantities of protein called leukocytic pyrogens are produced. According to most modern theories, these protein pyrogens trigger the biochemical reactions in the brain that alter the body's temperature set point. After this point, changes that occur throughout the system and raise the body's internal temperature depend on a component of the bacterial cell wall called endotoxin. By the end of the 1960's, researchers had drawn attention to at least twenty effects that activated endotoxins may have on the host organism. Key effects include enhancement of the production of new white blood cells (leukocytosis), enhancement of various forms of immunological resistance, reduction of serum iron levels, and lowering of blood pressure.

Most, if not all, of these effects brought about by endotoxins are accompanied by higher levels of heat throughout the body, the definition of fever. Closer biochemical examination of the source of the added heat yielded the suggestion, made by P. B. Beeson in 1948, that the host's endotoxin-affected cells begin to pro-

Effects of Fever

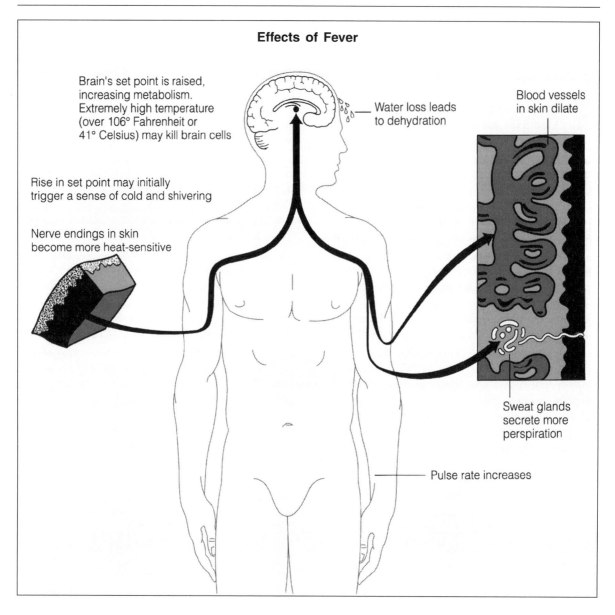

Brain's set point is raised, increasing metabolism. Extremely high temperature (over 106° Fahrenheit or 41° Celsius) may kill brain cells

Rise in set point may initially trigger a sense of cold and shivering

Nerve endings in skin become more heat-sensitive

Water loss leads to dehydration

Blood vessels in skin dilate

Sweat glands secrete more perspiration

Pulse rate increases

duce a distinct form of protein, now called endogenous pyrogens. Pyrogens are thought to induce the first stage of fever by interacting with cells in tissues very close to the brain, specifically in the brain stem itself. Laboratory experiments in the first half of the twentieth century allowed researchers to produce almost immediate fever reactions when they injected pyrogen protein material into rabbits. Studies of the induced febrile state in laboratory animals, and therefore presumably also in humans, linked fever to immunological (virus-resistant and bacteria-resistant) reactions, not necessarily in the initially affected tissues around the brain but in various places throughout the organism.

Although scientific research has produced many hypotheses concerning the origins of fever in the body, experts admit that the process is not well understood. Matthew J. Kluger, in *Fever: Its Biology, Evolution, and Function* (1979), claims that "the precise mechanism behind endogenous pyrogens' effect on the thermoregulatory set-point is unknown."

TREATMENT AND THERAPY

The febrile response has been noted in five of the seven extant classes of vertebrates on earth (Agnatha, such as lampreys, and Chondrichthyes, such as sharks, are excluded). Scientists have determined that its function as a reaction to bacterial infection can be traced back as far as 400 million years in primitive bony fishes. The question of whether the natural phenomenon of fever actually aids in combating disease in the body, however, has not been fully resolved.

In ancient and medieval times, it was believed that fever served to "cook" and separate out one of the four essential body "humors"—blood, phlegm, yellow bile, and black bile—that had become excessively dominant. Throughout the centuries, such beliefs even caused some physicians to try to induce higher internal body temperatures as a means of treating disease. Use of modern antipyretic drugs to reduce fever remained unthinkable until the nineteenth century.

It was the German physician Carl von Liebermeister who, by the end of the nineteenth century, set some of the guidelines that are still generally observed in deciding whether antipyretic drugs should or should not be used to reduce a naturally occurring fever during illness. Liebermeister insisted that the phenomenon of fever was not one of body temperature gone "out of control" but rather a sign that the organism was regulating its own temperature. He also demonstrated that part of the process leading to increased internal temperature could be seen in reactions that actually reduce heat loss at the body's surface, notably decreases in skin blood flow and evaporative cooling through perspiration. Liebermeister determined that one of the positive effects of higher temperatures inside the body was to impede the growth of harmful microorganisms. At the same time, however, other side effects of fever during illness were deemed to be negative, such as loss of appetite and, in some cases, actual degeneration of key internal organs. Liebermeister's generation of physicians, therefore, tended to rely on antipyretic drugs only when high fevers persisted for long periods of time. Moderate fevers or even high fevers, if they did not continue too long, were deemed to contribute to the overall process of natural body resistance to disease.

In fact, a limited school of physicians followed the teaching of 1927 Nobel laureate Julius Wagner-Jauregg, who claimed that "fever therapy" methods should be adopted for the treatment of certain diseases. Wagner-Jauregg himself had pioneered this theory by inoculating victims of neurosyphilis with fever-producing malaria. Part of his argument in favor of this experimental therapy was that malaria, with its accompanying fever, was a treatable disease (through the use of quinine) and could be controlled at regular intervals

during its "service" as a fighter against a disease that still had no known cure. Later use of fever therapy for treatment of other sexually transmitted diseases, specifically gonorrhea, proved to be moderately successful. When typhoid vaccine was used to induce fevers in some patients, however, side effects such as hypotension (low blood pressure) or cardiovascular shock introduced what some considered to be dangerous risk factors. Nevertheless, certain fields of medicine, especially those involved with eye diseases and related eye ailments, have proved that fever-inducing agents (specifically those contained in typhoid and typhoid-paratyphoid vaccines) also induce beneficial secretion of the anti-inflammatory hormone cortisol.

By the second half of the twentieth century, the medical use of antipyretic drugs, containing such components as salicylates and indomethacin, had become widespread. This phenomenon was not caused by any compelling reversal of earlier general assumptions that moderate levels of fever, being a natural body reaction, were not necessarily harmful to patients suffering from a wide variety of diseases. Rather, physicians may have opted to use such drugs as much for their pain-relieving qualities as for their fever-reducing characteristics. Although patients receiving such drug treatment notice a diminishing of severe pains or general aching, the cause of the disease has not been combated merely by the removal of such symptoms as fever and pain.

Modern medical science has tended to support further study of particular circumstances in which induced fevers can actually produce disease-combating reactions. A newly emerging field by the late 1970's, for example, involved studying the benefits of higher temperatures in newborn infants fighting viral infections. Although specific circumstances and the nature of disease prevent a generalized conclusion in terms of the use of induced fevers as a form of treatment, researchers have shown that an elevated body temperature serves to increase the speed at which white blood cells, the body's natural enemies against disease, move to infected areas.

PERSPECTIVE AND PROSPECTS

Although doctors have been aware of the symptoms of fever since the beginnings of medical history, centuries passed before its importance as an indicator of disease was accepted. A certain degree of sophistication in the study of fevers became possible largely as a result of the development of the common thermometer, in a rudimentary form in the seventeenth century and then with greater technical accuracy in the eighteenth century. Systematic use of the thermometer in the eighteenth century enabled doctors to observe such phenomena as morning remission and evening peaking of fever intensity. Studies involving the recording of temperature in healthy individuals also yielded important discoveries. One such discovery was made in 1774, when use of the thermometer showed that, even in a room heated to the boiling point of water (100 degrees Celsius), healthy subjects maintained an internal body heat that was very close to the normal 37-degree level.

Medical reports as late as the end of the eighteenth century, however, indicate that even internationally recognized pioneers of science were still not close to understanding the causes of fever. The English doctor John Hunter, for example, declared himself opposed to the prevailing view that rising body heat came from the circulation of warmer blood throughout the body. Hunter suspected that the warmth was produced by an entirely different agent that was independent of the circulatory system. He never learned what that agent might be, however, and failed in defense of his theory that the source of added body heat was in the stomach. Even the famous French chemist Antoine-Laurent Lavoisier erred when he tried to explain fever in terms of some form of chemical "combustion" involving hydrogen and carbon. Lavoisier identified the lungs as the possible location for this spontaneous production of internal body heat.

Although these theories were identified as erroneous, the late eighteenth and early nineteenth centuries left one legacy that would develop into the twentieth century and is still practiced by physicians: systematic thermometry. In essence, thermometry involves the tracing of the upward or downward direction of fever during illness in order to judge the course of the disease and the effects brought about by different stages of treatment. In many diseases, for example, clinical records of the full course of previous cases can be studied by doctors responsible for treating an individual patient. With thermometry, the doctor is able to determine how far the body's struggle against a certain disease has progressed. If thermometry shows a marked departure from what clinical records have charted as the normal course of disease under certain forms of treatment, then the physician may look for signs of another disease.

—Byron D. Cannon, Ph.D.

See also Avian influenza; Bacterial infections; Common cold; Heat exhaustion and heatstroke; Hyperthermia and hypothermia; Influenza; Kawasaki disease;

Reye's syndrome; Rheumatic fever; Scarlet fever; Sweating; Typhoid fever; Typhus; Viral infections; Yellow fever; *other specific diseases.*

FOR FURTHER INFORMATION:

Kemper, Kathi J. *The Holistic Pediatrician: A Pediatrician's Comprehensive Guide to Safe and Effective Therapies for the Twenty-five Most Common Ailments of Infants, Children, and Adolescents.* Rev. ed. New York: Quill, 2002. Integrates mainstream and alternative medicine to aid parents in dealing with the most common childhood health problems such as fever, diaper rash, ear infections, and allergies.

Kluger, Matthew J. *Fever: Its Biology, Evolution, and Function.* Princeton, N.J.: Princeton University Press, 1979. An accessible book-length study of the phenomenon of fever. Although some parts of the discussion are more technical in nature, the general level is comprehensible.

Kluger, Matthew J., Tamas Bartfai, and Charles A. Dinarello, eds. *Molecular Mechanisms of Fever.* New York: New York Academy of Sciences, 1998. The authors place major emphasis on advances using molecular tools such as cytokine knockout mice, cloned cytokines, descriptions of molecular pathways for signal transduction, and heat shock proteins.

Litin, Scott C., ed. *Mayo Clinic Family Health Book.* 4th ed. New York: HarperResource, 2009. Perhaps the best general medical text for the layperson, this book covers the entire medical field. While the information is derived from a wide variety of highly technical sources, the articles are written to be easily understood by a general audience.

Mackowiak, Philip A., ed. *Fever: Basic Mechanisms and Management.* 2d ed. Philadelphia: Lippincott-Raven, 1997. This text explains the physiology behind fever and addresses ways to treat it. Includes a bibliography and an index.

Nathanson, Laura Walther. *The Portable Pediatrician: A Practicing Pediatrician's Guide to Your Child's Growth, Development, Health, and Behavior from Birth to Age Five.* 2d ed. New York: HarperCollins, 2002. An engaging, easy-to-read guide for parents to assess their child's development, medical symptoms, and behavioral problems.

FIBER
BIOLOGY
ANATOMY OR SYSTEM AFFECTED: Gastrointestinal system, intestines

SPECIALTIES AND RELATED FIELDS: Alternative medicine, family practice, gastroenterology, geriatrics and gerontology, internal medicine, nursing, nutrition, preventive medicine, sports medicine

DEFINITION: Plant fiber components include hemicelluloses and pectin and are long, threadlike structures. Animal fiber is composed of protein collagen or segments of loose connective tissue in skin and organ tissue.

STRUCTURE AND FUNCTIONS

Dietary fiber helps regulate the passage of food material through the gastrointestinal tract and influences absorption of various nutrients. It represents the content of substances that cannot be broken down by human digestive enzymes or absorbed by the gastrointestinal tract. Nearly all dietary fiber content is contributed by the insoluble structural matter of plants. Cellulose is an insoluble unbranched glucose polymer that can absorb relatively large volumes of water. Hemicellulose is the name for a wide variety of polymers of five carbon sugars. Pectin is a water-soluble polymer that forms gels and binds water, cations, and bile acids. Gums and mucilages are highly branched polysaccharides that form gels and bind water and other organic material. Increased fiber intake may promote health by promoting normal elimination of waste products of digestion, by promoting satiety, by helping control serum cholesterol, and by other mechanisms. Greatly increased fiber intake, however, may reduce absorption of some nutrients.

DISORDERS AND DISEASES

The ingestion of too much fiber can result in the formation of an obstructing bolus in a narrowed intestinal or esophageal lumen. The purpose of a low-fiber or fiber-restricted diet is to help prevent this occurrence and to rest the gastrointestinal tract. In acute phases of ulcerative colitis, a fiber-restricted diet lessens the pain and stress of defecation by decreasing the weight and bulk of the stool and delaying intestinal transit time.

A low-fiber diet contains approximately 2 grams of crude fiber. Foods included are refined bread and cereal products, cooked fruits and vegetables that are low in fiber, and juices. Nuts, legumes, and whole-grain bread and cereal products are restricted. Minimal-fiber diets consist of strained fruit and vegetable juices and white potatoes without skins. Milk is limited to two cups per day, as it indirectly contributes to fecal residue even though it contains no fiber. Continued use of a low-

fiber diet in refined carbohydrates, however, is believed to cause diverticular disease of the colon. Reduced bulk causes the colonic lumen to narrow.

A high-fiber diet contains increased amounts of foods containing cellulose, hemicelluloses, lignin, and pectin and reduced amounts of refined carbohydrates. Insoluble fibers increase volume and weight of the residue to maintain the normal size of the colonic lumen and increase gastrointestinal mobility. Soluble fibers, such as gums and pectins, reduce the rate of intestinal absorption, altering the metabolic effects. High-fiber intake necessitates increased fluids.

Certain individuals should not be encouraged to increase the amount of fiber in their diet. Those who have had gastric surgery, vagotomy, pyloroplasty or Roux-en-Y and some diabetics with gastroparesis diabeticorum have less acid secretion or decreased gastrointestinal motility and may encounter bezoar formation, a compacted mass that does not pass into the intestine. The high-fiber diet has been recommended, however, in the treatment or prevention of dumping syndrome, hyperlipidemia, gallstones, diabetes, and many other diseases and disorders.

—Jane C. Norman, Ph.D., R.N., C.N.E.

See also Carbohydrates; Colitis; Constipation; Diarrhea and dysentery; Dietary reference intakes (DRIs); Digestion; Enzymes; Food biochemistry; Food Guide Pyramid; Gastroenterology; Gastroenterology, pediatric; Gastrointestinal disorders; Gastrointestinal system; Gluten intolerance; Malabsorption; Metabolism; Nutrition; Peristalsis; Phytonutrients; Protein.

FOR FURTHER INFORMATION:

Dudek, Susan G. *Nutrition Essentials for Nursing Practice.* Philadelphia: Lippincott, Williams and Wilkins, 2006.

Kirschmann, John D. *Nutrition Almanac.* New York: McGraw-Hill, 2006.

Nix, Staci. *Williams' Basic Nutrition and Diet Therapy.* New York: Elsevier Health Sciences, 2008.

Sizer, Frances. *Nutrition: Concepts and Controversies.* New York: Cengage Learning, 2007.

Whitney, Eleanor Noss. *Understanding Nutrition with Nutrition Explorer.* New York: Cengage Learning, 2007.

FIBROCYSTIC BREAST CONDITION
DISEASE/DISORDER

ALSO KNOWN AS: Fibrocyctic breast changes, benign breast disease, benign breast lesions, diffuse cystic mastopathy, mammary dysplasia, nonmalignant breast neoplasms

ANATOMY OR SYSTEM AFFECTED: Breasts, endocrine system, skin

SPECIALTIES AND RELATED FIELDS: Gynecology, histopathology, oncology

DEFINITION: The most common type of noncancerous breast condition, affecting approximately 60 percent of all women, the majority of whom are premenopausal. Because of its widespread incidence, the condition is now considered to be a normal physiologic variant. It is characterized by stromal tissue and glandular (lobules and ducts) changes in the breast or breasts that result in lumpiness, thickening, and localized edema (swelling).

KEY TERMS:

collecting duct: a tubular canal that transports milk from the milk duct to the nipple

lobule: a small gland that, when sent appropriate hormonal cues, produces milk

mammary gland: a group of milk-producing cells consisting of lobules and ducts

milk duct: a tubular canal that transports milk from the lobule to the collecting duct

stroma: the deeper layer of breast tissue

CAUSES AND SYMPTOMS

Fibrocystic breast change is the most common type of noncancerous breast condition. Its incidence rate in females is estimated to be more than 60 percent. Therefore, although once classified as a disease, it is now considered to be a normal physiologic variant. It occurs more commonly in females between the ages of thirty and fifty. Its cause is hypothesized to be an excess of circulating estrogen.

Female breast development begins at puberty, triggered by an increase in estrogen level. The four main components of the mature female breast are adipose tissue (fat), ducts (milk ducts and collecting ducts), groups of lobules (referred to as lobes), and connective tissue consisting of a matrix of suspensory ligaments (strong fibrous bands). Each breast contains approximately fifteen to twenty lobes that radiate from the nipple area in a spokelike pattern, with the highest distribution being in the upper outer quadrant of each breast. Breast lobe consistency tends to be firm and slightly nodular, but may vary by breast or by individual, while breast fat is almost always soft. Breasts of younger women primarily consist of glandular tissue. Aging changes result in shrinkage of glandular tissue and re-

placement with fat, which causes the breast to become softer and less well supported.

Symptoms of fibrocystic breast change result from hormone-induced alterations in the stromal (deeper layer) tissue, glands (lobules) and ducts within the breast. Those changes include possible fibrosis (formation of fibrous tissue like that of scar tissue) and/or formation of cysts, as fluid accumulates inside the glands. Small amounts of accumulated fluid result in microscopic cysts (microcysts); larger amounts of accumulated fluid result in palpable macrocysts that may grow to an inch or more in size. The two major types of breast cysts are type I, characterized by high concentrations of androgen and estrogen conjugates, epidermal growth factor, and potassium and low concentrations of sodium and chloride; and type II, characterized by high concentrations of sodium and chloride and lower concentrations of androgen and estrogen conjugates, epidermal growth factor, and potassium.

Symptoms of fibrocystic breast change include dense and irregular lumpiness in breast tissue, discomfort, dull pain, localized edema (swelling) and feeling of fullness, tenderness, and possible nipple discharge. Symptoms may vary in intensity throughout the menstrual cycle, peak just prior to menstruation, and range from mild to severe. Symptoms and signs of fibrocystic change may remit after menopause because of decreased amounts of glandular tissue in the breast and decreased levels of estrogen and progesterone.

TREATMENT AND THERAPY

Treatment is not for the condition itself but rather for the symptoms. For those women who are asymptomatic, no treatment beyond monitoring via breast self-

---

INFORMATION ON FIBROCYSTIC BREAST CONDITION

CAUSES: Possibly hormonal variations during the menstrual cycle; excess amount of circulating estrogen

SYMPTOMS: Dense, irregular lumpiness in breast tissue, discomfort and tenderness, dull pain, localized edema (swelling), feeling of fullness, possible nipple discharge

DURATION: Varies; usually cyclic

TREATMENTS: Symptom dependent, from breast self-examination and properly fitting support bra to hormone therapy

examination is required. For those women who are symptomatic, treatment options range from use of a properly fitting support bra to use of hormone therapy—via oral contraceptives, androgens, or tamoxifen (a drug that blocks estrogen activity)—which has the potential to cause side effects. Cysts may require fine needle aspiration or ultrasonogrphy to determine whether a biopsy is needed.

Anecdotal evidence suggests that avoidance of methylxanthine-containing items such as coffee, tea, chocolate, and certain sodas; reduction in sodium intake; use of vitamin supplements; and/or use of herbal supplements may ameliorate symptoms caused by fibrocystic changes. However, these findings have not been clinically proven.

PERSPECTIVE AND PROSPECTS

The preferred term for fibrocystic breast disease is now "fibrocystic breast changes" or "fibrocystic breast condition." It may also be referred to as benign breast disease, benign breast lesions, diffuse cystic mastopathy, mammary dysplasia, or nonmalignant breast neoplasms. Cohort studies of risk factors associated with this condition have been conducted for up to thirty years. A family history of fibrocystic breast condition is believed to be the highest risk factor. Consumption of a high-fat diet may be a cofactor. No association has been found between incidence rate of this condition and alcohol consumption or cigarette smoking.

Breast tissue changes as a result of fibrocystic breast condition may make breast examination and mammography interpretation more difficult. However, while presence of type I macrocytes—a fibrocystic change characterized by high concentrations of androgen and estrogen conjugates, epidermal growth factor, and potassium—may be linked to a moderate increase in breast cancer risk, most fibrocystic changes associated with fibrocystic breast condition (fibrosis, microcysts, and type II macrocysts) are not associated with an increased risk of breast cancer.

—*Cynthia L. De Vine*

See also Breast biopsy; Breast disorders; Breasts, female; Cyst removal; Cysts; Hormones; Lesions; Mammography; Menopause; Women's health.

FOR FURTHER INFORMATION:

Ajao, O. G. "Benign Breast Lesions." *Journal of the National Medical Association* 71, no. 9 (1979): 867-868.

Bruzzi P., L. Dogliotti, and C. Naldoni, et al. "Cohort Study of Association of Risk of Breast Cancer with Cyst Type in Women with Gross Cystic Disease of the Breast." *BMJ* 314 (1997): 925-928.

Dixon, J. M., A. B. Lumsden, and W. R. Miller. "The Relationship of Cyst Type to Risk Factors for Breast Cancer and the Subsequent Development of Breast Cancer in Patients with Breast Cystic Disease." *European Journal of Cancer and Clinical Oncology* 21 (1985): 1047-1050.

Guray, M. Sahin. "Benign Breast Diseases: Classification, Diagnosis, and Management." *Oncologist* 11 (2006): 435-449.

Haagensen, C. D., C. Bodian, and D. E. Haagensen, Jr., eds. *Breast Carcinoma: Risk and Detection*. Philadelphia: W. B. Saunders, 1981.

Hartmann, L. C., T. A. Sellers, M. H. Frost, et al. "Benign Breast Disease and the Risk of Breast Cancer." *New England Journal of Medicine* 353 (2005): 229-237.

Kamel, O. W., R. L. Kempson, and M. R. Hendrickson. "In situ Proliferative Epithelial Lesions of the Breast." *Pathology* 1 (1992): 65-102.

Miller, W. R., et al. "Using Biological Measurements: Can Patients with Benign Breast Disease Who Are at High Risk for Breast Cancer Be Identified?" *Cancer Detection and Prevention* 16 Suppl. (1992): 13-20.

Santen, R. J., and R. Mansel. "Benign Breast Disorders." *New England Journal of Medicine* 353 (2005): 275-285.

Schnitt, S. J., and J. L. Connolly. "Pathology of Benign Breast Disorders." In *Diseases of the Breast*, edited by J. R. Harris et al. 3d ed. Philadelphia: Lippincott Williams & Wilkins, 2004.

Washington C., et al. "Loss of Heterozygosity in Fibrocystic Change of the Breast: Genetic Relationship Between Proliferative Lesions and Associated Carcinomas." *American Journal of Pathology* 157, no. 1 (2000): 323-329.

FIBROMYALGIA

DISEASE/DISORDER

ALSO KNOWN AS: Fibromyalgia syndrome

ANATOMY OR SYSTEM AFFECTED: Brain, head, muscles, musculoskeletal system, nerves, nervous system, psychic-emotional system

SPECIALTIES AND RELATED FIELDS: Rheumatology

DEFINITION: A connective, soft tissue disease involving chronic, spontaneous, and widespread musculoskeletal pain, as well as recurrent fatigue and sleep disturbance.

KEY TERMS:

connective tissue: the supporting framework of the body, particularly tendons and ligaments

fibrositis: an earlier, less common term for fibromyalgia

flare-up: an episode of heightened pain and debilitation in fibromyalgia; sometimes flare-ups do not have an immediate, precipitating cause that is identifiable, while other times they are associated with humidity, cold, physical exertion, or psychological stress

functional somatic syndromes: a continuum or spectrum of disorders (such as chronic fatigue syndrome, Epstein-Barr virus, and primary headaches) characterized by complex interactions between symptoms and patients' personal stress

tender points: specific, precise, and localized areas of moderately to severely intense pain

---

INFORMATION ON FIBROMYALGIA

CAUSES: Unknown; possibly injury or trauma to central nervous system, changes in muscle and connective tissue metabolism, or infectious agent

SYMPTOMS: Severe muscle pain; joint and muscle stiffness; tender points in knee, hips, spine, shoulders, and neck; fatigue; weakness; sometimes concurrent irritable bowel syndrome (IBS) and migraine or tension headaches

DURATION: Chronic with acute episodes

TREATMENTS: Alleviation of symptoms through medications, physical therapy, massage therapy, acupuncture, behavioral therapy

---

CAUSES AND SYMPTOMS

The cause of fibromyalgia is unknown. Some researchers believe that an injury or trauma to the central nervous system causes the disorder. Other researchers believe that changes in muscle and connective tissue metabolism produce decreased blood flow, beginning a pathological cycle of weakness, fatigue, and decreased strength that eventually results in the full-blown syndrome. Still others believe that an as-yet-undiscovered virus or infectious agent attacks people who are naturally susceptible to the infection, who then develop the syndrome.

The most salient feature of fibromyalgia syndrome is pain. Described by sufferers as "having no boundaries," the pain is characteristically variable. The same sufferer experiences pain ranging from deep muscle aching to throbbing, stabbing, or shooting pains to a burning sensation that has been called "acid running through blood vessels." The pain frequently causes joint and muscle stiffness. Pain and stiffness may be worse in the morning and may be more intense in the joints and muscle groups that are used more often. Patients may have tender points, as in the knee, hips, spine, shoulders, and neck. There are typically eighteen potential tender points, and at least eleven must be painful for a diagnosis of fibromyalgia to be made.

Sufferers also experience fatigue and weakness, ranging from mild to debilitating. Patients liken the fatigue to having their arms and legs tied to concrete, and many feel that they are living in a kind of mental fog, unable to focus or concentrate. Between 40 and 70 per-

cent of patients also have some variation of irritable bowel syndrome (IBS): frequent abdominal cramping, nausea, and chronic constipation or diarrhea. About half of all sufferers also experience concurrent migraine or tension headaches. The condition is often mental as well as physical, as sufferers may also suffer from major depressive disorder and anxiety.

Less common, but readily found, are a constellation of symptoms that, in order of prevalence, include jaw, face, and head pain, which is easily misdiagnosed as temporomandibular joint syndrome (TMJ); hypersensitivities to odors, bright lights, and even fibromyalgia medications; painful menstruation; memory problems; and muscle twitching. Weather (particularly exposure to cold), normal hormonal fluctuation, stress, anxiety, depression, and physical exertion can aggravate fibromyalgia and produce flare-ups.

TREATMENT AND THERAPY

Because the cause of fibromyalgia is unknown, only its symptoms can be addressed. The treatment plan must be individualized and flexible, and it is considered long-term management. Rigid, stereotyped approaches can be worse than no management at all.

Because difficulty sleeping and pain can be both contributors to and outcomes of fibromyalgia, traditional treatment approaches focus on improving quality of sleep and reducing pain. Physicians commonly prescribe medications that increase the neurotransmitters serotonin and norepinephrine, which modulate sleep, pain, and the immune system. Amitriptyline (Elavil), paroxetine (Paxil), doxepin (Sinequan), cyclobenzaprine (Flexeril), clonazepam (Klonopin), and similar medications may be prescribed in low doses; they benefit one-third to one-half of patients. Alone or in combination, these medicines improve sleep staging, elevate mood, and relax overtense, stiff, and spasm-prone muscle groups. Other medications, such as Lyrica (pregabalin) and Neurontin (gabapentin)—both originally developed for epilepsy, diabetes pain, and neuropathic pain—have been shown to reduce fibromyalgia pain in some patients.

More comprehensive are approaches that use medications as part of a well-rounded treatment plan. Physical therapy, massage therapy, acupuncture, and behavioral health are other treatment options. Physical therapy and aerobic exercises such as swimming and walking reduce muscle tenderness and pain while improving muscle conditioning and fitness. Because of fibromyalgia sufferers' sensitivity to cold and frequent stiffness, applied heat and therapeutic massage can render short-term relief. Though acupuncture is less well studied, anecdotal accounts claim its effectiveness, making it a sought-after therapy. Psychological counseling, or psychotherapy, can be effective for patients as well.

Perspective and Prospects

Until the 1990's, fibromyalgia syndrome—or fibrositis, as it was then more often called—was not widely accepted by primary care specialists as a legitimate condition. Difficult to diagnose, it was often mistaken as chronic fatigue syndrome (itself a condition not widely recognized in primary care medicine), a sort of chronic pain syndrome, or some condition that was completely psychosomatic (that is, all in the patient's head). Fibromyalgia syndrome was often thought of as a "garbage can diagnosis": a little bit of everything, but not a real syndrome that could be treated. Sufferers had difficulty finding sympathetic medical help and were often at odds with family, friends, and coworkers who misattributed the causes of this connective, soft tissue disease whose existence could not be proven.

Advances in rheumatological research and the American College of Rheumatology's establishment of diagnostic criteria for fibromyalgia have made it a legitimate medical condition for which treatment can be sought. Previously, those with fibromyalgia often suffered from this painful, fatiguing condition and felt blamed for causing it—or worse, for "making it up." Even today, the Fibromyalgia Network, a grassroots informational clearinghouse, underscores research that proves fibromyalgia syndrome is real.

Despite differing theories about the cause of fibromyalgia, ongoing research has produced some results that all investigators consider reliable. This syndrome seems to involve a relationship among the nervous system, the endocrine system, and sleep. When sleep electroencephalograms (EEGs) for patients known to have fibromyalgia are compared with those for nonpatient subjects, disturbances in the non-rapid eye movement (non-REM) stages become evident. There are five well-known and easily recognized stages of sleep: four non-REM stages and then an REM stage. Most people effortlessly progress through non-REM and REM stages. When they reach stage 4, a non-REM stage, they have reached sleep at its deepest. This is the stage during which tissue repair, antibody production, and possibly neurotransmitter regulation occur. Fibromyalgia EEGs show that these patients revert to stage 2 after stage 3, without having reached stage 4. Specialists refer to this sleep disorder as the alpha-EEG anomaly.

This EEG finding corresponds directly with fibromyalgia patients' anecdotal reports that they frequently do not feel rested or refreshed after a night's sleep. This result also contributes to an understanding of why sufferers are fatigued so often. The disturbance of non-REM sleep helps to produce the symptoms of insufficient sleep: tiredness, reduced mental acuity, irritability, and autoimmune susceptibilities. The various stages of sleep also have corresponding hormonal activity, with different hormones and different levels released during each. Stages 3 and 4 are when growth hormones, including insulin growth factor (IGF), are primarily released. Fibromyalgia patients have low IGF levels.

A few other characteristic findings in these patients are not related to sleep. First, the neurotransmitter cerebrospinal fluid P (CSF P), also called substance P, is found in fibromyalgia patients at three times the normal level. Significantly, CSF P is associated with enhanced pain perception. Second, sufferers have low cortisol levels, suggesting that the hypopituitary-adrenal axis is adversely altered. Among much else, this axis mediates the fight-or-flight response and relaxation. Third, using an office procedure called tilt table testing, fibromyalgia symptoms can be provoked, accompanied by a rapid lowering of blood pressure in those with fibromyalgia but not in those without the disease. These findings all provide evidence that problems in the autonomic and endocrine systems cause fibromyalgia. What would set these problems into motion in the first place, however, is unknown, although many sufferers have experienced significant physical and/or psychological trauma before any syndrome-specific symptoms began.

—*Paul Moglia, Ph.D.*

See also Anxiety; Chronic fatigue syndrome; Depression; Fatigue; Headaches; Irritable bowel syndrome (IBS); Migraine headaches; Muscle sprains, spasms, and disorders; Muscles; Pain; Pain management; Sleep; Sleep disorders; Stress; Stress reduction.

FOR FURTHER INFORMATION:

Fibromyalgia Health Center. http://www.webmd.com/fibromyalgia.

Fibromyalgia Network. http://www.fmnetnews.com.

Goldenberg, Don L. *Fibromyalgia: A Leading Expert's Guide to Understanding and Getting Relief from the Pain That Won't Go Away.* Berkeley, Calif.: Berkeley Publishing Group, 2002.

Jones, Kim D., and Janice H. Hoffman. *Fibromyalgia.* Santa Barbara, Calif.: Greenwood Press/ABC-CLIO, 2009.

McCarberg, Bill. H., and Daniel J. Clauw, eds. *Fibromyalgia.* New York: Informa Healthcare, 2009.

National Fibromyalgia Association. http://www.fmaware.org.

Pellegrino, Mark. *Inside Fibromyalgia.* Columbus, Ohio: Anadem, 2001.

Wallace, Daniel J., and Daniel J. Clauw, eds. *Fibromyalgia and Other Central Pain Syndromes.* Philadelphia: Lippincott Williams & Wilkins, 2005.

Wallace, Daniel J., and Janice Brock Wallace. *All About Fibromyalgia: A Guide for Patients and Their Families.* 2d ed. New York: Oxford University Press, 2007.

Winfield, John Buckner. "Fibromyalgia." http://emedicine.medscape.com/article/329838-overview.

FIFTH DISEASE

DISEASE/DISORDER

ALSO KNOWN AS: Erythema infectiosum

ANATOMY OR SYSTEM AFFECTED: Nose, skin, throat

INFORMATION ON FIFTH DISEASE

CAUSES: Viral infection

SYMPTOMS: "Slapped cheek" rash, fever, sore throat, achiness, malaise

DURATION: Ten to fourteen days

TREATMENTS: Alleviation of symptoms through bed rest, administration of liquids

---

SPECIALTIES AND RELATED FIELDS: Family medicine, pediatrics

DEFINITION: An infectious disease of children characterized by an erythematous (reddish) rash and low-grade fever.

CAUSES AND SYMPTOMS

Fifth disease is caused by infection with the human parvovirus (HPV) B19. The disease is more prevalent during late winter or early spring. Fifth disease is most commonly observed in young children, with the peak attack rate between five and fourteen years of age. Adults may become infected, but they rarely show evidence of disease.

The virus is spread from person to person through nasal secretions or sneezing. Following an incubation period of several days, a rash develops on the face, which has the appearance of slapped cheeks. The bright red color fades as the rash spreads over the rest of the body. An erythematous, pimply eruption may also appear on the trunk or extremities. A mild fever, sore throat, and nasal stuffiness may also be apparent. The rash generally lasts from ten days to two weeks. Often, it will fade only to reappear a short time later. Sunlight may aggravate the skin during this period, also causing a reappearance of the rash.

The diagnosis of fifth disease is primarily clinical, based on the symptoms. Laboratory tests for the virus are generally not performed.

TREATMENT AND THERAPY

No antibiotic therapy is available for fifth disease. Since the disease is rarely serious, treatment is mainly symptomatic. Bed rest and the administration of liquids, as commonly used in treating mild illness in children, are generally sufficient. Isolation is unnecessary since transmission is unlikely following appearance of the rash.

PERSPECTIVE AND PROSPECTS

Fifth disease was first described during the late nineteenth century as the fifth in the series of erythematous illnesses often encountered by children; the others are measles, mumps, chickenpox, and rubella. HPV B19 was isolated in 1975 and shown to be the etiological agent of the disease in the mid-1980's.

The disease is common and generally benign. HPV B19 has been implicated, however, in certain forms of hemolytic anemias and arthritis in adults, and research continues on the virus.

—*Richard Adler, Ph.D.*

See also Childhood infectious diseases; Fever; Rashes; Sneezing; Sore throat; Viral infections.

For Further Information:

Behrman, Richard E., Robert M. Kliegman, and Hal B. Jenson, eds. *Nelson Textbook of Pediatrics.* 18th ed. Philadelphia: Saunders/Elsevier, 2007.

Burg, Fredric D., et al., eds. *Treatment of Infants, Children, and Adolescents.* Philadelphia: W. B. Saunders, 1990.

Kemper, Kathi J. *The Holistic Pediatrician: A Pediatrician's Comprehensive Guide to Safe and Effective Therapies for the Twenty-five Most Common Ailments of Infants, Children, and Adolescents.* Rev. ed. New York: Quill, 2002.

Kumar, Vinay, Abul K. Abbas, and Nelson Fausto, eds. *Robbins and Cotran Pathologic Basis of Disease.* 8th ed. Philadelphia: Saunders/Elsevier, 2010.

Sompayrac, Lauren. *How Pathogenic Viruses Work.* Boston: Jones and Bartlett, 2002.

Fingernail removal. *See* Nail removal.

First aid

Treatment

Also known as: Emergency aid

Anatomy or system affected: All

Specialties and related fields: All

Definition: The National First Aid Science Advisory Board defines "first aid" as "assessments and interventions that can be performed by a bystander (or by the victim) with minimal or no medical equipment."

Introduction

In 2005, the American Red Cross and the American Heart Association created the National First Aid Science Advisory Board (NFASAB) to review scientific literature on first aid. The board's review found few published studies on first aid practices and concluded that most of them are based on professional experience and expert opinion. The board then published evidence-based first aid guidelines that can be used to update training programs.

First aid administered at the scene of an accident can be lifesaving. As a general rule, a victim should not be moved if a spinal injury is suspected. Advanced first aid training should include the proper use of immobilization devices for suspected spinal injuries.

Common first aid breathing emergencies include asthma attacks, allergic anaphylaxis, seizures, and choking. A first aid responder to an asthma attack can assist a victim in administering his or her prescribed medication, usually an inhaler, while waiting for professional aid. For anaphylaxis due to allergies to insect stings or food, first aid responders should be trained how to administer epinephrine (if state law permits) in an emergency or how to assist a victim to self-administer. Seizure treatment should focus on preventing injury and keeping the airway open. However, restraining a victim during a seizure is not recommended as it can cause bruising or injury. Placing an object in the mouth can damage teeth or obstruct airways and is also not recommended. Choking can occur in adults and children when an object gets stuck in the throat and cuts off air. Techniques for choking first aid include using the heel of the hand to administer five firm blows between a person's shoulder blades, or if that fails to dislodge the object, administering the Heimlich maneuver. Both techniques can injure a person if not done correctly. Standard first aid training should include common breathing emergency techniques.

Common injury-related first aid includes bleeding control and wound management. Excessive bleeding should be controlled by applying pressure over the bleeding area until the bleeding stops. Gauze or other clean soft material can be placed over the wound while applying pressure but should not be removed prematurely. The use of pressure points and the elevation of a limb to aid in controlling excessive bleeding are not well studied and should not be used instead of the proven method of applied pressure to the wound. The safety and effective use of tourniquets is also under review.

Cuts, scrapes, and puncture wounds should all be cleaned with cool water. Soap and a soft cloth should be used to clean around the wound and sterile tweezers to remove any dirt that remains in the wound after rinsing with water. Bleeding can help clean out a shallow wound and usually stops in a few minutes. Deeper cuts may required gentle, firm pressure with gauze or other sterile material. If the wound is on the leg or arm, after bleeding has been controlled raising it above your head may help but should not be used if it interferes with applying firm gentle pressure, the most effective method to stop bleeding. The wound should be covered if it will get dirty or rub against something; otherwise a shallow wound can be uncovered to help it dry and heal faster. Bandages should be changed at least every day. Large area scrapes need to be kept moist and covered to avoid scarring. Antibiotic cream can help prevent infections; triple antibiotic cream is recommended as the most effective.

Burn first aid training includes how to identify first, second, and third grade burns. Serious burns can result from exposure to fire, heat sources, sun, electricity, chemicals, or radiation. A serious burn can be any burn more than several inches in diameter or a burn that turns the skin white or looks charred. Stabilizing treatment includes soaking the burned area in cool water (five minutes for a first-degree burn, fifteen minutes for a second-degree burn), then treating with a skin ointment like aloe or antibacterial cream and covering the burn area with loose gauze to keep air off and keep the area clean. Over-the-counter pain or anti-inflammatory medicine may help reduce pain and swelling. Direct contact of ice cubes to skin is not recommended. Burn blisters should not be popped or removed.

First aid for muscle injuries includes applying a cold pack for no more than twenty minutes to the injury to reduce hemorrhage, edema, pain, and disability. Use of compression bandage to reduce edema has not been well studied. If an injured extremity is blue or extremely pale, then immediate medical care is needed.

There are many toxic or poisonous substances in the home and workplace. First aid training includes understanding emergency procedures for different classes of poisons. Government-sponsored poison control centers are a good resource. Poisoning can occur by swallowing a poisonous substance, breathing in poisonous air, or though skin contact. Poison control centers can provide advice. First aid training for poison response includes strategies for stabilizing the victim, identification of the poison, and minimizing the responder's exposure to poisonous substances. For ingested poisons, some commonsense approaches or older methods are not recommended. Inducing vomiting with syrup of ipecac is not recommended, nor is administering charcoal. If poisons have been inhaled, then removing the person to a place with fresh air as fast as possible is essential.

Standard first aid includes recognition and treatment of insect, snake, and animal bites. Some insect bites or stings, such as from bees, wasps, yellow jackets, and fire ants, can cause localized pain and swelling or, if a person is allergic, can cause more serious reactions including life-threatening swelling of airway passages (anaphylaxis). Only two spiders cause serious reactions: the black widow and the brown recluse. First aid

training should include treatment for insect bites or stings, including tick bites, as well as animal bites, including assessment for possible rabies infection. Poisonous snake bites are a medical emergency. First aid recommendations focus on limiting the spread of venom in the bloodstream by not moving the affected area. It is not advised to try to suck out the venom or cut out the area bitten.

Wilderness first aid requires some additional skills and supplies. Stabilizing an injured person and assisting them in evacuating a remote area are critical skills. Components of wilderness first aid training can include treatment of hyperthermia and frostbite, treatment of altitude sickness, specific knowledge of marine hazards such as stinging jellyfish, knowledge of emergency treatment for diarrhea and dehydration, as well as knowledge of how to make splints and other supports from available materials. Hikers and explorers should learn specifics about first aid for the area where they will be traveling.

DISCUSSION

First aid training is often available through local Red Cross chapters or local community or health centers. Key components of first aid training should include knowing how to get help, knowing how to position a victim, and knowing how to handle medical emergencies. Key medical emergencies include breathing difficulties, anaphylaxis, and seizures. Key injury emergencies include bleeding; wounds and abrasions; burns; spine injuries; musculoskeletal injuries such as sprains, strains, and fractures; and dental injuries. Key environmental emergencies include hypothermia, drowning, poisoning, and snakebites. More complex first aid training may include safe handling of bloodborne pathogens and administration of oxygen and cardiopulmonary resuscitation (CPR). Specific first aid training, such as wilderness first aid and travel first aid, are offered by a number of organizations.

The most common first aid courses offer home first aid classes for parents and other caregivers. Basic first aid training for the home includes how to respond to common illnesses and conditions such as croup, stroke, angina, asthma, diabetes, epilepsy, meningitis, anaphylaxis, heart attack, and febrile convulsions. It can also include how to identify and respond to common household poisonings, eye injury, head injury, crush injury, spinal injury, and the effects of temperature extremes. Other topics include how to respond to minor injuries and illness such as fever, cramps, blisters, fainting, earache, vomiting, headache, diarrhea, toothache, sore throat, abdominal pain, crushed fingers, burns and scalds, allergic reactions, stings, splinters, and small wounds and grazes.

First aid kits are a key component of any first aid effort. First aid kits should be available in every home, school, worksite, and vehicle. A standard kit should include a first aid manual; bandages, including elastic bandages and sterile gauze; adhesive tape; disinfectants such as antiseptic wipes or solutions (for example, alcohol) and antibiotic ointment; over-the-counter pain and anti-inflammatory medicine such as acetaminophen and ibuprofen; tools such as tweezers, sharp scissors, and safety pins; a thermometer; and plastic gloves.

PERSPECTIVE AND PROSPECTS

First aid has been a part of organized Western medicine for more than 140 years, when it was expanded from efforts to tend to wounded soldiers. It began as basic training for soldiers to tend war casualties. The term "first aid" was coined from the terms "first response" and "National Aid" in 1863 by British Army officer Peter Shephard, who together with his colleague Francis Duncan, developed the first civilian training course in first aid. Participants received a certificate and volunteered to help care for wounded soldiers.

First aid became an established form of emergency care in the late nineteenth century. In Great Britain, the St. John Ambulance Brigade was established in 1873 to provide first aid to the public, and the St. John Ambulance Association was established in 1877 to train civilians in first aid care. The primary focus was on providing aid to industrial workers. As part of the St. John Ambulance Association program, first aid volunteers also helped in public disaster response. Both these groups have their roots in the Order of St. John, a religious order that provided medical services to soldiers as early as the twelfth century. St. John Ambulance remains one of the largest providers of first aid, and it operates in thirty-nine countries.

At about the same time that the Order of St. John was establishing first aid classes, the International Red Cross committee was working to provide humanitarian aid to soldiers worldwide. In 1863, Henry Dunant founded the International Committee of the Red Cross as a reaction to the mass war casualties that he witnessed during a business trip to Italy and the lack of medical and humanitarian care available to wounded soldiers. This was the beginning of international efforts to establish Red Cross Societies around the world. In the United States, Clara Barton, a nurse and teacher, became president of the American Red Cross in 1881. She expanded basic first aid training for soldiers to include training for industrial accidents and disaster relief. Today, National Red Cross Societies exist in most countries.

—*Sandra Ripley Distelhorst*

See also Accidents; Bites and stings; Bleeding; Burns and scalds; Cardiopulmonary resuscitation (CPR); Choking; Concussion; Critical care; Critical care, pediatric; Drowning; Electrical shock; Emergency medicine; Emergency medicine, pediatric; Fracture and dislocation; Fracture repair; Frostbite; Heart attack; Heat exhaustion and heatstroke; Hyperthermia and hypothermia; Laceration repair; Paramedics; Poisoning; Resuscitation; Shock; Snakebites; Sports medicine; Unconsciousness; Wounds.

FOR FURTHER INFORMATION:

American College of Emergency Physicians. *ACEP First Aid Manual.* 2d ed. New York: DK, 2004.

American Medical Association Handbook of First Aid and Emergency Care. New York: Random House Reference, 2009.

American Red Cross and Kathleen A. Handal. *The American Red Cross First Aid and Safety Handbook.* Boston: Little, Brown, 1992.

Weiss, Eric A. *A Comprehensive Guide to Wilderness and Travel Medicine.* 3d ed. Oakland, Calif.: Adventure Medical Kits, 2005.

FISTULA REPAIR

PROCEDURE

ANATOMY OR SYSTEM AFFECTED: Abdomen, anus, bladder, blood, gallbladder, gastrointestinal system, intestines, reproductive system, urinary system, uterus

SPECIALTIES AND RELATED FIELDS: Gastroenterology, general surgery, pediatrics, proctology

DEFINITION: The removal of any abnormal passage associated with body sites or tissues.

KEY TERMS:

anorectal: associated with the anal portion of the large intestine

arteriovenous: associated with arteries and/or veins

Crohn's disease: a chronic inflammation of the bowel, often as a result of an autoimmune disease

crypt: a pit or depression in the body

fistulectomy: the surgical elimination of a fistula

INDICATIONS AND PROCEDURES

A fistula represents any abnormal opening or passage between internal organs or between an internal organ and the surface of the body. Fistulas can occur nearly anywhere in the body, but they are most commonly associated with the anorectal portion of the anatomy. Some fistulas may result from congenital defects, while others may be created surgically in association with specific procedures. For example, an arteriovenous fistula may be created to allow the insertion of a cannula (tube) for hemodialysis.

Anorectal fistulas usually begin as an abscess within the anal region or internal crypt that then spreads to adjacent tissue or to the surface of the body. Pain, itching, or tenderness in the region is often the first sign of a problem. The discomfort may be aggravated by bowel movements. Since infection is common, the opening may become purulent (pus-producing).

Treatment of anorectal fistulas usually requires surgery. A crypt hook may be used if the site of the original crypt must be located, an observation which is often unnecessary. The crypt may also be observed through an anoscope, or as part of a proctoscopic examination. Often, digital examination of the anal canal may detect a nodule, representing the abscess itself.

Any abscess must first be drained and treated. If the fistula is small, it may heal itself. The surgical procedure, commonly referred to as a fistulectomy, is a relatively simple operation carried out under general anesthesia. The fistula must be reduced or removed. Surgical repair begins at the primary opening, and generally the entire tract is opened, both to allow for proper drainage of infectious material and to promote healing. If the surgery is carried out properly, the incision should heal relatively quickly.

Difficult labor in women may create a variety of fistulas. A vesicovaginal fistula, created between the uri-

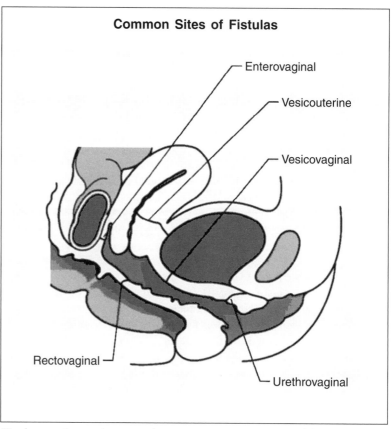

Common Sites of Fistulas

Enterovaginal

Vesicouterine

Vesicovaginal

Rectovaginal

Urethrovaginal

Fistulas are abnormal passages between organs or an organ and the outside of the body. They are more common in the rectal and genital regions of women, such as between the intestines and vagina (enterovaginal), the bladder and uterus (vesicouterine), the bladder and vagina (vesicovaginal), the urethra and vagina (urethrovaginal), and the rectum and vagina (rectovaginal).

nary bladder and the vagina, may be indicated by the presence of urine in the vaginal tract. As with any opening to the surface of the body, infection may develop. Likewise, a rectovaginal fistula, between the rectum and vagina, was formerly a possible serious complication of difficult childbirth. As with any fistulas, such openings have to be opened, drained, and sutured for healing.

Fistula formation may also be internal, as in biliary fistulas between the gallbladder and intestine. Such connections can occur as a consequence of gallstones, ulcers, or tumor formation. Often, the major symptom may be an intestinal blockage resulting from the stone or tumor itself. Bile may leak from the gallbladder into the peritoneum or body cavities, resulting in infection. Therapy for such fistula formation first requires an analysis of the channel itself. If the fistula is external, contrast material may be injected into the site to analyze the tract. If the fistula is internal, the extent of the tract may require cholangiography, the injection of a radiopaque material to outline the bile duct. General surgery is required for the proper correction of any underlying problem.

USES AND COMPLICATIONS

Surgical repair of a fistula has a number of functions, in addition to the elimination of the fistula itself. The goal of repair is to support the healing process, while at the same time attempting to maintain the normal function (and appearance, when applicable) of the tissue.

The anal fistula represents one of the more common types. Frequently, it begins as an abscess or break in the anal or rectal wall. Not infrequently, the underlying cause may be inflammation of the colon as a result of ulcerative colitis or Crohn's disease, an autoimmune disease which can cause ulceration of the intestinal wall. The fistula itself may become chronically infected, resulting in pain and discomfort. Cancer development in the area of the fistula, while uncommon, has been known to occur.

The major complication of anorectal surgery to repair the fistula is delayed healing. If not completely drained or covered, the area may continue to become infected. If the fistula is deep, damage to muscles during surgical repair may result in incontinence. Assuming that the fistula does not recur and postoperative care is properly provided, however, the prognosis is generally excellent.

Surgical procedures can also be used in the intentional formation of a fistula. For example, a site must be prepared for insertion of a cannula to carry out hemodialysis, the removal of waste from the blood under conditions of renal insufficiency. Generally, such a fistula between an artery and a vein is prepared one to two months prior to insertion of the cannula. The fistula is created either by grafting a section of bovine carotid artery into the site or by using a graft prepared from synthetic material. Proper circulation through the fistula must be monitored to ensure that infection does not develop.

PERSPECTIVE AND PROSPECTS

The development and widespread use of antibiotics in the mid-twentieth century provided a means for the effective treatment of the major complication associated with fistula development: infection. Fistulas may result in abscess formation or may be secondary to problems elsewhere, as with Crohn's disease. Better treatment of those infections associated with fistula formation, such as tuberculosis, has reduced their incidence. Likewise, proper prenatal care has largely controlled fistula development secondary to difficult labor in women.

—*Richard Adler, Ph.D.*

See also Abscess drainage; Abscesses; Anus; Childbirth complications; Colon; Colorectal surgery; Crohn's disease; Gallbladder; Gastroenterology; Gastroenterology, pediatric; Gastrointestinal disorders; Gastrointestinal system; Grafts and grafting; Gynecology; Infection; Intestines; Proctology; Rectum; Reproductive system; Stone removal; Stones; Tumor removal; Tumors; Ulcer surgery; Ulcers; Urinary system; Urology; Urology, pediatric.

FOR FURTHER INFORMATION:

American Medical Association. *American Medical Association Family Medical Guide.* 4th rev. ed. Hoboken, N.J.: John Wiley & Sons, 2004. An excellent reference for the beginner. The scientific accuracy of the text is not compromised by its accessibility.

Doherty, Gerard M., and Lawrence W. Way, eds. *Current Surgical Diagnosis and Treatment.* 12th ed. New York: Lange Medical Books/McGraw-Hill, 2006. A reference work on general surgery for physicians, this tome is nevertheless comprehensible to laypersons familiar with medical terminology. Presents succinct overviews of the stoma procedures and their potential complications and contains finely detailed illustrations.

Peikin, Steven R. *Gastrointestinal Health.* Rev. ed. New York: Quill, 2001. Examines a range of gastrointestinal ailments in depth, including diarrhea and colitis, and offers tips for managing them via diet, stress management, and drugs.

Saibil, Fred. *Crohn's Disease and Ulcerative Colitis: Everything You Need to Know.* Rev. ed. Toronto, Ont.: Firefly Books, 2009. A leading expert on IBD, Saibil covers topics such as signs and symptoms, how the gastrointestinal system works normally and how IBD affects it, procedures and instruments used to diagnose IBD, effects of diet, children and IBD, and effects on sexual activity and childbearing.

Tierney, Lawrence M., Stephen J. McPhee, and Maxine A. Papadakis, eds. *Current Medical Diagnosis and Treatment 2007.* New York: McGraw-Hill Medical, 2006. This text, updated yearly, is the point of reference for physicians and other health care practitioners. It incorporates each year's biomedical research discoveries that have immediate, relevant, and applicable use for the patient.

FLAT FEET

DISEASE/DISORDER

ALSO KNOWN AS: Pes planus, talipes planus
ANATOMY OR SYSTEM AFFECTED: Feet, ligaments, muscles, musculoskeletal system
SPECIALTIES AND RELATED FIELDS: Orthopedics, podiatry
DEFINITION: A congenital or acquired flatness of the longitudinal arch of the foot.

CAUSES AND SYMPTOMS

Congenital flat feet are considered to be hereditary. Acquired flat feet can be caused by stretching of the arch ligaments and a weakness of the muscles found in the arches; this produces flexible flat feet. Rigid flat feet are caused by changes in the shape of the foot bones or a short Achilles tendon. Other causes of flat feet include injury and a lack of muscle tone or weak foot muscles that cannot sustain the body's weight.

All infants appear to be flat-footed because of a pad of fat under each instep. Arch formation in the feet takes place once they begin walking. Flat feet are often detected by parents when an infant experiences delays in learning how to walk.

Flat feet usually are painless and do not contribute to changes in posture or the ability to walk. Adolescents and adults are occasionally prone to fallen arches, or temporary foot strain caused by an activity that overstretches the ligaments in the arch; this condition is accompanied by pain. Rigid flat feet caused by a short Achilles tendon and spastic flat feet caused by a deformity of the heel result in pain and clumsiness in walking.

TREATMENT AND THERAPY

Flexible, pain-free flat feet require no treatment. Special orthopedic shoes with arch supports do not change the shape of the feet over time, while foot exercises and prescribed changes in gait are hard to enforce in children.

In cases of fallen arches accompanied by fatigue or pain, however, rest, foot exercises, and the use of arch supports are recommended. If the Achilles tendon is too short or tight, it can be stretched by placing the foot in a cast. Severe cases of flat feet require surgery that

INFORMATION ON FLAT FEET
CAUSES: Congenital weakness of muscles in arches, changes in shape of foot bones, short Achilles tendon, injury
SYMPTOMS: Delays in learning how to walk, pain, clumsiness in walking
DURATION: Typically short-term
TREATMENTS: Depends on severity; ranges from orthopedic shoes with arch supports, foot exercises, and rest to casts or surgery

removes excess bone or reconstructs the soft tissue of the foot.

—*Rose Secrest*

See also Arthritis; Bone disorders; Bones and the skeleton; Feet; Foot disorders; Lower extremities; Orthopedics; Orthopedics, pediatric; Podiatry.

FOR FURTHER INFORMATION:

Copeland, Glenn, and Stan Solomon. *The Foot Doctor: Lifetime Relief for Your Aching Feet.* Rev. ed. Toronto, Ont.: Macmillan Canada, 1996.

Currey, John D. *Bones: Structures and Mechanics.* Princeton, N.J.: Princeton University Press, 2002.

Lippert, Frederick G., and Sigvard T. Hansen. *Foot and Ankle Disorders: Tricks of the Trade.* New York: Thieme, 2003.

Lorimer, Donald L., et al., eds. *Neale's Disorders of the Foot.* 7th ed. New York: Churchill Livingstone/Elsevier, 2006.

Van De Graaff, Kent M. *Human Anatomy.* 6th ed. New York: McGraw-Hill, 2002.

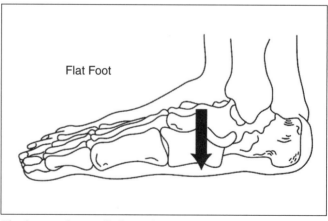

Flat feet, or abnormally flat arches, can arise from muscle weakness, improper walking, or developmental defects.

SALEM HEALTH

MAGILL'S MEDICAL GUIDE

ENTRIES BY ANATOMY OR SYSTEM AFFECTED

ALL

Accidents
African American health
Aging
Aging: Extended care
Alternative medicine
American Indian health
Anatomy
Antibiotics
Anti-inflammatory drugs
Antioxidants
Asian American health
Autoimmune disorders
Autopsy
Biological and chemical weapons
Bionics and biotechnology
Biophysics
Birth defects
Burkitt's lymphoma
Cancer
Carcinogens
Carcinoma
Chemotherapy
Chronobiology
Clinical trials
Cloning
Congenital disorders
Critical care
Critical care, pediatric
Cryotherapy and cryosurgery
Cushing's syndrome
Death and dying
Diagnosis
Dietary reference intakes (DRIs)
Disease
Domestic violence
Drug resistance
Embryology
Emergency medicine
Emergency medicine, pediatric
Emergency rooms
Emerging infectious diseases
Environmental diseases
Environmental health
Enzyme therapy
Epidemics and pandemics
Epidemiology
Family medicine
Fascia
Fatigue

Fever
First aid
Food Guide Pyramid
Forensic pathology
Gangrene
Gene therapy
Genetic diseases
Genetics and inheritance
Genomics
Geriatrics and gerontology
Grafts and grafting
Growth
Healing
Herbal medicine
Histology
Holistic medicine
Homeopathy
Hydrotherapy
Hyperadiposis
Hyperthermia and hypothermia
Hypertrophy
Hypochondriasis
Iatrogenic disorders
Imaging and radiology
Immunopathology
Infection
Inflammation
Internet medicine
Intoxication
Invasive tests
Ischemia
Leptin
Macronutrients
Magnetic resonance imaging
  (MRI)
Malignancy and metastasis
Malnutrition
Massage
Meditation
Men's health
Metabolic disorders
Metabolic syndrome
Mold and mildew
Mucopolysaccharidosis (MPS)
Multiple births
Münchausen syndrome by proxy
Neonatology
Noninvasive tests
Nursing
Occupational health

Oncology
Opportunistic infections
Over-the-counter medications
Pain
Pain management
Palliative medicine
Paramedics
Parasitic diseases
Pathology
Pediatrics
Perinatology
Physical examination
Physician assistants
Physiology
Phytochemicals
Plastic surgery
Polypharmacy
Positron emission tomography
  (PET) scanning
Prescription drug abuse
Preventive medicine
Progeria
Prognosis
Prostheses
Protein
Proteomics
Psychiatry
Psychiatry, child and adolescent
Psychiatry, geriatric
Psychosomatic disorders
Puberty and adolescence
Radiation therapy
Radiopharmaceuticals
Reflexes, primitive
Retroviruses
Safety issues for children
Safety issues for the elderly
Screening
Self-medication
Sexually transmitted diseases
  (STDs)
Side effects
Signs and symptoms
Single photon emission
  computed tomography
  (SPECT)
Staphylococcal infections
Stem cells
Stevens-Johnson syndrome
Streptococcal infections

Motor skill development
Necrosis
Neurofibromatosis
Niemann-Pick disease
Nuclear medicine
Nuclear radiology
Orthopedic surgery
Orthopedics
Orthopedics, pediatric
Osgood-Schlatter disease
Osteochondritis juvenilis
Osteogenesis imperfecta
Osteomyelitis
Osteonecrosis
Osteopathic medicine
Osteoporosis
Paget's disease
Periodontitis
Physical rehabilitation
Pigeon toes
Podiatry
Polydactyly and syndactyly
Prader-Willi syndrome
Rheumatology
Rickets
Rubinstein-Taybi syndrome
Sarcoma
Scoliosis
Slipped disk
Spinal cord disorders
Spine, vertebrae, and disks
Sports medicine
Teeth
Temporomandibular joint (TMJ)
  syndrome
Tendon disorders
Tendon repair
Upper extremities

BRAIN
Abscess drainage
Abscesses
Acidosis
Addiction
Adrenal glands
Adrenoleukodystrophy
Agnosia
Alcoholism
Altitude sickness
Alzheimer's disease
Amnesia
Anesthesia
Anesthesiology
Aneurysmectomy

Aneurysms
Angiography
Anosmia
Antianxiety drugs
Antidepressants
Aphasia and dysphasia
Aromatherapy
Attention-deficit disorder (ADD)
Auras
Batten's disease
Biofeedback
Body dysmorphic disorder
Brain
Brain damage
Brain disorders
Brain tumors
Caffeine
Carbohydrates
Carotid arteries
Chiari malformations
Chronic wasting disease (CWD)
Cluster headaches
Cognitive development
Coma
Computed tomography (CT)
  scanning
Concussion
Cornelia de Lange syndrome
Corticosteroids
Craniotomy
Creutzfeldt-Jakob disease (CJD)
Cytomegalovirus (CMV)
Defibrillation
Dehydration
Dementias
Developmental stages
Dizziness and fainting
Down syndrome
Drowning
Dyskinesia
Dyslexia
Electroencephalography (EEG)
Embolism
Embolization
Emotions: Biomedical causes
  and effects
Encephalitis
Endocrine glands
Endocrinology
Endocrinology, pediatric
Enteroviruses
Epilepsy
Failure to thrive
Fetal alcohol syndrome

Fetal surgery
Fetal tissue transplantation
Fibromyalgia
Fragile X syndrome
Frontotemporal dementia
  (FTD)
Galactosemia
Gigantism
Gulf War syndrome
Hallucinations
Head and neck disorders
Headaches
Hearing
Huntington's disease
Hydrocephalus
Hypertension
Hypnosis
Hypotension
Hypothalamus
Infarction
Intraventricular hemorrhage
Jaundice
Kinesiology
Kluver-Bucy syndrome
Lead poisoning
Learning disabilities
Leukodystrophy
Light therapy
Listeria infections
Malaria
Marijuana
Melatonin
Memory loss
Meningitis
Mental retardation
Migraine headaches
Narcolepsy
Narcotics
Nausea and vomiting
Neuroimaging
Neurology
Neurology, pediatric
Neurosurgery
Nicotine
Niemann-Pick disease
Nuclear radiology
Parkinson's disease
Pharmacology
Pharmacy
Phenylketonuria (PKU)
Pick's disease
Pituitary gland
Poliomyelitis
Polycystic kidney disease

Positron emission tomography
   (PET) scanning
Prader-Willi syndrome
Prion diseases
Psychiatric disorders
Psychiatry
Psychiatry, child and adolescent
Psychiatry, geriatric
Rabies
Restless legs syndrome
Reye's syndrome
Rocky Mountain spotted fever
Sarcoidosis
Schizophrenia
Seizures
Shock therapy
Shunts
Sleep
Sleep disorders
Sleeping sickness
Sleepwalking
Stammering
Strokes
Sturge-Weber syndrome
Subdural hematoma
Synesthesia
Syphilis
Tetanus
Thrombolytic therapy and TPA
Thrombosis and thrombus
Tics
Tinnitus
Tourette's syndrome
Toxicology
Toxoplasmosis
Transient ischemic attacks (TIAs)
Trembling and shaking
Tumor removal
Tumors
Unconsciousness
Vagus nerve
Vertigo
Weight loss medications
Wilson's disease
Yellow fever

BREASTS
Abscess drainage
Abscesses
Breast biopsy
Breast cancer
Breast disorders
Breast-feeding
Breast surgery

Breasts, female
Cyst removal
Cysts
Fibrocystic breast condition
Gender reassignment surgery
Glands
Gynecology
Gynecomastia
Klinefelter syndrome
Mammography
Mastectomy and lumpectomy
Mastitis
Tumor removal
Tumors

CELLS
Acid-base chemistry
Antibodies
Bacteriology
Batten's disease
Biological therapies
Biopsy
Cells
Cholesterol
Conception
Cytology
Cytomegalovirus (CMV)
Cytopathology
Dehydration
DNA and RNA
E. coli infection
Enzymes
Fluids and electrolytes
Food biochemistry
Gaucher's disease
Genetic counseling
Genetic engineering
Glycolysis
Gram staining
Gulf War syndrome
Host-defense mechanisms
Immunization and vaccination
Immunology
In vitro fertilization
Karyotyping
Kinesiology
Laboratory tests
Lipids
Magnetic field therapy
Microbiology
Microscopy
Mutation
Pharmacology
Pharmacy

Phlebotomy
Plasma
Pus
Toxicology

CHEST
Anatomy
Antihistamines
Asthma
Bacillus Calmette-Guérin (BCG)
Bones and the skeleton
Breasts, female
Bronchiolitis
Bronchitis
Bypass surgery
Cardiac rehabilitation
Cardiology
Cardiology, pediatric
Chest
Choking
Common cold
Congenital heart disease
Coughing
Croup
Cystic fibrosis
Defibrillation
Diaphragm
Electrocardiography (ECG or EKG)
Embolism
Emphysema
Gulf War syndrome
Heart
Heart transplantation
Heart valve replacement
Heartburn
Heimlich maneuver
Hiccups
Interstitial pulmonary fibrosis (IPF)
Legionnaires' disease
Lung cancer
Lungs
Pacemaker implantation
Pityriasis rosea
Pleurisy
Pneumonia
Pneumothorax
Pulmonary diseases
Pulmonary medicine
Pulmonary medicine, pediatric
Respiration
Respiratory distress syndrome
Resuscitation
Sarcoidosis
Sneezing

Thoracic surgery
Trachea
Tuberculosis
Wheezing
Whooping cough

CIRCULATORY SYSTEM

Aneurysmectomy
Aneurysms
Angina
Angiography
Angioplasty
Antibodies
Antihistamines
Apgar score
Arrhythmias
Arteriosclerosis
Atrial fibrillation
Biofeedback
Bleeding
Blood and blood disorders
Blood pressure
Blood testing
Blood vessels
Blue baby syndrome
Bypass surgery
Cardiac arrest
Cardiac rehabilitation
Cardiac surgery
Cardiology
Cardiology, pediatric
Cardiopulmonary resuscitation
   (CPR)
Carotid arteries
Catheterization
Chest
Cholesterol
Circulation
Claudication
Congenital heart disease
Coronary artery bypass graft
Decongestants
Deep vein thrombosis
Defibrillation
Dehydration
Diabetes mellitus
Dialysis
Disseminated intravascular
   coagulation (DIC)
Diuretics
Dizziness and fainting
Ebola virus
Echocardiography
Edema

Electrocardiography (ECG or EKG)
Electrocauterization
Embolism
End-stage renal disease
Endarterectomy
Endocarditis
Ergogenic aids
Exercise physiology
Facial transplantation
Food allergies
Heart
Heart attack
Heart disease
Heart failure
Heart transplantation
Heart valve replacement
Heat exhaustion and heatstroke
Hematology
Hematology, pediatric
Hemorrhoid banding and removal
Hemorrhoids
Hormones
Hyperbaric oxygen therapy
Hypercholesterolemia
Hypertension
Hypotension
Intravenous (IV) therapy
Ischemia
Juvenile rheumatoid arthritis
Kidneys
Kinesiology
Klippel-Trenaunay syndrome
Liver
Lymph
Lymphatic system
Marburg virus
Marijuana
Mitral valve prolapse
Motor skill development
Nosebleeds
Obesity
Obesity, childhood
Osteochondritis juvenilis
Pacemaker implantation
Palpitations
Phlebitis
Phlebotomy
Placenta
Plaque, arterial
Plasma
Preeclampsia and eclampsia
Pulmonary edema
Pulse rate
Resuscitation

Reye's syndrome
Rheumatic fever
Sarcoidosis
Scleroderma
Septicemia
Shock
Shunts
Smoking
Sports medicine
Stenosis
Stents
Steroid abuse
Strokes
Sturge-Weber syndrome
Systems and organs
Testicular torsion
Thrombocytopenia
Thrombolytic therapy and TPA
Thrombosis and thrombus
Transfusion
Transient ischemic attacks (TIAs)
Transplantation
Typhus
Uremia
Varicose vein removal
Varicose veins
Vascular medicine
Vascular system
Vasculitis
Venous insufficiency

EARS

Adenoids
Adrenoleukodystrophy
Agnosia
Altitude sickness
Antihistamines
Audiology
Auras
Biophysics
Cartilage
Cornelia de Lange syndrome
Cytomegalovirus (CMV)
Deafness
Decongestants
Dyslexia
Ear infections and disorders
Ear surgery
Ears
Earwax
Fragile X syndrome
Hearing
Hearing aids
Hearing loss

Hearing tests
Histiocytosis
Leukodystrophy
Ménière's disease
Motion sickness
Myringotomy
Nervous system
Neurology
Neurology, pediatric
Osteogenesis imperfecta
Otoplasty
Otorhinolaryngology
Pharynx
Plastic surgery
Quinsy
Rubinstein-Taybi syndrome
Sense organs
Speech disorders
Tinnitus
Vasculitis
Vertigo
Wiskott-Aldrich syndrome

ENDOCRINE SYSTEM
Addison's disease
Adrenal glands
Adrenalectomy
Adrenoleukodystrophy
Assisted reproductive technologies
Bariatric surgery
Biofeedback
Breasts, female
Carbohydrates
Congenital adrenal hyperplasia
Congenital hypothyroidism
Contraception
Corticosteroids
Diabetes mellitus
Dwarfism
Eating disorders
Emotions: Biomedical causes and
    effects
End-stage renal disease
Endocrine disorders
Endocrine glands
Endocrinology
Endocrinology, pediatric
Ergogenic aids
Failure to thrive
Fibrocystic breast condition
Gender reassignment surgery
Gestational diabetes
Gigantism
Glands

Goiter
Hashimoto's thyroiditis
Hormone therapy
Hormones
Hot flashes
Hyperhidrosis
Hyperparathyroidism and
    hypoparathyroidism
Hypoglycemia
Hypothalamus
Klinefelter syndrome
Liver
Melatonin
Nonalcoholic steatohepatitis (NASH)
Obesity
Obesity, childhood
Overtraining syndrome
Pancreas
Pancreatitis
Parathyroidectomy
Pituitary gland
Placenta
Plasma
Polycystic ovary syndrome
Postpartum depression
Prader-Willi syndrome
Prostate enlargement
Prostate gland
Prostate gland removal
Sexual differentiation
Small intestine
Steroid abuse
Steroids
Sweating
Systems and organs
Testicular cancer
Testicular surgery
Thymus gland
Thyroid disorders
Thyroid gland
Thyroidectomy
Turner syndrome
Weight loss medications

EYES
Adenoviruses
Adrenoleukodystrophy
Agnosia
Albinos
Antihistamines
Astigmatism
Auras
Batten's disease
Behçet's disease

Blindness
Blurred vision
Botox
Cataract surgery
Cataracts
Chlamydia
Color blindness
Conjunctivitis
Corneal transplantation
Cornelia de Lange syndrome
Cytomegalovirus (CMV)
Dengue fever
Diabetes mellitus
Dyslexia
Enteroviruses
Eye infections and disorders
Eye surgery
Eyes
Face lift and blepharoplasty
Galactosemia
Glaucoma
Gonorrhea
Gulf War syndrome
Jaundice
Juvenile rheumatoid arthritis
Keratitis
Kluver-Bucy syndrome
Laser use in surgery
Leukodystrophy
Macular degeneration
Marfan syndrome
Marijuana
Microscopy, slitlamp
Motor skill development
Multiple chemical sensitivity
    syndrome
Myopia
Ophthalmology
Optometry
Optometry, pediatric
Pigmentation
Ptosis
Refractive eye surgery
Reiter's syndrome
Rubinstein-Taybi syndrome
Sarcoidosis
Sense organs
Sjögren's syndrome
Strabismus
Sturge-Weber syndrome
Styes
Tears and tear ducts
Toxoplasmosis
Trachoma

Endocrine disorders
Endocrine glands
Endocrinology
Endocrinology, pediatric
Epstein-Barr virus
Gender reassignment surgery
Gigantism
Glands
Goiter
Gynecomastia
Hashimoto's thyroiditis
Hormone therapy
Hormones
Hyperhidrosis
Hyperparathyroidism and
    hypoparathyroidism
Hypoglycemia
Hypothalamus
Internal medicine
Liver
Mastectomy and lumpectomy
Melatonin
Metabolism
Mumps
Neurosurgery
Nuclear medicine
Nuclear radiology
Obesity
Obesity, childhood
Orchiectomy
Ovaries
Pancreas
Parathyroidectomy
Pituitary gland
Prader-Willi syndrome
Prostate enlargement
Prostate gland
Prostate gland removal
Semen
Sexual differentiation
Steroids
Styes
Sweating
Testicular cancer
Testicular surgery
Thymus gland
Thyroid disorders
Thyroid gland
Thyroidectomy

GUMS
Abscess drainage
Abscesses
Cavities

Cleft lip and palate
Cleft lip and palate repair
Crowns and bridges
Dengue fever
Dental diseases
Dentistry
Dentistry, pediatric
Dentures
Endodontic disease
Fluoride treatments
Gingivitis
Gulf War syndrome
Gum disease
Jaw wiring
Mouth and throat cancer
Nicotine
Nutrition
Oral and maxillofacial surgery
Orthodontics
Periodontal surgery
Periodontitis
Root canal treatment
Scurvy
Teeth
Teething
Tooth extraction
Toothache
Wisdom teeth

HAIR
Albinos
Cornelia de Lange syndrome
Dermatitis
Dermatology
Eczema
Gray hair
Hair
Hair loss and baldness
Hair transplantation
Klinefelter syndrome
Lice, mites, and ticks
Nutrition
Pigmentation
Radiation sickness
Radiation therapy

HANDS
Amputation
Arthritis
Bones and the skeleton
Bursitis
Carpal tunnel syndrome
Casts and splints
Cerebral palsy

Cornelia de Lange syndrome
Corns and calluses
Cysts
Dyskinesia
Fracture and dislocation
Fracture repair
Fragile X syndrome
Frostbite
Ganglion removal
Methicillin-resistant *Staphylococcus
    aureus* (MRSA) infections
Nail removal
Nails
Neurology
Neurology, pediatric
Orthopedic surgery
Orthopedics
Orthopedics, pediatric
Osteoarthritis
Polydactyly and syndactyly
Rheumatoid arthritis
Rheumatology
Rubinstein-Taybi syndrome
Scleroderma
Skin lesion removal
Sports medicine
Tendinitis
Tendon disorders
Tendon repair
Thalidomide
Upper extremities
Vasculitis
Warts

HEAD
Altitude sickness
Aneurysmectomy
Aneurysms
Angiography
Antihistamines
Botox
Brain
Brain disorders
Brain tumors
Cluster headaches
Coma
Computed tomography (CT)
    scanning
Concussion
Cornelia de Lange syndrome
Craniosynostosis
Craniotomy
Dengue fever
Dizziness and fainting

Dyskinesia
Electroencephalography (EEG)
Embolism
Epilepsy
Esophagus
Facial transplantation
Fetal tissue transplantation
Fibromyalgia
Hair loss and baldness
Hair transplantation
Head and neck disorders
Headaches
Hydrocephalus
Lice, mites, and ticks
Meningitis
Migraine headaches
Nasal polyp removal
Nasopharyngeal disorders
Neuroimaging
Neurology
Neurology, pediatric
Neurosurgery
Oral and maxillofacial surgery
Pharynx
Polyps
Rhinoplasty and submucous
  resection
Rubinstein-Taybi syndrome
Seizures
Shunts
Sports medicine
Strokes
Sturge-Weber syndrome
Subdural hematoma
Tears and tear ducts
Temporomandibular joint (TMJ)
  syndrome
Thrombosis and thrombus
Tinnitus
Unconsciousness
Whiplash

HEART
Acidosis
Aneurysmectomy
Aneurysms
Angina
Angiography
Angioplasty
Anxiety
Apgar score
Arrhythmias
Arteriosclerosis
Atrial fibrillation

Biofeedback
Bites and stings
Blood pressure
Blood vessels
Blue baby syndrome
Bypass surgery
Caffeine
Cardiac arrest
Cardiac rehabilitation
Cardiac surgery
Cardiology
Cardiology, pediatric
Cardiopulmonary resuscitation
  (CPR)
Carotid arteries
Catheterization
Circulation
Congenital heart disease
Cornelia de Lange syndrome
Coronary artery bypass graft
Defibrillation
DiGeorge syndrome
Diuretics
Echocardiography
Electrical shock
Electrocardiography (ECG or EKG)
Embolism
End-stage renal disease
Endocarditis
Enteroviruses
Exercise physiology
Fatty acid oxidation disorders
Glycogen storage diseases
Heart
Heart attack
Heart disease
Heart failure
Heart transplantation
Heart valve replacement
Hemochromatosis
Hypertension
Hypotension
Infarction
Internal medicine
Intravenous (IV) therapy
Juvenile rheumatoid arthritis
Kinesiology
Lyme disease
Marfan syndrome
Marijuana
Methicillin-resistant *Staphylococcus
  aureus* (MRSA) infections
Mitral valve prolapse
Nicotine

Obesity
Obesity, childhood
Pacemaker implantation
Palpitations
Plaque, arterial
Plasma
Prader-Willi syndrome
Pulmonary edema
Pulse rate
Respiratory distress syndrome
Resuscitation
Reye's syndrome
Rheumatic fever
Rubinstein-Taybi syndrome
Sarcoidosis
Scleroderma
Shock
Sports medicine
Stenosis
Stents
Steroid abuse
Strokes
Thoracic surgery
Thrombolytic therapy and TPA
Thrombosis and thrombus
Toxoplasmosis
Transplantation
Ultrasonography
Uremia
Yellow fever

HIPS
Aging
Arthritis
Arthroplasty
Arthroscopy
Bone disorders
Bones and the skeleton
Chiropractic
Dwarfism
Fracture and dislocation
Fracture repair
Hip fracture repair
Hip replacement
Liposuction
Lower extremities
Orthopedic surgery
Orthopedics
Orthopedics, pediatric
Osteoarthritis
Osteochondritis juvenilis
Osteonecrosis
Osteoporosis
Physical rehabilitation

Colorectal surgery
Constipation
Crohn's disease
Diarrhea and dysentery
Digestion
Diverticulitis and diverticulosis
E. coli infection
Eating disorders
Endoscopy
Enemas
Enterocolitis
Fiber
Fistula repair
Food poisoning
Gastroenteritis
Gastroenterology
Gastroenterology, pediatric
Gastrointestinal disorders
Gastrointestinal system
Gluten intolerance
Hemorrhoid banding and removal
Hemorrhoids
Hernia
Hernia repair
Hirschsprung's disease
Ileostomy and colostomy
Indigestion
Infarction
Internal medicine
Intestinal disorders
Intestines
Irritable bowel syndrome (IBS)
Kaposi's sarcoma
Kwashiorkor
Lactose intolerance
Laparoscopy
Malabsorption
Malnutrition
Metabolism
Nutrition
Obesity
Obesity, childhood
Obstruction
Peristalsis
Pinworm
Polyps
Proctology
Rectum
Rotavirus
Roundworm
Salmonella infection
Small intestine
Soiling
Sphincterectomy

Stomach, intestinal, and pancreatic
  cancers
Tapeworm
Toilet training
Trichinosis
Tumor removal
Tumors
Typhoid fever
Ulcer surgery
Ulcers
Vasculitis
Worms

JOINTS
Amputation
Arthritis
Arthroplasty
Arthroscopy
Braces, orthopedic
Bursitis
Carpal tunnel syndrome
Cartilage
Casts and splints
Chlamydia
Collagen
Corticosteroids
Cyst removal
Cysts
Endoscopy
Exercise physiology
Fracture and dislocation
Fragile X syndrome
Gout
Gulf War syndrome
Hammertoe correction
Hammertoes
Hip fracture repair
Juvenile rheumatoid arthritis
Klippel-Trenaunay syndrome
Kneecap removal
Ligaments
Lyme disease
Methicillin-resistant *Staphylococcus*
  aureus (MRSA) infections
Motor skill development
Orthopedic surgery
Orthopedics
Orthopedics, pediatric
Osteoarthritis
Osteochondritis juvenilis
Osteomyelitis
Osteonecrosis
Physical rehabilitation
Reiter's syndrome

Rheumatoid arthritis
Rheumatology
Rotator cuff surgery
Sarcoidosis
Scleroderma
Spondylitis
Sports medicine
Systemic lupus erythematosus
  (SLE)
Temporomandibular joint (TMJ)
  syndrome
Tendinitis
Tendon disorders
Tendon repair
Von Willebrand's disease

KIDNEYS
Abdomen
Abscess drainage
Abscesses
Adrenal glands
Adrenalectomy
Babesiosis
Carbohydrates
Corticosteroids
Cysts
Dialysis
Diuretics
End-stage renal disease
Galactosemia
Hantavirus
Hematuria
Hemolytic uremic syndrome
Hypertension
Hypotension
Infarction
Internal medicine
Intravenous (IV) therapy
Kidney cancer
Kidney disorders
Kidney transplantation
Kidneys
Laparoscopy
Lithotripsy
Metabolism
Methicillin-resistant *Staphylococcus*
  aureus (MRSA) infections
Nephrectomy
Nephritis
Nephrology
Nephrology, pediatric
Nuclear medicine
Nuclear radiology
Polycystic kidney disease

Preeclampsia and eclampsia
Proteinuria
Pyelonephritis
Renal failure
Reye's syndrome
Rocky Mountain spotted fever
Sarcoidosis
Scleroderma
Stone removal
Stones
Toilet training
Transplantation
Ultrasonography
Uremia
Urinalysis
Urinary disorders
Urinary system
Urology
Urology, pediatric
Vasculitis

KNEES
Amputation
Arthritis
Arthroplasty
Arthroscopy
Bone disorders
Bones and the skeleton
Bowlegs
Braces, orthopedic
Bursitis
Cartilage
Casts and splints
Endoscopy
Exercise physiology
Fracture and dislocation
Joints
Kneecap removal
Knock-knees
Liposuction
Lower extremities
Orthopedic surgery
Orthopedics
Orthopedics, pediatric
Osgood-Schlatter disease
Osteoarthritis
Osteonecrosis
Physical rehabilitation
Rheumatoid arthritis
Rheumatology
Sports medicine
Tendinitis
Tendon disorders
Tendon repair

LEGS
Amputation
Arthritis
Arthroplasty
Arthroscopy
Bone disorders
Bones and the skeleton
Bowlegs
Bursitis
Casts and splints
Cerebral palsy
Cornelia de Lange syndrome
Deep vein thrombosis
Dwarfism
Dyskinesia
Fracture and dislocation
Fracture repair
Gigantism
Hemiplegia
Hip fracture repair
Kneecap removal
Knock-knees
Liposuction
Lower extremities
Methicillin-resistant *Staphylococcus aureus* (MRSA) infections
Muscle sprains, spasms, and disorders
Muscles
Muscular dystrophy
Numbness and tingling
Orthopedic surgery
Orthopedics
Orthopedics, pediatric
Osteoarthritis
Osteoporosis
Paralysis
Paraplegia
Physical rehabilitation
Pigeon toes
Pityriasis rosea
Poliomyelitis
Quadriplegia
Rheumatoid arthritis
Rheumatology
Rickets
Sciatica
Sports medicine
Tendinitis
Tendon disorders
Tendon repair
Thalidomide
Varicose vein removal
Varicose veins

Vasculitis
Venous insufficiency

LIGAMENTS
Bones and the skeleton
Casts and splints
Collagen
Connective tissue
Flat feet
Joints
Kidneys
Ligaments
Muscle sprains, spasms, and disorders
Muscles
Orthopedic surgery
Orthopedics
Orthopedics, pediatric
Osteogenesis imperfecta
Physical rehabilitation
Slipped disk
Spleen
Sports medicine
Tendon disorders
Tendon repair
Whiplash

LIVER
Abdomen
Abdominal disorders
Abscess drainage
Abscesses
Alcoholism
Amebiasis
Babesiosis
Bile
Blood and blood disorders
Chyme
Circulation
Cirrhosis
Corticosteroids
Cytomegalovirus (CMV)
Edema
Embolization
Endoscopic retrograde cholangiopancreatography (ERCP)
Fatty acid oxidation disorders
Fetal surgery
Galactosemia
Gastroenterology
Gastroenterology, pediatric
Gastrointestinal disorders
Gastrointestinal system
Gaucher's disease

Glycogen storage diseases
Hematology
Hematology, pediatric
Hemochromatosis
Hemolytic disease of the newborn
Hepatitis
Histiocytosis
Internal medicine
Jaundice
Jaundice, neonatal
Kaposi's sarcoma
Liver
Liver cancer
Liver disorders
Liver transplantation
Malabsorption
Malaria
Metabolism
Methicillin-resistant *Staphylococcus aureus* (MRSA) infections
Niemann-Pick disease
Nonalcoholic steatohepatitis (NASH)
Polycystic kidney disease
Reye's syndrome
Schistosomiasis
Shunts
Thrombocytopenia
Transplantation
Wilson's disease
Yellow fever

LUNGS
Abscess drainage
Abscesses
Acute respiratory distress syndrome (ARDS)
Adenoviruses
Allergies
Altitude sickness
Anthrax
Antihistamines
Apgar score
Apnea
Asbestos exposure
Aspergillosis
Asphyxiation
Asthma
Bacterial infections
Bronchi
Bronchiolitis
Bronchitis
Cardiopulmonary resuscitation (CPR)

Chest
Childhood infectious diseases
Choking
Chronic obstructive pulmonary disease (COPD)
Coccidioidomycosis
Common cold
Coronaviruses
Corticosteroids
Coughing
Croup
Cystic fibrosis
Cytomegalovirus (CMV)
Diaphragm
Diphtheria
Drowning
Edema
Embolism
Emphysema
Endoscopy
Exercise physiology
Fetal surgery
Hantavirus
Heart transplantation
Heimlich maneuver
Hiccups
Histiocytosis
H1N1 influenza
Hyperbaric oxygen therapy
Hyperventilation
Hypoxia
Infarction
Influenza
Internal medicine
Interstitial pulmonary fibrosis (IPF)
Intravenous (IV) therapy
Kaposi's sarcoma
Kinesiology
Legionnaires' disease
Lung cancer
Lung surgery
Lungs
Marijuana
Measles
Mesothelioma
Multiple chemical sensitivity syndrome
Nicotine
Niemann-Pick disease
Oxygen therapy
Plague
Pleurisy
Pneumonia

Pneumothorax
Pulmonary diseases
Pulmonary edema
Pulmonary hypertension
Pulmonary medicine
Pulmonary medicine, pediatric
Respiration
Respiratory distress syndrome
Resuscitation
Rhinoviruses
Sarcoidosis
Scleroderma
Severe acute respiratory syndrome (SARS)
Smoking
Sneezing
Thoracic surgery
Thrombolytic therapy and TPA
Thrombosis and thrombus
Toxoplasmosis
Transplantation
Tuberculosis
Tularemia
Tumor removal
Tumors
Vasculitis
Wheezing
Whooping cough
Wiskott-Aldrich syndrome

LYMPHATIC SYSTEM
Adenoids
Angiography
Antibodies
Bacillus Calmette-Guérin (BCG)
Bacterial infections
Biological therapies
Blood and blood disorders
Blood vessels
Breast cancer
Breast disorders
Breasts, female
Bruises
Burkitt's lymphoma
Cancer
Cervical, ovarian, and uterine cancers
Chemotherapy
Circulation
Colon cancer
Coronaviruses
Corticosteroids
DiGeorge syndrome
Edema

Multiple sclerosis
Muscle sprains, spasms, and
  disorders
Muscles
Muscular dystrophy
Necrotizing fasciitis
Neurology
Neurology, pediatric
Numbness and tingling
Orthopedic surgery
Orthopedics
Orthopedics, pediatric
Osgood-Schlatter disease
Osteopathic medicine
Overtraining syndrome
Palsy
Paralysis
Paraplegia
Parkinson's disease
Physical rehabilitation
Poisoning
Poliomyelitis
Ptosis
Quadriplegia
Rabies
Respiration
Restless legs syndrome
Rheumatoid arthritis
Rotator cuff surgery
Seizures
Speech disorders
Sphincterectomy
Sports medicine
Steroid abuse
Strabismus
Tattoos and body piercing
Temporomandibular joint (TMJ)
  syndrome
Tendon disorders
Tendon repair
Tetanus
Tics
Torticollis
Tourette's syndrome
Trembling and shaking
Trichinosis
Upper extremities
Weight loss and gain
Yellow fever

MUSCULOSKELETAL SYSTEM
Acupressure
Amputation
Amyotrophic lateral sclerosis

Anatomy
Anesthesia
Anesthesiology
Arthritis
Ataxia
Atrophy
Back pain
Bed-wetting
Bell's palsy
Beriberi
Biofeedback
Bone cancer
Bone disorders
Bone grafting
Bone marrow transplantation
Bones and the skeleton
Botulism
Bowlegs
Braces, orthopedic
Breasts, female
Cartilage
Casts and splints
Cells
Cerebral palsy
Chest
Childhood infectious diseases
Chiropractic
Chronic fatigue syndrome
Claudication
Cleft lip and palate
Cleft lip and palate repair
Collagen
Congenital hypothyroidism
Connective tissue
Craniosynostosis
Cysts
Dengue fever
Depression
Diaphragm
Dwarfism
Ear surgery
Ears
Ehrlichiosis
Electromyography
Emotions: Biomedical causes
  and effects
Ergogenic aids
Ewing's sarcoma
Exercise physiology
Feet
Fetal alcohol syndrome
Fibromyalgia
Flat feet
Foot disorders

Fracture and dislocation
Fracture repair
Gigantism
Glycolysis
Guillain-Barré syndrome
Hammertoe correction
Hammertoes
Head and neck disorders
Heel spur removal
Hematology
Hematology, pediatric
Hematomas
Hemiplegia
Hip fracture repair
Hip replacement
Hyperparathyroidism and
  hypoparathyroidism
Jaw wiring
Joints
Juvenile rheumatoid arthritis
Kinesiology
Kneecap removal
Knock-knees
Kyphosis
Ligaments
Lower extremities
Marfan syndrome
Marijuana
Mastectomy and lumpectomy
Methicillin-resistant *Staphylococcus
  aureus* (MRSA) infections
Motor neuron diseases
Motor skill development
Multiple sclerosis
Muscle sprains, spasms, and
  disorders
Muscles
Muscular dystrophy
Myasthenia gravis
Neurology
Neurology, pediatric
Nuclear medicine
Nuclear radiology
Numbness and tingling
Orthopedic surgery
Orthopedics
Orthopedics, pediatric
Osteochondritis juvenilis
Osteogenesis imperfecta
Osteomyelitis
Osteonecrosis
Osteopathic medicine
Osteoporosis
Paget's disease

Palsy
Paralysis
Paraplegia
Parkinson's disease
Periodontitis
Physical rehabilitation
Pigeon toes
Poisoning
Poliomyelitis
Prader-Willi syndrome
Precocious puberty
Quadriplegia
Rabies
Radiculopathy
Respiration
Restless legs syndrome
Rheumatoid arthritis
Rheumatology
Rickets
Sarcoma
Scoliosis
Seizures
Sleepwalking
Slipped disk
Speech disorders
Sphincterectomy
Spinal cord disorders
Spine, vertebrae, and disks
Sports medicine
Systemic lupus erythematosus
    (SLE)
Systems and organs
Teeth
Tendinitis
Tendon disorders
Tendon repair
Tetanus
Tics
Tourette's syndrome
Trembling and shaking
Trichinosis
Upper extremities
Weight loss and gain
Yellow fever

NAILS
Anemia
Dermatology
Fungal infections
Malnutrition
Nail removal
Nails
Nutrition
Podiatry

NECK
Asphyxiation
Back pain
Botox
Braces, orthopedic
Carotid arteries
Casts and splints
Chiari malformations
Choking
Congenital hypothyroidism
Dyskinesia
Endarterectomy
Esophagus
Goiter
Hashimoto's thyroiditis
Head and neck disorders
Heimlich maneuver
Hyperparathyroidism and
    hypoparathyroidism
Laryngectomy
Laryngitis
Mouth and throat cancer
Otorhinolaryngology
Paralysis
Parathyroidectomy
Pharynx
Quadriplegia
Spine, vertebrae, and disks
Sympathectomy
Thyroid disorders
Thyroid gland
Thyroidectomy
Tonsillectomy and adenoid removal
Tonsillitis
Torticollis
Trachea
Tracheostomy
Vagus nerve
Whiplash

NERVES
Agnosia
Anesthesia
Anesthesiology
Back pain
Bell's palsy
Biofeedback
Brain
Carpal tunnel syndrome
Cells
Creutzfeldt-Jakob disease (CJD)
Cysts
Dyskinesia
Electromyography

Emotions: Biomedical causes and
    effects
Epilepsy
Facial transplantation
Fibromyalgia
Guillain-Barré syndrome
Hearing
Hemiplegia
Huntington's disease
Leprosy
Leukodystrophy
Listeria infections
Local anesthesia
Lower extremities
Marijuana
Motor neuron diseases
Motor skill development
Multiple chemical sensitivity
    syndrome
Multiple sclerosis
Nervous system
Neuralgia, neuritis, and neuropathy
Neuroimaging
Neurology
Neurology, pediatric
Neurosurgery
Numbness and tingling
Palsy
Paralysis
Paraplegia
Parkinson's disease
Physical rehabilitation
Poliomyelitis
Ptosis
Quadriplegia
Radiculopathy
Sarcoidosis
Sciatica
Seizures
Sense organs
Shock therapy
Skin
Spina bifida
Spinal cord disorders
Spine, vertebrae, and disks
Sturge-Weber syndrome
Sympathectomy
Tics
Tinnitus
Touch
Tourette's syndrome
Upper extremities
Vagotomy
Vasculitis

NERVOUS SYSTEM

Abscess drainage
Abscesses
Acupressure
Addiction
Adenoviruses
Adrenoleukodystrophy
Agnosia
Alcoholism
Altitude sickness
Alzheimer's disease
Amnesia
Amputation
Amyotrophic lateral sclerosis
Anesthesia
Anesthesiology
Aneurysmectomy
Aneurysms
Anosmia
Antidepressants
Anxiety
Apgar score
Aphasia and dysphasia
Apnea
Aromatherapy
Ataxia
Atrophy
Attention-deficit disorder (ADD)
Auras
Autism
Back pain
Balance disorders
Batten's disease
Behçet's disease
Bell's palsy
Beriberi
Biofeedback
Botulism
Brain
Brain damage
Brain disorders
Brain tumors
Caffeine
Carpal tunnel syndrome
Cells
Cerebral palsy
Chagas' disease
Chiari malformations
Chiropractic
Chronic wasting disease (CWD)
Claudication
Cluster headaches
Cognitive development
Coma

Computed tomography (CT) scanning
Concussion
Congenital hypothyroidism
Craniotomy
Creutzfeldt-Jakob disease (CJD)
Cysts
Deafness
Defibrillation
Dementias
Developmental disorders
Developmental stages
Diabetes mellitus
Diphtheria
Disk removal
Dizziness and fainting
Down syndrome
Dwarfism
Dyskinesia
Dyslexia
E. coli infection
Ear surgery
Ears
Ehrlichiosis
Electrical shock
Electroencephalography (EEG)
Electromyography
Emotions: Biomedical causes and effects
Encephalitis
Endocrinology
Endocrinology, pediatric
Enteroviruses
Epilepsy
Eye infections and disorders
Eyes
Facial transplantation
Fetal alcohol syndrome
Fetal tissue transplantation
Fibromyalgia
Frontotemporal dementia (FTD)
Gigantism
Glands
Guillain-Barré syndrome
Hallucinations
Hammertoe correction
Head and neck disorders
Headaches
Hearing aids
Hearing loss
Hearing tests
Heart transplantation
Hemiplegia
Histiocytosis

Huntington's disease
Hydrocephalus
Hypnosis
Hypothalamus
Insect-borne diseases
Intraventricular hemorrhage
Irritable bowel syndrome (IBS)
Kinesiology
Lead poisoning
Learning disabilities
Leprosy
Light therapy
Listeria infections
Local anesthesia
Lower extremities
Lyme disease
Malaria
Maple syrup urine disease (MSUD)
Marijuana
Memory loss
Meningitis
Mental retardation
Mercury poisoning
Migraine headaches
Motor neuron diseases
Motor skill development
Multiple chemical sensitivity syndrome
Multiple sclerosis
Myasthenia gravis
Narcolepsy
Narcotics
Nausea and vomiting
Nervous system
Neuralgia, neuritis, and neuropathy
Neurofibromatosis
Neuroimaging
Neurology
Neurology, pediatric
Neurosurgery
Niemann-Pick disease
Nuclear radiology
Numbness and tingling
Orthopedic surgery
Orthopedics
Orthopedics, pediatric
Overtraining syndrome
Paget's disease
Palsy
Paralysis
Paraplegia
Parkinson's disease
Pharmacology

Appetite loss
Aromatherapy
Asperger's syndrome
Attention-deficit disorder (ADD)
Auras
Autism
Bariatric surgery
Biofeedback
Bipolar disorders
Body dysmorphic disorder
Bonding
Brain
Brain disorders
Bulimia
Chronic fatigue syndrome
Club drugs
Cluster headaches
Cognitive development
Colic
Coma
Concussion
Corticosteroids
Death and dying
Delusions
Dementias
Depression
Developmental disorders
Developmental stages
Dizziness and fainting
Domestic violence
Down syndrome
Dyskinesia
Dyslexia
Eating disorders
Electroencephalography (EEG)
Emotions: Biomedical causes and
    effects
Endocrinology
Endocrinology, pediatric
Facial transplantation
Factitious disorders
Failure to thrive
Fibromyalgia
Frontotemporal dementia (FTD)
Gender identity disorder
Grief and guilt
Gulf War syndrome
Hallucinations
Headaches
Hormone therapy
Hormones
Hydrocephalus
Hypnosis
Hypochondriasis

Hypothalamus
Kinesiology
Klinefelter syndrome
Learning disabilities
Light therapy
Marijuana
Memory loss
Menopause
Mental retardation
Midlife crisis
Migraine headaches
Miscarriage
Morgellons disease
Motor skill development
Narcolepsy
Narcotics
Neurology
Neurology, pediatric
Neurosis
Neurosurgery
Nicotine
Nightmares
Obesity
Obesity, childhood
Obsessive-compulsive disorder
Overtraining syndrome
Palpitations
Panic attacks
Paranoia
Pharmacology
Pharmacy
Phobias
Pick's disease
Postpartum depression
Post-traumatic stress disorder
Prader-Willi syndrome
Precocious puberty
Prescription drug abuse
Psychiatric disorders
Psychiatry
Psychiatry, child and adolescent
Psychiatry, geriatric
Psychoanalysis
Psychosis
Psychosomatic disorders
Puberty and adolescence
Rabies
Rape and sexual assault
Restless legs syndrome
Schizophrenia
Seasonal affective disorder
Separation anxiety
Sexual dysfunction
Sexuality

Shock therapy
Sibling rivalry
Sleep
Sleep disorders
Sleepwalking
Soiling
Speech disorders
Sperm banks
Stammering
Steroid abuse
Stillbirth
Stress
Strokes
Stuttering
Substance abuse
Suicide
Synesthesia
Tics
Tinnitus
Toilet training
Tourette's syndrome
Weight loss and gain
Wilson's disease

REPRODUCTIVE SYSTEM
Abdomen
Abdominal disorders
Abortion
Acquired immunodeficiency
    syndrome (AIDS)
Adrenoleukodystrophy
Amenorrhea
Amniocentesis
Anatomy
Anorexia nervosa
Assisted reproductive technologies
Breast-feeding
Breasts, female
Candidiasis
Catheterization
Cervical, ovarian, and uterine
    cancers
Cervical procedures
Cesarean section
Childbirth
Childbirth complications
Chlamydia
Chorionic villus sampling
Circumcision, female, and genital
    mutilation
Circumcision, male
Conception
Congenital adrenal hyperplasia
Contraception

Hypoxia
Influenza
Internal medicine
Interstitial pulmonary fibrosis (IPF)
Kinesiology
Laryngectomy
Laryngitis
Legionnaires' disease
Lung cancer
Lung surgery
Lungs
Marijuana
Measles
Mesothelioma
Methicillin-resistant *Staphylococcus aureus* (MRSA) infections
Monkeypox
Mononucleosis
Multiple chemical sensitivity syndrome
Nasopharyngeal disorders
Nicotine
Niemann-Pick disease
Obesity
Obesity, childhood
Otorhinolaryngology
Oxygen therapy
Pharyngitis
Pharynx
Plague
Plasma
Pleurisy
Pneumonia
Pneumothorax
Poisoning
Pulmonary diseases
Pulmonary edema
Pulmonary hypertension
Pulmonary medicine
Pulmonary medicine, pediatric
Respiration
Resuscitation
Rheumatic fever
Rhinitis
Rhinoviruses
Roundworm
Sarcoidosis
Severe acute respiratory syndrome (SARS)
Sinusitis
Sleep apnea
Smallpox
Sneezing
Sore throat

Strep throat
Systems and organs
Thoracic surgery
Thrombolytic therapy and TPA
Thrombosis and thrombus
Tonsillectomy and adenoid removal
Tonsillitis
Tonsils
Toxoplasmosis
Trachea
Tracheostomy
Transplantation
Tuberculosis
Tularemia
Tumor removal
Tumors
Vasculitis
Voice and vocal cord disorders
Wheezing
Whooping cough
Worms

SKIN
Abscess drainage
Abscesses
Acne
Acupressure
Acupuncture
Adenoviruses
Adrenoleukodystrophy
Age spots
Albinos
Allergies
Amputation
Anesthesia
Anesthesiology
Anthrax
Anxiety
Athlete's foot
Auras
Bacillus Calmette-Guérin (BCG)
Bariatric surgery
Batten's disease
Bedsores
Behçet's disease
Biopsy
Birthmarks
Bites and stings
Blisters
Blood testing
Body dysmorphic disorder
Boils
Botox

Bruises
Burns and scalds
Candidiasis
Canker sores
Casts and splints
Cells
Chagas' disease
Chickenpox
Cleft lip and palate repair
Cold sores
Collagen
Corns and calluses
Corticosteroids
Cryotherapy and cryosurgery
Cyanosis
Cyst removal
Cysts
Dengue fever
Dermatitis
Dermatology
Dermatology, pediatric
Dermatopathology
Diaper rash
Ebola virus
Eczema
Edema
Electrical shock
Electrocauterization
Enteroviruses
Face lift and blepharoplasty
Facial transplantation
Fibrocystic breast condition
Fifth disease
Food allergies
Frostbite
Fungal infections
Glands
Gluten intolerance
Grafts and grafting
Gulf War syndrome
Hair
Hair loss and baldness
Hair transplantation
Hand-foot-and-mouth disease
Heat exhaustion and heatstroke
Hematomas
Hemolytic disease of the newborn
Histiocytosis
Hives
Host-defense mechanisms
Human papillomavirus (HPV)
Hyperhidrosis
Impetigo
Insect-borne diseases

STOMACH
Abdomen
Abdominal disorders
Abscess drainage
Abscesses
Acid reflux disease
Adenoviruses
Allergies
Bariatric surgery
Botulism
Bulimia
Burping
Bypass surgery
Campylobacter infections
Chyme
Clostridium difficile infection
Coccidioidomycosis
Colitis
Crohn's disease
Digestion
Eating disorders
Endoscopic retrograde
  cholangiopancreatography (ERCP)
Endoscopy
Esophagus
Food biochemistry
Food poisoning
Gastrectomy
Gastroenteritis
Gastroenterology
Gastroenterology, pediatric
Gastrointestinal disorders
Gastrointestinal system
Gastrostomy
Gluten intolerance
Halitosis
Heartburn
Hernia
Hernia repair
Indigestion
Influenza
Internal medicine
Kwashiorkor
Lactose intolerance
Malabsorption
Malnutrition
Metabolism
Motion sickness
Nausea and vomiting
Nutrition
Obesity
Obesity, childhood
Peristalsis
Poisoning

Poisonous plants
Pyloric stenosis
Radiation sickness
Rotavirus
Roundworm
Salmonella infection
Small intestine
Stomach, intestinal, and pancreatic
  cancers
Ulcer surgery
Ulcers
Vagotomy
Vitamins and minerals
Weaning
Weight loss and gain

TEETH
Braces, orthodontic
Cavities
Cornelia de Lange syndrome
Crowns and bridges
Dental diseases
Dentistry
Dentistry, pediatric
Dentures
Endodontic disease
Fluoride treatments
Forensic pathology
Fracture repair
Gastrointestinal system
Gingivitis
Gum disease
Jaw wiring
Lisping
Nicotine
Nutrition
Oral and maxillofacial surgery
Orthodontics
Osteogenesis imperfecta
Periodontal surgery
Periodontitis
Plaque, dental
Prader-Willi syndrome
Root canal treatment
Rubinstein-Taybi syndrome
Teeth
Teething
Temporomandibular joint (TMJ)
  syndrome
Thumb sucking
Tooth extraction
Toothache
Veterinary medicine
Wisdom teeth

TENDONS
Carpal tunnel syndrome
Casts and splints
Collagen
Connective tissue
Cysts
Exercise physiology
Ganglion removal
Hammertoe correction
Joints
Kneecap removal
Orthopedic surgery
Orthopedics
Orthopedics, pediatric
Osgood-Schlatter disease
Physical rehabilitation
Sports medicine
Tendinitis
Tendon disorders
Tendon repair

THROAT
Acid reflux disease
Adenoids
Antihistamines
Asbestos exposure
Auras
Bulimia
Catheterization
Choking
Croup
Decongestants
Drowning
Epiglottitis
Epstein-Barr virus
Esophagus
Fifth disease
Gastroenterology
Gastroenterology, pediatric
Gastrointestinal disorders
Gastrointestinal system
Goiter
Head and neck disorders
Heimlich maneuver
Hiccups
Histiocytosis
H1N1 influenza
Laryngectomy
Laryngitis
Mouth and throat cancer
Nasopharyngeal disorders
Nicotine
Nosebleeds
Otorhinolaryngology

Pharyngitis
Pharynx
Pulmonary medicine
Pulmonary medicine, pediatric
Quinsy
Respiration
Rhinitis
Rhinoviruses
Smoking
Sore throat
Strep throat
Tonsillectomy and adenoid
    removal
Tonsillitis
Tonsils
Tracheostomy
Voice and vocal cord disorders

URINARY SYSTEM
Abdomen
Abdominal disorders
Abscess drainage
Abscesses
Adenoviruses
Adrenalectomy
Bed-wetting
Bladder cancer
Bladder removal
Candidiasis
Catheterization
Circumcision, male
Cystitis
Cystoscopy
Cysts
Dialysis
Diuretics
E. coli infection
End-stage renal disease
Endoscopy
Fetal surgery
Fistula repair
Fluids and electrolytes
Geriatrics and gerontology
Hematuria
Hemolytic uremic syndrome
Hermaphroditism and
    pseudohermaphroditism
Host-defense mechanisms
Hyperplasia

Hypertension
Incontinence
Internal medicine
Kidney cancer
Kidney disorders
Kidney transplantation
Kidneys
Laparoscopy
Lithotripsy
Nephrectomy
Nephritis
Nephrology
Nephrology, pediatric
Pediatrics
Penile implant surgery
Plasma
Proteinuria
Pyelonephritis
Reiter's syndrome
Renal failure
Reye's syndrome
Schistosomiasis
Stone removal
Stones
Systems and organs
Testicular cancer
Toilet training
Transplantation
Trichomoniasis
Ultrasonography
Uremia
Urethritis
Urinalysis
Urinary disorders
Urinary system
Urology
Urology, pediatric

UTERUS
Abdomen
Abdominal disorders
Abortion
Amenorrhea
Amniocentesis
Assisted reproductive technologies
Cervical, ovarian, and uterine
    cancers
Cervical procedures
Cesarean section

Childbirth
Childbirth complications
Chorionic villus sampling
Conception
Contraception
Culdocentesis
Dysmenorrhea
Ectopic pregnancy
Electrocauterization
Embolization
Endocrinology
Endometrial biopsy
Endometriosis
Fistula repair
Gender reassignment surgery
Genetic counseling
Genital disorders, female
Gynecology
Hermaphroditism and
    pseudohermaphroditism
Hyperplasia
Hysterectomy
In vitro fertilization
Infertility, female
Internal medicine
Laparoscopy
Menopause
Menorrhagia
Menstruation
Miscarriage
Multiple births
Myomectomy
Obstetrics
Pap test
Pelvic inflammatory disease
    (PID)
Placenta
Pregnancy and gestation
Premature birth
Premenstrual syndrome (PMS)
Prostate enlargement
Reproductive system
Sexual differentiation
Sperm banks
Sterilization
Stillbirth
Tubal ligation
Ultrasonography
Uterus

ENTRIES BY SPECIALTIES AND RELATED FIELDS

ALL
Accidents
African American health
American Indian health
Anatomy
Asian American health
Biostatistics
Clinical trials
Diagnosis
Disease
Emergency rooms
First aid
Geriatrics and gerontology
Health maintenance organizations (HMOs)
Iatrogenic disorders
Imaging and radiology
Internet medicine
Invasive tests
Laboratory tests
Men's health
Neuroimaging
Noninvasive tests
Pediatrics
Physical examination
Physiology
Polypharmacy
Preventive medicine
Prognosis
Proteomics
Screening
Self-medication
Signs and symptoms
Syndrome
Systems and organs
Telemedicine
Terminally ill: Extended care
Veterinary medicine
Women's health

ALTERNATIVE MEDICINE
Acidosis
Acupressure
Acupuncture
Allied health
Alternative medicine
Antioxidants
Aphrodisiacs
Aromatherapy
Biofeedback

Biological therapies
Chronobiology
Club drugs
Colon therapy
Enzyme therapy
Fiber
Healing
Herbal medicine
Holistic medicine
Hydrotherapy
Hypnosis
Magnetic field therapy
Marijuana
Massage
Meditation
Melatonin
Nutrition
Oxygen therapy
Pain management
Stress reduction
Supplements
Yoga

ANESTHESIOLOGY
Acidosis
Acupuncture
Anesthesia
Anesthesiology
Catheterization
Cesarean section
Critical care
Critical care, pediatric
Defibrillation
Dentistry
Hyperbaric oxygen therapy
Hyperthermia and hypothermia
Hypnosis
Hypoxia
Intravenous (IV) therapy
Local anesthesia
Oral and maxillofacial surgery
Pain management
Pharmacology
Pharmacy
Pulse rate
Surgery, general
Surgery, pediatric
Surgical procedures
Surgical technologists
Toxicology

AUDIOLOGY
Adrenoleukodystrophy
Aging
Aging: Extended care
Audiology
Biophysics
Deafness
Dyslexia
Ear infections and disorders
Ear surgery
Ears
Earwax
Hearing
Hearing aids
Hearing loss
Hearing tests
Ménière's disease
Motion sickness
Neurology
Neurology, pediatric
Otoplasty
Otorhinolaryngology
Sense organs
Speech disorders
Tinnitus
Vertigo

BACTERIOLOGY
Amebiasis
Anthrax
Antibiotics
Antibodies
Bacillus Calmette-Guérin (BCG)
Bacterial infections
Bacteriology
Biological and chemical weapons
Blisters
Boils
Botulism
Campylobacter infections
Cells
Childhood infectious diseases
Cholecystitis
Cholera
Clostridium difficile infection
Cystitis
Cytology
Cytopathology
Diphtheria
Drug resistance

Prostate gland
Puberty and adolescence
Pulse rate
Radiopharmaceuticals
Sexual differentiation
Sexual dysfunction
Sleep
Stem cells
Steroids
Testicles, undescended
Testicular cancer
Thymus gland
Thyroid disorders
Thyroid gland
Thyroidectomy
Toxicology
Tumors
Turner syndrome
Vitamins and minerals
Vitiligo
Weight loss and gain
Weight loss medications

ENVIRONMENTAL HEALTH
Acidosis
Allergies
Asbestos exposure
Asthma
Babesiosis
Bacteriology
Biological and chemical weapons
Blurred vision
Cholera
Cognitive development
Coronaviruses
Elephantiasis
Enteroviruses
Environmental diseases
Environmental health
Epidemiology
Food poisoning
Frostbite
Gastroenteritis
Gulf War syndrome
Hantavirus
Heat exhaustion and heatstroke
Holistic medicine
Hyperthermia and hypothermia
Insect-borne diseases
Interstitial pulmonary fibrosis
 (IPF)
Lead poisoning
Legionnaires' disease
Lice, mites, and ticks

Lung cancer
Lungs
Lyme disease
Malaria
Mercury poisoning
Mesothelioma
Microbiology
Mold and mildew
Multiple chemical sensitivity
 syndrome
Nasopharyngeal disorders
Occupational health
Parasitic diseases
Pigmentation
Plague
Poisoning
Poisonous plants
Pulmonary diseases
Pulmonary medicine
Pulmonary medicine, pediatric
Salmonella infection
Skin cancer
Snakebites
Stress
Stress reduction
Toxicology
Trachoma
Tropical medicine
Tularemia
Typhoid fever
Typhus

EPIDEMIOLOGY
Acquired immunodeficiency
 syndrome (AIDS)
Amebiasis
Anthrax
Bacillus Calmette-Guérin (BCG)
Bacterial infections
Bacteriology
Biological and chemical weapons
Biostatistics
Carcinogens
Childhood infectious diseases
Cholera
Clostridium difficile infection
Coronaviruses
Creutzfeldt-Jakob disease (CJD)
Disease
E. coli infection
Ebola virus
Elephantiasis
Emerging infectious diseases
Environmental diseases

Environmental health
Epidemics and pandemics
Epidemiology
Food poisoning
Forensic pathology
Gulf War syndrome
Hantavirus
Health Canada
Hepatitis
H1N1 influenza
Influenza
Insect-borne diseases
Laboratory tests
Legionnaires' disease
Leprosy
Lice, mites, and ticks
Malaria
Marburg virus
Measles
Mercury poisoning
Methicillin-resistant *Staphylococcus
 aureus* (MRSA) infections
Microbiology
Multiple chemical sensitivity
 syndrome
Necrotizing fasciitis
Occupational health
Parasitic diseases
Pathology
Plague
Pneumonia
Poisoning
Poliomyelitis
Prion diseases
Pulmonary diseases
Rabies
Rhinoviruses
Rocky Mountain spotted fever
Rotavirus
Salmonella infection
Severe acute respiratory syndrome
 (SARS)
Sexually transmitted diseases
 (STDs)
Stress
Trichomoniasis
Tropical medicine
Typhoid fever
Typhus
Viral hemorrhagic fevers
Viral infections
World Health Organization
Yellow fever
Zoonoses

ETHICS

Abortion
Animal rights vs. research
Assisted reproductive technologies
Circumcision, female, and genital
 mutilation
Circumcision, male
Cloning
Defibrillation
Ergogenic aids
Ethics
Euthanasia
Fetal surgery
Fetal tissue transplantation
Gender identity disorder
Gene therapy
Genetic engineering
Genomics
Gulf War syndrome
Health Canada
Health care reform
Hippocratic oath
Law and medicine
Living will
Malpractice
Marijuana
Münchausen syndrome by proxy
Palliative medicine
Sperm banks
Stem cells
Xenotransplantation

EXERCISE PHYSIOLOGY

Acidosis
Back pain
Biofeedback
Blood pressure
Bone disorders
Bones and the skeleton
Cardiac rehabilitation
Cardiology
Carotid arteries
Circulation
Defibrillation
Dehydration
Echocardiography
Electrocardiography (ECG or EKG)
Ergogenic aids
Exercise physiology
Fascia
Glycolysis
Heart
Heat exhaustion and heatstroke
Hypoxia

Kinesiology
Ligaments
Lungs
Massage
Metabolism
Motor skill development
Muscle sprains, spasms, and
 disorders
Muscles
Nutrition
Orthopedic surgery
Orthopedics
Orthopedics, pediatric
Overtraining syndrome
Oxygen therapy
Physical rehabilitation
Physiology
Pulmonary diseases
Pulmonary medicine
Pulmonary medicine, pediatric
Pulse rate
Respiration
Sports medicine
Stenosis
Steroid abuse
Sweating
Tendinitis
Vascular system

FAMILY MEDICINE

Abdominal disorders
Abscess drainage
Abscesses
Acne
Acquired immunodeficiency
 syndrome (AIDS)
Alcoholism
Allergies
Alzheimer's disease
Amyotrophic lateral sclerosis
Anemia
Angina
Anosmia
Antianxiety drugs
Antidepressants
Antihistamines
Anti-inflammatory drugs
Antioxidants
Arthritis
Athlete's foot
Atrophy
Attention-deficit disorder (ADD)
Bacterial infections
Bed-wetting

Bell's palsy
Beriberi
Biofeedback
Birthmarks
Bleeding
Blisters
Blood pressure
Blurred vision
Body dysmorphic disorder
Boils
Bronchiolitis
Bronchitis
Bunions
Burkitt's lymphoma
Burping
Caffeine
Candidiasis
Canker sores
Carotid arteries
Casts and splints
Chagas' disease
Chickenpox
Childhood infectious diseases
Chlamydia
Cholecystitis
Cholesterol
Chronic fatigue syndrome
Cirrhosis
Clinics
Clostridium difficile infection
Cluster headaches
Coccidioidomycosis
Cold sores
Common cold
Constipation
Contraception
Corticosteroids
Coughing
Cryotherapy and cryosurgery
Cytomegalovirus (CMV)
Death and dying
Decongestants
Deep vein thrombosis
Defibrillation
Dehydration
Dengue fever
Depression
Diabetes mellitus
Diaper rash
Diarrhea and dysentery
Digestion
Dizziness and fainting
Domestic violence
Earwax

FORENSIC MEDICINE
Autopsy
Blood and blood disorders
Blood testing
Bones and the skeleton
Cytopathology
Dermatopathology
DNA and RNA
Forensic pathology
Genetics and inheritance
Genomics
Hematology
Histology
Immunopathology
Laboratory tests
Law and medicine
Pathology

GASTROENTEROLOGY
Abdomen
Abdominal disorders
Acid reflux disease
Acidosis
Adenoviruses
Amebiasis
Amyotrophic lateral sclerosis
Anal cancer
Anthrax
Anus
Appendectomy
Appendicitis
Bariatric surgery
Bile
Bulimia
Bypass surgery
Campylobacter infections
Celiac sprue
Cholecystectomy
Cholecystitis
Cholera
Chyme
Clostridium difficile infection
Colic
Colitis
Colon
Colonoscopy and sigmoidoscopy
Colorectal cancer
Colorectal polyp removal
Colorectal surgery
Computed tomography (CT)
    scanning
Constipation
Critical care
Critical care, pediatric

Crohn's disease
Cytomegalovirus (CMV)
Diarrhea and dysentery
Digestion
Diverticulitis and diverticulosis
E. coli infection
Emergency medicine
Endoscopic retrograde
    cholangiopancreatography (ERCP)
Endoscopy
Enemas
Enterocolitis
Enzymes
Epidemics and pandemics
Esophagus
Failure to thrive
Fiber
Fistula repair
Food allergies
Food biochemistry
Food poisoning
Gallbladder
Gallbladder cancer
Gallbladder diseases
Gastrectomy
Gastroenteritis
Gastroenterology
Gastroenterology, pediatric
Gastrointestinal disorders
Gastrointestinal system
Gastrostomy
Giardiasis
Glands
Gluten intolerance
Heartburn
Hemochromatosis
Hemolytic uremic syndrome
Hemorrhoid banding and removal
Hemorrhoids
Hernia
Hernia repair
Hirschsprung's disease
Ileostomy and colostomy
Indigestion
Infarction
Internal medicine
Intestinal disorders
Intestines
Irritable bowel syndrome (IBS)
Lactose intolerance
Laparoscopy
Lesions
Liver
Liver cancer

Liver disorders
Liver transplantation
Malabsorption
Malnutrition
Metabolism
Nausea and vomiting
Nonalcoholic steatohepatitis (NASH)
Noroviruses
Nutrition
Obstruction
Pancreas
Pancreatitis
Peristalsis
Poisonous plants
Polycystic kidney disease
Polyps
Proctology
Pyloric stenosis
Rectum
Rotavirus
Roundworm
Salmonella infection
Scleroderma
Shigellosis
Small intestine
Soiling
Stenosis
Stevens-Johnson syndrome
Stomach, intestinal, and pancreatic
    cancers
Stone removal
Stones
Tapeworm
Taste
Toilet training
Trichinosis
Ulcer surgery
Ulcers
Vagotomy
Vagus nerve
Vasculitis
Von Willebrand's disease
Weight loss and gain
Wilson's disease
Worms

GENERAL SURGERY
Abscess drainage
Adenoids
Adrenalectomy
Amputation
Anesthesia
Anesthesiology
Aneurysmectomy

Fetal surgery
Fragile X syndrome
Fructosemia
Galactosemia
Gaucher's disease
Gender identity disorder
Gene therapy
Genetic counseling
Genetic diseases
Genetic engineering
Genetics and inheritance
Genomics
Grafts and grafting
Hematology
Hematology, pediatric
Hemophilia
Hermaphroditism and
    pseudohermaphroditism
Huntington's disease
Hyperadiposis
Immunodeficiency disorders
In vitro fertilization
Karyotyping
Klinefelter syndrome
Klippel-Trenaunay syndrome
Laboratory tests
Leptin
Leukodystrophy
Malabsorption
Maple syrup urine disease (MSUD)
Marfan syndrome
Mental retardation
Metabolic disorders
Motor skill development
Mucopolysaccharidosis (MPS)
Muscular dystrophy
Mutation
Neonatology
Nephrology
Nephrology, pediatric
Neurofibromatosis
Neurology
Neurology, pediatric
Niemann-Pick disease
Obstetrics
Oncology
Osteogenesis imperfecta
Ovaries
Pediatrics
Phenylketonuria (PKU)
Polycystic kidney disease
Polydactyly and syndactyly
Polyps
Porphyria

Prader-Willi syndrome
Precocious puberty
Reproductive system
Retroviruses
Rh factor
Rhinoviruses
Rubinstein-Taybi syndrome
Sarcoidosis
Screening
Severe combined immunodeficiency
    syndrome (SCID)
Sexual differentiation
Sexuality
Sperm banks
Stem cells
Synesthesia
Tay-Sachs disease
Tourette's syndrome
Transplantation
Turner syndrome
Wiskott-Aldrich syndrome

GERIATRICS AND GERONTOLOGY
Age spots
Aging
Aging: Extended care
Alzheimer's disease
Arthritis
Assisted living facilities
Atrophy
Bed-wetting
Blindness
Blood pressure
Blurred vision
Bone disorders
Bones and the skeleton
Brain
Brain disorders
Cartilage
Cataract surgery
Cataracts
Chronic obstructive pulmonary
    disease (COPD)
Corns and calluses
Critical care
Crowns and bridges
Deafness
Death and dying
Dementias
Dentures
Depression
Domestic violence
Dyskinesia

Emergency medicine
End-stage renal disease
Endocrinology
Euthanasia
Family medicine
Fatigue
Fiber
Fracture and dislocation
Fracture repair
Gray hair
Hearing aids
Hearing loss
Hip fracture repair
Hip replacement
Hormone therapy
Hormones
Hospitals
Incontinence
Joints
Memory loss
Nursing
Nutrition
Ophthalmology
Orthopedics
Osteoporosis
Pain management
Palliative medicine
Paramedics
Parkinson's disease
Pharmacology
Pick's disease
Psychiatry
Psychiatry, geriatric
Radiculopathy
Rheumatology
Safety issues for the elderly
Sleep disorders
Spinal cord disorders
Spine, vertebrae, and disks
Suicide
Vision disorders
Wrinkles

GYNECOLOGY
Abortion
Amenorrhea
Amniocentesis
Assisted reproductive technologies
Biopsy
Bladder removal
Breast biopsy
Breast cancer
Breast disorders
Breast-feeding

Thrombocytopenia
Thrombolytic therapy and TPA
Thrombosis and thrombus
Transfusion
Uremia
Vascular medicine
Vascular system
Von Willebrand's disease

HISTOLOGY
Autopsy
Biopsy
Cancer
Carcinoma
Cells
Cytology
Cytopathology
Dermatology
Dermatopathology
Fluids and electrolytes
Forensic pathology
Healing
Histology
Laboratory tests
Microscopy
Nails
Necrotizing fasciitis
Pathology
Tumor removal
Tumors

IMMUNOLOGY
Acquired immunodeficiency
    syndrome (AIDS)
Adenoids
Adenoviruses
Allergies
Antibiotics
Antibodies
Antihistamines
Arthritis
Aspergillosis
Asthma
Autoimmune disorders
Bacillus Calmette-Guérin (BCG)
Bacterial infections
Biological and chemical weapons
Biological therapies
Bionics and biotechnology
Bites and stings
Blood and blood disorders
Boils
Bone cancer
Bone grafting

Bone marrow transplantation
Breast cancer
Cancer
Candidiasis
Carcinoma
Cervical, ovarian, and uterine
    cancers
Childhood infectious diseases
Chronic fatigue syndrome
Colorectal cancer
Coronaviruses
Corticosteroids
Cytology
Cytomegalovirus (CMV)
Dermatology
Dermatopathology
DiGeorge syndrome
Emerging infectious diseases
Endocrinology
Endocrinology, pediatric
Epidemics and pandemics
Epstein-Barr virus
Facial transplantation
Food allergies
Fungal infections
Gluten intolerance
Grafts and grafting
Healing
Hematology
Hematology, pediatric
Histiocytosis
Hives
Homeopathy
Host-defense mechanisms
Human immunodeficiency virus
    (HIV)
Hypnosis
Immune system
Immunization and vaccination
Immunodeficiency disorders
Immunology
Immunopathology
Impetigo
Juvenile rheumatoid arthritis
Kawasaki disease
Laboratory tests
Leprosy
Liver cancer
Lung cancer
Lymph
Lymphatic system
Microbiology
Multiple chemical sensitivity
    syndrome

Myasthenia gravis
Nicotine
Noroviruses
Oncology
Opportunistic infections
Oxygen therapy
Palliative medicine
Pancreas
Prostate cancer
Pulmonary diseases
Pulmonary medicine
Pulmonary medicine, pediatric
Rheumatology
Rhinitis
Rhinoviruses
Sarcoidosis
Sarcoma
Scleroderma
Serology
Severe combined immunodeficiency
    syndrome (SCID)
Side effects
Skin cancer
Small intestine
Stem cells
Stevens-Johnson syndrome
Stomach, intestinal, and pancreatic
    cancers
Stress
Stress reduction
Systemic lupus erythematosus (SLE)
Thalidomide
Thymus gland
Transfusion
Transplantation
Tropical medicine
Wiskott-Aldrich syndrome
Xenotransplantation

INTERNAL MEDICINE
Abdomen
Abdominal disorders
Acidosis
Adenoids
Adrenal glands
Amebiasis
Anatomy
Anemia
Angina
Antianxiety drugs
Antibodies
Anti-inflammatory drugs
Antioxidants
Anus

Physical examination
Physician assistants
Polycystic ovary syndrome
Pulse rate
Radiculopathy
Surgery, general
Surgery, pediatric
Surgical procedures
Surgical technologists
Well-baby examinations

NUTRITION
Aging: Extended care
Anorexia nervosa
Antioxidants
Appetite loss
Bariatric surgery
Bedsores
Beriberi
Bile
Breast-feeding
Bulimia
Carbohydrates
Cardiac rehabilitation
Cholesterol
Colon
Dietary reference intakes (DRIs)
Digestion
Eating disorders
Exercise physiology
Fatty acid oxidation disorders
Fiber
Food allergies
Food biochemistry
Food Guide Pyramid
Fructosemia
Galactosemia
Gastroenterology
Gastroenterology, pediatric
Gastrointestinal disorders
Gastrointestinal system
Geriatrics and gerontology
Gestational diabetes
Gluten intolerance
Glycogen storage diseases
Hyperadiposis
Hypercholesterolemia
Irritable bowel syndrome (IBS)
Jaw wiring
Kwashiorkor
Lactose intolerance
Leptin
Leukodystrophy
Lipids

Macronutrients
Malabsorption
Malnutrition
Metabolic disorders
Metabolic syndrome
Metabolism
Nursing
Nutrition
Obesity
Obesity, childhood
Osteoporosis
Phytochemicals
Pituitary gland
Plasma
Polycystic ovary syndrome
Protein
Scurvy
Small intestine
Sports medicine
Supplements
Taste
Tropical medicine
Ulcers
Vagotomy
Vitamins and minerals
Weaning
Weight loss and gain
Weight loss medications

OBSTETRICS
Amniocentesis
Apgar score
Assisted reproductive technologies
Birth defects
Breast-feeding
Breasts, female
Cervical, ovarian, and uterine
  cancers
Cesarean section
Childbirth
Childbirth complications
Chorionic villus sampling
Conception
Congenital disorders
Cytomegalovirus (CMV)
Disseminated intravascular
  coagulation (DIC)
Down syndrome
Ectopic pregnancy
Embryology
Emergency medicine
Episiotomy
Family medicine
Fetal alcohol syndrome

Fetal surgery
Gamete intrafallopian transfer
  (GIFT)
Genetic counseling
Genetic diseases
Genetics and inheritance
Genital disorders, female
Gestational diabetes
Gonorrhea
Growth
Gynecology
Hemolytic disease of the newborn
In vitro fertilization
Incontinence
Intravenous (IV) therapy
Invasive tests
Karyotyping
Listeria infections
Miscarriage
Multiple births
Neonatology
Nicotine
Noninvasive tests
Obstetrics
Ovaries
Perinatology
Pituitary gland
Placenta
Polycystic ovary syndrome
Postpartum depression
Preeclampsia and eclampsia
Pregnancy and gestation
Premature birth
Pyelonephritis
Reproductive system
Rh factor
Rubella
Sexuality
Sperm banks
Spina bifida
Stillbirth
Teratogens
Toxemia
Toxoplasmosis
Trichomoniasis
Ultrasonography
Urology
Uterus

OCCUPATIONAL HEALTH
Acidosis
Agnosia
Altitude sickness
Asbestos exposure

Stress
Sunburn
Testicular cancer
Thalidomide
Thymus gland
Toxicology
Transplantation
Tumor removal
Tumors
Uterus
Wiskott-Aldrich syndrome

OPHTHALMOLOGY
Adrenoleukodystrophy
Aging: Extended care
Albinos
Anti-inflammatory drugs
Astigmatism
Batten's disease
Behçet's disease
Biophysics
Blindness
Blurred vision
Botox
Cataract surgery
Cataracts
Color blindness
Conjunctivitis
Corneal transplantation
Eye infections and disorders
Eye surgery
Eyes
Geriatrics and gerontology
Glaucoma
Juvenile rheumatoid arthritis
Keratitis
Kluver-Bucy syndrome
Laser use in surgery
Macular degeneration
Marfan syndrome
Microscopy, slitlamp
Myopia
Ophthalmology
Optometry
Optometry, pediatric
Prostheses
Ptosis
Refractive eye surgery
Reiter's syndrome
Rubinstein-Taybi syndrome
Sarcoidosis
Sense organs
Stevens-Johnson syndrome
Strabismus

Sturge-Weber syndrome
Styes
Subdural hematoma
Tears and tear ducts
Trachoma
Vasculitis
Vision
Vision disorders

OPTOMETRY
Aging: Extended care
Astigmatism
Biophysics
Blurred vision
Cataracts
Eye infections and disorders
Eyes
Geriatrics and gerontology
Glaucoma
Keratitis
Myopia
Ophthalmology
Optometry
Optometry, pediatric
Ptosis
Refractive eye surgery
Sense organs
Styes
Tears and tear ducts
Vision disorders

ORGANIZATIONS AND PROGRAMS
Allied health
American Medical Association (AMA)
Assisted living facilities
Blood banks
Centers for Disease Control and Prevention (CDC)
Clinical trials
Clinics
Department of Health and Human Services
Education, medical
Food and Drug Administration (FDA)
Gates Foundation
Health Canada
Health maintenance organizations (HMOs)
Hospice
Hospitals
Managed care

Medical College Admission Test (MCAT)
Medicare
National Cancer Institute (NCI)
National Institutes of Health (NIH)
Sperm banks
Stem cells
World Health Organization

ORTHODONTICS
Bones and the skeleton
Braces, orthodontic
Dental diseases
Dentistry
Dentistry, pediatric
Jaw wiring
Nicotine
Orthodontics
Periodontal surgery
Teeth
Teething
Tooth extraction
Wisdom teeth

ORTHOPEDICS
Amputation
Arthritis
Arthroplasty
Arthroscopy
Atrophy
Back pain
Bariatric surgery
Bone cancer
Bone disorders
Bone grafting
Bones and the skeleton
Bowlegs
Braces, orthopedic
Bunions
Bursitis
Cancer
Cartilage
Casts and splints
Chiropractic
Connective tissue
Craniosynostosis
Disk removal
Dwarfism
Ewing's sarcoma
Fascia
Feet
Flat feet
Foot disorders
Fracture and dislocation

Poliomyelitis
Polydactyly and syndactyly
Porphyria
Prader-Willi syndrome
Precocious puberty
Premature birth
Progeria
Psychiatry, child and adolescent
Puberty and adolescence
Pulmonary medicine, pediatric
Pulse rate
Pyloric stenosis
Rashes
Reflexes, primitive
Respiratory distress syndrome
Reye's syndrome
Rheumatic fever
Rhinitis
Rickets
Roseola
Rotavirus
Roundworm
Rubella
Rubinstein-Taybi syndrome
Safety issues for children
Scarlet fever
Seizures
Severe combined immunodeficiency
    syndrome (SCID)
Sexuality
Sibling rivalry
Soiling
Sore throat
Steroids
Stevens-Johnson syndrome
Strep throat
Streptococcal infections
Sturge-Weber syndrome
Styes
Sudden infant death syndrome
    (SIDS)
Surgery, pediatric
Tapeworm
Tay-Sachs disease
Teething
Testicles, undescended
Testicular torsion
Thumb sucking
Toilet training
Tonsillectomy and adenoid removal
Tonsillitis
Tonsils
Trachoma
Tropical medicine

Urology, pediatric
Weaning
Well-baby examinations
Whooping cough
Wiskott-Aldrich syndrome
Worms

PERINATOLOGY
Amniocentesis
Assisted reproductive technologies
Birth defects
Breast-feeding
Cesarean section
Childbirth
Childbirth complications
Chorionic villus sampling
Congenital hypothyroidism
Critical care, pediatric
Embryology
Fatty acid oxidation disorders
Fetal alcohol syndrome
Glycogen storage diseases
Hematology, pediatric
Hydrocephalus
Karyotyping
Metabolic disorders
Motor skill development
Neonatology
Neurology, pediatric
Nursing
Obstetrics
Pediatrics
Perinatology
Pregnancy and gestation
Premature birth
Reflexes, primitive
Shunts
Stillbirth
Sudden infant death syndrome
    (SIDS)
Trichomoniasis
Umbilical cord
Uterus
Well-baby examinations

PHARMACOLOGY
Acid-base chemistry
Acidosis
Aging: Extended care
Anesthesia
Anesthesiology
Antianxiety drugs
Antibiotics
Antibodies

Antidepressants
Antihistamines
Anti-inflammatory drugs
Bacteriology
Blurred vision
Chemotherapy
Club drugs
Corticosteroids
Critical care
Critical care, pediatric
Decongestants
Digestion
Diuretics
Drug resistance
Dyskinesia
Emergency medicine
Emergency medicine, pediatric
Enzymes
Epidemics and pandemics
Ergogenic aids
Fluids and electrolytes
Food biochemistry
Genetic engineering
Genomics
Geriatrics and gerontology
Glycolysis
Herbal medicine
Homeopathy
Hormones
Laboratory tests
Marijuana
Melatonin
Mesothelioma
Metabolism
Narcotics
Nicotine
Oncology
Over-the-counter medications
Pain management
Pharmacology
Pharmacy
Poisoning
Polycystic ovary syndrome
Prader-Willi syndrome
Prescription drug abuse
Psychiatry
Psychiatry, child and adolescent
Psychiatry, geriatric
Rheumatology
Self-medication
Side effects
Sports medicine
Steroid abuse
Steroids

PREVENTIVE MEDICINE

Acidosis
Acupressure
Acupuncture
Aging: Extended care
Alternative medicine
Antibodies
Aromatherapy
Assisted living facilities
Bacillus Calmette-Guérin (BCG)
Biofeedback
Braces, orthopedic
Caffeine
Cardiac surgery
Cardiology
Chiropractic
Cholesterol
Chronobiology
Disease
Echocardiography
Electrocardiography (ECG or EKG)
Environmental health
Exercise physiology
Family medicine
Fiber
Genetic counseling
Geriatrics and gerontology
Holistic medicine
Host-defense mechanisms
Hypercholesterolemia
Immune system
Immunization and vaccination
Immunology
Mammography
Massage
Meditation
Melatonin
Mesothelioma
Noninvasive tests
Nursing
Nutrition
Occupational health
Osteopathic medicine
Over-the-counter medications
Pharmacology
Pharmacy
Physical examination
Phytochemicals
Polycystic ovary syndrome
Preventive medicine
Psychiatry
Psychiatry, child and adolescent
Psychiatry, geriatric
Rhinoviruses

Screening
Serology
Spine, vertebrae, and disks
Sports medicine
Stress
Stress reduction
Tendinitis
Tropical medicine
Yoga

PROCTOLOGY

Anal cancer
Anus
Bladder removal
Colon
Colonoscopy and sigmoidoscopy
Colorectal cancer
Colorectal polyp removal
Colorectal surgery
Crohn's disease
Diverticulitis and diverticulosis
Endoscopy
Fistula repair
Gastroenterology
Gastrointestinal disorders
Gastrointestinal system
Genital disorders, male
Geriatrics and gerontology
Hemorrhoid banding and removal
Hemorrhoids
Hirschsprung's disease
Internal medicine
Intestinal disorders
Intestines
Irritable bowel syndrome (IBS)
Palliative medicine
Physical examination
Proctology
Prostate cancer
Prostate gland
Prostate gland removal
Rectum
Reproductive system
Urology
Polyps

PSYCHIATRY

Addiction
Adrenoleukodystrophy
Aging
Aging: Extended care
Alcoholism
Alzheimer's disease
Amnesia

Amyotrophic lateral sclerosis
Anorexia nervosa
Antianxiety drugs
Antidepressants
Anxiety
Appetite loss
Asperger's syndrome
Attention-deficit disorder (ADD)
Auras
Autism
Bariatric surgery
Bipolar disorders
Body dysmorphic disorder
Bonding
Brain
Brain damage
Brain disorders
Breast surgery
Bulimia
Chronic fatigue syndrome
Circumcision, female, and genital
  mutilation
Club drugs
Corticosteroids
Delusions
Dementias
Depression
Developmental disorders
Developmental stages
Domestic violence
Dyskinesia
Eating disorders
Electroencephalography (EEG)
Emergency medicine
Emotions: Biomedical causes
  and effects
Factitious disorders
Failure to thrive
Family medicine
Fatigue
Frontotemporal dementia
  (FTD)
Gender identity disorder
Gender reassignment surgery
Grief and guilt
Gynecology
Hallucinations
Huntington's disease
Hypnosis
Hypochondriasis
Hypothalamus
Incontinence
Intoxication
Kluver-Bucy syndrome

PSYCHOLOGY

Stress reduction
Sturge-Weber syndrome
Stuttering
Substance abuse
Sudden infant death syndrome (SIDS)
Suicide
Synesthesia
Temporomandibular joint (TMJ) syndrome
Tics
Toilet training
Tourette's syndrome
Weight loss and gain
Yoga

PUBLIC HEALTH

Acquired immunodeficiency syndrome (AIDS)
Acute respiratory distress syndrome (ARDS)
Adenoviruses
Aging: Extended care
Allied health
Alternative medicine
Amebiasis
Anthrax
Antibodies
Asbestos exposure
Assisted living facilities
Babesiosis
Bacillus Calmette-Guérin (BCG)
Bacteriology
Beriberi
Biological and chemical weapons
Biostatistics
Blood banks
Blood testing
Botulism
Carcinogens
Chagas' disease
Chickenpox
Childhood infectious diseases
Chlamydia
Cholera
Chronic obstructive pulmonary disease (COPD)
Clinics
Club drugs
Common cold
Coronaviruses
Corticosteroids
Creutzfeldt-Jakob disease (CJD)
Dengue fever

Department of Health and Human Services
Dermatology
Diarrhea and dysentery
Diphtheria
Domestic violence
Drug resistance
E. coli infection
Ebola virus
Elephantiasis
Emergency medicine
Environmental diseases
Epidemics and pandemics
Epidemiology
Fetal alcohol syndrome
Food poisoning
Forensic pathology
Gonorrhea
Gulf War syndrome
Hantavirus
Health Canada
Health care reform
Hepatitis
H1N1 influenza
Hospitals
Human immunodeficiency virus (HIV)
Immunization and vaccination
Influenza
Insect-borne diseases
Kwashiorkor
Lead poisoning
Legionnaires' disease
Leishmaniasis
Leprosy
Lice, mites, and ticks
Lyme disease
Macronutrients
Malaria
Malnutrition
Managed care
Marburg virus
Marijuana
Measles
Medicare
Meningitis
Methicillin-resistant Staphylococcus aureus (MRSA) infections
Microbiology
Monkeypox
Multiple chemical sensitivity syndrome
Mumps
Necrotizing fasciitis

Nicotine
Niemann-Pick disease
Nursing
Nutrition
Occupational health
Osteopathic medicine
Parasitic diseases
Pharmacology
Pharmacy
Physical examination
Physician assistants
Pinworm
Plague
Pneumonia
Poliomyelitis
Polycystic ovary syndrome
Prion diseases
Protozoan diseases
Psychiatry
Psychiatry, child and adolescent
Psychiatry, geriatric
Rabies
Radiation sickness
Rape and sexual assault
Retroviruses
Rhinoviruses
Roundworm
Rubella
Salmonella infection
Schistosomiasis
Screening
Serology
Severe acute respiratory syndrome (SARS)
Sexually transmitted diseases (STDs)
Shigellosis
Sleeping sickness
Smallpox
Syphilis
Tapeworm
Tattoos and body piercing
Tetanus
Toxicology
Toxoplasmosis
Trichinosis
Trichomoniasis
Tropical medicine
Tuberculosis
Tularemia
Typhoid fever
Typhus
Whooping cough
World Health Organization

Endarterectomy
Exercise physiology
Glands
Healing
Hematology
Hematology, pediatric
Hemorrhoid banding and removal
Hemorrhoids
Histology
Hypercholesterolemia
Hyperlipidemia
Infarction
Ischemia
Klippel-Trenaunay syndrome
Lesions
Lipids
Lymphatic system
Mitral valve prolapse
Necrotizing fasciitis
Nicotine
Osteochondritis juvenilis
Phlebitis
Plaque, arterial
Plasma
Podiatry
Preeclampsia and eclampsia
Progeria
Pulse rate
Shunts
Smoking
Stents
Strokes
Sturge-Weber syndrome
Thrombolytic therapy and TPA
Thrombosis and thrombus
Toxemia
Transfusion
Transient ischemic attacks (TIAs)

Varicose vein removal
Varicose veins
Vascular medicine
Vascular system
Venous insufficiency
Von Willebrand's disease

VIROLOGY
Acquired immunodeficiency
    syndrome (AIDS)
Biological and chemical weapons
Chickenpox
Childhood infectious diseases
Chlamydia
Chronic fatigue syndrome
Common cold
Coronaviruses
Creutzfeldt-Jakob disease (CJD)
Croup
Cytomegalovirus (CMV)
Dengue fever
Drug resistance
Ebola virus
Encephalitis
Enteroviruses
Epidemics and pandemics
Epstein-Barr virus
Fever
Gastroenteritis
Hantavirus
Hepatitis
Herpes
H1N1 influenza
Human immunodeficiency virus
    (HIV)
Human papillomavirus (HPV)
Infection
Influenza

Laboratory tests
Marburg virus
Measles
Microbiology
Microscopy
Monkeypox
Mononucleosis
Mumps
Noroviruses
Opportunistic infections
Parasitic diseases
Pelvic inflammatory disease (PID)
Poliomyelitis
Pulmonary diseases
Rabies
Retroviruses
Rheumatic fever
Rhinitis
Rhinoviruses
Roseola
Rotavirus
Rubella
Sarcoidosis
Serology
Severe acute respiratory syndrome
    (SARS)
Sexually transmitted diseases
    (STDs)
Shingles
Smallpox
Tonsillitis
Tropical medicine
Viral hemorrhagic fevers
Viral infections
Warts
Yellow fever
Zoonoses